PHARMACOLOGY

Edited by **Luca Gallelli**

Pharmacology
Edited by Luca Gallelli

Published by InTech
Janeza Trdine 9, 51000 Rijeka, Croatia

Publishing Process Manager Iva Simcic

Technical Editor Teodora Smiljanic

Cover Designer InTech Design Team

Additional hard copies can be obtained from orders@intechopen.com

Pharmacology, Edited by Luca Gallelli
p. cm.
ISBN 978-953-51-0222-9

For EU product safety concerns:
IN TECH d.o.o., Prolaz Marije Krucifikse Kozulić 3, 51000 Rijeka, Croatia,
info@intechopen.com or visit our website at intechopen.com.

Meet the editor

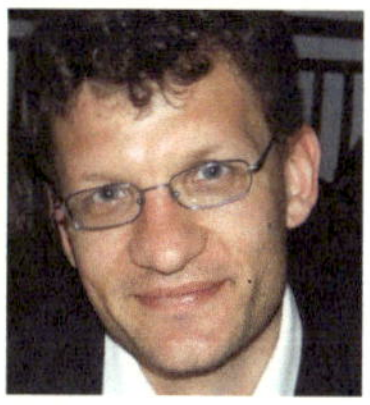

Dr Luca Gallelli obtained is first honour degree in Medicine and Surgery in 1997, Ph.D in in Pharmacology and Toxycology (Chemiotherapy) in 2001and Specialization in Clinical Pharmacology in 2005. He obtained a Grant for foreign country stay by SIF (Italian Society of Pharmacology) in 2000. From 2007 he is teaching Pharmacology nurse and medicine students and students which are specializing in Pharmacology, Respiratory Medicine and Forensic Medicine. Luca Gallelli has published 60 original research articles in international journals. He has also presented several papers in national and international symposia. He is a member of Italian Society of Pharmacology. Finally, he is referee for several international journal.

Contents

Preface

Pharmacology appeared as a science around the XIX century, based on an experimental approach and evolved over the years. Today it studies the clinical efficacy or toxicity of drugs in biological systems, as well as the role of genetic factors in the drug responses.

In this book we have tried to do a very detailed discussion on the receptors, pharmacogenetics and various other aspects, such as future applications in pharmacology.

The first section of the book contains chapters which are discussing the role of molecular pharmacology of several receptors (e.g. cannabinoid and GABA), while the second section describes experimental studies in immunopharmacology.

Today pharmacogenetics represents a new emerging branch of pharmacology which assesses the response to the drug based on genetic characteristics, therefore the third section is dedicated to this argument. The fourth section has been dedicated to clinical pharmacology and pharmacovigilance, while the fifth section is explaining the implication of pharmacology in diagnostic. The chapters whose main topic is related to etnopharmacology and toxicology are included in sixth section. Finally, the last section is dedicated to future applications.

Luca Gallelli
Department of Experimental and Clinical Medicine,
School of Medicine, University of Catanzaro,
Clinical Pharmacology Unit, Mater Domini Hospital,
Italy

Part 1

Pharmacodynamic

1

Metabotropic Receptors for Glutamate and GABA

Gregory Stewart, Julie Kniazeff, Laurent Prézeau, Philippe Rondard, Jean-Philippe Pin and Cyril Goudet
Institut de Génomique Fonctionnelle,
CNRS UMR5203 - INSERM U661 - Universités Montpellier 1&2
France

1. Introduction

G protein-coupled receptors (GPCRs) are the largest superfamily of transmembrane proteins and due to their ubiquitous expression and vast array of functions they present attractive targets for the treatment of a wide number of diseases and disorders. Accordingly, they represent up to 30% of targets of current therapeutics (Overington et al., 2006). Despite the capacity of GPCRs to modulate many (patho-)physiological functions there is a high attrition rate with regard to new compounds entering clinical trials. There are many reasons for the number of failed drug-like compounds such as non-specificity, unfavourable pharmacokinetic profile and lack of clinical efficacy. In this regard, molecules targeting neurotransmitter receptors in the CNS traditionally have poor side-effect profiles due to the high concentrations required to pass the blood-brain barrier. There remain many specific challenges in drug discovery such as promiscuous GPCR-effector coupling; differential cell- and tissue-specific effects; ligand-induced changes in receptor trafficking; and protein-protein interactions and receptor oligomerisation (Galandrin et al., 2007; Hanyaloglu and von Zastrow, 2008; Kniazeff et al., 2011; Wettschureck and Offermanns, 2005).

GPCRs are divided into three main classes (A-C) based on structural homology; however all GPCRs possess a 7-alpha-helical transmembrane-spanning (7TM) domain, which facilitates the transduction of extracellular signals into intracellular responses. GPCRs recognise a myriad of different stimuli from photons, amino acids and biogenic amines to large peptides and proteins. Class A (rhodopsin-like) GPCRs are among the best characterised and consist of a relatively short N-terminal domain, a 7TM domain connected by extracellular and intracellular loops, and an intracellular C-terminal domain (Fredriksson et al., 2003). Class B (secretin-like) GPCRs have comparatively long N-terminal domains with similar 7TM and C-terminal topography as Class A receptors. By far and away, Class C (glutamate-like) GPCRs have the most distinct topography compared the other GPCRs; they possess large, structured N-terminal domains, which form a venus-fly trap-like structure known as the venus-fly trap (VFT) domain. The VFT domain is often (with exceptions) connected to the 7TM domain via a cysteine-rich domain, and further to this the C-terminal domain is often comparatively longer than those of Class A GPCRs. Structurally, all GPCRs are similar in their 7TM domains, yet the activation mechanisms, at least by the endogenous ligand varies greatly across the classes. The orthosteric (endogenous ligand) binding site in Class A GPCRs lies in the 7TM helical bundle (with exceptions, e.g. CXCR4 chemokine receptor and relaxin family receptors (Allen et al., 2007; Sudo et al., 2003)); class B receptor ligands tend to bind in the large N-terminal domain and have been postulated to possess a bimodal receptor activation mechanism, whereby after the ligand binding event the ligand-N-terminal complex inserts into the 7TM helical bundle to elicit receptor activation (Hoare, 2005); class C receptor orthosteric ligands bind in the VFT domain and, through a series of conformational changes, are able to induce receptor activation via the 7TM domain (Pin et al., 2004)(Figure 1).

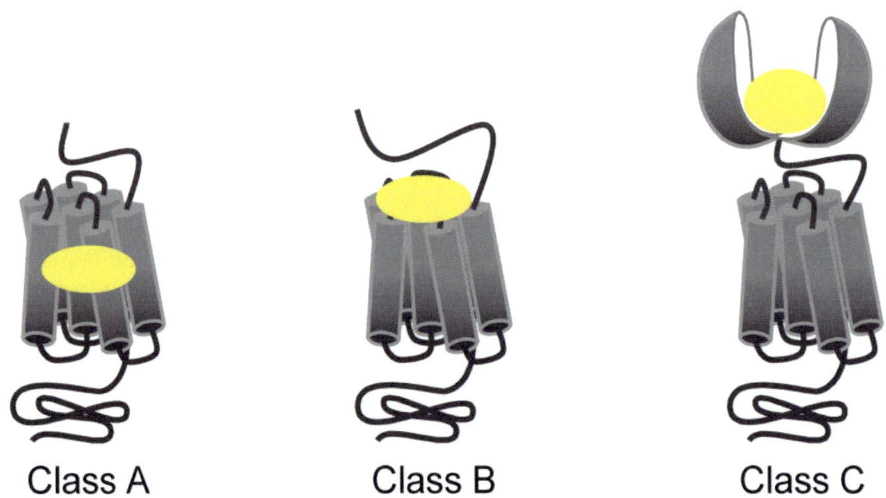

Fig. 1. Canonical orthosteric ligand-binding domains of the three classes of GPCRs. Highlighted in yellow are the typical binding regions of orthosteric ligands, in addition to the general architecture of the three major classes of GPCRs.

One large hindrance to drug discovery is the high degree of protein sequence and structural conservation between orthosteric sites of receptors of the same family, increasing the difficulty to specifically and selectively target a single receptor subtype. However, by their very nature GPCRs are highly dynamic proteins that are able to adopt a spectrum of conformational arrangements and it is this characteristic that allows GPCRs to be modulated by, not only a range of orthosteric ligands, but also ligands that bind in a topographically distinct region to the orthosteric binding pocket. These ligands are known as allosteric ligands and are able to modulate the affinity and/or efficacy of the orthosteric ligand, and indeed, possess their own efficacy in the absence of orthosteric ligand (Christopoulos and Kenakin, 2002; Conn et al., 2009a). This phenomenon presents a unique opportunity to exploit GPCRs as drug targets through offering novel and often less-conserved ligand binding sites across receptor subtypes.

Despite the best-characterised coupling partners of GPCRs being heterotrimeric G proteins, they are also well known to couple to a host of other intracellular proteins (e.g. arrestins and small G proteins (Burridge and Wennerberg, 2004; Lefkowitz, 1998)), thus adding an extra degree of complexity to the pluri-dimensional response of ligand-GPCR interactions. Furthermore, promiscuous coupling has been shown, in some cases, to be a concentration- and/or oligomerisation-dependent event (Sato et al., 2007; Scholten et al., 2011; Urizar et al., 2011).

Taken together, the ligand-receptor-effector combinations, receptor oligomerisation and allosteric modulation of GPCRs furnish a mode of fine-tuning functional outputs and potentially, therefore, clinical outcomes.

This chapter will focus on two major receptor types of Class C GPCRs, the metabotropic glutamate and metabotropic γ-amino-butyric acid (GABA) receptors, which are the GPCRs of the major excitatory and inhibitory neurotransmitters in the adult brain, respectively. These receptors represent major targets for many CNS disorders such as schizophrenia, Parkinson's disease, Alzheimer's disease, epilepsy and diseases of addiction (Conn et al., 2009a; Tyacke et al., 2010).

2. Metabotropic glutamate receptors

2.1 Phylogeny and structure/function of mGlu receptors

Metabotropic glutamate (mGlu) receptors are widely expressed in the CNS and are activated by the excitatory neurotransmitter, glutamate. These receptors play a vital role in the regulation on neuronal excitability and synaptic transmission (Conn and Pin, 1997). Consequently, these receptors are valuable targets for treating neurological disorders such as schizophrenia, Parkinson's disease and neuropathic pain, either by correcting neurological imbalances in non-glutamatergic systems or through treating disregulation of glutamatergic signalling.

The members of the mGlu receptor family are obligate dimers and long thought of as obligate homodimers, but have recently been demonstrated to selectively form heterodimers amongst other mGluR subtypes in HEK cells (Doumazane et al., 2011). This propensity may be of utility in texturing the glutamatergic response across diverse brain regions. mGlu receptors consist of 8 subtypes that are divided into three subgroups (I-III) based on sequence homology, function and pharmacological profile (Pin and Acher, 2002). Group I mGluRs ($mGlu_1$ and $mGlu_1$) are $G_{q/11}$-coupled thereby signalling through the phospholipase C-IP_3-Ca^{2+} axis; whereas Group II ($mGlu_2$ and $mGlu_3$) and Group III ($mGlu_4$, $mGlu_6$, $mGlu_7$ and $mGlu_8$) signal through inhibitory G proteins ($G_{i/o}$), which most likely serve as intermediaries between the receptor and ligand-gated ion channels, such as voltage-operated potassium channels (K_v2 channels) and voltage-operated calcium channels (Ca_v2 channels) (Doupnik, 2008; Herlitze et al., 1996; Peleg et al., 2002).

In drug discovery the understanding of the molecular mechanisms of ligand binding and receptor activation are paramount in order to investigate novel and improved methods for targeting these receptors therapeutically. In this regard, it is important to determine the overall receptor activation event by breaking it down into its fundamental component. Furthermore, to gather information about mGlu receptors, we must also use information gained from studies of other Class C GPCRs to form a global conformational image. Ligand binding in a VFT structure has been described with the periplasmic binding protein, which appears to be similar in class C receptors (O'Hara et al., 1993). The VFT remains in a state of equilibrium between two main conformations: open (o) and closed (c), known as the resting state. The orthosteric ligands bind primarily to the open VFT in lobe 1 and subsequently promote the closed conformation as interactions with lobe 2 stabilises this state. This suggests that, if agonists induce the closure of the VFT, orthosteric antagonists act to prevent the closure of the VFT, thereby blocking the appropriate mechanisms leading to 7TM activation (Bessis et al., 2000; Bessis et al., 2002; Kunishima et al., 2000; Tsuchiya et al., 2002). For a number of years, the question on how ligand binding in the VFT results in 7TM activation remained to be elucidated. The breakthrough came from the first crystal structures of a class C VFT dimer, from the mGlu1 receptor, crystallised in the presence and absence of glutamate (Kunishima et al., 2000). These structures confirmed the overall structure of the domain and, perhaps more importantly, the agonist binding mode in a single VFT domain. It also revealed large, structural rearrangements of the VFT dimer resulting in a change of the relative orientation of the two protomers. A general mechanism for VFT dimer conformational changes was proposed by the authors: two orientations of the VFT dimer exist and are in equilibrium: a resting (R) and an active (A) orientation. In the R orientation, the VFTs interact via lobe-I only, leaving the lobes-II separate from each other. In the A orientation, there is a reorganization of the VFTs relative orientation such that they also interact via each lobe-II. This large reorientation from R to A was proposed to induce the conformational changes required for 7TM activation. Resting and active designations were given to the different orientations as glutamate was proposed to stabilize the A form. The active and inactive property of the A and R orientations are further supported by mGlu1 structures obtained in the presence of an antagonist (MCPG) or in the presence of a potentiator (Gd^{3+}) in which the dimer orientation is R and A, respectively (Tsuchiya et al., 2002).

When considering the various conformations for the VFT and the VFT dimer, there are a total of six theoretical conformations that are possible: Roo, Rco and Rcc and Aoo, Aco and Acc, where A and R are indicative for the VFT dimer orientation and c and o for the VFT conformation. It is assumed that agonist binding to at least one of the VFT stabilizes the c form, which is the driving force leading to the VFT dimer reorientation from R to A. In agreement, only Roo, Rco, Aco and Acc are likely to exist. However, new crystal structures of the isolated VFT dimer in the 'forbidden' conformation Rcc (Muto et al., 2007) and Aoo (PDB accession number, 3KS9) were recently deposited in the protein data bank (PDB). In particular, the Aoo conformation appears to be highly unlikely to occur within a dynamic equilibrium as many residues of the same polarity from lobe 2 would be in close proximity to one another, so much so that this would likely destabilise this conformation through the repulsive forces exerted within lobe 2 (Tsuchiya et al., 2002). Whilst explanations for these surprising observations have not been provided, the absence of 7TM may have alleviated some conformational constraints that may otherwise be exerted on the VFT from the 7TM, acting as a structural tether that inhibits certain conformations.

A question arising upon closer analysis of the crystal structure is the number of agonists needed to activate a class C GPCR dimer. When considering the reorientation of the VFT from R to A as the sole mechanism responsible for 7TM activation, one may wonder whether there is a functional difference between Aco and Acc conformation. In other words, what would be the difference in binding one or two agonists? It was shown that in class C heterodimers a single subunit was responsible in binding the endogenous ligand (GABAB1 in GABAB receptor and T1R1 or T1R2 in the taste receptors)(Kniazeff et al., 2002; Nelson et al., 2001). This suggests that a single agonist molecule is sufficient to fully activate heterodimeric receptors in these cases.

As we have described above, an allosteric modulator binding in the 7TM affects both the G protein activation and agonist affinity for the VFT. Together with the fact that a conformational change in the VFT dimer activates the 7TM, this indicates that VFT and 7TM converse in both ways. The question that remains is how the stimulus is transduced through the VFT region to the 7TM domain?

In most of class C GPCRs, VFT and 7TM are connected with the CRD. The CRD is an 80 residues long domain containing 9 cysteines. This domain is present in mGlu, CaS, GPRC6A and T1R receptors, but not in $GABA_B$ receptors. The structure of this domain has been solved for $mGlu_3$ (Muto et al., 2007), and this domain appears to be a rigid 40Å long structure, which is most likely to form a physical gearing system between the VFT and 7TM domains. In agreement with these physical findings, both deletion of the CRD in mGlu or CaS receptors and mutations of T1R3 CRD abolish the agonist-induced receptor activation (Hu et al., 2000; Jiang et al., 2004). Furthermore, we have shown that the VFT and CRD domains in $mGlu_2$ are linked by a disulphide bridge between a cysteine at the bottom of the VFT and the only cysteine that is not engaged in intradomain disulphide bond within the CRD (Rondard et al., 2006). Rondard et al., had shown that the mutation of the residues involved in this interaction abolished agonist-mediated activation of the receptor. This supports the idea of a central role for the CRD in the transduction of the conformational changes from the VFT dimer to the 7TM in these receptors.

The exact mechanisms of 7TM activation Class C and indeed, mGlu receptors remain to be solved. This notwithstanding, there are approaches that can be employed in an attempt to determine the molecular mechanisms involved in the conformational changes that the 7TM domains undergoes upon activation. One of these approaches is entails the use of both positive and negative allosteric modulators. The first allosteric modulators of class C GPCRs to be described were found to be non-competitive antagonists or inverse agonists (Carroll et al., 2001; Litschig et al., 1999; Pagano et al., 2000). Other compounds have been described that potentiated the effect of the agonists (increased affinity and efficacy) (Felts et al., 2010; Hammond et al., 2010; Urwyler et al., 2001). These molecules are structurally distinct from the orthosteric agonists and antagonists, as reflected in their binding within the 7TM, in a binding region that is reminiscent of the orthosteric binding pocket in Class A receptors (Brauner-Osborne et al., 2007; Goudet et al., 2004). So far, no endogenous PAM or NAM binding in the 7TM pocket has been described. Selective pressure in the evolution of a site/pocket is often indicative of a biological function, but there is no conserved pocket located within the 7TM domain of mGluRs, making it less likely that there is an endogenous allosteric ligand that acts in that region. The absence of conservation allowed the discovery of molecules specific for a single subtype of mGlu receptor, as opposed to a ligand acting at the well conserved orthosteric binding site. If both PAM and NAM act at the 7TM, then their opposite effects are likely due to differences in the residues that the ligands are in contact with in the 7TM. Specifically, several studies indicate that PAM and NAM bind to overlapping but not identical sites (Miedlich et al., 2004; Petrel et al., 2004). Some of these interaction networks should stabilize the active conformation of the 7TM, whilst some others should lock the receptor in its inactive conformation. However, it was shown that structurally different molecules bind essentially at the same position in the 7TM, only the precise identity of the residues contacting the molecule may differ. It appears that the position of PAM/NAM binding site is largely conserved in the whole family and includes residues from TM3, 5, 6 and 7 (Hu et al., 2000; Miedlich et al., 2004; Pagano et al., 2000). However, in some cases, two distinct sites have been identified for PAMs, as exemplified at $mGlu_5$ (Chen et al., 2008). See Figure 2 for a schematic overview of mGlu receptor architecture and binding domains.

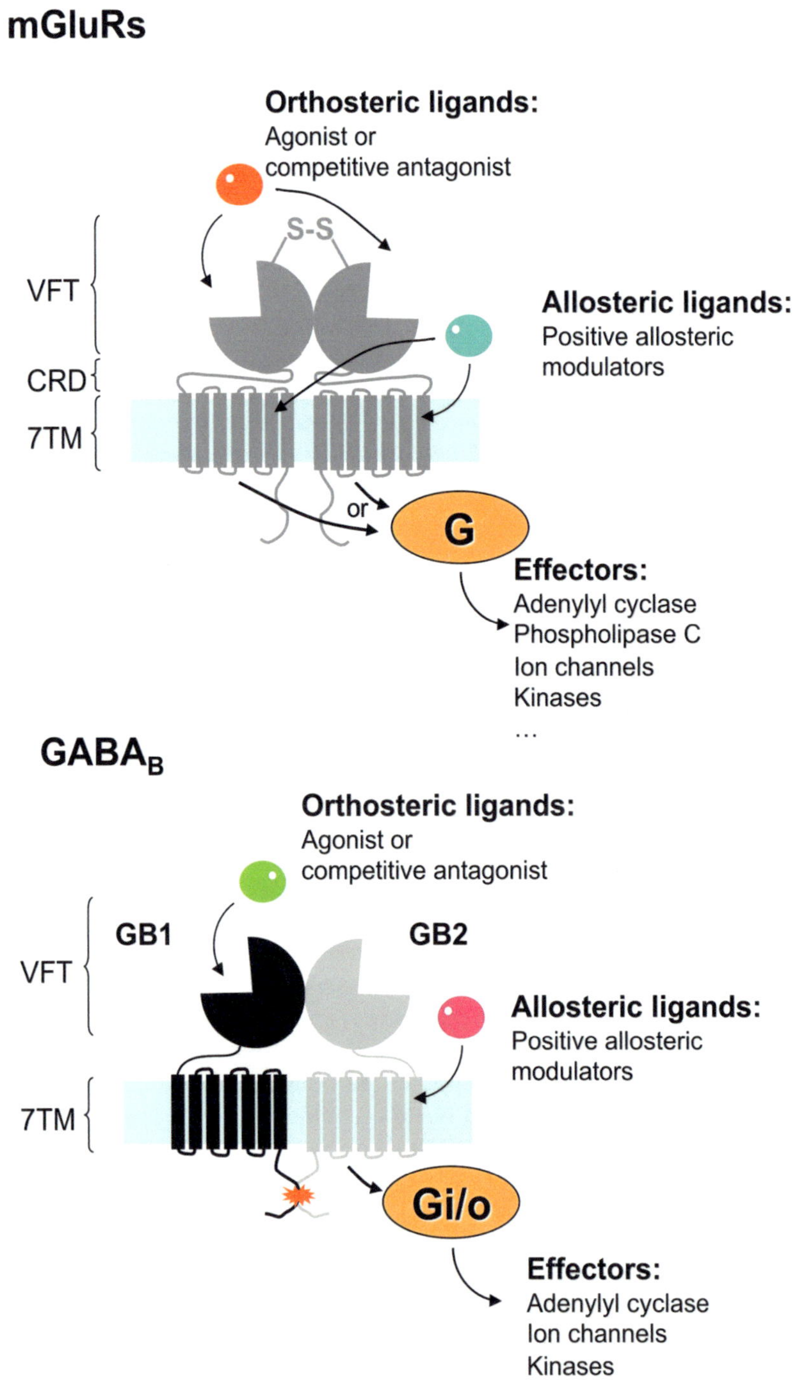

Fig. 2. Architecture, binding domains and dimerisation states of mGlu and $GABA_B$ receptors.

2.2 Protein-protein interactions of mGlu receptors

Studying molecular mechanisms and pharmacology of GPCRs in heterologous cells systems can be exceptionally useful due to the eradication of confounding factors such as multiple receptor subtypes; in addition the capacity to modulate receptor expression and function of specific signalling pathways with relative ease. However, these systems are rarely indicative of native systems and it needs to be recognised that various GPCR interactions exist *in vivo* that do not exist in heterologous cell systems for a myriad of reasons. One such interaction is that of protein-protein interactions, whereby the physical or functional interaction of a number of proteins can greatly alter its behaviour. An example of this occurrence is a fundamental component of some Class C GPCR pharmacology, such that receptor activity-modifying proteins (RAMPs) modulate the pharmacology of receptors such as the calcitonin and calcitonin receptor-like receptor (Sexton et al., 2006). mGlu receptors are also a family that are capable of interacting with non-mGluR proteins to form complexes.

2.2.1 $mGlu_1$–A_1 receptors

In cortical neurons, the simultaneous activation of adenosine A_1 and $mGlu_1$ receptors has been shown to synergistically decrease the neuronal toxicity due to application of NMDA (Ciruela et al., 2001). In astrocytes or in co-transfected HEK293 cells, activation of A_1 receptors elicits an increased $mGlu_1$ response via $G_{i/o}$ proteins (Ciruela et al., 2001; Toms and Roberts, 1999). That effect could be indicative of cross-talk and priming of the intracellular Ca^{2+} response; however, Hirono et al. (2001) did not observe any potentiation of the $mGlu_1$ response upon co-activation of the A_1 receptor in in cerebellar Purkinje cells, supporting the hypothesis of cooperativity (physical or otherwise) rather than cross-talk of the signalling pathways. Although both receptors are co-localized and coimmunoprecipitated from neurons and transfected HEK293 cells, the existence and the requirement of a direct physical interaction is yet to be clearly established (Ciruela et al., 2001).

2.2.2 $mGlu_5$–A_{2A}–D_2 receptors

The $mGlu_5$, adenosine A_{2A} and dopamine D_2 receptors are highly expressed in the striatum. These receptors have been proposed to play vital roles in the dysregulation of the motor coordination observed in the Parkinson's disease. Indeed, antagonists of both $mGlu_5$ and A_{2A} display anti-parkinsonian effects, while the dopamine D_2 receptor is the target of L-DOPA, which is used to treat parkinsonian symptoms. It has been suggested that these three receptors may act in concert in pairs or as a triplet via signalling cross-talk or otherwise, to influence the striatal function in motor coordination (Agnati et al., 2003; Cabello et al., 2009). Indeed, this cross-regulation was observed *in vivo*, where $mGlu_5$ antagonist-induced motor effects were augmented by A_{2A} receptor antagonists; and conversely these effects were diminished in A_{2A}-D_2 receptor double knock-out mice (Kachroo et al., 2005). The exact molecular mechanisms of the cross-regulation are not well understood, but DARPP-32 (dopamine- and cAMP-regulated neuronal phosphoprotein) may play a pivotal role. Adenosine A_{2A} receptors have been show to increase DARP-32 phosphorylation via the G_s signaling axis, whilst D_2 receptors counteract this effect via the $G_{i/o}$ pathway (Agnati et al., 2003); Furthermore, the co-activation of adenosine A_{2A} and dopamine D_2 receptors synergistically potentiated DARPP-32 phosphorylation *ex vivo* studies in striatum tissues. Notwithstanding, the regulation of intracellular Ca^{2+} and cAMP signals underpins other signalling interactions between these receptors (Ferre et al., 2002). Not only may this phenomenon be due to signalling cross talk amongst these receptors, but may be a result of physical interactions and allosteric regulation across heteromers. It A_{2A}–D_2 hetero-oligomers are mediated by electrostatic interactions between a basic-rich motif in the third intracellular loop of the D_2 receptor and an acidic/serine residue-containing motif in the C-terminus of the adenosine A_{2A} receptor (Azdad et al., 2009; Ciruela et al., 2004; Ferre et al., 2007). Additionally, are postulated to not only be co-expressed, but also to form hetero-oligomers in striatal neurons and in heterologous cells systems (Ferre et al., 2002). Recently, Cabello et al. (2009) demonstrated that $mGlu_5$, dopamine D_2 and adenosines A_{2A} receptors are localised within the same dendritic spines in glutamatergic striatal synapses, which led them to hypothesise that there may be hetero-oligomeric triplets of A_{2A}, $mGlu_5$ and D_2 receptors; this association was then investigated through the employment of various fluorescence techniques. Their data supported the formation of heterooligomers containing all three receptors and thus allosterically interacting with one another to influence either efficacy or affinity or both. It is noteworthy that additional cross-regulation between A_{2A} and $mGlu_5$ receptors has been reported in hippocampal neurons, where the inhibition of A_{2A} receptors decreased the $mGlu_5$-mediated potentiation of NMDA receptor responses (Tebano et al., 2006). However, the molecular mechanisms involved are yet to be elucidated.

2.2.3 $mGlu_2$–5-HT_{2A} receptors

One of the best-characterized receptor complex involving a Class C GPCR is the complex between $mGlu_2$ and the serotonin 5-HT_{2A} receptor. It is well documented that these receptors are both targeted by antipsychotic drugs such as 5-HT_{2A} receptor inverse agonists and $mGlu_2$ receptor agonists and PAMs (Benneyworth et al., 2008; Benneyworth et al., 2007). Furthermore, $5HT_{2A}$ receptors are the target of hallucinogenic substances, for example LSD and psilocybin, which induce hallucinogenic episodes that are thought to be similar to some of the symptoms in schizophrenics (Aghajanian and Marek, 1999). Indeed, non-hallucinogenic $5HT_{2A}$ agonists (5-HT included) activate the G_q signalling axis, whilst hallucinogenic compounds are proposed to additionally activate $G_{i/o}$ and Src tyrosine kinase pathways, in cortical neurons (Gonzalez-Maeso et al., 2007; Gonzalez-Maeso et al., 2003). Activation of $mGlu_2$ receptors in the prefrontal cortex by the $mGlu_2$ PAM, biphenyl-indanone A (BINA), abrogated the hallucinogenic effects of compounds such as (-)2,5-dimethoxy-4-bromoamphetamine, [(-)DOB] (Benneyworth et al., 2007); suggesting functional antagonism between $mGlu_2$ and $5HT_{2A}$ receptors in prefrontal cortex, an interaction that is possibly altered in schizophrenics (Gonzalez-Maeso et al., 2007). In fact, co-expression of both receptors revealed that the hallucinogen-induced G_i coupling of 5-HT_{2A} is ameliorated by $mGlu_2$ in basal conditions, but abolished when $mGlu_2$ is activated. The mechanism of this complex cross-talk remains to be fully unraveled, but it has been proposed to be the result of $mGlu_2$–5-HT_{2A} receptor oligomerisation. In cortical neurons, these receptors co-localise and co-immunoprecipitate (Gonzalez-Maeso et al., 2008). Indeed, biophysical approaches have been employed to demonstrate that these GPCRs are in fact in close enough proximity to be compatible with a physical association (Gonzalez-Maeso et al., 2008). Moreover, by adopting a chimeric approach between $mGlu_2$ and $mGlu_3$ (TM4 and TM5 substitution), the authors were able to demonstrate that $mGlu_3$ receptors with substituted TM domains were able to oligomerise with the 5-HT_{2A} receptor, further to exhibiting functional cross-talk (Gonzalez-Maeso et al., 2008). This supports the potential relationship between receptor oligomerisation and functional cross-talk. The study of the precise mechanism of this phenomenon is still ongoing, and can perhaps furnish novel approaches for targeting these receptors for the treatment of schizophrenia and other neuronal disorders.

2.2.4 $mGlu_5$-NMDA receptors

Another important interaction that further implicates the role of the glutamatergic system in schizophrenia is the interaction of the *N*-methly-D-aspartate (NMDA) receptor and $mGlu_5$. This GPCR-ion channel interaction has been relatively well characterised from a functional stand point, but the molecular mechanisms of the interaction are only beginning to be unfolded.

Indeed, in hippocampal neurons, $mGlu_{5a}$ co-localises with NMDA receptors, which mediates a slow excitatory postsynaptic current (Collingridge et al., 1983; Oliet et al., 1997). The activation of $mGlu_5$ receptors enhances the NMDA-evoked responses in different regions of the brain, such as the hippocampus, the striatum, the cortex, or the spinal cord (Aniksztejn et al., 1992; Harvey and Collingridge, 1993). Recently, Perroy et al., (2008) have shown that both receptors, indeed, interact via the C-terminal domain of $mGlu_{5a}$. Through use of the bioluminescence resonance energy transfer (BRET) approach, they demonstrated that a significant and specific BRET signal can be measured between the two receptors, and moreover that this signal was transiently increased by activation of either the $mGlu_{5a}$ receptor or the NMDA receptor; this suggests an allosteric interaction and ligand-dependent conformational rearrangement of the opposite protomer in the hetero-oligomer. Interestingly however, when co-expressed, the functional response of the either receptor was reduced, compared to the response when either receptor was expressed in isolation. Thus suggesting a reciprocal and constitutive suppression of the signalling between NMDA and $mGlu_{5a}$ receptors, which was suggested to be independent of the G protein coupling of $mGlu_{5a}$. The inhibitory reciprocal effect was dependent on the physical interaction between these receptors, given that the inhibition was abolished upon suppression of the C-terminal domain involved in receptor hetero-oligomerisation (Perroy et al., 2008).

2.3 Localisation and physiological function

Group I mGlu receptors ($mGlu_1$ and $mGlu_5$) are extensively expressed throughout neurons in the CNS and, in addition, $mGlu_5$ is expressed in glial cells. $mGlu_1$ is most abundantly expressed in Purkinje cells of the cerebellar cortex and in the olfactory bulb, in addition to strong expression in the hippocampus, substantia nigra and globus pallidus (Baude et al., 1993; Martin et al., 1992); and $mGlu_5$ is greatly expressed in corticolimbic regions, such as the striatum, hippocampus and cerebral cortex (Ferraguti and Shigemoto, 2006). For example in the hippocampus, $mGlu_1$ has been demonstrated to be involved in synaptic transmission and plasticity, in addition to neuronal excitability (Bortolotto et al., 1999), whilst in both $mGlu_1$ and $mGlu_5$ are required for the induction of long-term depression (LTD) in corticostriatal synapses (Sung et al., 2001). Through the use of knockout (KO) mice the putative function of mGluRs can be elucidated and, indeed, $mGlu_1$ and $mGlu_5$ KO mice have been studied. In $mGlu_1$ KO animals is a marked deficits in long-term potentiation (LTP) in hippocampal slices and in context-dependent fear conditioning task (Aiba et al., 1994a); suggesting reduced hippocampal-mediated learning and memory. Furthermore, these mice are also cerebellar-LTD deficient, suggesting that $mGlu_1$ receptors are important for LTD induction in the cerebellum and subsequently motor learning, as demonstrated by the ataxic gait of the $mGlu_1$ KO mice (Aiba et al., 1994b). Recently, mice have been generated whereby the $mGlu_5$ gene can be selectively disrupted in the central nucleus of the amygdala; these mice exhibited a lack of mechanical hypersensitivity induced by peripheral inflammation (Kolber et al., 2010), strongly suggesting a role of $mGlu_5$ in the regulation of inflammatory pain transmission. Both $mGlu_1$ and $mGlu_5$ KO mice exhibit deficiencies in prepulse inhibition of the startle reflex, which is an indicator of sensorimotor gating that is impaired in schizophrenic patients, a trait that can be reversed through treatment with antipsychotics (Brody et al., 2003; Brody et al., 2004).

$mGlu_2$ and $mGlu_3$ (Group II) are widely expressed in the CNS, of which $mGlu_2$ is more limited in expression compared to $mGlu_3$. $mGlu_2$ expression has been observed in Golgi cells of the cerebellar cortex and in mitral cells of the accessory olfactory bulb (Ohishi et al., 1998; Ohishi et al., 1994). $mGlu_3$ receptors have been observed in the olfactory tubercle, neocortex, limbic cortex, and is also present in Golgi cells of the cerebellar cortex (Tamaru et al., 2001). Similar to Group I mGlu receptors, KO mice have also been generated for Group II mGluRs, with both $mGlu_2$ and $mGlu_3$ KO mice exhibiting a loss of $mGlu_{2/3}$ agonist, LY354740-induced anxiolytic behaviour in an elevated plus maze test (Linden et al., 2005). Further to this, $mGlu_2$, but not $mGlu_3$ KO mice displayed a loss of Group II agonist-mediated antipsychotic behaviour (Fell et al., 2008; Woolley et al., 2008), highlighting the role of $mGlu_2$ in anxiety and psychotic behaviours. Interestingly, in addition to these functions, Group II mGlu receptors have also been demonstrated to modulate the release of other neurotransmitters, for example, LY354740 reduced KCl-induced [^{3}H]-GABA release in rat primary cortical cultures, this effect was then reversed with the $mGlu_{2/3}$ antagonist, LY341495 (Schaffhauser et al., 1998).

Group III mGluRs (consisting of $mGlu_4$, $mGlu_6$, $mGlu_7$ and $mGlu_8$) are mainly expressed on presynaptic neurons throughout the CNS, with the exception of $mGlu_6$, which is expressed postsynaptically on retinal ON bipolar cells (Nakajima et al., 1993). $mGlu_4$ is highly expressed in the cerebellum and consequently, $mGlu_4$ KO mice experience deficits in spatial memory (Gerlai et al., 1998) and learning of complex motor tasks (Pekhletski et al., 1996). $mGlu_6$ KO display deficits in ON response to light stimulation, yet the OFF response remained unchanged (Masu et al., 1995), highlighting the importance of $mGlu_6$ in synaptic neurotransmission in retinal ON bipolar cells. $mGlu_7$ deficient mice display learning and memory deficits, in addition to exhibiting an epileptic phenotype (Bushell et al., 2002; Sansig et al., 2001). Both $mGlu_7$ and $mGlu_8$ KO animals display increase anxiety (Cryan et al., 2003; Duvoisin et al., 2005).

As previously mentioned, the mGluR family of receptors are expressed widely through the CNS and exhibit a wide number of functions; moreover through KO studies, we can deduce the key roles played by each mGluR subtype and subsequently tailor our pharmacological armamentarium accordingly.

2.4 Pharmacology and clinical relevance

2.4.1 Ligands for group I mGlu receptors

The first selective orthosteric agonist at $mGlu_1$ and $mGlu_5$ receptors is (S)-3,5-dihydroxyphenylglycine, [(S)-3,5-DHPG], and this remains the case given that ligands such as quisqualate and [(1*S*,3*R*)-ACPD] also bind to ionotropic glutamate and other mGluR subtypes, respectively (Niswender and Conn, 2010). A range of other orthosteric ligands have been generated, but have limited use due to their low affinity and/or potency. As previously discussed, mGlu receptor subtype selectivity is difficult to obtain due to the high degree of sequence and structural homology between subtypes.

Therefore, one approach is to target non-canonical ligand-binding sites; from this strategy a major breakthrough in Group I mGlu receptor pharmacology was made, with the discovery of CPCCOEt, which was the first $mGlu_1$ negative allosteric modulator (NAM)(Annoura et al. 1996). CPCCOEt was later discovered to bind to an allosteric domain and this highlighted the capacity of ligands to bind in allosteric binding modes, thereby modulating orthosteric ligand function (Litschig et al., 1999). Thereafter, structurally distinct NAMs for $mGlu_1$ were also discovered such as BAY36-7620 and FTIDC (Carroll et al., 2001; Suzuki et al., 2007). $mGlu_5$ selective NAMs were also identified of which the two flagship molecules were MPEP and MTEP, both providing good potency and selectivity (Anderson et al., 2002; Gasparini et al., 1999).

In addition to NAMs, a wide variety of PAMs have also been identified and characterised. Two of these PAMs, Ro 67-4853 and Ro 01-6128 both potentiated DHPG-mediated VOCC inhibition responses in CA3 neurons, but did not exhibit any agonist activity of their own, suggesting their main characteristic is the allosteric potentiation of orthosteric ligand binding and/or efficacy (Knoflach et al., 2001). Interestingly, these PAMs were found to bind to a topographically distinct domain to the NAM binding region, when they failed to displace the well-characterised allosteric antagonist, R214127 (Hemstapat et al., 2006). These data suggest that $mGlu_1$ possesses multiple allosteric binding sites, in addition to its orthosteric ligand-binding site. Similar to $mGlu_1$, $mGlu_5$ PAMs have also been discovered, such as DFB, CPPHA, CDPPB, VU29, and ADX47273, with CDPPB also having some PAM activity at $mGlu_1$ (Conn et al., 2009b; Hemstapat et al., 2006).

2.4.2 $mGlu_1$ in anxiety and depression

Anxiety and depression are two of the most common mental disorders, with a lifetime prevalence of approximately 17% and 12%, respectively (Andrade et al., 2003; Depping et al., 2010). It has now been well documented that $mGlu_1$ receptors and the glutamatergic system represent tractable targets for treating these common disorders (Bittencourt et al., 2004; Paul and Skolnick, 2003).

Anxiety results from an imbalance between GABAergic and glutamatergic systems, either from overactive glutamatergic neurotransmission or inadequate GABAergic activity in hypothalamus, periaqueductal gray, hippocampus and prefrontal cortex (Engin and Treit, 2008). It is hypothesised that the antagonism of $mGlu_1$ receptors is capable of augmenting the GABAergic response, whilst concomitantly decreasing the NMDA receptor-mediated glutamatergic response in key brain regions involved in anxiety. It has been demonstrated that intraperitoneal administration of the $mGlu_1$ antagonist, 1-aminoindan-1,5-dicarboxylic acid (AIDA), rats exhibited anxiolytic-like behaviours in the conflict drinking test and in elevated plus maze tests (Klodzinska et al., 2004). This reinforces the results seen by Chojnacka-Wojcik et al., (1997) where intrahippocampal injection of the Group I mGlu receptor antagonist, (S)-4-carboxy-3-hydroxyphenyl-glycine (S-4C3H-PG), reduced anxiety-like behaviours in rats. The anxiolytic actions of $mGlu_1$ blockade were further confirmed through the study of the $mGlu_1$-selective antagonist, JNJ16259685 (Steckler et al., 2005). This study demonstrated that treatment with JNJ16259685 alleviated the suppression of the licking response in a conflict drinking test, which is consistent with other well characterized anxiolytic drugs (Petersen and Lassen, 1981). However, JNJ16259685 treatment did not induce anxiolytic-type behaviour in elevated plus maze tests, the authors thus postulating that the effects of JNJ16259685 be context specific (Steckler et al., 2005).

Depression is a complex disorder involving the interplay between different neurotransmitters, including noradrenaline, serotonin, dopamine and glutamate (Paul and Skolnick, 2003). Drugs for the treatment for depression are generally based on increasing the lifetime of biogenic amines, such as noradrenaline and serotonin, in the synaptic cleft, for example fluoxetine and escitalopram, which are inhibitors of serotonin- and serotonin and noradrenaline-reuptake transporters, respectively. Over the past decade, it has become more recognised that the glutamatergic system may also play a vital role in the regulation of depression, specifically NMDA receptors, where NMDA receptor expression was reduced in post-mortem depressive brains (Feyissa et al., 2009). This theory was retrospectively reinforced by evidence that NMDA receptor antagonists produce anti-depressant effects, whereby competitive and non-competitive antagonists of NMDA receptors, 2-amino-7-phosphonoheptanoic acid (AP-7) and Dizolcipine (MK-801) emulated anti-depressant effects of gold standard anti-depressants (Trullas and Skolnick, 1990). Given the regulatory link between $mGlu_1$ and NMDA receptors it was postulated that $mGlu_1$ receptor antagonists or NAMs could mimic the anti-depressant effect of NMDA receptor inhibitors. The $mGlu_1$ antagonist, JNJ-16567083 has been shown to be efficacious in despair-based animal models of depression, specifically forced swim test and tail suspension test (Belozertseva et al., 2007; Molina-Hernandez et al., 2008).

2.4.3 $mGlu_5$ and schizophrenia

Schizophrenia is a complex multi-faceted disease that manifests itself as a host of symptoms such as paranoia, social withdrawal and delusions, along with a number of cognitive deficits. Given that there is no single causative factor, there is some difficulty in finding a suitable target. Current first-line treatment involves broad-spectrum biogenic amine (e.g. dopamine, serotonin, acetylcholine) receptor antagonists, but these to not satisfactorily treat the cognitive symptoms. The underlying rationale of this approach is to decrease dopaminergic neurotransmission in thalamocortical and limbic circuits. One potential mode of treating schizophrenia lies within targeting GABAergic and glutamateric interneuons in pivotal cortical and limbic regions, specifically, the disregulation of the disinhibition of glutamatergic neurotransmission (Chavez-Noriega et al., 2002; Coyle, 2006). The blockade of *N*-methly-D-aspartate (NMDA) receptors on these interneurons results in a glutamatergic disinhibition, which in turn leads to an overexcitability of thalamocortical neurons, which is mostly mediated by DL-a-amino-3-hydroxy-5-methylisoxasole-4-propionate (AMPA) receptors in thalamocortical synapses. Within these regions NMDA and $mGlu_5$ receptors have been demonstrated to functionally and physically interact, i.e. the activation of $mGlu_5$ receptors increases the activity of NMDA receptors on GABAergic and glutamatergic neurons (Conn et al., 2009b); it is thus postulated that the activation of $mGlu_5$ can be employed as a means to decrease neuronal excitability in thalamocortical regions. This hypothesis is reinforced through knockout studies, whereby the knockout of $mGlu_5$ resulted in NMDA-dependent cognitive and learning deficits (Lu et al., 1997). Therefore, adopting an $mGlu_5$ agonist or PAM could alleviate the cognitive symptoms in schizophrenic patients; moreover, the use of a PAM will allow relatively specific $mGlu_5$ in the afflicted region whilst maintaining the spatio-temporal regulation of other $mGlu_5$-containing neurons. Indeed, the abovementioned $mGlu_5$ PAM, CDPPB, which has a suitable potency and solubility profile for *in vivo* studies, has been demonstrated to decrease amphetamine-induced disruption of prepulse inhibition (PPI) startle response and locomotor activity (Kinney et al., 2005); and to increase hippocampal synaptic plasticity, an important feature in cognition (Ayala et al., 2008; Conn et al., 2009b).

2.4.4 Group II mGlu receptor pharmacology

Group II mGlu receptors ($mGlu_2$ and $mGlu_3$) are generally localised presynaptically and negatively regulate cAMP signalling, and moreover, VOCCs. As with nearly all orthosteric mGlu pharmacological agents there is the underlying issue of selectivity. DCG-IV and LY379268 are reference Group II mGlu agonists, BINA and LY487379 are highly potent PAMs and the recently discovered MNI series of compounds (MNI-135, MNI-136 and MNI-137) are potent negative allosteric modulators (Galici et al., 2006; Hemstapat et al., 2006; Johnson et al., 2003; Linden et al., 2005; Schweitzer et al., 2000). Despite the large array of pharmacological tools available for Group II mGlu receptors, there remains a paucity of ligands that selectively differentiate between $mGlu_2$ and $mGlu_3$, which is due to the high degree of sequence homology between the two. Of lesser therapeutic relevance, there are also Group II mGlu receptor antagonists, such as 2*S*-2-amino-2-(1*S*,2*S*-2-carboxycyclopropan-1-yl)-3-(xanth-9-yl)propionic acid (LY341495) and (1*R*,2*R*,3*R*,5*R*,6*R*)-2-amino-3-(3, 4-dichlorobenzyloxy)-6-fluorobicyclo[3.1.0] hexane-2,6-dicarboxylic acid (MGS0039), which have been suggested to have some anti-depressant and anti-obsessive-compulsive characteristics; however they are mostly used and pharmacological tools (Palucha and Pilc, 2005; Shimazaki et al., 2004). Given the lack of selectivity across Group II mGlu receptors it is difficult to pharmacologically distinguish the roles of each receptor in various animal models of disease states without the use of knockout animals.

2.4.5 Group II mGlu receptors in addiction

Addiction is a unique disorder in that it is not only a physiological dependence, but is also a psychological dependence on, canonically, drugs of abuse. It is believed that $mGlu_2/mGlu_3$ receptor ligands could be capable of treating addiction to such substances as cocaine and nicotine. In fact, not only is it that $mGlu_2/mGlu_3$ receptor activation is involved in recovery of a dysfunctional system in the corticolimbic system, but it has been shown that the function of Group II mGlu receptors is impaired, either by receptor downregulation or dampening of the G protein-mediated signalling, after acute and chronic stimulation by nicotine, cocaine and ethanol (Bowers et al., 2004; Kenny and Markou, 2004; Neugebauer et al., 2000). Indeed, mechanistically, the decrease in function is hypothesised to be due to an alteration in expression of the activator of G protein signalling 3 (AGS3), whereby AGS3 is overexpressed during withdrawal of repeated dosing of cocaine (Bowers et al., 2004). The authors went on to postulate that AGS3 gates expression of cocaine-induced plasticity in prefrontal cortex, via the regulation of G protein signalling. Furthermore, the downregulation of $mGlu_2/mGlu_3$ receptors has been observed during cocaine withdrawal periods, specifically these receptors were downregulated in the shell and core of the nucleus accumbens (Ghasemzadeh et al., 2009). These alterations in expression and function in turn results in an impairment of long-term depression (LTD) in nucleus accumbens and prefrontal cortex in response to chronic morphine and cocaine exposure, respectively (Moussawi and Kalivas, 2010); similarly, a reduced activation of $mGlu_2/mGlu_3$ receptors resulted in a decrease in long-term potentiation (LTP) after self-administered cocaine withdrawal (Moussawi et al., 2009). Indeed, it is well documented that $mGlu_2/mGlu_3$ function is altered in the case of substance withdrawal, however the system is regulated in a manner of ways. Explicitly, Group II mGlu receptors are involved in the circuitry that leads to reward processing and addictive behaviour. The activation of $mGlu_2/mGlu_3$ receptors with the orthosteric agonist, LY379268 resulted in the attenuation of the reinstatement of cocaine-seeking behaviour after exposure, compared to a conventional reinforcer (in this case, sweetened condensed milk) (Baptista et al., 2004). The authors proposed that this was a cocaine-specific effect and was most likely related to the mechanism of action of cocaine itself. Functionally, this regulation may lie in the pre-activation of $mGlu_2$ receptors, whereby in $mGlu_2$ knockout mice there was an increased release of glutamate and dopamine in response to cocaine, in the nucleus accumbens (Morishima et al., 2005). Whilst this does provide some evidence on how glutamate is involved in reward circuitry, one must remain circumspect on their conclusions given any compensatory mechanisms are not accounted for.

2.4.6 Group III mGlu receptors and their ligands

For many years, much of the drug discovery efforts have been directed towards Group I and II receptors to exploit their roles in central nervous disorders such as schizophrenia and neuropathic pain. However, of late, efforts have been turned to developing selective ligands for Group III as novel targets for disorders, for example, Parkinson's disease. The prototypical Group III-selective orthosteric agonist is L-amino-4-phosphonobutyrate (L-AP4), yet this ligand is only selective for Group III mGlu receptors, not within the group. In an attempt to ameliorate the affinity and potency, a series of constrained cyclic forms of glutamate were generated and so was created aminocyclopentane-1,3,4-tricarboxylate (ACPT-I), which showed mildly enhanced potency at $mGlu_4$ and $mGlu_8$ compared to $mGlu_5$ and $mGlu_6$ (Acher et al., 1997; Schann et al., 2006). Similar to the agonists, there are only selective antagonists for Group III mGlu receptors, but not within the group. For example, there are the α-methyl analogues of L-AP4 and L-SOP, specifically MAP4 and MSOP, respectively, with affinity in the micromolar range (Wright et al., 2000). In addition to these, there are the hallmark antagonists of mGlu receptors such as DCG-IV and LY341495, which both have reasonable affinity for Group III mGlu receptors, but also have strong affinity at Group I and Group II receptors, respectively; notably, DCG-IV is also a Group II mGlu receptor agonist (Brabet et al., 1998). Allosteric modulators that act in the 7TM domain Group III mGlu receptors have also been characterised, specifically N-Phenyl-7-(hydroxyimino)cyclopropa[b]chromen-1acarboxamide (PHCCC) and cis-2-([(3,5-Dichlorophenyl)amino]carbonyl)cyclohexanecarboxylic acid (VU0155041), which are both PAMs at $mGlu_4$ (Niswender et al., 2008); 6-(4-Methoxyphenyl)-5-methyl-3-(4-pyridinyl)-isoxazolo[4,5-c]pyridine-4(5H)-one hydrochloride (MMPIP), a NAM for $mGlu_7$ (Niswender et al., 2010); however there remains a relative paucity of allosteric modulators for $mGlu_6$ and $mGlu_8$.

One pharmacological avenue that is only beginning to be explored at Class C GPCRs is that of extracellular domain allosteric modulators. For the umami taste receptors, it has been long known that purinergic ribonucleotides, such as inosine- and guanine-monophosphate molecules (IMP and GMP) were potent positive allosteric modulators of the L-glutamate action at the umami receptor (Yamaguchi and Ninomiya, 2000). Interestingly, mutants that altered the effects of glutamate effect were also enhanced by IMP and GMP (Zhang et al., 2008). By employing a chimeric approach along with mutagenesis and molecular modelling, sweet-umami receptors were analysed and the mode of binding and action of IMP was postulated; specifically, the residues lining the IMP binding pocket at the sweet-umami taste receptor, T1R1, were determined (Zhang et al., 2008). It was demonstrated that IMP binds to a novel site that is adjacent to the glutamate binding pocket, the authors thus proposed a model for ligand cooperativity for the mechanism of action of IMP in the T1R1 VFT. The binding of L-glutamate close to the hinge region of the VFT would stabilize the closed conformation of the domain; moreover, binding of 5' ribonucleotides to an adjacent site closer to the putative entrance of the VFT would further stabilize the closed conformation, thereby potentiating the affinity and/or efficacy of L-glutamate. At mGlu receptors, the glutamate-binding pocket is well conserved across the mGlu subtypes, encumbering the discovery selective orthosteric agonists and antagonists (Brauner-Osborne et al., 2007). However, recently, long alkyl chain containing derivatives of (R)-PCEP, a molecule discovered by virtual screening on the VFT of mGlu receptors, revealed a new binding pocket in $mGlu_4$ (Selvam et al., 2010). Indeed, these compounds not only bind in the glutamate-binding pocket itself, but may also interact with a novel, putative binding pocket adjacent to the glutamate-binding site. Given this new interacting region is formed with residues that are less conserved across the eight mGlu subtypes, this mode of targeting mGlu receptors may furnish compounds with greater selectivity. One such compound may already exist in LSP1-2111, with its L-AP4-like moiety and a 4-hydroxy-3-methoxy-5-nitro-phenyl moiety, it is possible that this molecule bridges across two distinct binding domains, in a similar fashion to bitopic ligands at muscarinic receptors (Antony et al., 2009; Valant et al., 2008; Valant et al., 2009). Accordingly, this ligand has superior selectivity at $mGlu_4$ and $mGlu_6$ over $mGlu_7$ and $mGlu_8$ (Beurrier et al., 2009).

For an overview of chemical structures of a small range of classical orthosteric mGlu receptor ligands, refer to Figure 3 below.

2.4.7 Group III mGlu receptors and Parkinson's disease

Parkinson's disease is one of the most common of neurological disorders, which is largely characterised by its effects on motor function, such as bradykinesia and dyskinesia; further to other non-motor symptoms, for example pain and gastrointestinal dysfunction. Parkinson's disease arises mostly due to a progressive degeneration of dopaminergic neurons in the substantia nigra, leading to excessive cholinergic neurotransmission in the striatum (Pisani et al., 2003). Subsequently, the inhibitory effect that dopamine provides in these circuits augments GABAergic firing in the striatopallidal pathway leading to excessive inhibition of GABAergic neurons in the subthalamic nucleus, in turn leading to the abnormal enhancement of glutamatergic neurons (Hirsch, 2000). Currently, the frontline treatment is levo-dopa, which compensates for the diminished dopaminergic function. However, the activation of presynaptic $mGlu_4$ specifically, may result in the diminution of

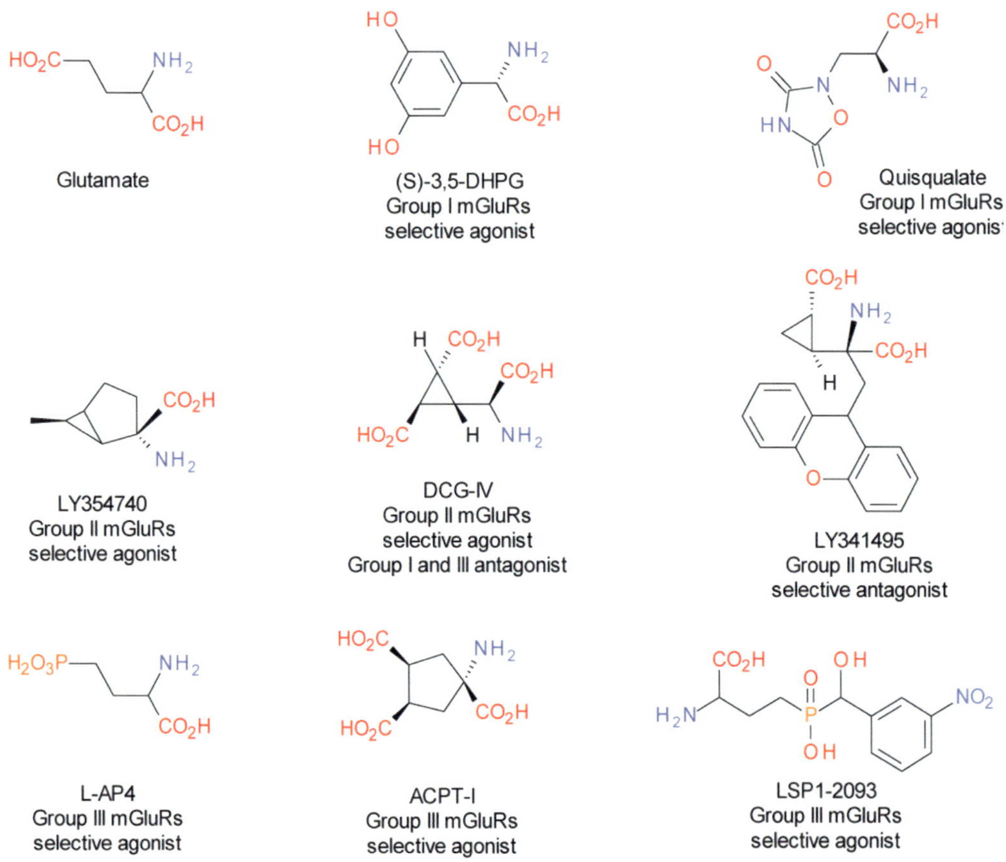

Fig. 3. Highlighting the structural diversity of agonist and antagonists of mGlu receptors.

increased GABAergic firing in striatopallidal projections. Indeed, compounds that have relatively good selectivity for $mGlu_4$ have been demonstrated to depress the GABA-mediated inhibitory synaptic transmission and relive motor symptoms in animal models of Parkinson's disease (Beurrier et al., 2009; Valenti et al., 2003). Given that the dopaminergic dysfunction in the substantia nigra and inhibition of GABA signalling by $mGlu_4$ in the globus pallidus are not inextricably linked there is potential that prolonged $mGlu_4$ receptor activation will result in less compensatory over-activation of the dopaminergic system, therefore maintaining the therapeutic activity of $mGlu_4$ targeting ligands (Nicoletti et al., 2011). Indeed, it has been shown that the *in vivo* treatment with the $mGlu_4$ PAM, PHCCC, reduced dopaminergic neurodegeneration in substantia nigral projections in an MPTP-induced Parkinsonism model (Battaglia et al., 2004; Maj et al., 2003). Along with PHCCC, a more recent PAM of $mGlu_4$ has been characterised and has demonstrated anti-parkinsonian effects (Niswender et al., 2008). VU0155041 is an allosteric agonist and positive allosteric modulator with potency nearly 10-fold of that of PHCCC, moreover, VU0155041 concentration-dependently diminished haloperidol-induced catalepsy and reversed reserpine-mediated akinesia in mice, with an effect that persisted longer than that of the reference Group III orthosteric agonist, L-AP4 (Niswender et al., 2008).

Despite receiving much of the attention within Group III mGlu receptors, $mGlu_4$ is not alone in its involvement in Parkinson's disease. There remains the possibility that post-synaptic $mGlu_7$ and $mGlu_8$ have some effect on the neuronal circuitry in question. The $mGlu_7$ allosteric agonist, *N,N'*-dibenzhydryl-ethane-1,2-diamine dihydrochloride (AMN082) may inhibit the release of [^{3}H]-D-aspartate in substantia nigral slices, suggesting that selective targeting of $mGlu_7$ may yield similar results to those at $mGlu_4$ (unpublished data; Duty, 2010). Despite there being a large amount of doubt surrounding the therapeutic potential of $mGlu_8$ for the treatment of Parkinson's disease, where the semi-selective $mGlu_8$ agonist was failed to reverse haloperidol-induced catalepsy (Lopez et al., 2007); administration of the mixed AMPA antagonist/$mGlu_8$ agonist, (*R,S*)-3-4-DCPG, decreased amphetamine- but not phencyclidine-induced hyperactivity (Ossowska et al., 2004). Concomitantly, (*R,S*)-3-4-DCPG actually enhanced haloperidol-induced catalepsy and induced catalepsy when administered alone. Taken together, and despite similar expression and function compared to $mGlu_4$, does not appear to be a good candidate target for the treatment of Parkinson's disease. Indeed, this scenario highlights the inherent difficulties that are encountered in the search for mGlu receptor subtype-selective therapeutics.

Taken together, it seems that the most appropriate and effective methods for targeting mGlu receptors is via their allosteric ligand-binding site, which increases subtype selectivity and does not impede normal neurotransmission. Refer to Figure 4 for the chemical structures of some allosteric ligands for mGlu receptors.

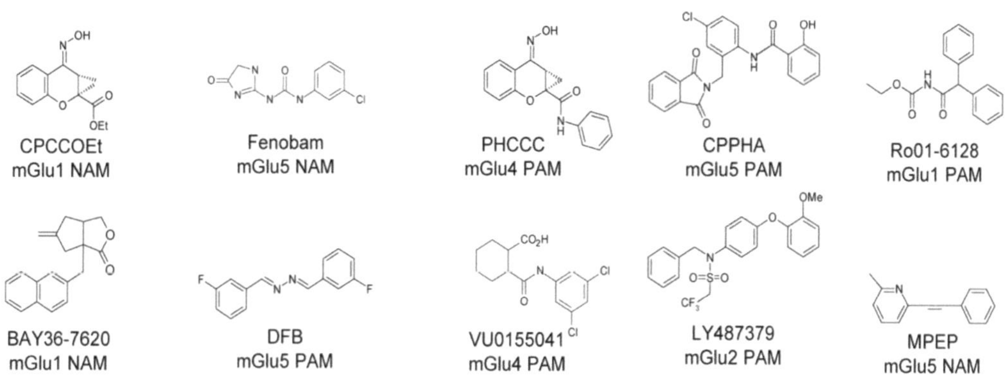

Fig. 4. Chemical structures of mGlu receptor allosteric ligands.

2.4.8 Clinical trials for mGlu receptor ligands

It is now well established that mGlu receptors are major targets for numerous central disorders and even for some in the periphery. Accordingly, there are a large number of clinical programs that are running at any one time (Table 1).

Gastro-(o)esophageal reflux disease (GERD) is a chronic condition, in which the major symptom is the abnormal reflux of stomach contents into the oesophagus. The inhibition of $mGlu_5$ is predicted to improve the tone of the cardiac sphincter, thus reducing reflux (Lehmann, 2008). In a recent phase II clinical study performed by Addex pharmaceuticals, reflux and other GERD symptoms are efficiently reduced by a NAM of $mGlu_5$. The same molecule has also entered into a different phase II study targeting migraine, which also yielded beneficial results. Since glutamate is the main neurotransmitter of the migraine circuit, then inhibition of postsynaptic $mGlu_5$ receptors that are present in this circuit would decrease glutamatergic neurotransmission and hence may pose a useful approach in migraine therapy. However, due to liver toxicity after long-term treatment with this particular molecule, the study was discontinued. Fragile X syndrome is the most common form of inherited mental retardation. Preclinical studies indicate that fragile X phenotypes are linked to an overactivity of $mGlu_5$ (Dolen et al., 2010), suggesting that antagonism of this receptor could be of therapeutic interest. Recently, fenobam, an $mGlu_5$ NAM also known for its anxiolytic properties, entered phase II clinical studies, which so far have demonstrated potential therapeutic benefits on Fragile X symptoms (Berry-Kravis et al., 2009).

Target	Ligand	Company	Trial Phase	Indication
$mGlu_{1/5}$	Antagonist	Forest Laboratories	Preclinical	Anxiety/Depression
$mGlu_2$	TS-032 (Agonist)	Pfizer	Preclinical	Schizophrenia
$mGlu_{2/3}$	ADX1149 (PAM)	Addex Pharmaceuticals	Phase I	Schizophrenia/ Alzheimer's/ Depression
$mGlu_{2/3}$	LY2140023 (Agonist)	Eli Lily	Phase II	Schizophrenia
$mGlu_{2/3}$	Agonist	Eli Lily	Phase III*	Anxiety
$mGlu_4$	PAM	Merck	Preclinical	Parkinson's disease
$mGlu_5$	ADX48621 (Antagonist)	Addex Pharmaceuticals	Phase I	Parkinson's disease
$mGlu_5$	AZD2516 (Antagonist)	Astra Zeneca	Phase I	Chronic pain
$mGlu_5$	AZD2066 (Antagonist)	Astra Zeneca	Phase II	Chronic pain/GERD
$mGlu_5$	NPL-2009	Neuropharm	Phase II	Fragile X syndrome

Table 1. mGlu receptor ligands currently undergoing clinical trials. Sources: ClinicalTrials.gov and EvaluatePharma.com. * - Trial discontinued.

$mGlu_2$ and $mGlu_3$ receptors are a major target for the treatment of anxiety and schizophrenia (Conn and Jones, 2009; Conn et al., 2009b). As a result, the activation of these receptors has been exploited for the treatment of said diseases in several clinical studies. Non-selective $mGlu_2$/$mGlu_3$ agonists have reached phase II clinical studies for the treatment of generalised anxiety disorders, but the trial was terminated due to risks of seizure observed in animals (Dunayevich et al., 2008). Allosteric ligands represent an alternative to the use of orthosteric ligands, since they do not interfere with the spatiotemporal profile of the endogenous ligand; therefore they are more targeted and usually produce less deleterious side effects. Recently, a phase I study on anxiety was started by Ortho-McNeil-Janssen Pharmaceuticals Inc. and Addex pharmaceuticals using ADX71149, an $mGlu_2$ PAM, but the conclusions remain known. Altered glutamatergic neurotransmission is also linked in part to schizophrenia and through a phase II study by Eli Lilly, the improvement of symptoms of schizophrenia with an $mGlu_2/mGlu_3$ agonist was similar to that demonstrated with olanzapine, a common antipsychotic drug; this drug was also tolerated by patients (Patil et al., 2007).

Preclinical studies strongly suggest that Group III mGlu receptors may play a vital role in the symptomatic control of Parkinson's disease. In particular, increasing $mGlu_4$ activity within the basal ganglia appears to be an interesting approach to reduce akinetic symptoms associated with Parkinson's disease (Beurrier et al., 2009; Lopez et al., 2007). However, to our knowledge, none of these compounds have reached phase I clinical trials.

3. Metabotropic GABA receptors

3.1 Structure/function of $GABA_B$ receptors

The metabotropic GABA ($GABA_B$) receptor is the only known GPCR that is responsive to GABA. Architecturally, it is not composed in the same manner as many other Class C GPCRs. Specifically, it consists of a ligand binding GB_1 subunit and a G protein coupling GB_2 subunit (Galvez et al., 2001; Kaupmann et al., 1998; Margeta-Mitrovic et al., 2001; White et al., 1998); each subunit consisting of a VFT and 7TM domains, but converse to mGlu receptors they lack a CRD (refer to Figure 2 for schematic overview). The two subunits are not covalently associated, but do interact via a coiled-coil domain in their C-terminal tails, which provides a solid hydrophobic interaction to maintain the integrity of the dimer (Kammerer et al., 1999). Through the use of circular dichroism spectroscopy the authors proposed a region in the C-terminal domains of GB_1 and GB_2 of approximately 30 amino acids, composed of roughly 5-7 heptads.

Discerning the number of ligands that bind to any one dimer at any one moment is often difficult, especially if there is the possibility for receptors to form higher-order oligomers. It has been shown that in class C heterodimers a single subunit was responsible for the binding of the endogenous ligand, in this case GB_1 in the $GABA_B$ receptor (Kniazeff et al., 2002). This suggests that a single agonist molecule is sufficient to fully activate heterodimeric receptors, but does not discount multiple binding sites on the same protomer. However, nearly nothing is known of the conformational movement of the GB_2 subunit, making it nearly impossible to distinguish between the conformational rearrangement and functional responses of Aco and Acc combinations. The only insights come from the $GABA_B$ receptor, whereby the introduction of several large residues, such as tryptophan in the crevice of GB_2 VFT leads to a decrease in G protein-mediated functional responses (Kniazeff et al., 2002).

It has always been questioned whether GPCRs remain in simple monomeric and dimeric forms or whether they self-associate into higher-order oligomers and, if so, what are the molecular determinants of these interactions. Recently, it has been demonstrated that $GABA_B$ are indeed capable of forming tetrameric complexes, which interact via their GB_1 subunits (Comps-Agrar et al., 2011; Maurel et al., 2008). By employing the use of a binding-null GB_1 subunit Comps-Agrar et al., (2011) demonstrated that $GABA_B$ receptor tetramers could be disrupted and that the resultant complexes are capable of binding approximately twice as much radioligand compared to the wild-type; in addition to increasing the apparent E_{max} in functional tests. The synthesis of this study was that $GABA_B$ receptors that are associated into a tetrameric assembly have reduced binding capacity and functional capability compared to $GABA_B$ receptors in dimeric form. Comps-Agrar et al., (2011) attempted to more precisely examine the structural determinants of the molecular construction of the $GABA_B$ receptor tetramer. They resolved that an important interaction between the VFTs of the GB_1 subunits occurs, and then experimentally demonstrated the disruption of this interaction through mutation and insertion of an *N*-glycosylation site ($G^{380}N$) increases the apparent B_{max} of fluorescent ligand binding and maximal function effect in intracellular calcium mobilisation assays. It is noteworthy that this study demonstrated that there is tetramerisation of GB_{1A} subunit-containing $GABA_B$ receptors, but not GB_{1B} subunit-containing receptors.

Stimulation of $GABA_B$ receptors results in the activation and dissociation of $G_{i/o}$ family G proteins, which in turn inhibit the function adeylyl cyclase thereby decreasing intracellular cAMP levels; activate Kir3 channels and inhibit Ca_v2 channels (Dunlap and Fischbach, 1981; Leaney and Tinker, 2000; Nishikawa et al., 1997). One of the major actions of $GABA_B$ receptor activation is the opening of Kir3 channels, where the increase in K^+ permeability through these channels hyperpolarises the cell thereby inhibiting the propagation of action potentials (Dascal, 1997; Misgeld et al., 1995).

Many GPCRs undergo rapid receptor phosphorylation and subsequent sequestration from the cell surface, commonly in an arrestin-dependent manner, followed by the recruitment of scaffolding proteins and by clathrin-mediated endocytosis (Shenoy and Lefkowitz, 2005). One interesting feature that is dissimilar to many GPCRs and is the subject of much debate is that $GABA_B$ receptors do not appear to undergo activation-dependent phosphorylation and internalisation. Indeed, it has been reported that these receptors are not phosphorylated by the canonical G protein-coupled receptor kinases (GRKs), yet are desensitised by GRK4 in the absence of any apparent phosphorylation (Perroy et al., 2003). It has been demonstrated in chick neurons that upon activation, $GABA_B$ receptors form a complex with Ca_v channels and arrestins, then are consequently internalised as a mechanism of rapid desensitisation of $GABA_B$ receptor signalling (Puckerin et al., 2006). This however, is conflicting with evidence provided by Fairfax et al., (2004) whereby $GABA_B$ receptors did not associate with arrestins and, indeed, the cAMP-dependent kinase- (PKA) mediated phosphorylation of the $GABA_B$ receptor at position Ser892 on the GB_2 subunit increases its cell-surface stability; rather than impeding its cellular function. It would appear in these cases that the phosphorylation state and the subsequent events may very well be cell type specific, which may be yet another degree of complexity for texturing $GABA_B$ receptor-mediated signalling. Interestingly, despite the lack of consistent evidence that $GABA_B$ receptors are phosphorylated as a consequence of receptor activation, there is an accumulating body of evidence that these receptors are phosphorylated mostly by second-messenger kinases. For example, protein kinase C (PKC) has been described to phosphorylate the GB_1 subunit $GABA_B$ receptors after the dissociation of the chaprone protein, *N*-ethylmaleimide-sensitive fusion (NSF) protein, in Chinese hamster ovary (CHO) cells (Pontier et al., 2006). More recently, there have been new developments on how $GABA_B$ receptors are phosphorylated and dephosphorylated in neurons. Recent evidence suggests that NMDA receptors can also act as regulators of $GABA_B$ receptor function, such that NMDA receptor activation, via calcium/calmodulin-dependent protein kinase, phosphorylates the GB_1 subunit at position Ser867, resulting in rapid receptor internalisation from dendritic spines and shafts in the hippocampus (Guetg et al., 2010). Similarly, prolonged NMDA receptor activation results in the rapid phosphorylation of Ser783 on GB_2 in an 5' adenosine-monophosphate-dependent protein kinase- (AMPK) dependent manner (Terunuma et al., 2010). The rapid phosphorylation by AMPK altered the endocytic sorting pathway from receptor recycling to endosomal degradation, Ser783 was then slowly dephosphorylated by protein phosphatase 2A, returning the system back to its receptor recycling processes. Although the modes of which $GABA_B$ receptors are phosphorylated and there consequences are not entirely clear, recently there has been a great deal of progress made in understanding how $GABA_B$ receptor phosphorylation is affected by distinct signalling systems and their consequences on receptor function.

3.2 Localisation and physiology of $GABA_B$ receptors

The $GABA_B$ receptor is extensively expressed throughout the central nervous system, specifically, hippocampus, cortex, thalamus and cerebellum (Bettler and Tiao, 2006; Billinton et al., 1999); and in parts of the peripheral nervous system. They are located both pre- and post-synaptically where they mediate activity of Ca_v and Kir3 channels, respectively (Dutar and Nicoll, 1988; Lopez-Bendito et al., 2004; Luscher et al., 1997). Presynaptic $GABA_B$ receptors can be found at both homo- and hetero-autoreceptors on GABA and, for example, glutamate nerve terminals, respectively (Thompson et al., 1993). Activation of these receptors leads to a hyperpolarisation of the nerve terminal thereby inhibiting further neurotransmitter release. Postsynaptically, $GABA_B$ receptors have been demonstrated to mediate slow inhibitory postsynaptic potentials (IPSPs) through the operation of Kir3 channels. It is noteworthy that in the human brain, there are two major isoforms of the $GABA_B$ receptors, those that contain a GB_{1A} subunits, and those that possess GB_{1B} subunits, notwithstanding there is no apparent difference in pharmacology or physiology between the two receptors in heterologous cell systems (Ulrich and Bettler, 2007). Despite a lack of obvious differences in function and pharmacology, there is indeed a differential expression pattern, such that GB_{1A} and GB_{1B} are both expressed on GABAergic nerve terminals, yet only GB_{1A} subunits are expressed on glutamatergic synaptic terminals (Kulik et al., 2003). By using different sets of complementary approaches, the authors showed that GB_{1A}-containing heterodimers mainly control presynaptic release of glutamate, whereas receptors possessing GB_{1B} subunits predominantly mediate post-synaptic inhibition.

3.3 $GABA_B$ receptor pharmacology and clinical relevance

Similar to mGlu receptors, $GABA_B$ receptors have two main ligand-binding domains, the orthosteric ligand-binding pocket located within the VFT of GB_1; and the allosteric ligand-binding domain, which is within the 7TM region, most likely within the 7TM bundle. There are surprisingly few $GABA_B$ receptor full agonists aside from GABA itself and the well-known baclofen (refer to Figure 5). There are some other agonists such as CGP27492, the tritiated form of which replaced [^{3}H]-baclofen as the radioligand agonist of choice, but was surrounded by controversy when it failed to reproduce the same physiological effects in some key assays (Froestl et al., 1995). A number of $GABA_B$ receptor partial agonists have been identified, the most famous of which is the endogenous metabolite of GABA, γ-hydroxybutyric acid (GHB), synthesised from GABA transaminase and semialdehyde reductase. Other partial agonists include CGP44532 and CGP35024, the latter is also a

$GABA_C$ receptor antagonist (Chebib et al., 1997). The number of antagonists is much greater than that of agonists, among these ligands there are the baclofen derivatives, saclofen and 2-OH saclofen; CGP54626, the most common of the antagonists; and CGP71872; the former two possessing high micromolar affinity, whilst the latter two exhibit low nanomolar affinity (Kaupmann et al., 1997).

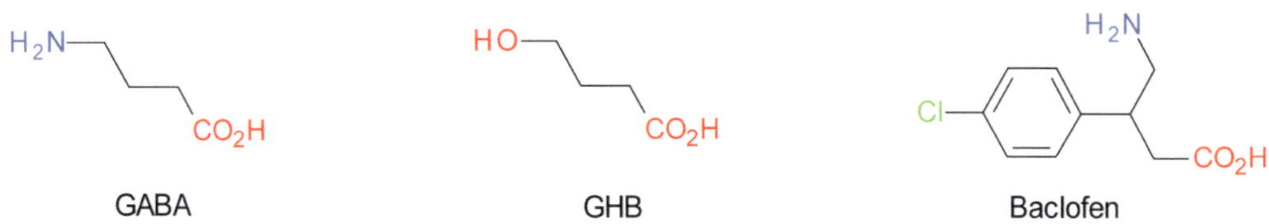

Fig. 5. Structural similarities across common $GABA_B$ receptor agonists.

As with many Class C GPCRs, there exist a number of allosteric modulators available for the $GABA_B$ receptor, yet all known modulators are PAMs, with no known NAMs, to date. Some PAMs of the $GABA_B$ receptor are CGP7930, GS39783 and the more recent, rac-BHFF (Malherbe et al., 2008; Pin and Prezeau, 2007)(Figure 6). These PAMs increase orthosteric agonist potency and maximal response in a system-dependent manner, whilst possessing partial agonism in their own right. Given that many PAMs will most often on activate their target receptor when the endogenous or orthosteric ligand is present, they offer an ideal approach for drug discovery given they maintain region-dependent transmission patterns, therefore theoretically limiting off-target effects and side effect profile.

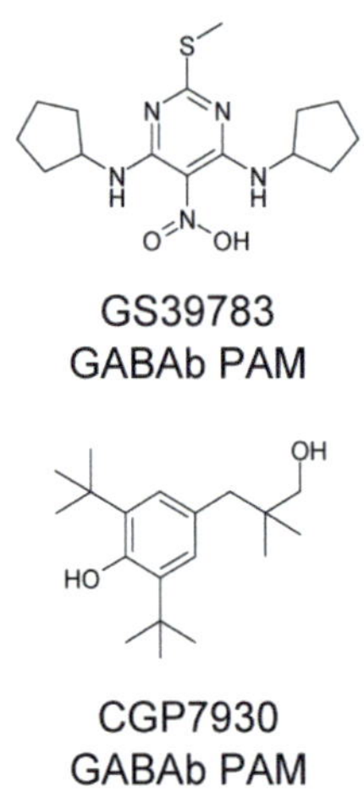

Fig. 6. Two of the best characterised positive allosteric modulators at the $GABA_B$ receptor.

3.3.1 Addiction and $GABA_B$ receptors

Today, there are two $GABA_B$ receptor ligands on the market, both agonist, but both treat largely different disorders. Baclofen, originally developed to treat epilepsy in the 1920s, was largely unsuccessful for the treatment of epileptic symptoms, but its potential was realised outside of epileptic patients. Among the more common uses for baclofen is the treatment of addiction of abusive substances. Specifically, alcohol dependence has received much attention with regard to GABAB receptors, such that baclofen administration in open-label trials reduced the number of heavy-drinking days and increased the number of abstinence days, in addiction to decreasing biological markers such as alanine aminotranferase and gamma glutamyl-transpeptidase, in some patients (Addolorato et al., 2000; Flannery et al., 2004). Baclofen was not only useful for the management of alcohol addiction, but may also be employed as a strategy against withdrawal and relapse (Addolorato et al., 2006). When compared with treatment of diazepam, baclofen was only slightly less efficient at reducing the symptoms of alcohol withdrawal, such as sweating, anxiety and agitation; however this suggests baclofen may be a useful treatment for alcohol withdrawal in patients that abuse other substances, for example, benzodiazepines.

Baclofen has also been investigated for its effects on relieving addiction to cocaine. In one study, users of freebase or crack cocaine who self-administered through inhalation of the drug (Haney et al., 2006). Users who were either treated with methadone or not were given varying doses of baclofen and subsequently were asked to choose to take either the available dose of cocaine or five dollar merchandise voucher. The group who were administered 60mg of baclofen and non-methadone treated demonstrated a decrease in the craving for the low dose of cocaine (12mg), whilst there was no change in the methadone-treated group. Interestingly, baclofen also decreased the effect of cocaine on heart rate, however the personal evaluation of the 'high' remained unchanged. These results suggest that in some specific cases that baclofen would have a positive effect on addiction, however these situations are also often confounded by psychological dependence and are by and large heavily dictated by the patient.

3.3.2 GHB and current therapeutic indications

As previously mentioned, GHB is a minor metabolite of GABA; however in the 1960s GHB was first developed as a therapeutic as a CNS depressor (Laborit et al., 1960). At the time, it was also used as an adjuvant for anesthetics and is still used in some countries as an intravenous anesthesia (Kleinschmidt et al., 1997). Nowadays, the therapeutic indications for GHB are cataplexy and excessive daytime sleepiness associated with sleep disorder narcolepsy. Narcolepsy is the condition characterised by interrupted nighttime sleep and excessive daytime sleep, in addition to this, approximately 70% of narcoleptics suffer from cataplexy, which is a sudden loss of muscle tone. The evidence of clinical efficacy of GHB is largely empirical through a number of studies on narcoleptic patients, daily doses of GHB was able to reduce the number of nocturnal sleep/awake transitions, cataplexy episodes and the frequency between wakefulness and REM sleep during the daytime (Pardi and Black, 2006; Scrima et al., 1990). Despite clinical evidence supporting the therapeutic benefits of GHB for these conditions, there is still much debate over the molecular mechanism of action of GHB. There is known to be at least two GHB-binding sites, a high-affinity site on an unidentified protein; and a low-affinity site, which is at the $GABA_B$ receptor (Kaupmann et al., 2003). However, there is evidence that the effects of GHB on stabilising patterns of somnolence are due to the subsequent actions at the $GABA_B$ receptor. Recently, Vienne et al., (2010) provided evidence that the effects on somnolence and circadian sleep organisation are dependent on $GABA_B$ receptors, whereby GHB and baclofen stabilised sleep/wake regulation in wild-type mice; these effects were lost in both GB_1-/- and GB_2-/- mice. This study suggests that the therapeutic benefits of GHB in narcoleptic patients may be mostly due to GHB-mediated activation of $GABA_B$ receptors.

3.3.3 $GABA_B$ receptors in pain

The importance of $GABA_B$ receptors in nociceptive processing was well documented in the early 90's in a series of preclinical studies in which the $GABA_B$ receptor agonist, baclofen, exhibited antinociceptive properties in models of acute (Malcangio et al., 1991) and chronic pain (Dirig and Yaksh, 1995; Smith et al., 1994). These effects are likely mediated by spinal and supraspinal $GABA_B$ receptors; where the supraspinal effects appear to reflect depression of ascending adrenergic and dopaminergic input to the brainstem, and facilitation of descending noradrenergic input to the spinal cord dorsal horn (Sawynok, 1984). Baclofen-induced antinociception at spinal cord level is attributed, at least partly, to the activation of presynaptic $GABA_B$ receptors localised on the nerve terminals of peptidergic primary afferents fibers (Price et al., 1984). In the substantia gelatinosa of the spinal cord, baclofen exhibits a greater effect on C-fibers than Aδ-fiber-evoked glutamate release, suggesting a preferential $GABA_B$ expression in C fibers afferent terminals (Ataka et al., 2000). Furthermore, baclofen inhibits electrically-evoked release of calcitonin gene-related peptide (CGRP) (Malcangio and Bowery, 1995) and substance P (Marvizon et al., 1999) from rat spinal cord slices. The decrease of dorsal horn neurons excitability and the regulation of intrinsic neuronal properties suggest additional postsynaptic sites for the action of baclofen on pain (Derjean et al., 2003; Kangrga et al., 1991). Taken together, the effects of activation of $GABA_B$ receptors on the inhibition of pain signalling suggest that it is a tractable target for combating neuropathic and potentially other types of pain.

4. Concluding remarks

The treatment of neurological disorders is perhaps one of the most difficult tasks in modern day medicine; the multi-factorial nature of disease and the availability of appropriate therapeutics continually hamper the drug discovery process. The initial step in surmounting these obstacles is the validation of a target, which is perpetually being revised and, has now furnished two invaluable targets in the mGlu and $GABA_B$ receptors. Both receptors, which present the major excitatory and inhibitory GPCR conduits, could be targeted for the treatment of a myriad of central and peripheral disorders. To better understand the function and physiology of these receptors it is paramount that we elucidate molecular mechanisms of receptor activation and ligand binding. There exists a large body of work the pharmacology of mGlu and $GABA_B$ receptors, yet we are only now scratching the surface, as recently there has been an influx on novel receptor-selective pharmacophores, especially for mGlu receptors. With a better pharmacological armamentarium we will be better equipped to delineate (patho)physiological phenomena as we progress development of better therapeutics.

5. References

Acher FC, Tellier FJ, Azerad R, Brabet IN, Fagni L and Pin JP (1997) Synthesis and pharmacological characterization of aminocyclopentanetricarboxylic acids: new tools to discriminate between metabotropic glutamate receptor subtypes. *J Med Chem* 40(19):3119-3129.

Addolorato G, Caputo F, Capristo E, Colombo G, Gessa GL and Gasbarrini G (2000) Ability of baclofen in reducing alcohol craving and intake: II--Preliminary clinical evidence. *Alcohol Clin Exp Res* 24(1):67-71.

Addolorato G, Leggio L, Abenavoli L, Agabio R, Caputo F, Capristo E, Colombo G, Gessa GL and Gasbarrini G (2006) Baclofen in the treatment of alcohol withdrawal syndrome: a comparative study vs diazepam. *Am J Med* 119(3):276 e213-278.

Aghajanian GK and Marek GJ (1999) Serotonin and hallucinogens. *Neuropsychopharmacology* 21(2 Suppl):16S-23S.

Agnati LF, Ferre S, Lluis C, Franco R and Fuxe K (2003) Molecular mechanisms and therapeutical implications of intramembrane receptor/receptor interactions among heptahelical receptors with examples from the striatopallidal GABA neurons. *Pharmacol Rev* 55(3):509-550.

Aiba A, Chen C, Herrup K, Rosenmund C, Stevens CF and Tonegawa S (1994a) Reduced hippocampal long-term potentiation and context-specific deficit in associative learning in mGluR1 mutant mice. *Cell* 79(2):365-375.

Aiba A, Kano M, Chen C, Stanton ME, Fox GD, Herrup K, Zwingman TA and Tonegawa S (1994b) Deficient cerebellar long-term depression and impaired motor learning in mGluR1 mutant mice. *Cell* 79(2):377-388.

Allen SJ, Crown SE and Handel TM (2007) Chemokine: receptor structure, interactions, and antagonism. *Annu Rev Immunol* 25:787-820.

Anderson JJ, Rao SP, Rowe B, Giracello DR, Holtz G, Chapman DF, Tehrani L, Bradbury MJ, Cosford ND and Varney MA (2002) [3H]Methoxymethyl-3-[(2-methyl-1,3-thiazol-4-yl)ethynyl]pyridine binding to metabotropic glutamate receptor subtype 5 in rodent brain: in vitro and in vivo characterization. *J Pharmacol Exp Ther* 303(3):1044-1051.

Andrade L, Caraveo-Anduaga JJ, Berglund P, Bijl RV, De Graaf R, Vollebergh W, Dragomirecka E, Kohn R, Keller M, Kessler RC, Kawakami N, Kilic C, Offord D, Ustun TB and Wittchen HU (2003) The epidemiology of major depressive episodes: results from the International Consortium of Psychiatric Epidemiology (ICPE) Surveys. *Int J Methods Psychiatr Res* 12(1):3-21.

Aniksztejn L, Otani S and Ben-Ari Y (1992) Quisqualate Metabotropic Receptors Modulate NMDA Currents and Facilitate Induction of Long-Term Potentiation Through Protein Kinase C. *Eur J Neurosci* 4(6):500-505.

Annoura H, Fukunaga A, Uesugi M, Tatsuoka T and Horikawa Y (1996) A novel class of antagonists for metabotropic glutamate receptors, 7-(hydroxyimino)cyclopropa[b]chromen-1a-carboxylates. *Bioorg. Med. Chem. Lett.* 6, 763-766

Antony J, Kellershohn K, Mohr-Andra M, Kebig A, Prilla S, Muth M, Heller E, Disingrini T, Dallanoce C, Bertoni S, Schrobang J, Trankle C, Kostenis E, Christopoulos A, Holtje HD, Barocelli E, De Amici M, Holzgrabe U and Mohr K (2009) Dualsteric GPCR targeting: a novel route to binding and signaling pathway selectivity. *Faseb J* 23(2):442-450.

Ataka T, Kumamoto E, Shimoji K and Yoshimura M (2000) Baclofen inhibits more effectively C-afferent than Adelta-afferent glutamatergic transmission in substantia gelatinosa neurons of adult rat spinal cord slices. *Pain* 86(3):273-282.

Ayala JE, Niswender CM, Luo Q, Banko JL and Conn PJ (2008) Group III mGluR regulation of synaptic transmission at the SC-CA1 synapse is developmentally regulated. *Neuropharmacology* 54(5):804-814.

Azdad K, Gall D, Woods AS, Ledent C, Ferre S and Schiffmann SN (2009) Dopamine D2 and adenosine A2A receptors regulate NMDA-mediated excitation in accumbens neurons through A2A-D2 receptor heteromerization. *Neuropsychopharmacology* 34(4):972-986.

Baptista MA, Martin-Fardon R and Weiss F (2004) Preferential effects of the metabotropic glutamate 2/3 receptor agonist LY379268 on conditioned reinstatement versus primary reinforcement: comparison between cocaine and a potent conventional reinforcer. *J Neurosci* 24(20):4723-4727.

Battaglia G, Busceti CL, Molinaro G, Biagioni F, Storto M, Fornai F, Nicoletti F and Bruno V (2004) Endogenous activation of mGlu5 metabotropic glutamate receptors contributes to the development of nigro-striatal damage induced by 1-methyl-4-phenyl-1,2,3,6-tetrahydropyridine in mice. *J Neurosci* 24(4):828-835.

Baude A, Nusser Z, Roberts JD, Mulvihill E, McIlhinney RA and Somogyi P (1993) The metabotropic glutamate receptor (mGluR1 alpha) is concentrated at perisynaptic membrane of neuronal subpopulations as detected by immunogold reaction. *Neuron* 11(4):771-787.

Belozertseva IV, Kos T, Popik P, Danysz W and Bespalov AY (2007) Antidepressant-like effects of mGluR1 and mGluR5 antagonists in the rat forced swim and the mouse tail suspension tests. *Eur Neuropsychopharmacol* 17(3):172-179.

Benneyworth MA, Smith RL and Sanders-Bush E (2008) Chronic phenethylamine hallucinogen treatment alters behavioral sensitivity to a metabotropic glutamate 2/3 receptor agonist. *Neuropsychopharmacology* 33(9):2206-2216.

Benneyworth MA, Xiang Z, Smith RL, Garcia EE, Conn PJ and Sanders-Bush E (2007) A selective positive allosteric modulator of metabotropic glutamate receptor subtype 2 blocks a hallucinogenic drug model of psychosis. *Mol Pharmacol* 72(2):477-484.

Berry-Kravis E, Hessl D, Coffey S, Hervey C, Schneider A, Yuhas J, Hutchison J, Snape M, Tranfaglia M, Nguyen DV and Hagerman R (2009) A pilot open label, single dose trial of fenobam in adults with fragile X syndrome. *J Med Genet* 46(4):266-271.

Bessis AS, Bertrand HO, Galvez T, De Colle C, Pin JP and Acher F (2000) Three-dimensional model of the extracellular domain of the type 4a metabotropic glutamate receptor: new insights into the activation process. *Protein Sci* 9(11):2200-2209.

Bessis AS, Rondard P, Gaven F, Brabet I, Triballeau N, Prezeau L, Acher F and Pin JP (2002) Closure of the Venus flytrap module of mGlu8 receptor and the activation process: Insights from mutations converting antagonists into agonists. *Proc Natl Acad Sci U S A* 99(17):11097-11102.

Bettler B and Tiao JY (2006) Molecular diversity, trafficking and subcellular localization of GABAB receptors. *Pharmacol Ther* 110(3):533-543.

Beurrier C, Lopez S, Revy D, Selvam C, Goudet C, Lherondel M, Gubellini P, Kerkerian-LeGoff L, Acher F, Pin JP and Amalric M (2009) Electrophysiological and behavioral evidence that modulation of metabotropic glutamate receptor 4 with a new agonist reverses experimental parkinsonism. *FASEB J* 23(10):3619-3628.

Billinton A, Upton N and Bowery NG (1999) GABA(B) receptor isoforms GBR1a and GBR1b, appear to be associated with pre- and post-synaptic elements respectively in rat and human cerebellum. *Br J Pharmacol* 126(6):1387-1392.

Bittencourt AS, Carobrez AP, Zamprogno LP, Tufik S and Schenberg LC (2004) Organization of single components of defensive behaviors within distinct columns of periaqueductal gray matter of the rat: role of N-methyl-D-aspartic acid glutamate receptors. *Neuroscience* 125(1):71-89.

Bortolotto ZA, Fitzjohn SM and Collingridge GL (1999) Roles of metabotropic glutamate receptors in LTP and LTD in the hippocampus. *Curr Opin Neurobiol* 9(3):299-304.

Bowers MS, McFarland K, Lake RW, Peterson YK, Lapish CC, Gregory ML, Lanier SM and Kalivas PW (2004) Activator of G protein signaling 3: a gatekeeper of cocaine sensitization and drug seeking. *Neuron* 42(2):269-281.

Brabet I, Parmentier ML, De Colle C, Bockaert J, Acher F and Pin JP (1998) Comparative effect of L-CCG-I, DCG-IV and gamma-carboxy-L-glutamate on all cloned metabotropic glutamate receptor subtypes. *Neuropharmacology* 37(8):1043-1051.

Brauner-Osborne H, Wellendorph P and Jensen AA (2007) Structure, pharmacology and therapeutic prospects of family C G-protein coupled receptors. *Curr Drug Targets* 8(1):169-184.

Brody SA, Conquet F and Geyer MA (2003) Disruption of prepulse inhibition in mice lacking mGluR1. *Eur J Neurosci* 18(12):3361-3366.

Brody SA, Dulawa SC, Conquet F and Geyer MA (2004) Assessment of a prepulse inhibition deficit in a mutant mouse lacking mGlu5 receptors. *Mol Psychiatry* 9(1):35-41.

Burridge K and Wennerberg K (2004) Rho and Rac take center stage. *Cell* 116(2):167-179.

Bushell TJ, Sansig G, Collett VJ, van der Putten H and Collingridge GL (2002) Altered short-term synaptic plasticity in mice lacking the metabotropic glutamate receptor mGlu7. *ScientificWorldJournal* 2:730-737.

Cabello N, Gandia J, Bertarelli DC, Watanabe M, Lluis C, Franco R, Ferre S, Lujan R and Ciruela F (2009) Metabotropic glutamate type 5, dopamine D2 and adenosine A2a receptors form higher-order oligomers in living cells. *J Neurochem* 109(5):1497-1507.

Carroll FY, Stolle A, Beart PM, Voerste A, Brabet I, Mauler F, Joly C, Antonicek H, Bockaert J, Muller T, Pin JP and Prezeau L (2001) BAY36-7620: a potent non-competitive mGlu1 receptor antagonist with inverse agonist activity. *Mol Pharmacol* 59(5):965-973.

Chavez-Noriega LE, Schaffhauser H and Campbell UC (2002) Metabotropic glutamate receptors: potential drug targets for the treatment of schizophrenia. *Curr Drug Targets CNS Neurol Disord* 1(3):261-281.

Chebib M, Vandenberg RJ, Froestl W and Johnston GA (1997) Unsaturated phosphinic analogues of gamma-aminobutyric acid as GABA(C) receptor antagonists. *Eur J Pharmacol* 329(2-3):223-229.

Chen Y, Goudet C, Pin JP and Conn PJ (2008) N-{4-Chloro-2-[(1,3-dioxo-1,3-dihydro-2H-isoindol-2-yl)methyl]phenyl}-2-hy droxybenzamide (CPPHA) acts through a novel site as a positive allosteric modulator of group 1 metabotropic glutamate receptors. *Mol Pharmacol* 73(3):909-918.

Chojnacka-Wojcik E, Tatarczynska E and Pilc A (1997) The anxiolytic-like effect of metabotropic glutamate receptor antagonists after intrahippocampal injection in rats. *Eur J Pharmacol* 319(2-3):153-156.

Christopoulos A and Kenakin T (2002) G protein-coupled receptor allosterism and complexing. *Pharmacol Rev* 54(2):323-374.

Ciruela F, Burgueno J, Casado V, Canals M, Marcellino D, Goldberg SR, Bader M, Fuxe K, Agnati LF, Lluis C, Franco R, Ferre S and Woods AS (2004) Combining mass spectrometry and pull-down techniques for the study of receptor heteromerization. Direct epitope-epitope electrostatic interactions between adenosine A2A and dopamine D2 receptors. *Anal Chem* 76(18):5354-5363.

Ciruela F, Escriche M, Burgueno J, Angulo E, Casado V, Soloviev MM, Canela EI, Mallol J, Chan WY, Lluis C, McIlhinney RA and Franco R (2001) Metabotropic glutamate 1alpha and adenosine A1 receptors assemble into functionally interacting complexes. *J Biol Chem* 276(21):18345-18351.

Collingridge GL, Kehl SJ and McLennan H (1983) Excitatory amino acids in synaptic transmission in the Schaffer collateral-commissural pathway of the rat hippocampus. *J Physiol* 334:33-46.

Comps-Agrar L, Kniazeff J, Norskov-Lauritsen L, Maurel D, Gassmann M, Gregor N, Prezeau L, Bettler B, Durroux T, Trinquet E and Pin JP (2011) The oligomeric state sets GABA(B) receptor signalling efficacy. *EMBO J* 30(12):2336-2349.

Conn PJ, Christopoulos A and Lindsley CW (2009a) Allosteric modulators of GPCRs: a novel approach for the treatment of CNS disorders. *Nat Rev Drug Discov* 8(1):41-54.

Conn PJ and Jones CK (2009) Promise of mGluR2/3 activators in psychiatry. *Neuropsychopharmacology* 34(1):248-249.

Conn PJ, Lindsley CW and Jones CK (2009b) Activation of metabotropic glutamate receptors as a novel approach for the treatment of schizophrenia. *Trends Pharmacol Sci* 30(1):25-31.

Conn PJ and Pin JP (1997) Pharmacology and functions of metabotropic glutamate receptors. *Annu Rev Pharmacol Toxicol* 37:205-237.

Coyle JT (2006) Glutamate and schizophrenia: beyond the dopamine hypothesis. *Cell Mol Neurobiol* 26(4-6):365-384.

Cryan JF, Kelly PH, Neijt HC, Sansig G, Flor PJ and van Der Putten H (2003) Antidepressant and anxiolytic-like effects in mice lacking the group III metabotropic glutamate receptor mGluR7. *Eur J Neurosci* 17(11):2409-2417.

Dascal N (1997) Signalling via the G protein-activated K+ channels. *Cell Signal* 9(8):551-573.

Depping AM, Komossa K, Kissling W and Leucht S (2010) Second-generation antipsychotics for anxiety disorders. *Cochrane Database Syst Rev*(12):CD008120.

Derjean D, Bertrand S, Le Masson G, Landry M, Morisset V and Nagy F (2003) Dynamic balance of metabotropic inputs causes dorsal horn neurons to switch functional states. *Nat Neurosci* 6(3):274-281.

Dirig DM and Yaksh TL (1995) Intrathecal baclofen and muscimol, but not midazolam, are antinociceptive using the rat-formalin model. *J Pharmacol Exp Ther* 275(1):219-227.

Dolen G, Carpenter RL, Ocain TD and Bear MF (2010) Mechanism-based approaches to treating fragile X. *Pharmacol Ther* 127(1):78-93.

Doumazane E, Scholler P, Zwier JM, Eric T, Rondard P and Pin JP (2011) A new approach to analyze cell surface protein complexes reveals specific heterodimeric metabotropic glutamate receptors. *FASEB J* 25(1):66-77.

Doupnik CA (2008) GPCR-Kir channel signaling complexes: defining rules of engagement. *J Recept Signal Transduct Res* 28(1-2):83-91.

Dunayevich E, Erickson J, Levine L, Landbloom R, Schoepp DD and Tollefson GD (2008) Efficacy and tolerability of an mGlu2/3 agonist in the treatment of generalized anxiety disorder. *Neuropsychopharmacology* 33(7):1603-1610.

Dunlap K and Fischbach GD (1981) Neurotransmitters decrease the calcium conductance activated by depolarization of embryonic chick sensory neurones. *J Physiol* 317:519-535.

Dutar P and Nicoll RA (1988) Pre- and postsynaptic GABAB receptors in the hippocampus have different pharmacological properties. *Neuron* 1(7):585-591.

Duty S (2010) Therapeutic potential of targeting group III metabotropic glutamate receptors in the treatment of Parkinson's disease. *Br J Pharmacol* 161(2):271-287.

Duvoisin RM, Zhang C, Pfankuch TF, O'Connor H, Gayet-Primo J, Quraishi S and Raber J (2005) Increased measures of anxiety and weight gain in mice lacking the group III metabotropic glutamate receptor mGluR8. *Eur J Neurosci* 22(2):425-436.

Engin E and Treit D (2008) The effects of intra-cerebral drug infusions on animals' unconditioned fear reactions: a systematic review. *Prog Neuropsychopharmacol Biol Psychiatry* 32(6):1399-1419.

Fairfax BP, Pitcher JA, Scott MG, Calver AR, Pangalos MN, Moss SJ and Couve A (2004) Phosphorylation and chronic agonist treatment atypically modulate GABAB receptor cell surface stability. *J Biol Chem* 279(13):12565-12573.

Fell MJ, Svensson KA, Johnson BG and Schoepp DD (2008) Evidence for the role of metabotropic glutamate (mGlu)2 not mGlu3 receptors in the preclinical antipsychotic pharmacology of the mGlu2/3 receptor agonist (-)-(1R,4S,5S,6S)-4-amino-2-sulfonylbicyclo[3.1.0]hexane-4,6-dicarboxylic acid (LY404039). *J Pharmacol Exp Ther* 326(1):209-217.

Felts AS, Lindsley SR, Lamb JP, Rodriguez AL, Menon UN, Jadhav S, Jones CK, Conn PJ, Lindsley CW and Emmitte KA (2010) 3-Cyano-5-fluoro-N-arylbenzamides as negative allosteric modulators of mGlu(5): Identification of easily prepared tool compounds with CNS exposure in rats. *Bioorg Med Chem Lett* 20(15):4390-4394.

Ferraguti F and Shigemoto R (2006) Metabotropic glutamate receptors. *Cell Tissue Res* 326(2):483-504.

Ferre S, Ciruela F, Quiroz C, Lujan R, Popoli P, Cunha RA, Agnati LF, Fuxe K, Woods AS, Lluis C and Franco R (2007) Adenosine receptor heteromers and their integrative role in striatal function. *ScientificWorldJournal* 7:74-85.

Ferre S, Karcz-Kubicha M, Hope BT, Popoli P, Burgueno J, Gutierrez MA, Casado V, Fuxe K, Goldberg SR, Lluis C, Franco R and Ciruela F (2002) Synergistic interaction between adenosine A2A and glutamate mGlu5 receptors: implications for striatal neuronal function. *Proc Natl Acad Sci U S A* 99(18):11940-11945.

Feyissa AM, Chandran A, Stockmeier CA and Karolewicz B (2009) Reduced levels of NR2A and NR2B subunits of NMDA receptor and PSD-95 in the prefrontal cortex in major depression. *Prog Neuropsychopharmacol Biol Psychiatry* 33(1):70-75.

Flannery BA, Garbutt JC, Cody MW, Renn W, Grace K, Osborne M, Crosby K, Morreale M and Trivette A (2004) Baclofen for alcohol dependence: a preliminary open-label study. *Alcohol Clin Exp Res* 28(10):1517-1523.

Fredriksson R, Lagerstrom MC, Lundin LG and Schioth HB (2003) The G-protein-coupled receptors in the human genome form five main families. Phylogenetic analysis, paralogon groups, and fingerprints. *Mol Pharmacol* 63(6):1256-1272.

Froestl W, Mickel SJ, Hall RG, von Sprecher G, Strub D, Baumann PA, Brugger F, Gentsch C, Jaekel J, Olpe HR and et al. (1995) Phosphinic acid analogues of GABA. 1. New potent and selective GABAB agonists. *J Med Chem* 38(17):3297-3312.

Galandrin S, Oligny-Longpre G and Bouvier M (2007) The evasive nature of drug efficacy: implications for drug discovery. *Trends Pharmacol Sci* 28(8):423-430.

Galici R, Jones CK, Hemstapat K, Nong Y, Echemendia NG, Williams LC, de Paulis T and Conn PJ (2006) Biphenyl-indanone A, a positive allosteric modulator of the metabotropic glutamate receptor subtype 2, has antipsychotic- and anxiolytic-like effects in mice. *J Pharmacol Exp Ther* 318(1):173-185.

Galvez T, Duthey B, Kniazeff J, Blahos J, Rovelli G, Bettler B, Prezeau L and Pin JP (2001) Allosteric interactions between GB1 and GB2 subunits are required for optimal GABA(B) receptor function. *EMBO J* 20(9):2152-2159.

Gasparini F, Lingenhohl K, Stoehr N, Flor PJ, Heinrich M, Vranesic I, Biollaz M, Allgeier H, Heckendorn R, Urwyler S, Varney MA, Johnson EC, Hess SD, Rao SP, Sacaan AI, Santori EM, Velicelebi G and Kuhn R (1999) 2-Methyl-6-(phenylethynyl)-pyridine (MPEP), a potent, selective and systemically active mGlu5 receptor antagonist. *Neuropharmacology* 38(10):1493-1503.

Gerlai R, Roder JC and Hampson DR (1998) Altered spatial learning and memory in mice lacking the mGluR4 subtype of metabotropic glutamate receptor. *Behav Neurosci* 112(3):525-532.

Ghasemzadeh MB, Mueller C and Vasudevan P (2009) Behavioral sensitization to cocaine is associated with increased glutamate receptor trafficking to the postsynaptic density after extended withdrawal period. *Neuroscience* 159(1):414-426.

Gonzalez-Maeso J, Ang RL, Yuen T, Chan P, Weisstaub NV, Lopez-Gimenez JF, Zhou M, Okawa Y, Callado LF, Milligan G, Gingrich JA, Filizola M, Meana JJ and Sealfon SC (2008) Identification of a serotonin/glutamate receptor complex implicated in psychosis. *Nature* 452(7183):93-97.

Gonzalez-Maeso J, Weisstaub NV, Zhou M, Chan P, Ivic L, Ang R, Lira A, Bradley-Moore M, Ge Y, Zhou Q, Sealfon SC and Gingrich JA (2007) Hallucinogens recruit specific cortical 5-HT(2A) receptor-mediated signaling pathways to affect behavior. *Neuron* 53(3):439-452.

Gonzalez-Maeso J, Yuen T, Ebersole BJ, Wurmbach E, Lira A, Zhou M, Weisstaub N, Hen R, Gingrich JA and Sealfon SC (2003) Transcriptome fingerprints distinguish hallucinogenic and nonhallucinogenic 5-hydroxytryptamine 2A receptor agonist effects in mouse somatosensory cortex. *J Neurosci* 23(26):8836-8843.

Goudet C, Gaven F, Kniazeff J, Vol C, Liu J, Cohen-Gonsaud M, Acher F, Prezeau L and Pin JP (2004) Heptahelical domain of metabotropic glutamate receptor 5 behaves like rhodopsin-like receptors. *Proc Natl Acad Sci U S A* 101(1):378-383.

Guetg N, Abdel Aziz S, Holbro N, Turecek R, Rose T, Seddik R, Gassmann M, Moes S, Jenoe P, Oertner TG, Casanova E and Bettler B (2010) NMDA receptor-dependent GABAB receptor internalization via CaMKII phosphorylation of serine 867 in GABAB1. *Proc Natl Acad Sci U S A* 107(31):13924-13929.

Hammond AS, Rodriguez AL, Townsend SD, Niswender CM, Gregory KJ, Lindsley CW and Conn PJ (2010) Discovery of a Novel Chemical Class of mGlu(5) Allosteric Ligands with Distinct Modes of Pharmacology. *ACS Chem Neurosci* 1(10):702-716.

Haney M, Hart CL and Foltin RW (2006) Effects of baclofen on cocaine self-administration: opioid- and nonopioid-dependent volunteers. *Neuropsychopharmacology* 31(8):1814-1821.

Hanyaloglu AC and von Zastrow M (2008) Regulation of GPCRs by endocytic membrane trafficking and its potential implications. *Annu Rev Pharmacol Toxicol* 48:537-568.

Harvey J and Collingridge GL (1993) Signal transduction pathways involved in the acute potentiation of NMDA responses by 1S,3R-ACPD in rat hippocampal slices. *Br J Pharmacol* 109(4):1085-1090.

Hemstapat K, de Paulis T, Chen Y, Brady AE, Grover VK, Alagille D, Tamagnan GD and Conn PJ (2006) A novel class of positive allosteric modulators of metabotropic glutamate receptor subtype 1 interact with a site distinct from that of negative allosteric modulators. *Mol Pharmacol* 70(2):616-626.

Herlitze S, Garcia DE, Mackie K, Hille B, Scheuer T and Catterall WA (1996) Modulation of Ca2+ channels by G-protein beta gamma subunits. *Nature* 380(6571):258-262.

Hirono M, Yoshioka T and Konishi S (2001) GABA(B) receptor activation enhances mGluR-mediated responses at cerebellar excitatory synapses. *Nat Neurosci* 4(12):1207-1216.

Hirsch EC (2000) Nigrostriatal system plasticity in Parkinson's disease: effect of dopaminergic denervation and treatment. *Ann Neurol* 47(4 Suppl 1):S115-120; discussion S120-111.

Hoare SR (2005) Mechanisms of peptide and nonpeptide ligand binding to Class B G-protein-coupled receptors. *Drug Discov Today* 10(6):417-427.

Hu J, Hauache O and Spiegel AM (2000) Human Ca2+ receptor cysteine-rich domain. Analysis of function of mutant and chimeric receptors. *J Biol Chem* 275(21):16382-16389.

Jiang P, Ji Q, Liu Z, Snyder LA, Benard LM, Margolskee RF and Max M (2004) The cysteine-rich region of T1R3 determines responses to intensely sweet proteins. *J Biol Chem* 279(43):45068-45075.

Johnson MP, Baez M, Jagdmann GE, Jr., Britton TC, Large TH, Callagaro DO, Tizzano JP, Monn JA and Schoepp DD (2003) Discovery of allosteric potentiators for the metabotropic glutamate 2 receptor: synthesis and subtype selectivity of N-(4-(2-methoxyphenoxy)phenyl)-N-(2,2,2- trifluoroethylsulfonyl)pyrid-3-ylmethylamine. *J Med Chem* 46(15):3189-3192.

Kachroo A, Orlando LR, Grandy DK, Chen JF, Young AB and Schwarzschild MA (2005) Interactions between metabotropic glutamate 5 and adenosine A2A receptors in normal and parkinsonian mice. *J Neurosci* 25(45):10414-10419.

Kammerer RA, Frank S, Schulthess T, Landwehr R, Lustig A and Engel J (1999) Heterodimerization of a functional GABAB receptor is mediated by parallel coiled-coil alpha-helices. *Biochemistry* 38(40):13263-13269.

Kangrga I, Jiang MC and Randic M (1991) Actions of (-)-baclofen on rat dorsal horn neurons. *Brain Res* 562(2):265-275.

Kaupmann K, Cryan JF, Wellendorph P, Mombereau C, Sansig G, Klebs K, Schmutz M, Froestl W, van der Putten H, Mosbacher J, Brauner-Osborne H, Waldmeier P and Bettler B (2003) Specific gamma-hydroxybutyrate-binding sites but loss of pharmacological effects of gamma-hydroxybutyrate in GABA(B)(1)-deficient mice. *Eur J Neurosci* 18(10):2722-2730.

Kaupmann K, Huggel K, Heid J, Flor PJ, Bischoff S, Mickel SJ, McMaster G, Angst C, Bittiger H, Froestl W and Bettler B (1997) Expression cloning of GABA(B) receptors uncovers similarity to metabotropic glutamate receptors. *Nature* 386(6622):239-246.

Kaupmann K, Malitschek B, Schuler V, Heid J, Froestl W, Beck P, Mosbacher J, Bischoff S, Kulik A, Shigemoto R, Karschin A and Bettler B (1998) GABA(B)-receptor subtypes assemble into functional heteromeric complexes. *Nature* 396(6712):683-687.

Kenny PJ and Markou A (2004) The ups and downs of addiction: role of metabotropic glutamate receptors. *Trends Pharmacol Sci* 25(5):265-272.

Kinney GG, O'Brien JA, Lemaire W, Burno M, Bickel DJ, Clements MK, Chen TB, Wisnoski DD, Lindsley CW, Tiller PR, Smith S, Jacobson MA, Sur C, Duggan ME, Pettibone DJ, Conn PJ and Williams DL, Jr. (2005) A novel selective positive allosteric modulator of metabotropic glutamate receptor subtype 5 has in vivo activity and antipsychotic-like effects in rat behavioral models. *J Pharmacol Exp Ther* 313(1):199-206.

Kleinschmidt S, Grundmann U, Janneck U, Kreienmeyer J, Kulosa R and Larsen R (1997) Total intravenous anaesthesia using propofol, gamma-hydroxybutyrate or midazolam in combination with sufentanil for patients undergoing coronary artery bypass surgery. *Eur J Anaesthesiol* 14(6):590-599.

Klodzinska A, Tatarczynska E, Stachowicz K and Chojnacka-Wojcik E (2004) The anxiolytic-like activity of AIDA (1-aminoindan-1,5-dicarboxylic acid), an mGLu 1 receptor antagonist. *J Physiol Pharmacol* 55(1 Pt 1):113-126.

Kniazeff J, Galvez T, Labesse G and Pin JP (2002) No ligand binding in the GB2 subunit of the GABA(B) receptor is required for activation and allosteric interaction between the subunits. *J Neurosci* 22(17):7352-7361.

Kniazeff J, Prezeau L, Rondard P, Pin JP and Goudet C (2011) Dimers and beyond: The functional puzzles of class C GPCRs. *Pharmacol Ther* 130(1):9-25.

Knoflach F, Mutel V, Jolidon S, Kew JN, Malherbe P, Vieira E, Wichmann J and Kemp JA (2001) Positive allosteric modulators of metabotropic glutamate 1 receptor: characterization, mechanism of action, and binding site. *Proc Natl Acad Sci U S A* 98(23):13402-13407.

Kolber BJ, Montana MC, Carrasquillo Y, Xu J, Heinemann SF, Muglia LJ and Gereau RWt (2010) Activation of metabotropic glutamate receptor 5 in the amygdala modulates pain-like behavior. *J Neurosci* 30(24):8203-8213.

Kulik A, Vida I, Lujan R, Haas CA, Lopez-Bendito G, Shigemoto R and Frotscher M (2003) Subcellular localization of metabotropic GABA(B) receptor subunits GABA(B1a/b) and GABA(B2) in the rat hippocampus. *J Neurosci* 23(35):11026-11035.

Kunishima N, Shimada Y, Tsuji Y, Sato T, Yamamoto M, Kumasaka T, Nakanishi S, Jingami H and Morikawa K (2000) Structural basis of glutamate recognition by a dimeric metabotropic glutamate receptor. *Nature* 407(6807):971-977.

Laborit H, Jouany JM, Gerard J and Fabiani F (1960) [Summary of an experimental and clinical study on a metabolic substrate with inhibitory central action: sodium 4-hydroxybutyrate]. *Presse Med* 68:1867-1869.

Leaney JL and Tinker A (2000) The role of members of the pertussis toxin-sensitive family of G proteins in coupling receptors to the activation of the G protein-gated inwardly rectifying potassium channel. *Proc Natl Acad Sci U S A* 97(10):5651-5656.

Lefkowitz RJ (1998) G protein-coupled receptors. III. New roles for receptor kinases and beta-arrestins in receptor signaling and desensitization. *J Biol Chem* 273(30):18677-18680.

Lehmann A (2008) Novel treatments of GERD: focus on the lower esophageal sphincter. *Eur Rev Med Pharmacol Sci* 12 Suppl 1:103-110.

Linden AM, Shannon H, Baez M, Yu JL, Koester A and Schoepp DD (2005) Anxiolytic-like activity of the mGLU2/3 receptor agonist LY354740 in the elevated plus maze test is disrupted in metabotropic glutamate receptor 2 and 3 knock-out mice. *Psychopharmacology (Berl)* 179(1):284-291.

Litschig S, Gasparini F, Rueegg D, Stoehr N, Flor PJ, Vranesic I, Prezeau L, Pin JP, Thomsen C and Kuhn R (1999) CPCCOEt, a noncompetitive metabotropic glutamate receptor 1 antagonist, inhibits receptor signaling without affecting glutamate binding. *Mol Pharmacol* 55(3):453-461.

Lopez S, Turle-Lorenzo N, Acher F, De Leonibus E, Mele A and Amalric M (2007) Targeting group III metabotropic glutamate receptors produces complex behavioral effects in rodent models of Parkinson's disease. *J Neurosci* 27(25):6701-6711.

Lopez-Bendito G, Shigemoto R, Kulik A, Vida I, Fairen A and Lujan R (2004) Distribution of metabotropic GABA receptor subunits GABAB1a/b and GABAB2 in the rat hippocampus during prenatal and postnatal development. *Hippocampus* 14(7):836-848.

Lu YM, Jia Z, Janus C, Henderson JT, Gerlai R, Wojtowicz JM and Roder JC (1997) Mice lacking metabotropic glutamate receptor 5 show impaired learning and reduced CA1 long-term potentiation (LTP) but normal CA3 LTP. *J Neurosci* 17(13):5196-5205.

Luscher C, Jan LY, Stoffel M, Malenka RC and Nicoll RA (1997) G protein-coupled inwardly rectifying K+ channels (GIRKs) mediate postsynaptic but not presynaptic transmitter actions in hippocampal neurons. *Neuron* 19(3):687-695.

Maj M, Bruno V, Dragic Z, Yamamoto R, Battaglia G, Inderbitzin W, Stoehr N, Stein T, Gasparini F, Vranesic I, Kuhn R, Nicoletti F and Flor PJ (2003) (-)-PHCCC, a positive allosteric modulator of mGluR4: characterization, mechanism of action, and neuroprotection. *Neuropharmacology* 45(7):895-906.

Malcangio M and Bowery NG (1995) Possible therapeutic application of GABAB receptor agonists and antagonists. *Clin Neuropharmacol* 18(4):285-305.

Malcangio M, Ghelardini C, Giotti A, Malmberg-Aiello P and Bartolini A (1991) CGP 35348, a new GABAB antagonist, prevents antinociception and muscle-relaxant effect induced by baclofen. *Br J Pharmacol* 103(2):1303-1308.

Malherbe P, Masciadri R, Norcross RD, Knoflach F, Kratzeisen C, Zenner MT, Kolb Y, Marcuz A, Huwyler J, Nakagawa T, Porter RH, Thomas AW, Wettstein JG, Sleight AJ, Spooren W and Prinssen EP (2008) Characterization of (R,S)-5,7-di-tert-butyl-3-hydroxy-3-trifluoromethyl-3H-benzofuran-2-one as a positive allosteric modulator of GABAB receptors. *Br J Pharmacol* 154(4):797-811.

Margeta-Mitrovic M, Jan YN and Jan LY (2001) Function of GB1 and GB2 subunits in G protein coupling of GABA(B) receptors. *Proc Natl Acad Sci U S A* 98(25):14649-14654.

Martin LJ, Blackstone CD, Huganir RL and Price DL (1992) Cellular localization of a metabotropic glutamate receptor in rat brain. *Neuron* 9(2):259-270.

Marvizon JC, Grady EF, Stefani E, Bunnett NW and Mayer EA (1999) Substance P release in the dorsal horn assessed by receptor internalization: NMDA receptors counteract a tonic inhibition by GABA(B) receptors. *Eur J Neurosci* 11(2):417-426.

Masu M, Iwakabe H, Tagawa Y, Miyoshi T, Yamashita M, Fukuda Y, Sasaki H, Hiroi K, Nakamura Y, Shigemoto R and et al. (1995) Specific deficit of the ON response in visual transmission by targeted disruption of the mGluR6 gene. *Cell* 80(5):757-765.

Maurel D, Comps-Agrar L, Brock C, Rives ML, Bourrier E, Ayoub MA, Bazin H, Tinel N, Durroux T, Prezeau L, Trinquet E and Pin JP (2008) Cell-surface protein-protein interaction analysis with time-resolved FRET and snap-tag technologies: application to GPCR oligomerization. *Nat Methods* 5(6):561-567.

Miedlich SU, Gama L, Seuwen K, Wolf RM and Breitwieser GE (2004) Homology modeling of the transmembrane domain of the human calcium sensing receptor and localization of an allosteric binding site. *J Biol Chem* 279(8):7254-7263.

Misgeld U, Bijak M and Jarolimek W (1995) A physiological role for GABAB receptors and the effects of baclofen in the mammalian central nervous system. *Prog Neurobiol* 46(4):423-462.

Molina-Hernandez M, Tellez-Alcantara NP, Perez-Garcia J, Olivera-Lopez JI and Jaramillo-Jaimes MT (2008) Antidepressant-like actions of minocycline combined with several glutamate antagonists. *Prog Neuropsychopharmacol Biol Psychiatry* 32(2):380-386.

Morishima Y, Miyakawa T, Furuyashiki T, Tanaka Y, Mizuma H and Nakanishi S (2005) Enhanced cocaine responsiveness and impaired motor coordination in metabotropic glutamate receptor subtype 2 knockout mice. *Proc Natl Acad Sci U S A* 102(11):4170-4175.

Moussawi K and Kalivas PW (2010) Group II metabotropic glutamate receptors (mGlu2/3) in drug addiction. *Eur J Pharmacol* 639(1-3):115-122.

Moussawi K, Pacchioni A, Moran M, Olive MF, Gass JT, Lavin A and Kalivas PW (2009) N-Acetylcysteine reverses cocaine-induced metaplasticity. *Nat Neurosci* 12(2):182-189.

Muto T, Tsuchiya D, Morikawa K and Jingami H (2007) Expression, purification, crystallization and preliminary X-ray analysis of the ligand-binding domain of metabotropic glutamate receptor 7. *Acta Crystallogr Sect F Struct Biol Cryst Commun* 63(Pt 7):627-630.

Nakajima Y, Iwakabe H, Akazawa C, Nawa H, Shigemoto R, Mizuno N and Nakanishi S (1993) Molecular characterization of a novel retinal metabotropic glutamate receptor mGluR6 with a high agonist selectivity for L-2-amino-4-phosphonobutyrate. *J Biol Chem* 268(16):11868-11873.

Nelson G, Hoon MA, Chandrashekar J, Zhang Y, Ryba NJ and Zuker CS (2001) Mammalian sweet taste receptors. *Cell* 106(3):381-390.

Neugebauer V, Zinebi F, Russell R, Gallagher JP and Shinnick-Gallagher P (2000) Cocaine and kindling alter the sensitivity of group II and III metabotropic glutamate receptors in the central amygdala. *J Neurophysiol* 84(2):759-770.

Nicoletti F, Bockaert J, Collingridge GL, Conn PJ, Ferraguti F, Schoepp DD, Wroblewski JT and Pin JP (2011) Metabotropic glutamate receptors: from the workbench to the bedside. *Neuropharmacology* 60(7-8):1017-1041.

Nishikawa M, Hirouchi M and Kuriyama K (1997) Functional coupling of Gi subtype with GABAB receptor/adenylyl cyclase system: analysis using a reconstituted system with purified GTP-binding protein from bovine cerebral cortex. *Neurochem Int* 31(1):21-25.

Niswender CM and Conn PJ (2010) Metabotropic glutamate receptors: physiology, pharmacology, and disease. *Annu Rev Pharmacol Toxicol* 50:295-322.

Niswender CM, Johnson KA, Miller NR, Ayala JE, Luo Q, Williams R, Saleh S, Orton D, Weaver CD and Conn PJ (2010) Context-dependent pharmacology exhibited by negative allosteric modulators of metabotropic glutamate receptor 7. *Mol Pharmacol* 77(3):459-468.

Niswender CM, Johnson KA, Weaver CD, Jones CK, Xiang Z, Luo Q, Rodriguez AL, Marlo JE, de Paulis T, Thompson AD, Days EL, Nalywajko T, Austin CA, Williams MB, Ayala JE, Williams R, Lindsley CW and Conn PJ (2008) Discovery, characterization, and antiparkinsonian effect of novel positive allosteric modulators of metabotropic glutamate receptor 4. *Mol Pharmacol* 74(5):1345-1358.

O'Hara PJ, Sheppard PO, Thogersen H, Venezia D, Haldeman BA, McGrane V, Houamed KM, Thomsen C, Gilbert TL and Mulvihill ER (1993) The ligand-binding domain in metabotropic glutamate receptors is related to bacterial periplasmic binding proteins. *Neuron* 11(1):41-52.

Ohishi H, Neki A and Mizuno N (1998) Distribution of a metabotropic glutamate receptor, mGluR2, in the central nervous system of the rat and mouse: an immunohistochemical study with a monoclonal antibody. *Neurosci Res* 30(1):65-82.

Ohishi H, Ogawa-Meguro R, Shigemoto R, Kaneko T, Nakanishi S and Mizuno N (1994) Immunohistochemical localization of metabotropic glutamate receptors, mGluR2 and mGluR3, in rat cerebellar cortex. *Neuron* 13(1):55-66.

Oliet SH, Malenka RC and Nicoll RA (1997) Two distinct forms of long-term depression coexist in CA1 hippocampal pyramidal cells. *Neuron* 18(6):969-982.

Ossowska K, Pietraszek M, Wardas J and Wolfarth S (2004) Potential antipsychotic and extrapyramidal effects of (R,S)-3,4-dicarboxyphenylglycine [(R,S)-3,4-DCPG], a mixed AMPA antagonist/mGluR8 agonist. *Pol J Pharmacol* 56(3):295-304.

Overington JP, Al-Lazikani B and Hopkins AL (2006) How many drug targets are there? *Nat Rev Drug Discov* 5(12):993-996.

Pagano A, Ruegg D, Litschig S, Stoehr N, Stierlin C, Heinrich M, Floersheim P, Prezeau L, Carroll F, Pin JP, Cambria A, Vranesic I, Flor PJ, Gasparini F and Kuhn R (2000) The non-competitive antagonists 2-methyl-6-(phenylethynyl)pyridine and 7-hydroxyiminocyclopropan[b]chromen-1a-carboxylic acid ethyl ester interact with overlapping binding pockets in the transmembrane region of group I metabotropic glutamate receptors. *J Biol Chem* 275(43):33750-33758.

Palucha A and Pilc A (2005) The involvement of glutamate in the pathophysiology of depression. *Drug News Perspect* 18(4):262-268.

Pardi D and Black J (2006) gamma-Hydroxybutyrate/sodium oxybate: neurobiology, and impact on sleep and wakefulness. *CNS Drugs* 20(12):993-1018.

Patil ST, Zhang L, Martenyi F, Lowe SL, Jackson KA, Andreev BV, Avedisova AS, Bardenstein LM, Gurovich IY, Morozova MA, Mosolov SN, Neznanov NG, Reznik AM, Smulevich AB, Tochilov VA, Johnson BG, Monn JA and Schoepp DD (2007) Activation of mGlu2/3 receptors as a new approach to treat schizophrenia: a randomized Phase 2 clinical trial. *Nat Med* 13(9):1102-1107.

Paul IA and Skolnick P (2003) Glutamate and depression: clinical and preclinical studies. *Ann N Y Acad Sci* 1003:250-272.

Pekhletski R, Gerlai R, Overstreet LS, Huang XP, Agopyan N, Slater NT, Abramow-Newerly W, Roder JC and Hampson DR (1996) Impaired cerebellar synaptic plasticity and motor performance in mice lacking the mGluR4 subtype of metabotropic glutamate receptor. *J Neurosci* 16(20):6364-6373.

Peleg S, Varon D, Ivanina T, Dessauer CW and Dascal N (2002) G(alpha)(i) controls the gating of the G protein-activated K(+) channel, GIRK. *Neuron* 33(1):87-99.

Perroy J, Adam L, Qanbar R, Chenier S and Bouvier M (2003) Phosphorylation-independent desensitization of GABA(B) receptor by GRK4. *EMBO J* 22(15):3816-3824.

Perroy J, Raynaud F, Homburger V, Rousset MC, Telley L, Bockaert J and Fagni L (2008) Direct interaction enables cross-talk between ionotropic and group I metabotropic glutamate receptors. *J Biol Chem* 283(11):6799-6805.

Petersen EN and Lassen JB (1981) A water lick conflict paradigm using drug experienced rats. *Psychopharmacology (Berl)* 75(3):236-239.

Petrel C, Kessler A, Dauban P, Dodd RH, Rognan D and Ruat M (2004) Positive and negative allosteric modulators of the Ca2+-sensing receptor interact within overlapping but not identical binding sites in the transmembrane domain. *J Biol Chem* 279(18):18990-18997.

Pin JP and Acher F (2002) The metabotropic glutamate receptors: structure, activation mechanism and pharmacology. *Curr Drug Targets CNS Neurol Disord* 1(3):297-317.

Pin JP, Kniazeff J, Goudet C, Bessis AS, Liu J, Galvez T, Acher F, Rondard P and Prezeau L (2004) The activation mechanism of class-C G-protein coupled receptors. *Biol Cell* 96(5):335-342.

Pin JP and Prezeau L (2007) Allosteric modulators of GABA(B) receptors: mechanism of action and therapeutic perspective. *Curr Neuropharmacol* 5(3):195-201.

Pisani A, Bonsi P, Centonze D, Gubellini P, Bernardi G and Calabresi P (2003) Targeting striatal cholinergic interneurons in Parkinson's disease: focus on metabotropic glutamate receptors. *Neuropharmacology* 45(1):45-56.

Pontier SM, Lahaie N, Ginham R, St-Gelais F, Bonin H, Bell DJ, Flynn H, Trudeau LE, McIlhinney J, White JH and Bouvier M (2006) Coordinated action of NSF and PKC regulates GABAB receptor signaling efficacy. *EMBO J* 25(12):2698-2709.

Price DD, Rafii A, Watkins LR and Buckingham B (1984) A psychophysical analysis of acupuncture analgesia. *Pain* 19(1):27-42.

Puckerin A, Liu L, Permaul N, Carman P, Lee J and Diverse-Pierluissi MA (2006) Arrestin is required for agonist-induced trafficking of voltage-dependent calcium channels. *J Biol Chem* 281(41):31131-31141.

Rondard P, Liu J, Huang S, Malhaire F, Vol C, Pinault A, Labesse G and Pin JP (2006) Coupling of agonist binding to effector domain activation in metabotropic glutamate-like receptors. *J Biol Chem* 281(34):24653-24661.

Sansig G, Bushell TJ, Clarke VR, Rozov A, Burnashev N, Portet C, Gasparini F, Schmutz M, Klebs K, Shigemoto R, Flor PJ, Kuhn R, Knoepfel T, Schroeder M, Hampson DR, Collett VJ, Zhang C, Duvoisin RM, Collingridge GL and van Der Putten H (2001) Increased seizure susceptibility in mice lacking metabotropic glutamate receptor 7. *J Neurosci* 21(22):8734-8745.

Sato M, Horinouchi T, Hutchinson DS, Evans BA and Summers RJ (2007) Ligand-directed signaling at the beta3-adrenoceptor produced by 3-(2-Ethylphenoxy)-1-[(1,S)-1,2,3,4-tetrahydronapth-1-ylamino]-2S-2-propan ol oxalate (SR59230A) relative to receptor agonists. *Mol Pharmacol* 72(5):1359-1368.

Sawynok J (1984) GABAergic mechanisms in antinociception. *Prog Neuropsychopharmacol Biol Psychiatry* 8(4-6):581-586.

Schaffhauser H, Knoflach F, Pink JR, Bleuel Z, Cartmell J, Goepfert F, Kemp JA, Richards JG, Adam G and Mutel V (1998) Multiple pathways for regulation of the KCl-induced [3H]-GABA release by metabotropic glutamate receptors, in primary rat cortical cultures. *Brain Res* 782(1-2):91-104.

Schann S, Menet C, Arvault P, Mercier G, Frauli M, Mayer S, Hubert N, Triballeau N, Bertrand HO, Acher F and Neuville P (2006) Design and synthesis of APTCs (aminopyrrolidinetricarboxylic acids): identification of a new group III metabotropic glutamate receptor selective agonist. *Bioorg Med Chem Lett* 16(18):4856-4860.

Scholten D, Canals M, Maussang D, Roumen L, Smit M, Wijtmans M, de Graaf C, Vischer H and Leurs R (2011) Pharmacological Modulation of Chemokine Receptor Function. *Br J Pharmacol.*

Schweitzer C, Kratzeisen C, Adam G, Lundstrom K, Malherbe P, Ohresser S, Stadler H, Wichmann J, Woltering T and Mutel V (2000) Characterization of [(3)H]-LY354740 binding to rat mGlu2 and mGlu3 receptors expressed in CHO cells using semliki forest virus vectors. *Neuropharmacology* 39(10):1700-1706.

Scrima L, Hartman PG, Johnson FH, Jr., Thomas EE and Hiller FC (1990) The effects of gamma-hydroxybutyrate on the sleep of narcolepsy patients: a double-blind study. *Sleep* 13(6):479-490.

Selvam C, Oueslati N, Lemasson IA, Brabet I, Rigault D, Courtiol T, Cesarini S, Triballeau N, Bertrand HO, Goudet C, Pin JP and Acher FC (2010) A virtual screening hit reveals new possibilities for developing group III metabotropic glutamate receptor agonists. *J Med Chem* 53(7):2797-2813.

Sexton PM, Morfis M, Tilakaratne N, Hay DL, Udawela M, Christopoulos G and Christopoulos A (2006) Complexing receptor pharmacology: modulation of family B G protein-coupled receptor function by RAMPs. *Ann N Y Acad Sci* 1070:90-104.

Shenoy SK and Lefkowitz RJ (2005) Receptor regulation: beta-arrestin moves up a notch. *Nat Cell Biol* 7(12):1159-1161.

Shimazaki T, Iijima M and Chaki S (2004) Anxiolytic-like activity of MGS0039, a potent group II metabotropic glutamate receptor antagonist, in a marble-burying behavior test. *Eur J Pharmacol* 501(1-3):121-125.

Smith GD, Harrison SM, Birch PJ, Elliott PJ, Malcangio M and Bowery NG (1994) Increased sensitivity to the antinociceptive activity of (+/-)-baclofen in an animal model of chronic neuropathic, but not chronic inflammatory hyperalgesia. *Neuropharmacology* 33(9):1103-1108.

Steckler T, Lavreysen H, Oliveira AM, Aerts N, Van Craenendonck H, Prickaerts J, Megens A and Lesage AS (2005) Effects of mGlu1 receptor blockade on anxiety-related behaviour in the rat lick suppression test. *Psychopharmacology (Berl)* 179(1):198-206.

Sudo S, Kumagai J, Nishi S, Layfield S, Ferraro T, Bathgate RA and Hsueh AJ (2003) H3 relaxin is a specific ligand for LGR7 and activates the receptor by interacting with both the ectodomain and the exoloop 2. *J Biol Chem* 278(10):7855-7862.

Sung KW, Choi S and Lovinger DM (2001) Activation of group I mGluRs is necessary for induction of long-term depression at striatal synapses. *J Neurophysiol* 86(5):2405-2412.

Suzuki G, Kimura T, Satow A, Kaneko N, Fukuda J, Hikichi H, Sakai N, Maehara S, Kawagoe-Takaki H, Hata M, Azuma T, Ito S, Kawamoto H and Ohta H (2007) Pharmacological characterization of a new, orally active and potent allosteric metabotropic glutamate receptor 1 antagonist, 4-[1-(2-fluoropyridin-3-yl)-5-methyl-1H-1,2,3-triazol-4-yl]-N-isopropyl-N- methyl-3,6-dihydropyridine-1(2H)-carboxamide (FTIDC). *J Pharmacol Exp Ther* 321(3):1144-1153.

Tamaru Y, Nomura S, Mizuno N and Shigemoto R (2001) Distribution of metabotropic glutamate receptor mGluR3 in the mouse CNS: differential location relative to pre- and postsynaptic sites. *Neuroscience* 106(3):481-503.

Tebano MT, Martire A, Pepponi R, Domenici MR and Popoli P (2006) Is the functional interaction between adenosine A(2A) receptors and metabotropic glutamate 5 receptors a general mechanism in the brain? Differences and similarities between the striatum and the hippocampus. *Purinergic Signal* 2(4):619-625.

Terunuma M, Vargas KJ, Wilkins ME, Ramirez OA, Jaureguiberry-Bravo M, Pangalos MN, Smart TG, Moss SJ and Couve A (2010) Prolonged activation of NMDA receptors promotes dephosphorylation and alters postendocytic sorting of GABAB receptors. *Proc Natl Acad Sci U S A* 107(31):13918-13923.

Thompson SM, Capogna M and Scanziani M (1993) Presynaptic inhibition in the hippocampus. *Trends Neurosci* 16(6):222-227.

Toms NJ and Roberts PJ (1999) Group 1 mGlu receptors elevate [Ca2+]i in rat cultured cortical type 2 astrocytes: [Ca2+]i synergy with adenosine A1 receptors. *Neuropharmacology* 38(10):1511-1517.

Trullas R and Skolnick P (1990) Functional antagonists at the NMDA receptor complex exhibit antidepressant actions. *Eur J Pharmacol* 185(1):1-10.

Tsuchiya D, Kunishima N, Kamiya N, Jingami H and Morikawa K (2002) Structural views of the ligand-binding cores of a metabotropic glutamate receptor complexed with an antagonist and both glutamate and Gd3+. *Proc Natl Acad Sci U S A* 99(5):2660-2665.

Tyacke RJ, Lingford-Hughes A, Reed LJ and Nutt DJ (2010) GABAB receptors in addiction and its treatment. *Adv Pharmacol* 58:373-396.

Ulrich D and Bettler B (2007) GABA(B) receptors: synaptic functions and mechanisms of diversity. *Curr Opin Neurobiol* 17(3):298-303.

Urizar E, Yano H, Kolster R, Gales C, Lambert N and Javitch JA (2011) CODA-RET reveals functional selectivity as a result of GPCR heteromerization. *Nat Chem Biol* 7(9):624-630.

Urwyler S, Mosbacher J, Lingenhoehl K, Heid J, Hofstetter K, Froestl W, Bettler B and Kaupmann K (2001) Positive allosteric modulation of native and recombinant gamma-aminobutyric acid(B) receptors by 2,6-Di-tert-butyl-4-(3-hydroxy-2,2-dimethyl-propyl)-phenol (CGP7930) and its aldehyde analog CGP13501. *Mol Pharmacol* 60(5):963-971.

Valant C, Gregory KJ, Hall NE, Scammells PJ, Lew MJ, Sexton PM and Christopoulos A (2008) A novel mechanism of G protein-coupled receptor functional selectivity. Muscarinic partial agonist McN-A-343 as a bitopic orthosteric/allosteric ligand. *J Biol Chem* 283(43):29312-29321.

Valant C, Sexton PM and Christopoulos A (2009) Orthosteric/allosteric bitopic ligands: going hybrid at GPCRs. *Mol Interv* 9(3):125-135.

Valenti O, Marino MJ, Wittmann M, Lis E, DiLella AG, Kinney GG and Conn PJ (2003) Group III metabotropic glutamate receptor-mediated modulation of the striatopallidal synapse. *J Neurosci* 23(18):7218-7226.

Vienne J, Bettler B, Franken P and Tafti M (2010) Differential effects of GABAB receptor subtypes, {gamma}-hydroxybutyric Acid, and Baclofen on EEG activity and sleep regulation. *J Neurosci* 30(42):14194-14204.

Wettschureck N and Offermanns S (2005) Mammalian G proteins and their cell type specific functions. *Physiol Rev* 85(4):1159-1204.

White JH, Wise A, Main MJ, Green A, Fraser NJ, Disney GH, Barnes AA, Emson P, Foord SM and Marshall FH (1998) Heterodimerization is required for the formation of a functional GABA(B) receptor. *Nature* 396(6712):679-682.

Woolley ML, Pemberton DJ, Bate S, Corti C and Jones DN (2008) The mGlu2 but not the mGlu3 receptor mediates the actions of the mGluR2/3 agonist, LY379268, in mouse models predictive of antipsychotic activity. *Psychopharmacology (Berl)* 196(3):431-440.

Wright RA, Arnold MB, Wheeler WJ, Ornstein PL and Schoepp DD (2000) Binding of [3H](2S,1'S,2'S)-2-(9-xanthylmethyl)-2-(2'-carboxycyclopropyl) glycine ([3H]LY341495) to cell membranes expressing recombinant human group III metabotropic glutamate receptor subtypes. *Naunyn Schmiedebergs Arch Pharmacol* 362(6):546-554.

Yamaguchi S and Ninomiya K (2000) Umami and food palatability. *J Nutr* 130(4S Suppl):921S-926S.

Zhang F, Klebansky B, Fine RM, Xu H, Pronin A, Liu H, Tachdjian C and Li X (2008) Molecular mechanism for the umami taste synergism. *Proc Natl Acad Sci U S A* 105(52):20930-20934.

2

Interactions Between Glutamate Receptors and TRPV1 Involved in Nociceptive Processing at Peripheral Endings of Primary Afferent Fibers

You-Hong Jin[1], Motohide Takemura[2],
Akira Furuyama[3] and Norifumi Yonehara[4]
[1]*Department of Anatomy the Affiliated Stomatological, Hospital of Nanchang University, Nanchang, Jiangxi Province,*
[2]*Department of Oral Anatomy and Neurobiology, Osaka University Graduate School of Dentistry,*
[3]*Departments of Oral Physiology*
[4]*Oral Medical Science (Division of Dental Pharmacology), Ohu University School of Dentistry, Koriyama, Fukushima,*
[1]*China*
[2,3,4]*Japan*

1. Introduction

Glutamate (Glu) is a main excitatory neurotransmitter in the central nervous system. Concerning the existence of Glu in the small-diameter afferent fibers, their central (Westlund et al., 1989; Keast and Stephensen, 2000) and peripheral (Westlund et al., 1992; Keast and Stephensen, 2000) processes as well as dorsal root ganglion (DRG) cells (Battaglia and Rustioni, 1988; Keast and Stephensen, 2000) contain Glu. Recently, Glu has been shown to have a role in transduction of sensory input at the periphery (Carlton, 2001).

Electron microscope studies demonstrate that Glu receptors are transported from the DRG cell bodies into central and/or peripheral primary afferent terminals (Liu et al., 1994). The N-methyl-D-aspartic acid (NMDA), α-amino-3-hydroxy-5methyl-4-isoxazole propionic acid (AMPA) and kainate receptors (NMDA/AMPA-kainate receptors) are localized on unmyelinated axons at the dermal-epidermal junction in the glabrous and hairy skin of the rat (Carlton et al., 1995; Coggeshall and Carlton, 1998), and in human hairly skin (Kinkelin et al., 2000). Approximately 20% of the fibers were immunostained in one of the receptor subtypes. As Sato et al. (1993) reported that virtually all DRG cells as well as their central (Laurie et al., 1995; Zou et al., 2002) and peripheral (Carlton et al., 1995) processes are positively labeled for the NMDA receptor, it is highly likely that two or more of the ionotropic Glu receptors are colocalized.

Behavioral evidence supports a role for peripheral Glu receptors in normal nociceptive transmission. Intraplantar injection of L-Glu into the hindpaw evokes hyperalgesia in rats (Follenfant and Nakamura-Craig, 1992; Carlton et al., 1995). Futhermore, intraplantar injection of the specific Glu receptors agonists NMDA, AMPA or kainate results in mechanical hyperalgesia and allodynia that can be blocked by appropriate antagonists (Zhou et al., 1996). Hyperalgesia is induced by binding the released glutamate to NMDA receptor (Leem et al., 2001; Du et al., 2003), group I mGluR (Bhave et al., 2001; Zhou et al., 2001; Hu et al., 2002; Walker et al., 2001; Lee et al., 2007), but not group II mGluR (Yang and Gereau IV, 2003).

In addition to these behavioral and anatomical data, Omote et al. (1998) showed that subcutaneous administration of inflammatory substances such as formalin induced the release of peripheral EAAs (Glu and aspartate) on the ipsilateral side. We have already reported that local application of capsaicin cream evoked a marked increase in Glu level in the s.c. perfusate. In addition, electrical stimulation of the sciatic nerve or noxious heat stimulation (50°C) also caused increase of Glu level in the s.c. space, and this capsaicin-evoked Glu release was significantly decreased by daily high-dose pretreatment with capsaicin for three consecutive days (Jin et al., 2006).

The capsaicin receptor, transient receptor potential vanilloid 1 (TRPV1), is located in a neurochemically heterogeneous population of small diameter primary afferent neurons (Tominaga et al., 1998). This receptor is sensitive to high temperature in the noxious range of 43°C to 50°C (Hardy, 1953; Beitel and Dubner, 1976; Caterina et al., 1997). Furthermore, repeated exposure to high-dose capsaicin selectively produces a prolonged influx of cations leading to desensitization of small-diameter sensory neurons to subsequent noxious stimulation (Yonehara et al., 1987; Lynn, 1990; Zhou et al., 1998; Caterina and Julius, 2001), while myelinated Aβ fibers are insensitive to capsaicin (Jancso et al., 1977; Nagy et al., 1983; Michael and Priestly, 1999).

There is an evidence suggesting possibility that capsaicin-evoked pain responses might be regulated by peripheral GluRs. In this connection, Lam et al. (2005) demonstrated that peripheral NMDA receptor modulate jaw muscle electromyographic activity induced by capsaicin injection into the temporomandibular joint of rats.

This study, therefore, has been done to elucidate at large in what manner Glu receptors and Glu existing in the peripheral endings of small-diameter afferent fibers and their extracellular space, respectively, are involved in development and/or maintenance of nociception evoked by capsaicin. Additionally, in order to demonstrate a link between the increase of Glu levels in the extracellular space following noxious stimulation and pain behavior, the changes in thermal withdrawal latency and the expression of c-Fos protein in the dorsal horn were determined following subcutaneous (s.c.) injection of drugs associated with Glu receptors with/without capsaicin.

2. Materials and methods

All surgical and experimental procedures for animals were reviewed and approved by the Ohu University Intramural Animal Care and Use Committee and conformed to the guidelines of the International Association for the Study of Pain (Zimmermann, 1983).

2.1 Experimental procedures

Adult male Sprague-Dawley rats weighing between 200-300 g (CLEA Japan, INC. Tokyo, Japan) were used in all experiments. Rats were on a 12 hrs light/dark cycle and received food and water ad libitum.

2.2 Release of Glu into the subcutaneous space

Animals were anesthetized with urethane (1 g/kg i.p.). A single loop catheter whose tip was covered with a 5000 molecular weight dialysis membrane (MS 0045, PSS® SELECT, Florida) was introduced into the s.c. space of the instep using a 2.2 mm outer diameter polyethylene tube as a guide. Ringer's solution was perfused at 15 μl/min through this catheter with a micro syringe pump (EP-60, Eicom, Kyoto, Japan) and perfusate was collected into the tubes placed in an ice bath at intervals of 20 min. The samples were kept at -80°C until analysis.

2.3 Amino acid analysis

Amino acids in the dialysate were analyzed by a high-performance liquid chromatography (HPLC) system for automated analysis of amino acids using o-phthalaldehyde derivatization and fluorescence detection. Amino acids were quantified by reverse-phase chromatography using a C_{18} octadecylsilyl (ODS) silica-gel column (EICOMPAK SC-50DS 2.1 mm x 150 mm) with pre-column (EICOM PREPAKSET-AC 3 mm x 4 mm). An HPLC system (HTEC500, EICOM) attaching this column consists of a pump connected with a degasser, a sampling injector with a sample processor and a cool pump, a fluorescence HPLC monitor and a personal computer with the data processor (Power Chrom; EPC-500, EICOM). The mobile phase used for separation of amino acids was 100 mM, pH 6 phosphate buffer containing 30% methanol and 10 μM EDTA. The flow rate was 0.23 ml/min. Peak areas of unknown substances were compared to those of control compounds for quantitation.

To determine the effect of drugs on the level of Glu, the average amounts of Glu concentration in two 20-min fractions collected over periods of 40 min before and after local application of capsaicin cream were obtained and expressed as percentages of the control value before stimulation.

2.4 Drug administration

While the animals were inside the small cage, drugs were administered into the s.c. left hindpaw in a volume of 50 μl using a 100 μl Hamilton syringe (Reno, NV, USA) with a 30-gauge needle without any anesthesia. The needle was inserted into the plantar skin proximal to the midpoint of the hindpaw. Capsazepine (30mg/kg) was injected in the volume of 50 μl into the s.c. of the neck.

2.5 Behavioral assessments

The Plantar Test (model 7370; Ugo Basile, Verese, Italy) was used in accordance with previously described methods (Yonehara et al., 1997) to determine whether the rats were hyperalgesic. In brief, prior to testing, the animals were placed in a small cage on a glass plate. They were not restrained and could move about and explore freely. Radiant heat was beamed onto the plantar surface of the hindpaw. The intensity of the beam was controlled and adjusted prior to the experiments, and the cutoff latency was set at 24 sec. The beam was applied to the test and control foot in turns and the latency of the withdrawal reflexes was recorded. The mean of the four responses was determined (Figs 4-8), and the ratio of the test foot latency divided by control foot latency, multiplied by 100, was calculated and termed the "percentage withdrawal latency" (Fig.3), at hourly intervals, from 1 hr before injection of the drugs to 6 h after the injection, except for 15 min after the injection

2.6 c-Fos immunohistochemistry

Two hours after the drug injection, animals were deeply anesthetized with sodium-pentobarbital and perfused transcardially with 100ml of 0.9% saline followed by 500 ml of 4% paraformaldehyde in 0.1 M phosphate buffer (PB; pH 7.4) and the spinal cord was taken out, postfixed in the same fixative overnight at 4°C, and then immersed into 20% sucrose in 0.1M PB at 4°C until it sank. Serial transverse 60 μm thick sections at L4-6 were cut using a freezing microtome and collected in 0.02 M phosphate buffered saline (PBS). Sections were washed in PBS for 30 min and blocked with 1% normal goat serum for 30 min and then incubated in a rabbit antibody against c-Fos (1:7000 dilution; Santa Cruz Biotech, Santa Cruz, CA, USA) for 60 min in room temperature and then for 12 hrs at 4°C. After washing in PBS for 30 min, sections were incubated in biotinylated goat anti-rabbit antiserum, and washed in PBS for 30 min and then immunohistochemically stained for 60 min using avidin-biotin-peroxidase complex (Vectastain, Vector Laboratories, Burlingame, CA, USA). To visualize peroxidase activity, sections were immersed in 0.05% diaminobenzidine tetrahydrochloride, 0.1% ammonium nickel sulfate and 0.01% hydrogen peroxide in 0.05 M Tris-HCl buffer (pH 7.2). Sections were washed in PBS for 30 min and then mounted on gelatin-coated slides, air-dried and coverslipped. The c-Fos-immunoreactive cells of 10 best-labeled sections were counted in the L5 spinal dorsal horn. In all these tests a double blind procedure was used to prevent the observers from knowing the experimental groups.

2.7 Drugs

The list of drugs and chemicals were as follows: as Glu receptors agonist, L-glutamic acid; selective NMDA receptor agonist, NMDA; AMPA receptor agonist, α-amino-3-hydroxy-4-isoxazoleproprionic acid (AMPA); selective group 1 mGlu receptor agonist, (S)-3,5-dihydroxyphenylglycine ((S)-3,5-DHPG); group II mGlu receptor agonist, (2S,1'S,2'S)-2-(carboxycyclopropyl) glycine (L-CCG-I); selective group III mGlu receptor agonist, L-(+)-2-amino-4-phosphonobutyric acid (L-AP4). The following drugs were used for Glu receptors antagonists, selective non-competitive NMDA receptor antagonist, (5S,10R)-(+)-5-Methyl-10,11-dihydro-5H-dibenzo[a,d] cyclo-hepten-5, 10-imine hydrogen maleate ((+)-MK-801 hydrogen maleate); competitive kainite/AMPA receptor antagonist, 6-Cyano-7-nitroquinoxaline-2,3-dione disodium (CNQX) and 2,3-Dioxo-6-nitro-1,2,3,4-tetrahydrobenzo[f]quinoxaline-7-sulfonamide disodium salt (NBQX); group 1 mGlu receptor selective non-competitive $mGlu_1$ receptor antagonist, 7-(hydroxyimino) cyclopropa[b]chromen-1a-carboxylate ethyl ester (CPCCOEt); group 1 mGlu receptor mGlu5 subtype-selective antagonist, 2-Methyl-6-(phenylethynyl)pyridine hydrochloride (MPEP); group II mGlu receptor antagonist, ((2S,3S,4S)-2-methyl-2-(carboxycyclopropyl)glycine

(MCCG); selective group III mGlu receptor antagonist, (RS)-α-methylserine-O-phoephate (MSOP). These compounds of Glu receptors were obtained from Tocris (Ballwin, MO, USA). 8-Methyl-N-vanillyl-6-noneamide (capsaicin) was obtained from Sigma Chemical Co. (USA). All other chemicals were obtained from Wako Pure Chemical Industries, Ltd. (Osaka, Japan).

In accordance with the product material safety data sheets, L-glutamate acid, L-CCG-I and L-AP4 were diluted in NaOH; and MK801, NMDA, (S)-3, 5,-DHPG, MCCG and MSOP were diluted in water. CNQX, CPCCOEt and MPEP were diluted in dimethyl sulphoxide. The other drugs except for these were dissolved in saline. Capsaicin was prepared as a 10 mg/ml solution in saline containing 10% ethanol and 10% Tween 80. The pH of all solutions was adjusted to 7.4. Capsazepine was dissolved in dimethyl formamide and then diluted with saline. O-phthalaldehyde was dissolved in methanol and adjusted to 4 mM with 0.1 M, pH 9.5 carbonate buffer.

2.8 Statistical analysis

All data are shown as mean ± S.E.M. In the study of Glu release, statistical analyses were performed using posthoc test of Fisher's protected least significant difference and $P<0.05$ was considered to be statistically significant. In the behavioral study, statistical analyses were performed with Dunnett's test for multiple comparison subsequent to analyses of variance. In the c-Fos immunohistochemichal study, a Student's test was used to test significant differences of the c-Fos expression between the treatments.

2.9 Abbreviations

AMPA; α-amino-3-hydroxy-4-isoxazole proprionic acid, Cap+MK801; Capsaicin combined with MK801, Cap+CNQX; Capsaicin combined with CNQX, Cap+NBQX; Capsaicin combined with NBQX, Cap+CPCCOEt; Capsaicin combined with CPCCOEt, Cap+MCCG; Capsaicin combined with MCCG, Cap+MSOP; Capsaicin combined with MSOP, CNQX; 6-Cyano-7-nitroquinoxaline-2,3-dione disodium, CPCCOEt; 7-(hydroxyimino) cyclopropa[b]chromen-1a-carboxylate ethyl ester, (S)-3,5-DHPG; (S)-3,5- dihydroxyphenylglycine, DRG; dorsal root ganglion, Glu, glutamate; L-CCG-I; (2S,1'S,2'S)-2-(carboxycyclopropyl) glycine, L-AP4; L-(+)-2-amino-4-phosphonobutyric acid, MCCG; (2S,3S,4S)-2-methyl-2-(carboxycyclopropyl) glycine, mGluRs; metabotropic glutamate receptors, (+)-MK-801; (5S,10R)-(+)-5-Methyl-10,11-dihydro-5H-dibenzo[a,d] cyclo-hepten-5, 10-imine hydrogen maleate, MPEP; 2-Methyl-6-(phenylethynyl) pyridine hydrochloride, MSOP; (RS)-α-methylserine-O-phoephate, NBQX; 2,3-Dioxo-6-nitro-1,2,3,4-tetrahydrobenzo[f]quinoxaline-7-sulfonamide disodium salt, NMDA; N-methyl-D-aspartic acid.

3. Results

3.1 Basal Glu release

The concentration of Glu in the perfusate was initially high, but gradually decreased with time reaching a stable level after 2 hrs of perfusion, which was then maintained for at least 4.5 h. Glu was present at 1.95 ± 0.25 μM (n=10, S.E.M.) in the resting state which is defined here as the mean of the two 20-min fraction collected from 80 min after starting perfusion to 120 min (fraction 5~6 in control group in Fig.1).

3.2 Effects of capsazepine on capsaicin-evoked Glu release

The s.c. injection of capsaicin (3 mM) in the vicinity of the perfusion side evoked a significant increase in Glu release (Fig.1). The average concentration of the released Glu was 4.86 ± 0.48 μM/20 min in 2 fractions collected after the injection of capsaicin. This augmentation of Glu release was last over 2 h. This effect was remarkably suppressed by preadministration of capsazepine (30 mg/kg, s.c.) 30 min before capsaicin injection (Fig.1). In the group of pretreatment with capsazepine, the average concentrations of the released Glu were 2.25 ± 0.4 μM/20 min and 2.36 ± 0.31 μM/20 min in 2 fractions collected after the injection of vehicle or capsaicin, respectively. S.c. injections of vehicle or capsazepine alone did not produce any significant changes in the levels of Glu in the perfusates.

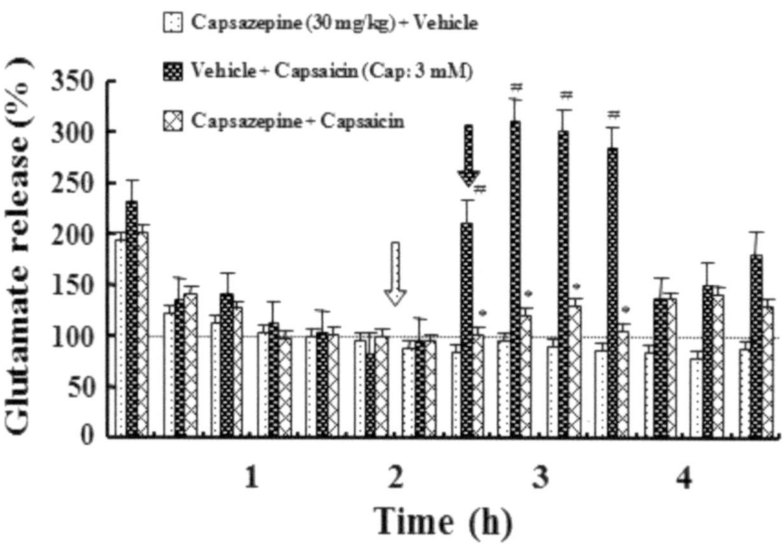

Fig. 1. Effect of capsazepine on the capsaicin-induced glutamate release. Capsazepine (s.c.) was injected subcutaneously into the neck 30 min before capsaicin treatment. Capsazepine (30 mg/kg) or vehicle for capsazepine, and capsaicin (3 mM) or vehicle for capsaicin were subcutaneously injected at the time indicated by the arrows, (⇩) and (⬇), respectively. All data are presented as the mean ± S.E.M. obtained from 10 animals. #P<0.05 compare with the value prior to s.c. administration of capsaicin+vehicle. *P<0.05 compared with capsaicin+vehicle (for capsazepine) group at each time measured.

3.3 Effects of iGluRs antagonists injection on capsaicin-evoked Glu release

The combined injection of capsaicin with MK801(1 mM) (Cap + MK-801) or NBQX (5 mM) (Cap + NBQX) into the perfusion region showed far less Glu release than injection of capsaicin alone (Fig 2-A). The average concentration of the released Glu was 1.20 ± 0.1 μM/ 20 min or 1.70 ± 0.1 μM/ 20min in 2 fractions collected after the co-injection of MK-801 or NBQX with capsaicin, respectively. These inhibitory effects of iGluRs antagonists sustained over 2.5 h.

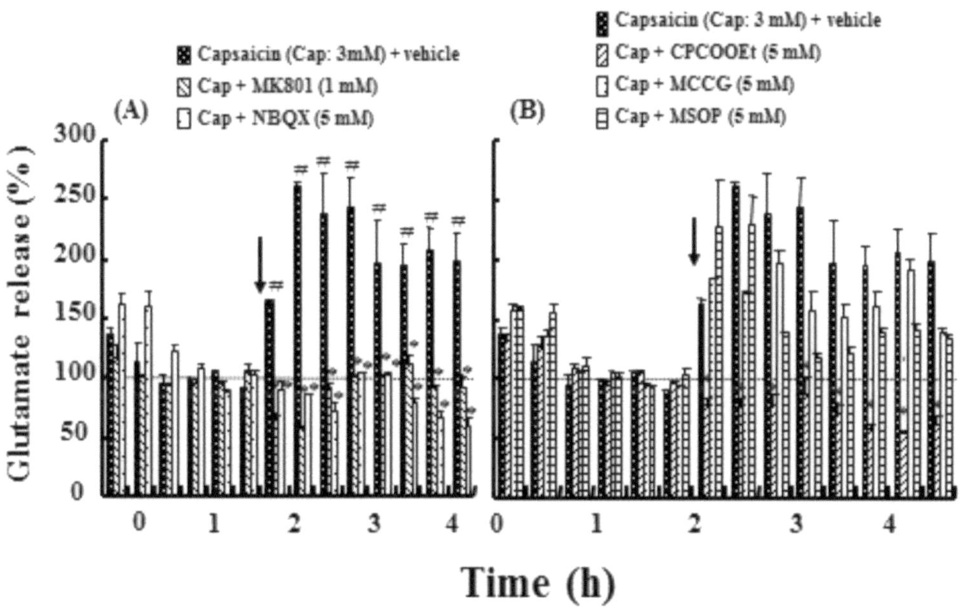

Fig. 2. Effect of the ionotropic (A) and metabotropic (B) glutamate receptor antagonists on the capsaicin-induced glutamate release. The glutamate receptor antagonists were subcutaneously injected together with capsaicin at the time indicated by the arrow. All data are presented as the mean ± S.E.M. obtained from 10 animals. #P<0.05 compare with the value prior to s.c. administration of capsaicin+vehicle. *P<0.05 compared with capsaicin+vehicle group at each time measured. MK801, selective non-competitive NMDA receptor antagonist; NBQX, competitive kainate/AMPA receptor antagonist; CPCOOEt, group 1 mGlu receptor selective non-competitive $mGlu_1$ receptor antagonist; MCCG, group II mGlu receptor antagonist; MSOP, selective group III mGlu receptor antagonist.

3.4 Effects of mGluRs antagonists injection on capsaicin-induced Glu release

At the doses employed, CPCCOEt (5 mM) (Cap + CPCCOEt) showed remarkable inhibition in capsaicin-evoked Glu release. The average concentration of the released Glu was 1.46 ± 0.1 μM/ 20 min after the co-injection of CPCCOEt with capsaicin. S.c. combined injection of MCCG (5 mM) (Cap + MCCG) or MSOP (5 mM) (Cap + MSOP) with capsaicin did not show significant decrease in Glu release compared to capsaicin injection alone. The average concentration of the released Glu was 3.68 ± 0.38 μM / 20 min or 4.31 ± 0.60 μM/ 20min in 2 fractions collected after the co-injection of MCCG or MSOP with capsaicin, respectively. (Fig. 2-B)

3.5 Effects of capsazepine on capsaicin-induced thermal hypersensitivity

The mean withdrawal latencies to stimulation with radiant heat at pre-injection were 11.2 ± 0.3 s and 11.2 ± 0.3 s (n=40) on the left and right side, respectively (Fig.3-A). The withdrawal latency did not significantly change after injection of vehicle or low dose of capsaicin (0.6 mM). A quarter and one h after injection of capsaicin (3 mM and 6 mM), withdrawal latency to irradiation decreased to much shorter than that of vehicle injection, which was recorded at the same interval (P<0.05), and then recovered gradually to the level of vehicle injection by 4 h after injection of capsaicin. Pretreatment of capsazepine (30 mg/kg, s.c.) produced a marked inhibition against capsaicin-induced thermal hyperalgesia (Fig.3-B). We did not observed any signs of motor deficiency or other side effects for any of the doses of any drugs in all paradigms described here and below.

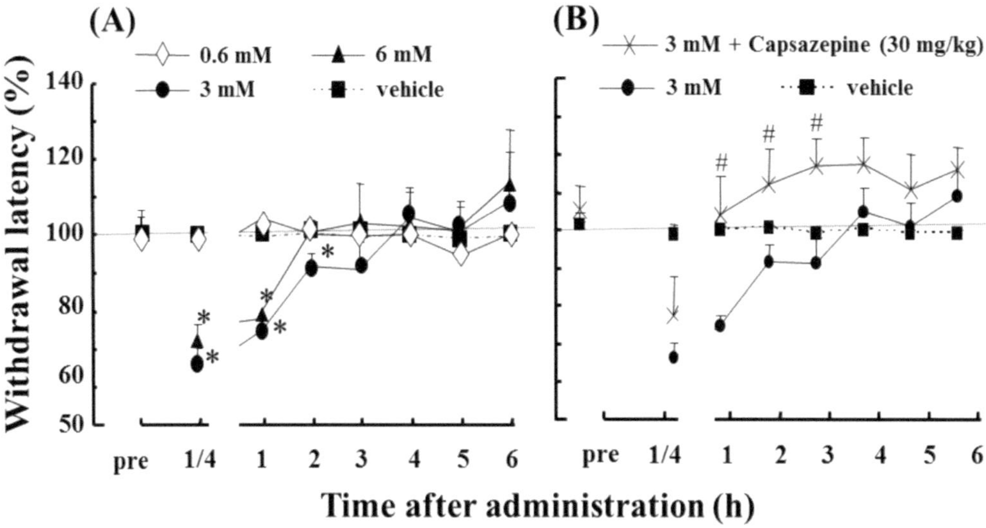

Fig. 3. Time course of withdrawal latencies in response to noxious heat stimulation after s.c. injection of capsaicin, and co-injection of capsazepine with capsaicin. The data for each group (10 animals) are presented as the means ± S.E.M. The withdrawal latency per animal at respective time points was calculated as the average of the latencies obtained from 3 consecutive stimuli applied at intervals of 5 min. The value at time zero (pre) was obtained 1 h prior to s.c. injection of capsaicin. * and # *P*<0.05 significantly different from vehicle-treated group and capsaicin-treated group (3 mM), respectively.

3.6 Thermal sensitivity after injection of iGluRs agonists

S.c. injections of Glu, NMDA or AMPA produced dose-dependent decreases in withdrawal latency on the ipsilateral side 15 min after s.c. injection, and lasted for a few hours (Fig. 4). S.c. injection of vehicle did not produced any changes in thermal-withdrawal latency.

3.7 Thermal sensitivity after injection of mGluRs agonists

S.c. injection of (s)-DHPG caused a dose-dependent decrease in withdrawal latencies on the ipsilateral side from 15 min to 6 h, but L-CCG-I and L-AP4 did not show any significant changes (Fig. 5).

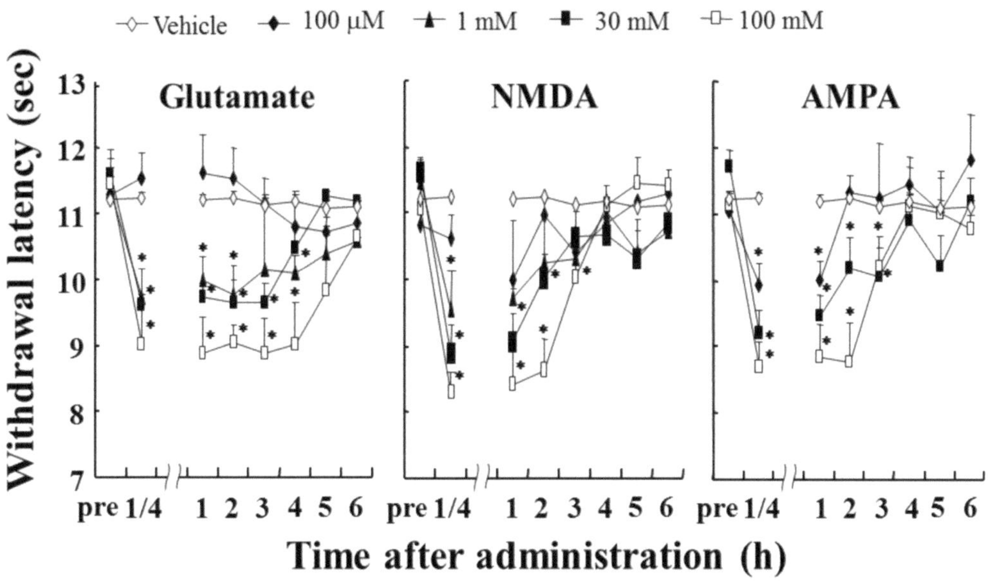

Fig. 4. Time course of withdrawal latencies in response to noxious heat stimulation after s.c. injection of various concentration of the ionotropic glutamate receptor agonists; glutamate, NMDA and AMPA. The data for each group (at least 10 animals) are presented as the means ± S.E.M. **P* <0.05 significantly different from vehicle-treated group.

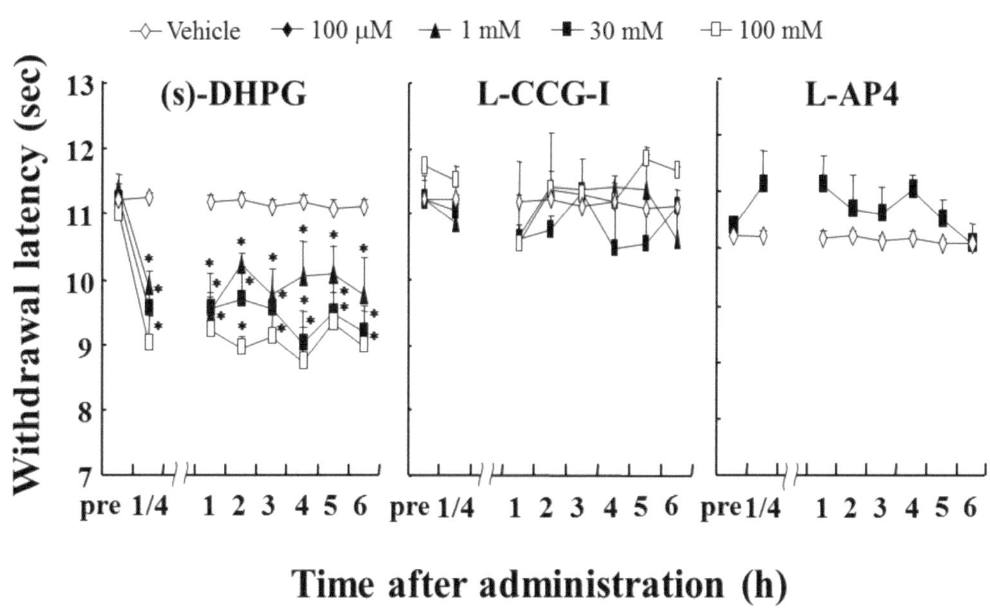

Fig. 5. Time course of withdrawal latencies in response to noxious heat stimulation after s.c. injection of various concentration of the metabotropic glutamate receptor agonists; (s)-DHPG, L-CCG-I and L-AP4. The data for each group (at least 10 animals) are presented as the means ± S.E.M. **P* <0.05 significantly different from vehicle-treated group.

3.8 Effect of iGluRs antagonists injection on capsaicin-induced thermal hypersensitivity

When MK801 or CNQX were injected together with capsaicin (Cap+MK801 or Cap+CNQX), a dose-dependent increase in withdrawal latency was observed. These analgesic effects of MK801 or CNQX on capsaicin-induced thermal hyperalgesia lasted for more than 6 h (Fig. 6). The single injection of MK801 or CNQX into the hindpaw did not show changes in withdrawal latencies compared to vehicle injection.

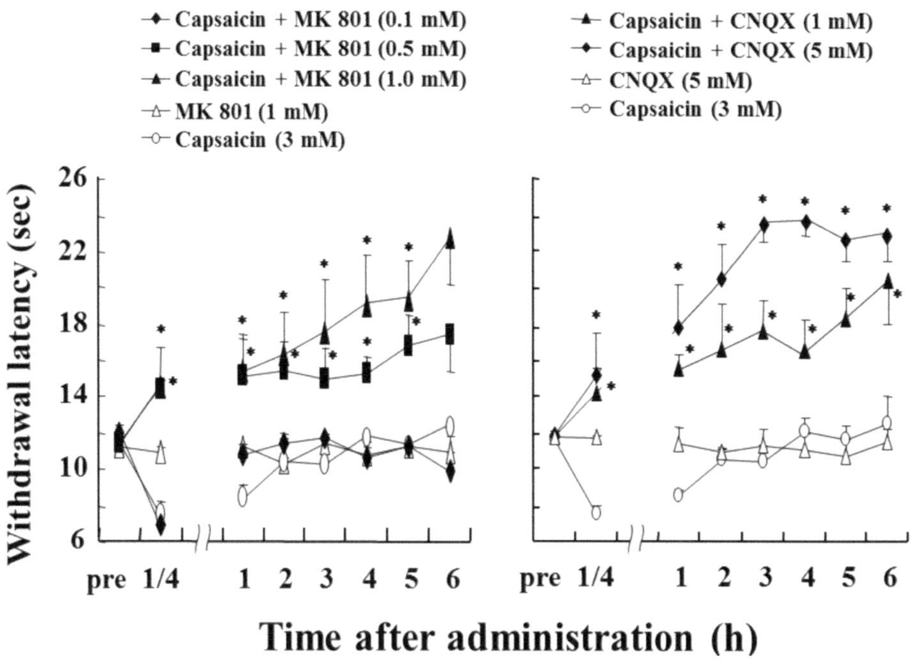

Fig. 6. Time course of withdrawal latencies in response to noxious heat stimulation after s.c. injection of capsaicin in combination with the ionotropic glutamate receptor antagonists; MK801 and CNQX. The data for each group (at least 10 animals) are presented as the means ± S.E.M. **P* <0.05 significantly different from capsaicin (3 mM)-treated group.

3.9 Effect of mGluRs antagonists injection on capsaicin-induced thermal hypersensitivity

Following s.c. injection of CPCCOEt (5 mM), MPEP (30 mM), MCCG (5 mM), and MSOP (5 mM) into hindpaw, there was no changes in withdrawal latencies compared to vehicle injection (Figs. 7 and 8). When CPCCOEt or MPEP were injected together with capsaicin (Cap+CPCCOEt or Cap+MPEP), withdrawal latencies showed a dose-dependent increase from 15 min to 2~3 h after the injection compared with when capsaicin was injected alone (P<0.05) (Fig. 7). The heat insensitivity evoked in ipsilateral side following Cap+CPCCOEt and Cap+MPEP injection continued for 5 h or more. S.c. injection of MCCG or MSOP combined with capsaicin did not show any significant changes in withdrawal latencies compared to capsaicin injection alone (Fig. 8).

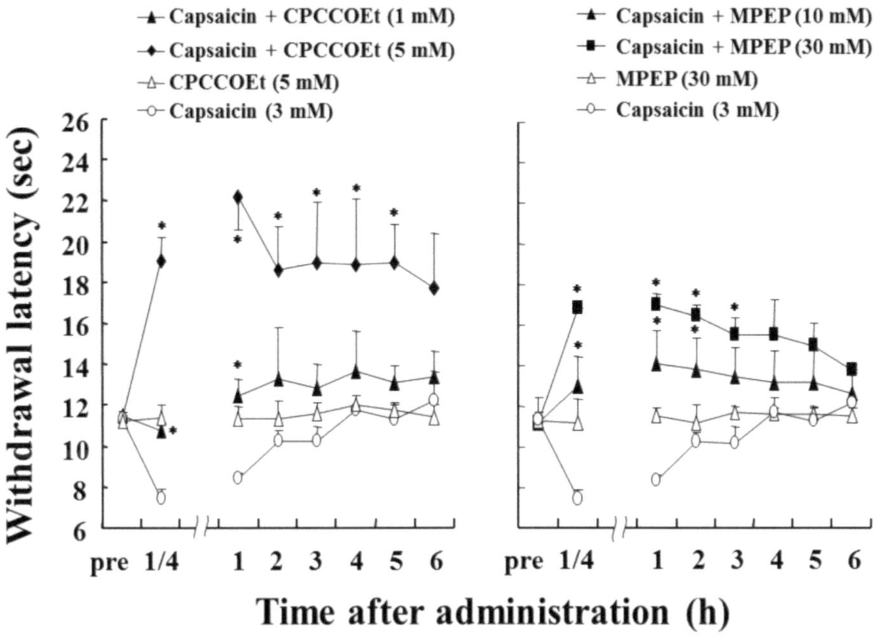

Fig. 7. Time course of withdrawal latencies in response to noxious heat stimulation after s.c. injection of capsaicin in combination with the metabotropic glutamate receptor antagonists; CPCCOEt and MPEP. The data for each group (at least 10 animals) are presented as the means ± S.E.M. *P <0.05 significantly different from capsaicin (3 mM)-treated group.

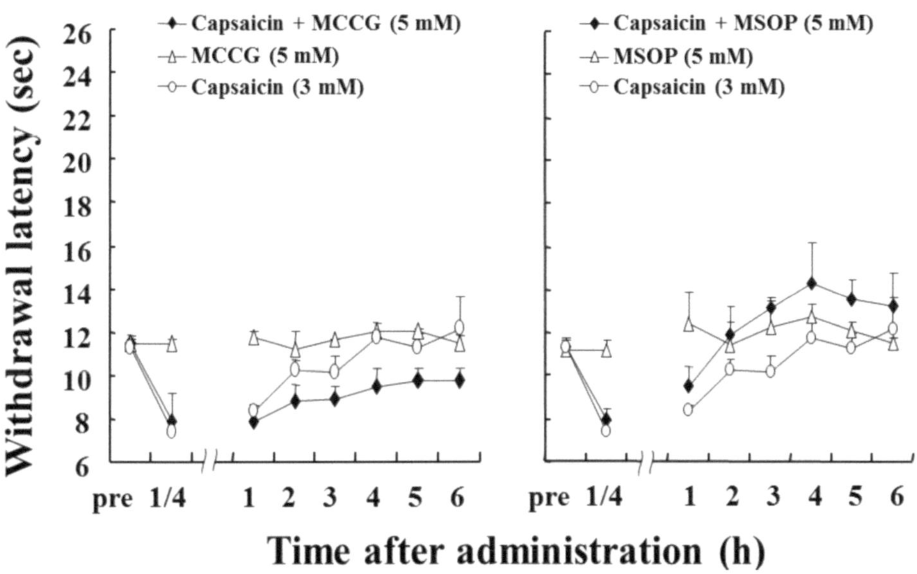

Fig. 8. Time course of withdrawal latencies in response to noxious heat stimulation after s.c. injection of capsaicin in combination with the metabotropic glutamate receptor antagonists; MCCG and MSOP. The data for each group (at least 10 animals) are presented as the means ± S.E.M

3.10 Basal c-Fos expression in dorsal horn after injection of vehicle, capsaicin and Glu into hindpaw

Immunoreactivity for c-Fos appeared gray-to-black and homogeneously labeled the oval or roundish nucleus of cells in spinal dorsal horn at L5 (Figs. 9-11). In all the experimental tests with injection of Glu, the maximum number of labeled cells occurred consistently in laminae I and II (I/II) of the spinal dorsal horn on the ipsilateral side (mean number ± S.E.M.=268 ± 21) (Figs. 9-11 and Table 1). Much smaller number of c-Fos immunopositive cells occurred in lamine III and IV (III/IV, 30 ± 7). The capsaicin-induced c-Fos expression in laminae I/II (489 ± 34) and laminae III/IV (63 ± 18) on the ipsilateral side was greater than that with Glu (Figs. 9, 10 and Table 1). The numbers of c-Fos-immunopositive cells on the contralateral side was modest either with glutamate (I/II, 16 ± 7; III/IV, 12 ± 6) or capsaicin (I/II, 44 ± 13; III/IV, 20 ± 9). In animals administered with vehicle, c-Fos-immunopositive cells were rarely distributed either in laminae I/II (60 ± 5) or in laminae III/IV (22 ± 8) on the ipsilateral side or on the contralateral side (I/II, 12 ± 4; III/IV, 7 ± 2) (Table 1).

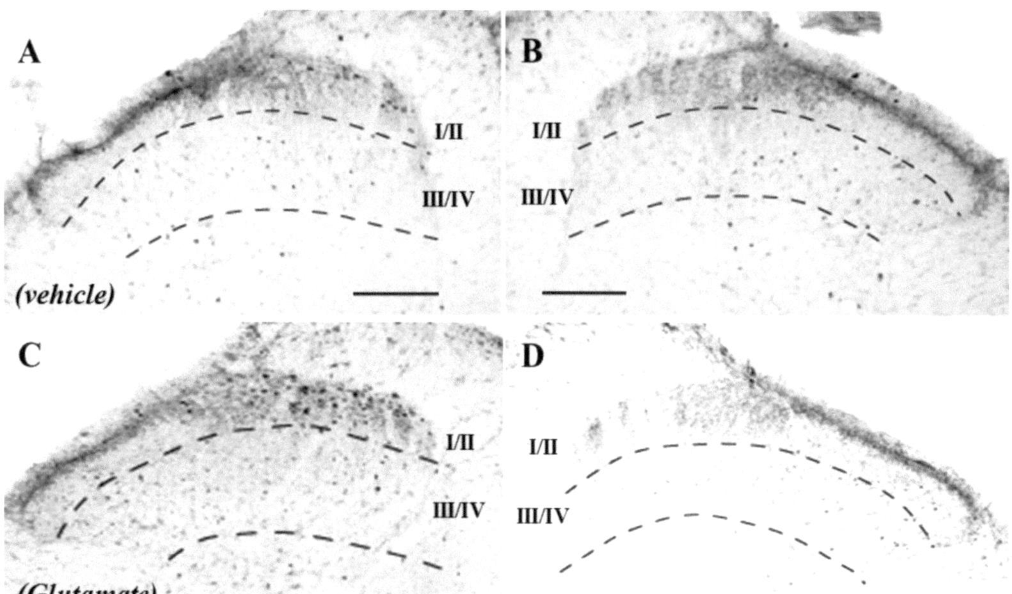

Fig. 9. Photomicrographs showing c-Fos-positive neurons in the dorsal horn of L5 2 h after hindpaw injection of vehicle and glutamate. A and C: ipsilateral side. B and D: contralateral side. Solid line indicates 100 μ m.

3.11 Effects of ionotropic Glu receptors antagonists injection on the capsaicin-induced c-Fos expression

Few c-Fos-immunopositive cells were found in laminae I/II and laminae III/IV of the ipsilateral dorsal horn after each single injection of ionotropic Glu receptors antagonists MK-801 (I/II, 79 ± 3; III/IV, 11 ± 7) and CNQX (I/II, 70 ± 8; III/IV, 7 ± 3) similar to vehicle injection (I/II, 60 ± 5; III/IV, 22 ± 8). The numbers of capsaicin-induced c-Fos-immunopositive cells in laminae I/II (489 ± 34), but not in laminae III/IV (63 ± 18), were significantly decreased (P<0,005), when MK801 and CNQX were injected with capsaicin (Cap+MK801, I/II, 227 ± 32, III/IV, 14 ± 4; Cap+CNQX, I/II, 205 ± 40, III/IV, 11 ± 7) (Fig. 10 and Table 1). The numbers of capsaicin-induced c-Fos-immunopositive cells on the contralateral sides did not significantly change by any of drugs with/without capsaicin.

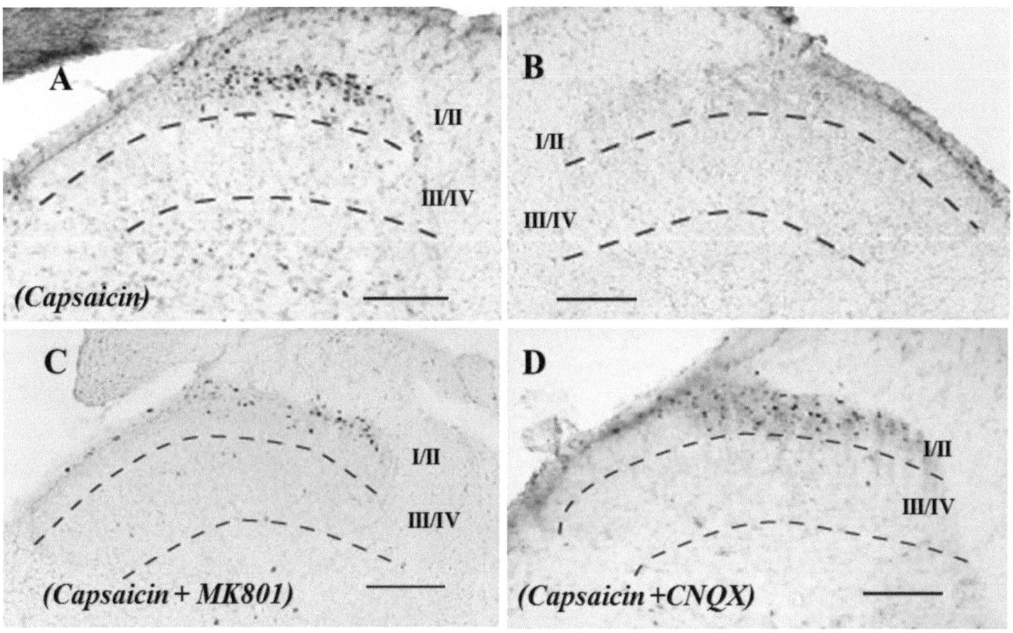

Fig. 10. Photomicrographs showing c-Fos-positive neurons in the dorsal horn of L5 2 h after hindpaw injection of capsaicin alone (A, B), combined with MK801 (C), and combined with MK801 CNQX (D). A, C and D: ipisilateral side. B: contralateral side. Solid line indicates 100 μm.

3.12 Effects of metabotropic glu antagonists injeection on the capsaicin-induced c-Fos expression

Few c-Fos-immunopositive cells in the ipsilateral laminae I/II and III/IV, and fewer cells in the contralateral sides, were observed with single injection of CPCCOEt (I/II, 59 ± 8, III/IV, 1 ± 1), MCCG (I/II, 63 ± 10, III/IV, 3 ± 2) and MSOP (I/II, 66 ± 16, III/IV, 5 ± 3). Co-injection of CPCCOEt with capsaicin (Cap+CPCCOEt) significantly decreased the number of capsaicin-induced c-Fos-immunopositive cells in the ipsilateral laminae I/II (236 ± 58), but not in laminae III/IV (6 ± 4) and contralateral laminae I/II and III/IV. There was no significant change in the number of c-Fos-immunopositive cells in the ipsilateral laminae I/II, and III/IV by administration of MCCG combined with capsaicin (Cap+MCCG) or by administration of MSOP combined with capsaicin (Cap+MSOP; I/II, 383 ± 21, III/IV, 22 ± 3) compared to single injection of capsaicin, respectively (Fig. 11 and Table 1).

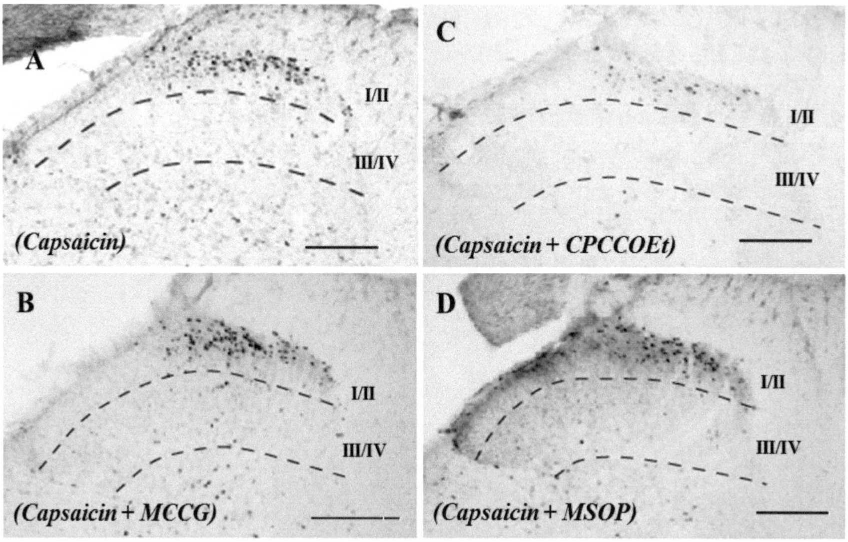

Fig. 11. Photomicrographs showing c-Fos-positive neurons in the dorsal horn of L5 2 h after hindpaw injection of capsaicin alone (A), combined with CPCCOEt (B), with MCCG (C), with MSOP (D). A, B, C and D: ipisilateral side. Solid line indicates 100 μm .

Group	Ipsilateral		Contralateral	
	I/II-layer	III/IV-layer	I/II-layer	III/IV-layer
Vehicle	60 ± 5	22 ± 8	12 ± 4	7 ± 2
Capsaicin(Cap)	489 ± 34*	63 ± 18	44 ± 13	20 ± 9
Glutamate	283 ± 18*	36 ± 5	19 ± 8	12 ± 6
MK801	79 ± 3	11 ± 7	33 ± 12	9 ± 5
CNQX	70 ± 8	7 ± 3	14 ± 7	3 ± 2
CPCCOEt	59 ± 8	6 ± 3	10 ± 4	6 ± 2
MCCG	63 ± 10	5 ± 2	28 ± 11	5 ± 2
MSOP	66 ± 16	5 ± 3	9 ± 4	5 ± 3
Cap + MK801	227 ± 32#	14 ± 4	8 ± 6	3 ± 2
Cap + CNQX	205 ± 40#	11 ± 7	22 ± 12	3 ± 2
Cap + CPCCOEt	236 ± 58#	17 ± 11	12 ± 7	4 ± 3
Cap + MCCG	560 ± 85	27 ± 10	24 ± 9	3 ± 1
Cap + MSOP	383 ± 21	22 ± 3	18 ± 13	4 ± 1

Table 1. Mean value of c-Fos-positive neurons in the dorsal horn of L5 2 h after s.c. injection of Glu receptors agonists and antagonists. The value in each group was represented mean ± S.E.M. obtained from at least 10 animals, and the difference of the means was analyzed with the Student's t-test. * Significant difference at $P< 0.05$ between vehicle and capsaicin, or glutamate-treated group. # Significant difference at $P< 0.05$ between capsaicin and capsaicin+MK801, or capsaicin+CNQX, or capsaicin+CPCCOEt-treated group

4. Discussion

We confirmed a large release of Glu immediately after the introduction of the catheter, followed by a rapid decrease, like in our previous study (Yonehara et al., 1987; Yonehara et al., 1992; Yonehara et al., 1995). Insertion of the polyethylene tube into the s.c. space of the rat instep did not evoke any inflammatory responses such as extravasation (Yonehara et al., 1995). All these data suggest that the basal levels of Glu in the s.c. perfusate were caused by neither acute noxious stimulation nor inflammation.

Topical application of capsaicin cream to the instep evoked a marked increase in Glu level in the s.c. perfusate, similar to the results in our previous study (Jin et al., 2006). In addition, electrical stimulation of the sciatic nerve or noxious heat stimulation (50°C) also caused an increase of Glu level in the s.c. space, and this capsaicin-evoked Glu release was significantly decreased by daily high-dose pretreatment with capsaicin for three consecutive days (Jin et al., 2006).

The TRPV1 is located in a neurochemically heterogeneous population of small diameter primary afferent neurons (Tominaga et al., 1998). Furthermore, repeated exposure to high-dose capsaicin selectively produces a prolonged influx of cations leading to desensitization of small-diameter sensory neurons to subsequent noxious stimulation (Yonehara et al., 1987; Lynn, 1990; Zhou et al., 1998; Caterina and Julius, 2001), while myelinated Aβ fibers are insensitive to capsaicin (Jancso et al., 1977; Nagy et al., 1983; Michael and Priestly, 1999). These findings and the present results suggest that the activation of capsaicin-sensitive afferent fibers by capsaicin causes release of Glu from the peripheral endings via activation of peripheral TRPV1, particularly from those of small-diameter fibers possibly through a mechanism such as the axon-reflex pathway, or autocrine and/or paracrine. It is reasonable to speculate that axon-reflex mechanism is involved in capsaicin-induced Glu release observed in Figs. 1 and 2, as only nociceptive afferent fibers have the axon-reflex mechanism which is localized on superficial tissues exposed to noxious influences (Celander and Folkow, 1953).

Amount of capsaicin-induced Glu release was remarkably decreased by concomitant administration of ionotropic Glu receptors antagonists; MK801 and NBQX, and mGluR I antagonist; CPCCOEt in the hindpaw, but not by administration of group II and III mGluR antagonist; MCCG and MSOP. These results suggest that peripheral ionotropic Glu receptors and group I mGluR appear to play a role in mediating capsaicin-evoked increases in Glu release. The Glu release through the activation of TRPV1 could then further activate ionotoropic Glu receptors and group I mGluR on the same neuronal terminal or adjacent neighboring peripheral terminals. In this connection, there were evidences supporting the co-localization of peripheral NMDA and TRPV1 receptors on the same primary afferent terminal (Lam et al., 2003; Lam et al., 2004).

Activation of peripheral Glu receptors could lead to enhance the Glu release in the peripheral tissues and might alter TRPV1 receptor responsiveness to reinforce nociceptive responses. As it is necessary to investigate the interaction between TRPV1 and glutamate receptors by using specific receptor antagonists of TRPV1 in detail, the mechanism to account for the antagonism of peripheral Glu receptors contributes to inhibit capsaicin-induced Glu release remains unanswered. However, it may be possible that glutamate receptors play a pivotal role for the activation of TRPV1 in the peripheral terminals. This idea is supported by the results that the intraplantar injection of ionotoropic Glu receptors and group I mGluR agonists evoked dose-dependent thermal hyperalgesia. Moreover, it is very interesting to note that injection of Glu receptors antagonists alone did not produce any changes on withdrawal latency, and intraplantar co-injection of ionotropic Glu receptors and group I mGluR antagonists with capsaicin not only antagonized capsaicin-induced hyperalgesia, but also resulted in remarkable longer withdrawal latency to heat irradiation.

Concerning the mechanism that ionotoropic Glu receptors and mGluR antagonists produced remarkable analgesic action in the presence of capsaicin, there is evidence that capsaicin injected into the rat temporomandibular joint evoked a dose-dependent increase in jaw muscle electromyographic activity. This capsaicin-evoked increase in electromyographic activity was attenuated by ipsilateral injection of NMDA receptor antagonists into the temporomandibular joint (Lam et al. 2005). This finding and our present results indicate that the activation of peripheral Glu receptors, especially ionotropic Glu receptors and group I mGluR could be indispensable in the mechanisms whereby capsaicin evokes nociceptive responses.

The ionotropic, and metabotropic subunits of Glu receptors are present in DRG cell bodies and on unmyelinated fibers in the glabrous skin of the mammalian foot (Carlton et al., 1995; Bhave et al., 2001; Carlton et al., 2001; Sato et al., 1993; Carlton et al., 2007). It is well established that the excitatory amino acids in the peripheral endings of small-diameter afferent fibers contribute to development and/or maintenance of pain in humans (Nordlind et al., 1993; Warncke et al., 1997) and in laboratory animals (Davidson et al., 1997; Cairns et al., 1998; Davidson et al., 1998). For example, peripherally applied NMDA and non-NMDA receptor antagonists attenuate or block nociceptive behaviors in several animal models of inflammation (Jackson et al., 1995; Lawand et al., 1997; Carlton et al., 1998).

In the present study, we examined the c-Fos expression in spinal cord dorsal horn following injection of drugs associated with glutamate receptors with/without capsaicin into the hindpaw. c-Fos is rapidly and transiently induced in cells of the spinal dorsal horn after noxious stimulation (Hunt et al., 1987, Strassman and Vos, 1993, Takemura et al., 2000), c-Fos has been widely used as a marker for analyzing nociceptive processing.

Our present data support the view that Glu receptors, in particular, ionotropic Glu receptors and group I mGluR existing in peripheral ending of capsaicin-sensitive afferent fibers play an important role on development and/or maintenance of pain following excitation of TRPV1. In addition, the formulation of the peripheral ionotoropic Glu receptors and group I mGluR antagonists that do not cross the blood brain barrier may be of potential benefit by reducing peripheral nociceptive excitability, and therefore they could provide a new therapeutic target to pain control in the periphery.

5. References

Battaglia, G., and Rustioni, A., 1988. Coexistence of glutamate and substance P in dorsal root ganglion neurons of the rat and monkey. J. Comp. Neurol. 277, 302-312.

Beitel, R.E., and Dubner, R., 1976. Response of unmyelinated (C) polymodal nociceptors to thermal stimuli applied to monkey's face. J. Neurophysiol. 39, 1160-1175.

Bhave, G., Karim, F., Carlton, S.M., and Gereau IV, R.W., 2001. Peripheral group I metabotropic glutamate receptors modulate nociception in mice. Nature 4, 417-423.

Cairns, B.E., Sessle, B.J., and Hu, J.W., 1998. Evidence that excitatory amino acid receptors within the temporomandibular joint region are involved in the reflex activation of the jaw muscles. J. Neurosci. 18, 8056-8064.

Carlton, S.M., Hargett, G.L., and Coggeshall, R.E., 1995. Localization and activation of glutamate receptors in unmyelinated axons of rat glabrous skin. Neurosci. Lett. 197, 25-28.

Carlton, S.M., Zhou, S., and Coggeshall, R.E., 1998. Evidence for the interaction of glutamate and NK1 receptors in the periphery. Brain Res. 790, 160-169.

Carlton, S.M., 2001. Peripheral excitatory amino acids. Current Opinion in Pharmacology, 1, 52-56.

Carlton, S.M., and Hargett, G.L., 2007. Colocalization of metabotropic glutamate receptors in rat dorsal root ganglion cells. J. Comp. Neurol. 501, 780-789.

Caterina, M.J., Schumacher, M.A., Tominaga, M., Rosen, T.A., Levine, J.D., and Julius, D., 1997. The capsaicin receptor: a heat-activated ion channel in the pain pathway. Nature. 389, 816-24.

Caterina, M.J., and Julius, D., 2001. The vanilloid receptor: a molecular gateway to the pain pathway. Annu. Rev. Neurosci. 24, 487-517.

Celander, O., and Folkow, B., 1953. The nature and the distribution of afferent fibers provided with the axon reflex arrangement. Acta Physiol. Scand. 29, 369-370.

Coggeshall, R.E., and Carlton, S.M., 1998. Ultrastructural analysis of NMDA, AMPA and kainate receptors on unmyelinated and myelinated axons in the periphery. J. Comp. Neurol. 391, 78-86.

Davidson, E.M., Coggeshall, R.E., and Carlton, S.M., 1997. Peripheral NMDA and non-NMDA glutamate receptors contribute to nociceptive behaviors in the rat formalin test. Neuroreport 8, 941-946.

Davidson, E.M., and Carlton, S.M., 1998. Intraplantar injection of dextrorphan, ketamine or memantine attenuates formalin-induced behaviors. Brain Res. 785, 136-142.

Du, J., Zhou, S., Coggeshall, R.E. and Carlton, S.M., 2003. *N*-methyl-d-aspartate-induced excitation and sensitization of normal and inflamed nociceptors. Neuroscience 118, 547–562.

Follenfant, R.L., and Nakamura-Craig, M., 1992. Glutamate induces hyperalgesia in the rat paw. Br. J. Pharmacol. 106, 49P

Hardy, J.D., 1953. Thresholds of pain and reflex ontraction as releated to noxious stimuli. J. Appl. Physiol. 5, 725-739.

Hu, H.-J., Bhave, G., and Gereau IV R.W., 2002. Prostaglandin and protein kinase A-dependent modulation of vanilloid receptor function by metabotropic glutamate receptor 5: Potential mechanism for thermal hyperalgesia. J Neurosci. 22, 7444–7452.

Hunt, S.P., Pini, A., and Evan, G., 1987. Induction of c-fos-like protein in spinal cord neurons following sensory stimulation. Nature 328, 632-634.

Jackson, D.L., Graff, C.B., Richardson, J.D., and Hargreaves, K.M., 1995. Glutamate participates in the peripheral modulation of thermal hyperalgesia in rats. Eur. J. Pharmacol. 284, 321-325.

Jancso, G., Kiraly, E., and Jancso-Gabor, A., 1977. Pharmacologically induced selective degeneration of chemosensitive primary sensory neurons. Nature 270, 741-743.

Jin, Y.H., Nishioka, H., Wakabayashi, K., Fujita, T., and Yonehara, N., 2006. Effect of morphine on the release of excitatory amino acids in the rat hind instep: pain is modulated by the interaction between the peripheral opioid and glutamate systems. Neuroscience 138, 1329-1339.

Keast, J.R., and Stephensen, T.M., 2000. Glutamate and aspartate immunoreactivity in dorsal root ganglion cells supplying visceral and somatic targets and evidence for peripheral axonal transport. J. Comp. Neurol. 424, 577-587.

Kinkelin, I., Brocker, E.-B., Koltzenburg, M., and Carlton, S.M., 2000. Localization of ionotropic glutamate receptors in peripheral axons of human skin. Neurosci. Lett. 283, 149-152.

Lam, D.K., Sessle, B.J. and Hu, J.W., 2003. Glutamate and capsaicin-induced activation primary afferents. (Abst) Program No. 294.6, Abstract Viewer/Itinerary Planner, Society for Neuroscience, Washington, DC (Online) .

Lam, D.K., Sessle, B.J. and Hu, J.W., 2004. Glutamate and capsaicin-evoked activity in deep craniofacial trigeminal nociceptive afferents. (Abst) Program No. 3817., Abstract Viewer/Itinerary Planner, International Association for Dental Research.

Lam, D.K., Sessle, B.J., Cairns, B.E. and Hu, J.W., 2005. Peripheral NMDA receptor modulation of jaw muscle elecromyographic activity induced by capsaicin injection into the temporomandibular joint of rats. Brain Res. 1046, 68-76.

Laurie, D.J., Putzke, J, Zieglgansberger, W, Seeburg, P.H. and Tolle, T.R., 1995. The distribution of splice variants of the NMDAR1 subunit mRNA in adult rat brain. Mol. Brain Res. 32, 94-108.

Lawand, N.B., Willis, W.D., and Westlund, K.N., 1997. Excitatory amino acid receptor involvement in peripheral nociceptive transmission in rats. Eur. J. Pharmacol. 324, 169-177.

Lee, K.S., Kim, J., Yoon, Y.W., Lee, M.G., Hong, S.K., Han, H.C., 2007. The peripheral role of group I metabotropic glutamate receptors on nociceptive behaviors in rats with knee joint inflammation. Neurosci. Lett. 416, 123–127.

Leem, J.W., Hwang, J.H., Hwang, S.J., Park, H., Kim, M.K., and Choi, Y., 2001. The role of peripheral N-methyl-d-aspartate receptors in Freund's complete adjuvant induced mechanical hyperalgesia in rats. Neurosci. Lett. 297, 155-158.

Liu, H., Wang, H., Sheng, M., Jan, L.Y., and Basbaum, A.I., 1994. Evidence for presynaptic N-methyl-D-aspartate autoreceptors in the spinal cord dorsal horn. Proc. Natl. Acad. Sci. USA 91, 8383-8387.

Lynn B., 1990. Capsaicin: Actions on nociceptive C-fibers and therapeutic potential. Pain 41, 61-69.

Michael, G.J., and Priestly, J.V., 1999. Differential expression of the mRNA for the vanilloid receptor subtype 1 in cells of the adult rat dorsal root and nodose ganglia and its downregulation by axotomy. J. Neurosci. 19, 1844-1854.

Nagy, J.I., Iversen, L.I., Goedert, M., Chapman, D., and Hunt, S.P., 1983. Dose-dependent effects of capsaicin on primary sensory neurons in the neonatal rat. J. Neurosci. 3, 399-406.

Nordlind, K., Johansson, O., Liden, S., and Hökfelt, T., 1993. Glutamate- and aspartate-like immunoreactivities in human normal and inflamed skin. Cell Path. Mol. Path. 64, 75-82.

Omote, K., Kawamata, T., Kawamata, M., and Namiki, A., 1998. Formalin-induced release of excitatory amino acids in the skin of the rat hindpaw. Brain Res. 787, 161-164.

Sato, K., Kiyama, H., Park, H.T., and Tohyama, M., 1993. AMPA, KA and NMDA receptors are expressed in the rat DRG neurones. Neuroreport 4, 1263-1265.

Strassman, A.M., and Vos, B.P., 1993. Somatotopic and laminar organization of Fos-like immunoreactivity in the medullary and upper dorsal horn induced by noxious facial stimulation in the rat. J. Comp. Neuro. 331, 495-516.

Takemura, M., Shimada, T., Sugiyo, S., Nokubi, T., and Shigenaga, Y., 2000. Mapping of c-Fos in the trigeminal sensory nucleus following high- and low-intensity afferent stimulation in the rat. Exp. Brain Res. 130, 113-123.

Tominaga, M., Caterina, M.J., Malmberg, A.B., Rosen, T.A., Gilbert, H., Skinner, K., Raumann, B.E., Basbaum, A.I., and Julius, D., 1998. The Cloned Capsaicin Receptor Integrates Multiple Pain-Producing Stimuli. Neuron 21, 531-543.

Walker, K., Reeve, A., Bowes, M., Winter J., Wotherspoon G., Davis A., Schmid, P., Gasparini, F., Kuhn R., and Urban, L., 2001. mGlu5 receptors and nociceptive function II. mGlu5 receptors functionally expressed on peripheral sensory neurones mediate inflammatory hyperalgesia. Neuropharmacol. 40, 10–19

Warncke, T., Jorum, E. and Stubhaug, A., 1997. Local treatment with the N-methyl-D-aspartate receptor antagonist ketamine, inhibits development of secondary hyperalgesia in man by a peripheral action. Neurosci. Lett. 227, 1-4.

Westlund, K.N., McNeill, D.L., and Coggeshall, R.E., 1989. Glutamate immnoreactivity in rat dorsal roots. Neurosci. Lett. 96, 13-17.

Westlund, K.N., Sun, Y.C., Sluka, K.A., Dougherty, P.M., Sorkin, L.S., and Willis, W.D., 1992. Neural changes in acute arthritis in monkeys. II. Increased glutamate immunoreactivity in the medial articular nerve. Brain Res. Rev. 17, 15-27.

Yanga, D., and Gereau IV, R.W., 2003. Peripheral group II metabotropic glutamate receptors mediate endogenous anti-allodynia in inflammation. Pain 106, 411–417.

Yonehara, N., Shibutani, T., and Inoki, R., 1987. Contribution of substance P to heat-induced edema in rat paw. J. Pharmacol. Exp. Ther. 242, 1071-1076.

Yonehara, N., Imai, Y., Chen, J.-Q., Takiuchi, S., and Inoki, R., 1992. Influence of opioids on substance P release evoked by antidromic stimulation of primary afferent fibers in the hind instep of rats. Regulatory Peptides 38, 13-22.

Yonehara, N., Saito, K., Oh-ishi, S., Katori, M., and Inoki, R., 1995. Contribution of bradykinin to heat-induced substance P release in the hind instep of rats. Life Science 56, 1679-1688.

Yonehara, N., Takemura, M., Yoshimura, M., Iwase, K., Seo, H.G., Taniguchi, N. and Shigenaga, Y., 1997. Nitric oxide in the rat spinal cord in Freund's adjuvant-induced hyperalgesia. Jpn. J. Pharmacol. 75, 327-335.

Zhou, L., Zhang, Q., Stein, C., and Schafer, M., 1998. Contribution of opioid receptors on primary afferent versus sympathetic neurons to peripheral opioid analgesia. J. Pharmacol. Exp. Ther. 286, 1000-1006.

Zhou, S., Bonasera, L., and Carlton, S.M., 1996. Peripheral administration of NMDA, AMPA or KA results in pain behaviors in rats. Neuroreport 7, 895-900.

Zhou, S., Komak, S., Du, J., and Carlton, S.M., 2001. Metabotropic glutamate 1a receptors on peripheral primary afferent fibers: their role in nociception. Brain Res. 913, 18-26.

Zou, X, Lin, Q, Willis, W.D., 2002. Role of protein kinase A in phosphorylation of NMDA receptor 1 subunits in dorsal horn and spinothalamic tract neurons after intradermal injection of capsaicin in rats. Neuroscience 115, 775-786.

Zimmermann, M., 1983. Ethical guidelines for investigations of experimental pain in conscious animals. Pain 16, 109-110.

3

Molecular Pharmacology of Nucleoside and Nucleotide HIV-1 Reverse Transcriptase Inhibitors

Brian D. Herman and Nicolas Sluis-Cremer
University of Pittsburgh, Department of Medicine, Division of Infectious Diseases, Pittsburgh, USA

1. Introduction

In 1985, 3'-azido-thymidine (AZT, zidovudine) was identified as the first nucleoside analog with activity against human immunodeficiency virus type 1 (HIV-1) (Mitsuya et al., 1985, 1987; Mitsuya & Broder, 1986), the etiologic agent of acquired immunodeficiency syndrome (Barre-Sinoussi et al., 1983; Gallo et al., 1984). This seminal discovery showed that HIV-1 replication could be suppressed by small molecule chemotherapeutic agents, and provided the basis for the field of antiviral drug discovery. Zidovudine was approved by the United States of America Food and Drug Administration for the treatment of HIV-1 infection in 1987. In the 26 years since, an additional seven nucleoside or nucleotide analogs have been approved, while several others are in clinical development. This chapter will provide a summary of the molecular pharmacology of these compounds.

2. Mechanism of action

Retroviruses such as HIV-1 carry their genomic information in the form of (+)strand RNA, but are distinguished from other RNA viruses by the fact that they replicate through a double-stranded DNA that is integrated into the host cell's genomic DNA (Temin & Mizutani, 1970; Baltimore, 1970; DeStefano et al., 1993). While the conversion of viral RNA into double-stranded DNA intermediate is a complex process, all chemical steps are catalyzed by the multi-functional viral enzyme reverse transcriptase (RT). HIV-1 RT exhibits two types of DNA polymerase activity, an RNA-dependent DNA polymerase activity that synthesizes a (-)strand DNA copy of the viral RNA, and a DNA-dependent DNA polymerase activity that generates the (+)strand DNA (Peliska & Benkovic, 1992; Cirno et al., 1995). RT also has ribonuclease H activity that degrades the RNA in the intermediate (+)RNA/(-)DNA duplex (Ghosh et al., 1997).

Once metabolized by host cell enzymes to their triphosphate forms (described in more detail below), nucleoside analogs inhibit HIV-1 reverse transcription. As such, they are typically referred to as nucleoside RT inhibitors (NRTI). NRTI-triphosphates (NRTI-TP) inhibit RT-catalyzed proviral DNA synthesis by two mechanisms (Goody et al., 1991). First, they are competitive inhibitors for binding and/or catalytic incorporation with respect to the analogous natural dNTP substrate. Second, they terminate further viral DNA synthesis due to the lack of a 3′-OH group. Chain termination is the principal mechanism of NRTI antiviral action (Goody et al., 1991). In theory, NRTI-TPs should be ideal antivirals. Each HIV virion carries only two copies of genomic RNA. There are about 20,000 nucleotide incorporation events catalyzed by RT during the synthesis of complete viral DNA, thus providing about 5000 chances for chain-termination by any given NRTI. Since HIV-1 RT lacks a formal proof-reading activity, a single NRTI incorporation event should effectively terminate reverse transcription. In reality, however, NRTIs are less potent than might be expected. The two primary reasons responsible for this are: (i) HIV-1 RT can effectively discriminate between the natural dNTP and NRTI-TP, and the extent of this discrimination is dramatically modulated by nucleic acid sequence (Isel et al., 2001); and (ii) HIV-1 RT can excise the chain-terminating NRTI-monophosphate (NRTI-MP) by using either pyrophosphate (pyrophophorolysis) or ATP as a substrate (Meyer et al., 1998; Goldschmidt & Marquet, 2004).

3. NRTI approved for clinical use

3.1 Zidovudine

Zidovudine was first synthesized in 1964 as a potential anticancer drug, but was not further developed for human use because of toxicity concerns. However, as described in the Introduction, it was found to have potent anti-HIV activity and, in 1987, was the first antiviral drug to be approved for clinical use. Zidovudine is a thymidine analog in which the 3′-OH group has been replaced with an azido (-N3) group (Figure 1). Zidovudine permeates the cell membrane by passive transport and not via a nucleoside carrier transporter (Zimmerman et al., 1987). It has good oral bioavailability and shows efficient penetration into the central nervous system. Zidovudine is efficiently metabolized to its 5′-MP form by cytosolic thymidine kinase (Ho & Hitchcock, 1989). The phosphorylation of zidovudine-MP to zidovudine-DP is catalyzed by thymidinylate monophosphate kinase (dTMP kinase; Furman et al., 1986). Interestingly, the apparent Michaelis constant (K_m) of zidovudine-MP for dTMP kinase is almost equivalent to that of dTMP, however its maximum kinetic rate (V_{max}) is only 0.3 % that of dTMP (Furman et al., 1986). Therefore, zidovudine-MP acts as a substrate inhibitor of dTMP kinase and limits its own conversion to the 5'-DP form. In this regard, there is a marked accumulation of zidovudine-MP and only low levels of the 5'-DP- and 5'-TP derivatives are detected in human T-lymphocytes (Balzarini et al., 1989). Cellular nucleoside diphosphate kinase (NDP kinase) is likely responsible for the further conversion of zidovudine-DP to zidovudine-TP. Zidovudine is metabolized to its 5′-O-glucuronide in the liver, kidney, and intestinal mucosa (Barbier et al., 2000). Because of the extensive glucuronidation of ZDV, other drugs that are also glucuronidated or that inhibit this process cause an increase in zidovudine plasma levels. Fourteen percent of the parent compound and 74% of the glucuronide have been recovered from the urine after oral administration in normal subjects (Ruane et al., 2004). Renal excretion of zidovudine is by both glomerular filtration and active tubular secretion. In some cells zidovudine can be metabolized to the highly toxic reduction product 3′-amino-thymidine (Weidner & Sommadossi, 1990).

3.2 Stavudine

Like zidovudine, stavudine (2′,3′-didehydro-3′-deoxythymidine, d4T) is a thymidine analog that undergoes metabolic activation by the sequential action of thymidine kinase and dTMP kinase (Figure 1). However, stavudine is inefficiently phosphorylated to its 5′-MP form by thymidine kinase (August et al., 1988; Zhu et al., 1990). As such, this first phosphorylation step is rate-limiting and most intracellular stavudine is not phophorylated (Balzarini et al., 1989). Maximal plasma concentrations of stavudine are achieved within 2 hours of oral administration and increase linearly as the dose increases, with an absolute bioavailability approaching 100 % (Rana & Dudley, 1997)). The drug distributes into total body water and appears to enter cells by non-facilitated diffusion (passive transport). Penetration into the central nervous system, however, is far less than zidovudine. Stavudine is cleared quickly with a terminal plasma half-life of 1-1.6 hours by both renal and nonrenal processes (Dudley et al., 1992).

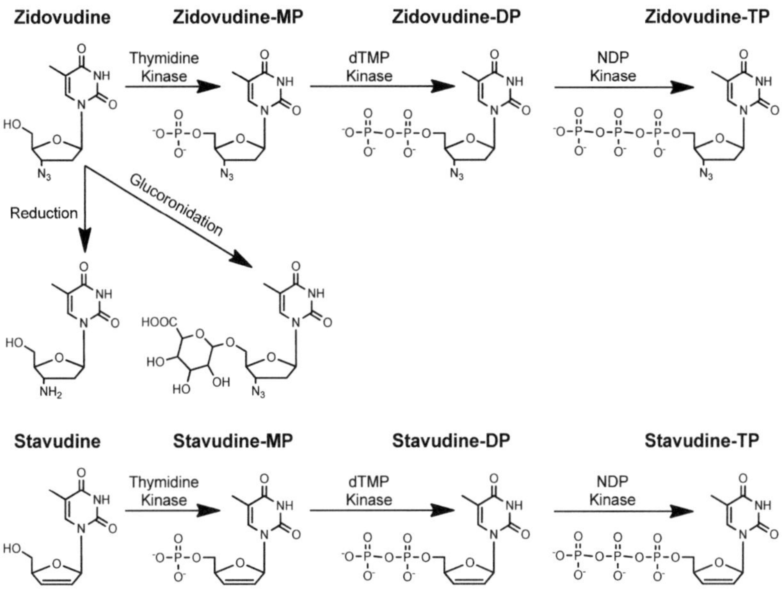

Fig. 1. Metabolic pathways of zidovudine and stavudine

3.3 Didanosine

Initially, 2′,3′-dideoxyadenosine (ddA) was evaluated as a clinical candidate but was ultimately discovered to cause nephrotoxicity. ddA is acid labile and oral administration leads to exposure to the acidic pH of the stomach and degradation to adenine (Masood et al., 1990). Adenine is further metabolized to 2,8-dihydroxyadenine which causes nephrotoxicity by crystallization in the kidney. Interestingly, ddA was shown to be metabolized to 2′,3′-dideoxyinosine (ddI, didanosine) by adenosine deaminase (Figure 2), and that much of the antiviral activity of ddA resides in didanosine (Cooney et al., 1987). Furthermore, the administration of didanosine avoids the production of adenine and the resulting nephrotoxicity. Didanosine is phosphorylated to didanosine-MP by cytosolic 5'-nucleotidase, which uses either inosine monophosphate (IMP) or guanosine monophosphate (GMP) as phosphate donors (Johnson & Fridland, 1989). Didanosine-MP is then converted to ddAMP by adenylosuccinate synthetase and 5' adenosine monophosphate-activated protein (AMP) kinase (Ahluwalia et al., 1987). The enzymes involved in phosphorylation of ddAMP to ddADP and ddATP have not been identified, although AMP kinase and NDP kinase have been proposed to play a role. ddATP is the active metabolite that is recognized by HIV-1 RT and incorporated into the nascent viral DNA chain causing chain-termination. No evidence has been provided for the formation of didanosine-DP or didanosine-TP. Didanosine is hydrolyzed to hypoxanthine by purine nucleoside phosphorylase (PNP) and further anabolized by hypoxanthine-guanine phosphoribosyl transferase to IMP (Ahluwalia et al., 1987). ATP and GTP are formed from IMP through the classical purine nucleotide biosynthetic pathways.

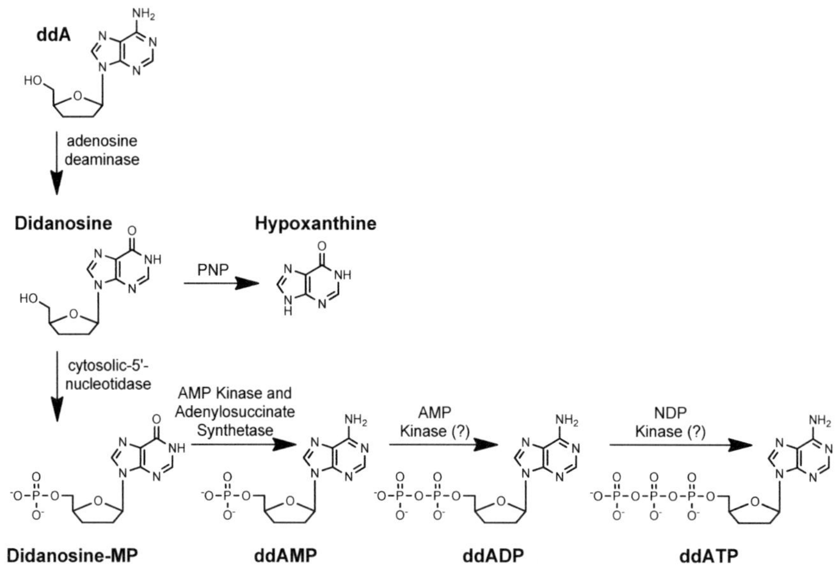

Fig. 2. Metabolic pathways of ddA and didanosine

3.4 Lamivudine and emtricitabine

The structurally related cytidine analogs lamivudine ((-)-3′-thia-2′,3′-dideoxycytidine; 3TC) and ematricitabine ((-)-3′-thia-5-flouro-2′,3′-dideoxycytidine; FTC) both contain the unnatural L-enantiomer ribose with a sulfur atom replacing the C3′ position (Figure 3). Emtricitabine has an additional 5-flouro moiety on the cytosine ring. Lamivudine and emtricitabine are both metabolized to their respective 5'-mono- and di- and triphosphate derivatives by deoxycytidine kinase, deoxycytidine monophosphate kinase, and 5′-nucleoside diphosphate kinase, respectively (Chang et al., 1992; Cammack et al., 1992; Stein & Moore 2001; Darque et al., 1999; Bang & Scott, 2003). There is no evidence that lamivudine or emtricitabine are deaminated to their uridine analogs by cellular cytidine or deoxycytidine deaminases (Starnes & Cheng, 1987). Formation of the free base by cellular pyrimidine phosphorylases has also not been observed. Lamivudine-DP and emtricitabine-TP accumulate to higher levels in peripheral blood mononuclear cells than their monophosphate forms. It has been suggested that conversion of lamivudine-DP to lamivudine-TP is rate limiting. Lamivudine and emtricitabine are rapidly absorbed through the GI tract with peek plasma levels of 85-93% achieved within 2 hours post oral administration. Lamivudine has a plasma half-life of 5-7 hours and is eliminated unmetabolized by active organic cationic excretion (Johnson et al., 1999). Emtricitabine persists in plasma with a half-life of 10 hours and is eliminated primarily in urine by glomerular filtration and active tubular secretion but approximately 14% is eliminated in feces. Oxidation of the 3′-thiol by unidentified enzymes yields 3′-sulfoxide diasteriomers and 2′-O-glucuronidation also occurs.

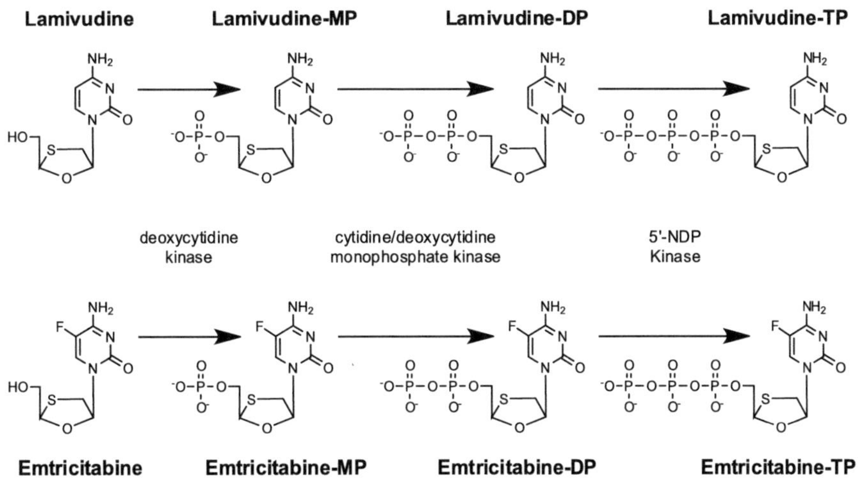

Fig. 3. Metabolic pathways of lamivudine and emtricitabine

3.5 Abacavir

Abacavir (1S,4R)-4-[2-amino-6-(cyclopropylamino)-9H-purin-9-yl]cyclopent-2-en-1-yl]methanol) is a prodrug of carbovir (2-Amino-1,9-dihydro-9-[(1R,4S)-4-(hydroxymethyl)-2-cyclopenten-1-yl]-6H-purin-6-one), a deoxyguanosine analog (Figure 4; Daluge et al., 1997). Abacavir permeates T lymophoblastoid cell lines by passive diffusion. Abacavir is phosphorylated to abacavir-MP by adenosine phosphotransferase (Faletto et al., 1997). A yet unidentified cytosolic deaminase then converts abacavir-MP to carbovir-MP. Phosphorylation to the diphosphate derivative occurs via guanidinylate monophosphate kinase. The final phosphorylation step can be catalyzed by a number of cellular enzymes including 5′-nucleotide diphosphate kinase, pyruvate kinase, and creatine kinase (Faletto et al., 1997). A linear dose relationship with carbovir-mono-, di-, and tri- phosphate derivatives over a 1000-fold dose range in vitro suggests there are no rate limiting steps in abacavir anabolism. The active metabolite carbovir-TP has been shown to persist with an elimination half-life of greater than 20 hours (McDowell et al., 2000). Abacavir bioavailability is ~83 % and is rapidly absorbed after oral dosing reaching peak plasma levels within 1 hour (Chittick et al., 1999). However, abacavir is extensively catabolized in the liver and only 1.2% is excreted as unchanged abacavir in urine. Abacavir oxidation by alcohol dehyrogenases to form the 5′-carboxylic acid derivative represents 36% of metabolites recovered from urine, while the 5′-O-glucuronide corresponds to 30% of metabolites from urine (Chittick et al., 1999). Fecal excretion also accounts for approximately 16 % of the given dose. Abacavir is not metabolized by cytochrome P450 enzymes and does not inhibit these enzymes.

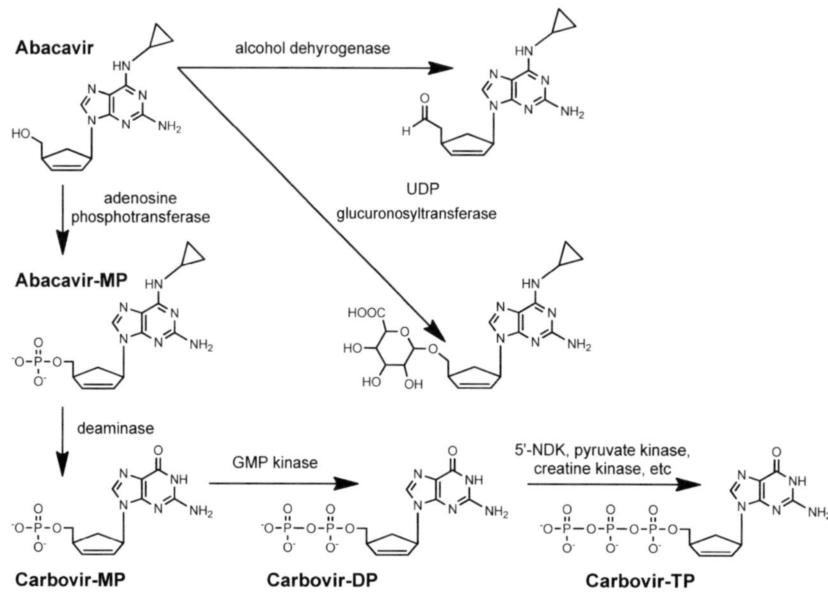

Fig. 4. Metabolic pathways for abacavir

3.6 Tenofovir and tenofovir disoproxil fumerate

The acyclic nucleoside phosphonate tenofovir (*R*-9-(2-phosphonylmethoxypropyl)-adenine) has no sugar ring structure but contains an acyclic methoxypropyl linker between the base N9 atom and a non-hydrolyzable C-P phosphonate bond. Thus tenofovir represents the only currently approved *nucleotide* HIV inhibitor. Tenofovir is poorly absorbed by the oral route and is therefore administered as a lipophilic orally bioavailable prodrug tenofovir disoproxil fumerate (TDF), a fumaric acid salt of the bis-isopropoxycarbonyloxymethyl ester of tenofovir (Figure 5). TDF is readily absorbed by the gastrointestinal epithelial cells with an oral bioavailability of 25% (Barditch-Crovo et al., 2001). Administration with a high fat meal increases absorption to 40%. Degradation of TDF to its monoester and subsequently to tenofovir occurs readily in the intestinal mucosa by the action of carboxylesterases and phosphodiesterases, respectively. The mono- or bis-ester forms of tenofovir are not observed in plasma suggesting efficient release of tenofovir following oral administration of TDF (Naesens et al., 1998). Following oral administration tenofovir has a long terminal half-life of 17 hours. The phosphonic acid linkage is chemically and metabolically stable and phosphorolysis back to the nucleoside does not occur (Naesens et al., 1998). Tenofovir is rapidly converted intracellularly to tenofovir-monophosphate and the active tenofovir-diphosphate forms by adenylate monophosphate kinase and 5'-nucleoside diphosphate kinase, respectively (Robbins et al., 1998). Tenofovir is not subject to intracellular deamination or deglycosylation. This stability results in a very long intracellular half-life for tenofovir-diphosphate of 15 hours in activated lymphocytes and 50 hours in resting lymphocytes (Robbins et al., 1998). Tenofovir is eliminated by glomerular filtration and active tubular secretion by organic anion transporter mediated uptake and MRP4 mediated efflux (Ray et al., 2006). At 72 hours post oral administration 70 - 80 % is recovered from urine as unchanged tenofovir. Tenofovir does not inhibit cytochrome P450 enzymes.

However, the mono- and di-phosphate forms both inhibit purine nucleoside phosphorylase which is responsible for base removal of didanosine to form hypoxanthine.

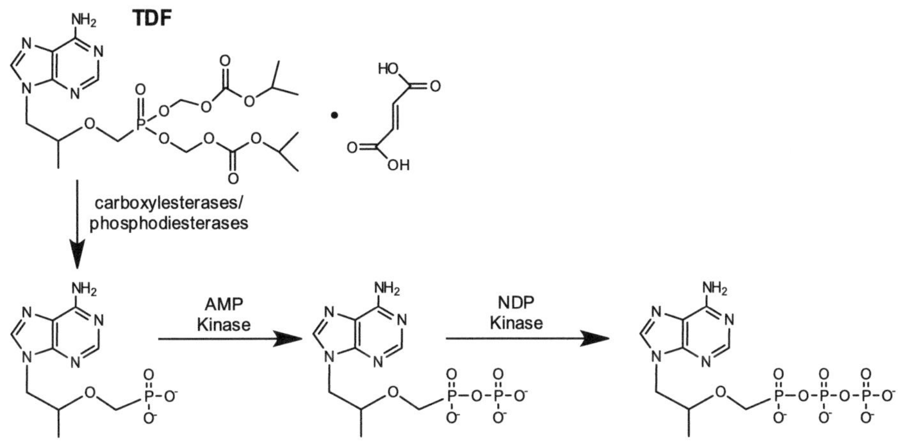

Tenofovir **Tenofovir-MP** **Tenofovir-DP**

Fig. 5. Metabolic pathways of tenofovir and TDF

4. NRTI in the pipeline

Despite the widespread clinical success of NRTI-containing therapy, the currently FDA approved NRTIs display important limitations including the selection of drug resistance mutations that display cross-resistance to other NRTI, toxicity-related adverse events, and drug-drug interactions (for review see Cihlar & Ray, 2010). Thus, there is a need for novel NRTI that overcome these limitations. Here we will discuss the pharmacology of several novel drug candidates.

4.1 Apricitabine

Apricitabine (ATC) is the (-)-enantiomer of 2′-deoxy-3′-oxa-4′-thiocytidine, a deoxycytidine analog that is currently in phase II/III clinical trials (Figure 6). Both the (+) and (-)-enantiomers of apricitabine demonstrate potent inhibition of HIV-1 replication, however the (+)-enantiomer demonstrated significant mitochondrial and cellular toxicity in pre-clinical studies that was not observed with the (-) enantiomer (de Muys et al., 1999; Taylor et al., 2000). Racemic conversion of (-)-apricitabine to (+)-apricitabine is not observed in vivo (Holdich et al., 2006). Orally administered ATC is absorbed quickly, reaching maximal plasma levels within 2 hours with a plasma half-life of 3 hours. Maximal peripheral blood mononuclear cell (PBMC) intracellular concentrations of apricitabine -TP are achieved 3.5 - 4 hours after oral administration in healthy and HIV-infected patients. The intracellular half-life is 6 - 7 hours (Sawyer & Struthers-Semple, 2006; Cahn et al., 2008; Holdich et al., 2007). Apricitabine is not metabolized by hepatocytes *in vitro*, however a deaminated metabolite was observed likely due to gastrointestinal metabolism (Nakatani-Freshwater et al., 2006). This metabolite is excreted renally and does not demonstrate antiviral or pharmacologic effects. Apricitabine had no effect on cytochrome P450 or glucouronidase but was a weak inhibitor of P-glycoprotein (Sawyer & Cox, 2006). The first phosphorylation of apricitabine is mediated by deoxycytidine kinase, the enzyme also responsible for the initial phosphorylation of lamivudine and emtricitabine (de Muys et al., 1999). The possibility of competition for deoxycytidine kinase was examined in PBMC. Co-administration of apricitabine with lamivudine or emtricitabine leads to a dose-dependent decrease in apricitabine phosphorylation, whereas lamivudine and emtricitabine phosphorylation was not affected by apricitabine (Bethell et al., 2007). In healthy volunteers given apricitabine and lamivudine, the intracellular PBMC levels of apricitabine-TP were decreased 75% compared to apricitabine alone (Holdich et al., 2006). Consequently, administration of apricitabine in combination with lamivudine or emtricitabine is not recommended. Similarly, lamivudine and emtricitabine co-administration is also contraindicated. Apricitabine-MP is sequentially phosphorylated to the di- and tri-phosphate forms by cytidine or deoxycytidine monophosphate kinase and 5′-nucleotide diphosphate kinase, respectively.

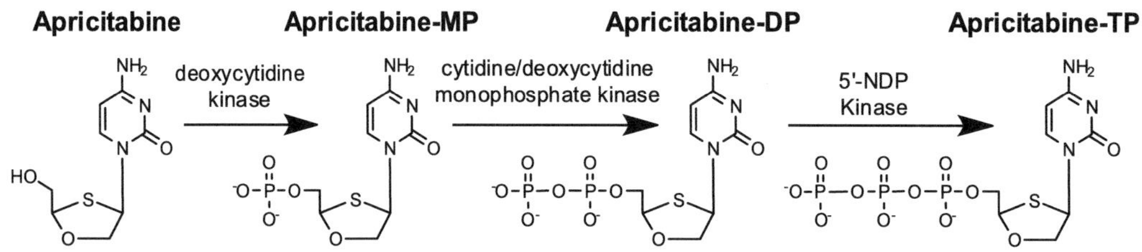

Fig. 6. Metabolic pathway of apricitabine

4.2 Festinavir

Festinavir (2′,3′-didehydro-3′-deoxy-4′-ethynylthymidine; 4′-Ed4T) is a 4′-ethynyl analog of stavudine that is 5-10 fold more potent (Figure 7) (Haraguchi et al., 2003; Nitanda et al., 2005). Festinavir shows decreased cellular toxicity compared to stavudine, with little or no inhibition of host polymerases (Yang et al., 2007; Dutschman et al., 2004). Stepwise phosphorylation of festinavir occurs via the same enzymes as stavudine. Thymidine kinase 1 phosphorylates festinavir to festinavir-MP with 4-fold greater efficiency than stavudine (Hsu et al., 2007). The efficiency of festinavir-MP phosphorylation by thymidinylate monophosphate kinase is approximately 10 % of that seen for stavudine-MP or zidovudine-MP. Conversion from festinavir-DP to festinavir-TP appears to be catalyzed by multiple enzymes including nucleoside diphosphate kinase, pyruvate kinase, creatine kinase, and 3-phosphoglycerate kinase (Hsu et al., 2007). In contrast to other thymidine analogs which are readily catabolized by thymidine phosphorylase, festinavir catabolism cannot be detected. Furthermore, festinavir efflux from the cell is much less efficient than that of zidovudine. The festinavir nucleoside form alone is effluxed by a yet to be identified cellular transporter, while zidovudine and zidovudine-MP are effluxed from the cell. A Phase 1a study investigated the pharmacokinetic profile of a single oral dose between 10 and 900 mg and found a linear dose response in plasma with no apparent effects from food (Paintsil et al., 2009). A Phase 1b/2a study of festinavir oral monotherapy in 32 patients was recently completed. The results indicated that festinavir was safe (few festinavir related adverse events), well tolerated, and demonstrated dose dependent decreases in viral load between 0.87 and 1.36 logs (Cotte et al., 2010).

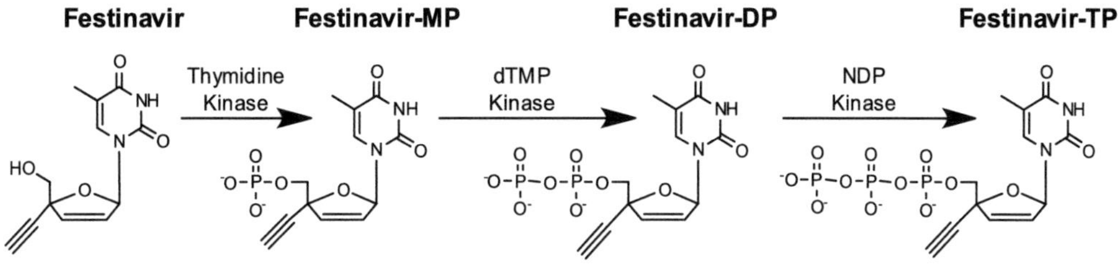

Fig. 7. Metabolic pathway of festinavir

4.3 Amdoxovir

The purine nucleoside analog 1-β-D-dioxolane guanosine (DXG) has potent activity against HIV and hepatitis B virus (Kim et al., 1993). However, it demonstrates poor solubility and limited oral bioavailability in monkeys (Chen et al., 1996). The analog 1-β-D-2,6-diaminopurine dioxolane (amdoxovir; Figure 8) also exhibits antiviral activity and is more water soluble and orally bioavailable (Chen et al., 1999; Kim et al., 1993)). Amdoxovir serves as a prodrug for DXG by deamination at the 6-position by adenosine deaminase (Gu et al., 1999). *In vitro,* amdoxovir bound adenosine deaminase as efficiently as adenosine, however amdoxovir was deaminated 540-fold slower than adenosine (Furman et al., 2001). Only DXG-triphosphate was detected in PBMC and CEM cells following exposure to DXG or amdoxovir (Rajagopalan et al., 1994; Rajagopalan et al., 1996). DXG is phosphorylated to DXG-MP by 5′-nucleotidase using IMP as a phosphate donor (Feng et al., 2004). DXG-diphosphate is then generated by guanosine monophosphate kinase (GMP kinase). DXG-DP acts as substrate for phosphorylation to the active DXG-TP for several enzymes including nucleotide diphosphate kinase (NDP kinase), 3-phosphoglycerate kinase (3-PG kinase, creatine kinase, and pyruvate kinase. Amdoxovir is rapidly converted to DXG in monkeys,

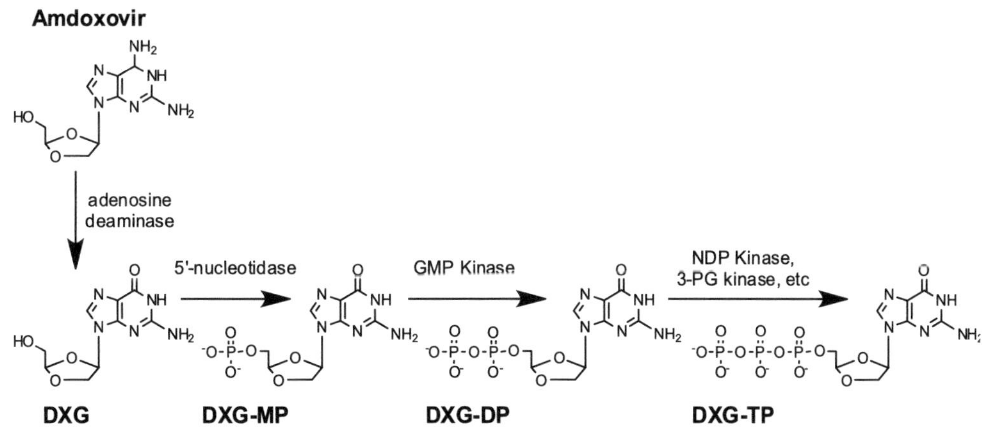

Fig. 8. Metabolic pathway of amdoxovir

woodchucks, and rats with approximately 61 % of the dose converted to DXG (Chen et al., 1996; Chen et al., 1999; Rajagopalan et al., 1996). The oral bioavailability of amdoxovir is estimated to be 30% (Chen et al., 1999). Following oral administration of amdoxovir to HIV-infected patients, peak plasma levels of amdoxivir and DXG were reached within 2 hours

(Thompson et al., 2005). Amdoxovir was eliminated from plasma with half-life of 1 - 2 hours by conversion to DXG, whereas DXG demonstrated a longer half-life of 4 - 7 hours. In animal studies amdoxovir toxicities included obstructive nephropathy, uremia, islet cell atrophy, hyperglycemia, and lens opacities (Rajagopalan et al., 1996). In a phase I/II clinical study 4 of 18 patients developed nongradeable lens opacities (Thompson et al., 2005). In other studies most adverse events were minor and included nausea, headache, and diarrhea (Gripshover et al., 2006; Murphy et al., 2008).

4.4 GS-7340

GS-7340 (9-[(R)-2-[[(S)-[[(S)-1-(isopropoxycarbonyl)ethyl]amino]phenoxyphosphinyl]-methoxy]propyl]adenine) is a novel isopropylalaninyl phenyl ester prodrug of tenofovir designed to increase intracellular delivery of the active tenofovir-DP metabolite by masking the charged phosphonate (Figure 9; Eisenberg et al 2001). Preclinical studies demonstrated 200-fold improved plasma stability and 400-fold increased accumulation of tenofovir and active tenofovir-DP in lymphatic tissues and peripheral blood mononuclear cells (PBMC) compared to tenofovir (Lee et al., 2005; Eisenberg et al., 2001). GS-7340 has 1000-fold improved potency *in vitro* over tenofovir. Following rapid target cell uptake, GS-7340 is hydrolyzed at the carboxy ester bond in lysozomes by the serine protease cathepsin A and other serine and cysteine proteases (Birkus et al., 2007; 2008). The resulting partially stable product spontaneously releases phenol by intramolecular cyclization and hydrolysis to a negatively charged, cell impermeable tenofovir-alanine intermediate (Balzarini et al., 1996). Formation of tenofovir-alanine is faster in resting PBMC compared to activated PBMC, while metabolism to parent tenofovir by a phosphoamidase and downstream phosphorylation to tenofovir-MP and tenofovir-DP is much faster in activated PBMC. A recent clinical study comparing 50 mg and 150 mg doses of GS-7340 with 300 mg TDF was conducted to determine the efficacy, safety and pharmacokinetics over 14 days (Markowitz et al., 2011). Viral loads were reduced -1.71-log and -1.57-log for 150 mg and 50 mg doses, respectively, compared to 0.94-log for TDF. PBMC levels of tenofovir were 4 – 33- times greater with GS-7340 than those for TDF at day 14 while plasma levels of tenofovir were decreased up to 88% at 24 hours with administration of GS-7340 compared to TDF. No serious adverse events were reported while the most frequent complaint was mild to moderate headache and nausea.

4.5 CMX-157

Like GS-7340, CMX-157 is an alternative prodrug of tenofovir designed to increase cell penetration by the natural lipid uptake pathways (Figure 9; Hostetler et al., 1997; Painter et al., 2004). CMX-157 contains a hexadecyloxypropyl (HDP) lipid conjugation which mimics lysophosphatidylcholine. CMX-157, unlike TDF is not cleaved to free tenofovir in the intestinal mucosa and thus circulates in plasma as the tenofovir-HDP lipid conjugate (Painter et al., 2007). Tenofovir-HDP is not a substrate for human organic anion transporters and therefore is subject to decreased renal excretion and increased intracellular drug exposure compared to TDF (Tippin et al., 2010). Free tenofovir is liberated intracellularly by hydrolytic removal of the HDP lipid by phospholipases. Intracellular activation to the active tenofovir-DP form is achieved in the same manner as TDF. CMX-157 delivers > 30-fold increased active metabolite tenofovir-DP in PBMC than tenofovir. Higher intracellular concentrations of CMX-157 provide >300-fold greater activity against clinical isolates than tenofovir with EC_{50} values < 1 nM (Lanier et al., 2010). It has additionally been proposed that CMX-157 may bind cell free virions by direct lipid insertion into the viral envelope resulting in facilitated delivery to target cells (Painter et al., 2007). CMX-157 recently completed a Phase I clinical trial to evaluate safety, tolerability and pharmacokinetics. CMX-157 was well tolerated with no drug-related adverse events. Plasma levels increased linearly with dose and active TFV-DP was detected up to six days post administration of a 400 mg dose suggesting the possibility of a once weekly dosing regimen.

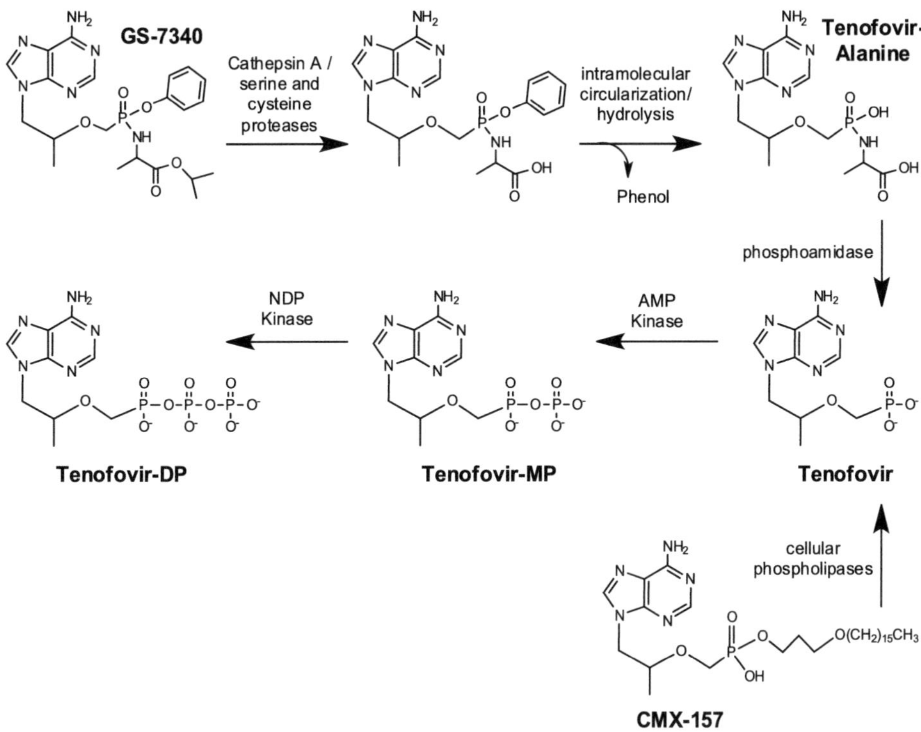

Fig. 9. Intracellular metabolism of GS-7340 and CMX-157

5. Conclusions

Nucleoside and nucleotide reverse transcriptase inhibitors have remained the backbone of antiretroviral therapy. The absolute dependence of NRTI on host cellular enzymes for activation is a unique property of this drug class. The eight approved NRTI and numerous experimental NRTI display great diversity for all of these factors, thus presenting pharmacological advantages and challenges that are unique to the NRTI class. The complex relationships between NRTIs and host cell enzymes have necessitated detailed studies of the *in vitro* and *in vivo* pharmacologic properties of novel NRTIs in pre-clinical development. Current drug discovery efforts increasingly utilize NRTI prodrugs in order to accelerate NRTI phosphorylation or otherwise improve pharmacologic properties. Further understanding of the cellular pharmacology of NRTI is crucial for the development of novel drugs for increased potency, improved safety and tolerability, and decreased resistance.

6. Acknowledgements

Research in the Sluis-Cremer laboratory was supported by grants AI081571, GM068406 and AI071846 from the National Institutes of Health (NIH), United States of America. Brian Herman was supported by an NIH training grant (T32 AAI 49820).

7. References

Ahluwalia, G., Cooney, D.A., Mitsuya, H., Fridland, A., Flora, K.P., Hao, Z., Dalal, M., Broder, S. & Johns, D.G. (1987). Initial studies on the cellular pharmacology of 2',3'-dideoxyinosine, an inhibitor of HIV infectivity. *Biochem. Pharmacol.* 36(22): 3797-800.

August, E.M., Marongiu, M.E., Lin, T.,S. & Prusoff, W.H. (1988). Initial studies on the cellular pharmacology of 3'-deoxythymidin-2'-ene (d4T): a potent and selective inhibitor of human immunodeficiency virus. *Biochem. Pharmacol.*, 37(23): 4419-22.

Baltimore, D. (1970) Viral RNA-dependent DNA polymerase. *Nature* 226: 1209-1211.

Balzarini, J., Herdewijn, P. & De Clercq, E. (1989). Differential patterns of intracellular metabolism of 2′,3′-didehydro-2′,3′-dideoxy-thymidine (D4T) and 3′-azido-2′,3′-dideoxythymidine (AZT), two potent anti-HIV compounds. *J. Biol. Chem.* 264: 6127-33.

Balzarini, J., Karlsson, A., Aquaro, S., Perno, C.F., Cahard, D., Naesens, L., De Clercq, E. & McGuigan, C. (1996). Mechanism of anti-HIV action of masked alaninyl d4T-MP derivatives. *Proc. Natl. Acad. Sci. U.S.A.* 93: 7295–7299.

Bang, L. & Scott, L.J. (2003). Emtricitabine: an antiretroviral agent for HIV infection. *Drugs.* 63: 2413–2424.

Barbier, O., Turgeon, D., Girard, C., Green, M.D., Tephly, T.R., Hum, D.W. & Bélanger, A. (2000). 3'-azido-3'-deoxythimidine (AZT) is glucuronidated by human UDP-glucuronosyltransferase 2B7 (UGT2B7). *Drug Metab. Dispos.* 28(5): 497-502.

Barditch-Crovo, P., Deeks, S.G., Collier, A., Safrin, S., Coakley, D.F., Miller, M., Kearney, B.P., Coleman, R.L., Lamy, P.D., Kahn, J.O., McGowan, I. & Lietman, P.S. (2001). Phase I/II trial of the pharmacokinetics, safety and antiretroviral activity of tenofovir disoproxil fumarate in human immunodeficiency virus-infected adults. *Antimicrob Agents Chemother.* 2001; 45: 2733-9.

Barre-Sinoussi, F., Chermann, J.C., Rey, F., Nugeyre, M.T., Chamaret, S., Gruest, J., Dauguet, C., Axler-Blin, C., Vezinet-Brun, F., Rouzioux, C., Rozenbaum,W., & Montagnier, L., (1983) Isolation of a T-lymphotropic retrovirus from a patient at risk for acquired immune deficiency syndrome (AIDS). *Science* 220: 868–871.

Bethell, R., de Muys, J., Lippens, J., Richard, A., Hamelin, B., Ren, C. & Collins, P. (2007). In vitro interactions between apricitabine and other deoxycytidine analogues. *Antimicrob. Agents Chemother.* 51: 2948 -53.

Birkus, G., Kutty, N., He, G.X., Mulato, A., Lee, W., McDermott, M. & Cihlar, T. (2008). Activation of 9-[(R)-2-[[(S)-[[(S)-1-(Isopropoxycarbonyl)ethyl]amino] phenoxyphosphinyl]-ethoxy]propyl]adenine (GS-7340) and other tenofovir phosphonoamidate prodrugs by human proteases. *Mol. Pharmacol.* 74(1): 92-100.

Birkus, G., Wang, R., Liu, X., Kutty, N., MacArthur, H., Cihlar, T., Gibbs, C., Swaminathan, S., Lee, W. & McDermott, M. (2007). Cathepsin A is the major hydrolase catalyzing the intracellular hydrolysis of the antiretroviral nucleotide phosphonoamidate prodrugs GS-7340 and GS-9131. *Antimicrob. Agents Chemother.* 51(2): 543-50.

Cahn, P., Rolon, M., Cassetti, I., Shiveley, L., Holdich, T. & Sawyer, J. (2008). Multiple-dose pharmacokinetics of apricitabine, a novel nucleoside reverse transcriptase inhibitor, in patients with HIV-1 infection. *Clin. Drug. Invest.* 28: 129 -38.

Cammack, N., Rouse, P., Marr, C.L., Reid, P.J., Boehme, R.E., Coates, J.A., Penn, C.R. & Cameron, J.M. (1992). Cellular metabolism of (-) enantiomeric 2,-deoxy-3,-thiacytidine. *Biochem. Pharmacol.* 43: 2059-2064.

Chang, C.N., Skalski, V., Zhou, J.H. & Cheng, Y.C. (1992). Biochemical pharmacology of (+)- and (-)-2',3'-dideoxy-3'-thiacytidine as anti-hepatitis B virus agents. *J. Biol. Chem.* 267(31): 22414-20.

Chen, H., Boudinot, F.D., Chu, C.K., Mcclure, H.M. & Schinazi, R.F. (1996). Pharmacokinetics of (-)-beta-D-2-aminopurine dioxolane and (-)-beta-D-2-amino-6-chloropurine dioxolane and their antiviral metabolite (-)-beta-D-dioxolane guanine in rhesus monkeys. *Antimicrob. Agents Chemother.* 40(10): 2332-6.

Chen, H., Schinazi, R.F., Rajagopalan, P., Gao, Z., Chu, C.K., McClure, H.M. & Boudinot, F.D. (1999). Pharmacokinetics of (-)-beta-D-dioxolane guanine and prodrug (-)-beta-D-2,6-diaminopurine dioxolane in rats and monkeys. *AIDS Res. Hum. Retroviruses.* 15(18): 1625-30.

Chittick, G.E., Gillotin, C., McDowell, J.A., Lou, Y., Edwards, K.D., Prince, W.T. & Stein, D.S. (1999). Abacavir: absolute bioavailability, bioequivalence of three oral formulations, and effect of food. *Pharmacotherapy.* 19(8): 932-42.

Cihlar, T. & Ray, A.S. (2010). Nucleoside and nucleotide HIV reverse transcriptase inhibitors: 25 years after zidovudine. *Antiviral Res.* 85(1):39-58.

Cirno, N.M., Cameron, C.E., Smith, J.S., Rausch, J.W., Roth, M.J., Benkovic, S.J. & Le Grice, S.F.J. (1995) Divalent cation modulation of the Ribonuclease h functions of human immunodeficiency virus reverse transcriptase. *Biochemistry* 34: 9936-9943.

Cooney, D.A., Ahiuwalia, G., Mitsuya, H., Fridland, A., Johnson, M., Hao, Z., Dalal, M., Balzarini, J., Broder, S. & Johns, D.G. (1987). Initial studies on the cellular pharmacology of 2′,3′-dideoxyadenosine, an inhibitor of HTLV-III infectivity. *Biochem. Pharmacol.* 36: 1765-1768.

Cotte, L., Dellamonica, P., Raffi, F., Yazdanpanah, L.Y., Molina, J. M., Boue, F., & Urata, Y. (2010). A Phase-Ib/IIa Dose-Escalation Study of OBP-601 (4'-ethynyl-d4T, Festinavir) in Treatment-Experienced, HIV-1-Infected Patients. *50th Interscience Conference on Antimicrobial Agents and Chemotherapy* (ICAAC 2010). Boston, MA. U.S.A. September 12-15, 2010.

Daluge, S.M., Good, S.S., Faletto, M.B., Miller, W.H., St Clair, M.H., Boone, L.R., Tisdale, M., Parry, N.R., Reardon, J.E., Dornsife, R.E., Averett, D.R. & Krenitsky, T.A. (1997). 1592U89, a novel carbocyclic nucleoside analog with potent, selective anti-human immunodeficiency virus activity. *Antimicrob. Agents Chemother.* 41(5): 1082-93.

Darque, A., Valette, G., Rousseau, F., Wang, L.H., Sommadossi, J.P. & Zhou, X.J. (1999). Quantitation of intracellular triphosphate of emtricitabine in peripheral blood mononuclear cells from human immunodeficiency virus-infected patients. *Antimicrob. Agents Chemother.* 43: 2245–2250.

de Muys, J.M., Gourdeau, H., Nguyen-Ba, N., Taylor, D.L., Ahmed, P.S., Mansour, T., Locas, C., Richard, N., Wainberg, M.A. & Rando, R.F. (1999). Anti-human immunodeficiency virus type 1 activity, intracellular metabolism, and pharmacokinetic evaluation of 2'-deoxy-3'-oxa-4'-thiocytidine. *Antimicrob. Agents. Chemother.* 43(8): 1835-44.

DeStefano, J.J., Bambara, R.A., & Fay, P.J. (1993) Parameters that influence the binding of human immunodeficiency virus reverse transcriptase to nucleic acid structures. *Biochemistry* 32: 6908-6915.

Dudley, M.N., Graham, K.K., Kaul, S., Geletko, S., Dunkle, L., Browne, M. & Mayer, K. (1992). Pharmacokinetics of stavudine in patients with AIDS or AIDS-related complex. *J. Infect. Dis.* 166: 480–485.

Dutschman, G.E., Grill, S.P., Gullen, E.A., Haraguchi, K., Takeda, S., Tanaka, H., Baba, M. & Cheng, Y.C. (2004). Novel 4′-substituted stavudine analog with improved antihumanimmunodeficiency virus activity and decreased cytotoxicity. *Antimicrob. Agents Chemother.* 48: 1640–1646.

Eisenberg, E.J., He, G.X. & Lee, W.A. (2001). Metabolism of GS-7340, a novel phenyl monophosphoramidate intracellular prodrug of PMPA, in blood. *Nucleosides Nucleotides Nucleic Acids.* 20: 1091-8.

Faletto, M.B., Miller, W.H., Garvey, E.P., St Clair, M.H., Daluge, S.M. & Good, S.S. (1997). Unique intracellular activation of the potent anti-human immunodeficiency virus agent 1592U89. *Antimicrob. Agents Chemother.* 41(5): 1099-107.

Feng, J.Y., Parker, W.B., Krajewski, M.L., Deville-Bonne, D., Veron, M., Krishnan, P., Cheng, Y.C. & Borroto-Esoda, K. (2004). Anabolism of amdoxovir: phosphorylation of dioxolane guanosine and its 5'-phosphates by mammalian phosphotransferases. *Biochem. Pharmacol.* 68(9): 1879-88.

Furman, P.A., Fyfe, J.A., St Clair, M.H., Weinhold, K., Rideout, J.L., Freeman, G.A., Lehrman, S.N., Bolognesi, D.P., Broder, S., Mitsuya H, et al. (1986). Phosphorylation of 3'-azido-3'-deoxythymidine and selective interaction of the 5'-triphosphate with human immunodeficiency virus reverse transcriptase. *Proc. Natl. Acad. Sci. U. S. A.* 83(21): 8333-7.

Furman, P.A., Jeffrey, J., Kiefer, L.L., Feng, J.Y., Anderson, K.S., Borroto-Esoda, K., Hill, E., Copeland, W.C., Chu, C.K., Sommadossi, J.P., Liberman, I., Schinazi, R.F. & Painter, G.R. (2001). Mechanism of action of 1-beta-D-2,6-diaminopurine dioxolane, a prodrug of the human immunodeficiency virus type 1 inhibitor 1-beta-D-dioxolane guanosine. *Antimicrob. Agents Chemother.* 45(1): 158-65.

Gallo, R.C., Salahuddin, S.Z., Popovic, M., Shearer, G.M., Kaplan, M., Haynes, B.F., Palker, T.J., Redfield, R., Oleske, J., Safai, B., et al., (1984) Frequent detection and isolation of cytopathic retroviruses (HTLV-III) from patients with AIDS and at risk for AIDS. *Science* 224, 500–503.

Ghosh M., Williams, J., Powell, M.G., Levin, J.G., & Le Grice, S.F.J. (1997) Mutating a conserved motif of the HIV-1 reverse transcriptase palm subdomain alters primer utilization. *Biochemistry* 36: 5758-5768.

Goldschmidt, V. & Marquet, R. (2004). Primer unblocking by HIV-1 reverse transcriptase and resistance to nucleoside RT inhibitors (NRTIs). *Int. J. Biochem. Cell Biol.* (9): 1687-705.

Goody, R.S., Müller, B. & Restle, T. (1991). Factors contributing to the inhibition of HIV reverse transcriptase by chain-terminating nucleotides in vitro and in vivo. *FEBS Lett.* 291(1):1-5.

Gripshover, B.M., Ribaudo, H., Santana, J., Gerber, J.G., Campbell, T.B., Hogg, E., Jarocki, B., Hammer, S.M. & Kuritzkes, D.R.; A5118 Team. (2006). Amdoxovir versus placebo with enfuvirtide plus optimized background therapy for HIV-1-infected

Gu, Z., Wainberg, M.A., Nguyen-Ba, N., L'Heureux, L., de Muys, J.M., Bowlin, T.L. & Rando, R.F. (1999) Mechanism of action and in vitro activity of 1',3'-dioxolanylpurine nucleoside analogues against sensitive and drug-resistant human immunodeficiency virus type 1 variants. *Antimicrob. Agents Chemother.* 43(10): 2376-82.

Haraguchi, K., Takeda, S., Tanaka, H., Nitanda, T., Baba, M., Dutschman, G.,E. & Cheng, Y.C. (2003). Synthesis of a highly active new anti-HIV agent 2',3'-didehydro-3'-deoxy-4'-ethynylthymidine. *Bioorg. Med. Chem. Lett.* 13(21): 3775-7.

Ho, H.,T. & Hitchcock, M.,J. (1989). Cellular pharmacology of 2',3'-dideoxy-2',3'-didehydrothymidine, a nucleoside analog active against human immunodeficiency virus. *Antimicrob. Agents Chemother.* 33(6): 844-9.

Holdich, T., Shiveley, L. & Sawyer, J. (2006). Pharmacokinetics of single oral doses of apricitabine, a novel deoxycytidine analogue reverse transcriptase inhibitor, in healthy volunteers. *Clin. Drug. Invest.* 26: 279 -86.

Holdich, T., Shiveley, L.A. & Sawyer, J. (2007). Effect of lamivudine on the plasma and intracellular pharmacokinetics of apricitabine, a novel nucleoside reverse transcriptase inhibitor, in healthy volunteers. *Antimicrob Agents Chemother.* 51: 2943 -2947.

Hostetler, K.Y., Beadle, J.R., Kini, G.D., Gardner, M.F., Wright, K.N., Wu, T.H. & Korba, B.A. (1997). Enhanced oral absorption and antiviral activity of 1-O-octadecyl-sn-glycero-3-phospho-acyclovir and related compounds in hepatitis B virus infection, in vitro. *Biochem. Pharmacol.* 53: 1815–1822.

Hsu, C.H., Hu, R., Dutschman, G.E., Yang, G., Krishnan, P., Tanaka, H., Baba, M. & Cheng, Y.C. (2007). Comparison of the phosphorylation of 4'-ethynyl 2',3'-dihydro-3'-deoxythymidine with that of other anti-human immunodeficiency virus thymidine analogs. *Antimicrob. Agents Chemother.* 51(5): 1687-93.

Johnson, M.A. & Fridland, A. (1989). Phosphorylation of 2',3'-dideoxyinosine by cytosolic 5'-nucleotidase of human lymphoid cells. *Mol. Pharmacol.* 36: 291-5.

Johnson, M.A., Moore, K.H., Yuen, G.J., Bye, A. & Pakes, G.E. (1999). Clinical pharmacokinetics of lamivudine. *Clin. Pharmacokinet.* 36(1):41-66.

Kim, H.O., Schinazi, R.F., Nampalli, S., Shanmuganathan, K., Cannon, D.L., Alves, A.J., Jeong, L.S., Beach, J.W. & Chu, C.K. (1993). 1,3-dioxolanylpurine nucleosides (2R,4R) and (2R,4S) with selective anti-HIV-1 activity in human lymphocytes. *J. Med. Chem.* 36(1): 30-37.

Lanier, E.R., Ptak, R.G., Lampert, B.M., Keilholz, L., Hartman, T., Buckheit, Jr., R.W., Mankowski, M.K., Osterling, M.C., Almond, M.R. & Painter, G.R. (2010). Development of hexadecyloxypropyl tenofovir (CMX157) for treatment of infection caused by wild-type and nucleoside/nucleotide-resistant HIV. *Antimicrob Agents Chemother.* 54(7): 2901-9.

Lee, W.A., He, G.X., Eisenberg, E., Cihlar, T., Swaminathan, S., Mulato, A. & Cundy, K.C. (2005). Selective intracellular activation of a novel prodrug of the human immunodeficiency virus reverse transcriptase inhibitor tenofovir leads to preferential distribution and accumulation in lymphatic tissue. *Antimicrob. Agents Chemother.* 49(5): 1898-906.

Markowitz, M., Zolopa, A., Ruane, P., Squires, K., Zhong, L., Kearney, B.P. & Lee, W. (2011). GS-7340 Demonstrates Greater Declines in HIV-1 RNA than Tenofovir Disoproxil Fumarate During 14 Days of Monotherapy in HIV-1 Infected Subjects. *18th Conference on Retroviruses and Opportunistic Infections* March 2, 2011 Boston, MA., Abstract # 152LB.

Masood, R.W., Ahluwalia, G.S., Cooney, D.A., Fridland, A., Marquez, V.E., Driscoll, J.S., Hao, Z., Mitsuya, H., Perno, C.F., Broder, S., et al. (1990). 2'-Fluoro-2',3'-dideoxyarabinosyladenine: a metabolically stable analogue of the antiretroviral agent 2',3'-dideoxyadenosine. *Mol. Pharmacol.* 37: 590-6.

McDowell, J.A., Lou, Y., Symonds, W.S. & Stein, D.S. (2000). Multiple-dose pharmacokinetics and pharmacodynamics of abacavir alone and in combination with zidovudine in human immunodeficiency virus-infected adults. *Antimicrob. Agents Chemother.* 44(8): 2061-7.

Meyer, P.R., Matsuura, S.E., So, A.G. & Scott, W.A. (1998). Unblocking of chain-terminated primer by HIV-1 reverse transcriptase through a nucleotide-dependent mechanism. *Proc. Natl. Acad. Sci. U.S.A.* 95(23): 13471-6.

Mitsuya, H., & Broder, S. (1986) Inhibition of the in vitro infectivity and cytopathic effect of human T-lymphotrophic virus type III/lymphadenopathy-associated virus (HTLV-III/LAV) by 2′,3′-dideoxynucleosides. *Proc. Natl. Acad. Sci. U.S. A.* 83: 1911–1915.

Mitsuya, H., Jarrett, R.F., Matsukura, M., Veronese, F.D., DeVico, A.L., Sarngadharan, M.G., Johns, D.G., Reitz, M.S., & Broder, S. (1987) Long-term inhibition of human T-lymphotropic virus type III/lymphadenopathy-associated virus (human immunodeficiency virus) DNA synthesis and RNA expression in T cells protected by 2′,3′-dideoxynucleosides in vitro. *Proc. Natl. Acad. Sci. U. S. A.* 84: 2033–2037.

Mitsuya, H., Weinhold, K.J., Furman, P.A., St Clair, M.H., Nusinoff-Lehrman, S., Gallo, R.C., Bolognesi, D., Barry, D.W., & Broder, S. (1985) 3′-azido-3′-deoxythymidine (BW A509U): an antiviral agent that inhibits the infectivity and cytopathic effect of human T-lymphotropic virus type III/lymphadenopathy-associated virus in vitro. *Proc. Natl. Acad. Sci. U. S. A.* 82: 7096–7100.

Murphy, R., Zala, C., Ochoa, C., Tharnish, P., Mathew, J., Fromentin, E., Asif, G., Hurwitz, S.J., Kivel, N.M., & Schinazi, R.F. (2008). Pharmacokinetics and potent anti-HIV-1 activity of amdoxovir plus zidovudine in a randomized double-blind placebo-controlled study. *15th Conference on Retroviruses and Opportunistic Infections.* February 3-6, 2008. Boston, MA. Abstract 794.

Naesens, L., Bischofberger, N., Augustijns, P., Annaert, P., Van den Mooter, G., Arimilli, M.N., Kim, C.U., De Clercq, E., (1998). Antiretroviral efficacy and pharmacokinetics of oral bis-(isopropyloxycarbonyloxymethyl)-9-(2-phosphonylmethoxypropyl)adenine in mice. *Antimicrob. Agents Chemother.* 42: 1568–1573.

Nakatani-Freshwater, T., Babayeva, M., Dontabhaktuni, A. & Taft, D.R. (2006). Effects of trimethoprim on the clearance of apricitabine, a deoxycytidine analog reverse transcriptase inhibitor, and lamivudine in the isolated rat perfused kidney. *J. Pharmacol. Exper. Ther.* 319: 941 -947.

Nitanda, T., Wang, X., Kumamoto, H., Haraguchi, K., Tanaka, H., Cheng, Y.C. & Baba, M. (2005). Anti-human immunodeficiency virus type 1 activity and resistance profile of 2′,3′-didehydro-3′-deoxy-4′-ethynylthymidine in vitro. *Antimicrob. Agents Chemother.* 49: 3355–3360.

Painter, G.R., Almond, M.R., Trost, L.C., Lampert, B.M., Neyts, J., De Clercq, E., Korba, B.E., Aldern, K.A., Beadle, J.R. & Hostetler, K.Y. (2007). Evaluation of hexadecyloxypropyl-9-R-[2-(phosphonomethoxy)propyl]-adenine, CMX157, as a potential treatment for human immunodeficiency virus type 1 and hepatitis B virus infections. *Antimicrob. Agents Chemother.* 51: 3505–3509.

Painter, G.R. & Hostetler, K.Y. (2004). Design and development of oral drugs for the prophylaxis and treatment of smallpox infection. *Trends Biotechnol.* 22: 423–427.

Paintsil, E., Mastuda, T., Ross, J., Schofield, J., Cheng, Y.C., Urata, Y., (2009). A Singledose escalation study to evaluate the safety, tolerability, and pharmacokinetics of OBP-601, a novel NRTI, in healthy subjects. In: *16th Conference on Retroviruses and Opportunistic Infections,* February 2009, Montreal, Canada. Abstract 568.

Peliska, J.A. & Benkovic, S.J. (1992) Mechanism of DNA strand transfer reactions catalyzed by HIV-1 reverse transcriptase. *Science* 258: 1112-1118.

Rajagopalan, P., Boudinot, F. D., Chu, C.K., McClure, H.M., & Schinazi, R.F. (1994). Pharmacokinetics of (2)-β-D-2,6-diaminopurine dioxolaneand its metabolite guanosine in rhesus monkeys. *Pharm. Res.* 11(Suppl.): 381–386.

Rajagopalan, P., Boudinot, F.D., Chu, C.K., Tennant, B.C., Baldwin, B.H. & Schinazi, R.F. (1996). Pharmacokinetics of (2)-β-D-2,6-diaminopurinedioxolane and its metabolite, dioxolane guanosine, in woodchucks (Marmotamonax). *Antivir. Chem. Chemother.* 7: 65–70.

Rana, K.Z. & Dudley, M.N. (1997). Clinical pharmacokinetics of stavudine. *Clin. Pharmacokinet.* 33:276–284.

Ray, A. S., Cihlar, T., Robinson, K. L., Tong, L., Vela, J. E., Fuller, M. D., Wieman, L. M., Eisenberg, E. J. & Rhodes, G. R. (2006). Mechanism of active renal tubular efflux of tenofovir. *Antimicrob. Agents Chemother.* 50: 3297–3304.

Robbins, B.L., Srinivas, R.V., Kim, C., Bischofberger, N., Fridland, A. (1998). Anti-human immunodeficiency virus activity and cellular metabolism of a potential prodrug of the acyclic nucleoside phosphonate 9-*R*-(2-phosphonomethoxypropyl)adenine (PMPA), bis(isopropyloxymethylcarbonyl)PMPA. *Antimicrob. Agents Chemother.* 42: 612–617.

Ruane, .P.J, Richmond, G.J., DeJesus, E., Hill-Zabala, C.E., Danehower, S.C., Liao, Q., Johnson, J. & Shaefer, M.S. (2004). Pharmacodynamic effects of zidovudine 600 mg once/day versus 300 mg twice/day in therapy-naïve patients infected with human immunodeficiency virus. *Pharmacotherapy.* 24(3): 307-12.

Sawyer, J. & Cox, S. (2006). In vitro pharmacology of Apricitabine, a new NRTI for HIV. *XVI International AIDS Conference,* August 2006, Toronto, Canada, abstract CDB0046.

Sawyer, J. & Struthers-Semple, C. (2006). Pharmacokinetics of apricitabine in healthy volunteers and HIV-infected individuals. *XVI International AIDS Conference,* August 2006, Toronto, Canada, Abstract TUPE0077.

Starnes, M.C. & Cheng, Y.C. (1987). Cellular metabolism of 2',3'-dideoxycytidine, a compound active against human immunodeficiency virus in vitro. *J Biol. Chem.* 262(3): 988-91.

Stein, D.S. & Moore, K.H. (2001). Phosphorylation of nucleoside analog antiretrovirals: a review for clinicians. *Pharmacotherapy.* (1):11-34.

Taylor, D.L., Ahmed, P.S., Tyms, A.S., Wood, L.J., Kelly, L.A., Chambers, P., Clarke, J., Bedard, J., Bowlin, T.L., Rando, R.F. (2000). Drug resistance and drug combination features of the human immunodeficiency virus inhibitor, BCH-10652 [(+/-)-2'-deoxy-3'-oxa-4'-thiocytidine, dOTC]. *Antivir. Chem. Chemother.* 11(4): 291-301.

Temin, H. & Mizutani, S. (1970) RNA-dependent DNA polymerase in virions of Rous sarcoma virus. *Nature* 226: 1211-1232.

Thompson, M.A., Kessler, H.A., Eron, J.J. Jr., Jacobson, J.M., Adda, N., Shen, G., Zong, J., Harris, J., Moxham, C. & Rousseau, F.S.; DAPD-101 Study Group. (2005). Short-term safety and pharmacodynamics of amdoxovir in HIV-infected patients. *AIDS* 19: 1607–1615.

Tippin, T.K., Lampert, B.M., Painter, G.R. & Lanier, E.R. (2010). CMX001 & CMX157 Are Not Substrates of Human Organic Anion Transporters hOAT1 and hOAT3. *FIP Pharmaceutical Sciences World Congress and AAPS Meeting* November 16, 2010 New Orleans, LA.

Weidner, D.,A. & Sommadossi, J.P. (1990). 3'-Azido-3'-deoxythymidine inhibits globin gene transcription in butyric acid-induced K-562 human leukemia cells. *Mol. Pharmacol.* 38(6): 797-804.

Yang, G., Dutschman, G.E., Wang, C.J., Tanaka, H., Baba, M., Anderson, K.S. & Cheng, Y.C. (2007). Highly selective action of triphosphate metabolite of 4'-ethynyl D4T: a novel anti-HIV compound against HIV-1 RT. *Antiviral Res.* 73: 185–191.

Zhu, Z., Ho, H.T., Hitchcock, M.J. & Sommadossi, J.P. (1990). Cellular pharmacology of 2',3'-didehydro-2',3'-dideoxythymidine (D4T) in human peripheral blood mononuclear cells. *Biochem. Pharmacol.* 39(9): R15-9.

Zimmerman, T.P., Mahony, W.B. & Prus, K.L. (1987). 3'-Azido-3'-deoxythymidine. An unusual nucleoside analogue that permeates the membrane of human erythrocytes and lymphocytes by nonfacilitated diffusion. *J. Biol. Chem.* 262: 5748-54.

4

Opioid Kappa Receptor Selective Agonist TRK-820 (Nalfurafine Hydrochloride)

Hideaki Fujii, Shigeto Hirayama and Hiroshi Nagase
School of Pharmacy, Kitasato University
Japan

1. Introduction

TRK-820 (nalfurafine hydrochloride) is a selective opioid κ receptor agonist (Fig. 1) that was launched as an antipruritic for hemodialysis patients in Japan in 2009. In general, clinically used opioids, such as morphine, exhibit potent antinociceptive effects and simultaneous severe adverse effects, including drug dependence, derived from the opioid μ receptor. To develop analgesics without drug dependence, κ receptor agonists are investigated. However, conventional κ agonists, arylacetamide derivatives, showed aversive effects like psychotomimetic effects, and have not yet been used clinically. On the other hand, the novel κ agonist TRK-820 has no dependent or aversive properties. TRK-820, which has a structure different from arylacetamides, was first developed as an analgesic for postoperative pain, but the indication was changed to pruritus (Nakao & Mochizuki, 2009; Nagase & Fujii, 2011). The rational drug design and synthesis of the compound have been reported (Kawai et al., 2008; Nagase et al., 1998; Nagase & Fujii, 2011); therefore, in this chapter, we will focus on its pharmacological properties.

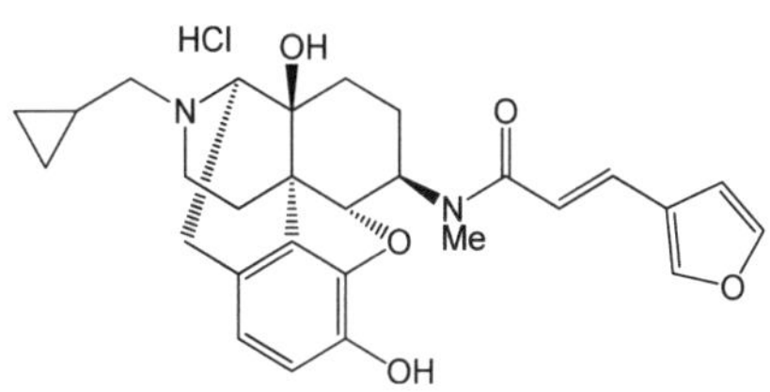

Fig. 1. Structure of nalfurafine hydrochloride (TRK-820)

2. Opioid receptor type selectivity (*In vitro*)

The binding affinities of TRK-820 were evaluated using various tritiated ligands and opioid receptors derived from various species (Table 1). The κ selectivity over the δ receptor (K_i ratio δ/κ) tended to be higher than over the μ receptor (K_i ratio μ/κ). Binding affinities for the L-type Ca^{2+} channel and 45 receptors, except the opioid receptors, were examined (Nakao & Mochizuki, 2009). Among the tested receptors, TRK-820 showed the strongest affinity for the muscarine M_1 receptor, but its K_i value was 1,700 nmol/L and approximately 7,000 times higher than that of the κ receptor. A comparison of the binding properties of TRK-820 and a conventional κ agonist, U-69,593, was noteworthy. In a competitive binding

K_i (nM)			K_i ratio		References
μ	δ	κ	μ/κ	δ/κ	
53	1200	3.5	15	343	Seki et al., 1999
5.2	161	0.075	69	2147	Wang, Y et al., 2005
0.71	49.9	0.36	2.0	139	Vanderah et al., 2008
2.21	484	0.244	9.1	1984	Nakao & Mochizuki, 2009
0.582	96.5	0.225	2.6	429	Nagase et al., 2010

Table 1. Binding affinities (K_i values) and selectivities (K_i ratios) of TRK-820 for the opioid receptors. Seki et al. used [^{3}H]bremazocine and the recombinant rat opioid receptors. Wang, Y et al. used [^{3}H]diprenorphine and recombinant rat μ, recombinant mouse δ, and recombinant human κ receptors. Vanderah et al. used [^{3}H]DAMDO, [^{3}H]*p*Cl-DPDPE, and [^{3}H]U-69,593 for the recombinant human μ, δ, and κ receptors, respectively. Nakao et al. used [^{3}H]diprenorphine and the recombinant human receptors. Nagase et al. used [^{3}H]DAMDO, [^{3}H]NTI, and [^{3}H]U-69,593 for the μ, δ, and κ receptors, respectively. Guinea pig forebrain or guinea pig cerebellum was used to assay the μ and δ receptor or κ receptor, respectively.

Assay	Selectivity		References
	μ/κ	δ/κ	
MVD	980	NC	Kawai et al., 2008
GPI	78.6	-	Kawai et al., 2008
cAMP (Sato et al.)	55	>6,667	Seki et al., 1999
cAMP (Nakao et al.)	203	2,610	Nakao & Mochizuki, 2009
[^{35}S]GTPγS	128	11,560	Wang, Y et al., 2005

Table 2. Selectivities of TRK-820 in various functional assays. Selectivity in MVD and GPI assays was obtained by *K*e ratios. The selectivity for the κ receptor over the δ receptor in the MVD assay was not calculated (NC) due to a lack of agonist activity for the δ receptor. The selectivity for the κ receptor over the δ receptor in the GPI assay was not obtained because GPI preparation contained only the μ and κ receptors. Seki et al. and Nakao et al. used the recombinant rat and human receptors in their assays, respectively. In the [^{35}S]GTPγS binding assay, recombinant rat μ, recombinant mouse δ, or recombinant human κ receptors were used.

assay using [^{3}H]TRK-820, TRK-820 completely replaced [^{3}H]TRK-820 binding, whereas U-69,593 did not replace it completely, with roughly 20% of [^{3}H]TRK-820 binding remaining. Moreover, Scatchard analysis of [^{3}H]TRK-820 and [^{3}H]U-69,593 binding using guinea pig cerebellum showed that TRK-820 had stronger binding affinity than U-69,593 (K_d values: 0.46±0.03 nM for [^{3}H]TRK-820, 1.17±0.14 nM for [^{3}H]U-69,593) and that the B_{max} value for [^{3}H]TRK-820 (284±43.3 fmol/mg protein) was significantly higher than the value for [^{3}H]U-69,593 (83.7±7.86 fmol/mg protein). Even in the presence of μ agonist DAMDO (100 nM) and δ agonist DPDPE (200 nM), the K_d and B_{max} values for [^{3}H]TRK-820 did not change (K_d = 0.51±0.03 nM, B_{max} = 265±27.2 fmol/mg protein) (Endoh et al., 2000). These results suggest that TRK-820 was selective ligand for the κ receptor and that its binding property for the κ receptor was different from that of the conventional κ agonist U-69,593. Many binding assays are carried out using [^{3}H]U-69,593 because it is commercially available. However, the binding property of TRK-820 is difficult to be definitively evaluated because [^{3}H]TRK-820 is not available now.

TRK-820 was selective for the κ receptor, but the selectivity over the μ receptor was apparently not as high in the binding assays. Contrarily TRK-820 showed more selectivities for the κ receptor in functional assays: MVD (mouse vas deference) and GPI (guinea pig ileum) assay (Nagase et al., 1998), cAPM assay (Nakao & Mochizuki, 2009; Seki et al., 1999), and [^{35}S]GTPγS binding assay (Wang, Y et al., 2005) (Table 2). The results of the cAMP assay (IC_{50} (μ) = 8.3±1.4 nM, I_{max} (μ) = 69±3%, IC_{50} (δ) > 1,000 nM, I_{max} (δ) not determined, IC_{50} (κ) = 0.15±0.07 nM, I_{max} (κ) = 81±3% by Seki et al.; IC_{50} (μ) = 1.66±0.09 nM, I_{max} (μ) = 53.2±1.3%, IC_{50} (δ) = 21.3±1.0 nM, I_{max} (δ) = 77.9±1.6%, IC_{50} (κ) = 0.00816±0.00138 nM, I_{max} (κ) = 91.3±0.5% by Nakao et al.) indicated that TRK-820 was a selective and potent full agonist for the κ receptor and partial agonist for the μ and δ receptors. The potency for the δ receptor was very low (Nakao & Mochizuki, 2009; Seki et al., 1999). The [^{35}S]GTPγS binding assay provided similar results (EC_{50} (μ) = 3.2±1.3 nM, E_{max} (μ) = 54±7%, EC_{50} (δ) = 289±60 nM, E_{max} (δ) = 51±6%, EC_{50} (κ) = 0.025±0.003 nM, E_{max} (κ) = 93±5%) (Wang, Y et al., 2005). Mizoguchi et al. exhibited partial agonist activity of TRK-820 for the μ receptor in both *in vitro* and *in vivo* assays (Mizoguchi et al., 2003). TRK-820 concentration- or dose-dependently attenuated [^{35}S]GTPγS binding by DAMGO or antinociception induced by intracerebroventricular (i.c.v.) administration of DAMGO. On the other hand, the effects of morphine alone or a mixture with TRK-820 were investigated using a mouse acetic acid-induced writhing test or warm water (50 °C) tail-withdrawal assay in rhesus monkeys (Ko & Husbands, 2009; Nagase, 2010). Isobologram analysis of the results showed that additive or synergetic effects for TRK-820 in combination with morphine in the antinociceptive effect were observed, indicating that TRK-820 had no μ antagonist activity, at least no antagonism against analgesic activity induced by morphine. Why the effects of TRK-820 against DAMGO differed from those against morphine is not clear.

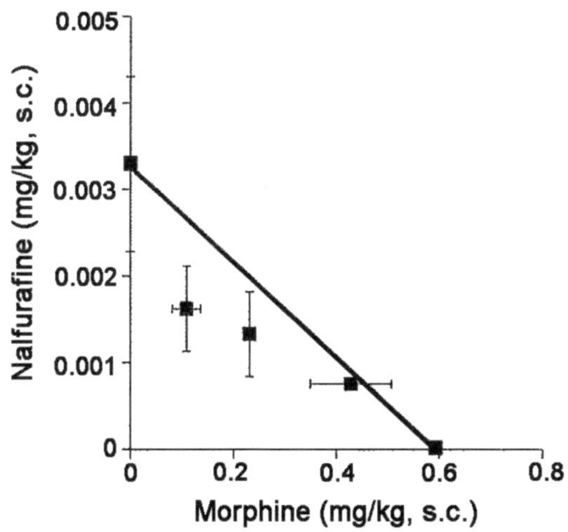

Fig. 2. Isobologram for the mixture of TRK-820- and morphine-induced antinociception in the mouse acetic acid-induced writhing test. Reprinted with permission from Nagase, 2010.

3. Analgesic effects

TRK-820 showed potent analgesic effects in some species (rodents and primates) with various stimuli: chemical, thermal, or mechanical stimuli and inflammatory, diabetic, herpetic, and postherpetic pain models. The antinociceptive effects of TRK-820 are summarized in Tables 3-7. Subcutaneous (s.c.) administration of TRK-820 produced dose-dependent and profound antinociceptive effects in the low temperature hot plate, tail flick, tail pressure, and tail pinch tests. However, TRK-820 was not as effective in high temperature hot plate tests (Table 3) (Endoh et al., 1999).

In a rat paw pressure test, TRK-820 given s.c. or intramuscularly (i.m.) induced dose-dependent and sufficient analgesic effects, which were suppressed by pre-treatment with selective κ antagonist nor-BNI (Table 3). The antinociceptive effect by TRK-820 (ED_{50} = 0.064 mg/kg, s.c.) was 170, 2, 20, and 78-fold more potent than U-50,488H, CI-977, morphine, and pentazocine, respectively (ED_{50} values : 11.0, 0.15, 1.3, and 5.0 mg/kg) (Endoh et al., 2000).

Compound	High temperture hot plate (55 °C)	Low temperature hot plate (51 °C)	Tail flick	Tail pressure	Tail pinch
TRK-820	32.0 % at 0.2	0.129	0.062	0.009	0.035
U-50,488H	63.8 % at 20	8.71	5.18	1.0	11.5
ICI-199,441	n.t.	0.065	0.042	0.024	0.051
U-69,593	n.t.	1.33	n.t.	0.48	2.8
CI-977	n.t.	n.t.	n.t.	n.t.	n.t.
PD-117302	n.t.	n.t.	n.t.	n.t.	n.t.
Pentazocine	44.6 % at 40	52.2	n.t.	n.t.	n.t.
Morphine	3.65	5.30	5.26	1.5	12.2

Compound	Paw pressure	Formalin test	Acetic acid-induced writhing test
TRK-820	0.064	0.0096	0.0033
U-50,488H	11.0	n.t.	1.16
ICI-199,441	0.074	0.0095	0.0071
CI-977	0.15	n.t.	0.0069
PD-117302	n.t.	n.t.	1.22
Pentazocine	5.0	n.t.	n.t.
Morphine	1.3	0.975	0.58

Table 3. ED_{50} values (mg/kg, s.c.) of the antinociceptive effects of some opioid agonists in various tests. U-50,488H, U-69,593, ICI-199,441, CI-977, and PD-117302 are conventional κ agonists. n.t. : not tested. Hot plate, tail flick, tail pressure, tail pinch, and acetic acid-induced writhing tests were performed in mice (Endoh et al., 1999). Paw pressure and formalin tests were performed in rats (Endoh et al., 2000).

In the formalin test, s.c. TRK-820 given 15 min prior to the formalin injection markedly inhibited the second phase of the nociceptive response induced by formalin in a dose-dependent manner. However, the analgesic effect of TRK-820 was low for the first phase of the formalin response. Similarly, a conventional κ agonist, ICI-199,441, also markedly inhibited the second phase. On the other hand, a μ agonist, morphine inhibited both phases in a dose-dependent manner. The antinociceptive potencies of TRK-820 and ICI-199,441 were almost equivalent (Table 3) (Endoh et al., 2000). A potent and dose-dependent antinociceptive effect of TRK-820 (i.m.) was also observed in cynomolgus monkeys. The analgesic effect of TRK-820 was 295 and 492-fold more potent than that of morphine in the 50 °C and 55 °C hot water tests, respectively, and 40 and 1000-fold more potent than that of U-50,488H and pentazocine in the 50 °C hot water test, respectively (Table 4) (Endoh et al., 2001).

Furthermore, the antinociceptive effects of TRK-820 administered s.c. and perorally (p.o.) were compared. The dose-dependent antinociception of TRK-820 (ED_{50} = 0.0033 mg/kg, s.c. and 0.032 mg/kg, p.o.) in the acetic acid-induced writhing test were inhibited by pre-treatment with nor-BNI. The antinociceptive effects induced by s.c. or p.o. administration of TRK-820 were 351 and 796-fold more potent than those induced by U-50,488H, respectively, and 175 and 187-fold more potent than those induced by morphine, respectively. Because the ED_{50} p.o./s.c. ratio for TRK-820 was the least among the tested compounds, TRK-820 was expected to be the most effective agent when administered p.o. (Table 5) (Endoh et al., 1999). Intravenous administration of TRK-820 was also reported to be effective in the same test (Vanderh et al., 2008).

The effect of repeated administration of some κ agonists and morphine on antinociceptive tolerance was examined by the acetic acid-induced writhing test in mice. After five

Compound	50 °C hot water	55 °C hot water
TRK-820	0.0078	0.012
Morphine	2.3	5.9
U-50,488H	0.31	n.t.
Pentazocine	> 10	n.t.

Table 4. ED_{50} values (mg/kg, i.m.) of antinociceptive effects induced by some opioid agonists in the hot water tail withdrawal test in cynomolgus monkeys. n.t. : not tested.

Compound	s.c.	p.o.	ED_{50} p.o./s.c. ratio
TRK-820	0.0033	0.032	9.7
U-50,488H	1.16	25.5	22.0
CI-977	0.0069	> 1.0	> 145
ICI-199441	0.0071	0.3	42.3
PD-117302	1.22	33.0	27.0
Morphine	0.58	6.01	10.4

Table 5. ED_{50} values (mg/kg, s.c. or p.o.) for antinociceptive effects induced by some opioid agonists in the acetic acid-induced writhing test in mice.

administrations of TRK-820 (0.1-0.8 mg/kg, s.c.), U-50,488H (10-80 mg/kg, s.c.), ICI-199,441 (0.025-0.2 mg/kg, s.c.), or morphine (1.25-10 mg/kg, s.c.) over three days, the development of tolerance to the antinociception induced by each compound at a fixed dose was assessed and tolerance ED_{50} was calculated. Comparing the ratio of tolerance ED_{50} to acute antinociceptive ED_{50} of each compound, TRK-820 was found to develop the least tolerance to antinociception (Table 6) (Suzuki et al., 2004).

An analgesic effect of TRK-820 (i.m.) was also examined using rats with arthritis induced by adjuvant. TRK-820 dose-dependently produced potent and equivalent antinociceptive activity in both arthritic and normal rats in the paw pressure test. Similar results were obtained when morphine was injected i.m. However, the analgesic effect of a conventional κ agonist, ICI-199,441, in the arthritic rats was less potent than in normal rats (Table 7) (Endoh et al., 2000).

Compound	Tolerance ED_{50}	Acute antinociceptive ED_{50}	Ratio of tolerance ED_{50}/acute antinociceptive ED_{50}
TRK-820	0.54	0.0033	163.6
U-50,488H	30.7	1.16	26.5
ICI-199,441	0.078	0.0071	11.0
Morphine	5.72	0.58	9.9

Table 6. ED_{50} values (mg/kg, s.c.) for tolerance and antinociceptive effects induced by some opioid agonists in the acetic acid-induced writhing test.

Compound	Normal rat	Arthritic rat	ED50 ratio of arthritic rat/ normal rat
TRK-820	0.055	0.095	1.7
ICI-199,441	0.047	0.24	5.1
Morphine	1.1	1.1	1.0

Table 7. ED_{50} values (mg/kg, i.m.) for antinociceptive effects induced by some opioid agonists in the paw pressure test in normal and arthritic rats.

In streptozotocin-induced diabetic mice, the antinociceptive effects induced by several κ agonists, including TRK-820, were compared in the tail flick test. Intrathecal (i.t.) and i.c.v. administration of TRK-820 produced dose-dependent antinociceptive effects in both diabetic and non-diabetic mice. However, antinociception induced by TRK-820 administered i.t. or i.c.v. in diabetic mice were less potent than antinociception in non-diabetic mice. However, the antinociceptive effects of CI-977 administered i.t., but not i.c.v., in diabetic mice were less potent than those in non-diabetic mice. On the other hand, the antinociceptive effects of ICI-199,441 and R-84760 injected i.c.v., but not i.t., in diabetic mice were less potent than those in non-diabetic mice. These results indicate that the antinociceptive effects of κ agonists in diabetic mice are altered in a region-specific manner in the central nervous system and by chemotypes of κ agonists (Ohsawa et al., 2005).

In acute herpetic and postherpetic pain models induced by herpes simplex virus type-1 infection in mice, TRK-820 dose-dependently and remarkably inhibited the allodynia and hyperalgesia stimulated by von Frey filaments (Takasaki et al., 2004, 2006). The effects of TRK-820, but not morphine, were not significantly different between herpetic and postherpetic pain (Takasaki et al., 2006). TRK-820 (0.1 mg/kg, s.c.) almost completely relieved both allodynia and hyperalgesia in herpetic pain, whereas a high dose of morphine (20 mg/kg, s.c.) did not produce complete inhibition. However, TRK-820 (0.01-0.1 mg/kg, s.c.) did not affect the spontaneous locomotor activity of normal mice (Takasaki et al., 2004). Moreover, repeated administration of TRK-820 (0.1 mg/kg, p.o., twice daily) produced constant inhibition of allodynia and hyperalgesia in herpetic pain. The effects of the fourth administration with TRK-820 were not significantly different from those of the first administration. On the other hand, the effects of morphine rapidly decreased after repeated administration (20 mg/kg, p.o., twice daily). The effects of the third and fourth administration of morphine were significantly weaker than those of the first administration. Pre-treatment with morphine (20 mg/kg, p.o., three times) did not affect the antinociceptive effect of TRK-820 (0.1 mg/kg, p.o.), whereas the effect of morphine (20 mg/kg, p.o.) was significantly reduced (Takasaki et al., 2006). These results indicate that TRK-820 is effective on both herpetic and postherpetic pain in mice. In addition, the analgesic dose of TRK-820 did not develop acute tolerance and induced cross-tolerance to morphine in herpetic pain.

4. Antipruritic effects

4.1 Preclinical studies

The p.o. administration of TRK-820 dose-dependently inhibited scratching behavior induced by histamine in mice, which is one of the representative pruritogenic substances, without obvious suppression of spontaneous locomotor activity. The antiscratching activity of TRK-820 with ED_{50} 7.3 μg/kg was antagonized by nor-BNI (Togashi et al., 2002). TRK-820 was effective in scratching induced by the other pruritogenic substances: substance P (Togashi et al., 2002; Umeuchi et al., 2003; Utsumi et al., 2004), chloroquine (Inan & Cowan, 2004), compound 48/80 (Wang, Y et al., 2005), agmatin (Inan & Cowan, 2006a), and 5'-GNTI (Inan et al., 2009a, 2011) (Table 8). 5'-GNTI-induced scratching was suppressed by both pre-treatment and post-treatment with TRK-820. Tolerance did not develop to the antiscratching effect of TRK-820 in the subchronic study (Inan et al., 2009a).

Pruritogenic substance	Antipruritic effect	References
Histamine	ED_{50} = 7.3 μg/kg, p.o.	Togashi et al., 2002
Substance P	ED_{50} = 19.6 μg/kg, p.o.	Togashi et al., 2002
Chloroquine	TRK-820 (120 μg/kg, p.o.) suppressed the scratching almost completely	Inan & Cowan, 2004
Compound 48/80	ED_{50} = 6.64 μg/kg, s.c.	Wang, Y et al., 2005
Agmatin	TRK-820 (0.02 mg/kg, s.c.) was effective	Inan & Cowan, 2006a
5'-GNTI	TRK-820 (20 μg/kg, s.c.) suppressed the scratching almost completely	Inan et al., 2009a

Table 8. The antipruritic effects of TRK-820 against itching behaviors induced by various pruritogenic substances.

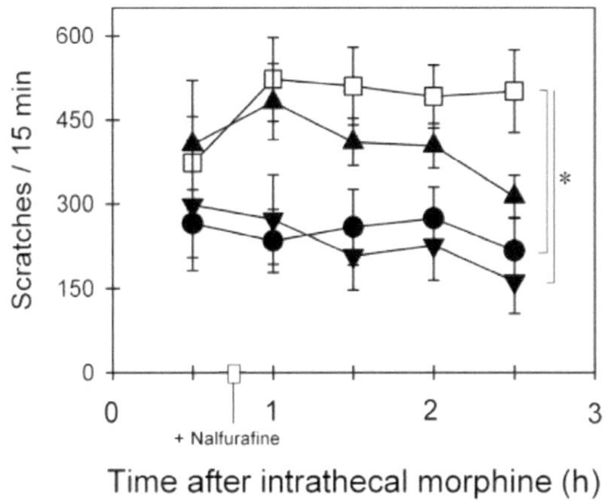

Fig. 3. Effects of TRK-820 on scratching induced by i.t. administration of morphine in rhesus monkeys. TRK-820 (0 (□), 0.1 (▲), 0.3 (•), and 1 (▼) μg/kg, i.m.) was given 45 min after the administration of morphine (0.03 mg, i.t.). * $p < 0.05$ between vehicle and time points 1 and 2.5 h. Reprinted with permission from Ko & Husbands, 2009.

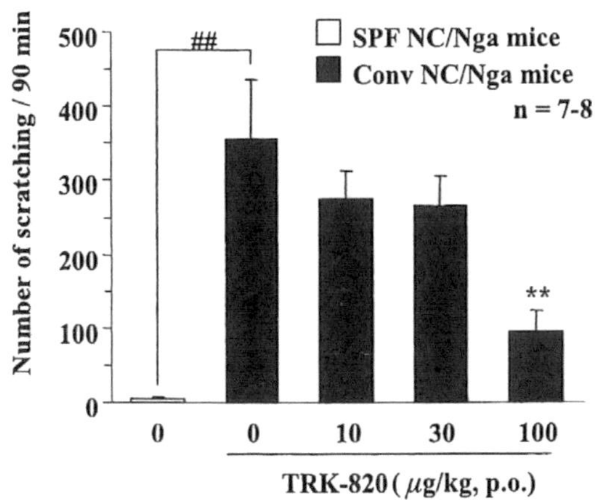

Fig. 4. Effects of TRK-820 on scratching behaviors observed in NC/Nag mice maintained in a conventional environment. $^{##}p < 0.01$, Welch test. $^{**}p < 0.01$ compared to NC/Nag mice not treated with TRK-820, parametric Dunnett multiple comparison test. Reprinted with permission from Nakao et al., 2008.

Although epidural or i.t. administration of a μ agonist like morphine is an important method for pain management, an itching sensation is the most common side effect (Ballantyne et al., 1988; Cousins & Mather, 1984). The effect of TRK-820 on morphine-induced scratching in mice or primates was also evaluated (Ko & Husbands, 2009; Utsumi et al., 2004; Wakasa et al., 2004). Intramuscular administration of TRK-820 (0.3–1 μg/kg) dose-dependently attenuated scratching induced by morphine (i.t.) in rhesus monkeys without affecting antinociception by morphine (Fig. 3) (Ko & Husbands, 2009).

TRK-820 reportedly exhibited antipruritic effects on spontaneous scratching behavior in aged MRL/*lpr* mice (a possible model for pruritus in autoimmune disease) (Umeuchi et al.,

2005) or NC/Nag mice maintained in a conventional environment (an animal model for atopic dermatitis) (Nakao et al., 2008), and scratching behavior secondary to cholestasis induced chronic ethynylestradiol injections in rats (Inan & Cowan, 2006b). Interestingly, TRK-820 was effective in scratching behaviors observed in conventional NC/Nag mice, which were considered a model of atopic dermatitis (Fig. 4).

4.2 Clinical studies

Wikström et al. (2005) and Kumagai et al. (2010) reported the results of randomized, double-blind, placebo-controlled clinical studies in which TRK-820 was administered to patients undergoing hemodialysis intravenously or orally (Fig. 5). In these studies, TRK-820 exhibited significant antipruritic effects without severe adverse drug reactions. These outcomes suggest that TRK-820 can be considered a safe agent.

TRK-820 is prescribed in Japan as an antipruritic for hemodialysis. Very recently, Kumagai et al. reported that TRK-820 has been prescribed for approximately 18,000 hemodialysis patients and effective in 70 to 80% (Kumagai et al., 2011).

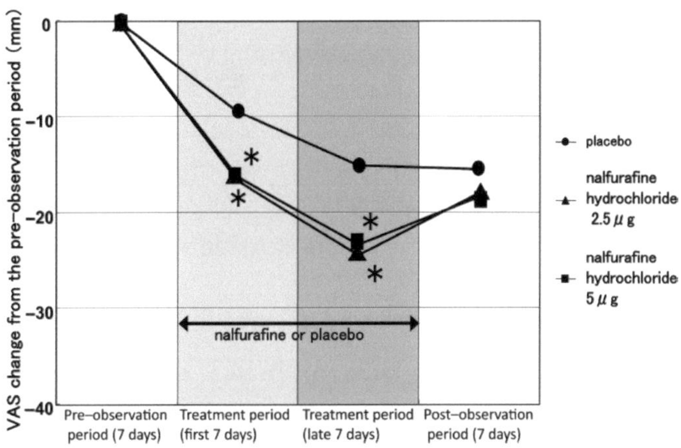

Fig. 5. Changes in VAS (visual analogue scale) values from the pre-observation period. All symbols show the mean values of VAS changes. *$p < 0.025$ compared to placebo, one-sided ANCOVA. Reprinted from Nagase & Fujii, 2011 with permission from Springer Science+Business Media. The VAS test consisted of a 100-mm horizontal line without scale markings. The patients were asked to mark the intensity of itching on the scale, with the right end of the line (100 mm) indicating the strongest possible itching and the left end (0 mm) indicating no itching.

5. Effects of TRK-820 on drug dependence

5.1 Effects of TRK-820 in the conditioned place preference (CPP) test

The μ agonists have a rewarding effect, which accounts for the abuse of morphine by humans. In animal models, the rewarding effects of μ agonists have been evaluated by the conditioned place preference (CPP) and self-administration paradigms (Di Chiara & North, 1992). In contrast to μ agonists, conventional κ agonists such as U-50,488H and U-69,593 generally lack a rewarding effect (Dykstra et al., 1997). However in the CPP test, animals avoid an environment associated with the administration of the κ agonists, indicating that these drugs have aversive effects (Barr et al., 1994; Funada et al., 1993). In contrast to conventional κ agonists, such as U-50,488H, TRK-820 (3.0-30 μg/kg, s.c.) did not induce significant place aversion in mice at doses producing significant antinociception (Fig. 6) (Nagase, 2010). Notably, TRK-820 exhibited neither preferential nor aversive properties. Recently, the peroral administration of TRK-820 (5.0 μg/day) was reported to show no signs of psychological or physical dependence in an open-labeled clinical trial for one year (Nagase & Fujii, 2011).

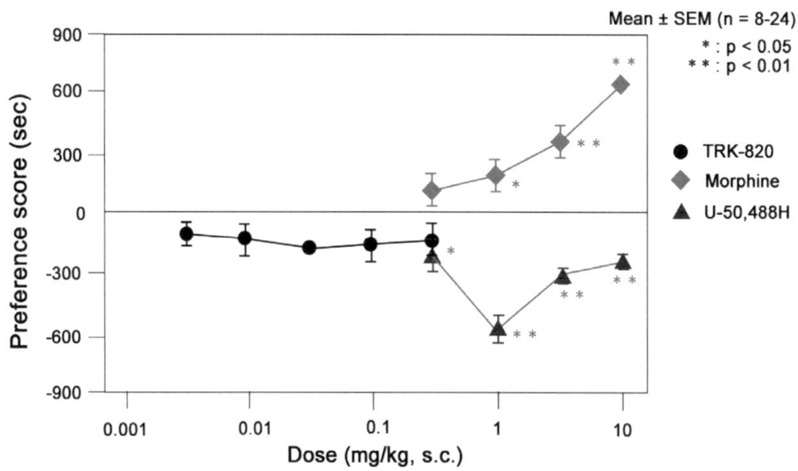

Fig. 6. The effect of TRK-820 in the CPP test. Reprinted with permission from Nagase, 2010.

5.2 The effects of TRK-820 on morphine and cocaine-induced rewarding effects

The mechanism of μ agonist-induced rewarding effects is outlined below. The activation of the μ receptor on γ-aminobutyric acid-containing interneurons is likely to disinhibit ventrotegmental area dopaminergic neurons, thereby increasing dopamine release in their terminal areas, including the nucleus accumbens (N.Acc). On the other hand, the activation of the κ receptor decreases dopamine release in the N.Acc (Di Chiara & Imperato, 1988; Spanagel et al., 1992). Therefore, κ agonists may be useful for treating morphine dependence. Indeed, the pretreatment with U-50,488H attenuated the morphine-induced place preference in mice (Funada et al., 1993). TRK-820 also significantly suppressed the place preference produced by morphine, and the effect of TRK-820 was antagonized by pre-treatment with nor-BNI (3.0 mg/kg, s.c.) in mice (Tsuji et al., 2001). In addition, TRK-820 was effective in reducing the rewarding effect produced by cocaine. TRK-820 (20 and 40 μg/kg, i.p.), at doses producing no aversive or sedative effects, suppressed the rewarding effect of cocaine (4.0 mg/kg, i.p.) in rats (Mori et al., 2002). U-50,488H and U-69,593 exhibited similar effects as TRK-820 (Shippenberg et al., 1996; Suzuki et al., 1992). Drug discrimination procedures provide relevant information about neuropharmacological mechanisms underlying the subjective effects of abused drugs, including cocaine, methamphetamine, and opioids, in animals. Therefore, the procedures are potentially useful for identifying candidate therapeutics for the management of drug abuse (Schuster & Johanson, 1988). Pre-treatment with TRK-820 (10 and 20 μg/kg, s.c.) significantly shifted the dose-response curve for cocaine (10 mg/kg, i.p.) to the right without changing the response rate. This attenuating effect of TRK-820 was completely reversed by pre-treatment with nor-BNI (10 mg/kg, s.c.) (Mori et al., 2002).

5.3 Effects of TRK-820 on the morphine withdrawal response

In humans, withdrawal from the chronic administration of opioids such as morphine results in characteristic behaviors, including anxiety, nausea, insomnia, hot and cold flashes, muscle aches, perspiration, and diarrhea. Such symptoms would pose clinical problems in patients receiving long-term treatment with opioids for pain relief. Rodents that are physically dependent on morphine elicit characteristic signs (jumping, wet dog shakes, rearing, diarrhea, ptosis, and forepaw tremor) when administrated naloxone. The withdrawal signs precipitated by naloxone are used as an index of the physical dependence on morphine. The effects of κ agonists TRK-820 and U-50,488H on the development of physical dependence on morphine were reported. Co-injection of TRK-820 (0.003-0.03 mg/kg, s.c.) during chronic morphine treatment dose-dependently suppressed naloxone-precipitated body weight loss, and the other withdrawal signs in morphine-dependent mice treated with TRK-820 (0.03 mg/kg, s.c.) were significantly fewer than those in untreated mice. In contrast to TRK-820, co-injection of U-50,488H (1.0-10 mg/kg, s.c.) did not inhibit naloxone-precipitated body weight loss and other withdrawal signs (Tsuji et al., 2000).

5.4 The effect of TRK-820 on the nicotine-withdrawal response

Nicotine withdrawal produces characteristic syndromes, including irritability, anxiety, depression, and craving for nicotine. Pre-treatment with TRK-820 (10 and 30 μg/kg, s.c.) or U-50,488H (0.01-1.0 mg/kg, s.c.) has been reported to decrease dose-dependently mecamylamine-precipitated nicotine-withdrawal aversion in nicotine-dependent rats (Ise et al., 2002).

6. Comparison of pharmacological properties between TRK-820 and conventional κ agonists

We described in the previous sections some pharmacological properties of TRK-820 that are different from conventional κ agonists, arylacetamides such as U-50,488H and U-69,593: binding properties (section 2) and exhibition of no preferential and no aversive effect in the CPP paradigm (section 5). As described below, drug discrimination procedures indicate conclusive difference between TRK-820 and arylacetamides.

6.1 Discriminative tests

Drug discrimination procedures have shown that the properties of TRK-820 differ from those of conventional κ agonists, such as U-50,488H. In the cross-substitution tests using rats, U-50,488H (1.0-3.0 mg/kg) substituted for the discriminative stimulus effects of TRK-820 (40 μg/kg, i.p.), whereas TRK-820 (10-76 μg/kg) did not completely substitute for those of U-50,488H (3.0 mg/kg, i.p.). E-2078 (0.3-3.0 mg/kg), but not R-84760 (0.01-0.3 mg/kg), substituted for the discriminative stimulus effects of both TRK-820 and U-50,488H. KT-90 (0.03-3.0 mg/kg), CI-977 (1-30 mg/kg), or ICI-199441 (3.0-56 mg/kg) substituted for the discriminative stimulus effects of U-50,488H, but not for those of TRK-820 (Mori et al., 2004).

In this study, cross-substitution between the discriminative effects of U-50,488H and TRK-820 was not observed. The κ agonists tested in this study, except E-2078, tended to substitute for the discriminative stimulus effects of U-50,488H rather than those of TRK-820. These results suggest that U-50,488H and TRK-820 have differential properties. Furthermore, non-competitive NMDA antagonists phencyclidine (PCP, 0.5-2.0 mg/kg) and MK-801 (10-80 μg/kg) dose-dependently generalized to the discriminative stimulus effects of U-50,488H (3.0 mg/kg, i.p.) in the cross-substitution tests. On the other hand, PCP and MK-801 at doses that generalized to the discriminative stimulus effects of U-50,488H did not generalize to those of TRK-820 (40 μg/kg, i.p.) (Mori et al., 2006). The outcomes clearly indicate different properties between TRK-820 and U-50,488H.

7. Other pharmacological effects

7.1 The effect of TRK-820 on a rat model of schizophrenia

The effects of TRK-820 on hyperlocomotion and stereotyped behaviors (head-weaving, sniffing, and turning) induced by PCP were evaluated. These behaviors are thought to resemble the schizophrenia-like effects in humans. TRK-820 (10–100 μg/kg, s.c.) dose-dependently inhibited PCP (10 mg/kg, i.p.)-induced hyperlocomotion, and this effect was antagonized with nor-BNI (20 mg/kg, s.c.). PCP-induced stereotyped behaviors were also inhibited by treatment with TRK-820 in a dose-dependent manner. These findings that TRK-820 potentially ameliorates abnormal behaviors induced by PCP suggest its therapeutic potential against the symptoms of schizophrenia (Yoshikawa et al., 2009).

7.2 The effect of TRK-820 on dyskinesia symptoms in a parkinsonian rat model

The effects of TRK-820 on rotational behavior were investigated in unilateral 6-hydroxydopamine (6-OHDA)-treated rats (hemi-parkinsonian rats), and on dyskinesia produced by administering L-DOPA to hemi-parkinsonian rats for 3 weeks (dyskinesia rats). TRK-820 significantly ameliorated abnormal behavior in hemi-parkinsonian rats at 30 μg/kg (s.c.), and L-DOPA induced dyskinesia at 10 and 30 μg/kg (s.c.). This effect was antagonized by pretreatment with nor-BNI (20 mg/kg, s.c.). Additionally, co-administration of TRK-820 (3 and 10 μg/kg, s.c.) with L-DOPA for 3 weeks suppressed the development of L-DOPA-induced dyskinesia. TRK-820 may be a suitable drug for the treatment of parkinsonian patients with dyskinesia symptoms (Ikeda et al., 2009).

7.3 The diuretic effect of TRK-820 in rats

Diuresis is a well-recognized effect of conventional κ agonists in animals and humans. A diuretic effect of TRK-820 in rats has also been reported. TRK-820 (0.005-0.02 mg/kg, s.c.) dose-dependently induced a diuretic effect without developing tolerance, and this effect was inhibited by selective κ antagonist 5′-GNTI (Inan et al., 2009b).

7.4 The effects of TRK-820 on endothelial cell differentiation and development of vasculature

The roles of the opioid κ system in vascular development were investigated (Yamamizu et al., 2011). U-50,488H and TRK-820 significantly inhibited endothelial cell differentiation and vascular formation through the inhibition of cAMP/PKA signaling.

8. Conclusion

TRK-820 was a selective κ agonist. However, its pharmacological properties were different from those of conventional arylacetamide κ agonists, including U-50,488H. A noteworthy feature of TRK-820 was that it showed no preferential or aversive properties, whereas U-50,488H produced aversion. This disparity of properties between TRK-820 and arylacetamide κ agonists was reported to stem from the difference in κ receptor subtypes each compound interacted with: arylacetamide κ agonists would interact with κ_1 receptor subtype, whereas TRK-820 may interact with another κ receptor subtype (perhaps κ_3) (Endoh et al., 1999; 2000; 2001; Tsuji et al., 2000a; 2000b). Although opioid receptors have been classified historically into three types (μ, δ, and κ types) and further divided into several subtypes from the pharmacological viewpoint (Dhawan et al., 1996), only the three major types have been cloned (Satoh & Minami, 1995). Much evidence has been compiled indicating that various receptors, including opioid receptors, exist as homo- or hetero dimers of the receptors (George et al., 2000, 2002; Gomes et al., 2000, 2004; Devi, 2001; Levac et al., 2002; Wang, D et al., 2005), and receptor dimerization has been invoked to explain the discrepancy between widely varied pharmacologies and the identification of only three opioid receptor types. Therefore, the disparity of properties between TRK-820 and arylacetamide κ agonists may stem from the difference in receptor dimers each compound interacts with. Both TRK-820 and arylacetamide κ agonists are expected to be useful tools for the investigation of receptor dimerization and/or κ receptor subtype. As mentioned in section 2, a binding assay using [^{3}H]TRK-820 and [^{3}H]U-69,593 is thought to be a facile and useful method for achieving that purpose. However, [^{3}H]TRK-820 is not currently available.

In addition to antipruritic and antinociceptive effects, TRK-820 exhibited various pharmacological effects, such as the treatment of the symptoms of schizophrenia or dyskinesia symptoms of parkisonian patients, or remedy for drug addiction. Moreover, TRK-820 has been already launched in Japan. TRK-820 is expected not only to be developed with the other indication, such as symptoms of schizophrenia or parkinson's disease, but also to be utilized to investigate pharmacology *via* the κ receptor.

9. References

Ballantyne, J.C.; Loach, A. B. & Carr, D. B. (1988). Itching after epidural and spinal opiates, *Pain*, 33, 2, 149-160, ISSN 0304-3959.

Barr, G. A.; Wang, S.; Carden, S. (1994). Aversive properties of the *κ* opioid agonist U50,488 in the week-old rat pup, *Psychopharmacology*, 113, 3-4, 422-428, ISSN 0033-3158.

Cousins, M.J. & Mather, L.E. (1984). Intrathecal and Epidural Administration of Opioids, *Anesthesiology*, 61, 3, 276-310, ISSN 0003-3022.

Devi, L. A. (2001). Heterodimerization of G-protein-coupled receptors: pharmacology, signaling and trafficking, *Trends Pharmacol. Sci.*, 22, 10, 532-537, ISSN 0165-6147.

Dhawan, B. N.; Cesselin, F.; Raghubir, R.; Reisine, T.; Bradley, P. B.; Portoghese, P. S. & Hamon, M. (1996). International Union of Pharmacology. XII. Classification of Opioid Receptors, *Pharmacol. Rev.*, 48, 4, 567-592, ISSN 0031-6997.

Di Chiara, G.; Imperato, A. (1988). Drugs abused by humans preferentially increase synaptic dopamine concentrations in the mesolimbic system of freely moving rats, *Proc. Natl. Acad. Sci. U. S. A.*, 85, 14, 5274-5278, ISSN 0027-8424.

Di Chiara, G.; North, R. A. (1992). Neurobiology of opiate abuse, *Trends Pharmacol. Sci.*, 13, 5, 185-193, ISSN 0165-6147.

Dykstra, L. A.; Preston, K. L.; Bigelow, G. E. (1997). Discriminative stimulus and subjective effects of opioids with *mu* and *kappa* activity: data from laboratory animals and human subjects, *Psychopharmacology*, 130, 1, 14-27, ISSN 0033-3158.

Endoh, T.; Matsuura, H.; Tajima, A.; Izumimoto, N.; Tajima, C.; Suzuki, T.; Saitoh, A.; Suzuki, T.; Narita, M.; Tseng, L. & Nagase, H. (1999). POTENT ANTINOCICEPTIVE EFFECTS OF TRK-820, A NOVEL κ-OPIOID RECEPTOR AGONIST, *Life Sci.*, 65, 16, 1685-1694, ISSN 0024-3205.

Endoh, T.; Tajima, A.; Suzuki, T.; Kamei, J.; Suzuki, T.; Narita, M.; Tseng, L. & Nagase, H. (2000). Characterization of the antinociceptive effects of TRK-820 in the rat, *Eur. J. Pharmacol.*, 387, 2, 133-140. ISSN 0014-2999.

Endoh, T.; Tajima, A.; Izumimoto, N.; Suzuki, T.; Saitoh, A.; Suzuki, T.; Narita, M.; Kamei, J.; Tseng, L. F.; Mizoguchi, H.; Nagase, H. (2001). TRK-820, a Selective κ-Opioid Agonist, Produces Potent Antinociception in Cynomolgus Monkeys, *Jpn. J. Pharmacol.*, 85, 3, 282-290, ISSN 0021-5198.

Funada, M.; Suzuki, T.; Narita, M.; Misawa, M.; Nagase, H. (1993). Blockade of morphine reward through the activation of κ-opioid receptors in mice, *Neuropharmacology*, 32, 12, 1315-1323, ISSN 0028-3908.

George, S. R.; Fan, T.; Xie, Z.; Tse, R.; Tam, V.; Varghese, G. & O'Dowd, B. F. (2000). Oligomerization of μ- and δ-Opioid Receptors. GENERATION OF NOVEL FUNCTIONAL PROPERTIES, *J. Biol. Chem.*, 275, 34, 26128-26135, ISSN 0021-9258.

George, S. R.; O'Dowd, B. F. & Lee, S. P. (2002). G-protein-coupled receptor oligomerization and its potential for drug discovery, *Nat. Rev. Drug Discov.*, 1, 10, 808-820, ISSN 1474-1776.

Gomes, I.; Jordan, B. A.; Gupta, A.; Trapaidze, N.; Nagy, V. & Devi, L. A. (2000). Heterodimerization of μ and δ Opioid Receptors: A Role in Opiate Synergy, *J. Neurosci.*, 20, 22, RC110, ISSN 0270-6474.

Gomes, I.; Gupta, A.; Filipovska, J.; Szeto, H. H.; Pintar, J.E. & Devi, L. A. (2004). A role for heterodimerization of μ and δ opiate receptors in enhancing morphine analgesia, *Proc. Nat. Acad. U.S.A.*, 101, 14, 5135-5139 ISSN 0027-8424.

Ikeda, K.; Yoshikawa, S.; Kurokawa, T.; Yuzawa, N.; Nakao, K.; Mochizuki, H. (2009). TRK-820, a selective kappa opioid receptor agonist, could effectively ameliorate L-DOPA-induced dyskinesia symptoms in a rat model of Parkinson's disease, *Eur. J. Pharmacol.*, 620, 1-3, 42-48, ISSN 0014-2999.

Inan, S. & Cowan, A. (2004). Kappa opioid agonists suppress chloroquine-induced scratching in mice, *Eur. J. Pharmacol.*, 502, 3, 233-237. ISSN 0014-2999.

Inan, S. & Cowan, A. (2006a). AGMATINE-INDUCED STEREOTYPED SCRATCHING IN MICE IS ANTAGONIZED BY NALFURAFINE, A KAPPA OPIOID AGONIST, *Pharmacologist*, 48, 1, 38, ISSN 0031-7004.

Inan, S. & Cowan, A. (2006b). Nalfurafine, a kappa opioid receptor agonist, inhibits scratching behavior secondary to cholestasis induced by chronic ethynylestradiol injections in rats, *Pharmacol. Biochem. Behav.*, 85, 1, 39-43. ISSN 0091-3057.

Inan, S.; Dun, N. J. & Cowan, A. (2009a). NALFURAFINE PREVENTS 5'-GUANIDINONALTRINDOLE- AND COMPOUND 48/80-INDUCED SPINAL c-fos EXPRESSION AND ATTENUATES 5'-GUANIDINONALTRINDOLE-

ELICITED SCRATCHING BEHAVIOR IN MICE, *Neuroscience*, 163, 1, 23-33, ISSN 0306-4522.

Inan, S.; Lee, D. Y. -W; Liu-Chen, L. Y.; Cowan, A. (2009b). Comparison of the diuretic effects of chemically diverse kappa opioid agonists in rats: nalfurafine, U50,488H, and salvinorin A, *Naunyn Schmiedebergs Arch. Pharmacol.*, 379, 3, 263-270, ISSN 0028-1298.

Inan, S.; Dun, N. J. & Cowan, A. (2011). Investigation of gastrin-releasing peptide as a mediator for 5'-guanidinonaltrindole-induced compulsive scratching in mice, *Peptides*, 32, 2, 286-292, ISSN 0196-9781.

Ise, Y.; Narita, M.; Nagase, H.; Suzuki, T. (2002). Modulation of κ-opioidergic systems on mecamylamine-precipitated nicotine-withdrawal aversion in rats, *Neurosci. Lett.*, 323, 2, 164-166, ISSN 0304-3940.

Kawai, K.; Hayakawa, J.; Miyamoto, T.; Imamura, Y.; Yamane, S.; Wakita, H.; Fujii, H.; Kawamura, K.; Matsuura, H.; Izumimoto, N.; Kobayashi, R.; Endo, T. & Nagase, H. (2008). Design, synthesis, and structure–activity relationship of novel opioid κ-agonists, *Bioorg. Med. Chem.*, 16, 20, 9188-9201. ISSN 0968-0896.

Ko, M. -C. & Husbands, S. M. (2009). Effects of Atypical *κ*-Opioid Receptor Agonists on Intrathecal Morphine-Induced Itch and Analgesia in Primates, *J. Pharmacol. Exp. Ther.*, 328, 1, 193-200. ISSN 0022-3565.

Kumagai, H.; Ebata, T.; Takamori, K.; Muramatsu, T.; Nakamoto, H. & Suzuki, H. (2010). Effect of a novel kappa-receptor agonist, nalfurafine hydrochloride, on severe itch in 337 haemodialysis patients: a Phase III, randomized, double-blind, placebo-controlled study, *Nephrol. Dial. Transplant.*, 25, 4, 1251-1257, ISSN 0931-0509.

Kumagai, H.; Yamamoto, K.; Kushiyama, T.; Higashi, Y.; Takechi, H. & Suzuki, H. (2011). A novel *κ*-receptor agonist, nalfurafine, for severe itch in hemodialysis patients, *Kidney and Dialysis*, 70, 4, 651-657, ISSN 0385-2156.

Levac, B. A. R.; O'Dowd, B. F. & George, S. R. (2002). Oligomerization of opioid receptors: generation of novel signaling units, *Curr. Opin. Pharmacol.*, 2, 1, 76-81, ISSN 1471-4892.

Mori, T.; Nomura, M.; Nagase, H.; Narita, M.; Suzuki, T. (2002). Effects of a newly synthesized κ-opioid receptor agonist, TRK-820, on the discriminative stimulus and rewarding effects of cocaine in rats, *Psychopharmacology*, 161, 1, 17-22, ISSN 0033-3158.

Mori, T.; Nomura, M.; Yoshizawa, K.; Nagase, H.; Narita, M.; Suzuki, T. (2004). Differential properties between TRK-820 and U-50,488H on the discriminative stimulus effects in rats, *Life Sci.*, 75, 20, 2473-2482, ISSN 0024-3205.

Mori, T.; Nomura, M.; Yoshizawa, K.; Nagase, H.; Sawaguchi, T.; Narita, M.; Suzuki, T. (2006). Generalization of NMDA-Receptor Antagonists to the Discriminative Stimulus Effects of *κ*-Opioid Receptor Agonists U-50,488H, but Not TRK-820 in Rats, *J. Pharmacol. Sci.*, 100, 2, 157-161, ISSN 1347-8613.

Nagase, H.; Hayakawa, J.; Kawamura, K.; Kawai, K.; Takezawa, Y.; Matsuura, H.; Tajima, C. & Endo, T. (1998). DISCOVERY OF A STRUCTURALLY NOVEL OPIOID κ-AGONIST DERIVED FROM 4,5-EPOXYMORPHINAN, *Chem. Pharm. Bull.*, 46, 2, 366-369. ISSN 0009-2363.

Nagase, H. (2010). Design and Synthesis of a Novel Antipruritic Drug, Nalfurafine Hydrochloride and Its Pharmacological Feature, *Jpn. J. Pharm. Palliat. Care Sci.* 3, 4, 115-122. ISSN 1882-9783.

Nagase, H.; Watanabe, A.; Nemoto, T.; Yamaotsu, N.; Hayashida, K.; Nakajima, M.; Hasebe, K.; Nakao, K.; Mochizuki, H.; Hirono, S. & Fujii, H. (2010). Drug design and synthesis of a novel κ opioid receptor agonist with an oxabicyclo[2.2.2]octane skeleton and its pharmacology, *Bioorg. Med. Chem. Lett.* 20, 1, 121-124. ISSN 0960-894X.

Nagase, H. & Fujii, H. (2011). Opioids in Preclinical and Clinical Trials, In: *Chemistry of Opioid,* Nagase, H. (Ed.), 29-62, Springer, ISBN 978-3-642-18106-1, Heidelberg.

Nakao, K.; Ikeda, K.; Kurokawa, T.; Togashi, Y.; Umeuchi, H.; Honda, T.; Okano, K. & Mochizuki, H. (2008). Effect of TRK-820, a selective κ opioid receptor agonist, on scratching behavior in an animal model of atopic dermatitis, *Jpn. J. Neuropsychopharmacol.*, 28, 2, 75-83, ISSN 1340-2544.

Nakao, K. & Mochizuki, H. (2009). NALFURAFINE HYDROCHLORIDE: A NEW DRUG FOR THE TREATMENT OF UREMIC PRURITUS IN HEMODIALYSIS PATIENTS, *Drugs Today* 45, 5, 323-329. ISSN 1699-3993.

Ohsawa, M.; Kamei, J. (2005). Modification of *κ*-Opioid Receptor Agonist-Induced Antinociception by Diabetes in the Mouse Brain and Spinal Cord, *J. Pharmacol. Sci.*, 98, 1, 25-32, ISSN 1347-8613.

Satoh, M. & Minami, M. (1995). MOLECULAR PHARMACOLOGY OF THE OPIOID RECEPTORS, *Pharmacol. Ther.*, 68, 3, 343-364, ISSN 0163-7258.

Schuster, C. R.; Johanson, C. E. (1988). Relationship between the discriminative stimulus properties and subjective effects of drugs, *Psychopharmacol. Ser.* 4, 161–175, ISBN 0931-6795.

Seki, T.; Awamura, S.; Kimura, C.; Ide, S.; Sakano, K.; Minami, M.; Nagase, H. & Satoh, M. (1999). Pharmacological properties of TRK-820 on cloned μ-, δ- and κ-opioid receptors and nociceptin receptor, *Eur. J. Pharmacol.* 376, 1-2, 159-167. ISSN 0014-2999.

Shippenberg, T. S.; LeFevour, A.; Heidbreder, C. (1996). *κ*-Opioid Rreceptor Agonists Prevent Sensitization to the Conditioned Rewarding Effects of Cocaine, *J. Pharmacol. Exp. Ther.*, 276, 2, 545-554, ISSN 0022-3565.

Spanagel, R.; Herz, A.; Shippenberg, T. S. (1992). Opposing tonically active endogenous opioid systems modulate the mesolimbic dopaminergic pathway, *Proc. Natl. Acad. Sci. U. S. A.*, 89, 6, 2046-2050, ISSN 0027-8424.

Suzuki, T.; Shiozaki, Y.; Masukawa, Y.; Misawa, M.; Nagase, H. (1992). The Role of Mu- and Kappa-Opioid Receptors in Cocaine-Induced Conditioned Place Preference, *Jpn. J. Pharmacol.*, 58, 4, 435-442, ISSN 0021-5198.

Suzuki, T.; Izumimoto, N.; Takezawa, Y.; Fujimura, M.; Togashi, Y.; Nagase, H.; Tanaka, T.; Endoh, T. (2004). Effect of repeated administration of TRK-820, a κ-opioid receptor agonist, on tolerance to its antinociceptive and sedative actions, *Brain Res.*, 995, 2, 167-175, ISSN 0006-8993.

Takasaki, I.; Suzuki, T.; Sasaki, A.; Nakao, K.; Hirakata, M.; Okano, K.; Tanaka, T.; Nagase, H.; Shiraki, K.; Nojima, H.; Kuraishi, Y. (2004). Suppression of Acute Herpetic Pain Related Responses by the *κ*-Opioid Receptor Agonist (-)-17- Cyclopropylmethyl-3,14β-dihydroxy-4,5α-epoxy-6β-[N-methyl-3-trans-3-(3-furyl)Acrylamido]

Morphinan Hydrochloride (TRK-820) in Mice, *J. Pharmacol. Exp. Ther.*, 309, 1, 36-41, ISSN 0022-3565.

Takasaki, I.; Nojima, H.; Shiraki, K.; Kuraishi, Y. (2006). Specific down-regulation of spinal μ-opioid receptor and reduced analgesic effects of morphine in mice with postherpetic pain, *Eur. J. Pharmacol.*, 550, 1-3, 62-67, ISSN 0014-2999.

Togashi, Y.; Umeuchi, H.; Okano, K.; Ando, N.; Yoshizawa, Y.; Honda, T.; Kawamura, K.; Endoh, T.; Utsumi, J.; Kamei, J.; Tanaka, T. & Nagase, H. (2002). Antipruritic activity of the κ-opioid receptor agonist, TRK-820, *Eur. J. Pharmacol.*, 435, 2-3, 259-264. ISSN 0014-2999.

Tsuji, M.; Yamazaki, M.; Takeda, H.; Matsumiya, T.; Nagase, H.; Tseng, L. F.; Narita, M. & Suzuki, T. (2000a). The novel κ-opioid receptor agonist TRK-820 has no affect on the development of antinociceptive tolerance to morphine in mice, *Eur. J. Pharmacol.*, 394, 1, 91-95. ISSN 0014-2999.

Tsuji, M.; Takeda, H.; Matsumiya, T.; Nagase, H.; Yamazaki, M.; Narita, M. & Suzuki, T. (2000b). A NOVEL κ-OPIOID RECEPTOR AGONIST, TRK-820, BLOCKS THE DEVELOPMENT OF PHYSICAL DEPENDENCE ON MORPHINE IN MICE, *Life Sci.*, 66, 25, PL353-358, ISSN 0024-3205.

Tsuji, M.; Takeda, H.; Matsumiya, T.; Nagase, H.; Narita, M.; Suzuki, T. (2001). The novel κ-opioid receptor agonist TRK-820 suppresses the rewarding and locomotor-enhancing effects of morphine in mice, *Life Sci.*, 68, 15, 1717-1725, ISSN 0024-3205.

Umeuchi, H.; Togashi, Y.; Honda, T.; Nakao, K.; Okano, K.; Tanaka, T. & Nagase, H. (2003). Involvement of central μ-opioid system in the scratching behavior in mice, and the suppression of it by the activation of κ-opioid system, *Eur. J. Pharmacol.*, 477, 1, 29-35. ISSN 0014-2999.

Umeuchi, H.; Kawashima, Y.; Aoki, C. A.; Kurokawa, T.; Nakao, K.; Itoh, M.; Kikuchi, K.; Kato, T.; Okano, K.; Gershwin, M. E. & Miyakawa, H. (2005). Spontaneous scratching behavior in MRL/*lpr* mice, a possible model for pruritus in autoimmune diseases, and antipruritic activity of a novel κ-opioid receptor agonist nalfurafine hydrochloride, *Eur. J. Pharmacol.*, 518, 2-3, 133-139. ISSN 0014-2999.

Utsumi, J.; Togashi, Y.; Umeuchi, H.; Okano, K.; Tanaka, T. & Nagase, H. (2004). Antipruritic Activity of a Novel κ-Opioid Receptor Agonist, TRK-820, In: *Itch: Basic Mechanisms and Therapy* Yosipovitch, G.; Greaves, M. W.; Fleischer A. B. Jr.; McGlone, F. (Ed.) 107-114. ISBN 0-8247-4747-X.

Vanderah, T. W.; Largent-Milnes, T.; Lai, J.; Porreca, F.; Houghten, R. A.; Menzaghi, F.; Wisniewski, K.; Stalewski, J.; Sueiras-Diaz, J.; Galyean, R.; Schteingart, C.; Junien, J. -L.; Trojnar, J.; Riviere, P. J. -M.(2008). Novel D-amino acid tetrapeptides produce potent antinociception by selectively acting at peripheral κ-opioid receptors, *Eur. J. Pharmacol.*, 583, 1, 62-72, ISSN 0014-2999.

Wakasa, Y.; Fujiwara, A.; Umeuchi, H.; Endoh, T.; Okano, K.; Tanaka, T. & Nagase, H. (2004). Inhibitory effects of TRK-820 on systemic skin scratching induced by morphine in rhesus monkeys, *Life Sci.*, 75, 24, 2947-2957, ISSN 0024-3205.

Wang, D.; Sun, X.; Bohn, L. M. & Sadée, W. (2005). Opioid Receptor Homo- and Heterodimerization in Living Cells by Quantitative Bioluminescence Resonance Energy Transfer, *Mol. Pharmacol.*, 67, 6, 2173-2184, ISSN 0026-895X.

Wang, Y.; Tang, K.; Inan, S.; Siebert, D.; Holzgrabe, U.; Lee, D. Y. W.; Huang, P.; Li, J. -G.; Cowan, A. & Liu-Chen, L. -Y. (2005). Comparison of Pharmacological Activities of

Three Distinct κ Ligands (Salvinorin A, TRK-820 and 3FLB) on κ Opioid Receptors in Vitro and Their Antipruritic and Antinociceptive Activities in Vivo, *J. Pharmacol. Exp. Ther.*, 312, 1, 220-230. ISSN 0022-3565.

Wikström, B.; Gellert, R.; Ladefoged, S. D.; Danda, Y.; Akai, M.; Ide, K.; Ogasawara, M.; Kawashima, Y.; Ueno, K.; Mori, A. & Ueno, Y. (2005). κ-Opioid System in Uremic Pruritus: Multicenter, Randomized, Double-Blind, Placebo-Controlled Clinical Studies, *J. Am. Soc. Nephrol.*, 16, 12, 3742-3747, ISSN 1046-6673.

Yamamizu, K.; Furuta, S.; Katayama, S.; Narita, M.; Kuzumaki, N.; Imai, S.; Nagase, H.; Suzuki, T.; Narita, M.; Yamashita, J. K. (2011). The κ opioid system regulates endothelial cell differentiation and pathfinding in vascular development, *Blood,* 118, 3, 775-785, ISSN 0006-4971.

Yoshikawa, S.; Hareyama, N.; Ikeda, K.; Kurokawa, T.; Nakajima, M.; Nakao, K.; Mochizuki, H.; Ichinose, H. (2009). Effects of TRK-820, a selective kappa opioid receptor agonist, on rat schizophrenia models, *Eur. J. Pharmacol.*, 606, 1-3, 102-108, ISSN 0014-2999.

5

The Cannabinoid 1 Receptor and Progenitor Cells in the Adult Central Nervous System

Alexandra Sideris[1], Thomas Blanck[2] and Esperanza Recio-Pinto[3]
[1]*Department of Anesthesiology,*
[2]*Department of Anesthesiology, Department of Physiology and Neuroscience*
[3]*Department of Anesthesiology; Department of Pharmacology*
New York University Langone Medical Center, New York
USA

1. Introduction

The aims of this chapter are to: (1) examine the key developments leading up to the discovery the cannabinoid 1 receptor (CB1R) and (2) assess the potential therapeutic benefits of cannabinoid drugs with respect to neurogenesis in the adult brain and spinal cord. As one of the most abundant G-protein coupled receptors found in the central nervous system, localization of CB1R and its role in the mature and in the developing brain will be discussed. Pharmacological studies with cannabinergic drugs, and studies utilizing knock-out mice of various endocannabinoid system components will be reviewed in the context of adult brain neurogenesis. The apparent conflicting data reveal the complexity of endocannabinoid signaling in this process. Though many studies have focused on CB1R and neurogenesis in the brain, none have evaluated the potential ability for CB1R to modulate the fate, and specifically neuronal differentiation, of adult spinal cord progenitors. The implications for CB1R modulation of adult neurogenesis are pivotal for understanding the behavioral and cognitive effects of chronic marijuana use, but also for assessing the potential consequences of pharmacotherapeutics with CB1R agonists or antagonists

2. Discovery of an endogenous cannabinoid system

The history leading up to the discovery of the "endocannabinoid (eCB) system" is an interesting one, sprouting from a decades- long quest for the active constituents of the marijuana plant, *Cannabis sativa*. Though the cannabis plant has long been used for a variety of purposes dating back more than 4000 years (O'Shaughnessy 1842; Mechoulam and Hanus 2000), only recently was it found that delta 9- tetrahydrocannabinol (Δ^9-THC) was the ingredient responsible for the psychotropic effects associated and exploited with its use (Mechoulam and Gaoni 1965).

One of the original and most ancient uses of the *Cannabis sativa* plant was to induce a trance-like state, often an essential component to the elaborate religious rites in ancient cultures ranging from the Chinese, to the Ayurvedic Indians, to the Persians and Greeks (O'Shaughnessy 1842; Aldrich 2006). Herodotus referred to the use of the hemp plant by the

Scythians as incense in funeral rites, and also described the use of the hemp plant by the Phoenicians to make 'cordage' for building bridges (Herodotus 1824). The plant was extensively cultivated for its fiber which was used to make fabric for ship sails and clothing, but was also used for food, cooking oil, as a lubricant, and as an analgesic (Grinspoon 1993).

The earliest work to find the active ingredient began in the late 19th century after reports from Dr. O'Shaugnessy during his travels in India. In the true spirit of a responsible clinical researcher, before testing on humans, Dr. O'Shaugnessy described the use of hemp on various animals, a practice not standard for physicians at his time. Based on his findings, he believed that certain patients could benefit from the use of cannabis extracts (O'Shaughnessy 1842). His case studies described the use of the drug in humans for rheumatism, hydrophobia, cholera, tetanus, and infantile convulsions. He cautioned, however, of the "delirium occasioned by continued Hemp inebriation," which continues to be a great -but not insurmountable- obstacle for modern pharmacologists synthesizing drugs targeting the endocannabinoid system. He detailed the effects of cannabis preparations for a variety of ailments in a lecture given to the Medical College of Calcutta in 1839. Based on his work, a renewed interest in active cannabis extracts led to scientific inquiry in Europe and the United States, but an active component was not isolated mostly due to lack of effective techniques available at the time. It was not until 1965 that the major psychoactive constituent Δ^9-THC by Mechoulam's group (Mechoulam and Gaoni 1965). By the 1970s, many phytocannabinoids were characterized, and it was determined that they were lipid derivatives. Because of the lipophilic nature of these compounds, their mechanism of action was thought to be mediated by their ability to adhere to cellular membranes, much like the proposed mechanism of anesthetic action (Paton 1975). The isolation of Δ^9-THC was a key breakthrough in the discovery of an endogenous cannabinoid system because it allowed for the unexpected identification of a highly specific binding site in the body (Devane, Dysarz et al. 1988). This binding site was isolated and cloned in 1990, from both rat and human tissues (Matsuda, Lolait et al. 1990; Gerard, Mollereau et al. 1991) and was named the cannabinoid 1 receptor (CB1R).

Since it did not seem logical that the body would invest energy in the synthesis of receptors that specifically bind the constituents of this one plant, scientists began looking for compounds produced by the body that could also bind to CB1R. Binding studies with known neurotransmitters and hormones proved to be unfruitful, indicating that a unique ligand was utilizing this newly discovered CB1R. By using a highly specific probe for CB1R labeled with tritium (Devane, Breuer et al. 1992), competitive binding studies in pig brain fractions indicated the presence of endogenous compounds with cannabimimetic activity. Chromatography, nuclear magnetic resonance and mass spectrometry were used to identify arachidonoylethanolamide (Devane, Hanus et al. 1992). An amide group in this newly discovered compound and the historically acknowledged effect of cannabis use, led to the witty alternate name for the very first endocannabinoid 'anandamide', deriving from the Sanskrit word for 'bliss' (Devane, Hanus et al. 1992; Mechoulam 2000). Not only did anandamide work like Δ^9-THC in binding assays, it also mimicked its effects on motor functions, sedation and pain relief (Mechoulam 2000).

In 1993, shortly after the discovery of anandamide, another cannabinoid receptor was found and cloned from the periphery (rat spleen), and identified mostly on immune cells (Munro, Thomas et al. 1993). It was referred to as the CB2 receptor (CB2R). Two groups, made the separate discovery of another endocannabinoid, 2-arachidonoyl glycerol (2-AG), that was capable of binding to both the original CB1R, and to this novel CB2R receptor [(Mechoulam, Ben-Shabat et al. 1995; Sugiura, Kondo et al. 1995) and see **Figure 1** for a timeline].

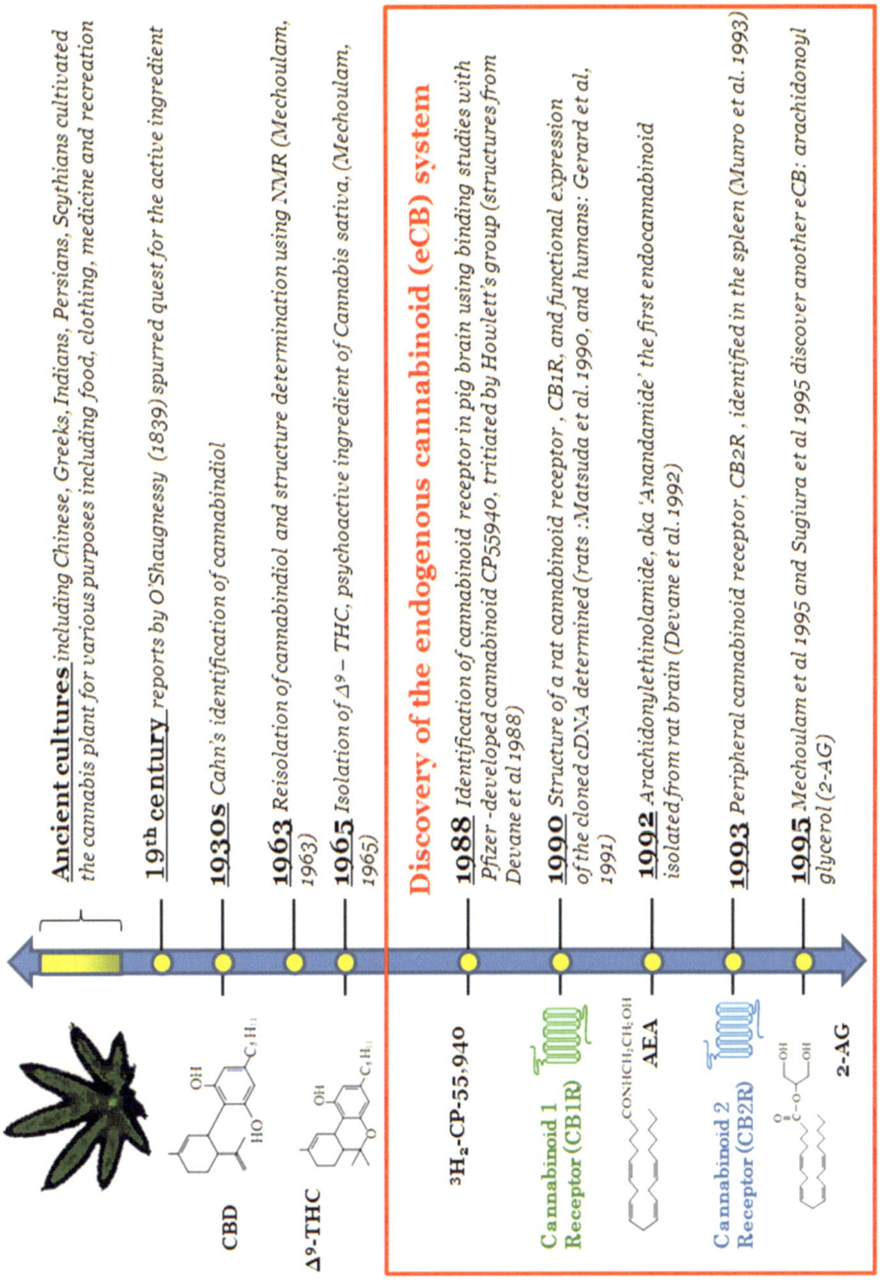

Fig. 1. **A Historical timeline of the eCB system.** Illustrated above are the major developments leading up to the discovery of an endogenous cannabinoid system, with the pivotal discoveries of the cannabinoid receptors, CB1R and CB2R, and the ligands AEA & 2-AG. Partly summarized from (Mechoulam and Hanus 2000). Receptors made with motifolio.com©.

By the end of the 20th century, the basic components of the endocannabinoid system- the receptors, endogenous ligands, and the enzymes responsible for their synthesis and degradation- were identified, paving the way for the groundbreaking discoveries that continually emerge, bringing forth the often surprising and unexpected ways in which this system works in the body.

3. CB1R localization in the central nervous system

With the discovery of the endocannabinoid system came the natural question as to what exactly these ligands and receptors are doing in the body. The location and density of CB1R could not only help explain some of the effects of cannabis use, but also has suggested the potential role of the endocannabinoids in learning, memory, motor function, emesis, reward behaviors and pain.

CB1R is a G-protein coupled receptor encoded by a single gene located on chromosome 4 in the mouse, 5 in the rat and 6 in humans. The mouse and rat display 95% nucleic acid homology, and 99.5% amino acid homology, while the mouse and human display 90% nucleic acid homology, and 97% amino acid homology (Onaivi, Leonard et al. 2002).

This receptor has been identified in both cortical and subcortical areas, the olfactory bulb, the retina, periaqueductal gray area, the cerebellum and the spinal cord (Mackie 2005). Original autoradiography studies revealed that the substantia nigra contains the highest density of CB1R in the central nervous system (CNS) (Herkenham, Lynn et al. 1991). The substantia nigra is a structure in the midbrain that plays an important role in movement, reward and addiction. CB1R is localized to the GABAergic (GABA = Gamma-aminobutyric acid) axons that project to the substantia nigra from the putamen. CB1R is also found in the caudate putamen, and on axons of medium spiny neurons projecting into the globus pallidus, on excitatory glutamatergic axons projecting from the sub-thalamic nucleus into the substantia nigra (Mailleux, Verslijpe et al. 1992; Sanudo-Pena, Tsou et al. 1997; Mackie 2005).

Much attention has been paid to the hippocampus and CB1R expression mainly because of the striking effects of marijuana on cognitive processes like memory. CB1R is widely distributed in the hippocampal structures. For example, high amounts of the receptor are found in the molecular and granule cell layer of the dentate gyrus (Mackie 2005), in the perisomatic region of CA1 indicative of expression that is post-synpaptic to basket cells, and may also be found on glutamatergic terminals of the perforant path (Kirby, Hampson et al. 1995). In the frontal cortex, double-immunocytochemical labeling experiments revealed GABAergic cholecystokinin (CCK) positive interneurons have somatic immunoreactivity for CB1R (Katona, Sperlagh et al. 1999; Tsou, Mackie et al. 1999). In terms of the laminar distribution within the neocortex high expression is found in layer II, upper III, layer IV and VI. Also it was found that the majority of cells in the neocortex which express the CB1R also express GAD65 (glutamic acid decarboxylase), the enzyme which converts L-glutamate to GABA, thus identifying inhibitory neurons in the CNS. In the cerebellum, there is a very high expression of CB1R in the molecular layer where the Purkinje neuron- parallel fiber synapse is found. Also, electrophysiological experiments infer that there are somatic CB1Rs on basket cells within the cerebellum. Therefore, there is strong evidence to suggest the presence of CB1R on GABAergic and glutamatergic neurons within the cerebellum (Mackie 2005).

Since it is believed that cannabis can be habit forming, evidence suggests that the brain area that processes addictive and reinforcing behaviors, the ventral tegmental area (VTA), contain GABAergic and glutamatergic terminals that express CB1R (Melis, Pistis et al. 2004). A potential, but yet unsubstantiated, role of CB1R in this area may be to facilitate other addictive behaviors such as alcoholism or illicit drug use (Mackie 2005). Cannabis and cannabinoid compounds have also been used as anti-emetics (Darmani 2001). Studies have illustrated that indeed the brain area responsible for emesis, the medullary nuclei of the brainstem (i.e. area postrema) contain high levels of the CB1R predominantly located on axon terminals. It is strongly believed that this anti-emesis may be attributed to CB1R activation in this area (Van Sickle, Oland et al. 2001; Van Sickle, Oland et al. 2003; Martin and Wiley 2004; Mackie 2005).

In the spinal cord, several studies have been published demonstrating that CB1R is found throughout the gray matter, but at higher densities in the dorsal areas relative to the ventral areas (Herkenham, Lynn et al. 1991; Tsou, Brown et al. 1998; Ong and Mackie 1999; Farquhar-Smith, Egertova et al. 2000; Mackie 2005; Hegyi, Kis et al. 2009). Many of our essential functions depend on an intact and healthy spinal cord, such as sensation (modulated primarily by the dorsal spinal cord) and locomotion (modulated primarily by the ventral spinal cord). This is evident particularly is diseases of the spinal cord or after traumatic injury, in which the most severe cases render the individual incapable of feeling or moving, or even death. At the spinal cord level, endocannabinoid tone and receptor expression appear to play a role in modulating movement (El Manira, Kyriakatos et al. 2008; El Manira and Kyriakatos 2010), but also nociception (Pernia-Andrade, Kato et al. 2009). Therefore, understanding the role of the eCB system in the adult spinal cord is clinically relevant, and deserves as much attention as other areas of the CNS.

Though strong evidence exists for neuronal CB1R expression, evidence also exists for its expression on astrocytes in the rat striatum (Rodriguez, Mackie et al. 2001), hippocampus (Navarrete and Araque 2008), and spinal cord (Salio, Doly et al. 2002). In addition, microglia derived from neonatal rat brains, were also found to be immunoreactive for CB1R (Waksman, Olson et al. 1999). RIP-positive or APC-positive oligodendrocytes in healthy adult rat brains and spinal cords, respectively, constitutively express CB1R (Molina-Holgado, Vela et al. 2002).

4. Role of CB1R activation in adult neurons

CB1R is included among the most abundant receptors in the brain, with picomolar ranges per milligram of tissue (as determined from rat brain (Herkenham, Lynn et al. 1991; Pazos, Nunez et al. 2005). Interestingly, compared to the abundance of CB1R, under physiological conditions, the amounts of eCBs (AEA and 2-AG) reach only into the low femtomolar range (Bisogno, Berrendero et al. 1999; Pazos, Nunez et al. 2005). This discrepancy - higher amounts of receptor and lower amounts of endogenous ligands- can be reconciled by understanding the function of the endocannabinoid system as an elegant and efficient negative feedback mechanism to control the levels of neurotransmitters released into the synaptic cleft.

Neurotransmitters are synthesized in the pre-synaptic neuron, and stored in vesicles ready to be released into the synaptic cleft after depolarization leads to an influx of calcium through voltage-dependent calcium channels. In contrast, eCBs are synthesized on demand in the post-synaptic neuron using lipid precursors from cell membranes (Di Marzo, Bifulco et al. 2004) - **Figure 2**.

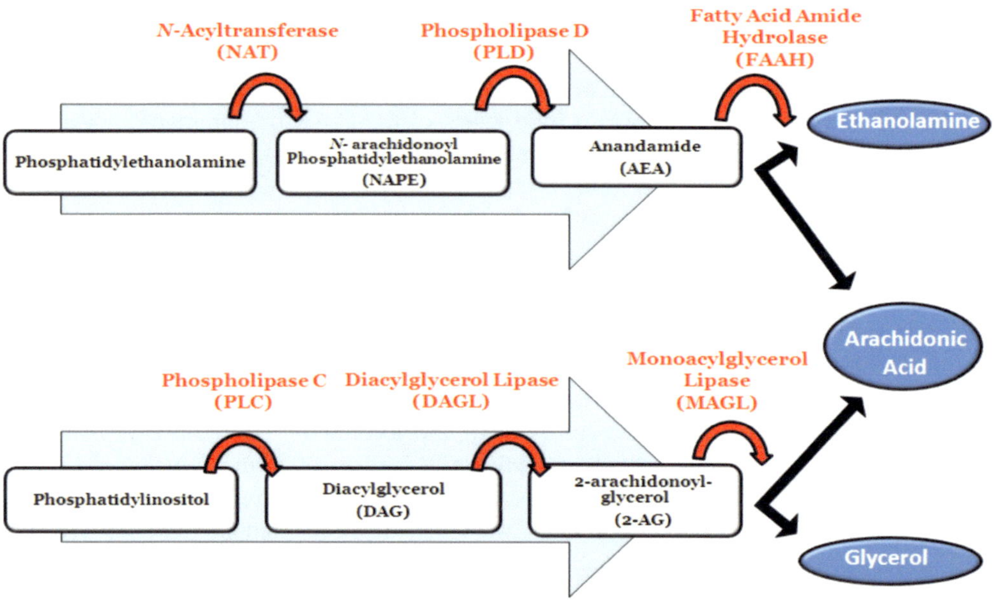

Fig. 2. The enzymes responsible for the synthesis and degradation of the two major eCBs, AEA and 2-AG. They are made on-demand from membrane lipid precursors in the post-synaptic neuron. The endocannabinoid membrane transporter (EMT) facilitates their re-uptake into either the post-synaptic (2-AG) or pre-synaptic (AEA) neuron for degradation by MAGL, or FAAH, respectively (Di Marzo, Bifulco et al. 2004; El Manira and Kyriakatos 2010)

Endocannabinoids readily pass through the post-synaptic membrane, travel retrogradely into the synaptic cleft, and bind to pre-synaptically located CB1Rs (Wilson and Nicoll 2002). As a G-protein coupled receptor, activation of CB1R by the endocannabinoids results in various cellular consequences, two of which are the ability to inhibit voltage-dependent calcium channels, or activate inwardly rectifying potassium channels. These processes affect the pre-synaptic neuron by ultimately decreasing the probability of neurotransmitter release (**Figure 3**).

The magnitude and duration of CB1R activation affects the machinery responsible for the release of several neurotransmitters such as glutamate, GABA, glycine, acetylcholine, noradrenaline and serotonin (Szabo and Schlicker 2005). Therefore, within a neuronal circuit, cells are able to regulate the strength of their synaptic inputs by on-demand release of eCBs which can then bind to CB1R (Freund, Katona et al. 2003). The high abundance of CB1Rs coupled with the relatively low-levels of detectable eCBs can be attributed to the fact that released ligand does not accumulate, but rather acts rapidly and transiently to mediate synaptic plasticity (Pazos, Nunez et al. 2005). In order to achieve such a highly efficient modulation of activity without accumulation of ligand, there must be a high density of receptors. This is precisely the state of the endocannabinoid system under physiological conditions.

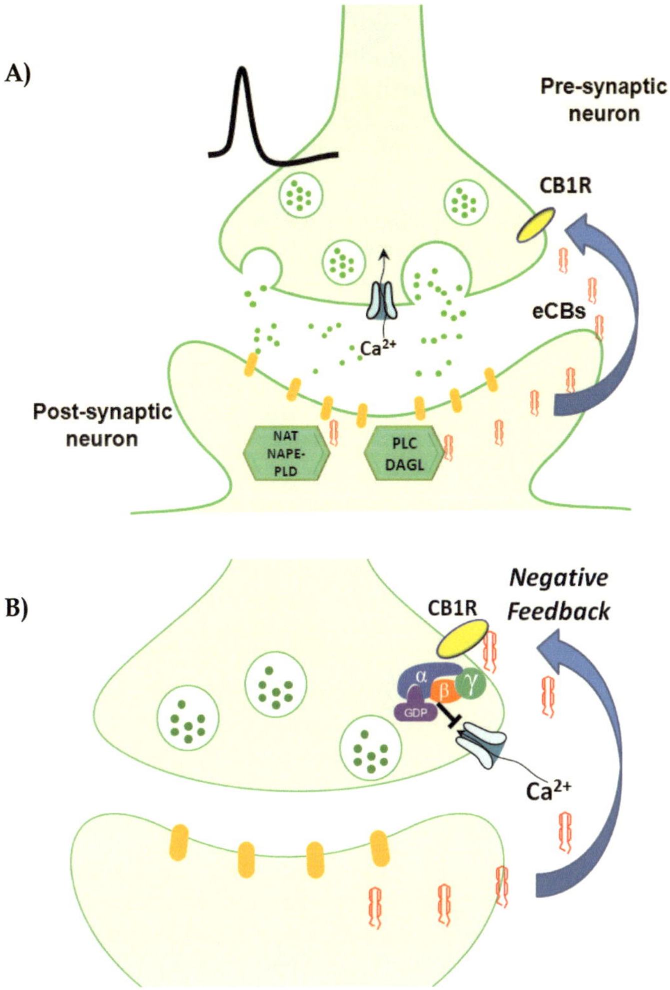

Fig. 3. **Endocannabinoids act as retrograde messengers in the CNS. (A)** Neurotransmitters bind to their postsynaptic receptors causing the synthesis of AEA or 2-AG via their synthetic enzymes, NAT/NAPE-PLD and PLC DAGL, respectively, before traveling retrogradely to bind to CB1Rs. **(B)** Inhibition of voltage-dependent calcium channels is one way by which neurotransmitter release probability is decreased. Binding of ligand to CB1R can result in the inactivation of N and P/Q- type, but not L-type calcium (Ca^{2+}) channels (Caulfield and Brown 1992; Mackie and Hille 1992; Mackie, Devane et al. 1993; Pertwee 1997). The particular channel involved is related to the brain region: in rat striatum, CB1Rs modulate N-type Ca^{2+} channels (Huang, Lo et al. 2001; Schlicker and Kathmann 2001) and not L, P or Q-type Ca^{2+} channels. In cultured rat hippocampal neurons, the CB1R modulates N- and Q-, but not P-type calcium channels (Sullivan 1999; Schlicker and Kathmann 2001). However, CB1R does not modulate any of the voltage- dependent Ca^{2+} channels found in the nucleus accumbens (Robbe, Alonso et al. 2001; Schlicker and Kathmann 2001). In contrast, newer evidence suggests that CB1R activation modulates all of the voltage-dependent Ca^{2+} channels found at the granule cell-Purkinje cell synapse of the cerebellum: the N-, P/Q- and R-type Ca^{2+} channels (Brown, Safo et al. 2004).

Furthermore, CB1R activation causes cAMP levels to drop because CB1R is negatively coupled to adenylate cyclase (AC) through heterotrimeric $G_{i/o}$ proteins, (Matsuda, Lolait et al. 1990; Munro, Thomas et al. 1993; Guzman, Sanchez et al. 2002). CB1R activation is also associated with activation of extracellular signal-related kinase (ERK) (Bouaboula, Poinot-Chazel et al. 1995; Wartmann, Campbell et al. 1995) c-Jun N-terminal kinase (Jnk) p38 mitogen activated-protein kinase (p38) (Rueda, Navarro et al. 2002), protein kinase B (Gomez del Pulgar, Velasco et al. 2000), and increased levels of the second messenger ceramide (Sanchez, Galve-Roperh et al. 1998; Guzman, Sanchez et al. 2002) (**Figure 4**). These pathways have been shown to modulate various cellular functions including cell fate, apoptosis and survival in different cell types (Guzman, Sanchez et al. 2001).

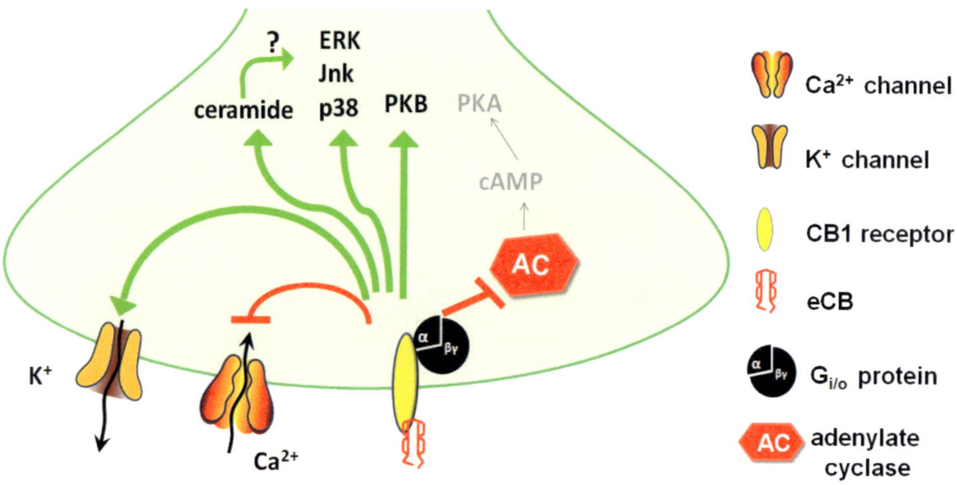

Fig. 4. **The effects of pre-synaptic CB1 receptor activation**. CB1R activation on pre-synaptic neurons inhibits voltage dependent calcium channels, and adenylate cyclase, but can also activate inwardly rectifying potassium channels, and the MAPK pathway. (Image adapted from DiMarzo et al. 2004, and Guzman et al. 2002. and created with motifolio.com©)

5. Role of cannabinoid receptors during pathological states

Because of the ubiquitous expression of the receptor throughout the CNS, several pre-clinical and clinical studies have addressed the potential therapeutic value in modulating the endocannabinoid system for analgesia, weight loss, appetite stimulation, neuroprotection after ischemic injuries, and for anti-emetic, anti-epileptic and anti-spasmodic purposes (Nogueiras, Diaz-Arteaga et al. 2009; Bisogno and Di Marzo 2010; Karst, Wippermann et al. 2010; Scotter, Abood et al. 2010). The premise of many of these therapeutic approaches lies in the neuromodulatory function of CB1R, or in the anti-inflammatory effects on CB2R activation.

During disease or following injury, cannabinoid receptor expression and levels of eCBs are altered. For example, after rat spinal cord injury, cannabinoid receptor expression is altered at the spinal level, but also in brain areas: in the spinal cord, CB1R becomes expressed in reactive astrocytes, and CB2R becomes strongly upregulated in microglia, astrocytes and macrophages. In the brain, CB1R is upregulated in thalamic and hippocampal areas, while downregulated in the amygdala and Periaqueductal Gray Area (Garcia-Ovejero, Arevalo-Martin et al. 2009; Knerlich-Lukoschus, Noack et al. 2011). In healthy spinal cords, several studies indicate that there are very low levels of CB2R, but peripheral nerve injury, for example, leads to significant upregulation of this receptor, corresponding to significant microglial activation in the spinal cord (Zhang, Hoffert et al. 2003; Romero-Sandoval, Nutile-McMenemy et al. 2008). Microglial cells contribute to the inflammatory response by producing and secreting the pro-inflammatory cytokines that contribute to excitotoxic damage in the CNS, but also to the differentiation of pathogenic lymphocytes entering the CNS (Arevalo-Martin, Garcia-Ovejero et al. 2008). Activation of CB2R in cultured microglial cells inhibits these inflammatory cytokines, making CB2R activation an anti-inflammatory target. However, the potential role of CB2R in microglial cells following injury is not clear. Cultured rat microglial cells can produce the eCBs 2-AG and AEA, which in turn auto-stimulate their CB2Rs to induce proliferation (Carrier, Kearn et al. 2004).

Whether these changes reflect an adaptive defense mechanism or contribute to pathology is still a matter of debate. These studies implicate CB1R and CB2R as double edged swords for CNS insult, and whether their activation promotes protection or contributes to damage likely depends on the etiology and progression of the disease or injury, but also in the localization of each receptor on specific cell types.

6. Adult CNS progenitor cells and CB1R

Progenitor cells in the adult CNS are promising targets as endogenous repair mechanisms following insult, and their proliferation and differentiation may provide an avenue to do so. The functional significance of constitutive or pathologically-induced neurogenesis in the adult brain has been associated with wide ranging processes such as memory formation and consolidation, depression, anxiety, and seizure- like activity (Ming and Song 2011). Endocannabinoid system elements have recently been discovered in adult brain progenitor cells (Aguado, Monory et al. 2005; Aguado, Palazuelos et al. 2006; Palazuelos, Aguado et al. 2006). There is an emerging and critical role for the eCB system and specifically, CB1R in adult brain progenitor cells, revealing a novel strategy to help the brain repair itself (Galve-Roperh, Aguado et al. 2007).

In the adult brain, the subgranular zone (SGZ) of the hippocampus, and the subventricular zone (SVZ) contain two different populations of progenitor cells. The first population is referred to as the type 1 or type B cells (SGZ and SVZ, respectively). These cells resemble their developmental counterparts, the radial glia. They are characterized by their slow proliferation kinetics, their morphological hallmarks (tiny processes extending from their somata in the SVZ), and these cells express both Nestin and Glial Fibrillary Acidic Protein (GFAP). The type 2 or C cells (SGZ and SVZ, respectively) are actively dividing, non-radial cells that maintain their Nestin expression, but do not express GFAP. They are occasionally positive for the immature neuronal marker Doublecortin (DCX). Ablation studies indicate that these two different populations are distinct in their characteristics, but they are developmentally connected to one another. The type 1, B cells give rise to the type 2, C cells, and if the latter are destroyed, they can eventually be replenished by the former (Suh, Deng et al. 2009). These progenitor cells give birth to new neurons continually throughout adulthood, in a process known as adult neurogenesis.

It is imperative to distinguish these progenitor populations when assessing the role of the various eCB components in the neurogenic process. This distinction is rarely made in the literature, and yet it is very plausible that the various eCB system components affect these progenitor populations differently. The results from the following studies indicate that the distinct processes involved in adult brain neurogenesis cannot be grouped together with regards to endocannabinoid modulation.

The role of the eCB system, and in particular CB1R, on adult brain neurogenesis is not clear, partly because the separation between effects on progenitor proliferation and neuronal differentiation have not always been made. A study published in 2004 concluded that that there is defective neurogenesis in the CB1R knockout (KO) mouse (Jin, Xie et al. 2004). A major limitation to this study is that the authors equated changes in BrdU (thymidine analog) incorporation with changes in neurogenesis. Their data strongly support the view that CB1R is critical in progenitor proliferation in the hippocampus, but nothing more can be deduced with regards to which progenitor population is affected, nor about neuronal differentiation and maturation of the remaining progenitor cells.

Pharmacological studies in wild-type mice support the conclusions from CB1R KO mice. Treatment with CB1R agonists (either with the endocannabinoid anandamide, the synthetic agonists WIN 55, 212-2 or HU-210) increased the number of BrdU positive(+)/NeuN negative(-) hippocampal cells, but decreased the number of co-labeled, newly generated BrdU(+)/NeuN(+) neurons *in vivo* (Rueda, Navarro et al. 2002; Aguado, Palazuelos et al. 2006; Galve-Roperh, Aguado et al. 2006). Furthermore, these studies showed that a CB1R antagonist, SR141716, reversed the agonist actions- the number of co-labeled cells increased, while BrdU(+)/NeuN(-) cells decreased. Similarly, in a study by Jiang et al, 2005, CB1R activation resulted in increased BrdU(+) cells, which was interpreted as enhanced neurogenesis by cannabinoids; however, the authors themselves never show increases in co-labeled cells, and also point out that relative to no treatment, CB1R agonists do not change the percentage of cells expressing immature neuronal markers (Jiang, Zhang et al. 2005).

Adult hippocampal progenitor cells from mouse brains express CB1R *in vitro* and *in vivo* (Aguado, Monory et al. 2005; Aguado, Palazuelos et al. 2006). CB1R activation induced proliferation of these progenitors assessed by quantifying the amount of cells expressing Nestin and incorporating the thymidine analog BrdU. Interestingly, these studies showed CB1R and FAAH are selectively enriched in type 1 (Nestin(+)/GFAP(+)) progenitors *in vivo* compared to type 2 (Nestin(+)/ GFAP(-)) (Aguado, Palazuelos et al. 2006). Utilizing various markers for immature neurons and glia, CB1R activation appears to promote astroglial differentiation, while inhibition of the receptor appears to promote neuronal differentiation (Aguado, Palazuelos et al. 2006). In contrast, a recent study indicated that CB1R was preferentially expressed on type 2b/3 cells that are also expressing DCX, suggesting that CB1Rs have a role in later stages of neuronal differentiation, and migration of the nascent neuron (Wolf, Bick-Sander et al. 2010). This study examined the levels of DCX expressing cells in the hippocampi of CB1R KO mice, and also in Nestin-GFP reporter mice treated with the CB1R antagonist AM251. According to the authors, genetic deletion of CB1R resulted in increased proliferation but decreased net neurogenesis relative to wild-type mice. But, administration of the CB1R specific antagonist AM251 to wild-type mice promoted proliferation of type 2b/3 DCX(+) cells 7 days after BrdU administration (**Figure 5**).

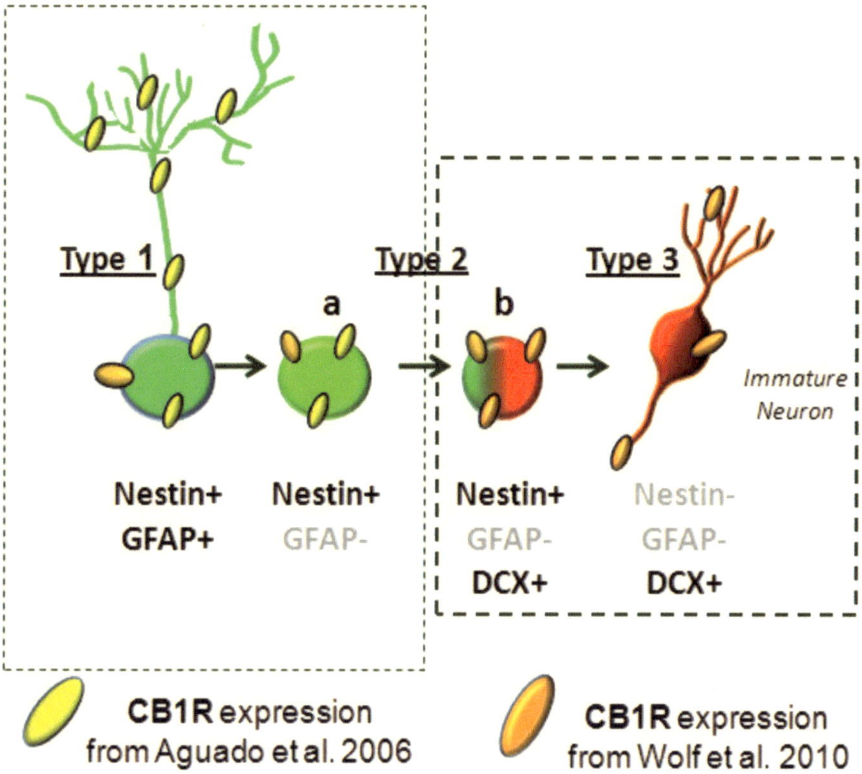

Fig. 5. CB1R is expressed throughout neuronal development (Harkany, Guzman et al. 2007; Harkany, Keimpema et al. 2008), and also at all stages of adult hippocampal neurogenesis. It is not clear whether CB1R is enriched in certain progenitor populations, and if so, how endogenous cannabinoids differentially affect these populations. Equally compelling is how exogenous CB1R agonists or antagonists may affect these different populations, and what the functional outcomes of such interventions may be. Image created with motifolio.com©.

Clarification through additional studies must be made to reconcile these seemingly disparate results. Species, sex and strain of the animals used, chronic versus acute treatment with cannabinergic drugs, specificity, dose/concentration of cannabinergic drugs, BrdU injection protocol and immunohistochemical markers must all be considered when interpreting the many studies published on CB1R's role on adult hippocampal neurogenesis. Table 1 summarizes several knock-out mice that have been developed that target endocannabinoid system components, and the consequences on progenitor proliferation, neuronal differentiation and glial differentiation.

✓ = successful induction; ✗ = impaired induction; nc = no change; N.D. = Not determined		CB1 -/- (Cannabinoid 1 Receptor)	CB2-/- (Cannabinoid 2 Receptor)	FAAH -/- (Fatty Acid Amide Hydrolase)	DAGLαβ -/- [d] (Diacyl-glycerol Lipase) *in vivo*, SVZ	DAGLαβ -/- [d] (Diacyl-glycerol Lipase) *in vivo*, Hippocampus
Neural Progenitor Proliferation	Embryonic/ Postnatal	✗ *in vivo* P2 hippocampus[a]	✗ *in vitro*,[c]	N.D.	N.D.	
	Adult	✗ *in vivo* 3 months old hippocampus[a]	✗ *in vitro* & *in vivo*[c]	✓ *in vivo*, 3 months old hippocampus[a]	α-/- ✗	✗
					β-/- nc	✗
Glial differentiation or Gliogenesis	Embryonic/ Postnatal	✗ *in vivo* P2 hippocampus[a]	N.D.	N.D.	N.D.	
	Adult	✗ *in vivo*, 3 months old hippocampus[a]	N.D.	✓ *in vivo*, 3months old hippocampus[a]	N.D.	
Neuronal Differentiaiton or Neurogenesis	Embryonic/ Postnatal	✓ *in vivo*, P2 hippocampus[a]	N.D	N.D.	N.D.	
	Adult	✓ *in vivo* 3 months old hippocampus[a]	N.D	✗ *in vivo*, 3 months old hippocampus[a]	α-/- ✗	✗
		✗ *in vivo* hippocampus[b]			β-/- N.D.	N.D.

Table 1. **eCB Knock-out mice and adult CNS progenitor cells.** [a] (Aguado, Palazuelos et al. 2006); [b](Jin, Xie et al. 2004); [c](Palazuelos, Aguado et al. 2006); [d](Gao, Vasilyev et al. 2010); KO= Knockout; SVZ = subventricular zone. The apparent conflicting results in the adult CB1 -/- brains may be attributed to the interpretation of 'neurogenesis'(see Section 6).

7. Neurogenesis in the adult spinal cord

Compared to the brain, even though progenitor cells also exist in the adult spinal cord, the spinal cord environment does not seem to support robust constitutive neurogenesis, nor does it seem to support neurogenesis following region specific injury or disease. Though injury results in different functional consequences for the brain and spinal cord, it is not clear why one region of the CNS is capable of generating new neurons, while another area is not. There are several clinical examples where new neuron formation in the adult spinal cord could potentially ameliorate disease symptoms or progression, or replace damaged neurons following trauma. Replacement of dead or damaged neurons in the compromised spinal cord may be able to promote functional motor recovery, but also reduce pain (Hofstetter, Holmstrom et al. 2005; Scholz, Broom et al. 2005; Ohori, Yamamoto et al. 2006; Meisner, Marsh et al. 2010). Manipulating the spinal cord environment to coerce neurogenesis from endogenous progenitors is a promising therapeutic intervention, which may bypass the many obstacles inherent to transplantation of exogenous stem/progenitor cells (Obermair, Schroter et al. 2008).

Several models propose distinct locations for the endogenous spinal cord progenitors, and how they respond to physiological and pathological stimuli (Namiki and Tator 1999; Horner, Power et al. 2000; Horky, Galimi et al. 2006; Meletis, Barnabe-Heider et al. 2008; Hamilton, Truong et al. 2009; Barnabe-Heider, Goritz et al. 2010; Hugnot and Franzen 2011). The overwhelming majority of progenitor cells do not differentiate into neurons *in vivo*. Nevertheless, these progenitors have neurogenic potential revealed from *in vitro* studies, but also from *in vivo* transplantation studies. Progenitors isolated from all levels and areas of the adult spinal cord can give rise to neurons in culture (Weiss, Dunne et al. 1996; Yamamoto, Yamamoto et al. 2001). When spinal cord progenitors were transplanted into the hippocampus- a pro-neurogenic environment, they readily formed neurons (Shihabuddin, Horner et al. 2000). These studies imply that the spinal cord environment is restricting the neurogenic potential of the endogenous progenitors, and astrocytes may be one of the culprits (Song, Stevens et al. 2002).

New evidence is emerging to challenge the idea that new neurons cannot be generated in the adult spinal cord. Direct injury to the spinal cord results in massive progenitor proliferation leading to astrocyte differentiation, and a massive inflammatory response which contributes to glial scar formation (Barnabe-Heider, Goritz et al. 2010; Wang, Cheng et al. 2011). This injured environment has been demonstrated as non-neurogenic (Yamamoto, Nagao et al. 2001; Hannila, Siddiq et al. 2007); however, there are instances in which an environment filled with inflammatory cytokines can still elicit neurogenesis in the adult spinal cord. For example, in an experimental rat model of multiple sclerosis (experimental autoimmune encephalomyelitis), newly generated neurons migrated towards the neuroinflammatory lesion (Danilov, Covacu et al. 2006). Also there are instances of indirect injury to the adult spinal cord, such as dorsal rhizotomy (cutting of the dorsal root at the cervical spinal level) in which neurogenesis is observed in the dorsal horn at the corresponding spinal level (Vessal, Aycock et al. 2007). Recent papers showed that in non-injured, intact adult spinal cords, immature neurons can be found in the area surrounding the central canal (Shechter, Ziv et al. 2007; Marichal, Garcia et al. 2009), but also throughout the spinal cord, with a preferential dorsal gray matter localization and exclusive GABAergic phenotype (Shechter, Ziv et al. 2007; Shechter, Baruch et al. 2011). The exact roles of these immature neurons in the healthy spinal cord have not been determined, but may indicate physiological roles for new GABAergic neurons in nociception (Shechter, Baruch et al. 2011), and also for movement. The existence of these cells is exciting, as it sets the tone for more intensive studies to characterize their function and promote their differentiation.

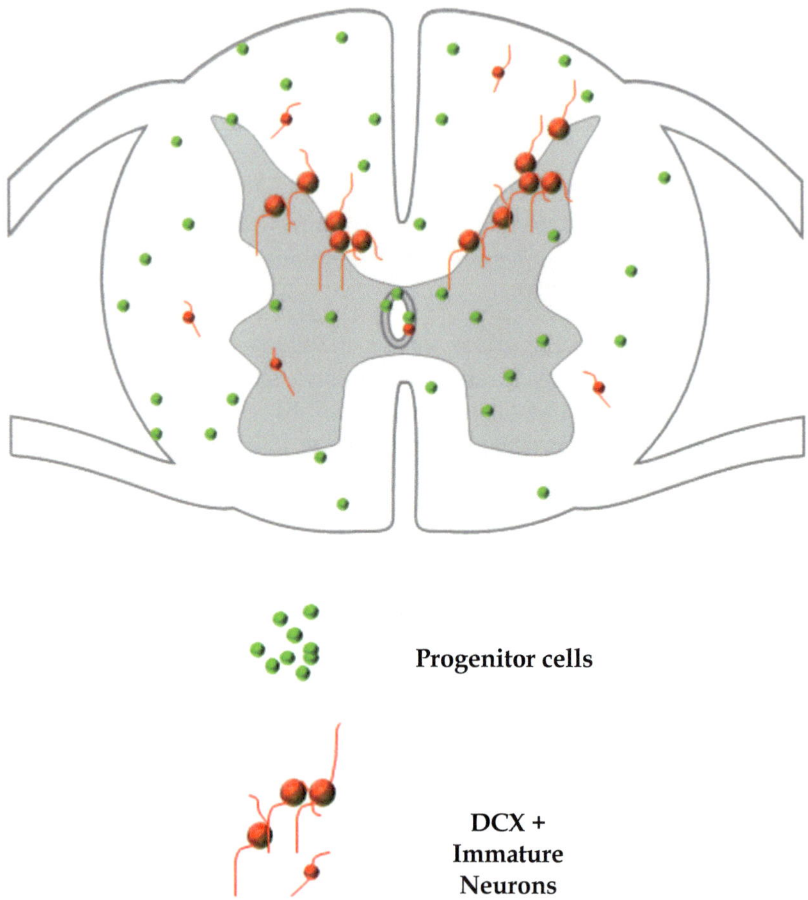

Fig. 6. Transverse section of an adult mouse spinal cord, depicting a model for progenitor cell and immature neuron location. Based on the work by Shechter et al, 2007, 2011, the majority of the GABAergic, BrdU(+)/ DCX(+) immature neurons reside in the gray matter of the dorsal horn. Under physiological conditions, the levels of these cells depend on the type of and exposure to sensory environmental enrichment. Image generated with motifolio.com©.

8. CB1R and adult spinal cord neurogenesis

Taking the adult brain as an example of endocannabinoid system involvement in progenitor cell proliferation and differentiation, there is a possibility that the spinal cord progenitors may also be modulated by this system. There is an overwhelming lack of published studies addressing the presence and roles of the endocannabinoid system in adult spinal cord progenitor cells. Of particular importance is that CB1R is widely distributed on cells throughout the spinal cord, but also in lamina X, which includes the putative progenitor cell niche. We have identified CB1R on adult spinal cord-derived Nestin(+) progenitor cells in primary cultures (**Figure 7**).

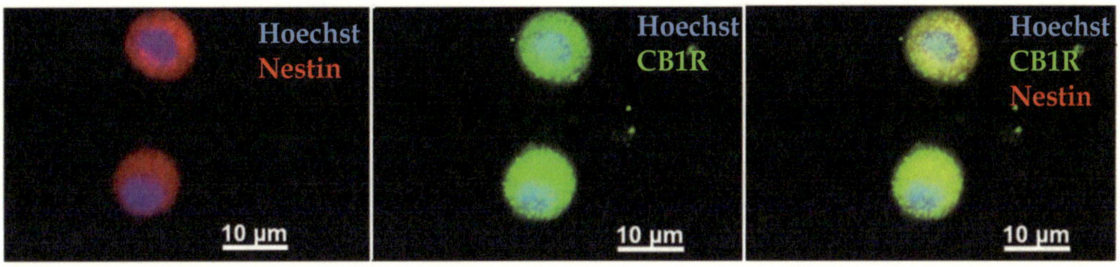

Fig. 7. Primary adult spinal cord cultures from rats contain Nestin(+) progenitor cells (red), which also express CB1R (green). The role of CB1R on these progenitors has not been examined, and further studies are needed to determine how the receptor is involved in progenitor cell quiescence, proliferation or differentiation. Image obtained after 6 days *in vitro* with 63X objective.

In response to injury, not only do progenitor cells proliferate in the spinal cord (Frisen, Johansson et al. 1995; Johansson, Momma et al. 1999; Namiki and Tator 1999; Shibuya, Miyamoto et al. 2002), but levels of endocannabinoids, receptors and enzymes are also altered as described earlier (in Section 4). Rigorous studies are needed to address if and how adult spinal cord progenitor cells respond to endogenous cannabinoid tone or to exogenously administered cannabinoids. Does endocannabinoid tone contribute to the non-neurogenic spinal cord environment? Are endo/exo-cannabinoids capable of promoting spinal cord neurogenesis or gliogenesis? These are just a few critical and novel avenues for potentially promoting neurogenesis in the adult spinal cord.

9. The effect of chronic cannabinergic drug use on the CNS- implications for the treatment of chronic pain

Cannabis is used both acutely and chronically for recreational or medicinal purposes. There is controversy regarding medical marijuana because of the documented cognitive side effects of chronic recreational use (Jager and Ramsey 2008; Hester, Nestor et al. 2009; Battisti, Roodenrys et al. 2010). However, all drugs come with a risk-benefit consideration, and a plethora of historical and emerging evidence indicates that the medicinal value of cannabis cannot be ignored. Many studies have demonstrated that endocannabinoids and application of exogenous cannabinoids (usually mixed CB1R/CB2R agonists) reduce pain sensation (Guindon and Hohmann 2009). Presently, such an approach is becoming more clinically accepted for treating chronic pain states (Aggarwal, Carter et al. 2009; Karst, Wippermann et al. 2010; Lynch and Campbell 2011). While CB2R activation attenuates nociception mostly by modulating the inflammatory response (Guindon and Hohmann 2008), the role of CB1R is more complex because its location on various cells along the pain pathways appears to contribute differently to nociception. Moreover, many cannabinergic drugs are not only mixed agonists, but may bind non-specifically to other receptors, including TRP-channels (Patwardhan, Jeske et al. 2006; Patil, Patwardhan et al. 2011).

The use of several CB1R knock-outs (global and conditional) has helped to clarify the role of these receptors in nociception. Recent worked demonstrated that cannabinoids mediate analgesia by activating CB1Rs located on peripheral nociceptors (dorsal root ganglia sensory neurons) (Agarwal, Pacher et al. 2007). Interestingly, by using *in vitro* spinal cord slices and *in vivo* recordings of dorsal horn neurons, activation of CB1Rs on spinal cord dorsal horn neurons actually enhances (not reduces) nociceptive responses (Pernia-Andrade, Kato et al. 2009; Zhang, Chen et al. 2010). Stimulation of spinal cord CB1Rs inhibits the release of GABA, glycine (Pernia-Andrade 2009), and opioids, while enhancing the release of substance P (Zhang, Chen et al. 2010). Therefore, CB1R activation may contribute to nociception by increasing excitability at the spinal cord level. Consequently, CB1R antagonists have shown anti-nociceptive efficacy in several experimental pain models (Costa, Trovato et al. 2005; Croci and Zarini 2007; Pernia-Andrade, Kato et al. 2009). On the contrary, another recent study also using *in vivo* recordings demonstrated that blocking spinal CB1Rs enhanced the evoked response of the spinal cord dorsal horn neurons in neuropathic rats, indicative of a pro-nociceptive role of the receptor (Sagar, Jhaveri et al. 2010). One explanation for these different results could be attributed to the anesthetic used. Pernia-Andrade et al 2009 used a mixture of pentobarbital with pancuronium (a muscle relaxant), while Sagar et al.'s study only used isoflurane. The use of a muscle relaxant would allow the use of lower levels of the anesthetic to achieve immobility (required for the *in vivo* recordings). It is possible that the level of anesthesia used in Sagar et al's 2010 recordings may have depressed the neuronal activity relevant to pain sensation. Consistent with this possibility is that there was no difference in the firing rate of dorsal horn neurons in anesthetized neuropathic and sham operated animals at various levels of stimulation.

The chronic use of mixed cannabinoid drugs should be further investigated in light of the fact that the majority readily cross the blood-brain barrier. These compounds may be capable of providing pain relief, but they may also be affecting other important cellular functions, such as neurogenesis in the brain and spinal cord. Neurogenesis from endogenous progenitor cells is associated with a wide range of functions, and perturbations of this process are correlated with disease symptoms. Interference of physiological neurogenesis may be a highly undesirable side-effect of chronic endocannabinoid system manipulation by the use of CB1R/CB2R agonists or antagonists. For example, following peripheral nerve injury or direct spinal cord injury, a specific loss of inhibitory GABAergic interneurons in the spinal cord dorsal horn is postulated to be a major contributor to chronic pain (Moore, Kohno et al. 2002; Scholz, Broom et al. 2005; Meisner, Marsh et al. 2010). Replacement of these neurons through neurogenesis is an attractive therapeutic strategy because it attempts to go beyond the management of symptoms; it targets an underlying biological phenomenon of neuronal death following injury. Given the controversy regarding how cannabinoids modulate neurogenesis, it is possible that while treatment with mixed cannabinoids can ameliorate pain, long term usage may prevent the replacement of damaged inhibitory neurons by blocking neurogenesis, and thus contribute to an underlying etiology of chronic pain. Hence understading the role of the individual CBRs in adult neurogenesis, but also during pain states, could help discern how to more susccesfully use these agents clinically.

10. Conclusions

CB1R expression on adult CNS-derived progenitor cells is not only indicative of endogenous cannabinoid modulation, but also points to potential consequences of cannabinoid pharmacotherapy on progenitor proliferation and differentiation- whether beneficial or deleterious. The complex results published about adult brain progenitors and the lack of data on adult spinal cord progenitors demonstrate that extensive basic research is still needed to understand how the endocannabinoid system affects these cells normally and in response to injury and disease.

11. References

Agarwal, N., P. Pacher, et al. (2007). "Cannabinoids mediate analgesia largely via peripheral type 1 cannabinoid receptors in nociceptors." Nat Neurosci 10(7): 870-879.

Aggarwal, S. K., G. T. Carter, et al. (2009). "Medicinal use of cannabis in the United States: historical perspectives, current trends, and future directions." J Opioid Manag 5(3): 153-168.

Aguado, T., K. Monory, et al. (2005). "The endocannabinoid system drives neural progenitor proliferation." Faseb J 19(12): 1704-1706.

Aguado, T., J. Palazuelos, et al. (2006). "The endocannabinoid system promotes astroglial differentiation by acting on neural progenitor cells." J Neurosci 26(5): 1551-1561.

Aldrich, M. R. (2006). "The Remarkable W.B. O'Shaughnessy" Retrieved January 29, 2011, from http://antiquecannabisbook.com/chap2B/Shaughnessy/Shaughnessy.htm.

Arevalo-Martin, A., D. Garcia-Ovejero, et al. (2008). "CB2 cannabinoid receptors as an emerging target for demyelinating diseases: from neuroimmune interactions to cell replacement strategies." Br J Pharmacol 153(2): 216-225.

Barnabe-Heider, F., C. Goritz, et al. (2010). "Origin of new glial cells in intact and injured adult spinal cord." Cell Stem Cell 7(4): 470-482.

Battisti, R. A., S. Roodenrys, et al. (2010). "Chronic use of cannabis and poor neural efficiency in verbal memory ability." Psychopharmacology (Berl) 209(4): 319-330.

Bisogno, T., F. Berrendero, et al. (1999). "Brain regional distribution of endocannabinoids: implications for their biosynthesis and biological function." Biochem Biophys Res Commun 256(2): 377-380.

Bisogno, T. and V. Di Marzo (2010). "Cannabinoid receptors and endocannabinoids: role in neuroinflammatory and neurodegenerative disorders." CNS Neurol Disord Drug Targets 9(5): 564-573.

Bouaboula, M., C. Poinot-Chazel, et al. (1995). "Activation of mitogen-activated protein kinases by stimulation of the central cannabinoid receptor CB1." Biochem J 312 (Pt 2): 637-641.

Brown, S. P., P. K. Safo, et al. (2004). "Endocannabinoids inhibit transmission at granule cell to Purkinje cell synapses by modulating three types of presynaptic calcium channels." J Neurosci 24(24): 5623-5631.

Carrier, E. J., C. S. Kearn, et al. (2004). "Cultured rat microglial cells synthesize the endocannabinoid 2-arachidonylglycerol, which increases proliferation via a CB2 receptor-dependent mechanism." Mol Pharmacol 65(4): 999-1007.

Caulfield, M. P. and D. A. Brown (1992). "Cannabinoid receptor agonists inhibit Ca current in NG108-15 neuroblastoma cells via a pertussis toxin-sensitive me[illegible]ism." Br J Pharmacol 106(2): 231-232.

Costa, B., A. E. Trovato, et al. (2005). "Effect of the cannabinoid CB1 receptor antagonist, SR141716, on nociceptive response and nerve demyelination in rodents with chronic constriction injury of the sciatic nerve." Pain 116(1-2): 52-61.

Croci, T. and E. Zarini (2007). "Effect of the cannabinoid CB1 receptor antagonist rimonabant on nociceptive responses and adjuvant-induced arthritis in obese and lean rats." Br J Pharmacol 150(5): 559-566.

Danilov, A. I., R. Covacu, et al. (2006). "Neurogenesis in the adult spinal cord in an experimental model of multiple sclerosis." Eur J Neurosci 23(2): 394-400.

Darmani, N. A. (2001). "Delta(9)-tetrahydrocannabinol and synthetic cannabinoids prevent emesis produced by the cannabinoid CB(1) receptor antagonist/inverse agonist SR 141716A." Neuropsychopharmacology 24(2): 198-203.

Devane, W. A., A. Breuer, et al. (1992). "A novel probe for the cannabinoid receptor." J Med Chem 35(11): 2065-2069.

Devane, W. A., F. A. Dysarz, 3rd, et al. (1988). "Determination and characterization of a cannabinoid receptor in rat brain." Mol Pharmacol 34(5): 605-613.

Devane, W. A., L. Hanus, et al. (1992). "Isolation and structure of a brain constituent that binds to the cannabinoid receptor." Science 258(5090): 1946-1949.

Di Marzo, V., M. Bifulco, et al. (2004). "The endocannabinoid system and its therapeutic exploitation." Nat Rev Drug Discov 3(9): 771-784.

El Manira, A. and A. Kyriakatos (2010). "The role of endocannabinoid signaling in motor control." Physiology (Bethesda) 25(4): 230-238.

El Manira, A., A. Kyriakatos, et al. (2008). "Endocannabinoid signaling in the spinal locomotor circuitry." Brain Res Rev 57(1): 29-36.

Farquhar-Smith, W. P., M. Egertova, et al. (2000). "Cannabinoid CB(1) receptor expression in rat spinal cord." Mol Cell Neurosci 15(6): 510-521.

Freund, T. F., I. Katona, et al. (2003). "Role of endogenous cannabinoids in synaptic signaling." Physiol Rev 83(3): 1017-1066.

Frisen, J., C. B. Johansson, et al. (1995). "Rapid, widespread, and longlasting induction of nestin contributes to the generation of glial scar tissue after CNS injury." J Cell Biol 131(2): 453-464.

Galve-Roperh, I., T. Aguado, et al. (2007). "The endocannabinoid system and neurogenesis in health and disease." Neuroscientist 13(2): 109-114.

Galve-Roperh, I., T. Aguado, et al. (2006). "Endocannabinoids: a new family of lipid mediators involved in the regulation of neural cell development." Curr Pharm Des 12(18): 2319-2325.

Gao, Y., D. V. Vasilyev, et al. (2010). "Loss of Retrograde Endocannabinoid Signaling and Reduced Adult Neurogenesis in Diacylglycerol Lipase Knock-out Mice." J Neurosci 30(6): 2017-2024.

Garcia-Ovejero, D., A. Arevalo-Martin, et al. (2009). "The endocannabinoid system is modulated in response to spinal cord injury in rats." Neurobiol Dis 33(1): 57-71.

Gerard, C. M., C. Mollereau, et al. (1991). "Molecular cloning of a human cannabinoid receptor which is also expressed in testis." Biochem J 279 (Pt 1): 129-134.

Gomez del Pulgar, T., G. Velasco, et al. (2000). "The CB1 cannabinoid receptor is coupled to the activation of protein kinase B/Akt." Biochem J 347(Pt 2): 369-373.

Grinspoon, L. (1993). Marihuana, the forbidden medicine. New Haven, Yale University Press.

Guindon, J. and A. G. Hohmann (2008). "Cannabinoid CB2 receptors: a therapeutic target for the treatment of inflammatory and neuropathic pain." Br J Pharmacol 153(2): 319-334.

Guindon, J. and A. G. Hohmann (2009). "The endocannabinoid system and pain." CNS Neurol Disord Drug Targets 8(6): 403-421.

Guzman, M., C. Sanchez, et al. (2001). "Control of the cell survival/death decision by cannabinoids." J Mol Med 78(11): 613-625.

Guzman, M., C. Sanchez, et al. (2002). "Cannabinoids and cell fate." Pharmacol Ther 95(2): 175-184.

Hamilton, L. K., M. K. Truong, et al. (2009). "Cellular organization of the central canal ependymal zone, a niche of latent neural stem cells in the adult mammalian spinal cord." Neuroscience 164(3): 1044-1056.

Hannila, S. S., M. M. Siddiq, et al. (2007). "Therapeutic approaches to promoting axonal regeneration in the adult mammalian spinal cord." Int Rev Neurobiol 77: 57-105.

Harkany, T., M. Guzman, et al. (2007). "The emerging functions of endocannabinoid signaling during CNS development." Trends Pharmacol Sci 28(2): 83-92.

Harkany, T., E. Keimpema, et al. (2008). "Endocannabinoid functions controlling neuronal specification during brain development." Mol Cell Endocrinol 286(1-2 Suppl 1): S84-90.

Hegyi, Z., G. Kis, et al. (2009). "Neuronal and glial localization of the cannabinoid-1 receptor in the superficial spinal dorsal horn of the rodent spinal cord." Eur J Neurosci 30(2): 251-262.

Herkenham, M., A. B. Lynn, et al. (1991). "Characterization and localization of cannabinoid receptors in rat brain: a quantitative in vitro autoradiographic study." J Neurosci 11(2): 563-583.

Herodotus (1824). The History of Herodotus. R. Larcher, Mitford, Schweighaeuser. Oxford, Talboys and Wheeler. Volume 2.

Hester, R., L. Nestor, et al. (2009). "Impaired error awareness and anterior cingulate cortex hypoactivity in chronic cannabis users." Neuropsychopharmacology 34(11): 2450-2458.

Hofstetter, C. P., N. A. Holmstrom, et al. (2005). "Allodynia limits the usefulness of intraspinal neural stem cell grafts; directed differentiation improves outcome." Nat Neurosci 8(3): 346-353.

Horky, L. L., F. Galimi, et al. (2006). "Fate of endogenous stem/progenitor cells following spinal cord injury." J Comp Neurol 498(4): 525-538.

Horner, P. J., A. E. Power, et al. (2000). "Proliferation and differentiation of progenitor cells throughout the intact adult rat spinal cord." J Neurosci 20(6): 2218-2228.

Huang, C. C., S. W. Lo, et al. (2001). "Presynaptic mechanisms underlying cannabinoid inhibition of excitatory synaptic transmission in rat striatal neurons." J Physiol 532(Pt 3): 731-748.

Hugnot, J. P. and R. Franzen (2011). "The spinal cord ependymal region: a stem cell niche in the caudal central nervous system." Front Biosci 16: 1044-1059.

Jager, G. and N. F. Ramsey (2008). "Long-term consequences of adolescent cannabis exposure on the development of cognition, brain structure and function: an overview of animal and human research." Curr Drug Abuse Rev 1(2): 114-123.

Jiang, W., Y. Zhang, et al. (2005). "Cannabinoids promote embryonic and adult hippocampus neurogenesis and produce anxiolytic- and antidepressant-like effects." J Clin Invest 115(11): 3104-3116.

Jin, K., L. Xie, et al. (2004). "Defective adult neurogenesis in CB1 cannabinoid receptor knockout mice." Mol Pharmacol 66(2): 204-208.
Johansson, C. B., S. Momma, et al. (1999). "Identification of a neural stem cell in the adult mammalian central nervous system." Cell 96(1): 25-34.
Karst, M., S. Wippermann, et al. (2010). "Role of cannabinoids in the treatment of pain and (painful) spasticity." Drugs 70(18): 2409-2438.
Katona, I., B. Sperlagh, et al. (1999). "Presynaptically located CB1 cannabinoid receptors regulate GABA release from axon terminals of specific hippocampal interneurons." J Neurosci 19(11): 4544-4558.
Kirby, M. T., R. E. Hampson, et al. (1995). "Cannabinoids selectively decrease paired-pulse facilitation of perforant path synaptic potentials in the dentate gyrus in vitro." Brain Res 688(1-2): 114-120.
Knerlich-Lukoschus, F., M. Noack, et al. (2011). "Spinal cord injuries induce changes in CB1 cannabinoid receptor and C-C chemokine expression in brain areas underlying circuitry of chronic pain conditions." J Neurotrauma 28(4): 619-634.
Lynch, M. E. and F. Campbell (2011). "Cannabinoids for Treatment of Chronic Non-Cancer Pain; a Systematic Review of Randomized Trials." Br J Clin Pharmacol.
Mackie, K. (2005). "Cannabinoid receptor homo- and heterodimerization." Life Sci 77(14): 1667-1673.
Mackie, K., W. A. Devane, et al. (1993). "Anandamide, an endogenous cannabinoid, inhibits calcium currents as a partial agonist in N18 neuroblastoma cells." Mol Pharmacol 44(3): 498-503.
Mackie, K. and B. Hille (1992). "Cannabinoids inhibit N-type calcium channels in neuroblastoma-glioma cells." Proc Natl Acad Sci U S A 89(9): 3825-3829.
Mailleux, P., M. Verslijpe, et al. (1992). "Initial observations on the distribution of cannabinoid receptor binding sites in the human adult basal ganglia using autoradiography." Neurosci Lett 139(1): 7-9.
Marichal, N., G. Garcia, et al. (2009). "Enigmatic central canal contacting cells: immature neurons in "standby mode"?" J Neurosci 29(32): 10010-10024.
Martin, B. R. and J. L. Wiley (2004). "Mechanism of action of cannabinoids: how it may lead to treatment of cachexia, emesis, and pain." J Support Oncol 2(4): 305-314; discussion 314-306.
Matsuda, L. A., S. J. Lolait, et al. (1990). "Structure of a cannabinoid receptor and functional expression of the cloned cDNA." Nature 346(6284): 561-564.
Mechoulam, R. (2000). "Looking back at Cannabis research." Curr Pharm Des 6(13): 1313-1322.
Mechoulam, R., S. Ben-Shabat, et al. (1995). "Identification of an endogenous 2-monoglyceride, present in canine gut, that binds to cannabinoid receptors." Biochem Pharmacol 50(1): 83-90.
Mechoulam, R. and Y. Gaoni (1965). "Hashish. IV. The isolation and structure of cannabinolic cannabidiolic and cannabigerolic acids." Tetrahedron 21(5): 1223-1229.
Mechoulam, R. and Y. Gaoni (1965). "A Total Synthesis of Dl-Delta-1-Tetrahydrocannabinol, the Active Constituent of Hashish." J Am Chem Soc 87: 3273-3275.
Mechoulam, R. and L. Hanus (2000). "A historical overview of chemical research on cannabinoids." Chem Phys Lipids 108(1-2): 1-13.

Meisner, J. G., A. D. Marsh, et al. (2010). "Loss of GABAergic interneurons in laminae I-III of the spinal cord dorsal horn contributes to reduced GABAergic tone and neuropathic pain after spinal cord injury." J Neurotrauma 27(4): 729-737.

Meletis, K., F. Barnabe-Heider, et al. (2008). "Spinal cord injury reveals multilineage differentiation of ependymal cells." PLoS Biol 6(7): e182.

Melis, M., M. Pistis, et al. (2004). "Endocannabinoids mediate presynaptic inhibition of glutamatergic transmission in rat ventral tegmental area dopamine neurons through activation of CB1 receptors." J Neurosci 24(1): 53-62.

Ming, G. L. and H. Song (2011). "Adult neurogenesis in the mammalian brain: significant answers and significant questions." Neuron 70(4): 687-702.

Molina-Holgado, E., J. M. Vela, et al. (2002). "Cannabinoids promote oligodendrocyte progenitor survival: involvement of cannabinoid receptors and phosphatidylinositol-3 kinase/Akt signaling." J Neurosci 22(22): 9742-9753.

Moore, K. A., T. Kohno, et al. (2002). "Partial peripheral nerve injury promotes a selective loss of GABAergic inhibition in the superficial dorsal horn of the spinal cord." J Neurosci 22(15): 6724-6731.

Munro, S., K. L. Thomas, et al. (1993). "Molecular characterization of a peripheral receptor for cannabinoids." Nature 365(6441): 61-65.

Namiki, J. and C. H. Tator (1999). "Cell proliferation and nestin expression in the ependyma of the adult rat spinal cord after injury." J Neuropathol Exp Neurol 58(5): 489-498.

Navarrete, M. and A. Araque (2008). "Endocannabinoids mediate neuron-astrocyte communication." Neuron 57(6): 883-893.

Nogueiras, R., A. Diaz-Arteaga, et al. (2009). "The endocannabinoid system: role in glucose and energy metabolism." Pharmacol Res 60(2): 93-98.

O'Shaughnessy, W. B. (1842). On the preparations of the Indian Hemp, or Gunjah. Transactions of the Medical and Physical Society of Calcutta. Calcutta, William Rushton and Co. VIII: 40.

Obermair, F. J., A. Schroter, et al. (2008). "Endogenous neural progenitor cells as therapeutic target after spinal cord injury." Physiology (Bethesda) 23: 296-304.

Ohori, Y., S. Yamamoto, et al. (2006). "Growth factor treatment and genetic manipulation stimulate neurogenesis and oligodendrogenesis by endogenous neural progenitors in the injured adult spinal cord." J Neurosci 26(46): 11948-11960.

Onaivi, E. S., C. M. Leonard, et al. (2002). "Endocannabinoids and cannabinoid receptor genetics." Prog Neurobiol 66(5): 307-344.

Ong, W. Y. and K. Mackie (1999). "A light and electron microscopic study of the CB1 cannabinoid receptor in the primate spinal cord." J Neurocytol 28(1): 39-45.

Palazuelos, J., T. Aguado, et al. (2006). "Non-psychoactive CB2 cannabinoid agonists stimulate neural progenitor proliferation." Faseb J 20(13): 2405-2407.

Patil, M., A. Patwardhan, et al. (2011). "Cannabinoid receptor antagonists AM251 and AM630 activate TRPA1 in sensory neurons." Neuropharmacology 61(4): 778-788.

Paton, W. D. (1975). "Pharmacology of marijuana." Annu Rev Pharmacol 15: 191-220.

Patwardhan, A. M., N. A. Jeske, et al. (2006). "The cannabinoid WIN 55,212-2 inhibits transient receptor potential vanilloid 1 (TRPV1) and evokes peripheral antihyperalgesia via calcineurin." Proc Natl Acad Sci U S A 103(30): 11393-11398.

Pazos, M. R., E. Nunez, et al. (2005). "Functional neuroanatomy of the endocannabinoid system." Pharmacol Biochem Behav 81(2): 239-247.

Pernia-Andrade, A. J., A. Kato, et al. (2009). "Spinal endocannabinoids and CB1 receptors mediate C-fiber-induced heterosynaptic pain sensitization." Science 325(5941): 760-764.

Pertwee, R. G. (1997). "Pharmacology of cannabinoid CB1 and CB2 receptors." Pharmacol Ther 74(2): 129-180.

Robbe, D., G. Alonso, et al. (2001). "Localization and mechanisms of action of cannabinoid receptors at the glutamatergic synapses of the mouse nucleus accumbens." J Neurosci 21(1): 109-116.

Rodriguez, J. J., K. Mackie, et al. (2001). "Ultrastructural localization of the CB1 cannabinoid receptor in mu-opioid receptor patches of the rat Caudate putamen nucleus." J Neurosci 21(3): 823-833.

Romero-Sandoval, A., N. Nutile-McMenemy, et al. (2008). "Spinal microglial and perivascular cell cannabinoid receptor type 2 activation reduces behavioral hypersensitivity without tolerance after peripheral nerve injury." Anesthesiology 108(4): 722-734.

Rueda, D., B. Navarro, et al. (2002). "The endocannabinoid anandamide inhibits neuronal progenitor cell differentiation through attenuation of the Rap1/B-Raf/ERK pathway." J Biol Chem 277(48): 46645-46650.

Sagar, D. R., M. D. Jhaveri, et al. (2010). "Endocannabinoid regulation of spinal nociceptive processing in a model of neuropathic pain." Eur J Neurosci.

Salio, C., S. Doly, et al. (2002). "Neuronal and astrocytic localization of the cannabinoid receptor-1 in the dorsal horn of the rat spinal cord." Neurosci Lett 329(1): 13-16.

Sanchez, C., I. Galve-Roperh, et al. (1998). "Involvement of sphingomyelin hydrolysis and the mitogen-activated protein kinase cascade in the Delta9-tetrahydrocannabinol-induced stimulation of glucose metabolism in primary astrocytes." Mol Pharmacol 54(5): 834-843.

Sanudo-Pena, M. C., K. Tsou, et al. (1997). "Endogenous cannabinoids as an aversive or counter-rewarding system in the rat." Neurosci Lett 223(2): 125-128.

Schlicker, E. and M. Kathmann (2001). "Modulation of transmitter release via presynaptic cannabinoid receptors." Trends Pharmacol Sci 22(11): 565-572.

Scholz, J., D. C. Broom, et al. (2005). "Blocking caspase activity prevents transsynaptic neuronal apoptosis and the loss of inhibition in lamina II of the dorsal horn after peripheral nerve injury." J Neurosci 25(32): 7317-7323.

Scotter, E. L., M. E. Abood, et al. (2010). "The endocannabinoid system as a target for the treatment of neurodegenerative disease." Br J Pharmacol 160(3): 480-498.

Shechter, R., K. Baruch, et al. (2011). "Touch gives new life: mechanosensation modulates spinal cord adult neurogenesis." Mol Psychiatry 16(3): 342-352.

Shechter, R., Y. Ziv, et al. (2007). "New GABAergic interneurons supported by myelin-specific T cells are formed in intact adult spinal cord." Stem Cells 25(9): 2277-2282.

Shibuya, S., O. Miyamoto, et al. (2002). "Embryonic intermediate filament, nestin, expression following traumatic spinal cord injury in adult rats." Neuroscience 114(4): 905-916.

Shihabuddin, L. S., P. J. Horner, et al. (2000). "Adult spinal cord stem cells generate neurons after transplantation in the adult dentate gyrus." J Neurosci 20(23): 8727-8735.

Song, H., C. F. Stevens, et al. (2002). "Astroglia induce neurogenesis from adult neural stem cells." Nature 417(6884): 39-44.

Sugiura, T., S. Kondo, et al. (1995). "2-Arachidonoylglycerol: a possible endogenous cannabinoid receptor ligand in brain." Biochem Biophys Res Commun 215(1): 89-97.

Suh, H., W. Deng, et al. (2009). "Signaling in adult neurogenesis." Annu Rev Cell Dev Biol 25: 253-275.

Sullivan, J. M. (1999). "Mechanisms of cannabinoid-receptor-mediated inhibition of synaptic transmission in cultured hippocampal pyramidal neurons." J Neurophysiol 82(3): 1286-1294.

Szabo, B. and E. Schlicker (2005). "Effects of cannabinoids on neurotransmission." Handb Exp Pharmacol(168): 327-365.

Tsou, K., S. Brown, et al. (1998). "Immunohistochemical distribution of cannabinoid CB1 receptors in the rat central nervous system." Neuroscience 83(2): 393-411.

Tsou, K., K. Mackie, et al. (1999). "Cannabinoid CB1 receptors are localized primarily on cholecystokinin-containing GABAergic interneurons in the rat hippocampal formation." Neuroscience 93(3): 969-975.

Van Sickle, M. D., L. D. Oland, et al. (2001). "Cannabinoids inhibit emesis through CB1 receptors in the brainstem of the ferret." Gastroenterology 121(4): 767-774.

Van Sickle, M. D., L. D. Oland, et al. (2003). "Delta9-tetrahydrocannabinol selectively acts on CB1 receptors in specific regions of dorsal vagal complex to inhibit emesis in ferrets." Am J Physiol Gastrointest Liver Physiol 285(3): G566-576.

Vessal, M., A. Aycock, et al. (2007). "Adult neurogenesis in primate and rodent spinal cord: comparing a cervical dorsal rhizotomy with a dorsal column transection." Eur J Neurosci 26(10): 2777-2794.

Waksman, Y., J. M. Olson, et al. (1999). "The central cannabinoid receptor (CB1) mediates inhibition of nitric oxide production by rat microglial cells." J Pharmacol Exp Ther 288(3): 1357-1366.

Wang, Y., X. Cheng, et al. (2011). "Astrocytes from the contused spinal cord inhibit oligodendrocyte differentiation of adult oligodendrocyte precursor cells by increasing the expression of bone morphogenetic proteins." J Neurosci 31(16): 6053-6058.

Wartmann, M., D. Campbell, et al. (1995). "The MAP kinase signal transduction pathway is activated by the endogenous cannabinoid anandamide." FEBS Lett 359(2-3): 133-136.

Weiss, S., C. Dunne, et al. (1996). "Multipotent CNS stem cells are present in the adult mammalian spinal cord and ventricular neuroaxis." J Neurosci 16(23): 7599-7609.

Wilson, R. I. and R. A. Nicoll (2002). "Endocannabinoid signaling in the brain." Science 296(5568): 678-682.

Wolf, S. A., A. Bick-Sander, et al. (2010). "Cannabinoid receptor CB1 mediates baseline and activity-induced survival of new neurons in adult hippocampal neurogenesis." Cell Commun Signal 8: 12.

Yamamoto, S., M. Nagao, et al. (2001). "Transcription factor expression and Notch-dependent regulation of neural progenitors in the adult rat spinal cord." J Neurosci 21(24): 9814-9823.

Yamamoto, S., N. Yamamoto, et al. (2001). "Proliferation of parenchymal neural progenitors in response to injury in the adult rat spinal cord." Exp Neurol 172(1): 115-127.

Zhang, G., W. Chen, et al. (2010). "Cannabinoid CB1 receptor facilitation of substance P release in the rat spinal cord, measured as neurokinin 1 receptor internalization." Eur J Neurosci 31(2): 225-237.

Zhang, J., C. Hoffert, et al. (2003). "Induction of CB2 receptor expression in the rat spinal cord of neuropathic but not inflammatory chronic pain models." Eur J Neurosci 17(12): 2750-2754.

6

Peroxisome Proliferator Activated Receptor Alpha (PPARα) Agonists: A Potential Tool for a Healthy Aging Brain

Jennifer Tremblay-Mercier
Université de Sherbrooke, Research Center on Aging
Canada

1. Introduction

1.1 Definitions and considerations

Cognitive decline related to advancing age includes many sub-categories of diseases, some more or less well defined and understood. First, there is "normal" cognitive decline, which is gradual and progressive during aging and seems inevitable. When cognitive decline is large enough to disrupt the activities of daily life, a state of dementia is diagnosed. There are several types of dementia according to the etiology of cognitive decline: vascular dementia, which results from a circulatory disorder causing an obstruction of cerebral blood vessels which leads to the progressive degeneration of brain cells due to a lack of oxygen. Vascular dementia represents 20% of all cases of dementia. Lewis body dementia is an accumulation of α-synuclein protein within the cell and it represents 5 to 15% of neurodegenerative diseases. Frontotemporal dementia as the name suggests, is a degeneration of the region of the frontal and temporal anterior cortex. The reasons for this degeneration are not fully understood. Alzheimer's disease (AD) represents the majority of cases of dementia (65%) although its etiology is not known exactly, or rather multi-factorial.

The most accepted theory in the medical community to explain the origin of AD is currently the accumulation of β-amyloid protein in the form of plaques accompanied by neurofibrillary tangles of tau protein that cause neuronal death and loss of brain matter. However, this theory is challenged for many reasons. The high profile failures of anti-amyloid interventions and lack of agreement on which form the β-amyloid is toxic and the mechanism by which this occurs force the scientific community to consider amyloid only as one part of a multi-factorial disease process including a variety of aggravating factors. A recent paper entitled "Changing perspectives on Alzheimer's Disease: Thinking outside the amyloid Box" resume this thinking (D'Alton & George, 2011).

1.2 Alzheimer's disease diagnosis

The clinical diagnosis of AD is based on clinical examination and confirmed by neuropsychological tests and is diagnosed through exclusion. That means if the person presents a certain profile of cognitive decline and does not match certain criteria (Table 1) the patient is put into the broad category of "probable" AD (Whitehouse, 2008). Within this category there are "typical" Alzheimer and those who are called "atypical" which means that their profile may include some features of vascular dementia or components of Lewis Body dementia. In 2011, the use of brain imaging (Positrons Emission Tomography (PET) and Magnetic Resonance Imaging (MRI)) can optimize the basic clinical diagnosis (clinical and neuropsychological data) of atypical profile, if this kind of technological platform is available. However, it is only at death that the diagnosis can be confirmed by neuropathological brain examination of the abundance of β-amyloid plaques and neurofibrillary tangle, even if the amyloid theory is increasingly questioned. Not surprisingly, neuropathological diagnosis of post-mortem brain does not always correlate with the clinical diagnosis. One classic example is the "Nun Study" from Chicago (Snowdon et al., 1997), in this study, several participants showed abundant neurofibrillary tangles and β-amyloid plaques at the post-mortem analysis, but had not received a clinical diagnosis of AD and were mentally intact during their life. The opposite was also seen i.e. that a person with a clinical AD diagnostic presented an intact brain (no neuropathology) at death.

Diagnosis of probable AD will be posed only :
IF THE PATIENT DOES NOT PRESENT:
Hypothyroidism; other metabolic problem
Vascular problem
Vitamine deficit (Vitamin B12)
Hypercalcemia
Hydrocephalus
Head injury
Psychiatric disorders (depression, schizophrenia)
Structural brain lesion (tumor, injury, blood clot)
Other degenerative disease (Parkinson disease)
Simulation or factitious disorder
Dehydration or other sources of confusion / delirium
Brain infection (HIV, encephalitis, meningitis, syphilis)
Chronic effects of various substances (alchool, drugs)

Table 1. Alzheimer's Disease: diagnosis of exclusion (Adapted from Whitehouse, 2008)

The mismatch between clinical diagnosis and aβ and tau neuropathology at death shakes the causation link and suggests the importance of other aspects in the etiology of the cognitive decline associated with aging.

1.3 Physiopathology: Focus on brain metabolism

In addition to the abnormal protein (aβ, tau, α-synuclein) present in the demented brains, there is also a decrease in brain glucose metabolism in the majority of dementia. The brain is one of the most metabolically active organs. Despite representing about 2% of adult body weight, the brain uses about 23 % of the body's total energy needs. The brain gets its energy from glucose to 97% making it the main energy substrate. Every day, an average human brain consumes approximately 16% of the total oxygen consumption and metabolizes approximately 110 to 145 g of glucose. Over 90% of used glucose is oxidized to ensure the supply of ATP which is vital for the cells and maintenance of synaptic transmission (Henderson, 2008). The determination of the brain glucose metabolism pattern is used in the differential diagnosis of dementia using Position Emission Tomography (PET) imaging with an analog of glucose; ^{18}fluorodeoxyglucose (^{18}FDG). The cerebral glucose hypometabolism in cases of AD has been known since the 1980s with the beginning of PET imaging and represents about 20% reduction but varies between 8 and 49% (reviewed in Cunnane et al., 2011).

In the case of AD, several evidences shows that brain glucose hypometabolism is present in certain regions well before the first clinical signs of cognitive decline, so it is not simply the result of neuronal loss but rather would be responsible for this loss. For example, in a clinical study containing 20 AD patients and 20 young adults (20-39 years old) at risk of developing AD (carrier of the Apolipoprotein E4 allele; ApoE4), small areas of cortical glucose hypometabolism were present in the young participants, especially in the posterior cingulate, parietal, temporal and prefrontonal cortex. These hypometabolic regions were the same in the AD patients but in a more extensive way. This reduction in brain glucose metabolism may be the earliest brain abnormalities yet found in living persons at risk for AD (Reiman et al., 2004).

It is still unclear as to whether or not healthy aging (no cognitive impairment) is associated with reduction in brain glucose metabolism. Cunnane and collegues reviewed the literature on this specific question and they found out that eight studies showed that cerebral glucose metabolism does not decline with healthy aging and nine studies have demonstrated that it does in a proportion of about 18% (Cunnane et al., 2011.)

The reason for this alteration in brain glucose metabolism is not clearly elucidated. It could be a problem in the glucose transport, glucose availability, or a dysfunction in the production of energy derived from glucose. Mitochondria play a central role in producing ATP as the central source of cellular energy, so a dysfunction at the mitochondria level is conceivable.

The brain uses glucose as main energy source but can also use ketones as an alternative energy source in situations of glucose deprivation (fasting, intense physical activity). Ketones refer to 3 molecules: acetoacetate, β-hydroxybutyrate (β-OHB) and acetone. In starvation conditions, up to 60% of the human brain energy requirements can be met by ketones (Owen, 1967). Whether ketone brain metabolism is also decreasing in healthy aging or in AD is not yet known, but Cunnane's team developed a ketone radiotracer (^{11}C-acetoacetate) especially to be able to study brain ketone metabolism in the elderly; studies are ongoing. Based on the fact that ketones are energetic molecules and used by the brain as an alternative to glucose, some studies have demonstrated the ability of ketones to improve some cognitive dysfunction in diabetic hypoglycemia (Page et al., 2009) and even in case

AD (Henderson et al., 2009). Although brain ketone metabolism is less known in the elderly population, fundamental and clinical studies suggests that they could represents an interesting therapeutic potential for cognitive decline (reviewed in Veech et al., 2001)

1.4 Risk factors: Importance of the metabolic condition

In addition to understanding the physiopathology underlying the cognitive decline it is important to know the factors that increase the risk of being affected by a decline in cognitive function to help prevent them. Aging is the main factor and it often say that it is inevitable. It is true that the passage of time cannot be slowing down, but individuals can play a role in modifying their "biological" age or their metabolic condition. Effectively, aging naturally tends to reduce the cognitive functioning but also worsen the metabolic condition. At advanced age, the prevalence of hypertension, dyslipidemia, inflammation, atherosclerosis and diabetes increase. To prevent these metabolic problems, it is highly documented that the adoption of a healthy lifestyle (physical activities and equilibrate diet) through the lifespan is an efficient way (Colcombe et al., 2003, Peters, 2009.) It turns out that having a bad metabolic condition raises up the risk to develop a cognitive disorder (Frisardi et al., 2010) Peripheral problems and brain disorders are often dissociated but a close relationship exist between these two entities.

Having type II diabetes is associated with the increased risk of developing a cognitive disorder. More than 80% of AD patients have type II diabetes or present an abnormal glucose level. Insulin resistance and hyperinsulinemia, two characteristics of type II diabetes, have been shown to have a high correlation with memory impairment and risk for AD. The rising insulin level that occurs with aging is also a strong predicator of cognitive impairments, in non-diabetics. (Landreth et al., 2008). The Italian Longitudinal study on aging shows that patients with mild cognitive impairment who were also afflict by metabolic syndrome had a higher risk of progression to dementia compared with those without metabolic syndrome. Hypertriglyceridemia was the major component of metabolic syndrome related to dementia (Solfrizzi et al., 2009). Genetic studies and epidemiological observations strongly suggest a relationship between dyslipidemia and AD. Elevated serum cholesterol levels have been reported to correlate with an increased incidence of AD (Landreth et al., 2008). Longitudinal studies have reported that obesity and chronic hypertension are also associated with higher risk of cognitive decline (reviewed in Frisardi et al., 2010).

Then, improvement in those metabolic parameters could modify the individual risk for dementia. Preventive activities during the lifespan are primordial but changing individual behaviour is a long term challenge for the public health. The use of metabolic regulator as a secondary prevention may become essential in individuals at middle age who presents a poor metabolic condition (high blood glucose, deteriorated lipids profile, hypertension, etc.) not only to prevent heart diseases but precisely to delay the first signs of cognitive decline. Given that tertiary prevention of AD dementia which refers to anticholinesterase drugs is known to modestly delay progression of dementia because its probaby too late to correct the existing damage, primary and secondary prevention are essentials (Haan & Wallace 2004) (figure 1).

It is well known that if you want to avoid a pulmonary cancer you should not smoke cigarettes, but the population feels armed less in front of neurodegenerative disorders and should not: progression to dementia can be prevented or modified (Haan et Wallace 2004).

2. PPARα

2.1 Mecanisms, pathways, activators

Peroxisome Proliferator Activated Receptor alpha (PPARα) is a nuclear receptor present in tissues where fatty acids catabolism is at elevated rate, especially in liver but also in heart, kidney, skeletal muscles, enterocytes and astrocytes. This receptor is activated by fatty acids and their derivates and among the synthetic ligands; by compounds of the fibrate family. PPARα regulates gene expression by associating with his ligand in the cytoplasm of cells; the complex then migrates into the nucleus and binds with the 9-cis retinoic acid receptor (RXR). The heterodimer (PPARα/RXR) recognizes specific response elements (peroxisome proliferator response element; PPRE) presents in the promoter regions of genes and binds to activate or repress (figure 2).

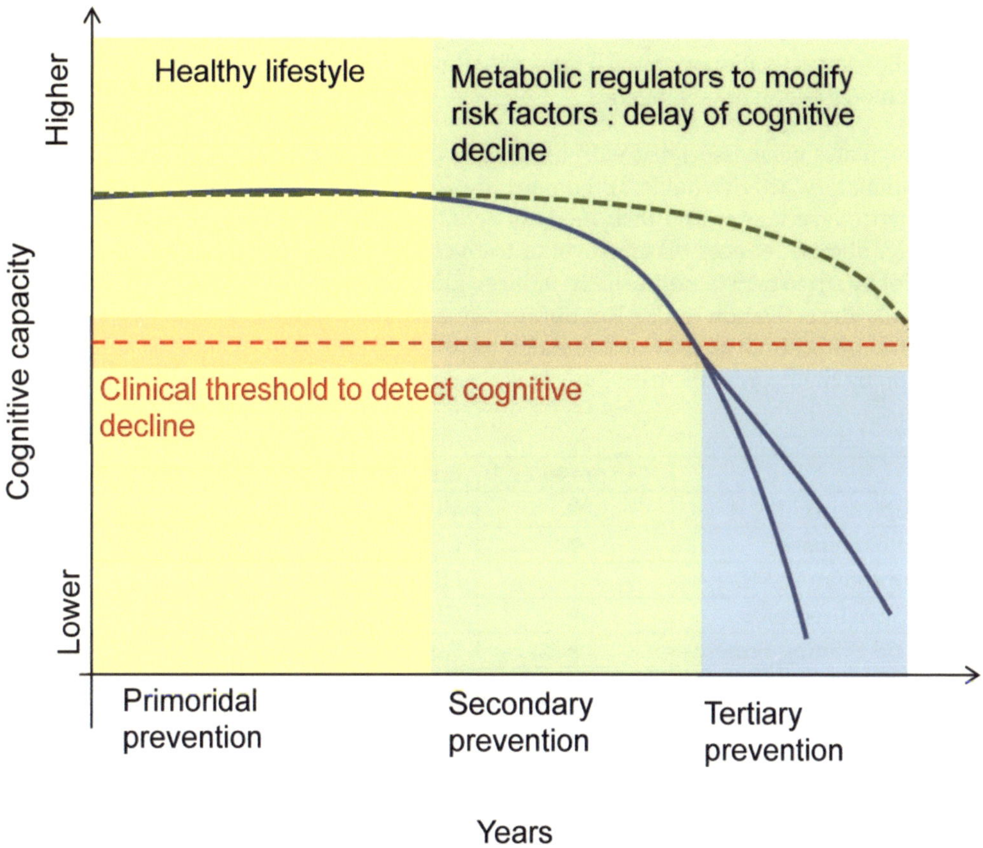

Fig. 1. Schematic cognitive capacity during life. Primordial and secondary preventions, by regulating metabolic condition, may maintain cognitive capacity above the clinical threshold of cognitive decline. Tertiary prevention can modestly help to delays progression of dementia once it is installed. Progression of cognitive capacity in Alzheimer's disease (___) and in cognitively healthy elderly (_ _).

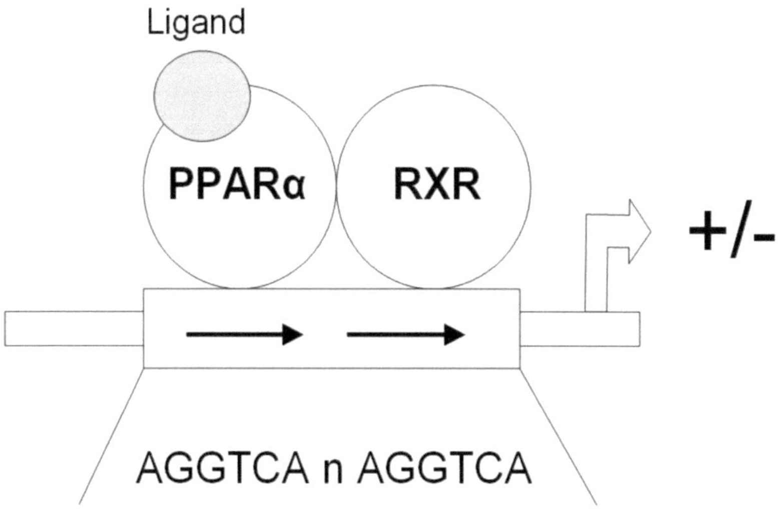

Fig. 2. Following activation with the ligand, PPARα binds a specific DNA sequence (PPRE) in the promoter region of target genes.

PPARα regulates gene associated with lipids, glucose and energy metabolism and exert an anti-inflammatory activity (table 2). Fibrates are first-line drugs used for over 40 years to treat hypertriglyceridemia and their mode of action is entirely via the activation of PPARα. Effectively, fibrates reduces plasma level of triglycerides by 30-50%, slightly increase HDL-cholesterol by up to 5-15 % and usually reduces LDL-cholesterol by 15 to 20% (Chapman et al., 2006). By the activation of PPARα, fibrates are effective to stimulate lipolysis, to increase cellular and mitochondrial fatty acid uptake, to promote fatty acid oxidation, to reduce TG production by the liver, to increase the VLDL clearance and to increase the HDL-cholesterol synthesis.

Genes	Expression	Functions
Apolipoprotein CIII	↓	VLDL clearance inhibition
Lipoprotein Lipase	↑	Lipolysis
Apolipoprotein AI AII	↑	HDL cholesterol synthesis
SR-BI/CLA-1 receptor	↑	Cholesterol efflux
Fatty Acid Binding Protein	↑	Fatty acids entry into the cell
AcylCoA Synthase	↑	Fatty acids entry into the mitochondria
AcetylCoA carboxylase	↓	Fatty acids synthesis
Fibrinogen	↓	Blood clotting
C reactive protein	↓	Inflammation
Interleukin 6	↓	Inflammation
Cyclooxygenase-2	↓	Arachidonic acid metabolism
VCAM-1	↓	Adhesion molecules

Table 2. Target genes regulated by PPARα (Goldenberg et al., 2008). Abbreviations: VLDL: very low density lipoprotein. SR-BI/CLA1: class B scavenger receptor. VCAM-1: vascular cell adhesion molecule 1.

Clofibrate is a first generation fibrate and was used for numerous years before the arrival of the second generation comprising bezafibrate and fenofibrate which are more selective and causes fewer side effects (figure 3). Clofibric acid and fenobibric acid (active metabolites of clofibrate and fenofibrate) activate PPARα and PPARγ but they are 10 times more selective to PPARα. Bezafibrate activates PPARα but can also be linked to PPARγ and PPARδ.

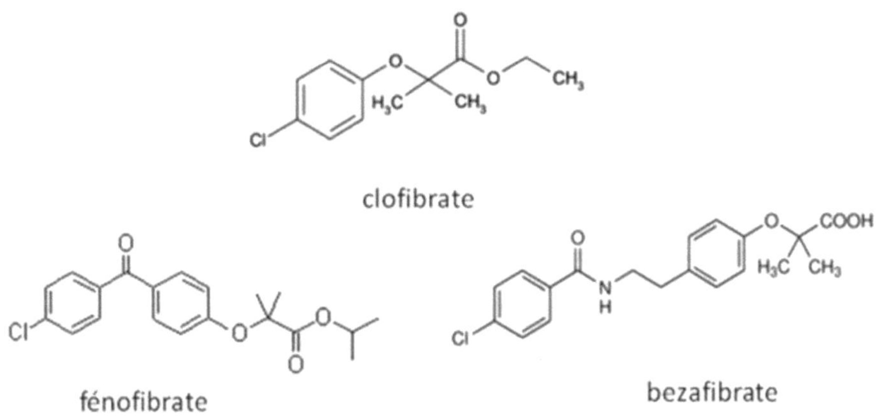

Fig. 3. Structures of clofibrate, fenofibrate and bezafibrate.

2.2 How can PPARα stimulation help cognitive functioning?

The impact of PPARα agonists on cognition was not deeply investigated at a large scale level but some observational studies are interesting. In a large Europeean study (8582 subjects) fibrate use tended ($p=0.07$) to be associated with a reduction in the prevalence of dementia. Dementia included AD (65%), vascular dementia (12%), mixed dementia (11%) and other form of dementia (11.7%). Prevalence of dementia was 1.5% among fibrates user and 2.3% among non-user (Dufouil et al., 2005). In another observational study Rodriguez et al, showed that in a population of 845 individuals, 20.1% of the cohort were demented (based on Clinical dementia Rating) and the proportion of lipid lowering drugs user within the demented population was lower compared to the non-demented (3.5% versus 10.8%) which suggest that lipid lowering drugs may be protective (Rodriguez et al., 2002). In an older study, reducing triglycerides with gemfibrozil (a fibrate) appeared to improve cerebral perfusion and cognitive performance compared to untreated group (Rogers RL et al., 1989). Next sections will focused on how fibrates intake can be protective for the aging brain.

2.3 Insulin resistance

Insulin is produce by the pancreas and control blood glucose level by allowing the transport of glucose molecules from the circulation into cells. Insulin resistance occur when the cells (insulin receptors) are progressively unable to have a proper insulin response resulting in an inadequate entry of glucose in the cells. By a compensatory mechanism, pancreas will secretes more insulin. If the higher amount of insulin is still inefficient to control blood glucose, the person with high insulin and high glucose level will present a situation of pre-diabetes and insulin resistance. Eventually, pancreas will decrease the insulin secretion, consequence of a pancreatic cell stress and damage, and insulin level will gradually drop and glucose will stay high: type II diabetes is then diagnose. If not treated well, diabetic patient will present high circulating glucose level that can causes deleterious effects including cardiovascular disease, kidney disease, nerve damage, retinopathy, etc. This condition will also lead to deficits in cellular energy production, increased oxidative stress and reduced neuronal survival.

For a long period of time, brain glucose metabolism was known to be independent of insulin action since brain glucose transporters (GLUT-1 and GLUT-3) are insensitive to insulin. Recent literature shows that GLUT-4 responds to insulin and that insulin is produce within the brain in various regions especially in the hippocampus which is associated with learning and memory. Insulin receptors are also presents in the brain (de la Monte et al., 2006). Given that brain cells are dependent on a high glucose supply, brain and peripheral insulin may then play an essential role in brain glucose homeostasis.

Evidences showed a physiological link between insulin and cognition. Reports have documented that brain insulin receptor signaling is reduced in AD brain (reviewed in Rupinder K et al., 2011). Production as well as neuronal insulin receptors was also greatly lower in AD brain compared to age-matched controls (Zhu et al., 2005). Interestingly, in AD patients, peripheral administration of insulin improved memory and cognition, reduced brain atrophy and dementia severity (Burns et al., 2007). In an experimental animal model, intracerebral streptozotocine injection was used to deplete brain insulin, but not pancreatic insulin. This brain specific depletion was associated with progressive neurodegeneration with similar features of AD. This same experiment demonstrates that early treatment with PPARα agonist can effectively prevent this experimentally induced neurodegeneration and the related deficits in learning and memory. This same research team also showed that AD is associated with major impairements in insulin gene expression and that abnormality increase with the severity of dementia. They suggest that AD brain may represent a brain specific form of diabetes; type 3 diabetes (de la Monte et al, 2006).

Hyperlipidemia and fatty acids overload (lipotoxicity) contribute to insulin resistance phenomenon (Reviewed in Carpentier, 2008). By their reducing action on triglycerides and their role in enhancement of fatty acids β-oxidation, PPARα activators should improve insulin sensibility. At human level, findings from a study deriving from Bezafibrate Infarction Prevention trial (BIP) suggest that treatment with fibrate reduce the incidence by 30% and delay the onset of type II diabetes. However, there is not a clear consensus regarding the direct impact of fibrate on insulin sensibility, but from studies reviewed, 10 showed an improvement (Tenenbaum et al., 2007, Cree et al., 2007, Kim et al., 2003, Damci et al., 2003, Jonkers et al., 2001, Idzio-Wallus, 2001, Yong et al., 1999, Kobayashi et al., 1988, Murakami et al. 1984, Ferrari et al., 1977) and 6 a reduction in sensibility or no change (Anderlova et al., 2007, Rizos et al., 2002, Whitelaw et al., 2002, Asplund-Carlson, 1996, Sane et al., 1995, Skrha et al., 1994) . In a recent study (2010) bezafibrate treatment for 12 weeks in a mild hypertriglyceridemic population showed a postprandial insulin response 26% lower after bezafibrate, suggesting the beneficial impact of fibrate on insulin sensitivity (figure 4; Tremblay-Mercier et al., 2010). Further clinical studies measuring insulin sensibility are warranted to confirm the real insulin-sensitizing potential of fibrates and the subsequent impact on brain glucose metabolism and further impact on cognition.

2.4 Ketone production

Ketones are the alternative fuel for the brain when glucose availability is low to insure an optimal brain functioning. They are the product of triglycerides lipolysis, β-oxidation of fatty acids and ketogenesis (figure 5). The majoritary of ketones are synthesised in the liver. Studies have shown that astocytes have the capacity to produce ketones from fatty acids and the ketogenic system (Auestad et al. 1991; Guzman & Blazquez, 2001). Acetyl CoA resulting from the β-oxidation of fatty acids, undergo the Krebs cycle but if the metabolic context is favorable for the ketone body formation, acetyl CoA will be redirected in the ketogenesis pathway.

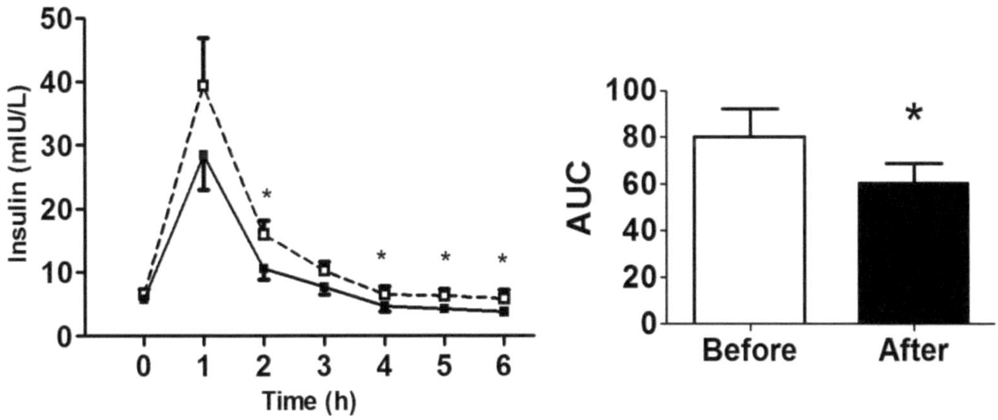

A B

Fig. 4. A) Insulin concentration (mIU/L) during 6 hours. Breakfast was taken between time 0 and time 1 with no further meal. Before (-□-) and after (-■-), 12 weeks on bezafibrate. B) Area under the curve of the insulin curves were lower after bezafibrate treatment. Data are expressed by mean ± SEM. n=12, * p≤0.05. (Adapted from Tremblay-Mercier, 2010)

Under normal conditions (regular meals) ketogenesis is at a low rate (ketone bodies concentration <0.1 mmol/L), because a slight rise in blood glucose and the following increase in insulin concentration inhibits lipolysis and ketogenesis. After their production, β-OHB and acetoacetate will reach skeletal muscles, brain and heart by the systemic circulation to provide energy. Ketones will then be retransformed into acetyl CoA by the reaction called ketolysis (figure 6). Liver cannot use ketones as energetic molecules because the enzyme β-ketoacyl-CoA transferase is not present in the liver, so ketolysis can not occur (figure 6). Ketones pass through the blood brain barrier (BBB) by facilitated transport following the concentration gradient by the monocarboxylate transporter 1 (MCT-1), as well as pyruvate and lactate. The rate of cerebral ketone metabolism depends primarily on the concentration in blood. Cerebral ketone metabolism is also regulated by the permeability of the BBB, which depends on the abundance of MCT-1. An increase in ketone body concentration up regulates the expression of MCT-1 transporter (Leino et al. 2001; Pifferi et al., 2011).

In vitro experiments show that β-OHB protects hippocampal neurons in culture against the toxicity of the protein β-amyloid 1-42, found in the senile plaques in AD patients. This protective effect may be partly due to the fact that the ketone metabolism does not require the action of the enzyme pyruvate dehydrogenase (PDH) which is affected by the toxic effect of β-amyloid protein and essential for the conversion of glucose into energy (Kashiwaya et al., 2000). Rats and human studies also showed that ketones decreased damages associated with free radical (Sullivan et al., 2004)

Ketone production can be stimulated by fasting but also by the administration of a ketogenic diet. This classic ketogenic diet contains a 4:1 ratio by weight of lipids to combined glucose and protein; this high fat intake forces the body to burn fatty acids rather than glucose. The therapeutic ketogenic diet was developed for treatment of pediatric epilepsy refractory to anticonvulsant in the 1920s. This diet is very effective to treat epilepsy in 30-50% of cases but is very hard to apply in a daily basis and causes significant side effects (Cross et al., 2007). Another dietary way to stimulate ketogenesis is by the ingestion of medium chain triglycerides (MCTs), which provokes an acute elevation in ketone body concentration. Those triglycerides are composed of saturated fatty acids from 6 to 12 carbons and are absorbed across the intestinal barrier and directly enter the portal vein. This allows for much quicker absorption and utilization of MCTs compared to long chain triglycerides. MCTs are transported into the mitochondria independent of the carnitine palmitoyltransferase (CPT), which is necessary for the mitochondrial absorption of long chain fatty acids. After a single dose of MCTs, a significant raise (176%) in ketone bodies concentration occur within one hour but rapidly drops to baseline values (within 2 hours) so the effect is transient (Courchesne-Loyer et al., in preparation).

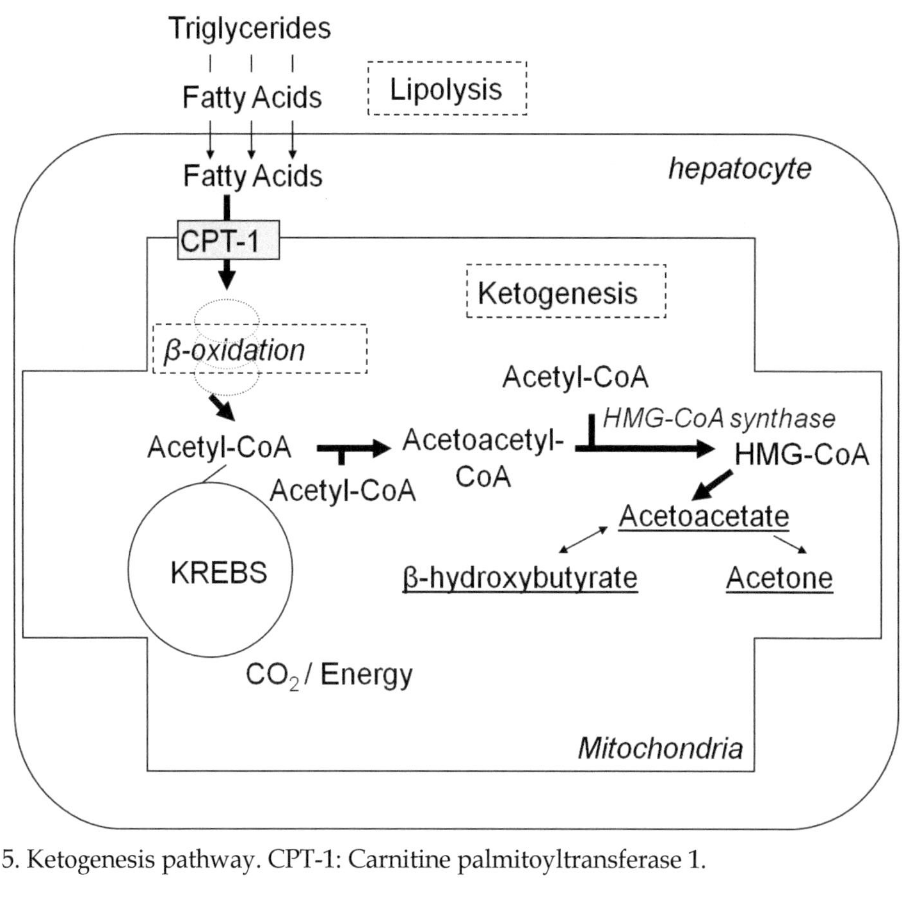

Fig. 5. Ketogenesis pathway. CPT-1: Carnitine palmitoyltransferase 1.

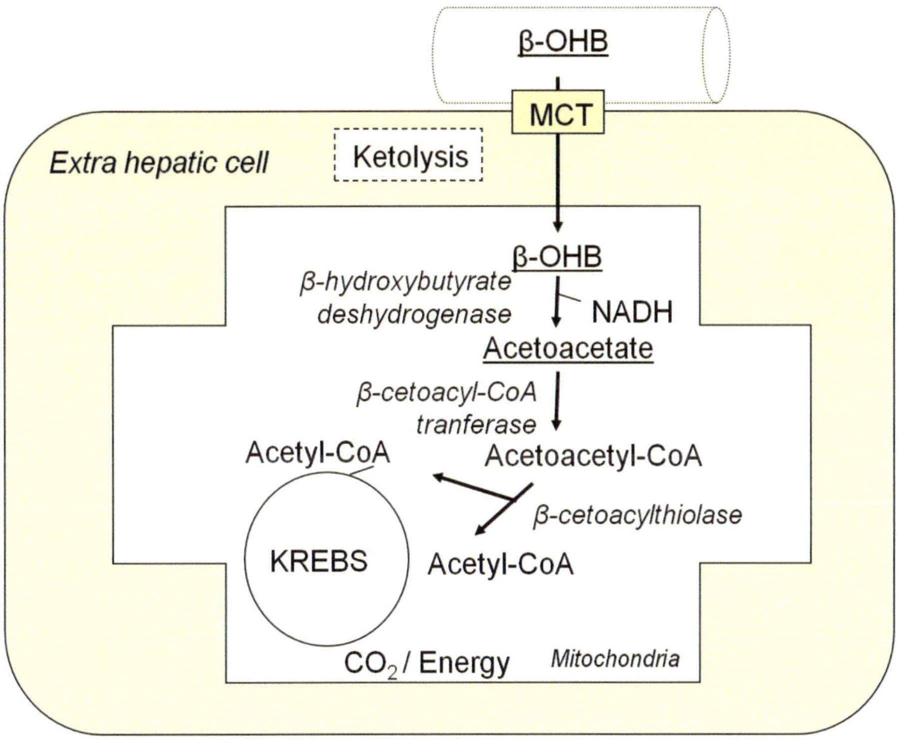

Fig. 6. Ketolysis pathway. β-OHB: β-hydroxybutyrate

Several human studies show that a slight raise in ketones concentration can maintain normal brain function even when plasma glucose would normally be low enough to result in acute cognitive and functional deficits. For example, Page and colleagues in 2009, administered MCTs to type 1 diabetics patient in hypoglycemic crisis and they observed an acute improvement in cognitive functions. Levels of ketones after the ingestion of MCTs were about 0.3-0.4 mM and were sufficient to have an impact on cognitive functioning (Page et al. 2009). Another team showed that a daily supplementation with MCTs for 90 days increased the ketogenic response to 400% and showed a score improvement at different cognitive tests in AD patients (Henderson et al, 2009). In 2004, Reger and colleagues conducted a study with 20 AD patients and showed that high β-OHB concentrations obtained after MCTs administration are positively correlated with ameliorations in the paragraph recall test which is involving memory cognitive function (figure 7).

Ketogenic diet and MCT ingestion, provides low glucose, low insulin environment and/or susbtrates for ketogenesis and are effective in raising ketones concentrations but need a change in eating habits. Another way to increase ketone bodies production without modifying eating habits is to up regulate the enzymes implicated in the pathway. As mentioned earlier fibrate drugs, via PPARα, stimulates the transcription of genes encoding for triglyceride lipolysis and fatty acid β-oxidation. As well, fibrate increase the transcription for the key enzyme in the ketogenesis which is the HMG CoA synthase. This enzyme catalyses the reaction between acetoacetyl CoA and acetyl CoA to form HMG-CoA (figure 4). Few studies on rats have demonstrated an increase in the production of ketone

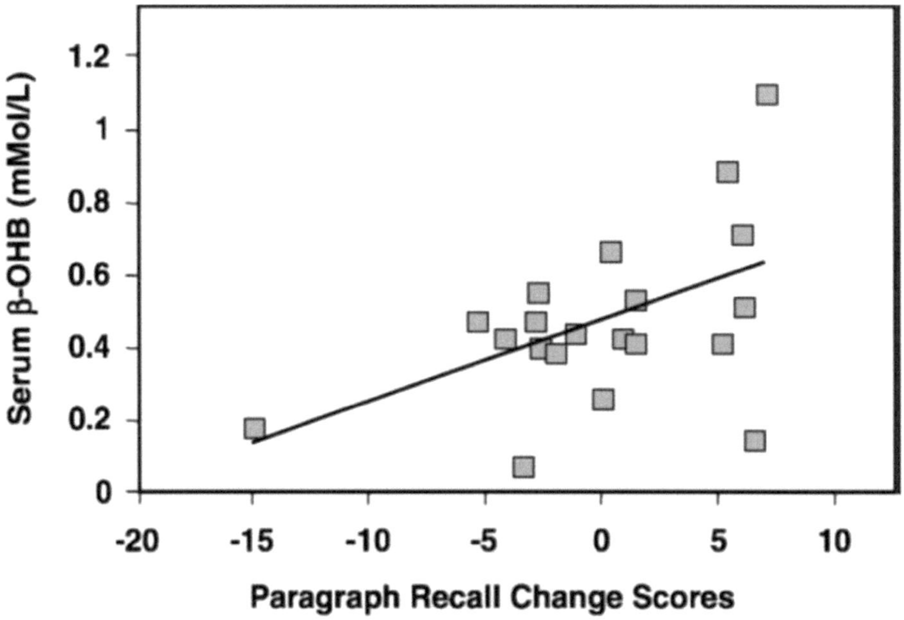

Fig. 7. Relationship between β-hydroxybutyrate (β-OHB) levels at the time of cognitive testing and the change in paragraph recall; $r = 0.50$, $P = 0.02$ (Reger et al., 2004).

bodies by the liver following a fibrate treatment which concord with studies on hepatocytes. In rats treated with clofibrate, PPARα stimulation leads to an upregulation of MCT-1 (König et al., 2008). At the human level the first study to investigate ketone metabolism following a fibrate therapy was done at the Research Center on Aging in Sherbrooke, Quebec, Canada. This study suggests that treatment with bezafibrate has a mild ketogenic potential; postprandial β-OHB response was 58% higher after bezafibrate treatment for 12 weeks. With bezafibrate treatment, the level of ketones (β-OHB) was low during fasting (early in the morning) but was rising during the experimental day to reach 0.3-0.4 mM β-OHB at the end of the day (Tremblay-Mercier et al., 2010). Perhaps in conjunction with a fibrate, joint administration of a dose of MCT, would maintain a moderate level of circulating ketones to insure the delivery to the brain to maintain the energetic homeostasis (Tremblay-Mercier et al., 2010). Preliminary results concerning cerebral ketone metabolism with the tracer ^{11}C-acetoacetate shows that brain ketones uptake is proportional to physiologic plasma ketones concentration as expected by anterior studies (Cunnane et al,. 2011). Further studies with this tracer will help to better understand the impact of fibrate on ketogenesis and the repercussion on brain metabolism in elderly and in cognitively impaired patients.

2.5 Mitochondrial function

Mitochondria are the central organelle in the generation of cellular energy via the Krebs cycle and the electron transport chain. They may be a key players in the cerebral low glucose metabolism observed in AD. Effectively, in the diseased brain, the numbers of neuronal mitochondria are greatly reduced. Several studies have demonstrated aberrations in the electron transport complexes and Krebs cycle in AD (Atamna & Frey, 2007). Mitochondrial perturbations are also seen in normal aging. Those perturbations decrease activities of complex I and IV of the electron transport chain which lead to an elevated reactive oxygen species production. Increased free radicals and peroxidative damage is also seen in AD (Cunnane et al., 2011). Mitchondria dysfunction seems to contribute to the early stage and to the development of various neurodegenerative diseases (Gibson et al., 2010). Numerous studies have suggested that the activation of PPAR may improve mitochondrial functions. PPARγ stimulation is likely to be more effective than PPARα in inducing mitochondrial biogenesis and seems to be effective to potentiate glucose utilization leading to improved cellular and cognitive function (Rupinder et al., 2011). Fibrates are more selective to PPARα but they also have an action on PPARγ. PPARα play a role in the oxidative stress observed in aging. Effectively, level of PPARα correlated negatively with lipid peroxide levels which are actually reduced following a bezafibrate administration (Pineda Torra et al., 1999). Therapeutic strategies targeted at preventing, delaying or treating mitochondrial dysfunction should contribute to the prevention or treatment of age related neurodegeneratives diseases (Atamna & Frey, 2007), and fibrates may be an interesting target to consider.

2.6 Cardiovascular condition /inflammation

There is a close link between cardiovascular condition and cognitive status. High blood pressure, obesity, hyperlipidemia and diabetes are among the principal risk factors for cardiovascular disease. Having those conditions also increase the risk of developing cognitive decline. Vascular risk factors may impair cognitive functions and are related to the occurrence of AD, hypertension and type II diabetes present the strongest association, especially when these factors are assessed in middle age. Atherosclerosis is also believed to be involved in development of dementia, particularly, vascular dementia. Some investigations have shown the importance of inflammation in the pathogenesis of AD, (Akiyama et al., 2000). Hypercholesterolemia, oxidative stress and inflammation have emerged as the dominant mechanism in the development of both atherosclerosis and AD (Steinberg, 2002).Genetic studies and epidemiological observations strongly suggest a relationship between dyslipidemia and AD. Elevated serum cholesterol levels have been reported to correlate with an increased incidence of AD.

Based on its efficiency to reduce plasma triglycerides and to increase HDL cholesterol and it lowering action on LDL-cholesterol, major randomized intervention trials involving fibrate therapy were done to evaluate the drug efficiency to prevent cardiac events. These studies showed that a treatment with a fibrate has beneficial effects by reducing myocardial infarction and coronary event (Goldenberg et al., 2008). The Bezafibrate Infarction Prevention (BIP) trial in 2000 showed that bezafibrate also prevent atherosclerosis and significantly attenuates the risk of long term major cadiovascular events (Tennenbaum et al., 2005). PPARα is also involved in the anti-inflammatory response by his inhibition of NFκB transcription and by decreasing the production of pro-inflammatory IL-6, prostaglandins and C- reactive protein. Fibrates are known to be efficient molecules to prevent cardiovascular disease, knowing that cardiovascular disease and cognitive decline share the same risk factors, preventing cardiovascular disease with fibrate therapy should help preserving cognitive functioning during aging.

3. Conclusions

Fibrates act as synthetic ligands for PPARα and are commonly used to treat hypertriglyceridemia and to prevent coronary heart disease. PPARα is also involved in the anti-inflammatory response and in improvement of mitochondrial function. Fibrate therapy reduces the incidence and delays the onset of type II diabetes and seems to improve insulin sensibility in humans (Goldenberg et al., 2008). A recent clinical study suggests that in hypertriglyceridemic individuals, bezafibrate increase the production of ketone bodies, the alternative energy source for the brain (Tremblay-Mercier et al., 2010). Thus, by reducing triglycerides, enhancing glucose availability, providing alternative brain fuel and improving cardiovascular profile, PPARα agonist could have relevant impact on the maintenance of a good cognitive health later in life (figure 8). Fibrate therapy may have potential as pharmacological agents aiming to reduce the risk of AD and future research are needed to determine if secondary prevention with fibrate therapy is able to delay the apparition of cognitive decline.

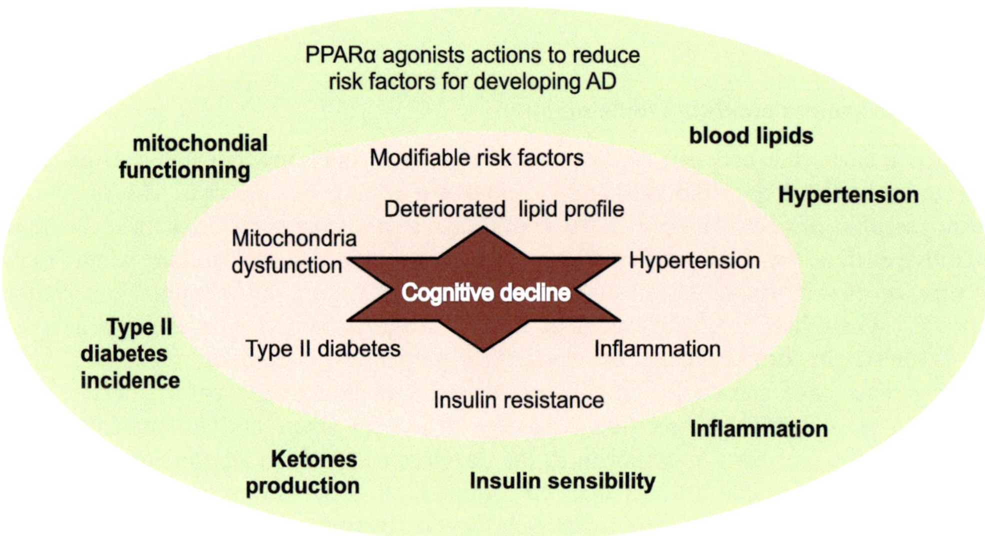

Fig. 8. Summary diagram on the PPARα agonist's action on modifiable risk factors for cognitive decline.

4. Acknowledgment

This chapter was possible because of the collaboration of Stephen Cunnane's laboratory, and was based on this following work:

Tremblay-Mercier, J. (2009) Étude des fibrates en tant qu'agent stimulateurs de la synthèse des cétones, des substrats énergétiques pour le cerveau vieillissant. Master's thesis, the Medecine and Health Science Faculty of Université de Sherbrooke , Sherbrooke, Qc, Canada, 19 January 2009.

Tremblay-Mercier, J., Tessier, D. Plourde, M. Fortier, M. Lorrain, D. Cunnane, S.C. (2010). Bezafibrate mildly stimulates ketogenesis and fatty acid metabolism in hypertriglyceridemic subjects. *J Pharmacol Exp Ther,* Vol. 334 No.1 pp. 341-346.

5. References

Akiyama, H. Barger, S. Barnum, S. (2000) Inflammation and Alzheimer's disease. *Neurobiol Aging,* Vol. 2, No. 3, pp. 383-421.

Anderlova, K. Dolezalova, R. Housova, J. Bosanska, L. Haluzikova, D. Kremen, J. Skrha, J. Haluzik, M. (2007) Influence of PPAR-alpha agonist fenofibrate on insulin sensitivity and selected adipose tissue-derived hormones in obese women with type 2 diabetes. *Physiol Res* Vol. 56 pp. 579-86.

Asplund-Carlson, A. (1996) Effects of gemfibrozil therapy on glucose tolerance, insulin sensitivity and plasma plasminogen activator inhibitor activity in hypertriglyceridaemia. *J Cardiovasc Risk,* Vol.3, pp.385-390.

Atamna, H. Frey, WH. (2007) Mechanism of mitochondrial dysfunction and energy deficiency in Alzheimer's disease. *Mitochondrion,* Vol. 7, pp. 297-310, ISSN 1567-7249

Auestad, N. Korsak, R. A. Morrow, J.W. Edmond J. (1991). Fatty acid oxidation and ketogenesis by astrocytes in primary culture. *J Neurochem,*Vol. 56, No. 4, (April 1991) pp. 1376-1386.

Blennow, K., M. J. de Leon, et al. (2006). Alzheimer's disease, *Lancet,* Vol. 368 No. 9533 (July 2006) pp. 387-403.

Burns, J.M. Donnelly, J.E. Anderson, H.S. Mayo, M.S. Spencer-Gardner, L. Thomas, G. Cronk, B.B. Haddad, Z. Klima, D. Hansen, D. Brooks, W.M. (2007) Peripheral insulin and brain structure in early Alzheimer disease. Neurology, Vol. 969, pp. 1094-1101

Carpentier, A. (2008) Postprandial fatty acid metabolism in the development of lipotoxicity and type 2 diabetes, *Diabetes & Metabolism,* Vol. 34. Pp. 697-107 ISSN 1262-3636

Colcombe, S. Erikson, K. Raz, N. Webb, A.G. Cohen, N.J. McAuley, E. Kramer, A.F. (2003) Aerobic fitness reduces brain tissue loss in ageing humans. *Journal of Gerontology,* Vol. 58, pp. 176-180. Courchesne-Loyer et al., in preparation

Cree, M.G. Newcomer, B.R. Read, L.K. Sheffield-Moore, M. Paddon-Jones, D. Chinkes, D. Aarsland, A. Wolfe, R.R. (2007) Plasma triglycerides are not related to tissue lipids and insulin sensitivity in elderly following PPAR-alpha agonist treatment. *Mech Ageing Dev* Vol.128, pp.558-565.

Cross, H. Ferrie, C. Lascelles, K. Livingstone, J. Mewasingh, L. (2007) Old versus new anti-epileptic drug; the SANAD study. *Lancet,* Vol. 370, pp. 314-16.

Cunnane, S. Nugent, S. Roy, M., Courchesne-Loyer, A. Croteau, E., Tremblay, S. Castellano, A. Pifferi, F. Bocti, C. Paquet, N. Begdouri, H. Bentourkia, M. Turcotte, E. Allard, M. Barbeger-Gateau, P. Fulop, T. Rapoport, S. (2011). Brain fuel metabolism, aging, and Alzheimer's disease. *Nutrition* Vol. 27, No.1, pp. 3-20, ISSN 0899-9007.

D'Alton S.,George D. (2011) Changing perspectives on Alzheimer's Disease: Thinking outside the amyloid Box, *Journal of Alzheimer's Disease,* Vol. 24, (February 2011) pp. 1-11, ISSN 1384-2877.

Damci, T. Tatliagac, S. Osar, Z. Ilkova, H. (2003) Fenofibrate treatment is associated with better glycemic control and lower serum leptin and insulin levels in type 2 diabetic patients with hypertriglyceridemia. *Eur J Intern Med,* Vol.14: 357-360.

de la Monte, S.M. Tong, M. Lester-Coll, N. Plater, M. Jr. Wands, J.R. (2006) Therapeutics rescue of neurodegeneration in experimental type 3 diabetes: relevance to Alzheimer's disease. *Journal of Alzheimers Disease,* Vol. 10, No. 1, pp.89-109.

Dufouil, C. Richard, F. Fievet, N. Dartigues, J. F. Ritchie, K. Tzourio, C. Amouyel, P. Alperovitch, A. (2005) APOE genotype, cholesterol level, lipid-lowering treatment, and dementia: the Three-City Study. *Neurology* Vol. 64, pp.1531-8.

Ferrari, C. Frezzati, S. Romussi, M. Bertazzoni, A. Testori, G.P. Antonini, S. Paracchi, A. (1977) Effects of short-term clofibrate administration on glucose tolerance and insulin secretion in patients with chemical diabetes or hypertriglyceridemia. *Metabolism*, Vol 26, pp. 129-39.

Frisardi, V. Solfrizzi, V. Seripa, D. Capurso, C. Santamato, A. Sancarlo, D. Vendemiale, G. Pilotto, A. Panza, F. (2010) Metabolic-cognitive syndrome: A cross-talk between metabolic syndrome and Alzheimer's disease. *Ageing Research Reviews*, Vol. 9, No. 4 (October 2010) pp.399-417, ISSN 1568-1637.

Gibson, G.E. Starkov, A. Blass, J.P. Ratan, R.R, Beal, M.F. (2010) Cause and consequence: mitochondrial dysfunction initiates and propagates neuronal dysfunction, neural death and behavorial abnormalities in age-associated neurodegenerative diseases, Biochim Biophys Acta, Vol. 1802, pp. 122-34.

Goldenberg, I. Benderly, M. Goldbourt, U. (2008) Update on the use of fibrates: focus on bezafibrate. *Vascular Heath and risk management*. Vol. 4 No. 1 pp. 131-41

Guzman, M. Blazquez, C. (2001) Is there an astrocyte-neurone ketone body shuttle? TRENDS Endocrinology & Metabolism, Vol.12 No. 4 (May/June 2001) pp.169-73.

Haan, M. Wallace, R. (2004) Can dementia be prevented? Brain aging in a population-Based Context, Annu. Rev. Public Health, Vol. 25, pp. 1-24. ISSN 0163-7525.

Henderson, S. T. (2008). Ketone bodies as a therapeutic for Alzheimer's disease. *Neurotherapeutics*, Vol. 5, No. 3, pp. 470-480.

Idzior-Wallus, B, (2001) Fibrate influence on lipids and insulin resistance in patients with metabolic syndrome (In Polish) *Przegl Lek*, Vol. 58 pp. 924-27

Jonkers, I. J. de Man, F. H. van der Laarse, A. Frolich, M.. Gevers Leuven, J. A M. Kamper, A. Blauw G. J. Smelt, A. H. (2001) Bezafibrate reduces heart rate and blood pressure in patients with hypertriglyceridemia. *J Hypertens*, Vol. 19 pp. 749-55

Kashiwaya, Y. Takeshima, T. Nozomi, M. Kenji, N. Kieran, C. Veech, R.L. (2000).D-beta-hydroxybutyrate protects neurons in models of Alzheimer's and Parkinson's disease. *Proc Natl Acad Sci U S A*, Vol. 97 No. 10, (May 2000) pp. 5440-5444.

Kim, H. Haluzik, M. Asghar, Z. Yau, D. Joseph, J.W. Fernandez, A.M. Reitman, M.L. Yakar, S. Stannard, B. Heron-Milhavet,. Wheeler, M.B. Leroith, D. (2003) Peroxisome proliferator activated receptor-α agonist treatment in a transgenic model of type 2 diabetes reverses the lipotoxic state and improves glucose homeostasis. *Diabetes*, Vol. 52, pp. 1770-78.

Kobayashi, M. Shigeta, Y. Hirata, Y . Omori, Y. Sakamoto, N. Nambu, S. Baba, S. (1988) Improvement of glucose tolerance in NIDDM by clofibrate. Randomised double-blind study. *Diabetes Care*, Vol. 11 pp. 495-499.

König, B. Koch, A. Giggel, K. Dordschbal, B. Eder, K. Stangl, G. (2008) Monocarboxylate transporter (MCT)-1 is up-regulated by PPARα. Biochimica et Biophysica Acta, Vol. 1780, pp. 899-904. ISSN 0304-4165

Landreth, G. Jiang, Q. Mandrekar, S. Heneka, M. (2008) PPARγ agonists as therapeutics for the treatement of Alzheimer's disease, *Neurotherapeutic*, Vol. 5 No. 3, pp 481-89.

Leino, R.L. Gerhart, D.Z. Duelli, R. Enerson, B.E. Drewes L.R. (2001) Diet-induced ketosis increases monocarboxylate transporter (MCT1) levels in rat brain. *Neurochem Int* Vol. 38, pp. 519-27.

Murakami, K. Nambu, S. Koh, H. Kobayashi, M. Shigeta, Y. (1984) Clofibrate enhances affinity of insulin receptors in non-insulin dependent diabetes mellitus. *Br J Clin Pharmacol*, Vol. 17, pp. 89-91 et al. 1984

Owen, O.E. Morgan, H.G. Kemp, J.M. Sullivan, M. Herrera, G. Cahill, F. Jr. (1967) Brain metabolism during fastinf . J Clin Invest, Vol. 46, pp. 1589-95.

Page, K. A. Williamson, A. Yu, N. McNay, E.C. Dzuira, J. McCrimmon, R.J. Sherwin, R.S.(2009). Medium-chain fatty acids improve cognitive function in intensively treated type 1 diabetic patients and support in vitro synaptic transmission during acute hypoglycemia. *Diabetes*, Vol. 58 No. 5, pp. 1237-1244.

Pifferi, F. Tremblay, S. Croteau, E. Fortier, M, Tremblay-Mercier, J. Lecomte, R. Cunnane, S.C. (2011) Mild experimental ketosis increases brain uptake of 11C-acetoacetate and 18F-fluorodeoxyglucose: a dual-tracer PET imaging study in rats.*Nutr Neurosci*, Vol. 14, No. 2 (March 2011) pp. 51-8.

Peters, R. (2009). The prevention of dementia. Int. J. Geriatr. Psychiatry. Vol. 24 pp. 452-458.

Reger, M. A. Henderson S. T. Hale, C. Cholerton, B. Baker, L.D. Watson, G.S. Hyde, K. Chapman, D. Craft, S. (2004) Effects of beta-hydroxybutyrate on cognition in memory-impaired adults, *Neurobiol Aging*, Vol.25, No. 3, pp. 311-314.

Reiman, E. M. Chen, K. Alexander, G. E. Caselli, R.. Bandy J. D. Osborne, D. Saunders, A. M. Hardy, J. (2004) Functional brain abnormalities in young adults at genetic risk for late-onset Alzheimer's dementia. *Proc Natl Acad Sci U S A*, Vol. 101, pp. 284-9.

Rizos, E. Kostoula, A. Elisaf, M. Mikhailidis, D.P. (2002) Effect of ciprofibrate on C-reactive protein and fibrinogen levels. *Angiology*, Vol.53, pp. 273-277.

Rodriguez, E.G. Dodge, H.H. Birzescu, M.A. Stoehr, G.P. Ganguli, M. (2002) Use of lipid-lowering drugs in older adults with and without dementia: a community-based epidemiological study. *Journal of American Geriatrics Society*, Vol. 50, No.11 (November 2002) pp. 1852-6.

Rogers, R.L. Meyer, J.S. McClintic, K. Mortel, K.F. (1989) Reducing hypertriglyceridemia in elderly patients with cerebrovascular disease stabilizes or improves cognition and cerebral perfusion. *Angiology*, Vol. 40, pp. 260-9.

Sane, T. Knudsen, P. Vuorinen-Markkola, H. Yki-Jarvinen, H. Taskinen, M.R. (1995) Decreasing triglyceride by gemfibrozil therapy does not affect the glucoregulatory or antilipolytic effect of insulin in nondiabetic subjects with mild hypertriglyceridemia. *Metabolism*, Vol. 44, pp. 589-596.

Škrha, J. Šindelka, G. Haas, T. Hilgertová, J. Justaová, V. (1994) Relation between hypertriacylglycerolemia and the action of insulin in type 2 diabetes mellitus (in Czech). *Čas Lék Česk*, Vol. 133, pp. 496-499.

Snowdon, D.A. (1997) Aging and Alzheimer's disease: lessons from the Nun Study. *Gerontologist*, Vol. 37, No. 2, pp. 150-6.

Solfrizzi, V. Scafato, E. Capurso, C. D'Introno, A. Colacicco, A.M. Frisardi, V. Vendemiale, G. Baldereschi, M. Crepaldi, G. Di Carlo, A. Galluzzo, L. Gandin, C. Inzitari, D. Maggi, S. Capurso, A. Panza, F. for the Italian Longitudinal Study on Aging Working Group(2009). Metabolic syndrom, mild cognitive impairment, and progression to dementia, The Italian Longitudinal Study on Aging. *Neurobiol. Aging*, Vol. 12, 10.106/j.neurobiolaging.2009.12.012.

Steinberg, D. (2002) Atherogenesis in perspective: hypercholesterolemia and inflammation as partners in crime. *Nat Med*, Vol. 8, pp. 1211-7.

Sullivan, P. G. Rippy, N. A, Dorenbos, K. Concepcion, R. C. Agarwal, A. K. Rho, J. M. (2004) The ketogenic diet increases mitochondrial uncoupling protein levels and activity. *Ann Neurol* Vol. 55, pp. 576-80.

Tenenbaum, A. Motro, M. Fisman, E.Z. Tanne, D. Valentina, B. Behar, S. (2005) Bezafibrate for the secondary prevention of myocardial Infarction in patients with metabolic syndrome. *Arch Intern Med*, Vol. 165, pp. 1154-1160.

Tenenbaum, H. Behar, S. Boyko, V. Adler, Y. Fisman, EZ. Tanne, D. Lapidot, M. Schwammenthal, E. Feinberg, M. Matas, Z. Motro, M. Tenenbaum, A. (2007) Longterm effect of bezafibrate on pancreatic beta-cell function and insulin resistance in patients with diabetes. *Atherosclerosis*, Vol. 194 pp. 265-271.

Pineda-Torra, I. Gervois, P. Staels, B. (1999) Peroxisome proliferator-activated receptor alpha in metabolic disease, inflammation, atherosclerosis and aging. *Curr Opin Lipidol*, Vol. 10, No. 2, pp. 151-159.

Tremblay-Mercier, J., Tessier, D. Plourde, M. Fortier, M. Lorrain, D. Cunnane, S.C. (2010). Bezafibrate mildly stimulates ketogenesis and fatty acid metabolism in hypertriglyceridemic subjects. *J Pharmacol Exp Ther*, Vol. 334 No.1 pp. 341-346

Veech, R. L. Chance, B. Kashiwaya, Y. Lardy, H.A.Cahill, F.Jr. (2001). Ketone bodies, potential therapeutic uses. *IUBMB Life* Vol. 51, No. 4, pp. 241-47. ISSN 1521-6543.

Yong, Q.W. Thavintharan, S. Cheng, A, Chew, L.S. (1999) The effect of fenofibrate on insulin sensitivity and plasma lipids profile in non-diabetic males with low high density lipoprotein/dyslipidaemic syndrome. *Ann Acad Med Singapore*. Vol. 28, pp. 778-782.

Whitehouse P.J, George, D., (2008) *The Myth of Alzheimer's: What You Aren't Being Told About Today's Lost Dreaded Diagnosis*, (Solal) St Martin's press, ISBN 978-2-35327-080-4, New York, USA.

Whitelaw, D.C. Smith, J.M. Nattrass, M. (2002) Effects of gemfibrozil on insulin resistance to fat metabolism in subjects with type 2 diabetes and hypertriglyceridaemia. *Diabetes Obes Metab*, Vol. 4, pp. 187-194.

Zhu, X. Perry, G. Smith, M.A. (2005) Insulin signaling, diabetes mellitus, and risk of Alzheimer's disease: a population based study of the oldest old. *Int Psychogeriatr*, Vol. 14, pp. 239-48.

Part 2

Experimental Study

7

The Influence of Cyclophosphamide on Immune Function of Murine Macrophages

Krzysztof Bryniarski
Jagiellonian University Medical College, Department of Immunology, Krakow, Poland

1. Introduction

1.1 The structure of cyclophosphamide (CY) and its active metabolites acrolein (ACR) and phosphoramide mustard (PM)

Cyclophosphamide (CY), an alkylating compound is commonly used as a cytoreductive agent in the treatment of cancer (blood, breast, ovary) because of its ability to interfere with DNA synthesis and its pharmacological action on dividing cells (Ben Efraim 2001). Its action is however more complex since it exerts a strong influence on the immune system. Studies on cyclophosphamide are conducted for a long time, but its effect on macrophages (Mf) was not yet definite, therefore this study was attempted.

CY is *in vitro* inactive by itself, and is converted *in vivo* into two ultimately biologically active alkylating metabolites: phosphoramide mustard (PM) and acrolein (ACR).The first step of that complicated pathway of CY metabolism occurs in the liver and results in the formation of derivative hydroperoxycyclophosphamide and then it is followed by several enzymatic reactions that format carbonamide, aldehyde and carboxylacide inactive structures or lead to non-enzymatic formation of phosphoramide mustard and acrolein, active metabolites of cyclophosphamide which were tested in our immune research. Instead of highly unstable phosphoramide mustard (PM), we used nitrogen mustard (NM, mechlorethamine) (see **Fig 1**.) which is structurally and functionally related to PM, previously shown *in vitro* and *in vivo* to have the same activity as CY (Bryniarski et al. 1996).

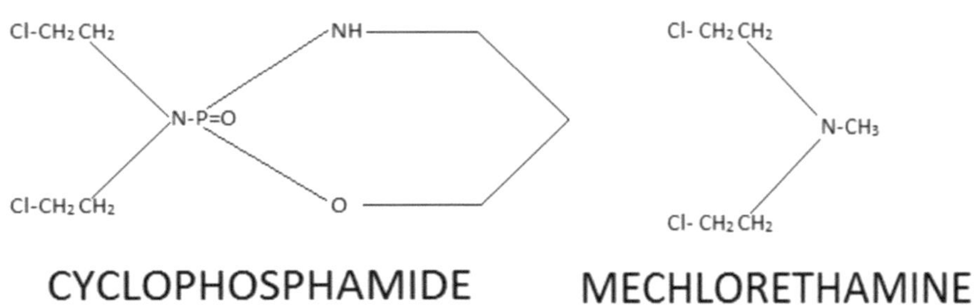

Fig. 1. The chemical structure of cyclophosphamide and nitrogen mustard

2. Differences of CY dose treatment used in the treatment of malignant diseases and autoimmune diseases in comparison to immune regulation

Immunoregulatory function of CY is observed in doses 20-100 mg/kg in mice, which can be calculated in human treatment as below 2mg/kg (less than 100 mg/m^2). The higher doses of cyclophosphamide above 100mg/m^2 (2-3mg/kg) in humans mainly used in several pulses or as prolonged treatments are used in anticancer therapy of peripheral blood cancers and lymphoma (Audia et al. 2007; Vitolo et al. 2008) as well as in metastases of breast, ovarian and bronchial cancers (Snowden et al. 1997; Audia et al. 2007; Burger 2007) trophoblastic tumors (Cole et al. 2008), leiomyosarcoma (Durhan et al. 2009), pheochromocytoma (Adjalle et al. 2009), rhabdomyosarcoma (Breitfeld & Mayer 2005).

Much higher doses of CY (50mg/kg per 3 days) are proposed to be used in treatment of Graft Versus Host Disease (GVHD) after allogenic hematopoetic stem cells transplantation (alloHSCT) for treatment of hematologic malignancies (Luznik & Fuchs 2010). Post-transplantation CY promotes tolerance in alloreactive host and donor T cells leading to suppression of both graft rejection and GVHD after alloHSCT.

In autoimmune diseases like sclerosis multiplex (MS), lupus nephritis or immune mediated neuropathies, CY is the medicament used for pulsed first treatment as well for the retreatment in several doses mainly higher than 100 up to 1600 mg/m^2. It is proved that CY treatment seems to give better therapeutic effect in patients in earlier stages of MS where inflammation predominates over degenerative processes in the central nervous system (CNS). There is no evidence of efficacy in primary progressive MS or later stages of secondary progressive MS. In these high doses of CY therapy, patients show low pro-inflammatory cytokine secretion which activates anti-inflammatory cytokine secretion, what is suggested in an elegant review by Weiner and Cohen as one of curative effects in MS neurodegenerative disease (Weiner & Cohen 2002). That high dose treatment can express quite a different suppressor effect on the immune system mediated by B and T lymphocytes that mediate two branches of humoral and cellular immune responses. High doses of CY used for the treatment of malignant or autoimmune diseases express more toxic effects on the immune system by elimination of different currently activated subpopulations of immune cells and lead to inhibition of inflammatory reactions which diminish the formation of degenerative lesions.

Cyclophosphamide is commonly used in multiagent chemotherapy rather than intravenous (i.v.) monotherapy for treatment of malignancies, therefore its dose can be relatively lesser than in case of single use (because of the effect of summarizing or multiplying of drug activity and toxicity). It also must be taken into consideration what kind of regulatory therapeutic effect is desired - the activating effect based on elimination of natural suppression in case of low doses treatment, or suppressor effect on the immune cells, maintained mainly by cytotoxic effect which appears in case of treatment with high doses of CY. It is estimated that the therapeutic dose of endoxan equals about 25-50% of toxic dose. The control of unwanted and unexpected toxic effects must be also taken into consideration in case of establishing any kind of CY therapy. Between the most frequent unwanted toxic effects observed in case of CY treatment is gonadal disfunction observed in man in a lower cumulative dose in man (60 g/m^2) less expressed in female (Vitolo et al. 2008). Moreover, apart from alopecia and nausea, the other toxic effects are infections and hemorrhagic cystitis. There is also an increased risk of cancer and bladder toxicity which appears in the cumulative life-time dose exceeding 80-100 g (which is about 50 doses of 1000 mg/m^2 during life-time) (Weinar & Cohen 2002) .

3. Immunoregulatory activities of cyclophosphamide treatment – The evidence performed in mice by the low dose cyclophosphamide treated macrophages

Macrophages (Mf) carry out the fundamental protective function of phagocyting and killing invading organisms and release a vast number of factors involved in host defense and inflammation. Moreover they play a critical role in the induction, regulation and expression of both cellular and humoral responses. These highly diversified functions are accompanied by heterogeneous morphology and biochemical and phenotypical characteristics.

3.1 Methods for estimation of macrophage activity in innate and in adaptive humoral and cellular immune responses

My experimental studies were aimed at the establishing the influence of low dose of CY treatment (20-50 mg/kg) on the macrophages (Mf) - the important cells involved in an innate and humoral or cellular adaptive immune responses in mice. The innate immune response was measured by both the capacity of reactive oxygen intermediates production and secretion by phagocytic activating macrophages and by the ability of production of proinflammatory cytokines (IL-1β, IL-6 and TNF-α) (Marcinkiewicz et al. 1994). The ability of cyclophosphamide treated Mf (MfCY) to secrete regulatory cytokine (proinflammatory IL-12 and inhibitory TGF-β and IL-10) was also tested in their supernatant over the Mf culture and was estimated by ELISA (total concentration) (Bryniarski 2004 & 2009), or in bioassays which utilize proliferation effect of particular cytokine by cytokine-dependent cell lines and measures exclusively bioactive form of particular cytokine (Marcinkiewicz et al. 1994 & Bryniarski et al. 1996). The cell surface markers of tested Mf were estimated cytofluorimetrically in FACS (Szczepanik et al. 1993 & Bryniarski et al. 2009), but the phenotypical differences between functionally differentiated macrophages were estimated by measuring the pattern of esterase activity (Czajkowska et al. 1995).

The induction of cellular response was tested in contact hypersensitivity against TNP/PCL hapten (Szczepanik et al. 1993, Bryniarski et al. 2004) which activates CD4 Th1 subpopulation of lymphocytes and macrophages and is classified by Pichler as a classical type IVa delayed type hypersensitivity (Lerch & Pichler 2004; Posadas & Pichler 2007). Humoral activity against corpuscular antigen was tested in plaque forming assay (PFA) from Mf pulsed with sheep red blood cells and cultured 4 days in the presence of naïve B cells. The antigen presenting activity was estimated as a number of plaque forming cells PFC/10^6 splenocytes (Bryniarski et al. 2004).

3.2 Treatment of donors of macrophages with low dose of CY uncovers the subpopulation of peritoneal macrophages that induce CHS response in mice

Application of hapten on the skin is a classical way to immunize for contact sensitivity reaction, but animals can also be sensitized by subcutaneous injection of hapten substituted peritoneal macrophages. However, if haptenated macrophages are injected i.v. a long-lasting unresponsiveness ensues, in which the activity of Th1 immune effector lymphocytes is obliterated by simultaneously recruited CD8⁺suppressor cells. When subsequently skin sensitized, such animals have significantly diminished CHS reactions. Moreover this state of unresponsiveness can be adoptively transferred to naïve syngeneic animals by lymphoid cells.

The CHS reaction to trinitrophenyl (TNP/PCL) hapten is activated by CD4 Th1 lymphocytes which recognize TNP/PCL hapten on the surface of MHC class II expressed by hapten-labeled macrophages. After 5 days the sensitized recipients of TNP-Mf are able to reduce the CHS reaction when challenged by applying a very low dose of the same hapten (TNP/PCL) on the ear skin. The CHS reaction develops 24 h after challenge (with hapten) as ear swelling CHS response and is measured with the engineering micrometer and expressed in units of ear swelling (Szczepanik et al. 1993). When the donors of macrophages are injected intravenously (i.v.) with low dose of cyclophosphamide (20-100mg/kg) a day before cell harvesting, then the cells are labeled with hapten and injected i.v. into naïve recipients instead of unresponsiveness strong contact hypersensitivity develops 24 h after the challenge with the same hapten. Moreover it was shown that in vivo CY treatment activates strong functional diversification of macrophage subpopulations in mice. Thus result of in vivo CY treatment, hapten-conjugated Mf (TNP-MfCY) when injected i.v. into naïve recipients TNP-MfCY activate strong contact hypersensitivity (CHS) reaction against hapten, instead of unresponsiveness induced by TNP-Mf mediated by $CD8^+$ T suppressor lymphocytes, which inhibit hapten specific CHS response (**Fig. 2**).

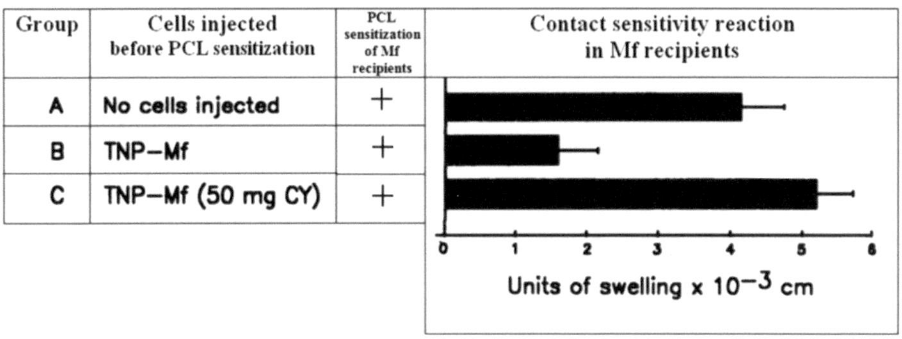

CBA/J mice were injected i.v. with 1 x 10^6 TNP-Mf from donors treated (group C) or untreated (group B) with CY. Seven days later these animals and a group of naïve mice (group A) were skin sensitized with PCL and tested for contact hypersensitivity (CHS) after additional 4 days. Statistical significance group B ve groups A & C $p<0.002$

Fig. 2. Peritoneal macrophages from cyclophosphamide-treated mice do not induce suppressor cells.

It was shown by us that CY sensitive subpopulation of peritoneal macrophages responsible for induction of suppressor cells has higher density when separated in discontinuous gradient of Ficoll than population activating CHS response. Moreover it has also strong adherent and higher phagocyting properties and has high expression of FcγRI and FcγRII (33-44%) in comparison to the low density cell fraction, which is CY resistant. The latest fraction of cells is weakly phagocytic and adherent, has less FcγR (22-26%). It is widely known that antigen presenting cells (APC) are macrophages, dendritic cells and B lymphocytes. First two populations can phagocyte, but last is inactive in this activity. For two reasons it seems unlikely that previously described light fraction of cells are contaminated with dendritic cells.

First almost all of them labeled with macrophage specific F4/80 antibody, second, as shown previously by Steinman and Cohn peritoneal exudate cells induced by thioglycolate, although contaminated by several cell types do not contain dendritic cells (Szczepanik et al. 1993). Both subpopulations of tested macrophages express no significant differences in Mac-1 (30-50%) and Mac-3 (33-46%) markers and no differences were found between CY-treated and untreated mice in a surface expression of I-A (7-14%) and I-E (3-6%) antigens. We were not able to associate the differences in surface markers expression in both populations of macrophages with variety of their bioactivity and immune function (Szczepanik et al. 1993). We also found that Mf CY express slightly higher percentage of molecules important in the stimulation of phagocytosis (CD14 and CD23) and molecules basic for activation of antigen-presenting immune response (CD80/CD86 and MHC class II) in comparison to control oil-induced peritoneal macrophages. Results are shown in **Table 1**.

Macrophages	CD23/Mac3	CD80/Mac3	CD86/Mac3	CD14/Mac3	DR/Mac3
Mf	62.0	50.0	51.6	59.3	45.4
Mf CY [50mg/kg]	73.7	68.4	71.6	71.7	59.0

Oil-induced macrophages were labeled for direct immunofluorescence with monoclonal antibodies specific against specific macrophage antigen (Mac3-FITC) and cell surface markers (CD23-PE, CD80-PE, CD86-PE, CD14-PE, MHCII DR-PE). Results are expressed as a percent of double positive cells. The measurement was performed on the FASC Cytoron-Absolute.

Table 1. Expression of selected surface markers on macrophages isolated from oil-induced peritoneal cavity from donors treated or not treated with cyclophosphamide in dose 50 mg/kg.

In following experiment we have shown (Bryniarski et al. 2009) that cyclophosphamide in vivo as well as its both tested metabolic products in vitro - acrolein (ACR) and mechloretamine (NM) (nitrogen mustard – an analogue of phosphoramide mustard) make TNP-substituted Mf (TNP-Mf) immunogenic for the induction of CHS response. The results are shown in **Table 2**.

Group	Mice injected with	CHS response [U x 10^{-2} mm] ± SD
A	TNP-Mf	0.2 ± 0.84
B	TNP-Mf CY	4.8 ± 0.68
C	TNP-Mf ACR	5.3 ± 1.12
D	TNP-Mf NM	5.2 ± 0.66
E	TNP-Mf ACR & NM	5.5 ± 0.90

The following abbreviations are used: TNP-Mf - TNP substituted Mf from control mice; TNP-Mf CY - Mf from mice treated with CY (50 mg/kg); TNP-Mf ACR – normal Mf treated in vitro with 10^{-7} M ACR; TNP-Mf NM - normal Mf treated in vitro with 10^{-7} M ACR; TNP-Mf ACR & NM - Mf treated with both metabolites.

CBA/J mice were injected i.v. with $1x10^6$ TNP-substituted Mf . Seven days after TNP-Mf injection the mice were tested for CHS reaction which is expressed in units x 10^{-2} mm ± SD. The negative values (ear swelling in control, unimmunized mice) were substracted from experimental values. The statistical significance (a posteriori Bonferroni test): Group A vs. Groups B, C, D, E $p<0.001$. Each group consisted of five mice.

Table 2. Immunognecity of oil-induced peritoneal macrophages untreated or treated in vivo with 50 mg/kg CY or in vitro with acrolein (ACR) or mechloretamine (NM).

3.3 The phenotypical differences between functionally differentiated macrophages estimation of activity IL-6 and a heterogeneity of α- and β- naphtyl acetate esterase isoenzymes

Some differences were shown when a population of different immune functions were tested by unspecific esterase activity, which is regarded to play a role in intracellular processing and trafficking of antigen (Czajkowska et al. 1995). In these experimental works we tested two different, but phenotypically indistinguishable macrophage clones 59 and 63 obtained from Martin Dorf and coworkers from Harvard University, Boston, MA. Both are adherent and phagocytic, produce IL-1 and IL-6 and constitutively express a number of identical cell surface markers, including Ia. However they differ functionally and while clone 59 presents antigen to Th1 lymphocytes, clone 63 induces suppressor T lymphocytes. These obvious functional differences in antigen presenting capacities between the seemingly phenotypically identical cell lines were identified by us in testing them for activity of nonspecific α- and β- naphtyl acetate esterase isoenzymes and secretion of IL-6 in case of cell lines stimulated with mechloretamine (NM)– the alkylating agent relating to cyclophosphamide. The isoenzymatic patterns of α-esterase express strong differences in line 59 treated with MN in comparison to background non-activated cells. In line 59, NM treatment increases the heterogeneity and activity of esterase in both pH 7.5 and pH 5.8. In contrast to line 59 no differences in the isoenzymatic pattern of α–esterase in NM-treated and untreated 63 line cells were found. The β-esterase activity was also tested but no significant differences were found between untreated and MN-treated cell lines.

The results in **Table 3** show that CHS inducing clone 59 produces little IL-6 and NM does not activate its production in comparison to basal activity. In contrary clone 63 is a high producer of IL-6 and stimulated by NM.

Groups	Clone 59 IL-6 [ng/mL] X ± SD	Clone 63 IL-6 [ng/mL] X ± SD
Mf	62 ± 9.6	111 ± 9.3
Mf & NM 10^{-6} M	27 ± 4.3	358 ± 3.1
Mf & NM 10^{-8} M	35 ± 4.7	226 ± 1.5
Mf & NM 10^{-10} M	21 ± 5.5	209 ± 2.1

$2x10^7$ Mf were treated with NM at concentrations from 10^{-10} to 10^{-6} M for 40 min at 0^0C then thoroughly washed out from NM with phosphate buffered saline (PBS). Cells cultured in RPMI 1640 medium supplemented with 5% fetal calf serum (FCS) at concentration 10^6 Mf per mL in 24 wells flat bottom plates at 37^0C at 5% CO_2. The concentration of IL-6 was estimated in bioassay with B9 cell line with (data not shown, but all results were estimated less than 2ng/mL) or without mAb anti-IL-6 and expressed in ng/mL.

Table 3. The production of IL-6 by Mf cell line 59 and 63 treated with different concentration of nitrogen mustard

Our experiments show that two macrophage lines differ in isoenzyme patterns such that α and β esterases of line 59 which induces immunity, are more heterogeneous than esterase of line 63, which induces suppression. Both cell lines, when non activated with NM however produce comparable amounts of IL-6 (Czajkowska et al. 1995). We have shown previously the peritoneal macrophages (Bryniarski et al. 1996), like line 63 cells, when tagged with the antigen, induce T suppressor cells, however, when treated with NM, a pharmacological derivative of cyclophosphamide, produce high amounts of IL-6, also change their functional (suppressive) properties to activation the hapten specific CHS immune response (Bryniarski et al. 2009).

It was also shown that NM, changed the isoenzyme pattern in line 59, which was accompanied by somewhat decreased production of IL-6, while esterases of line 63 were not affected by NM, which however activated the production of IL-6. NM, like other alkylating factors, binds covalently and non-selectively to variety of molecules including amino acids, proteins and DNA. Since the Mf were incubated with NM at 0^{0}C the possibility of its intracellular penetration was negligible and we presume that under such condition NM binds mainly to cell surface proteins. We suggested that the translation of intracellular membrane signal acts in a different way, which can result in a different production of IL-6 by line 59 and 63 cells and their isoenzyme patterns after NM stimulation (Czajkowska et al. 1995).

3.4 Proinflammatory cytokine secretion by functionally different subpopulation of Mf treated with CY or its derivatives ACR or NM

CY influence on the cytokine releasing activity by the functionally different subpopulation of macrophages was examined by Marcinkiewicz and Bryniarski (Marcinkiewicz et al. 1994 and Bryniarski et al. 1996 & 2009). They have shown that low dose of CY treatment activates Mf to production and secretion of mainly IL-6 while simultaneously diminish TNF-α and IL-1β production (Marcinkiewicz et al. 1994). The strong activation of IL-6 production was observed in case of peritoneal macrophage stimulation with mechloretamine (NM) the analogue of nitrogen mustard (Bryniarski et al. 1996). This is a common phenomenon which is observed in NM-treated oil-induced and thioglycolate peritoneal macrophages obtained from different mouse strains (CBA/J, Balb c, C57/BL6 and SWISS) and tested in bioassay with IL-6 dependent B9 cells as well as in IL-6 ELISA assay (Bryniarski et al. 1996 & 2009).

3.4.1 Production of cytokines by control Mf or Mf from animals treated *in vivo* with CY or Mf treated *in vitro* by its metabolites

Control Mf or Mf from CY-treated animals (50 mg/kg) or Mf incubated *in vitro* with ACR (10^{-7} M) or NM (10^{-6} M) were cultured for 24 or 48 h in RPMI 1640 medium and the production of five different cytokines was measured in the resultant supernatants by ELISA. These results are shown in **Table 4**. Mf from CY treated animals (Group B) and Mf treated *in vitro* with NM (Group D) showed an increased production of pro-inflammatory IL-6 and IL-12, and a decreased production of anti-inflammatory IL-10 and TGF-β cytokines compared to the control group (Group A). Mf treated with ACR (Group C) manufactured more IL-6 and less TGF-β than control cells (Group A), but the production of IL-12 remained unchanged. Treatment with CY or its derivatives did not influence TNF-α production although in Group B, there it was somewhat lower than in the control group.

Cell cultured		Cytokine production [pg/ml]				
		TNF-α	IL-6	IL-10	IL-12	TGF-β
A	Mf	250 ± 5	283 ± 7	61 ± 3	213 ± 3	109 ± 2
B	Mf CY [50 mg/kg]	182 ± 4	467 ± 4	22 ± 4	455 ± 14	50 ± 4
C	Mf ACR [10^{-6} M]	287 ± 21	982 ± 25	33 ± 2	167 ± 10	33 ± 3
D	Mf NM [10^{-7} M]	245 ± 30	1500 ± 100	47 ± 4	460 ± 28	59 ± 17

Five x10^5 control Mf or cells from cyclophosphamide-treated animals (Mf CY) or Mf treated with acrolein (Mf ACR) or nitrogen mustard (Mf NM) *in vitro* (for details see legend to Table 3) were cultured in 1 ml of RPMI 1640 medium supplemented with 5% FCS for 24h (TNF-α and IL-6) or 48h (other cytokines) and concentrations of cytokines were measured by ELISA assays. Table 2 shows the results of one representative experiment out of three as the mean of three estimations ± SD.

Table 4. Cytokine production by macrophages (Mf) from naïve mice, or animals treated with cyclophosphamide (CY) *in vivo* or acrolein (Mf ACR) or nitrogen mustard (Mf NM) *in vitro*.

3.4.2 High tolerogenicity of TNP-Mf *in vivo* can be reversed by administration into recipients of anti-IL-10 and/or anti-TGF-β mAbs

Since inefficient immunogenicity of administered intravenously control TNP-Mf as compared with CY-treated cells may be due to the different cytokine sets that they produce, we injected these cells into recipients that simultaneously received an *i.v.* injection of 500 µg of anti-IL-10, anti-TGF-β or a mixture of both antibodies. The CHS reaction was measured 7 days later. **Figure 3** shows that TNP-Mf

Group	Treatment of recipients with monoclonal antibody		Cyclophosphamide treatment of donors of Mf
	mAb αIL-10	mAb αTGF-β	
A	–	–	–
B	–	–	+
C	+	–	–
D	–	+	–
E	+	–	+
F	+	+	–
G	+	+	+

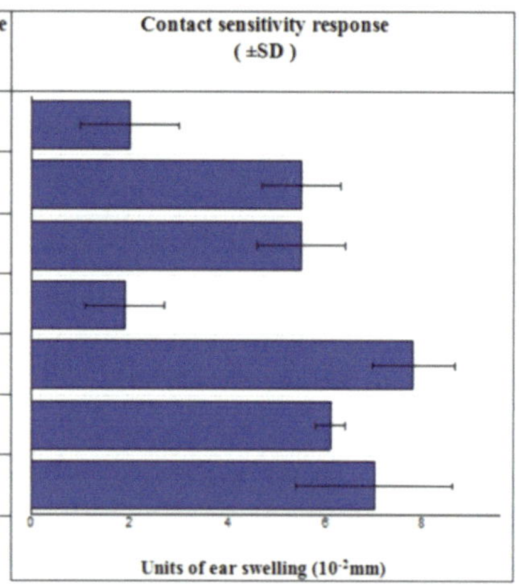

CBA/J mice were injected i.v. with 1x10^6 TNP substituted Mf (groups A, C, D and F) or TNP-Mf CY (groups B, E, G). In the groups C and E the mice simultaneously received i.v. 500 µg of anti-IL-10 mAb and in group D, 500 µg anti-TGFβ mAb, and in groups F & G both mAbs were given. Seven days later the CHS response was measured (see legend to Table 2). Statistiacally significant (a posteriori Bonferroni test) Group A ve groups B, C and F $p<0.002$; group A ve groups E and G $p<0.001$; Group B ve groups C, F and G →NS; group B ve D $p<0.02$

Fig. 3. Tolerance induced by intravenous injection of TNP-Mf can be reversed by simultaneous administration of anti-IL-10 and/or anti-TGF-β mAbs. Comparison with in vivo CY treatment (50 mg/kg) of TNP-Mf (TNP-Mf CY) combined with administration with mAbs anti-IL10 or/and anti-TGF-β.

obtained from naïve donors were non-immunogenic (Group A) but from CY-treated donors (Group B) induced CHS response, while animals treated with anti-IL-10 alone (Group C & E) or together with anti-TGF-β (Group F & G) from both donors produced a significant CHS reaction. Anti-TGF-β alone (Group D) had no influence on the level of the CS reaction.

3.5 Production of the reactive oxygen intermediates by Mf CY or macrophages treated with low doses of ACR or NM

The testing of innate immune response mediated by macrophages can be estimated by reactive oxygen intermediates (ROI's) production. We use the luminol-dependent chemiluminescence as a measure of activity in Mf stimulated by opsonized zymosan particles. **Figure 4** shows that Mf from animals treated with 20 or 50 mg/kg of CY produce a significantly increased level of ROI's while the dose of 100 mg/kg remains without effect and 200 mg/kg diminished the production of ROI's below the control level. A marked increase of ROI's level was induced by in vitro incubation Mf in a low concentration of NM (10^{-7} or 10^{-6} M) while 10^{-5} M had a slightly inhibitory effect. ACR at concentration 10^{-7} M and 10^{-6} M had no effect when compared with control Mf, whereas 10^{-5} M was inhibitory.

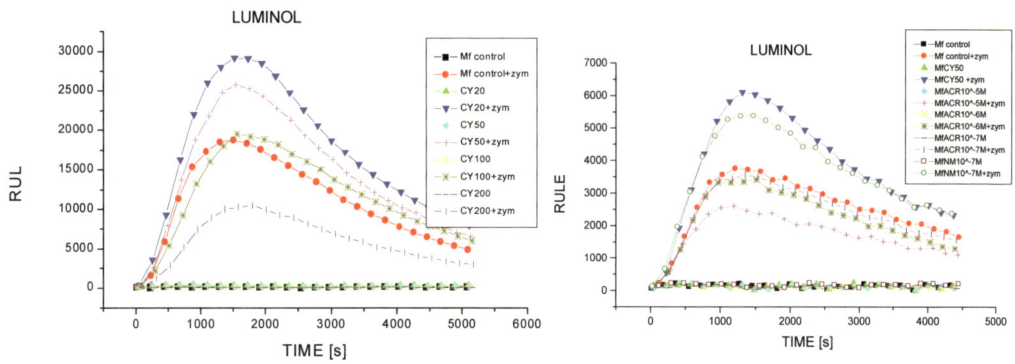

Production of reactive oxygen intermediates (ROI's) by macrophages is dependent upon the dose of cyclophosphamide (CY) used to treat donors. The highest activity is observed with doses 20-50 mg/kg. The higher dose of CY (200 mg/kg) decreases ROI's production by Mf in comparison with control cells (Mf). The low concentration of nitrogen mustard (NM) used to treat Mf increases the production of ROI's to a similar level as in vivo treatment of Mf–donors with CY (50 mg/kg). Treatment by 10^{-5}M NM was slightly inhibitory (results not shown). Treatment of Mf with acrolein (ACR) (10^{-5}-10^{-7} M) reduces the secretion of ROI's in a dose dependent manner in comparison to the control group (Mf). Zym - zymosan

Fig. 4. Influence of in vivo treatment with cyclophosphamide (CY) and in vitro treatment with nitrogen mustard or acrolein on the production of reactive oxygen intermediates (ROI's)by murine peritoneal Mf.

3.6 Testicular macrophages (TMf) and their immune response in the reaction with CY

Residual testicular macrophages (TMf) that are present in interstitial tissue of male gonads are regarded as essential cells for male reproductive function involved in the regulation of hormonal balance in the testis. TMf by released products and also directly by cell-to-cell contacts participate in the process of steroidogenesis by Leydig cells. They also influence the behavior of Sertoli cells by releasing mediators and regulate spermatogenesis in testis.

Apart from that function TMf play an important role in their functional contribution of anatomical blood-testis barrier formed by Sertoli cells (Bryniarski et al 2004).

3.6.1 Induction of contact hypersensitivity by TMf and effect of CY-treatment

Similarly to peritoneal macrophages testicular macrophages can be purified by glass adherence or fractionation on discontinuous gradient (Bryniarski 2004). Results in **Table 5** show that TNP substituted TMf (TNP-TMf) when injected i.v. into naïve recipient induce unresponsiveness since the following PCL skin sensitization fail to induce CHS reaction (group B), but TNP-TMf obtained from donors treated with low dose of CY under the seen conditions express strong CHS reaction comparable with control mice actively immunized with PCL (group C ve group A).

Groups	Cells injected i.v. before PCL sensitization	PCL sensitization	CHS reaction in TMf recipients in units of swelling x 10^{-2} mm
A	No cells injected	+	8.2 ± 1.25
B	TNP-TMf	+	2.5 ± 0.80
C	TNP-TMf (50 mg CY)	+	7.5 ± 1.54

Purified TMf obtained from CY-untreated (group B) or CY-treated donors (group B) when substituted with TNP hapten (TNP-TMf) were injected i.v. into mice. Seven days later all TMf recipients and naïve mice (group A) were skin sensitized with 5% PCL and 4 days later challenged on ear skin with 0.4% PCL. 24 h later CHS ear swelling response was measured with engineers micrometer and results expressed in units of swelling x 10^{-2}mm. Statistics: group A ve group B $p<0.001$, group B ve group C $p<0.01$.

Table 5. Testicular macrophages (TMf) from cyclophosphamide-treated mice do not induce suppressor cells in contrast to non-CY treated donors.

Our further experiments show that the tolerogenic activity of TNP-TMf is mediated by the high cytokine secretory activity mainly TGF-β. This cytokine is a very basic tool for functional strategy of TMf within testis and generates the state of organ as immune privileged site.

The methods used by us for obtaining enriched populations of TMf form mixture of testicular interstitial cells lead to separation of TMf into two functionally different cellular fractions - low density (fractions between interfaces of Percoll gradient 21/27 - 33/39) and high density (over 39/45). Low density fraction produces significantly more TGF–β than heavier cells and are CY-sensitive, while high density cells are not (Bryniarski et al. 2004). Our later experiments show that elimination of TGF-β activity by injection of anti-TGF-β mAb, but not anti-IL-10 mAb completely removed unresponsiveness obtained in TNP-TMf recipients after i.v. injection. The other adequate results implementing experiments with anti-TGF-β mAbs are shown in our paper (Bryniarski 2004).

Our experiment with TMf shows that injected intravenously induced CHS response in recipients pre-treated with CY. We found them also actively presenting corpuscular antigen (SRBC) in humoral response (Bryniarski et al. 2004). Again the low density subpopulation of TMf failed to induce CHS when injected i.v. into recipients, but in fact induced the state of tolerance in which subsequent skin application of hapten did not lead to development of contact sensitization. More interestingly, pretreatment of TMf donors with CY made the whole TMf population immunogenic. The mechanisms of action of CY are not cleared, but it has been argued that CY metabolites bind to sulfhydryl groups on antigen presenting cells (APC) changing their function (Bryniarski et al. 2004).

4. Discussion

Our results show that cyclophosphamide in vivo and both its metabolic highly reactive alkylating products -αβ-unsaturated aldehyde acrolein (ACR) and nitrogen mustard a derivative of phosphoramide mustard second metabolic agent formed in CY metabolism, activate TNP substituted Mf that leads to activation of CHS reaction mediated by Mf and hapten specific Th1 lymphocytes. We are tempted to suggest that this activity is mediated by the net of different proinflammatory (TNF-α, IL-1β, IL-6) and suppressory (IL-10 and TGF-β) cytokines secreted by Mf which can uncovering TNP-specific immunization activated by TNP substituted Mf and change their potential from inhibition of unresponsiveness (untreated Mf) into Mf immunogenicity (treated with CY or with CY metabolites).

4.1 CY and its action on CHS

Low dose of CY activates mainly of subpopulation of oil- or thioglycolate- induced peritoneal macrophages which are able to present hapten and subsequently activate trigger of Th1 mediated immune CHS response and diminishes the bioactivity of high density subpopulation of macrophages. That subpopulation induces specific immunologic unresponsiveness as a result of activating a network excess of efferent suppressor cells and mainly cooperates with T suppressor $CD8^+$ hapten specific cells (Treg) and mediates the hapten specific tolerance. (Szczepanik et al. 1993; Marcinkiewicz et al. 1994, Bryniarski et al. 2004 & 2009). The question arises as to how treatment with ACR or NM converts tolerogenic Mf into immunogenic Mf. One possibility is that these CY metabolites disrupt the function of the Mf subpopulation that induces Treg cells. Alternatively they can enhance the activity of Mf subpopulation responsible for the induction of Th1 cells that mediates CHS reaction. Finally these two possibilities are not mutually exclusive and the increased production of IL-12 and IL-6, and the simultaneously decreased production of anti-inflammatory IL-10 and TGF-β cytokines, make these later assumptions most likely.

4.2 CY regulates cytokine network released by Mf

One of the most strongly expressed of CY and their derivatives treatment of macrophages is the activation of IL-6 production (Bryniarski 1996, 2009) . Our results do not address directly the questions by which mechanisms NM modifies the macrophages to produce more IL-6. IL-6 gene expression can be induced by a variety of physiological (cytokines, growth factor, bacterial products) and non-physiological stimuli (certain toxins, medicaments, prostaglandin E1), by at least three different signals pathways (diacyloglycerol, cAMP- and Ca^{2+}- activated pathways). At the DNA level three functional promoter domains were described in conserved region of IL-6 promoter (MRE, NF-IL6 and NFκB). Exactly how transduction pathways are assigned seems unknown with the possible exception of protein kinase C signal which seems to focus on MRE region (Bryniarski et al. 1996). Since NM binds to both DNA and proteins, it could stimulate IL-6 production directly by alkylating any domain of promoter region, or indirectly, by the alkylation of cell surfaces or by both mechanisms simultaneously.

IL-6 is one of the major mediators of the immune response, with pleotropic and sometimes opposed effects on many different targets. It has been shown for instance that IL-6 enhances the cytotoxic activity of NK cells, thus may potentially augment the host defenses and contribute to anti-tumor effects of alkylating agents. Nonetheless, in case of the IL-6 dependent tumours like myelomas or plasma cell leukemias increased IL-6 level could be deleterious. The increased production of IL-6 may be responsible for observed paradoxical effects of CY which under certain conditions enhances, rather than suppresses both the humoral and cell mediated immune responses (Bryniarski et al.1996).

Apart from the influence of CY and its metabolites on the IL-6 production the inhibition of IL-10 and TGF-β production by macrophages was also observed. The results presented above in Table 4 and Fig.3 clearly suggest that the state of tolerance or unresponsiveness observed after TNP-Mf i.v. injection seems to be mediated by the network of pro- and anti-inflammatory cytokines secreted from macrophages and also tentatively delivered by natural regulatory cells. It is highly unlikely that low concentration of cytokine metabolites (10^{-7} and 10^{-6}M) have a direct cytotoxic effect on the Treg-inducing Mf since the cell viability remains unchanged during 24 h culture. Our interpretation is also supported by finding that shifting the balance between pro- and anti-inflammatory cytokines allows for deliberate manipulation of the outgoing response. IL-10 and TGF-β, which are anti-inflammatory cytokines, inhibit the activity of Th1 cells and Mf and down-regulate their function. As shown in Figure 3, administration of anti-IL-10 and/or anti-TGF-β mAbs into animals which received non-immunogenic TNP-Mf restores their immune potential although to different degrees. It indicates that the key suppressive cytokine is IL-10, a finding that is supported by other groups (Bryniarski et al. 2009). In a symmetrical situation, as we have shown previously, administration of anti-IL-12 antibodies inhibits the function of immunogenic TNP-Mf *in vivo* (Bryniarski et al. 2009). The increased production of IL-12 and IL-6 by macrophages indicates that the cell surface signal delivered by ACR or NM activates the transcription factor NF-κB required for the release of inflammatory cytokines (Bryniarski et al. 2009). As reported by other groups, ACR, when allowed free access to the interior of the cell, can either block or enhance the activity of NF-κB in alveolar macrophages depending on the design of cell treatment (Bryniarski et al. 2009).

4.3 CY modulates oxygen radicals formation by macrophages

Our results indicate that CY upregulates not only the specific immune response, by converting non-immunogenic (tolerogenic) Mf into antigen-presenting cells but also positively influences a typical parameter of innate immunity - production of oxygen radicals. In up-regulating the immune function of Mf, ACR and NM had much the same effect. This was however not the case with regard to the production of ROI's by these cells. Using the low concentrations of metabolites, NM was highly stimulatory while ACR did not influence the formation of oxygen radicals above the level observed in control Mf (high concentration of both metabolites were inhibitory). One possibility is that the ACR and NM bind to different targets on the cell surface. NADPH oxidase catalyzing the generation of ROI is composed of several cytosolic and membrane-bound proteins which, after the cell receives a proper signal (e.g. phagocytosis), translocate to form an active enzyme. We propose a possible explanation that under our experimental conditions, ACR, in contrast to NM, does not bind efficiently to important docking proteins to trigger the increased production of ROI. Conflicting results regarding ROI production were also published by other groups. Some reports describe the inhibitory activity of ACR, and others indicate an increased production of radicals. In effect, one can conclude that experimental conditions were the key (Bryniarski at al. 2009).

Our experimental data showed that untreated and in vivo CY treated populations of peritoneal macrophages produce the similar level of nitrogen oxide (Marcinkiewicz et al. 1994) which does not allow to speculate on its function in the immune regulatory system mediated by macrophage stimulated with CY.

4.4 Immunomodulation in chemotherapy with low doses of CY

Our data show that chemotherapy by CY or its products may activate the immune system by modulating cytokine networks and activation of Mf. This may lead to an enhancement of antigen-specific cell mediated immunity but also to activation of mechanisms of innate immunity mediated by Mf, like the production of ROI. Additionally, in animal models derivatives of different mustards led to decreased secretion of IL-10 and TGF-β by tumor cells and to their elimination. These and other similar experiments in humans support the notion that, at a correct dosage, CY and its metabolites can be a promising accessory tool in anti-tumor therapy.

The mechanism of CY influences macrophage immune function in as was shown previously in case of peritoneal Mf and TMf and seems to be the effect of network of different related factors. The analysis shows as the most important the influence of CY on the secretory activity of Mf which is the inhibition of IL-10 (in case of peritoneal Mf) and TGF-β (mainly in case of TMf) with parallel activation of proinflammatory cytokines secretion mainly IL-6, and to a lesser degree IL-12. Both cytokine signals lead to activation of antigen presentation in Mf. The other important factor mediated by CY treatment is an influence on the activation of a cell surface markers expression responsible for uptaking antigen into APC (FcγR I, FcγRII, CD23 - FcεRII/III) and their following presentation to T lymphocytes subpopulations (CD80/CD86, MHC class II, CD14-LPS receptor).

4.5 Influence of CY on testicular macrophages

Although our experiments indicate that in the testis - immune privileged organ - some subpopulations of Mf are potentially able to present antigen if they would sneak through the blood-testis barrier, they also suggest how this potential activity is under control of other Mf and Sertoli cells. Our previous observations have shown that TMf are poor producers of oxygen radicals and nitric oxide both involved in the mechanisms of natural immunity which may be an evolutionary adaptation to diminish the risk of DNA mutations during spermatogenesis. Additionally we showed that specific immune responses controlled by the male gonads minimize the risk of development of autoimmune reactions and are potentially deleterious to testicular functions (Bryniarski 2004). Testicular Mf are good producers of TGF-β, which allows them to play an important functional population of testicular interstitial tissue cells that preserves state of tolerance in testes an immune privilege organs.

That state of tolerance eliminates the cellular immune response from the testis and in consequence makes an extremely dangerous the viral infection as well as in malignances taking place in testis. CY treatment often change TMf activity from unresponsiveness into actively antigen presenting cells which in consequence help to undertake anticancer response but also often can leads to activation an autoimmune response and immunological infertility as a consequences of chemotherapy.

5. Conclusions

The influence of CY on Mf can be summarized as a sum of several different mechanisms mediated by macrophages such as secretion of a specific pattern of cytokines and enhances expression of cell surface markers that can stimulate antigen presenting function by macrophages and last not least production of ROI's. On the other side there are several observations that low dose CY treatment has a direct influence of the different regulatory cells in immune system. One of them is a negative activation of $CD8^+$ T lymphocytes leading to elimination of their effector mediators - suppressor cytokines secretion mainly TGF-β and IL-10, which negatively regulate the cellular immune response, but do not express any negative effect of humoral response. That state of abrogation of unresponsiveness is also observed experimentally when the TNP-substituted Mf obtained from oil-induced donors are injected into CY treated recipients of cells (see **Figure 5**) group C. In that case instead of unresponsiveness expressed by control group (group A) strong CHS response appears 24 h after challenge. This phenomenon clearly shows the influence of CY on the suppressor network of T reg cells. This also clearly shows that CY-manipulation leads to manifold effects in which manifold can be described as wiped out or misdirected. In the literature there are two papers suggesting depletion activity of CY on Treg CD4 CD25 T lymphocytes and Treg CD4 CD25 $FoxP3^+$ lymphocytes (Ghiringhelli et al. 2004 & Zhao et al. 2010)

Group	Cyclophosphamide treatment of donors of TNP-Mf	Cyclophosphamide treatment of recipients of TNP-Mf
A	-	-
B	+	-
C	-	+
D	+	+

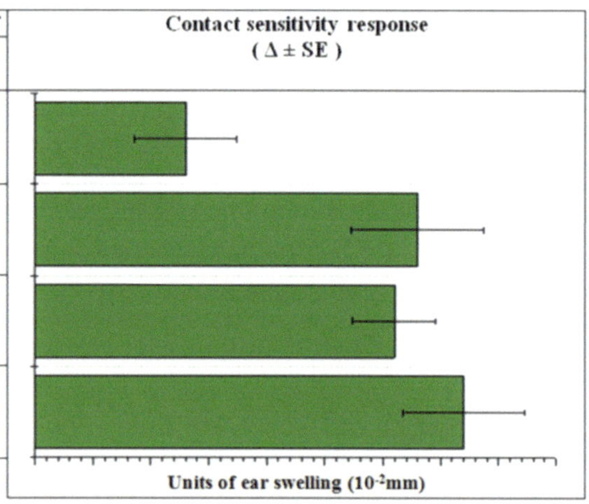

$1x10^6$ TNP substituted Mf (groups A and C) or TNP-Mf CY (groups B and D) were injected i.v. into naive (groups A and B) or treated with low dose of CY CBA/J mice. Seven days later the CHS response was measured (see legend to Table 2). Statistical significance (a posteriori Bonferroni test) Group A ve groups B, C and D p<0.001.

Fig. 5. Alleviation of suppression of contact sensitivity response induced by low dose treatment with cyclophosphamide applied either to macrophage donors or recipients.

A single administration of low dose of CY (50 mg/kg) into either donors or recipients restores the ability of Mf to induce significant CS reaction as a result of: i.) elimination of suppressive properties of Mf; ii.) and/or depletion of population of regulatory T cells in recipients or iii.) elimination of their suppressive activities. In vitro studies with metabolites of CY in contrast to studies in vivo allow identifying the factors which express direct action on selected populations of cells in contrary to experimental research in vivo which is able to identify parallel with direct also indirect effects of cyclophosphamide action on other than macrophages cell populations (T reg cells) that may change and modulate the activity of macrophages and their influence on the immune response. We propose the schemes which summarize the influence of low doses of CY on the immune response in mice (**Figures 6a-6c**).

Figure 6 a-c. The network of the CY influence on the macrophage and regulatory T cells in mice.

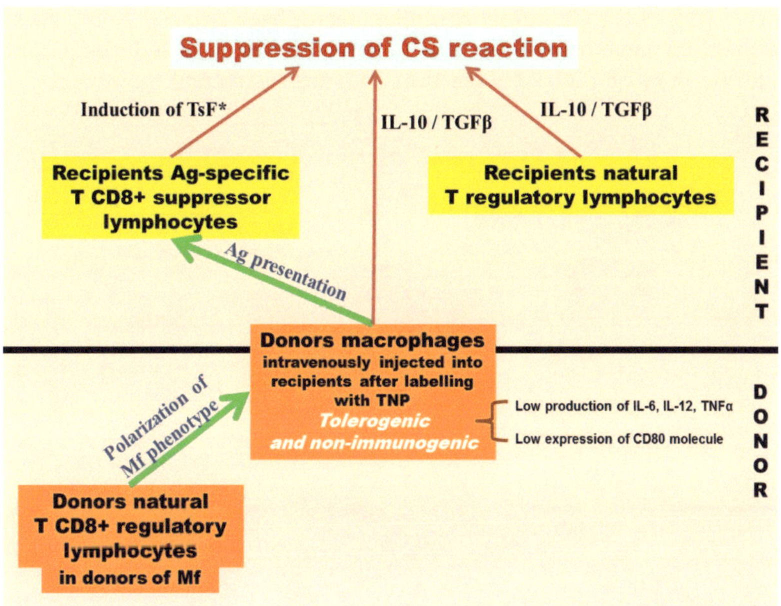

* Induction of T suppressor factor (see the reference by Bryniarski et al. 2-nd European Congress of Immunology Berlin 2009)

Fig. 6.a. Activation of unresponsiveness in recipients after i.v. injection of TNP substituted Mf - lack of CHS reaction.

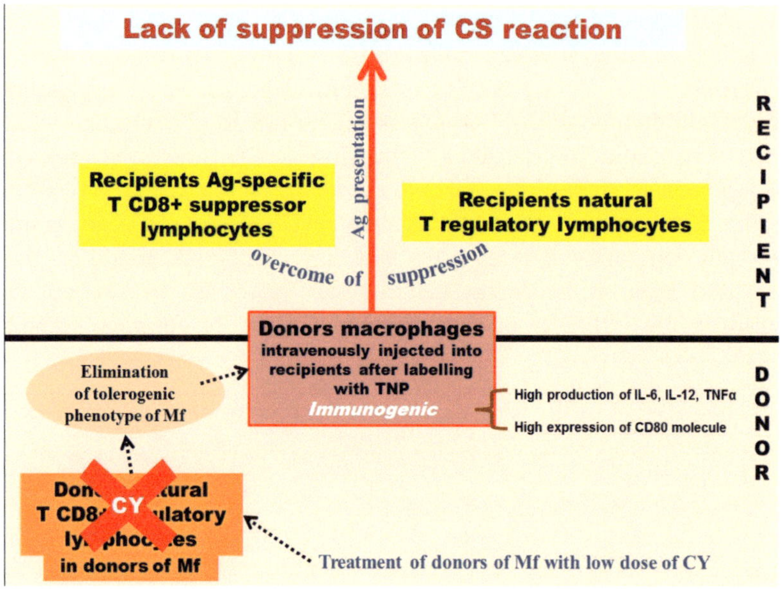

Fig. 6.b. The network of the CY influence on the macrophage and regulatory cells in mice. The i.v. injection into naïve recipient of TNP substituted Mf harvested from CY treated donors results in a state of high CHS reaction 24 h after challenge.

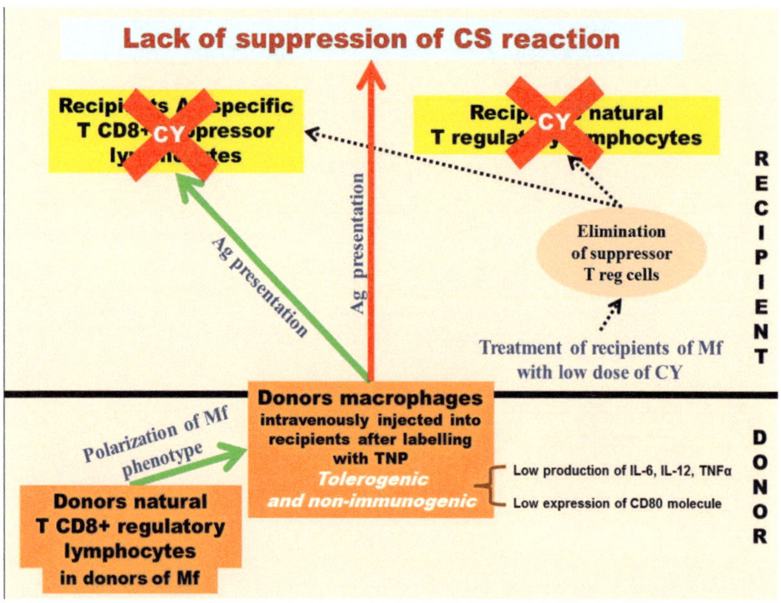

Fig. 6.c. The network of the CY influence on the macrophage and regulatory cells in mice. The i.v. injection of TNP substituted Mf harvested from naïve donors into recipients previously treated with low dose of CY results in expression of high CHS reaction 24 h after challenge with PCL hapten. The activation of CHS is the effect of blocking of natural reg T cells or antigen specific Ts cells.

6. Acknowledgments

The work is supported by grant No K/ZDS/001429 to KB. The author expresses gratitude to Ms. Katarzyna Nazimek M.Sc. for precious help in preparing the Figures and Tables.

7. References

Adjalle, R. Plouin, P. F. Pacak, K. & Lehnert, H. (2009). Treatment of malignant pheochromocytoma. *Horm Metabol Res.* Vol. 41, pp. 687-696.

Audia, S. Nicolas, A. Cathelin, D Larmonier N, Ferrand C, Foucher P, Fanton A, Bergoin E, Maynadie M, Arnould L, Bateman A, Lorcerie B, Solary E, Chauffert B, Bonnotte B.(2007). Increase of $CD4^{+}CD25^{high}$ regulatory T cells in the peripheral blood of patient with metastatic carcinoma: a phase I clinical trial using cyclophosphamide and immunotherapy to eliminate $CD4^{+}CD25^{+}$ T lymphocytes. *Clinical and Experimental Immunology.* Vol. 150, pp. 532-30.

Ben-Efraim, S. (2001). Immunomodulating anticancer alkylating drugs targets and mechanisms of activity. Curr Drug Targ Vol. 2, pp. 197-212.

Breitfeld, P. P. & Meyer, W. H. (2005). Rhabdomyosarcoma: New windows of opportunity. *The Oncologist.* Vol. 10, pp. 518-527.

Bryniarski, K. Ptak, M. & Ptak, W. (1996). The in vivo and in vitro effects of an alkylating agent, mechlormethamine, on IL-6 production in mice and the role of macrophages. *Immunopharmacology.* Vol. 34, pp. 73-78.

Bryniarski, K. Szczepanik, M. Maresz, K. Ptak, M. & Ptak, W. (2004). Subpopulations of mouse testicular macrophages and their immunoregulatory function. *American Journal of Reproductive Immunology.* Vol. 52, pp. 27-35.

Bryniarski, K. Szczepanik, M. Ptak, M. Zemelka, M. & Ptak, W. (2009). Influence of cyclophosphamide and its metabolic products on the activity of peritoneal macrophages in mice. *Pharmacological Reports.* Vol. 61, pp. 550-557.

Bryniarski, K. Ptak, M. Sikora, E. Szczepanik, M. Guerrier-Takada, C. Altman, S. Askenase, P.W. Ptak, W. (2009) Role of low molecular weight RNA in contact sensitivity response. Medimond International Proceedings ECI Berlin 2009 pp 183-186.

Burger, R. A. (2007). Experience with Bevacizumab in the management of epithelial ovarian cells. *Journal of Clinical Oncology.* Vol. 25 (20) Jul.10, pp. 2902-2908.

Cole, M. E. Broaddus, R. Thaker, P. Lauden, C. & Freedman, R. S. (2008). Placenta - side of trophoblastic tumors: case of resistant pulmonary metastasis. *Nature, Clinical Practice, Oncology.* Vol. 5, (3), pp. 171-175.

Czajkowska, B. Ptak, M. Bobek, M. Bryniarski, K. & Szczepanik, M. (1995). Different isoenzyme patterns of nonspecific esterases and the level of IL-6 production as markers of macrophage functions. *Folia Histologica et Biologica* Vol. 33, (2), pp. 111-115.

Durhan, N. Singh, S. Singh Kadin, Y. Durhan, V. Rajotia & N. Sangwen N. (2009). Primary leiomyosarcoma of broad ligament: case report and review of literature. *Arch Gynocol Obstet.* Vol. 279, pp. 705-708.

Ghiringhelli, F. Larmounier, N. Schmidt, E. Parcellier, A. Cathelin, D. Garrido, C. Chauffert, B. Solary, E. Bonnotte, B. & Martin F. (2004). $CD4^{+}CD25^{+}$ regulatory T cells suppress tumor immunity but are sensitive to cyclophosphamide which allows immunotherapy of established tumors to be curative. *European Journal of Immunology*. Vol. 34 pp.336-344.

Lerch,M. & Pichler, W. J. (2004). The immunological and clinical spectrum of delayed drug-induced exanthems. *Current Opinion in in Allergy and Clinical Immunology*. Vol. 4, pp. 411-419.

Luznik, L. & Fusch, E. J. (2010). High-dose post-transplantation cyclophosphamide to promote graft-host tolerance after allogenic hematopoetic stem cell transplantation. *Immunological Research*. Vol. 47 (1-3), pp. 65-77.

Marcinkiewicz, J. Bryniarski, K. & Ptak, W. (1994). Cyclophosphamide uncovers two separate macrophage subpopulations with opposite immunogenic potential and different patterns of monokine production. *Cytokine*. Vol. 6 (5), pp. 472-477.

Posadas, S. J. & Pichler, W. J. (2007). Delayed drug hypersensitivity reactions - new concepts. *Clinical and Experimental Allergy*. Vol. 37, pp. 989-999.

Snowden, J. A. Angel, C. A. Winfield, D. A. Pringle, J. H. West, K. P. (1997). Angiotropic lymphoma: report of a case with histiocytic features. *Journal of Clinical Pathology* Vol. 50, pp. 67-70.

Suzuki, R. (2010). Treatment of advanced NK/T cell lymphoma: Nasal type and aggressive NK-cell leukemia. *Int J Hematol*. Vol. 92, pp. 697-701.

Szczepanik, M. Bryniarski, K. Pryjma, J. & Ptak, W. (1993). Distinct population of antigen-presenting macrophages are required for induction of effector and regulatory cells in contact sensitivity response in mice. *Journal of Leukocyte Biology* Vol. 53 (3), pp. 320-326.

Vitolo, V. Ferreri, A. J. M. & Zucca, E. (2008). Primary testicular lymphoma. *Critical Review in Oncology/Hematology*.Vol.65, pp. 183-189.

Weiner, H. L. and Cohen, J. A. (2002). Treatment of multiple sclerosis with cyclophosphamide: critical review of clinical and immunologic effects. *Multiple Sclerosis*. Vol. 8, pp. 142 -154.

Zhao, J. Cao, Y. Lei, Z. Yang, Z. Zhang, B. & Huang B. (2010). Selective depletion of $CD4^+CD25^+FoxP3^+$ regulatory T cells by low-dose cyclophosphamide is explained by reduced intracellular ATP levels. *Cancer Research*. Vol. 70, (12), pp. 4850-4858.

8

Modification of Interleukin-10 with Mannose-6-Phosphate Groups Yields a Liver-Specific Cytokine with Antifibrotic Activity in Rats

Heni Rachmawati[1,2], Adriana Mattos[2],
Catharina Reker-Smit[2], Klaas Poelstra[2] and Leonie Beljaars[2]
[1]*Pharmaceutics, Bandung Institute of Technology, Bandung*
[2]*University of Groningen, Dept. of Pharmacokinetics, Toxicology and Targeting,*
[1]*Indonesia*
[2]*The Netherlands*

1. Introduction

Cytokines and other biological compounds are considered as future drugs and they are of particular interest for the treatment of chronic diseases. These endogenous compounds, that normally mediate local cellular communications, are very promising candidates to generate new drugs because of their high potency (pM-nM concentrations) and their fundamental roles in pathological processes. However, the therapeutic application of cytokines is limited, because several problems are encountered with their application *in* vivo (Schooltink and Rose-John 2002; Standiford 2000; Vilcek and Feldmann 2004). For instance, some cytokines are efficiently degraded in plasma by various enzymes and cytokines are rapidly excreted by the kidneys. Consequently their residence time in the body and thus the exposure to the diseased cells is short (plasma half life is often minutes), which does not favour an optimal biological efficacy. Another major problem is the occurrence of side effects. Because cytokine receptors are ubiquitously expressed in all organs, unusual high plasma concentrations of the cytokine can lead to (unwanted) effects in various organs.

To overcome these problems, we use drug targeting techniques to selectively deliver the cytokine to a specific (diseased) cell (Allen and Cullis 2004; Beljaars, Meijer, Poelstra 2002). The challenge is to improve its distribution within the body and direct the cytokine to a cell of interest, while maintaining the biological activity of that particular cytokine after chemical modification. A conventional way to modify proteins is conjugation with polyethylene glycol (PEG) (Jevsevar, Kunstelj, Porekar 2010). The attachment of PEG moieties improves the pharmacokinetics. That is, PEG substitution prevents rapid renal elimination which results in compounds with prolonged plasma concentrations, thereby making a reduced number of doses possible. For instance, PEGasys (PEGylated interferon α2a), an example of a PEGylated cytokine that is now commonly used to treat patients infected with viral hepatitis, is dosed once a week while the unmodified interferon is dosed daily. This leads to an improvement in the compliance and quality of life in patients with chronic diseases. The side effects, however, are not diminished after PEGylation.

Our strategy of active drug targeting, in contrast to the abovementioned PEGylation approach, aims to improve pharmacokinetics and efficacy while simultaneously avoiding side-effects by cell-specific delivery of the cytokine to the diseased cell via receptor-mediated interaction. To that end, the cytokine is modified with homing devices that recognize receptors present on the diseased (target) cells. In the past, we designed sugars and receptor-recognizing peptides that interact with hepatic stellate cells (HSC) (Beljaars and others 1999; Beljaars and others 2000; Beljaars and others 2003). These cells play the central role in liver cirrhosis (Bataller and Brenner 2005; Friedman 2010; Schuppan and Afdhal 2008). Our newly designed homing devices displayed affinity for the mannose 6-phosphate/insulin-like growth factor (M6P/IGF) II receptor, platelet derived growth factor (PDGF)-β or collagen type VI receptors, which are all essential during stellate cell functioning in fibrogenesis, and upregulate in the diseased liver.

Currently, it is accepted that liver cirrhosis is a fibrotic disease that is reversible (Iredale 2007). However, to date, no drug is marketed that is able to reverse the fibrotic process in patients (Pinzani, Rombouts, Colagrande 2005). The only treatment that is applied to these patients deals with the treatment of complications and with eradication of the cause (for instance removal of the hepatitis virus in case of HCV-induced cirrhosis). However, fibrosis often progresses to end-stage liver failure leaving a liver transplantation as the only available option. Therefore, worldwide research focuses on the identification of compounds that are able to reverse the disease, but unfortunately many potential interventions fail in clinical trials (Pinzani, Rombouts, Colagrande 2005). We hypothesize that this failure may be due to an inadequate pharmacokinetic profile of the potential drugs or due to the occurrence of side-effects of these drugs preventing the administration of effective doses, which may be solved by applying drug targeting techniques.

The selective delivery of cytokines to the cells that control pathological processes is quite relevant. PEGylation of cytokines like interferon α, TNFα, and IL-2 has provided substantial benefits, but in that approach cytokines are not actively delivered to the site of action. In the present study, we will show an example of this second approach using the cytokine interleukin-10 (IL10). IL10 has potent immunosuppressive and anti-inflammatory effects (Di Marco and others 1999; Khan and others 2002; Kitching and others 2000; Oberholzer, Oberholzer, Moldawer 2002) and also direct antifibrotic properties in HSC (Cuzzocrea and others 2001; Demols and others 2002; Gloor and others 1998; Louis and others 1998; Louis and others 2003; Thompson and others 1998; Wang and others 1998). Several of these studies showed beneficial effects of IL10 therapies in animal models and clinical trials during various diseases. However, other studies demonstrated only a limited effect of IL10 or even showed disappointing results (Chadban and others 1997; Colombel and others 2001; Herfarth and Scholmerich 2002). This variable efficacy might be due to the low concentration of IL10 at the target sites. Recombinant IL10 is a low molecular weight protein that is rapidly cleared from the circulation through glomerular filtration. The plasma half-life of IL10 is only 2 min (Rachmawati and others 2004). The ultimate concentrations at the site of action therefore could be too low to result in clear effects. Dose escalation of systemically administered IL10 leads to adverse effects due to its inherent biological actions (Fedorak and others 2000; Schreiber and others 2000). In accordance with this, clinical studies reported beneficial effects of long-term IL10 therapy to treat HCV-associated liver fibrosis but this was accompanied by an immunosuppressive action, as noted in a flare-up of the viral burden, and low therapeutic efficacy (Nelson and others 2000)(Meijer and others

2001). Liver-selective delivery of this cytokine may prevent these clinical problems and create biological effects within relevant cells.

Upregulation of mannose-6-phosphate/IGF-II receptors during liver injury on HSC (de Bleser and others 1995) offers an excellent target for receptor-mediated antifibrotic drug delivery as shown with albumin substituted with mannose-6-phosphate groups (Beljaars and others 1999). We therefore modified IL10 with the sugar mannose-6-phosphate (M6P) to selectively deliver this cytokine to HSC in fibrotic livers (Rachmawati and others 2007). We showed that after modification of IL10 with mannose 6-phosphate (M6P) a compound was generated that binds to the M6P/IGF-II receptor which is highly present on activated HSC. Our chemically engineered cytokine, M6P-IL10, displayed good pharmacological activity in vitro in freshly isolated HSC. We now performed biodistribution studies of radiolabeled-M6P-modified IL10 using gamma-camera techniques to examine the active delivery of this compound to the diseased tissue. Furthermore, we studied the pharmacological activities of this conjugate in rats at an early stage of liver fibrosis and compared this to the effects of unmodified IL10.

2. Results

2.1 Synthesis of M6P-IL10

Mannose-6-phosphate-residues were coupled to the amino acid lysine in recombinant human IL10 as described (Rachmawati and others 2007). The product was first characterized by Western Blotting techniques using a rabbit polyclonal anti-IL10 antibody (Santa Cruz Biotechnology, USA). Western Blot analysis of unmodified IL10 yielded two bands corresponding to a molecular weight (MW) of 18.5 and 37 kD (fig.1) representing the monomeric and the homodimeric form of IL10 (Reineke and others 1998). The prepared conjugate M6P-IL10 revealed a shift in these bands: both bands had a higher MW (resp. approximately 20 and 40 kD) than unmodified IL10 indicating covalent binding of M6P to the cytokine.

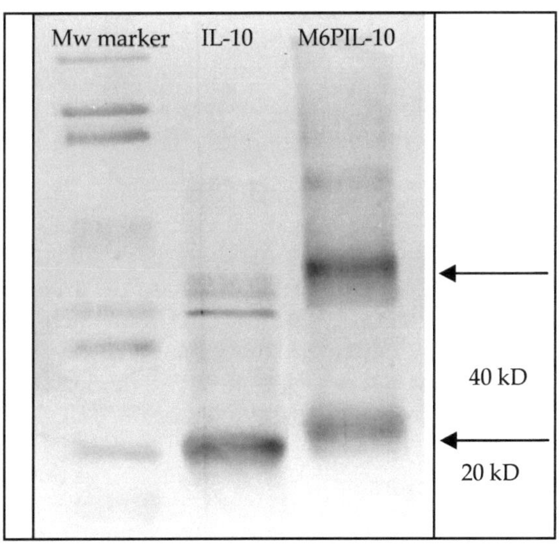

Fig. 1. Western blot analysis of M6P-IL10 and IL10. Note the increase in molecular weight of the monomeric (± 20 kD) and the homodimeric (± 40 kD) forms of M6P-IL10 compared with the monomeric and homodimeric forms of native IL10 (respectively, 18.5 kD and 37 kD).

2.2 Body distribution of IL10 and M6P-IL10

To visualize the body distribution of IL10 and M6P-IL10 with a gamma camera, both proteins were labeled with Iodine-123 (^{123}I). Fibrotic rats were monitored during the course of their disease by subjecting them to gamma camera analysis, just prior to BDL and one, two and three weeks after BDL (respectively, normal, BDL-1, BDL-2, and BDL-3, n=3). Anaesthetized rats were placed on a low-energy all-purpose collimator of a gamma-camera and received an intravenous tracer dose. The results are shown in figure 2. Already two min after iv injection of [^{123}I]M6P-IL10, the gamma-camera detected high levels of radioactivity within the livers (white intensity) and low levels in the kidneys (yellow-red intensity). Hepatic levels of [^{123}I]M6P-IL10 remained high for at least 30 min. The results of the distribution studies were similar in various stages of liver fibrosis (BDL-1, BDL- 2 and BDL-3). In contrast, native [^{123}I]IL10 rapidly accumulated in the kidneys (white intensity) with low uptake in livers (fig.2a), which is in agreement with previous studies (Andersen and others 1999; Rachmawati and others 2004).

Subsequently, we quantitatively measured the distribution of [^{125}I]IL10 and [^{125}I]M6P-IL10 ten minutes after intravenous injection in rats with end-stage liver fibrosis (BDL-3 weeks). Native [^{125}I]-IL10 accumulated in the kidneys in these rats (Fig 2b). Only, 15% and 30% of the dose was found in livers of normal and BDL-3 rats respectively. The rest was dispersed throughout the body or present in the blood. In contrast, [^{125}I]M6P-IL10 accumulated for nearly 60% of the dose within the livers in BDL-3 rats. Uptake in kidneys was only 20%. Differences in blood- , liver- and kidney-concentrations between IL10 and M6P-IL10 were significant ($p<0.05$).

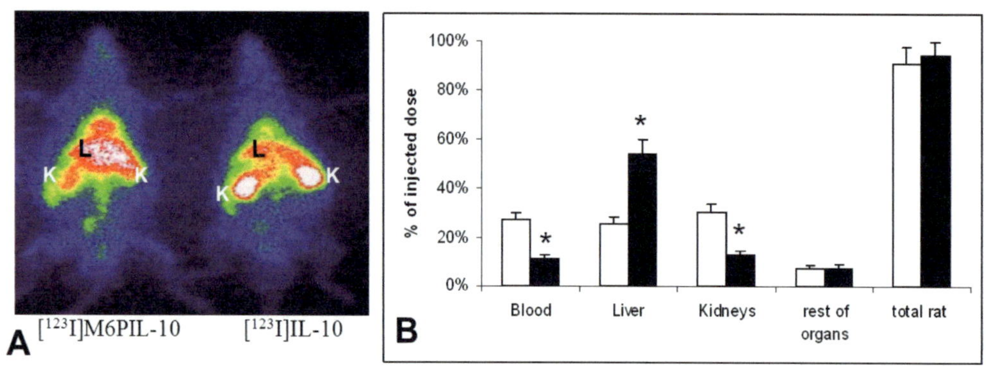

Fig. 2. Organ Distribution of M6P-IL10 and IL10. **A**: Gamma-camera images of [^{123}I]IL10 and [^{123}I]M6P-IL10 distribution in BDL-1 rats. Pictures show an overlay of recordings from t=20 to t=30 minutes after i.v. injection of radiolabeled proteins. The images show a high accumulation of M6P-IL10 in the liver (L) in contrast to IL10, which is mostly distributed to the kidneys (K). **B:** Quantitative measurement of organ uptake of [^{125}I]-labeled IL10 (white bars) and M6P-IL10 (black bars) in BDL-3 rats 10 minutes after i.v. administration of the radiolabeled proteins. N = 3 per group (* $p<0.05$ compared with IL-10 distribution)

2.3 Identification of target receptors

(Modified) IL10 could not be detected within livers by immunohistochemistry, most likely due to the very low dose administered (2-2.5 μg). Therefore, several receptor antagonists were applied to identify the target receptors responsible for the uptake of the proteins in different organs in order to obtain information about the hepatocellular distribution. Rats were pre-treated with either succinylated human serum albumin (sucHSA) to block the scavenger receptor, or with mannose-6-phosphate-HSA, to block the M6P/IGFII receptor. These receptor antagonists (i.v. dose of 5 mg/kg) were administered 5 min. prior to the i.v. injection of a tracer amount of radiolabeled IL10 or M6P-IL10. Control animals received pre-treatment with unmodified HSA (5 mg/kg).

Kidney accumulation of [^{125}I]IL10 or [^{125}I]M6P-IL10 was not influenced by administration of any of the proteins (fig. 3). Uptake of [^{125}I]IL10 in the livers was also not influenced by any of the proteins, but remained approximately 20% of the dose in all groups. However, liver uptake of M6P-IL10 was reduced from 54 ± 6% in rats receiving only M6P-IL10, to 29± 4% by sucHSA ($p<0.05$) and to 24 ± 8% by M6P-HSA pre-administration ($p<0.05$). Co-administration of both sucHSA and M6P-HSA did not have an additive effect (24 ± 5% liver uptake). Unmodified HSA did not affect liver uptake of M6P-IL10 at all (57 ± 13% liver uptake).

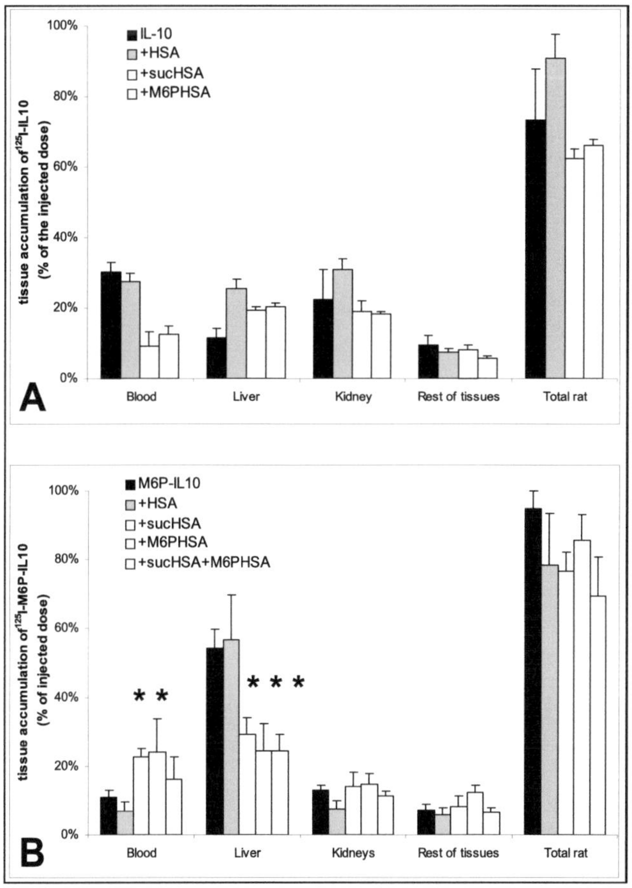

Fig. 3. Organ distribution of [^{125}I]IL10 (fig. **A**) and [^{125}I]M6P-IL10 (fig. **B**) in BDL-3 rats 10 min. after i.v. administration of the radiolabeled proteins. Five min. before administration of these proteins, HSA, sucHSA, M6PHSA or the combination of two proteins was administered to test receptor specificity. Note that sucHSA and M6PHSA influenced liver uptake and blood concentrations of M6P-IL10, whereas IL10 distribution was not affected by any of the proteins. N=4-6 per group. * =$p<0.05$ compared with HSA pre-administration.

2.4 Effects of IL10 and M6P-IL10 in vitro

The in vitro activities of IL10 and M6P-IL10 were studied in culture-activated primary HSC. The presence of IL10 receptors and M6P/IGFII-receptors on these cells was verified by immunohistochemical methods. No effect of IL10 or M6P-IL10 was found on HSC proliferation as assessed by Alamar blue assays (data not shown).

We also examined type I collagen deposition in cultures of HSC treated with IL10 or M6P-IL10 using immunostaining methods. Deposition of type I collagen was clearly detectable in HSC cultures at day-7 (fig 4A) and this staining was reduced in cultures treated for 24 hr with IL10 (Fig 4B) and in cultures treated with M6P-IL10 (fig 4C).

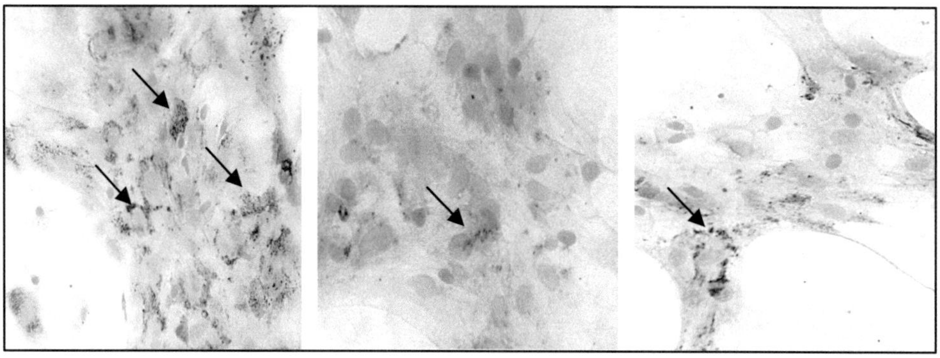

Fig. 4. Type I collagen deposition in cultures of primary isolated rat HSC's as detected with immunostaining methods. Collagen staining (using a goat polyclonal anti-collagen I antibody) is present on HSC's after 7 days in culture (**A**, arrows). Deposition of collagen is attenuated by 24 hr incubation with 12.5 ng/ml IL10 (**B**) or M6P-IL10 (**C**). Original magnification 200x.

2.5 Effects of IL10 and M6P-IL10 *in vivo*

2.5.1 Experimental design

Bile duct ligated rats were randomly divided into three groups: BDL rats received either vehicle (PBS, N = 5), or IL10 (N = 5) or M6P-IL10 (N = 5). Untreated normal rats (N = 3) served as reference group. Animals received a bolus iv dose (8 µg/kg/day) of (modified-) IL10 at day 4, 5 and 6 after BDL. At day 7, animals were sacrificed and samples of blood and various organs were harvested.

2.5.2 Effect of IL10 and M6P-IL10 on liver function

Plasma levels of markers reflecting liver injury and cholestasis in BDL-1 rats receiving IL-10 or M6PIL-10 were not significantly different from untreated BDL rats (table 1).

2.5.3 Effect of IL10 and M6P-IL10 on inflammatory parameters

To study the effects of IL10 and M6P-IL10 on inflammation, staining for reactive oxygen species (ROS)-production and IL10 receptor expression was performed. The number of 3,3'-diaminobenzidine (DAB)-positive cells in the liver was high around necrotic areas and in portal areas. DAB staining reflects ROS production (Poelstra and others 1990) by activated neutrophils, eosinophils and macrophages.

Parameters	PBS-treated rats	IL10-treated rats	M6PIL-10-treated rats
Alkaline Phosphatase (U/L)	*493.8 ± 71.2*	*476.2 ± 53.8*	*450.6 ± 16.13*
AST (U/L)	*350.0 ± 166.6*	*354.0 ± 118.8*	*301.0 ± 109.64*
ALT (U/L)	*92.2 ± 27.44*	*90.2 ± 24.9*	*84.0 ± 17.0*
Total bilirubin (μmol/L)	*191.2 ± 43.13*	*231.6 ± 21.9*	*194.8 ± 68.6*
GGT (U/L)	*65.0 ± 56.0*	*74.0 ± 75.95*	*34.8 ± 23.34*

Table 1. Plasma levels of markers reflecting liver injury and cholestasis in BDL-1 rats treated with PBS, IL10 or M6P-IL10. Values represent the mean ± SD of 5 rats per group.

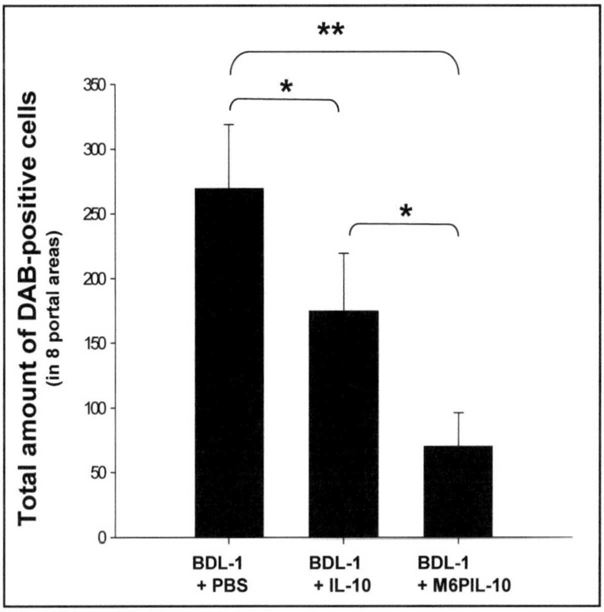

Fig. 5. Effect of IL-10- and M6PIL-10-treatment on the number of DAB-positive cells in livers of BDL-1 rats. Both treatments significantly reduced the number of DAB-positive cells in the portal areas compared with PBS-treated rats. *= $p<0.05$; **=$p<0.01$

IL10 and M6P-IL10 strongly attenuated the staining for DAB (Fig. 5). Quantitative evaluation of this staining by counting the number of positive cells/area showed that DAB staining was reduced by 35% in rats receiving IL10 ($p<0.05$ compared with untreated BDL-1 rats, Fig 5b), whereas the number of DAB-positive cells per area in M6P-IL10-treated rats was reduced by 74% compared with untreated rats ($p<0.05$). Thus, both IL10 and M6P-IL10 exerted anti-inflammatory effects within the liver and M6P-IL10 was superior in this respect.

Staining for IL10 receptors (with anti-IL-10 receptor IgG (Santa Cruz Biotech)) on liver sections of BDL-1 rats revealed occasional positive cells: some cells around the proliferating bile ducts and around hepatic arteries were positive. Based on the localization and the positivity for α-smooth muscle actin or HIS-48, these cells were identified as fibroblasts, HSC and neutrophils. In BDL-1 rats that received IL10, hepatic IL10 receptor expression was strongly reduced, in particular around the portal areas (fig.6). In contrast, in BDL-1 rats receiving M6P-IL10, IL10 receptor expression was still present.

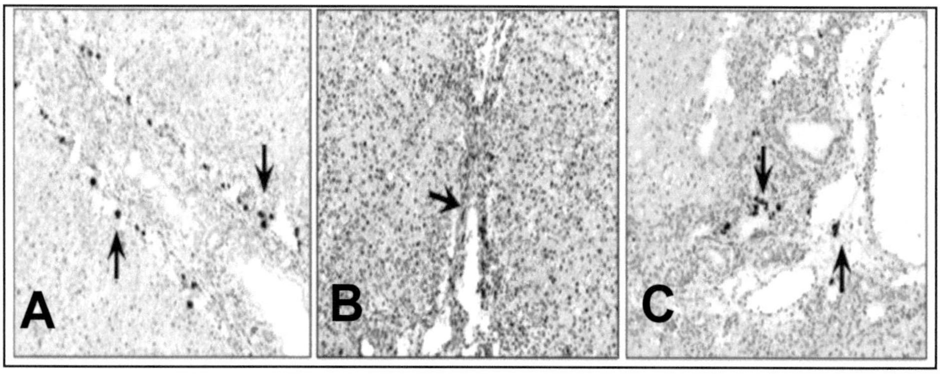

Fig. 6. Intrahepatic staining for IL10 receptor expression in fibrotic livers. In PBS-treated BDL-1 rats, positive cells were found around bile ducts (fig. **A,** arrows). In rats treated with IL10, only occasional IL10 receptor-positive cells were found (fig. **B**) whereas the portal areas contained many IL10 receptor positive cells in BDL-1 rats treated with M6P-IL10 (fig. **C**). Original magnification 100x.

2.5.4 Antifibrotic effects of IL10 and M6P-IL10

Characteristic for fibrosis is deposition of extracellular matrix in tissues. Collagen type I and III are the most important extracellular matrix proteins present in a fibrotic liver. Therefore, we assessed the effect of M6P-IL10 and IL10 administration on the deposition of collagen. First, we evaluated the deposition of fibrous tissue by histochemical staining with Sirius Red (figure 7A). This staining was strongly enhanced in BDL-1 rats compared with normal rats. The portal-to-portal bridging was already apparent in the untreated group at this time point. However, in IL10-treated rats, the portal-portal fibrous bridges were observed in only one out of five rats and bridging was not seen in any of the M6P-IL10-treated rats. The matrix deposition around portal areas was clearly reduced by the treatments compared to untreated group. This reduction was confirmed by immunostaining for collagen type III using goat anti-collagen III IgG (SouternBiotech, USA) antibodies. The strong staining seen in BDL-1 rats was reduced by IL10 and M6P-IL10 (fig. 7B).

With ImageJ software, the effects of IL10 and M6PIL10 on the deposition of fibrous tissue were quantified. In normal livers, 1.0 ± 0.45 % of the total liver area was positive for Sirius Red. This positive area increased to 4.6 ± 1.0% of the livers of BDL-1 rats ($p<0.001$ compared with normal rats, Fig. 7C). In IL10-treated BDL-1 rats the Sirius Red-positive area per liver changed to 3.6 % ± 1.6 (not significant compared with untreated BDL-1 rats). In M6P-IL10-treated BDL-1 rats, Sirius Red-staining changed to 3.4 ± 1.1 % of liver area ($p< 0.05$ compared with untreated BDL-1 rats, Fig. 7C). The effect of IL10 and M6P-IL10 on the fibrotic process was also assessed by staging the lesions via a semiquantitative scoring system; the Histologic Activity Index-Knodell (Ishak and others 1995). Grading of the fibrotic lesions in these livers by the HAI-Knodell's index revealed a reduction of the fibrotic index from 3.2 ± 0.8 in untreated BDL-1 rats to 2.6 ± 0.9 and 2.2 ± 0.45 ($p<0.05$) in rats receiving IL10 and M6P-IL10, respectively (fig. 7D).

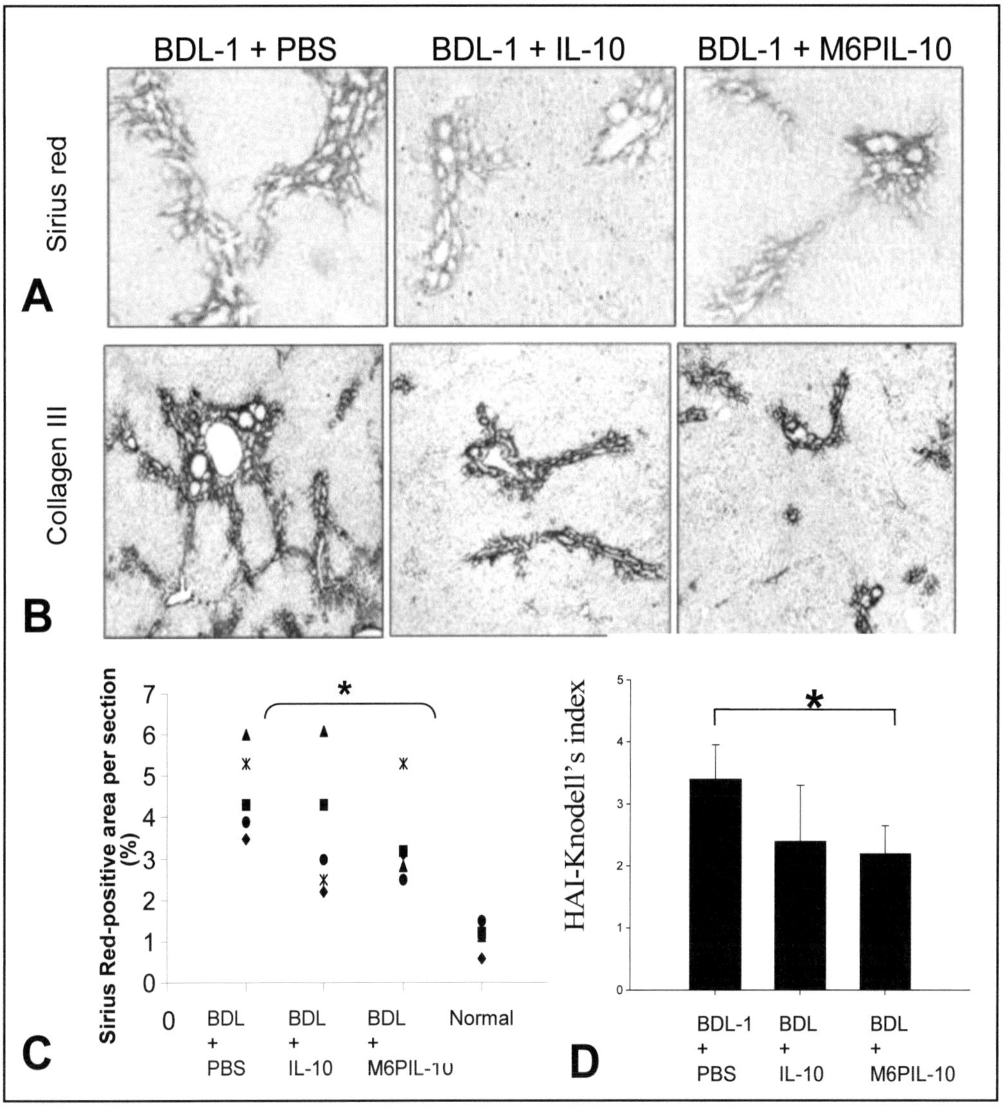

Fig. 7. Collagen deposition in BDL rats after treatment with M6P-IL-10 or IL-10. A. Representative photomicrographs of Sirius Red (fig. **A**) and collagen type III staining (fig. **B**) in livers of BDL-1 rats treated with PBS, IL-10 or M6PIL-10 (magnification 10x4). Figure **C** depicts the quantitative analysis of the Sirius Red stainings in the livers of the different groups as measured by Image J software. The individual values of each rat are shown in the graph. Figure **D** shows the semiquantitative grading of the fibrotic process in BDL-1 rats with the Histological Activity Index-Knodell method. N=5 per group, * = $p<0.05$ compared with PBS-treated BDL rats.

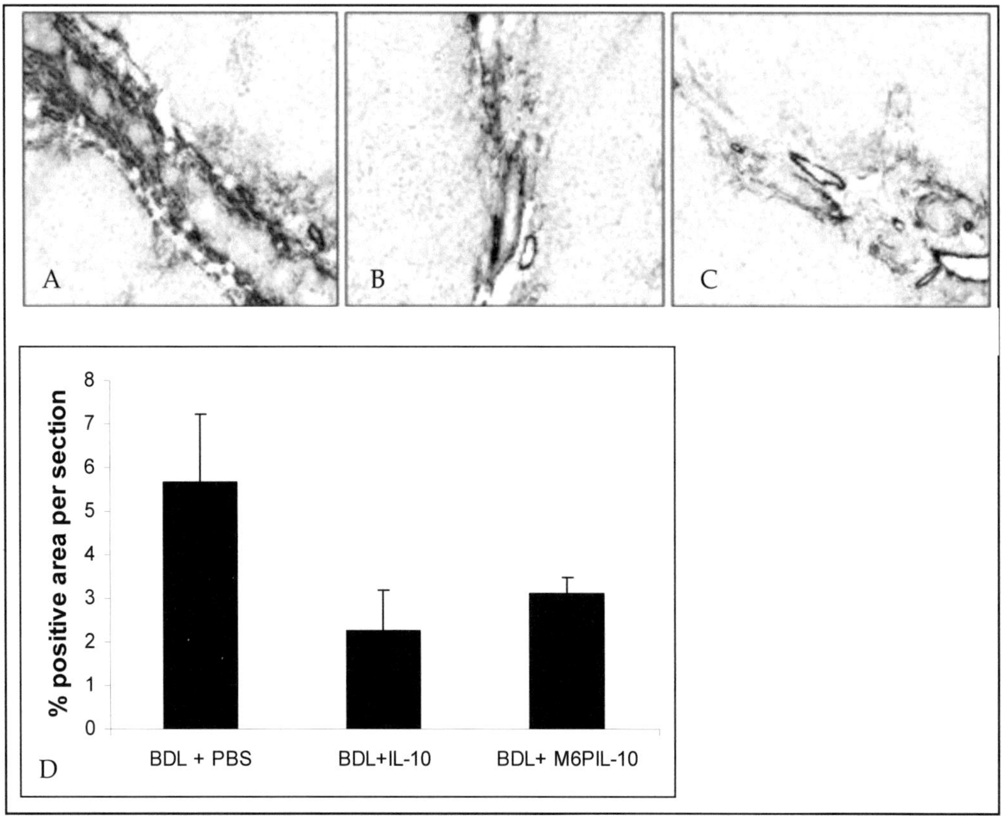

Fig. 8. Representative photomicrographs of immunohistochemical staining for α-smooth muscle actin (αSMA) in livers of BDL-1 rats treated with PBS (fig. **A**) or IL10 (fig. **B**) or M6P-IL10 (fig. **C**). Figure **D** depicts the quantitative analysis of the intrahepatic αSMA staining with Image J software (n=5 animals per group). *=p<0.05, Original magnification 100x.

Subsequently, we evaluated the in vivo effects of M6P-IL10 and IL10 on α-smooth muscle staining (α-SMA), that reflects the proportion of activated HSC and myofibroblasts. These cells are responsible for the production of collagen. One week after BDL, staining for α-SMA was highly increased around portal ducts and in fibrotic septa compared with normal rats. IL10 and M6P-IL10 clearly diminished this α-SMA staining (fig.8). Quantitative evaluation of this staining using ImageJ software (fig.8B), demonstrated a significant reduction by 54% ± 17% and 33% ± 19% after treatment with IL10 or M6P-IL10, respectively compared to PBS-treated BDL rats (p<0.05).

3. Conclusion/discussion

This study demonstrates that chemical modification of a cytokine, in our study IL10 modified with M6P groups, leads to a compound with improved biodistribution and pharmacological activity *in vivo* in a rat model of liver fibrosis. M6P is a homing device with high affinity for the M6P/IGF-II receptor which is upregulated on the cell membrane of HSCs during liver diseases (de Bleser and others 1995). Upregulation of this receptor on HSC during liver fibrosis yields an excellent target for receptor-mediated drug delivery. The delivery of antifibrotic compounds to the major pathogenic cells in the liver by modification with M6P groups is a rational and new approach to treat this chronic disease (Schuppan and Popov 2009).

Chemical modification of a cytokine can influence the biological activity, in particular when essential amino acids necessary for interaction of the cytokine with its receptor are conjugated with homing devices or when the conformation of the protein is changed too much. Therefore, it is essential to test whether the prepared conjugate is pharmacologically active. In our study, we coupled several M6P groups to the lysine amino acids within the protein and some of these lysine-groups are present at the receptor-binding site of IL10 (Reineke and others 1998). Attachment of M6P-residues to these groups might therefore affect the biological activities of IL10. Studies on culture-activated primary HSC *in vitro* showed that M6P-IL10 reduced collagen deposition by these cells (fig 4) indicating that IL10-related activities are still intact in the modified cytokine. There was no effect of M6P-IL10 on HSC proliferation but native IL10 also did not affect growth of HSC. Previously, we demonstrated that M6P-IL10 was able to increase collagen degradation (by increasing the MMP13/TIMP ratio) in primary cultures of HSC (Rachmawati and others 2007). Based on its effects on collagen deposition, we conclude that M6P-IL10 is pharmacologically active within the target cell *in vitro*.

The key concept in active drug targeting is that the distribution within the body is confined to the diseased organ/cell-types. This will lead to more optimal effects and less side effects because uptake in other organs is avoided. In pharmacokinetic terms, this means that the Volume of Distribution (Vd) is decreased. The presented results of gamma-camera imaging studies and the biodistribution studies with radiolabeled IL10 and M6P-IL10 indicate a preferential homing of the modified cytokine to the fibrotic liver. The shift in biodistribution of IL10 from the kidney to the liver after coupling of M6P is in accordance with the high liver uptake of M6P modified proteins found in previous studies with HSA as the core protein (Beljaars and others 1999; van Beuge and others 2011). These studies showed uptake of M6PHSA within HSC. The cells responsible for the uptake of M6P-IL10 within the liver could not be directly identified due to the low amount of cytokines administered. Both proteins are only available in the microgram scale and immunohistochemical detection of proteins requires injection of milligrams per rat. Therefore, receptor antagonists were applied to identify the target receptors. These studies indicated that liver uptake of M6P-IL10 was receptor-mediated since the uptake was not attenuated by the control protein HSA whereas sucHSA and M6P-HSA, both ligands for receptors, significantly reduced its uptake. The fact that sucHSA and M6P-HSA both had an effect indicates that M6P-IL10 binds to at least two receptors: the scavenger receptor and the M6P/IGFII receptor, respectively. Involvement of the scavenger receptor, which recognizes strongly anionic compounds, can be explained by the negative charges introduced by phosphate groups (PO_4^{3-}). This was also found in another study in which liposomes were modified with M6P sugars (Adrian and others 2006). The combination of M6PHSA and sucHSA did not completely block the liver uptake which suggests the involvement of yet another receptor, possibly the IL10 receptor which is also present in the liver (fig 6). Based on the expression of M6P/IGF II receptors, scavenger receptors and IL10 receptors, the putative target cells for M6P-IL10 are HSC's, portal fibroblasts, endothelial cells, Kupffer cells and neutrophils within the liver. Antifibrotic effects of IL10 are anticipated in all these cells.

To test whether M6P-IL10 is effective *in vivo*, we now administered (modified-)IL10 to bile duct ligated rats after the initiation of the fibrotic process, i.e. from day 4 till day 7 after BDL. In this time frame, pro-inflammatory activity is high in the liver and fibrosis is initiated (39-43). In addition, M6P/IGF-II receptor expression on HSC is enhanced at day 4 (Greupink and others 2006), which ensures targeting to this receptor at this time point. During the first week after BDL, enhanced IL10 receptor expression was noted (fig 6), also providing a rationale for the start of treatment at day 4.

Treatment with IL-10 or M6P-IL10 had significant effects on the inflammatory activity within the liver. A reduction in the number of infiltrating cells as reflected by DAB-positive cells was noted. These data indicate that M6P-IL10 is pharmacologically active *in vivo*. Based on inflammatory cell influx, its effect may even be superior to native IL10. Of particular interest is the reduction in IL-10 receptor expression after treatment with IL10, but not after treatment with M6P-IL10. The down regulation of the target receptor during treatment is relevant for IL10-based therapies. This may contribute to the lack of effectiveness of such therapies (Chadban and others 1997; Colombel and others 2001; Herfarth and Scholmerich 2002).

Next to the anti-inflammatory effects, we evaluated the effects of M6P-IL10 on fibrogenesis *in vivo*. The target cell of IL10 is the (activated) HSC, the extracellular matrix producing hepatic cell, and therefore antifibrotic effects are primarily anticipated in HSC and the most important feature in this respect is collagen deposition. Our results showed a clear reduction in collagen deposition in these livers after treatment with M6P-IL10 (figure 7). This reduction was established with various methods. The lack of portal-to-portal bridging was evident in nearly all the livers of the cytokine-treated animals. In addition, IL10 and M6P-IL10 also significantly reduced αSMA staining which reflects a reduction in the activation of HSC in these livers. These results indicate that our modified IL10 is pharmacologically active *in vivo*.

Although cytokines are interesting compounds which may yield potent new drugs, so far only a relatively few are approved and clinically used. The number is still disappointing low regarding the large number of endogenous cytokines. The main reasons for this are the poor stability and poor pharmacokinetic profile of cytokines. To overcome these pharmacokinetic problems, we apply drug targeting techniques to selectively deliver the cytokine to a specific (diseased) cell. In the current study, we demonstrate the possibilities of this strategy with successful *in vivo* application of a modified IL10. Recently, we also reported on the cell-specific delivery of another very interesting cytokine with antifibrotic activities, that is interferon-gamma (IFNγ) (Bansal and others 2011). This study shows that HSC-targeted IFNγ, in contrast to unmodified IFNγ, blocked liver fibrogenesis in a chronic CCL4 mice model of liver fibrosis, by specifically acting on the key pathogenic cells within the liver. Furthermore, we clearly demonstrated that the targeted IFNγ was devoid of side effects. In addition, others show beneficial effects of a targeted cytokine by means of coupling receptor specific ligands to the cytokine (Curnis and others 2000; Curnis and others 2005; Fournier, Aigner, Schirrmacher 2011; Jazayeri and Carroll 2008; Nissim and others 2004) often focussing on the treatment of tumours. These approaches may lead to a more optimal use of cytokines for therapeutic purposes.

In summary, we demonstrated potent pharmacological effectivity of a novel liver-specific form of the cytokine IL10. After conjugation with M6P, the novel cytokine efficiently accumulates in the liver and attenuates the fibrotic process *in vivo*. Further dose-response studies are required to examine whether M6P-IL10 is more effective than the native product and exerts less adverse effects. Furthermore, targeting of potentially interesting cytokines to the liver is promising and it may lead to the generation of a therapeutic antifibrotic compound which has not been realized so far.

4. Acknowledgment

We thank Dr. M.N. Lub-de Hooge, Mr. Hans Pol and Mr. Hans ter Veen (Department of Nuclear Medicine, University Medical Center Groningen, The Netherlands) for their radiolabelling of proteins and help during the gamma-camera studies.

5. References

Adrian JE, Poelstra K, Scherphof GL, Molema G, Meijer DK, Reker-Smit C, Morselt HW, Kamps JA. 2006. Interaction of targeted liposomes with primary cultured hepatic stellate cells: Involvement of multiple receptor systems. J Hepatol 44(3):560-7.

Allen TM and Cullis PR. 2004. Drug delivery systems: Entering the mainstream. Science 303(5665):1818-22.

Andersen SR, Lambrecht LJ, Swan SK, Cutler DL, Radwanski E, Affrime MB, Garaud JJ. 1999. Disposition of recombinant human interleukin-10 in subjects with various degrees of renal function. J Clin Pharmacol 39(10):1015-20.

Bansal R, Prakash J, Post E, Beljaars L, Schuppan D, Poelstra K. 2011. Novel engineered targeted interferon-gamma blocks hepatic fibrogenesis in mice. Hepatology 54(2):586-96.

Bataller R and Brenner DA. 2005. Liver fibrosis. J Clin Invest 115(2):209-18.

Beljaars L, Meijer DK, Poelstra K. 2002. Targeting hepatic stellate cells for cell-specific treatment of liver fibrosis. Front Biosci 7:e214-22.

Beljaars L, Weert B, Geerts A, Meijer DK, Poelstra K. 2003. The preferential homing of a platelet derived growth factor receptor-recognizing macromolecule to fibroblast-like cells in fibrotic tissue. Biochem Pharmacol 66(7):1307-17.

Beljaars L, Molema G, Schuppan D, Geerts A, De Bleser PJ, Weert B, Meijer DK, Poelstra K. 2000. Successful targeting to rat hepatic stellate cells using albumin modified with cyclic peptides that recognize the collagen type VI receptor. J Biol Chem 275(17):12743-51.

Beljaars L, Molema G, Weert B, Bonnema H, Olinga P, Groothuis GM, Meijer DK, Poelstra K. 1999. Albumin modified with mannose 6-phosphate: A potential carrier for selective delivery of antifibrotic drugs to rat and human hepatic stellate cells. Hepatology 29(5):1486-93.

Chadban SJ, Tesch GH, Lan HY, Atkins RC, Nikolic-Paterson DJ. 1997. Effect of interleukin-10 treatment on crescentic glomerulonephritis in rats. Kidney Int 51(6):1809-17.

Colombel JF, Rutgeerts P, Malchow H, Jacyna M, Nielsen OH, Rask-Madsen J, Van Deventer S, Ferguson A, Desreumaux P, Forbes A, et al. 2001. Interleukin 10 (tenovil) in the prevention of postoperative recurrence of crohn's disease. Gut 49(1):42-6.

Curnis F, Gasparri A, Sacchi A, Cattaneo A, Magni F, Corti A. 2005. Targeted delivery of IFNgamma to tumor vessels uncouples antitumor from counterregulatory mechanisms. Cancer Res 65(7):2906-13.

Curnis F, Sacchi A, Borgna L, Magni F, Gasparri A, Corti A. 2000. Enhancement of tumor necrosis factor alpha antitumor immunotherapeutic properties by targeted delivery to aminopeptidase N (CD13). Nat Biotechnol 18(11):1185-90.

Cuzzocrea S, Mazzon E, Dugo L, Serraino I, Britti D, De Maio M, Caputi AP. 2001. Absence of endogeneous interleukin-10 enhances the evolution of murine type-II collagen-induced arthritis. Eur Cytokine Netw 12(4):568-80.

de Bleser PJ, Jannes P, van Buul-Offers SC, Hoogerbrugge CM, van Schravendijk CF, Niki T, Rogiers V, van den Brande JL, Wisse E, Geerts A. 1995. Insulinlike growth factor-II/mannose 6-phosphate receptor is expressed on CCl4-exposed rat fat-storing cells and facilitates activation of latent transforming growth factor-beta in cocultures with sinusoidal endothelial cells. Hepatology 21(5):1429-37.

Demols A, Van Laethem JL, Quertinmont E, Degraef C, Delhaye M, Geerts A, Deviere J. 2002. Endogenous interleukin-10 modulates fibrosis and regeneration in experimental chronic pancreatitis. Am J Physiol Gastrointest Liver Physiol 282(6):G1105-12.

Di Marco R, Xiang M, Zaccone P, Leonardi C, Franco S, Meroni P, Nicoletti F. 1999. Concanavalin A-induced hepatitis in mice is prevented by interleukin (IL)-10 and exacerbated by endogenous IL-10 deficiency. Autoimmunity 31(2):75-83.

Fedorak RN, Gangl A, Elson CO, Rutgeerts P, Schreiber S, Wild G, Hanauer SB, Kilian A, Cohard M, LeBeaut A, et al. 2000. Recombinant human interleukin 10 in the treatment of patients with mild to moderately active crohn's disease. the interleukin 10 inflammatory bowel disease cooperative study group. Gastroenterology 119(6):1473-82.

Fournier P, Aigner M, Schirrmacher V. 2011. Targeting of IL-2 and GM-CSF immunocytokines to a tumor vaccine leads to increased anti-tumor activity. Int J Oncol 38(6):1719-29.

Friedman SL. 2010. Evolving challenges in hepatic fibrosis. Nat Rev Gastroenterol Hepatol 7(8):425-36.

Gloor B, Todd KE, Lane JS, Rigberg DA, Reber HA. 1998. Mechanism of increased lung injury after acute pancreatitis in IL-10 knockout mice. J Surg Res 80(1):110-4.

Greupink R, Bakker HI, van Goor H, de Borst MH, Beljaars L, Poelstra K. 2006. Mannose-6-phosphate/insulin-like growth factor-II receptors may represent a target for the selective delivery of mycophenolic acid to fibrogenic cells. Pharm Res 23(8):1827-34.

Herfarth H and Scholmerich J. 2002. IL-10 therapy in crohn's disease: At the crossroads. treatment of crohn's disease with the anti-inflammatory cytokine interleukin 10. Gut 50(2):146-7.

Iredale JP. 2007. Models of liver fibrosis: Exploring the dynamic nature of inflammation and repair in a solid organ. J Clin Invest 117(3):539-48.

Ishak K, Baptista A, Bianchi L, Callea F, De Groote J, Gudat F, Denk H, Desmet V, Korb G, MacSween RN. 1995. Histological grading and staging of chronic hepatitis. J Hepatol 22(6):696-9.

Jazayeri JA and Carroll GJ. 2008. Fc-based cytokines : Prospects for engineering superior therapeutics. BioDrugs 22(1):11-26.

Jevsevar S, Kunstelj M, Porekar VG. 2010. PEGylation of therapeutic proteins. Biotechnol J 5(1):113-28.

Khan AQ, Shen Y, Wu ZQ, Wynn TA, Snapper CM. 2002. Endogenous pro- and anti-inflammatory cytokines differentially regulate an in vivo humoral response to streptococcus pneumoniae. Infect Immun 70(2):749-61.

Kitching AR, Tipping PG, Timoshanko JR, Holdsworth SR. 2000. Endogenous interleukin-10 regulates Th1 responses that induce crescentic glomerulonephritis. Kidney Int 57(2):518-25.

Louis H, Le Moine O, Goldman M, Deviere J. 2003. Modulation of liver injury by interleukin-10. Acta Gastroenterol Belg 66(1):7-14.

Louis H, Van Laethem JL, Wu W, Quertinmont E, Degraef C, Van den Berg K, Demols A, Goldman M, Le Moine O, Geerts A, et al. 1998. Interleukin-10 controls neutrophilic infiltration, hepatocyte proliferation, and liver fibrosis induced by carbon tetrachloride in mice. Hepatology 28(6):1607-15.

Meijer DK, Beljaars L, Molema G, Poelstra K. 2001. Disease-induced drug targeting using novel peptide-ligand albumins. J Control Release 72(1-3):157-64.

Nelson DR, Lauwers GY, Lau JY, Davis GL. 2000. Interleukin 10 treatment reduces fibrosis in patients with chronic hepatitis C: A pilot trial of interferon nonresponders. Gastroenterology 118(4):655-60.

Nissim A, Gofur Y, Vessillier S, Adams G, Chernajovsky Y. 2004. Methods for targeting biologicals to specific disease sites. Trends Mol Med 10(6):269-74.

Oberholzer A, Oberholzer C, Moldawer LL. 2002. Interleukin-10: A complex role in the pathogenesis of sepsis syndromes and its potential as an anti-inflammatory drug. Crit Care Med 30(1 Supp):S58-63.

Pinzani M, Rombouts K, Colagrande S. 2005. Fibrosis in chronic liver diseases: Diagnosis and management. J Hepatol 42 Suppl(1):S22-36.

Poelstra K, Hardonk MJ, Koudstaal J, Bakker WW. 1990. Intraglomerular platelet aggregation and experimental glomerulonephritis. Kidney Int 37(6):1500-8.

Rachmawati H, Reker-Smit C, Lub-de Hooge MN, van Loenen-Weemaes A, Poelstra K, Beljaars L. 2007. Chemical modification of interleukin-10 with mannose 6-phosphate groups yields a liver-selective cytokine. Drug Metab Dispos 35(5): 814-21.

Rachmawati H, Beljaars L, Reker-Smit C, Van Loenen-Weemaes AM, Hagens WI, Meijer DK, Poelstra K. 2004. Pharmacokinetic and biodistribution profile of recombinant human interleukin-10 following intravenous administration in rats with extensive liver fibrosis. Pharm Res 21(11):2072-8.

Reineke U, Sabat R, Volk HD, Schneider-Mergener J. 1998. Mapping of the interleukin-10/interleukin-10 receptor combining site. Protein Sci 7(4):951-60.

Schooltink H and Rose-John S. 2002. Cytokines as therapeutic drugs. J Interferon Cytokine Res 22(5):505-16.

Schreiber S, Fedorak RN, Nielsen OH, Wild G, Williams CN, Nikolaus S, Jacyna M, Lashner BA, Gangl A, Rutgeerts P, et al. 2000. Safety and efficacy of recombinant human interleukin 10 in chronic active crohn's disease. crohn's disease IL-10 cooperative study group. Gastroenterology 119(6):1461-72.

Schuppan D and Popov Y. 2009. Rationale and targets for antifibrotic therapies. Gastroenterol Clin Biol 33(10-11):949-57.

Schuppan D and Afdhal NH. 2008. Liver cirrhosis. Lancet 371(9615):838-51.

Standiford TJ. 2000. Anti-inflammatory cytokines and cytokine antagonists. Curr Pharm Des 6(6):633-49.

Thompson K, Maltby J, Fallowfield J, McAulay M, Millward-Sadler H, Sheron N. 1998. Interleukin-10 expression and function in experimental murine liver inflammation and fibrosis. Hepatology 28(6):1597-606.

van Beuge MM, Prakash J, Lacombe M, Post E, Reker-Smit C, Beljaars L, Poelstra K. 2011. Increased liver uptake and reduced hepatic stellate cell activation with a cell-specific conjugate of the rho-kinase inhibitor Y27632. Pharm Res 28(8):2045-54.

Vilcek J and Feldmann M. 2004. Historical review: Cytokines as therapeutics and targets of therapeutics. Trends Pharmacol Sci 25(4):201-9.

Wang SC, Ohata M, Schrum L, Rippe RA, Tsukamoto H. 1998. Expression of interleukin-10 by in vitro and in vivo activated hepatic stellate c

Part 3

Pharmacogenetic

9

Pharmacogenetics: The Scientific Basis

Bosun Banjoko
Obafemi Awolowo University, Ile-Ife, Nigeria

1. Introduction

The history of genetic variations in drug responses can be traced to the 1950s with the observations that muscle relaxant suxamethonium chloride and drugs metabolized by N-acetyl transferase exhibit differences in response in patients. One in 3500 caucasians was found to possess the less efficient variant of the enzyme, butyryl chlolinesterase that metabolizes suxamethonium chloride; an anaesthetic agent.As a consequence, the drug's effect is prolonged with slower recovery from surgical paralysis.

The term pharmacogenetics evolved from the combination of two areas of study namely pharmacology and genetics. Pharmacology is the study of how drugs work in the body and genetics is the study of how characteristics that result from the action of genes acting together are inherited and how they function in the cells of the body . Therefore, pharmacogenetics refers to genetic differences in metabolic pathways which can affect individual responses to drugs both in terms of therapy and adverse effects. Pharmacogenetics helps our understanding of why some individuals respond to drugs and others do not and why some require higher or lower doses to achieve optimal therapeutic responses.

In addition, pharmacogenetic information helps the physician to identify those patients who will respond favourably to therapy or develop side effects.

A recent offshoot of pharmacogenetics, termed pharmacogenomics is the study of drug response in the context of the entire genome. Pharmacogenomics facilitates information on variations in all the genes in a group of individuals simultaneously to determine the basis of variants in drug response. It is therefore not uncommon to find the two being used interchangeably.However for the purpose of this chapter, pharmacogenetics will be the focus.

Individual variation in response to drug ranges from failure to respond to drug therapy to drug to drug interactions when several drugs are taken simultaneously. The clinical consequences range from patients' discomfort through serious clinical illness to the occasional fatality. Approximately 7% of patients are affected by adverse drug reactions, increasing the overall hospital costs by 19% and drug costs by 15%. Some 0.3% of adverse drug reactions have fatal outcome (Topic 2010).

1.1 Individual variation in drug effects

Variation in drug metabolism and drug response among individuals of the same body weight and on the same drug dose can be due to temporary causes such as transient enzyme inhibition, induction or permanent causes such as genetic mutation, gene deletion or amplification. (Shenfield 2004).

Genetic variability is known to affect drug absorption, drug metabolism and drug interactions with receptors. These therefore form the basis for slow or rapid drug absorption, poor, efficient or ultrarapid drug metabolism and poor or efficient receptor interactions.

A genetic mutation frequency exceeding 10% of a population is considered a genetic polymorphism (Meyer 2000). Genetic polymorphism based on drug metabolizing ability is related to four phenotypic classes. The phenotype of extensive or normal drug metabolizers (EM) is characteristic of the normal population .Individuals are either homozygous or heterozygous for wild type allele. Those individuals who are heterozygous for the wild type allele may have intermediate metabolizer phenotype (IM) and may require lower than average drug dose for optimal therapeutic response. Those individuals with mutation or deletion of both alleles for the determinant of phenotypic response can be classified as poor metabolizers (PM) and therefore prone to accumulation of drug substrates in their systems with attendant effects. The fourth class, termed the ultrarapid metabolizers (UM) possess enhanced drug metabolism capabilities due to gene amplification and are prone to drug failure because drug concentrations at normal doses are expected to be too low for therapeutic effects (Meyer 2000, Davies 2006).

There are ethnical and racial differences in the frequency of variant alleles and up to 10 - 20% of patients belong to the risk groups. (Evans 1986, Banjoko & Akinlade 2010).

1.2 Mechanism of genetic polymorphism

Pharmacogenetic polymorphism can manifest at the pharmacokinetic and pharmacodynamics levels. The pharmacokinetic level deals with gene polymorphism that modify concentrations of drugs and its metabolites at the site of their molecular action (polymorphism of drug metabolizing enzymes, drug transporters) whereas the pharmacodynamics level deal with polymorphism of action not related to its concentration (receptors, ion channels). Genetic variations are the result of multiple mechanism such as insertion, deletion, variable tandem repeats and microsatellites but the most frequent polymorphism are point mutation or single nucleotide polymorphism (SNPS). Some of the polymorphism are without consequences but others cause synthesis of altered proteins, truncated proteins, unstable proteins or proteins at the level of expression.

Genotype is the detailed gene structure of an individual whereas the more commonly measured phenotype is the outcome of metabolism of a drug in an individual. Since genotype is the result of interactions between genetic make up and the environment, it is not always concordant with phenotype.

1.3 Consequences of pharmacogenetics

The underpinning factors for the growing importance of pharmacogenetics are the necessity to prevent adverse drug reaction, obtain maximum benefits from drug therapy and reduce therapeutic failure.

Adverse drug reactions are thought to kill many hospitalized patients worldwide. In the US alone, the estimate of deaths attributable to drug reactions is about 100,000 annually and it is believed that many of these reactions are due to genetic variations. Thus many deaths are avoidable if genetic testing or genomic information of patients are available and utilized prior to therapy.

Pharmacogenetics will therefore permit gene profiling to answer questions about drug responses and promote the design of better and safer drugs. In addition, individualized dosing has the potential of better therapeutic outcome. Therefore pharmacogenetics is expected to revolutionise drug dosing and therapy .However, there are still many challenges to overcome. These include cost implications, standardization , quality control of testing, and relevance of biomarkers and tests. Nevertheless, the advent of pharmacogenetics and establishment of guidelines by regulatory bodies like Food and Drugs Administration (FDA) European Medicines Agency (EMEA) and American Association of Clinical Chemists (AACC) are expected to impact individualized dosing of many drugs.

1.4 Confounding issues in pharmacogenetics

The understanding that drug response may be multifactoral helps us to recognize the importance of examining more than the classical "single gene-single protein concept which gave birth to pharmacogenomics. In addition, there are more evidences that modifications besides outright mutation of genes, for example, methylation of promoter region by epigenetic factor impact gene expression and drug responses. Moreover, genotype is not the only determinant of phenotype. For example, individuals whose genotypes falls extensive metabolizers via CYP2D6 can display a phenotype that would characterize them as poor metabolizers if they are co-administered low doses of quinidine which is a potent inhibitor of CYP2D6 . Therefore, differences in phenotype does not necessarily translate into difference in pharmacologic response between subjects. In the same fashion, mutation of the genes may not necessarily translate into effect on drug metabolism (Henningson et al 2005).

Because of significant racial differences in genetic composition, it is important that caution is exercised in the interpretation of genetic testing. For example different genotypes may give rise to the same phenotype.In addition, there are varieties of mutations in NAT2 that give rise to slow acetylator status.

Furthermore the historical use of wild-type alleles and mutant alleles may not necessarily hold true for all the races hence the migration to the term reference and mutant alleles.

2. Basic genetics

Genetics is the study concerned with hereditary and variation. One of the most fundamental properties of all living organisms is the ability to reproduce. All organisms therefore inherit the genetic information specifying their structure and function from their parents. In the same manner, all cells arise from pre - existing cells, so the genetic material must be replicated and passed from a parent to progeny cell at each cell division. The hereditary molecules that are transmitted from one generation to the next i.e. inherited are called genes. These molecules (genes) reside in the deoxyribonucleic acid (DNA) that exist within all cells. The DNA in conjunction with a protein matrix forms nucleoprotein and become organized into structures called chromosomes located in the nucleus or nuclear region of cells. The genes contains coded information for the synthesis of proteins and some ribonucleic acids (RNA). Occasionally, a change may occur spontaneously in some part of the DNA. This change is called mutation and may result in an alteration of the code designated for a particular function resulting in production of a defective protein.

A mutation may lead to a change in the physical appearance of an individual or change in some other measurable attributes of the organism called a character or trait. Through the process of mutation, a gene may be changed into two or more alternative forms called alleles. Each gene occupies a specific position on the chromosomes called the gene locus. All allelic forms of a gene therefore are found at corresponding positions on genetically similar (homologous) chromosomes.

All the genes on a chromosomes are said to be linked to one another and to belong to the same linkage group. Since a gene can be changed to alternative forms by the process of mutation, a large number of alleles are theoretically possible in a population of individuals. Whenever more than two alleles are identified at a gene locus in a population, such is described as multiple allele series.

Genetic information is stored and transmitted in the four letter alphabet and language of DNA (A,C,G,T) and ultimately expressed in the twenty letter alphabet of proteins. Protein biosynthesis is called translation because it involves the biochemical translation of information between languages.

A capital letter is commonly used to designate the allele that is dominant to other alleles in the series. For example letter "R" for a character is dominant over 'r' which is an allele that is recessive to all others in the series .Intermediate in their degree of dominance between the two extremes are usually assigned the lower case letter with superscript which in this example is r*. Many genes may contribute to a single character or trait (polygenic traits) or traits exhibiting continuous variation. In addition, each gene may have multiple phenotypic effects (pleiotropy).

Each character is controlled by a pair of genes. The progeny or offspring are therefore hybrids of the parents, inheriting a pair of gene, one each from each parent. For example for trait for tallness being represented by letter T, possible genetic composition are TT, Tt, and tt whereby T allele is dominant over t. It is expected that an offspring with tt genetic composition will be short while those with TT or Tt will be tall.

The genetic composition of a trait is referred to as the genotype and the physical appearance corresponding to the genotype, in this example tallness is called the phenotype.With different generations of offsprings i.e. the filial generations, different genotypes and corresponding phenotypes are obtainable.

The originator of the classical principles of genetics is Macgregor Mendel who made public the result of his study of peas breeding in 1865. Mendel studied the inheritance of a number of well defined traits in the pea such as seed colour and was able to deduce general rules for their transmission. He was the first to observe that each trait was determined by a pair of inherited factors later termed the genes. Mendel's findings provided the template for determination of genotypes and phenotypes of different genetic diseases of humans, animals and plants and notable examples include: sickle cell disease, albinism and thalassaemias.

By 1900, Mendel's laws of inheritance were well established and are thus stated:

Law of segregation: Each parent possesses 2 copies of a unit of inheritance (now called the gene) for each trait. However, only one of these two genes (an allele) is transmitted through a gamete to the offspring.

Law of independent assortment: says segregation of one gene pair occurs independently of any other gene pair.

2.1 Chromosomes, genes and inheritance

Chromosomes are known to be carrier of genes. Most cells of higher plants and animals are diploid. i.e. they contain two copies of each chromosome. Formation of the germ cells; the sperm and egg involves a unique type of cell division termed meiosis. In this process, only one member of each chromosome pair is transmitted to each progeny cell. Therefore, the sperm and egg are haploid containing only one copy of each chromosome. The fusion of these two haploid cells at fertilization result in a new diploid organism; the offspring which consists of one member of each chromosome pair. Behaviour of chromosome pairs is directly related to their genes indicating a strong relationship between genes and chromosomes.

Genetic alterations i.e. mutation which is the basis of genetic diseases was first identified in the experiment with *Drosophilia melanogaster* (the fruit fly) in the early 1900. Mutations in drosophila was observed to involve such phenotypes like eye colour and wing shape. Experimented evidences revealed that the genes governing these traits are inherited independently of each other, suggesting that these genes are located on different chromosomes that segregate independently during meiosis. Other genes are inheritable as paired characteristics and such are said to be linked to each other by virtue of being located on the same chromosome. The frequency of recombination between two linked genes depends on distance between them on the chromosomes. In addition, genes that are close to each other recombine less frequently than do genes further apart. Thus the differences with which the different genes recombine can be used to determine their relative position on the chromosome allowing the construction of a genetic map.

2.2 Genes, proteins and enzymes

Genes act by determining the structure of proteins which are responsible for directing cell metabolism through the activities of enzymes. Many genes encode enzymes that are important for catalysing biological synthesis (anabolic) and degradation (catabolic reactions) within a cell. These reactions grouped together into a series of reactions are called biochemical pathways and commence with the enzymes acting on their corresponding substrate.

The first indication linking genes and enzymes can be traced to 1909 when it was observed that patients suffering from phenylketonuria were suspected to have a genetic defect in the metabolism of the amino acid for phenylalanine.This line of thought was supported by the experiment of George Beadle and Edward Tatum in 1941 with the fungus; *Neurospora cassa*. Using mutant strains of the organism, they observed that each mutant required specific nutritional supplement such as a particular aminoacid for growth.Furthermore, the requirement for a specific nutritional supplement correlates with the failure of the mutant to synthesize that particular compound. Thus each mutant resulted in a deficiency in a specific metabolic pathway. Since metabolic pathways are known to be controlled by enzymes, these findings gave rise to the one - gene - one enzyme hypothesis which by implication means that each gene specified the structure of a single enzyme. However, the revelation that genes not only codes for proteins and enzymes but tRNAs resulted in this hypothesis being modified to one - gene - one - polypeptide concept.

Transfer RNA's (tRNAs) serve as adaptations between aminoacids and messenger RNA (mRNA) during translation. Prior to its use in protein synthesis, each aminoacid is attached by a specific enzyme to its appropriate tRNA. Base pairing between a recognition sequence in each tRNA and a complimentary sequence on the mRNA then directs the attached aminoacid to its correct position on the mRNA template.

2.3 Genetic polymorphism

Genetic polymorphism can be defined as differences in DNA sequence among individuals, groups or population. Genetic mutation can create genetic variance in a population and this can manifest in different ways. Somatic cell mutation can create a genetic variation in a cell population which may induce cancer and tumour when such mutation takes place in repressor genes controlling cell cycles such as p53 gene. On the other hand,germ line cell mutation can cause genetic diseases such as sickle cell disease, thalassemia, Parkinson's disease as well as defect of biochemical pathway that influence drug - receptor interaction with attendant deleterious effects on patients. Point mutation such as a single base nucleotide substitution (SNP) are common particularly with adverse drug reactions. Mutation that occurs in germ line cell would be inherited by the progeny and these mutated genes can spread in a population through the fertilization process. Mutations that occur in coding frame of DNA region that are responsible for synthesis of specific products could give rise to genetic disease. Similarly, mutation that affects enzymes responsible for biotransformation of drugs particularly C450 gene family and pharmacokinetic and pharmacodynamic gene functions can result in adverse drug reactions or drug inefficacy. These reasons make phamacogenetics an important area of study.

3. Basic pharmacology

Pharmacology is the study that deals with interaction of endogenously administered chemical molecules termed drugs with living systems. It involves such studies like (i) Pharmacokinetics (ii) Pharmacodynamics (iii) Toxicology

i. **Pharmacokinetics** : Pharmacokinetics is the quantitative study of drug movement from administration throughout out the body till excretion. All pharmacokinetic processes involve transport of the drug across cell membrane,. absorption, distribution and excretion
ii. **Pharmacodynamics**: Pharmacodynamics coined from two Greek words pharmacon; drugs and dynamis: power, involves the physiological and biochemical effect of drugs and their mechanism of action at organ, systemic, subcellular and macromolecular levels. The pharmacodynamic process describes all those matters concerned with the pharmacological action of a drug, whether they be determinants of the therapeutic effect or of the toxic effect.

iii. **Toxicology:** This is the study of poisonous effects of drugs and other chemicals. Although a speciality on it's own, it is nevertheless still considered under pharmacology with regards to adverse drug effects.

3.1 Principles of drug actions

There are eight main drug actions and these are:

Stimulation: Through direct receptor agonism and downstream effect e.g. adrenaline stimulates heart, pilocarpine stimuates salivary glands. However, excessive stimulation is often followed by depression of that function e.g. high dose of picrotoxin, a CNS stimulant, produces convulsions followed by coma and respiratory depression.

Depression: Through direct receptor agonism and down stream effect e.g. barbiturates depress CNS while quinines depresses the heart. The action of this mechanism is selective.

Blocking/Antagonizing action: The drugs binds the receptor but does not activate it.

Stabilizing action: In this case, the drugs seem to act neither as a stimulant nor as a depressant but to stabilize general receptor activation like buprenorphine in opioid dependence or aripiprazole in schizophrenia.

Replacement: Refers to the use of natural metabolites including hormones and vitamins in deficiency stages e.g. levodopa in Parkinsonism, insulin in diabetes mellitus, iron in anemia and oestrogen replacement in women of menopausal age.

Direct beneficial chemical reaction: As in use of antioxidants like Vitamins C,E and *B*-carotene for free radical scavenging

Cytotoxic action: Selective cytotoxic action for parasite, bacterial or cancer cells, attenuating them without significantly affecting the host cells e.g. use of antibiotics like penicillin, zidovudin and cyclophosphamide

Irritation: A none selective often noxious effect applicable to less specialized cells, for example the epithelial, connective tissue cells). Mild irritation may stimulate associated function e.g. bitters increase salivary and gastric secretions which results in increased blood flow to the site. However, strong irritation may result in inflammation, corrosion, necrosis and morphological damage with resultant diminution or loss of function. Therefore caution should be exercised in the administration because of tendency of excessive ingestion.

4. Metabolism of drug and other xenobiotics

Metabolism of drugs and other xenobiotics involves activities that modify the chemical structure of the substances which are foreign to the body's internal mileu. These reactions often act to detoxify poisonous compounds; however in some cases, the intermediate metabolite can themselves be toxic

The purpose of biotransformation is to convert lypophilic compounds to hydrophilic ones which will facilitate their excretion. The consequences of biotransformation is changes in pharmacokinetic characteristics.

Xenobiotics metabolism can be divided into three phases. In phase 1, enzymes such as cytochrome p450 oxidases introduce an active or polar group into the xenobiotics. These modified compounds are then conjugated to polar compounds in phase II reactions. The main enzyme that catalyses the reactions in phase II is glutathione S-transferase since it acts on a wide range of substrates.

The final phase; phase III may involve further metabolism of conjugates of phase II reactions like the processing of glutathione conjugates to acetylcysteine (mercapturic acic) conjugates before being recognized by efflux transporters and pumped out of the cells (Boyland & Chassaud 1969, Thomalley 1990)

Peculiar to all organisms is the possession of cell membranes which serve as hydrophobic permeability barriers to control access to their internal environment. Polar compounds cannot diffuse across these cell membranes, and the uptake of useful molecules is mediated through transport proteins that specifically select substrates from the extracellular mixture. The implication of this structure is that most hydrophilic molecules cannot enter the cells since they need to be recognized by specific transporters (Mizuno et al 2003).

The detoxification of reactive by-products is via a different mechanism. Because these species are derived from normal cellular constituents, they usually share the same polar characteristics therefore, specific designated enzymes can metabolize them. A notable example of these specific detoxification system is the glyoxalase system which catalyses the removal of the reactive aldehyde, methylglyoxal (Thormalley 1990) and the various antioxidant systems that eliminate reactive oxygen species (Sies 1997).

4.1 Phase I reactions

In Phase I reactions, a variety of enzymes act to introduce reactive and polar groups into their substrates. This is basically a functionalization reaction. One of the most common modifications in this phase is hydroxylation, a reaction catalysed by the cytochrome P-450 dependent mixed function oxidase system. These enzymes complexes act to incorporate an atom of oxygen into nonactivated hydrocarbons, which can result in either the introduction of hydroxyl groups, or Nitrogen, Oxygen.and Sulphate- dealkylation of substrates (Schlichting et al 2000).Of all the enzymes involved in drug metabolism, the cytochrome P450.(CYP450) is regarded as the most important because many drugs are substrates for the enzymes of the group. In all, CYP3A4, CYP2D6, CYP2C9, CYP219, CYP2B6 and CYP1A2 subtypes play the most critical role and account for more than 90% of drugs metabolized by CYP 450 enzymes (Evans & Relling 1999). These enzymes have proven genetic polymorphism with associated drug responses (Hiratsuka et al 2002, Wong et al 2005, McAlpine et al 2011) and racial variations (Meyer 2004 & Suarez - Kurtz 2005).

Phenotypes of P450 are divided into four groups and these are; the extensive metabolizers (EM)who show low metabolic activities, the poor metabolisers(PM)who carry gene alterations on both alleles which are inherited in an autosomal manner, the intermediate metabolizers (IM) with metabolic capacity in between those of PM and EM and finally the ultra rapid metabolizers (UM)who show higher metabolic capacity than the EM. (Murphy 2001, Hiratsuka et al 2005). Genetic variations have been observed particularly with CYP 2D6, CYP2C9 and CYP2C19 genotypes (Ingelman - Sundberg 1999, Hiratsuka 2006). With regards to CYP2D6,five to ten percent of caucasians are poor metabolizers and have little enzyme activities. In addition, there is a distinct racial diversity in the frequency of the classes. Examples of CYP450 catalyzed drug metabolic reactions include

i. **Hydroxylation**: S-mephenytoin CYP3A4 4-OH-S-mephenytoin
ii. **Epoxidation:** Carbamazepine CYP3A4/5 10,11 Epoxide
iii. **Oxygenation**: Amines CYP 2D6 Hydroxylamines
iv. **O-dealkylation**: Dextromethorphan CYP2D6 Dextrophan
v. **N-demethylation**: Caffeine CYP2E1 Theobromine
vi. **N-demethylation:** Caffeine CYP1A2 Paraxanthine
vii. **N-demethylation** Caffeine CYP2E1 Theophylline
viii. **Oxidative Group Transfer**: Parathion CYP2B6 Paraoxon
ix. **Dehydrogenation:** Acetaminophen CYP2E1 N-Aacetyl benzoquinoneimine
x. **Ester Cleavage**: Loratidine CYP3A4, CYP2D6 Desacetylated Loratidine
xi. **Reduction**: Paraquat FLAVOPROTEIN REDUCTASE paraquat radicals

4.1.1 Non P450 enzyme catalysis

Besides the CYP 450 enzymes, other enzymes that participate in drug biotransformations include; monoamineoxidases, peroxidases, lactoperoxidases myeloperoxidases, prostaglandin-H-synthetase and flavin-containing monooxygenases.(FMO).Examples of the reactions they catalyse include:

i. **Hydrolysis:** hydrolysis of peptide bond of Insulin
ii. **Reduction**: Chloral Hydrate ALC. DEHYDROGENASE Trichloroethanol
iii. **Oxidoreduction**: Alcohol ALC.DEHYDROGENASE Aldehyde

4.2 Phase II reactions

In phase II reactions, the activated xenobiotic metabolites are conjugated with charged species such as glutathione (GSH), sulfate, glycine or glycuronic acid and increased risk of early renal complications in type 2 diabetes mellitus (Banjoko & Akinlade 2010). These reactions are catalysed by substrate specific transferases which in total can metabolize almost any hydrophobic compound that contains nucleophilic or electrophilic group.

One of the most important of this group is the glutathione S-transferase (GSTs). The addition of large anionic groups such as glutathione detoxifies reactive electrophiles and produces more polar metabolites that cannot diffuse across membranes and may therefore be actively transported.

4.2.1 Glutathione conjugation

Glutathione is a tripeptide of glycine, cysteine and glutamic acid formed by the action of glutamylcysteine synthetase (glutathione synthetase).The enzyme glutathione transferase catalyses the conjugation of modified xenobiotic with glutathione. A large number of drugs are conjugated by glutathione during metabolism. Inhibitors of the enzyme include Buthione - S - Sulfoxine. Two types of reactions are common with glutathione. The first is displacement of halogen, sulfate, sulfonate or phosphonitro group. The second is the addition of glutathione to activated double bond or strained ring system. Some of the conjugation reactions include:

i. N - acetylbenzoquinoneimine, an activated metabolic of acetaminophen.
ii. O - demethylation of organophosphates
iii. Activation of trinitroglycine to oxidized glutathione (GSSG) dinitroglycerine and Nitric oxide (NO) a vasodilator.

Distinct cytosolic and microsomal glutathione -S transferases have been identified. In all, four classes of soluble glutathione S transferase are known to exist. The enzyme also exhibit genetic polymorphism and overexpression of the enzyme leads to e.g. resistance of insects to DDT, corn to atrazine and cancer cells to chemotherapy. The enzyme also participates in reduction of hydroperoxides and prostaglandin metabolism. Inducers of the enzyme include 3-methylcholanthrene, phenobarbital, corticosteroids and antioxidants. GST exhibit specie specificity; for example, aflatoxin B_1 is not carcinogenic in mice because it conjugates with glutathione very rapidly in them. Conjugates are excreted intact in bile or converted to mercapturic acid in kidney and excreted in urine in a reaction catalysed by glutamyl transpeptidase an aminopeptidase

4.2.2 Uridyl Diphosphate Glucuronyl transferase (UDPG transferase)

The reaction of UDP Glucuronyl transferase results in the formation of O^-, N^-, S and C^- glucuronides. Six forms of this enzyme have been identified in the liver. The cofactor for its reaction is UDP - glucuronic acid. Inducers include phenobarbital, indoles, 3 methyl cholanthrene and cigarette smoke. Some of its substrate are dextrophan, methalidone, morphine, p-nitrophenol, valproic acid, non steroidal anti-inflamatory drugs, bilirubin and steroid hormones. In Criggler Najjar syndrome; a severe form of bilirubinaemia, the enzyme is inactive hence inducers have no effect. However, in Gilbert's syndrome; a mild form of hyperbilirubinaemia, phenobarbital can increase the rate of bilirubin glucuronidation to normal functions . Other substrates of the enzymes include, morphine and chloramphenicol. Conjugates of UDPG transferase are excreted in bile and urine. An S-glucuronidase from the gut microflora cleaves the glucuronic acid, the glycone formed can be reabsorbed to undergo enterohepatic cycling. Other associated reactions include metabolic activation of 2, 6 dinitrotoluene by S-glucuronidase; whereby the latter removes glucuronic acid from N-glucuronide. The nitrogroup is then reduced by microbial N-reductase and the resultant hepatocarcinogen may be reabsorbed.

4.2.3 Sulfation

The sulfation process is catalysed by sulfotransferases which are widely distributed in the body. The co-factor for their reaction is 3^1 phosphoadenosine 5 phosphosulfate (PAPS). Their conjugation result in highly water soluble sulfate esters which are eliminated in urine and bile. Examples of substances for sulfation include phenols, catecholamines and hydroxylamines. Sulfation is a high affinity, low capacity pathway which is limited by low PAPS level. Acetaminophen is a drug that undergoes both sulfation and glucuronidation. At low doses, sulfation predominates but at high doses glucuronidation predominates. Four sulfotransferases in human liver cytosol have been identified to date. Aryl sulfatases in gut microflora remove sulfate groups in a sort of enterohepatic recycling. Sulfation decreases pharmacologic and toxic activities but can also cause activation of chemically unstable groups to carcinogens, for example hydroxylamine.

4.2.4 Methylation

This is a common minor pathway of xenobiotic biotransformation which generally decreases water solubility. Enzymes that catalyse the reactions are called methyltransferases and the co-factor is S-adenosylmethionine (SAM). In methylation, a methyl group (CH_3) is transferred to O, N, S or C molecule on the substrates which include phenols, catecholamines and heavy metals like Hg, As and Se. There are several methyltransferases in human tissues examples of which are phenol - O - methyltransferases, catechol - O - methyltransferase, O-methyl transferase and S-methyl transferase. Genetic polymorpohism has been observed in thiopurine metabolism in a reaction catalysed by a member of this group of enzymes. High activity allele causes increased toxicity and low activity allele causes decreased efficacy.

4.2.5 Acetylation

This is the major route of biotransformation of aromatic amines and hydrazines. The reaction is catalysed by N - acetyl transferases (NAT) enzyme and the co factor acetyl-coenzyme-A. The process generally causes a decrease in water solubility. Substrates of the enzyme include sulfanilamide, isoniazid, dapsone and caffeine. In humans three phenotypic forms have been identified and these are slow, intermediate and rapid acetylators (Evans 1999, Murphy 2001). Various mutations of the enzyme result in decreased enzyme activity or stability. Like every other entity exhibiting genetic polymorphism, there are various ethnic and tribal variations. For example, 70% of slow acetylator status was observed in Middle Eastern population, 50% in Caucasians and 25% in Asians (Hiratsuka 2006, Evans and Relling 1989). Drug toxicities in slow acetylators include nerve damage from dapsone and bladder cancer in cigarette smokers due to increased levels of hydroxylamines (Ohno and Yamaguchi 2000, Evans 1999, Hiratsuka et al 2006).

4.2.6 Amino acid conjugation

This is an alternative pathway to glucuronidation. Amino acid conjugation operate with two principles. The first is that carboxylic group (COOH) group of a substrate is conjugated with an amino (NH_2) group of glycine, serine, glutamine requiring co enzyme-A activation. Notable example is the conjugation of benzoic acid with glycine to form hippuric acid. Benzoic acid is commonly used as a preservative in carbonated drinks. Alternatively aromatic NH_2 or NHOH conjugate with COOH of serine proteins requiring ATP activation. This metabolic pathway demonstrate specie specificity in accepting amino acid. For example, in mammals, benzoic acid is conjugated by glycine whereas for the same substrate in birds, ornithine acts. Dogs and cats utilize taurine to conjugate bile acids while other non human primates utilize glutamine for conjugation. Metabolic activation of serine or proline results in N-esters of hydroxylamine which are unstable and may degrade to reactive electrophile.

4.2.7 Ribonucleoside/nucleoside synthesis

This pathway is important for the activation of many purine and pyrimidine antimetabolites used in cancer chemotherapy

4.3 Phase III reactions

Phase III reactions can be described as a stage of further modification and excretion. Although many authors do not regard this phase as a distinct phase, current knowledge of efflux transporters tend to support the categorization. A common example is the processing of glutathione conjugates to acetylcysteine (mercapturic acid) conjugates (Boyland and Chassaud 1969). In this scenario, glutamate and glycine residing in the glutathione molecule are removed by gamma-glutamyltranspeptidase and dipeptidases. Finally, the cysteine residue in the conjugate is acetylated .The conjugates and their metabolites can then be excreted from cells in phase III of their metabolism with anionic groups acting as affinity taps for a variety of membrane transporters of the multidrug resistance protein (MRP) family (Homolya et al 2003). These proteins are members of the family of ATP-binding cassette transporters and can facilitate the ATP dependent transport of a large varieties of hydrophobic ions (Konig et al 1999) and thus act to remove phase II products to the extracellular medium, where they may be further metabolized and excreted (Commandeur et al 1995).

Since the discovery of permeability glycoprotein (P - glycoprotein) complex; an initial member of the ATP binding cassette (ABC) family of drug transporters by Juliano and Ling in 1976, (Juliano and Ling 1976) research into this group of proteins has been gaining wide interests. Some of the membrane transporters confer on the cells the ability to be resistant not only to the selective agent but also to a broad spectrum of structurally and functionally distinct antibiotics and alkaloids.This phenotypic character is referred to as multiple drug resistance (MDR). The MDR genotype/phenotype relationship is complex with over 18 ABC genes associated with human disease (Dean and Annilo 2005).

In addition to the ABC transporters, other important drug/xenobiotic transporters include the organic cation transporters of the SLC 22A super family and the organic anion transporting peptides of the SLC21 superfamily (Hagenbuch 2010). It is expected that with the growing interests in this phase of drug metabolism, investigations on the transcriptional regulatory control of this important transport system in target organs such as the liver, kidney and central nervous system will become intense in the next few decades (Omiecinski 2011).

5. Target genes of pharmacogenetics

About 20 kinds of enzymes are involved in metabolism of drugs. The cytochrome enzyme (CYP450) is regarded as the most important enzyme in drug metabolism. About 15 types of this group have been identified in human beings where they catalyse the biotransformation of many xenobiotics. Other enzymes include thiopurine methyl transferase (TMPT) which metabolizes 6- mercaptopurine and azathioprine, uridyl diphosphate glucuronyl transferase (UDGT) responsible for the conjugation of bilirubin, N - acetyltransferase (NAT2) responsible for metabolism of sulpha containing drugs and caffeine, catachol - o - methyl transferase (COMT) responsible for the metabolism of levodopa and dihydropyrimidine dehydrogenase (DPD) a rate limiting enzyme for the metabolism of 5 - florouracil (5 FU). Genetic polymorphism has been identified in many of these enzymes with varying degrees of drug response (Evans & Relling 1999, Furuta et al 2001, McAlpine et al 2001,Suzuki et al 2011) Of all the enzymes involved in drug metabolism, the cytochrome P450.(CYP450) is regarded as the most important because many drugs are substrates for the enzyme of the group. CYP3A4, CYP2D6, CYP2C9, CYP219, CYP2B6 and CYP1A2 play the most critical role and account for more than 90% of drugs metabolized by P450 (Evans & Relling 1999). These enzymes have proven genetic polymorphism with associated drug responses (Hiratsuka et al 2002, Wong et al 2005, McAlpine et al 2011) and racial variations (Meyer 2004 & Suarez - Kurtz 2005). As discussed earlier, genetic polymorphism can manifest at both pharmacokinetic and pharmacodynamic levels whereby many genetic variants of respective enzymes, membrane transporters, receptors and ion channels have been dectected (Wiesler et al 2008, Phipps - Green et al 2010 & Bouamar et al 2011)

5.1 Pharmacokinetic related genes

5.1.1 Genes of phase i reaction enzymes

Genetic variations have been observed particularly with CYP2D6, CYP2C9 aand CYP2C19 genotypes (Ingelman - Sundberg 1999, Hiratsuka 2006) and therefore will be further elucidated.

i. **CYP2D6:** With regards to this CYP subtype, 5 - 10% of Caucasians are poor metabolizers and have little enzyme activity and there is a distinct racial diversity in the frequency of the classes. About 50 genetic polymorphisms of CYP2D6 have been reported. The popular ones are CYP2D6*3, CYP2D6*4 and CYP2D6*5. More than 90% of PMs in Caucasians are ascribable to these three genetic polymorphism (Daly et al 1996,& Suzuki et al 2011). In blacks, the common variant is CYP2D*17 (Evans 1989)
ii. **CYP2C9:** is involved in the metabolism of an epileptic agent; phenytoin and an anticoagulant; warfarin. To date, 12 CYP2C9 variants have been reported. For example in cases with phenytoin, oral clearance decreased to one quarter in subjects with homozygous polymorphism for CYP2CP*3 (Kidd et al 1999 , Scodo et al 2002, Linder et al 2009). Many studies focused on CYP2C9 polymorphism to link variability with warfarin therapy. However only about 10% of dosage variation can be attributed to CYP2C9 polymorphism. It is thought that environmental and genetic factors can influence warfarin response therefore dosage is individualized based on sex, age, vitatmin K intake, and disease states. Warfarin dosing can be challenging because of its narrow therapeutic index and the serious risk of bleeding in overdosage. Warfarin exerts its anticoagulant effects by inhibiting hepatic vitamin K epoxide reductase; an enzyme involved in the vitamin K epoxide reductase complex sub unit 1 (VKORC1). The gene that encodes this enzyme has been identified and is believed to contribute to the variability in warfarin response (Scodo et al 2002, Aquilante et al 2006, Linder et al 2009, Guengerich 2001).
iii. **The CYP2C19:** enzyme metabolizes many drugs including the proton pump inhibitor; citalopram (lelexa) diazepam (valium) and imipramine (toranil). More than 16 variants of CYP2C19 associated with deficient, reduced, normal or increased activity have been identified. The most common genotypic variants for poor metabolizers are CYP2C19*2 and CYP2C19*3. The CYP2C19*17 variant is associated with ultrarapid metabolizers and seems to be common in Swedes (18%), Ethiopians (18%) and Chinese (4%). (Sum et al 2006). The proton pump inhibitor omeprazole (prilosec) is primarily metabolized by CYP2C19 to its inactive metabolite 5 - hydroxyl-omeprazole. Individuals who are CYP2C19 poor metabolizers can have five fold higher blood concentrations of omeprazole and experience superior acid suppression and higher cure rate than the rest

of the population. Conversely, blood concentrations of omeprazole are predicted to be 40% lower in ultrarapid metabolizers than the rest of the population and are therefore at risk of therapeutic failure. (Sum et al 2006)

5.1.2 Genes of phase II reaction enzymes

N - Acetyl Transferase: Activities of human hepatic drug metabolizing enzymes was earlier been recognized as a cause of inter - individual variation in the metabolism of drugs. Therefore acetylation of many drugs like isoniazid caffeine, nitrozepam and sulphonamide exhibit genetic polymorphism. The N - acetyl transferase (NAT) enzyme is controlled by two genes, (NAT 1) and (NAT 2) of which NAT2 A and B are responsible for clinically significant metabolic polymorphism. (Heiss 1988, Grant et al 1990). Three phenotypes have been recognized with activities of NAT2 and these are rapid acetylator (RA), intermediate acetylator (IA) and slow acetylator (SA) status (Cranswick 2005). The frequency of slow acetylator in Caucasians and Negro populations is 50% and 10% in Oriental groups. (.Evans D.A 1989) Slow acetylator phenotype is preponderant among different Arab populations irrespective of geographical location of the country. (Woolhouse et al 1997, At- Moussa et al 2002 & Desoky et al 2005). Three genetic polymorphisms NAT2*5, NAT2*6, NAT2*7 but not NAT2*4 (wild type allele) are responsible for almost all SAs in the Japanese (Huang et al 2002) Drug induced hepatitis caused by isoniazid occurs often in SA than RA (Ohno et al 2000) and Type II diabetes SA may be predisposed to progression to renal complications than their RA counterparts (Banjoko & Akinlade 2010).

Thiopurine - S -Methyl Transferase (TPMT: Catalyses the S - Methylation of the thiopurine agents, azathioprine, mercaptopurine and thiogleamine. These agents are commonly used for a diverse range of medical indications including leukaemia, rheumatic diseases and organ transplant. The principal cytotoxic mechanism of these agents is mediated via incorporation of thioguanine nucleotides (TGN) into DNA. Thiopurines are inactive prodrugs that require metabolism to thioguanine nucleotides to exert cytotoxicity. This activation is catalyzed by a multienzyme pathway which include hypoxanthine phosphoribosyl transeferase (HPRT), oxidation by xanthine oxidase (XO) or methylation by TPMT. During metabolism, hypoxanthine-guanine phosphoribosyl transferase (HPGRT) converts 6-mercaptopurine to cytotoxic6-thioguanine nucleotide analogues, while thiopurine methyl transferase (TPMT) inactivates 6-mercaptopurine through methylation to form 6 -methylmercaptopurine. However, TMPT is the major pathway and it is highly variable and polymorphic. More than 12 TPMT alleles have been identified. The most common ones are TPMT*2, TPMT*3A, TPMT*3C, with all three associated with lower enzyme activity attributable to enhanced rates of proteolysis of the variant proteins (Donnan et al 2011, Haghuid et al 2011, Guengerich 2001). Caucasian infant patients with acute myeloid leukaemia carrying TPMT*2, TPMT*3A, TPMT*3B, TPMT*3C showed significantly higher concentrations of the thiopurine intermediate metabolite 6-mercaptopurine in their red cells that requires dose reduction or termination of thiopurine administration due to adverse effects such as myelosuppression (Relling et al 1999, Tavadia et al 2001).

Dihydro Pyrimidine Dehydrogenase (DPD): Dihydro pyrimidine dehydrogenase (DPD) is a rate limiting enzyme for the metabolism of the anti cancer drug; 5 fluorouracil (5FU). With DPD being responsible for over 50% of its biotransformation. Other substrates for DPD are carmofur, tegafur and doxifluridine. The gene encoding for DPD is DPDY and about 13 genetic variants have been reported (McLeod et al 1998, Collie - Duguid et al 2000). The genetic variant that is responsible for decreased DPD activity has been reported to be DPYD*2 with a polymorphism at the splicing recognition site. (Wei at al 1996) Administration of 5 - FU to the patients with decreased enzyme activity results in adverse effects such as leukocytopenia, stomatitis, diarrhea, nausea and vomiting (Etienne et al 1994)

Glutathione - S - Tranferase (GST): GSTs and the human genes encoding these enzymes are highly polymorphic with about 50% and 25% of most populations having a mutation or complete deletion of these gene respectively rendering them deficient or lacking the enzyme. Major racial and ethnic differences exist and GST M and GST T1 are the major genes. Other GSTs include GST P1 and GST*A which are also subject to genetic polymorphism and have been implicated in resistance to anti cancer drugs. High GST activity has been associated with decreased risk of haematologic relapse, central nervous system response and improved prednisolone response. (Commandeur et.al 1995) Inherited GST - P1 allele encoding for the 11e 105 Val. amino acid substitution, has been associated with improved overall breast cancer survival compared with patients who have at least one wild type GST P1 allele. Conversely in patients with acute myeloid leukaemia treated with high doses of combination therapy, the homozygous GST - T1 deletion is associated with a higher risk of toxic death during remission. (Arruda et. al 2001)

Uridyl Diphosphate Glucuronyl Transferase (UGT): The UDP - glucuronyl transferase (UGT) belongs to a super family of membrane bound proteins localized in the endoplamic reticulum and are responsible for glucuronidation of many xenobiotics and endobiotics. The UGT genes have been classified into families and sub families based on evolutionary divergence with all known human UGT's being in the UGT1A 2A and 2B sub families. (Mackenzie et al 1997, Randominska - Pandya et al 1999, Tukey & Strassburg 2000). To date, polymorphism in UGTA1 have been more studied extensively and seem to have clinical significance. The anticancer drug irinotecan is metabolized by the enzyme and polymorphism resembling condition seen in Gilbert's syndrome characterised by total lack of UGT enzyme due to deletion of the gene which leads to fifty fold reduction in irinotecan metabolism and such patients can be at risk of toxicity (Huang et al 2002 Desai et al 2003).

5.1.3 Phase III reactions: Transporter genes

Membrane transporters as mentioned earlier are heavily involved in drug clearance and alter drug disposition by actively transporting drugs between organs and tissues. Therefore polymorphisms in the genes encoding these proteins may have significant effects on the absorption, distribution, metabolism and excretion of xenobiotics and may alter the pharmacodynamics of these agents. Uptake transporters are required for the uptake of some drugs into the cell whereas efflux transporters are responsible for pumping some drugs out of cells or preventing them from ever getting in. Transporters are also thought to be involved in drug - drug reactions.

The most important families of the transporters include (i) ATP binding cassette (ABC) family whose genes include important members like the multi drug resistance gene also classified as ABCB 1 i.e. (ABCB1/MDR1), ABCC1, ABCC2, uric acid transporter (ABCG2), breast cancer resistance protein BCRP also classified ABCG2 i.e. (BCRP/ABCG2).(ii) The solute transporter superfamily (SLC) which include the organic anion transport polypeptide

(SLC 21/OATP), organic cation transporter SLC 22 OCT), zwitterion/cation transporter (OCTNs), folate transporter(SLC19A1), neurotransmitter transporter(SLC6,SLC17,&SLC18)and serotonin transporter (5HTT).Genetic polymorphism in drug transporter genes have increasingly been recognized as a possible mechanism accounting for variation in drug response because these transporters play important roles in the gastrointestinal absorption, biliary and renal elimination and distribution to target sites of their substrates. (Meier et al 2007, Shu et al 2007, Choi & Song 2008)

5.1.3.1 The ABC family genes

ABCB1: Refers to ATP binding cassette (ABC) sub family B member 1, or MDR 1 also designated cluster of differentiation (CD243) is the permeability glycoprotein (P - glycoprotein).ABC genes are divided into seven distinct sub families (ABC1, MDR/TAP, MRP, ALD, OABP, CaCW 20 andWhite). Members of the MDR/TAP sub- family are involved in multi drug resistance. The protein encoded by this gene is an ATP dependent drug efflux pump of xenobiotics with broad substrate specificity. It is responsible for decreased drug accumulation in multi drug resistant cells and often mediates the development of resistance to cancer cells (Viguie 1998). This protein also function as a transporter in the blood brain barrier (Viguie 1998, Phipps - Green et al 2010). It likely evolved as a defense mechanism against harmful substances. Some of the functions of protein encoded by ABCB 1 gene include regulation of distribution and bioavailability of drugs, removal of metabolites and xenobiotics from cells into urine, bile and intestinal lumen, transport of compounds out of the brain across the blood - brain barrier, digoxin uptake, prevention of invermectin entry into the central nervous system and protection of hamatopoietic cells from toxins (Dean 2002.) Mutation of ABCB1 gene will therefore result in disruption of these functions. The activity of the transporter can be determined by both membrane ATPase and cellular calcein assays. Drug resistance had been observed in M89T, L662R, R669 and S1141T variants of the gene and decreased drug efficacy in W1108R variant. In addition, genetic variation in ABCB1 has been associated with both toxicity and drug response in 5Fluoro-uracil (Gonzalez - Haba et al 2011) and pacilitaxel therapy (Henningson et al 2011).

ABCC 1 genes: Multidrug resistant protein 1 (MRP1) an ATP bounding cassette transporter encoded by ABCC 1 gene is expressed in many tissues and function as an efflux transporter for glutathione, glycine and sulphate conjugates as well as unconjugated substrates. An evaluation of single nucleotide polymorphism (SNP) revealed 7 mutations in the gene (Colombo et al 2005) while in a Japanese study, 86 genetic variants were identified (Fukushina - Uesaka et al 2007). Mutations in ABC transporters cause or contribute to many different Mendelian and complex disorders including adrenoleukodystrophy, cystic fibrosis and retinal degeneration (Dean & Annilo 2005). There has been no evidence of clinical significance in studies of the variants. (Colombo et al 2005, Pauli Magrus & Kroetz 2005 & Fukushina -Uesaka 2007).

ABCC2 gene: ABBCC2 genes codes for the ABCC2 or MRP2 protein. (MRP2) is an export pump expressed at tissue barriers. Genetic variants 24 e>T, 1249Ca>A and 3972 > T had been observed and are thought to cause inter individual differences of bioavailability of various endogenous and exogenous compounds (Colombo et al 2005, Laechelt et al 2011). About 27 other variants have also been detected (Colombo et al 2005). A haplotype dependent influence on transport capacity of ABCC2 had been observed but seems to be mainly based on post transcriptional modifications rather than transport rates (Laechelt et al 2011).

TheABCG2 gene encodes an inhibitor of breast cancer resistance protein (BCRP) (ABCG2) protein, another member of the ABC transporter. The protein confers protection against the development of breast cancers. Evaluation of single nucleotide polymorphism identified 16 variants (Morisaki et al 2005, Colombo et al 2005). Genetic polymorphism in ABCG2 might alter the transport activity of some drugs causing therapy in drugs like irinotecan, to cause severe myelosuppression (Choi et al 2009, Hampras et al 2010). A polymorphism, C421A observed in human placenta is not a genetic variant acting in cis but is considered to influence the translational efficiency (Kobayeshi et al 2005). Another genetic variant (ABCG2) (rs 2231142, Q141K) encoding a uric acid transporter is associated with gout in diverse populations (Phipps - Green et al 2010)

5.1.3.2 Solute Carrier Superfamily: (SLC) Genes

The solute carrier (SLC) superfamily of transporters consists of more than 300 members subdivided into 47 families. They are expressed in most tissues but primarily in liver, lungs, kidney and intestine.

i. **OATP/SLC21:** Organic anion transporter facilitates movement of anion across the cell membrane.OATP1B and OATP1B3 are human hepatocyte transporters that mediate the uptake of various endogenous and exogenous substrates. Genetic variation was observed in the SLCO1B1 and SLCO1B3 genes which encode OATP1B1 and OATP1B3 proteins. Forty nine (49) and 41 nucleotide sequence variants leading to 10 and 9 in SLCO1B1 and SLCO1B3 genes respectively were identified (Bowin et al 2010). Furthermore, in OATPC (SLC21A6) and OATP3 (SLC22A8) genes, polymorphism did not appear to be associated with changes in renal and tubular secretory clearance in the latter but the former was associated with differences in the disposition kinetics of pravastin. Individualswith the OATP - C*15 allele (ASP 130 Ala 174) had a reduced total and non renal clearance compared with those of OATPC*15 allele (ASP130Val 174) (Nishizato Y et al 2003).
ii. **SLC 19A1 (Folate Transporter)member 1:** The SLC19A1 are the proteins responsible for the transport of folate. Transport of folate into the mammalian cells can occur via receptor mediated (folate receptor 1) or carrier mediated (SLC19A1) mechanism. Methotrexate is an antifolate chemotherapeutic agent that is actively transported by the carrier mediated uptake system. Individuals carrying a specific polymorphism of SLC19A1 gene ї.e (C80GG) have lower levels of folate. (Whetsine 2003, Matherly et al 2007) and those carrying the C80AA genotype treated with methrotrexate have higher levels of this antifolate chemotherapeutic agent. This underpins requirements for personalized dosing with the drug based on patients genotype
iii. **OCT/SLC22:** Most solute carrier transporters are localized at either the basolateral or apical plasma membrane of polarized cells but some are also expressed in mitochondria and other organelles (Wojtal et al 2009). The genes encoding the three organic cation transporter isoforms OCT1, OCT2 and OCT 3 are clustered together on the long arm of chromosome 8 in humans and carry out functions of transport of small organic cations with different molecular structures independent of sodium gradient. These organic

cation substrate include drugs like metformin, procainamide and cimetidine as well as endogenous compounds like dopamine and norepinephrine and toxic substances like tetraethylammonium bromide (TEA) (Kang et al 2007).

5.2 Pharmacodynamic related genes

i. **Receptors:** Many receptors are involved with several signaling pathways. Example of which is epidermal growth factor receptor(EGFR). This receptor has been implicated in the oncogenesis and progression of several solid tumours thereby being identified as a suitable target for anticancer treatment. Polymorphism has been observed in the development of cancer on dinucleotide repeats in intron 1 of the EGFR gene and this has correlated with EGFR expression with therapeutic implication for treatment with tyrosinase kinase inhibitor. A higher proportion of Asians do overexpress EGFR that may influence their responses to tyrosine kinase inhibitor (Tan et al 2004).
   G-protein Coupled Receptors (GPCR):Over 50% of all drug targets have G-protein coupled receptors (GPCR). Genes of GPR has more coding regions than non - GPCR genes making them more important for pharmacological investigations.
   GABAA Receptor Mutation in GABAA receptor ion channel may be a reason for the diminished protection of anti epileptic drugs.
   Insulin Receptor(INSR): The receptor is important in the management of diabetes mellitus patients and mutation of the gene encoding the receptor will result in poor response particularly in type 2 diabetes.Mutation of the gene has also been suspected to contribute to genetic susceptibility to the polycystic ovarian syndrome(Siega et al2002)
   B2 Receptor: B2 agonist; albuterol (Proventil) is used to control acute attacks of asthma and are prescribed as needed .Patients with β_2 receptor arginine genotype experience poor asthma control with frequent symptoms and a decreasing scores of poor exploratory volume compared with those with glycine genotype (Cowburn et al 1998, de Maat et al 1999). Seventeen (17%) of whites and 20% of blacks carry the arginine genotype (Wechsler et al 2005)
ii. **Ion Channels:** Many genes encode for different ion channels including those of the central nervous system which include KCNJ10, KCNJ3, CLCN2, GABRA1, SCN1B and SCN1A. Some polymorphism of this channel has been linked to idiopathic generalized epilepsy (Lucarini et al 2007)
   The 5-HT3 receptor is a ligand-gated ion channel composed of five subunits. To date, five different human subunits are known; 5-HT3A-E, which are encoded by the serotonin receptor genes HTR3A, HTR3B, HTR3C, HTR3D and HTR3E, respectively. Functional receptors are pentameric complexes of diverse composition. Different receptor subtypes seem to be involved in chemotheraphy-induced nausea and vomiting (CINV), irritable bowel syndrome and psychiatric disorders. 5-HTR3A and HTR3B polymorphisms may also contribute to the etiology of psychiatric disorders and serve as predictors in CINV and in the medical treatment of psychiatric patients. (Niesler et al 2008).
iii. **Enzymes:** Polymorphism of pharmacokinetic enzymes no doubt influence the pharmacodynamics of drugs. However there are few enzymes that influence drugs at the point of actions one of these enzymes is the tyrosine kinase which modulate receptor activities. Therefore polymorphism in tyrosine kinase gene will affect drugs at the target point.

Another important enzyme of drug target is vitamin K epoxide reductase complex subunit 1(VKORC1). This enzyme is the drug target for warfarin an anticoagulant with a narrow therapeutic window and with serious consequences of bleeding in the event of an overdose. Variation in maintenance dose of warfarin is largely attributable to genetic variants in the genes that encode the drug target VKORC1 the major metabolizing enzyme. The two genetic polymorphisms explain 30 - 40% of the total variation in those on therapy.

Angiotensin converting enzyme (ACE) genes encode for ACE, a target for ACE inhibitors which improves symptom and survival in cases of heart failure. Genetic polymorphism is suspected to be causing greater effects of the drug in Europeans than Afro-Americans. Pre-treatment genetic screening is therefore apt to improve therapy

iv. **Neurotransmitter Transporters:** Neurotransmitter transporters namely SLC6, SLC17 and SLC18 families are primarily expressed in the neurons of the central and peripheral nervous system. These transporters are the sites of action of various drugs of abuse e.g cocaine, amphetamine and other clinically approved drugs like desipramine, reserpine, benztropine and tiagabine. Genetic variation in the SLC6, SLC17 and SLC18 encoding genes may result in altered expression and function of these proteins. In particular, antidepressants and antiepileptic drugs target these neurotransmitters as part of their primary mechanism of action. Therefore genetic variations may affect the efficacy of such drugs.

6. Pharmacogenetic testing

A genetic test is the analysis of human DNA, RNA chromosomes, proteins or certain metabolites in order to detect alterations related to a heritable disorder. This can be accomplished by directly examining the DNA or RNA that makes up a gene (Direct testing), looking at markers co-inherited with a disease causing gene (linkage testing), assaying certain metabolites (biochemical testing), or examining the chromosomes (cytogenetic testing). Although genetic testing shares some features common with other kinds of laboratory testing, it is however unique in many ways and therefore requires special consideration .Pharmacogenetic testing can therefore be defined as utilization of aforementioned genetic biomarkers related to drug metabolism and effects. A biomarker can be described as a characteristic that is objectively measured and evaluated as an indicator of normal biological processes to a therapeutic intervention (EMEA 2006)

Methods of Pharmacogenetic testing depends on the biomarker to be assessed. These vary from simple spectrophotometric estimation of metabolites to DNA sequences, use of PCR and DNA probes, enzymes linked immunosorbent assay, cell culture, gel electrophoresis high performance liquid chromatography and DNA hybridization techniques. It is not uncommon to use combined techniques to study clinical relevance of pharmacogenetic testing.

Because information on pharmacogenetics is still evolving, there is a necessity for guidelines to be adopted for ethical reasons, economic considerations and patient benefit. Overall, the quest for pharmacogenetic information is likely to grow. As a matter of fact some drugs already carry labels addressing such.

6.1 European medicines agency guideline for pharmacogenetic testing

The guidelines for European Medicines Agency (EMEA) was desighned by the Agency's committee for Human Medicinal Products (CHMP). The rationale for this guidelines include standardization, data analysis, interpretation, evaluation of clinical relevance, ethical consideration and setting the stage for technical, scientific and regulatory issues. The guidelines addresses the following among other issues.

i. Chosen design and rationale
ii. the population selected for pharmacogenetic studies (i.e. species, age, gender and other variable related to the phenotype e.g. for human exposure ethnic group)
 *In the target population or relevant animal model
 *In the study population e.g. matched groups (responders/non responders, presence/absence of adverse events)
iii. The population size selected for PG studies and a discussion on the power to detect an association in appropriate
iv. Predictive values (positive and negative) of the PG biomarkers as per clinical trials experience
v. Assumptions on clinical utility e.g. benefit In using predictive pharmacogenetics testing versus other predictive biomarkers, use of a pharmacogenetic biomarker as a segregation marker or as a stratification tool for a subpopulation in a general matching population.

6.2 Pharmacogenetic testing and clinical benefits

The overall purpose of PG testing is clinical benefits. Pharmacogenetic testing have resulted in some clinical benefit so far, some of which can be life saving. It was observed that roughly about 106,000 deaths and 2.2 million serious events caused by adverse drug reactions were reported yearly (Lazarom 1998) and 5 - 7% of hospital admissions in US and Europe lead to the withdrawal of 4% of new medicines with attendant financial loss. Since such drugs were linked to metabolizing enzymes with known polymorphism,prudence dictates suggestion of pharmacogenetic testing in indicated instances Pharmacogenetics testing is expectedly becoming commonly required particularly with drugs with low therapeutic window (Phillips et al 2001). However, the decision to use pharmacogenetic testing will be influenced by the relative costs of genotyping technologies and the cost of providing a treatment to a patient with an incompatible genotype.

Notable clinical benefits of pharmacogenetic testing have been observed in NAT2 genotyping for isoniazid treatment (Hiratsuka et al 2002, Weishilboum et al 2003, Gardiner and Begg 2006) andCYP2C19 genotyping for omeprazole treatment (Desta et al 2002).

Others are TPMT genotyping for 6-mercaptopurine and azathioprine treatment (Relling et al 1999, Gardener and Begg 2006) mtDNA A155G genotyping for aminoglycoside treatment (Cortopassi and Hatchin 1994, Usami et al 1999) CYP 2D6 genotyping for codeine treatment (Bradford 2002) Hepatitis C genotype for pegylated interferon - alpha - 2a or pegylated - interferon - alpha - 2b treatment. (Ingelman - Sundberg et al 2009, Thomas et al 2009) and Dihydropyrimidine dehydrogenese (DPI) testing for 5-fluoro-Uracil (5FU) treatment (Gionzalez and Fernandez -Salguero, 1995, McMurrough et al 1996, Wei et al 1996, Van Kuilenburg et al 1998).

There are currently requirements of pharmacogenetic testing of specific drugs before they can be prescribed and these include cetuximab, trastuzumab, maraviroc and dasatinib. In December 2007, the FDA recommended testing for HLA-B* 1502 allele in patients with Asian ancestry before initiating carbamazepine therapy because of high risk of developing carbamazepine induced Steven's Johnson syndrome (SSS) or toxic epidermal necrolysis.

Pharmacogenetic testing is also recommended for patients treated with warfarin, thiopurine, valproic acid, irinotecan, abacavir or rasburicase.

Currently, drug labels contain information on pharmacogenetic tests which are classified as test required, test recommended and for information only.

7. Conclusion

With the application of molecular biology methods and completion of the human genome projects and establishment of guidelines for pharmacogenetics practices and applications, it is expected that the interwoven field of pharnmacogenetics and pharmacogenomics will revoluntionise personalized medicine. Furthermore the field of predictive medicine is expected to receive a boost from pharmacogenetic information with attendant reduction in morbidity and mortality particularly from adverse drug reactions and therapeutic failure. With more intense researches and genotyping profiling, the challenges of standardization and interpretation of pharmacogenetic testing are apt to be overcome. It is worthy of note that currently some drug labels carry information on pharmacogenetic testing and requirements for therapeutic use. The promise of pharmacogenetics is therefore improvement of the overall health being of the patients.

8. References

Ait Moussa L, Khassouni CE, Hue B, Jana M, Begand B, Soulaymani R (2002). Determination of the acetylator phenotype in Moroccan tuberculosis patients using isoniazid as metabolic probe *Critical Care Medicine 30 (2) 107 – 14*

Arruda VR, Lima CS, Grignoll CR, de Melo MB, Lorrand-Metze I, Alberto FL, Saad ST & Costa FF (2001) Increased risk of acute myeloid leukaemia in individuals with glutathione-S-transferase MU1(GST M1 and theca 19GST T10 gene defects .*European Journal of Haematology 66(6) 383-8*

Aquilante CL, Langace TY, Lopez Lm (2006) Influence of coagulation factor, vitamin K epoxide reductase complex subuniit 1 and cytochrome P4502C9 gene polymorphisms on warfarin dose requirements. *Clinical Pharmacology and Therapeutics 79 (4):291 – 302*

Banjoko, S.O. &Akinlade K.S. (2010) Acetylation Pharmacogenetics and renal function in diabetes mellitus patients. *Indian Journal of Clinical Biochemistry, 25(3) 289*

Boivin A A, Cardinal H, Barama A, Pichelte V, Hebert M J, Rocher M (2010) Organic Anion Transporting Polypeptide 1B1 (OATP1B1) and OATP1B3. genetic variability and haplotype analysis of the white Canadians. *Drug Metabolism and Pharmacokinetics 25 (5): 508 – 515*

Boyland E,& Chassaud LF, (1969) The role of glutathione and glutathione S transferase in mercapturic acid synthesis. *Advances in Enzymology Related Area of Molecular Biology 32 (1) : 173 – 219*

Choi MK, Song IS (2008) Organic cation transporters and their pharmacokinetic and pharmacodynamic consequences *Drug Metabolism and Pharmacokinetics 23: 243 – 253*

Collie - Dughid ES, Etienne MC, Milano G,& Mc Leod HL. (2000) Known variant of DPYD alleles do not explain DPD deficiency in cancer patients *Pharmacogenetics10:217 – 23*

Colombo S, Soranzo N, Rolger M, Sprenger R Bleiber G, Furrer H, Buclin T. Goldstein DB, Descoslerd L, Telenti A & Swiss HIV cohort (2005). Influence of ABCB1, ABCC 2 and ABCG 2 haplotypes on the cellular exposure of nelfinavir in vitro. *Pharmacogenetics & Genomics 15(9)599-60*

Commandeur JN, Stintes GT, and Vermeulen NP (1995) Enzymes and transport systems involved in the formation and disposition of glutathione S - conjugates. Role in bioactivation and detoxication mechanisms of xenobiotics *Pharmacology Review 47 (2) : 271 – 330*

Cowburn AS, Sladek, Soja J et al 5(1998) Overexpression of leukotriene C4 synthase in bronchial biopsies from patients with aspirin-intolerant asthma..*Journal of Clinical Investigations,101(4):834-836*

Cranswick N. and Mulholland K. (2005) Isoniazid treatment of Children. can genetic help guide treatment? *Archives of Diseases in Children 90:551 – 3*

Daly AK, Brockmoller J, Body F (1996) Nomenclature for human CYP2D6 alleles. *Pharmacogenetics 1996, 6: 193 – 201.*

Dasai AA, Innocent F, and Ratain MJ (2003) UGT pharmacogenomics. implications for cancer risk and cancer therapeutics. *Pharmacogenetics 13:517 – 523.*

de Maat MP, Jukema JW, Ye S et al (1999) Effect of the stromelysin-1 promoter on efficacy of provastatin in coronary atherosclerosis and restenosis *American Journal of Cardiology 83 (6): 852-856*

Dean M and Annilo T (2005) Evolution of the ATP - Binding Cassette (ABC) transporter superfamily in vertebrates. *Annual Review of Genomics and Human Genetics 6: 123 – 1.42*

Desta Z, Zhas X, Shin JG, Flockhart DA (2002) Clinical significance of the cytochrome P450 2C19 genetic polymorphism. *Clinical Pharmacokinetics 41 : 913 – 58*

Donnan JR, Ungar WS, Matthews M and Rahman PV Systematic review of thiopurine methyl transferase genotype and enzymatic testing strategies. *Therapeutic Drug Monitoring 33 (2): 192*

El. Desoky ES, Abdel Salam YM, Salama RH, El Akkah MA, Atansova S, Von Ahsen N (2005) NAT 2*5/*5 genotype (351T<C) is a potential risk factor for schistosomiasis associated bladder cancer in Egyptians. *Therapeutic Drug Monitoring 27(3) 297 – 304.*

Etienne MC, Lagrange JL, Dassonville O. (1994) Population study of dihydropyrimidine dehydrogenase in cancer patients. *Journal of Clinical Oncology 12:2248 – 53*

EuropeanMedicinesAgency(EmeA)(2006)*DocRefEMEA/CHMP/PGXWP/2027/2004*

Evans DA (1989) N – acetyl transferase, *Pharmacology and therapeutics, 42:157 – 234*

Evans WE (2004) Pharmacogenetics of thiopurine S - methyl transerase and thiopurine. *Therapeutic drug monitoring 26:186 – 9*

Evans WE, Relling MV (1999) Phrmacogenomics translating functional genomics into rational therapeutics *Science: 286 : 487 – 91*

Fukushima-Uesaka H, Saito Y, Tohkin M, Maekura K, Hasegawa R, Kawamoto M, Kamatani N(2007).Genetic variation and haplotype structures of the ABC transporter gene ABCC1 in a Japanese population.*Drug Metabolism & Pharmacokinetics, Feb 22(1):48-60*

Gardener SJ, Begg EJ (2006) Pharmacogenetics, drug-metabolizing enzymes and clinical practice. *Pharmacocology Review 58 (3): 521 – 90*

Gonzalez-Haba E, Garcia MI, Corte Joso L, Lopez –Lillo C, Barrue N, Garcia –Alfonsop, Alvarez S, Jimenez JL, Martin ML, Munoz-Fernandez MA, Sanjurjo M and Lopez-Fernandez LA (2011)ABCB 1 Polymorphism in fluoropyrimidine treatment. *Pharmacogenomics 11(12);1715-1723*

Goldstein DB, Tate SK, Sisodiya SM pharmacogenetics goes genomic (2003) *Nature Review of Genetics, 4: 937-4*

Grant DM (1990) Morike K, Eichelbaum M, Mayer V.A Acetylation Pharmacogenetics, the slow acetylators pharmacogenetics, the slow acetylators phenotypes is caused by decrease or absent arylamine N – acetyl transferase in human live. *Journal of Clinical Investigations .85(3):968-72*

Guengerkich FB (2001) Common and uncommon cytochrome p450 reactions related to metabolism and chemical toxicity. *Chemical Research &Toxicology 14 (6) 611 – 50*

Hagenbuch B (2010) Drug uptake systems in liver and kidney a historic perspective. *Clinical Pharmacology and Therapeutics 87 (1) 39 – 47.*

Haglund S, Vikingssons Soderman J, Huidorf U, Granno G, Donelius M, Coulthard S, Peterson C & Aliner S (2011) The role of Inosine 5^1 - Monophosphate Dehydrogenase in Thiopurine metabolism in patient with Inflammatory Bowel Disease. *Therapeutic Drug Monitoring 32(2):192-199*

Hampras S S, Sucheston L, Weiss Joli, Baer MR, Zirpoli G, Singh PK, Wetzler M, Chennamaneni R, Blanco JG, Ann Ford L, Moysich KB, (2010) Genetic Polymorphisms of ATP - binding cassette (ABC) proteins, overall survival and drug toxicity in patients with acute myeloid Leukaemia *International Journal of Molecular Epidemiology and Genetics 1 (3): 201-207*

Hanene C, Jihene I, Jamel A, Kamel A & Agnestl (2007) Association of polymorphism with genes of GST with asthma in Tunisian Children. *Mediators of Inflammation Dol:10.1155/2007/19567*

Henningson A, Marsh S, Loos WJ, Karlsson MO, Garba A, mross K, Mielke S, Vigano L, Locatelli A, Verweij, Sparreboom A, McLeod HL (2005)Associate of CYP2C8, CYP3A4, CYP3A5 and ABCBI polymorphism with the pharmacogenetic of paclitroxel in Clinical Cancer research Nov. 22: 8097 - 104ABCBI polymorphism in Fluoro pyramidine - Treated Patient .*Pharmacogenomics (2011) 11 (12) 1715 – 1723*

Hiratsuka M, Agatsuma Y, Omori F et al (2002) Allele and genotype frequencies of CYP2B6 and CYP3A5 in the Japanese population. *European Journal of Clinical Pharmacology 58 : 417 – 21*

Hiratsuka M, Kishikawa Y, Takekuma Y (2002) genotyping of the N-acetyl transferase-2polymorphism in the prediction of adverse drug reactions to isoniazid in Japanese patients. *Drug metabolism &Pharmacokinetics* 17:357-361

Hiratsuka M, sasaki T, Mizugaki M (2006) Genetic testing for Pharmacogenetics and its clinical application in drug therapy *Clinical Chimica Acta 363 177 – 185*

Huang Y, Galijatoric A, Nguyen N, Geske D, Beaton D, Green J (2002) Identification and Functional Characterization of UDP - glycuronyl transfeerase UGT1A8*1, UGT1A8*2, UGT1A8*3. *Pharmacogenetics 12:287 – 297.*

Huang, YS, Cher, HD, SUWJ (2002) Polymorphism of the N – acetyl transferase 2 gene as a susceptibility risk factor for anti tuberculosis drug induced hepatitis. *Hepatology 35: 839 – 83*

Ingelman – Sundberg M, Rodrighmez – Antona C, McHutchinson JG, Goldstein DB (2009) Genetic variation in IL28B predicts hepatitis C treatment induced viral clearance – *Nature 461 (7262) 399 – 401*

Juliano RL and Ling V (1976) A surface glycoprotein modulating drug permeability in Chinese hamster ovary cell mutants. *Biochemical & BiophysicaActa, 465 (1) 15 – 62.*

Kang HJ, Song I S, Shin H J, Kim WY, Lee CH, Shim JC, Zhou H H, Lee S S, Shin J. G (2007) Identification and Functional Characterization of genetic variant of human organic cation transporters in a Korean population. *Drug metabolism and Disposition 35: 667 – 675*

Kimura M, Leiri I, Mamiya K, Urae A, Hignchi S. Genetic polymorphism of cyto chrome P450s CYP2C19 and CYP2C9 in a Japanese population. *Therapeutic Drug Monitoring 20: 243 – 7.*

Klotz V (2007) The role of Pharmacogenetics in the metabolism of antiepileptic drugs: Pharcomacokinectic and therapeutic implications. *Clinical Pharmacokinetics* 46 (4): 27 – 9

Konig J, Nies AT, Cui Y, Leier I, Keppler D (1999) conjugate export pump of the multidrug resistance protein (MRP) family: localization substrate specificity and MRP 2 – mediated drug resistance. *Biochemica and BiophysicaActa* 1461 (2) 377

Kroetz DL, Yee SW, Griacomini KM (2010) The Pharmacogenetics of membrane transport project : research at the interface of genomics and transporter pharmacology *Clinical Pharmacology.& Therapeutics 87: 109 – 116*

Kweon YS, Lee HK, Lee CT, Lee KU, Pae CU (2005) Association of the serotonin transporter gene polymorphism with Korean male alcoholics *Journal of Psychiatry Research Jul, : 39 (4) : 371 – 376*

Laechelt S, Turrini SL, Ruehmkorf A, Siegmind W, Cascorbi I and Haenisehi S. (2011) Impact of ABCC2 haplotypes on transcriptional and post transcriptional gene regulation and function.*The Pharmacogenetics Journal 11,23-34*

Linder MW, Homme MB, Reynolds KK, Gage BF, Eby C, Silverstrov Natalia and Valdes R Jr (2009) Interactive Modeling for ongoing utility of Pharmacogenetic

Diagnostic Testing. Application for Wanfarin Therapy *Clinical chemistry 55 (10) 1861 - 1868*

Mackenzie P1, Owens IS, Burchell B, Brock KW, Bairoeh A, Belanger A (1997). The UDP glyceronyl transferase gene super family: recommended nomenclature update based on evolutionary divergence *Pharmacogenetics 7:255 – 259.*

Matherly L H, Hou Z, Deng Y (2007) Human reduced folate carrier: translation of basic biology to cancer. *Cancer Metastasis Review 26 (1): 111 - 12*

Mc Leod HL, Collie - Dugiud ES, Vreken P. et al (1998) Nomenclature for human DPYD alleles. *Pharmacogenetic 8:455 – 9*

McAlpine DE, Biernacka JM, Mrazdek D.A., O'Kane DJ, Stevens S.R, Longman LJ, coverson VI Bhagia J and Moyer TP (2011) Effect of cytochrome P450 Enzyme Polymorphism on Pharmacokinetics of venlafaxine *Therapeutic Drug Monitoring 33 (1) 14 – 20*

Mcleod HL (2005) Pharmacogenetic analysis of clinically relevant genetic polymorphism *Clinical Infectious Diseases, 41 suppl, 7:5449 – 52*

Meyer UA (2004) Pharmacogenetics: Five decades of therapeutic ;lessons from genetic diversity *Nature Review of Genetics 5: 669 – 676*

Meyer VA (2000) Pharmacogenetics and adverse drug reacgtions. *Lancet, 356: 1667-71*

Meier Y, Eloranta JJ, Darimont J, Ismair MG, Hiller C, Fried M, Kullak - Vblick GA, Varricka Sr (2007) Regional distribution of solute carrier MRNA expression along the human intestinal tract. *Drug metabolism and Disposition 35: 590 – 594.*

Morisaki K, Robey RW, Ozregy Laceka C, Honjo Y, Polgar O, Steadinain K, Sarkadi B, Bates SE (2005) Single Nucleotide Polymorphism modify the transporter activity of ABCG 2 *Cancer Chemotherapy and Pharmacology April 19 : 1 – 2*

Murphy PJ (2001) Xenobiotic mechanism a look from the past to future. *Drug Metabolism and Disposition 29 (6): 779 – 80*

Niesler B, Kapeller J, Hammer C and Rappold G (2008) Serotonin type 3 receptor genes: HTR 3A, B, C, D E, *Pharmacogenomics May (9) 5: 501 – 504*

Nilsson KW, Sjberg RL, Damberg M, Alm PO, Ohrvi KJ, Leppert J, lundstrom L, Oreland L (2005) Role of the serotonim transporter gene and family function in adolescent alcohol consumption. *Alcohol Clinical and Experimental Research. Apr 29 (4): 564 – 70*

Nishizato Y, Leiri I, Suzuki H, Kinura M, Kawabata K, Hirota K et al (2003) Polymorphism of OATP - C (SLC 21A6) and OAT3 (SLC22AB) genes. Consequences for Pravastin pharmacokinetics .*Clinical Pharmacology and Therapeutics June 73 (6): 554 –*

Ohno M, Yamaguchi I, (2000) slow N-acetyl transferase 2 genotype affects the incidence of isoniazid and rimfapicin induced hepatoroxity. *International Journal of Tuberculosis and lime Diseases 4: 256 – 61*

Omiecinski CJ, Vanden Heuvel JP, Perdew GH and Peters JM (2011) Xerobiotic Metabolism, disposition and regulation by receptors: from biochemical phenomenon to predictors of major toxicities. *Toxicological Science 120 (51) 549 – 575.*

Phillips KA, Veenstra DI, Oren E, Lee JK, Sadee W (2001) Potential role of Pharmacogenetics in reducing adverse drug reactions: a systemic review. *Journal of American Medical Association 286 (18) 2270 –*

Phipps Green A, Hollis Moffa HJE, Dalbeth N, merriman ME, Topless R, Gow PJ, Harrison AA, Highton J, Jones PBB, Stamp LK, Merrkiman TR (2010) A strong role for the ABCG2 gene in susceptibility to gout in New Zealand, Pacific island and Caucasian, but not Maori, case and control sample sets. *Human Molecular Genetics 19 (24): 4813 – 4819*

Radominska - Pandya, Zemik PJ, Little JM (1999) Structural and Functional Studies of UDP. glucuronyl transferases, *Drug Metabolism Review 31:817 – 899*

Roepke TK and Abbot GW (2006) Pharmacogenetics and cardiac ion channels. *Vascular Pharmacology Feb. 44 (2) 90 – 160*

Sakata T, Anzal N, Shis HJ, Noshire R, Hirata T, Yokoyama H, Kanai Y, Endou H (2004) Novel single nucleolide polymorphisms of organic Cation transporter 1 (SLC 22A 1) affecting transport functions. *Biochemistry and Biophysics Research Communication 313: 789 – 793*

Scordo MG, Pengo V, Spina E, Da2). Influence of CYP2C9 and CyP2C19 genetic polymorphism on warfarin maintenance dose and metabolic clearance. *Clinical Pharmacology and Therapeutics 72: 702 – 10*

Shar GM, Hammer EJ, Zhu H et al (2002) Maternal periconceptional vitamin use genetic variation of infant reduced folate carrier (ASOG) and risks of spina bifida: *America Journal of Medical Genetics 108 (1): 1 – 6*

Shenfield GM, (2004) Genetic polymorphosis, drug metabolism and drug concentrations, *Clinical Biochemistry Review; Nov 203 -6*

Shin J, Kayser SR, Langace T, (2009) Pharmacogenetics: from discovery to patient care pharmacogenetic test information on drug labels *American Journal of Health Systems Pharmacy 66 (7) : 66 – 637*

Shord SS (2010) Pharmacogenomic: A testing issue. *FDA Perspective on pharmacogenetic testing. PSWC 2010 New or Leans.*

Shu Y, Sheardown SA, Brown C, Owen RP, Zhang S, Castro RA, Lanculescu AG, Yive L, Lo JC, Bachard EG, Brett CM, Giacomini KM (2007) Effect of genetic variation in the organic cation transporter 1 (OCT 1) on metformin action. *Journal of Clinical Investigation 117: 1422 -1431*

Sies H (1997) Oxidative stress,oxidants and antioxidants. *Experimental Physiology 82 (2): 291 – 5*

Soldner A, Christians V, Susanto M, Wacher VJ, Silver man JA, benet LZ (1999) Grape fruit juice activates P-glucoprotein mediated drug transport *Pharmacology Research April 16 (4) 478 – 85.*

Steiner W (2010) Pharmacogenetics and psychoactive drug therapy: ready for the patient *Therapeutic Drug Monitoring 32 (4) 381 – 386*

Suarez - Kurtz G (2005) Pharmacogenomics in admixed population. Trends in *Pha.rmacological Science 26: 196 – 201*

Suzuki T, Mihara K, Nakemura A, Naga G, Kogenwa S, Nemoto K, Ohia I, Arakaki H, Uno T & Kondo T (2011) Effect of the CYP 206 10 Allele on the steady state plasma concentrations of Arupiprazole and its active metabolite dehydroaripiprazole, in Japanese Patients with Schizophrenia. *Therapeutic Drug Monitoring 33 (1) 21 – 24*

Taradia SM, Mydlarski PR, Reis MD et al (2000) screening for azathioprine toxicity: a pharmaco economic analysis based on a target case .*Journal of American Academy of Dermatology 42:628 – 32*

Thomalley PJ (1990) The glyoxalase s.ystem: new developments towards functional characterizations of a metabolic pathway fundamental to biological life. *Biochemistry Journal 269 (1) : 1 – 11*

Thomas DL, Thio CL, Martin MP, QiY, Ge D, O' Hiigin C, Kidd J, Kidd K, Khakoo S.I., Alexander G, Goedert JJ, Kurk GD, Donfield SM, Rosen HR, Tobler LH, Busch MP, McHwchison JG, Goldstein DB, Carrington M (2009) Genetic Variation in Il 28 B and spontaneous clearance of Hepatitis C. virus. *Nature 461 (7265): 798 – 801*

Tukey RH and Strassburg CP. (2000) Human UDP - Glucuronyltransferases: metabolism, expression and disease *Annual Review of Pharmacology and Toxicology 40: 581 – 616*

Tzevetkov MV, Vormfelde SV, Balen D, Meineke I, Schmidt T, Sehrt D, Sabolic I, Koepsell H, Brockmoller (2009) The effects of genetic polymorphism in the organic cation transporters OCT1; OCT2 and OCT 3 on the renal clearance of metformin. *Clinical Pharmacology and Therapeutics 66: 299 – 306*

Usami S, Abe, S, Shinkawa H, Inouse Y, Yamaguchu T (1999) Rapid mass screening method and counselling for the 1555A-G mitochondrial mutation *Journal of Human Genetics 44: 304 – 7*

Wechsler M E and Israel E. (2005) How pharmacogenomics will play a role in the management of asthma. *American Journal of Respiratory and Critical Medicine 172(1): 12-18.*

Weishilboum RC, Francis S, Weinshilboum (2003) Inheritance in drug response. *New England Journal of medicine 348 (6): 529 – 37*

Weix, Mc Leod Hc, Mc Murrough J, Caonzalez FJ, Fernandez - Salguero P. (1996) Molecular basis of the human dihydropyrimidine dehydrogenase deficiency and 5 fluorouracil toxicity. *Journal of Clinical Investigations 98:610 – 5*

Wherstine JR, Gifford AJ, Witt t et al (2002) single nucleotide polymorphism in the human reduced folate carrier : characterization of a high frequency G/A variant at position 80 and transport properties of the His (27) and Arg (27) carriers. *Clinical Cancer Research 7 (11) : 3416 – 22*

Whetstine JR, Flatley RM, Mattherly LH (2002) The human reduced folate carrier gene is ubiquitously and differentally expressed in normal human tissues, identification of seven non-coding exons and characterization of a novel promoter *Biochemistry Journal 367 (3) : 629 – 40*

Wojtal KA, Eloranta JJ, Hruz P, Gutmann H, Drewe J, Staumann A, Beglinger C, Fried M, Kullak-Ublick GA, Varricka SR (2009) Challenges in mRNA express ion levels in solute carrier transporters in inflammatory bowel disease patients. *Drug Metabolism and Disposition 37 : 1871 – 1877*

Wong M, Balleine RL, Collins M, Liddle C, Clarke CL, Caumey H (2004) CYP 3A5 genotype abd midazotam clearance in Australian patients receiving chemotherapy. *Clinical Pharmacology & Therapeutics 75 : 529 – 38*

Wool house WM, Qureshi MM, Bastaki SMA, Patel M, Abchilrazzaq, Y, Bayoumi RAL (1997). Polymorphic N - acetyltranseferase (NAT2) genotyping of Emiratis *Pharmacogenetics 7:73 – 82*

Yamaka Y, Hamada A, Nakashima R, Yuki M, Hirayama C, Kawaguchi T and Saito H (2011) Association of genetic polynmorphism in the influx transporter SLCOIB3 and the efflux transporter ABCB1 with Imatinib pharmacokinetics in patients with chronic myeloid leukaemia .*Therapeutic Drug Monitoring 33(2):244-250* .

Zhou Q, Kibat C, Cheung YB, Tan EH, Ang P, Balran C (2004) Pharmacogenetics of epidermal growth factor receptor (EGFR) gene in Chinese, Malay and Indian populations.*Journal of Clinical Oncology: ASCO Annual Meeting Proceedings (Post meeting Edition) 22 (145) : 3014*

10

Future of Pharmacogenetics in Cardiovascular Diseases

Rianne M.F. Van Schie#, Talitha I. Verhoef#
and Anke-Hilse Maitland-Van Der Zee et al.*
Utrecht University
The Netherlands

1. Introduction

Pharmacogenetics is the study of variations in DNA sequence as related to drug response (European Medicines Agency [EMA], 2007). Several gene-drug interactions have been discovered in the field of cardiovascular diseases (CVDs). These gene-drug interactions can help to identify nonresponse to drugs, estimate dose requirements or identify an increased risk of developing adverse drug reactions. An individualized approach based on pharmacogenetic testing will provide physicians and pharmacists with tools for decision making about pharmacotherapy. While pharmacogenetic testing is already part of everyday practice in oncology, it is not widely implemented in the field of CVDs. However, in the near future, pharmacogenetics will probably also play a valuable role in this field as well.

1.1 Complexity of pharmacogenetics of CVDs

Prophylaxis and treatment of CVD is complex. Patients often have more than one cardiovascular risk factor (e.g. hypertension and hypercholesterolemia) and/or CVD, or other comorbidities such as diabetes mellitus. Frequently, more than one drug is used by the patient and this may potentially lead to serious drug interactions with adverse health outcomes. Therefore, not only the comorbidities but also the interaction between co-medications should be taken into account if a pharmacogenetics based dosing strategy is developed.

1.2 The aim of this book chapter

The aim of this book chapter is to describe and explore several examples of gene-drug interactions in CVD, the factors that affect the implementation in clinical practice, the cost-effectiveness analysis of pharmacogenetic testing, and the development of new technologies that could improve research of pharmacogenetic interactions in CVD.

---

* Anthonius de Boer[1], Tom Schalekamp[1], Felix J.M. Van Der Meer[2],
William K. Redekop[3] and Rahber Thariani[4]
# These authors contributed equally
[1]*Utrecht University, The Netherlands*
[2]*Leiden University Medical Center, The Netherlands*
[3]*Erasmus University Rotterdam, The Netherlands*
[4]*University of Washington, USA*

2. Examples of pharmacogenetics for cardiovascular diseases

Cardiovascular drugs are widely used for prevention or treatment of CVD. Gene-drug interactions were demonstrated in the treatment with platelet inhibitors, anticoagulants, antihypertensive drugs and statins. The findings of the many studies that have been conducted on pharmacogenetics of antihypertensive drugs, are not suitable for clinical implementation, often because the results could not be replicated or the clinical relevance was low (Arnett & Claas, 2009). The most commonly prescribed drugs in the management of CVD with important gene-drug interactions are statins, clopidogrel and coumarin derivatives. These three drugs are candidates for pharmacogenetic testing in everyday practice and will be discussed in more detail below.

2.1 Statins

Patients with hypercholesterolemia have an increased risk of CVD. Statins are widely used to treat hypercholesterolemia and prevent CVD. This treatment, often accompanied by lifestyle changes, has been proven to be effective and safe, but the efficacy varies among patients (Pearson et al., 2000). The effect of statins depends on the statin concentration at the site of action, the liver. This concentration can be altered by several factors, like diet and concomitant medication (Romaine et al., 2010). Muscle symptoms are a common problem during statin use ranging from mild myalgia to severe rhabdomyolysis (Law & Rudnicka, 2006). Although muscle symptoms are generally not life-threatening, they can negatively affect the patient's quality of life and also his or her adherence to statin therapy (Peters et al., 2009).

Several transporters play a role in the access of statins in the liver. Multiple studies have demonstrated a role for statin transportation by the organic anion transporter polypeptide 1B1 (OATP1B1) (Niemi, 2007; Pasanen et al., 2006), which is encoded by the *SLCO1B1* gene. An impaired hepatic uptake of several statins has been shown for patients with a specific single nucleotide polymorphism (SNP) in this gene, namely the *SLCO1B1* c.521T>C SNP. A decreased effect of statins is therefore seen in patients with this variant allele. This effect was shown in users of atorvastatin, pitavastatin, pravastatin and rosuvastatin in some studies, while others could not find a significant or clinically relevant effect (SEARCH Collaborative Group, 2008; Voora et al., 2009).

The impaired hepatic uptake causes an increased plasma concentration of statins, which probably causes a higher rate of adverse events. Carriers of a c.521C allele show an increased risk of developing myopathy after simvastatin use. Because this SNP does not seem to influence plasma concentration of fluvastatin, this could be an alternative for patients at risk of simvastatin induced muscle symptoms (Niemi et al., 2006). Genotyping before starting statin therapy might help to choose the right statin. Carriers of a variant allele could then be identified and treated with a *SLCO1B1* genotype independent statin, for example fluvastatin. In this way, genotyping for this *SLCO1B1* SNP may increase the safety of statin therapy. This approach of determining the most optimal therapy has not yet been investigated in a clinical trial.

2.2 Clopidogrel

Clopidogrel is a platelet inhibitor (PI), used together with aspirin to treat patients after percutaneous coronary interventions. This dual antiplatelet therapy reduces the risk of stent thrombosis, myocardial infarction, stroke and cardiovascular death. Clopidogrel monotherapy may be used for secondary prevention of atherosclerotic complications, in case aspirin can not be used, for example due to allergy (Anderson et al., 2010).

Clopidogrel is administered to patients as a prodrug. It needs to be metabolized by several hepatic cytochrome P450 (CYP) enzymes in order to form the active platelet aggregation inhibiting metabolite. This is done in two steps. During the first step, the intermediate 2-oxo-clopidogrel metabolite is formed. In this step three isoenzymes (CYP1A2, CYP2B6 and CYP2C19) are involved. During the second step this metabolite is hydrolyzed into the active thiol derivative R-130964, which blocks the ADP P2Y12 receptors on the platelet surface, causing inhibition of platelet aggregation. This step is catalyzed by four isoenzymes (CYP2B6, CYP2C9, CYP2C19 and CYP3A4) (Yukhanyan et al., 2011).

Although the effectiveness of clopidogrel has been demonstrated in many trials, variation in response is still an issue. Some patients experience cardiovascular events despite dual antiplatelet therapy (Yukhanyan et al., 2011). This difference in risk of cardiovascular events is genetically determined. In addition, response-variability is also caused by a genetically determined difference in platelet aggregation (Harmsze et al., 2010a). The interindividual variability in response to clopidogrel can be explained by multiple genetic and environmental factors. Variation in response to clopidogrel related to genetic variability in the *CYP2C19* gene has been investigated thoroughly, as the CYP2C19 enzyme plays an important role in both metabolizing steps (Anderson et al., 2010). In several studies a relationship between carriage of a loss-of-function allele in the *CYP2C19* gene and the occurrence of adverse cardiovascular events has been demonstrated. Up to now, more than 33 alleles of the *CYP2C19* gene have been identified. Most of these are rare in the general population. The most common allele in the European population is *CYP2C19**1. The enzyme encoded by this allele enables extensive metabolizing of clopidogrel into the active metabolite. A common variant allele is the *2 allele. Patients carrying at least one of this variant allele have a decreased activity of the CYP2C19 enzyme. This leads to a reduced plasma concentration of the active metabolite and possibly to an increased risk of recurrent cardiovascular events. Knowledge of the *CYP2C19**2 genotype can explain approximately 12% of the variation in response to clopidogrel. An increased risk of stent thrombosis has been demonstrated in carriers of a *CYP2C19**3 allele. Both carriers of a *2 of a *3 allele have a decreased enzyme activity, resulting in a lower amount of active metabolite (Harmsze et al., 2010b). The *CYP2C19**17 allele however, encodes for a more active enzyme. Carriers of this allele therefore have an increased antiplatelet response to clopidogrel. This might be associated with an increased risk of bleeding (Yukhanyan et al., 2011; Zabalza et al., 2011).

Pharmacogenetic testing for the *2 or *3 variant alleles could identify patients that are less likely to respond to clopidogrel and who might benefit more from treatment with an alternative, more expensive PI such as prasugrel or ticagrelor. Prasugrel and ticagrelor have less variability in response than clopidogrel, mainly due to a smaller influence of genetic variations. However, patients using prasugrel or ticagrelor have an increased risk of bleeding compared to patients using clopidogrel (Jakubowski et al., 2011; Collet & O'Connor, 2011). At the moment, randomized controlled trials (RCTs) are ongoing to evaluate the (cost) effectiveness of pre-treatment genotyping (Crespin et al., 2011). Based on the results of these trials, physicians can decide whether or not to prescribe clopidogrel or another PI on the patient's genotype.

2.3 Coumarin derivatives

Oral anticoagulants of the coumarin type are used to treat and prevent thromboembolic events in patients with different conditions, including venous thromboembolism and atrial fibrillation (Ansell et al., 2008). The effect is monitored by the International Normalized Ratio (INR), which should be kept within a certain range (for example, the range for atrial fibrillation is between 2.0 and 3.0). Wide interpatient variability in dose requirement means that the dosage is difficult to predict and frequent monitoring of the INR is necessary. INR values below the therapeutic range increase the risk of thromboembolic events while a supratherapeutic INR leads to an increased risk of bleeding events. These bleeding events can range from minor bleedings to major, life-threatening bleedings such as intracranial hemorrhage (James et al., 1992).

The wide variability in dose requirement is caused by several factors. Dietary intake of Vitamin K, comorbidities (e.g. altered thyroid function), concomitant medication, sex, age, height and weight all influence the required coumarin dose. Also genetic factors are shown to have an important role (Custodio das Dores et al., 2007; Penning-van Beest et al., 2001; Torn et al., 2005). First the influence of the *CYP2C9* gene, encoding the main metabolizing enzyme, cytochrome P450 2C9 (CYP2C9) was discovered. Carriers of a *2 or *3 allele require a lower dose and have an increased risk of overanticoagulation, which is associated with an increased risk of bleedings (Schalekamp, 2004). A few years later was discovered that with the *VKORC1* gene, encoding the target enzyme vitamin K epoxide reductase multiprotein complex 1, even a larger part of dose requirement variability could be explained. *CYP2C9* and *VKORC1* together explain approximately half of the variation in coumarin dose requirement (Schalekamp & de Boer, 2010; van Schie et al., 2011).

Currently, most patients receive an identical initial coumarin dosage. After a few days, the response is evaluated by INR measurement. The dose can then be adapted to the patient's needs. If patients are genotyped before starting coumarin therapy, they can receive a genotype-guided dose from day 1 on. This is suggested to prevent overanticoagulation in carriers of a variant allele and to reach a stable dose earlier. RCTs are currently ongoing to provide evidence for the (cost) effectiveness of pre-treatment genotyping for coumarin derivatives (van Schie et al., 2009; French et al., 2010).

In addition to the three mentioned examples, we expect more pharmacogenetic interactions will be found to be clinically relevant in CVD therapy.

3. Pharmacogenetic testing

Pharmacogenetic testing is thought to increase the efficacy and safety of drugs. However, for CVD, pharmacogenetic testing is not yet established in daily practice. Currently ongoing RCTs will hopefully provide evidence to implement pharmacogenetic testing in daily practice. However, implementation of a pharmacogenetic approach of a treatment depends on many different factors that extend beyond the outcomes of RCTs. These factors will be discussed in this paragraph.

3.1 Clinical trials to provide evidence

At this moment, a pharmacogenetic approach to determine the appropriate therapy for an individual patient is not yet widely used. There are currently only a few therapies where genotyping is used to establish the right dose or make a decision about which drug to use. Pharmacogenetic testing has not yet been used extensively since physicians are still hesitant about genotyping. Although physicians are willing to customize the therapy for an individual patient based on the patient's genetic profile, their capacity to do so is limited by their time and complexity of the procedure (Levy & Young, 2008). However, genotyping may provide physicians with tools for optimizing drug treatment for the individual patient. In other words, it could provide the physician with information on the individual reaction of the patient to the medication or the dose, comparable to what liver- and kidney function tests provide them with. These function tests were implemented in clinical practice without evidence for their added value from clinical trials. However, it is unlikely that pharmacogenetic tests would be implemented without RCTs, because of considerable uncertainty surrounding their efficacy and overall health outcome impact. These RCTs are therefore needed to convince physicians of the added value of genotyping the patient.

Currently, a number of RCTs are underway to hopefully provide evidence of improved efficacy and safety by genotyping the patient and using this information to individualize the treatment. Use of the search term "pharmacogenetics" on clinicaltrials.gov, a website where clinical trials are registered, produced a list of 361 studies (performed on 15 August 2011). Of these studies, 117 studies were interventional studies seeking new volunteers. In contrast, use of the term "cardiovascular" produced a list of 20,123 studies. However, only 61 studies were found after combining the search term "pharmacogenetics" with "cardiovascular". Of those 61 studies, 4 were being performed for statins, 4 for clopidogrel and 18 for the coumarin derivatives. This suggests that pharmacogenetics is currently only a minor research field in clinical trials and that most of the activity in that field is on coumarin derivatives.

Although thorough research is currently being performed to investigate the added value of genotyping on the efficacy and safety of drugs, it is not feasible to conduct a clinical trial for each newly found gene-drug interaction. There are several reasons for this. The first reason is that it is not always ethical to perform a clinical trial, for example in a situation in which observational studies have already shown that patients will be at a risk for an adverse event if they have a certain genotype (Peters, 2010). Secondly, costs and resource use would be prohibitive (e.g. study personnel, insurance). Thirdly, clinical trials are time-consuming. The length of the actual follow-up period is only one factor here; clinical trials take substantial time to initiate (e.g. writing the protocol, instructing study personnel), perform and analyse. For obvious gene-drug interactions, it is not ethical to waste money and time for performing clinical trials instead of implementing them directly. This would mean that we expect, in the future, that some observational studies should provide sufficient evidence to implement the findings in clinical practice. However, replication of the results in observational pharmacogenetic studies is often not obtained. Therefore, strict guidelines should be developed to define which evidence is necessary to implement the investigated pharmacogenetic interaction into clinical practice. Factors to consider are:

- Have the results been replicated in different studies with independent researchers?
- Are the results valid for various countries and ethnicities?
- Is the estimated improvement large enough?
- Is the estimated improvement cost-effective (see also paragraph 4)?
- Is it feasible to implement it in clinical practice? For example:
    - Are the genotyping results available in time?

- Are all facilities available?
- Are the parties involved trained to perform the implementation?

3.2 Parties involved in implementation

Once studies have shown that a pharmacogenetic approach of determining the optimal treatment for a patient is superior to the conventional therapy, it can be implemented in clinical practice. There are multiple parties involved in the implementation of pharmacogenetic based therapies in everyday clinical situations. In this paragraph, we will discuss all different parties involved and their rationales.

3.2.1 Patients

Successful implementation of pharmacogenetic testing in everyday practice heavily depends on patient attitudes. Without the cooperation of patients, development of new pharmacogenetic strategies or guidelines is futile. Fortunately, research has shown that this group is willing to provide a sample for genotyping. Van Wieren-De Wijer e*t al.* examined the reasons for non-response in a pharmacogenetic case-control study. They approached 1871 myocardial infarction cases and 14,102 controls of which 794 and 4997 responded, respectively. Only 1.1% of the non-responding participants were unwilling to provide a DNA sample (van Wieren et al., 2009). Moreover, since this study used a case-control design where all cardiovascular events had occurred before testing, the participants could not benefit from the test outcome. In case their drug treatment would be personalized by their genetic profile, this percentage is expected to decrease.

3.2.2 Health care professionals

The attitude of health care providers towards pharmacogenetic guided therapies is important in making their decision about the treatment the patient will receive. Although the FDA updated the warfarin label already in 2008 (Teichert et al., 2009a; Food and Drug Administration [FDA], 2007), genotyping preceding the anticoagulation therapy with coumarin derivatives is not commonly performed. Currently, health care professionals' attitudes are reserved towards pharmacogenetic dosing. Not many therapies need pharmacogenetic testing at the moment, so health care professionals need to get familiarized with the idea of genetic testing, like they are familiarized with performing liver and kidney function tests. Different approaches are thought to help with familiarizing health care professionals with pharmacogenetic testing:

- Clinical trials are needed to convince the health care professional and make genetic testing as normal as liver and kidney function tests.
- Recommendations in guidelines and drug labels of pharmacogenetic testing to improve treatment quality are required, such as the FDA did for warfarin.
- Education of the health care profession on how to perform and use the pharmacogenetic tests is desired.
- Favourable experiences will stimulate the health care professional to use pharmacogenetic testing in everyday clinical practice.
- Facilities for genotyping need to be available at the right place and time.
- Consistency and standards for pharmacogenetic testing are needed.

The focus of the process should not only be on the physician but also pharmacists should be involved. To enhance the implementation of pharmacogenetic testing, the Royal Dutch Association for the Advancement of Pharmacy developed pharmacogenetic-based therapeutic (dose) recommendations (Swen et al., 2011; Wilffert et al., 2010). In addition, the pharmacist could be involved in genotyping the patient with easy to use point-of-care tests that will be available soon. The results of, for example, CYP-enzymes, could be used for decision making in multiple therapies. The pharmacist is not the only candidate to genotype the patient; others such the GP or a nurse in the hospital could also genotype the patient. Therefore, dissemination of the genotyping results (e.g., by means of electronic dossiers) is important.

3.2.3 Regulatory authorities

Regulatory authorities will also play an important role in the implementation of pharmacogenetic guided therapies in daily practice. They have the power to develop guidelines which health care professionals are obligated to follow. They can also adjust the label information of the medication.

In order to harmonize approaches to drug regulation, a guideline was developed to ensure that consistent definitions of terminology are applied across all constituents of the International Conference on Harmonisation (ICH) (EMA, 2007; FDA, 2008). This guideline contains nonbinding recommendations. The Committee for Human Medicinal Products (CHMP) facilitated an informal process of sharing scientific and technical information between applicants and regulators by releasing a concept paper on "Briefing Meetings on Pharmacogenetics". The Pharmacogenetics Working Party was set up to support discussions regarding the implementation of pharmacogenetic testing. In April 2006, a guideline on Pharmacogenetics Briefing Meetings was adopted by the CHMP. This guideline provides guidance for starting the discussion with the Pharmacogenetics Working Party and provides considerations on the submission of pharmacogenetic data in informal regulatory submissions. Briefing meetings take place when new pharmacogenetic information becomes available during the development of a new medicinal product or when a new indication is explored based on recent developments in pharmacogenetics (EMA, 2006). The Food and Drug Administration (FDA) developed a guideline called "Guidance for Industry, Pharmacogenomic Data Submissions". This guideline facilitates the scientific pharmacogenomics process and the use of pharmacogenomic data in drug development (U.S. Department of Health and Human Services et al., 2005). The FDA and European Medicinal Agency (EMA) have joint Voluntary Genomic Data Submissions (VGDSs). This is not part of the regulatory decision-making process, but gains an understanding of genomic data and provides options for sponsors to have joint FDA-EMA briefing meetings (Goodsaid, 2006). A consistent regulatory environment is also helpful in encouraging industry to develop pharmacogenetic products, and for consumers (including patients and physicians) to use the product.

3.2.4 Health insurance companies

Implementation of pharmacogenetic guided approaches to plan therapy will depend on whether it is reimbursed by health insurance companies. If the patient needs to pay for the genotyping kit, it is less likely that pharmacogenetic testing will be implemented in clinical practice than when health insurance companies will pay for it. However, these companies will likely only pay for genetic tests if their use leads to more cost-effective care. Health insurers would be very interested in genotyping if it improved treatment effectiveness but also reduced total health care costs (including the cost of genotyping). There are different ways in which genotyping results could lead to lower health care costs, for example:

- Fewer visits to the GP or hospital for therapy adjustments, i.e. improved patient response or efficacy
- Better prophylaxis resulting in lower costs
- Fewer side effects, especially serious side effects resulting in expensive hospital admissions.

In some cases, health insurers may reimburse genotyping even if it is believed to increase overall costs. For example, if the genotyping approach is more costly and more effective compared to the non-genotyping approach, the health insurer could consider the greater effectiveness worth the extra cost. All in all, this means that pharmaco-economic evaluations are of importance in pharmacogenetic studies. See also paragraph 4 on cost-effectiveness analysis.

3.2.5 Researchers (public and private industry)

Sound scientific research is needed to develop new strategies of pharmacogenetic guided therapies. Without research, new ideas of pharmacogenetic guided therapies will not arise. Both the public as well as the private industry could perform this research. There are different focus points that researchers could have. First, they could investigate new pharmacogenetic interactions. Interactions could be of different value. They could look for common SNPs that have a small effect, but since the SNPs are common, many patients might benefit. On the other hand, they could investigate rare SNPs that might cause major effects, in which case there could be a huge benefit for relatively few patients. However, this last area of research would require big sample sizes to have enough power to investigate the effect of a rare SNP. Second, studies to develop better and faster genotyping methods will be required if pharmacogenomic testing is to be used just as extensive as liver and kidney function tests. An example of a user-friendly and quick genotyping system is Optisense's Genie 1 with HyBeacon® assays (Howard et al., 2011). See also paragraph 5. Third, the industry could develop new drug therapies for a subpopulation. For example, a new drug that does not have the desired effect in the whole population might benefit patients with a certain genotype. Although only for this subpopulation, this new medication could then still enter the market. Forth, scientists should aim to develop genotype guided therapies that do not require large and time-consuming clinical trials. Currently, clinical trials are needed to convince health care professionals, but in the future, cohort studies could be used for the implementation of pharmacogenetic testing. It is important that the results are replicated in various external datasets before being implemented in clinical practice. After implementation, it remains important to validate the process and, if necessary, adjust the pharmacogenetic based guidelines if it does not seem to be working satisfactorily.

3.3 Facilities

Several facilities should be in place before pharmacogenetic testing can be implemented in clinical practice.

3.3.1 Availability of genotyping results

Genotyping results should be available quickly. If results are available before the therapy starts, they are of greater value than when they become available after treatment start. However, in the current clinical situation, health care professionals need to collect blood samples from a number of patients to be able to genotype a batch of samples. Therefore, it can sometimes take a few weeks before the genotype is known. Currently, new techniques are being developed, and will continue to be developed in the coming years, to make genotyping results more rapidly available (Howard et al., 2011). The need to collect samples from many patients will diminish, since one assay can be run using a Point-Of-Care Test (POCT) for a single patient. By increasing the number of tests needed, the availability of POCTs will increase (Huang, 2008) and the price per POCT assay will probably decrease (see also paragraph 5).

3.3.2 Authority guidelines

The authorities can assist in implementing pharmacogenetic testing in clinical practice by developing guidelines and ensuring that health care professionals follow them. In 2008, the FDA updated the warfarin label (Teichert et al., 2009a; Food and Drug Administration [FDA], 2007) and advised pharmacogenetic testing before the coumarin therapy starts. However, at that time no guidelines were provided as to how the dosages should be changed based on the genetic profile of the patient. This illustrates that guidelines should contain information on how to adjust drug therapy based on genotype. It also underlines the importance that different parties work closely together.

4. Cost-effectiveness analysis of pharmacogenetic testing

Many would argue that clinical practice guidelines should just focus on whether pharmacogenetic testing improves effectiveness and ignore cost considerations. However, decision making about the widespread use of genotyping also depends on its cost-effectiveness. This means that even if authorities were to recommend genotyping patients prior to cardiovascular therapy based on proof of effectiveness, the recommendation might not easily be implemented without the support of other stakeholders. One important stakeholder is the payer, such as a health insurance company and its attitude can be an instrumental factor in the successful implementation of pharmacogenetic testing. Health insurance companies may require proof of cost-effectiveness - and some estimates of budget impact - before considering reimbursement.

A cost-effectiveness analysis (CEA) compares the total costs and effectiveness of two or more different treatment strategies. All sorts of costs must be considered here, including not just the cost of genotyping, but also the cost of monitoring and the cost of cardiovascular events that occur later in time. While costs are all expressed in the same way (money!), effectiveness can be defined in different ways. The definition of effectiveness determines how cost-effectiveness is expressed. For example, effectiveness can focus on the risk of an adverse event and the difference in effectiveness between two treatments can be expressed as the absolute reduction in risk of an event. The cost-effectiveness of one treatment versus another will then be expressed as the extra cost to avoid one adverse event (calculated by dividing the difference in costs by the reduction in risk). However, since this expression of cost-effectiveness is very disease-specific, it is difficult, if not impossible, to compare the cost-effectiveness of different treatments for different diseases with each other and this comparability is valuable when making budget allocation decisions. For this reason, some authorities or health insurance companies require a cost-utility analysis. In a cost-utility analysis (CUA), the health gains acquired by a new treatment are expressed in Quality Adjusted Life Years (QALYs), which can be compared more easily with other treatments, also in other diseases, than the cost per adverse event avoided.

Several economic evaluations (such as CEAs and CUAs) have been performed for coumarin derivatives. The problem with these analyses is that no robust data on the effectiveness of genotyping are available yet; the large RCTs that can provide this data are still ongoing (van Schie et al., 2009; French et al., 2010). This current lack of evidence results in a wide variability in cost-effectiveness ratios among the studies that have been done, ranging from dominance (where use of genotyping reduces costs and increases health) to a very high incremental cost of $347,000 per QALY gained (Verhoef et al., 2010). The costs of genotyping are also not clear yet. In literature, the estimated cost of genotyping for *CYP2C9* ranges from $67 to $350 and the estimated cost of genotyping both *CYP2C9* and *VKORC1* ranges from $175 to $575. Recently, a Point-Of-Care Test (POCT) for genotyping *CYP2C9* and *VKORC1* has been developed. With this test, the patient's genotype can be determined in the physician's office within 2 hours and this is estimated to cost less than $50 per patient for both *CYP2C9* and *VKORC1* (Howard et al., 2011). The costs of genotyping are expected to decrease even further, with increased usage. This will also influence the chance that pharmacogenetic testing is cost-effective.

Decisions about whether or not to implement pharmacogenetic testing in clinical practice will differ among different countries. This difference can be caused by several factors. Firstly, the amount of money society is willing to pay varies among different countries. For example, this 'willingness to pay' is approximately $50,000 per QALY gained in the US or £20,000–30,000 (approximately $33,000-50,000) per QALY gained in the UK (National Institute for Health and Clinical Excellence [NICE], 2008). Secondly, the costs, not only of genotyping but also of the consequences like bleeding events, are not identical in all countries. Next to this, the effectiveness of genotyping can also be higher in one country than in another. This is for example possibly the case with coumarin derivatives. In some countries the standard care is already of very high quality, with specialized anticoagulation clinics to monitor the effect of the drug, while in other countries this is not the case and there is still room for further improvement.

As mentioned before, the use of pharmacogenetics in treatment with a certain drug can only be recommended if information on effectiveness and costs of genotyping is available, although it is not clear what level of evidence is needed for a valid decision. Obviously, it is impossible to obtain perfect evidence. Therefore, value of information (VOI) analyses could be performed to establish the cost-effectiveness of further research on the efficiency of the strategy. If the costs of performing this research are greater than the benefits of the additional information, then it would not be worthwhile to conduct this research (Sculpher & Claxton, 2005). The parameters that have the greatest influence on the uncertainty regarding the cost-effectiveness of genotyping should be the main focus of future studies in this area. The costs of conducting these studies should also be considered. However, this will also depend upon the regulatory environment, and VOI forms only a part of the picture.

5. Pharmacogenetic developments

Until now, only the most obvious gene-drug interactions have been detected since these are least complicated to detect when researchers are looking for causal SNPs. However, rare SNPs with large effects might as well be of importance, but it is a challenge to find large numbers of cases that are required to obtain enough power in pharmacogenetic studies when looking at smaller effects or lower allele frequencies (Daly, 2010). A trend is observed that larger studies are being performed and meta-analyses are carried out to investigate these less frequent genetic profiles. Several techniques are further developed and might lead to new insights in the pharmacogenetic research field. We will discuss them in this paragraph.

5.1 Candidate-gene studies

This type of study investigates the association between drug response and previously identified candidate genes. These candidate genes might play a relevant role in the pharmacokinetics or pharmacodynamics of the drug and might therefore be, for example, the metabolizing enzyme or the target protein. An example is the use of candidate gene approaches for the understanding of the overall drug response to coumarins. (Daly, 2010). In 1992, Rettie *et al.* indicated *CYP2C9* as main metabolizing enzyme of warfarin (Rettie et al., 1992). A few years later, Furuya *et al.* first reported that SNPs in this gene affect the stable coumarin maintenance dose (Furuya et al., 1995). A decade later, VKORC1 was identified as the target enzyme of the coumarins (Rost et al., 2004; Li et al., 2004) and studies confirming the association between *VKORC1* genotypes and stable coumarin maintenance dose followed. Another example is the role of the *CYP2C19* genotype on the clopidogrel (Hulot, 2006) therapy response and how the treatment with tamoxifen is influenced by the *CYP2D6* genotype (Hoskins, 2009).

5.2 Genome-wide association studies

Since 2007, genonome wide association (GWA) studies have become more frequently applied in the pharmacogenetics field. This resulted in novel identified associations between drug response and variations in DNA (Daly, 2010). In CVD, GWA studies resulted in confirmation of the already available knowledge, rather than in newly identified interactions. For clopidogrel, the influence of *CYP2C19* was confirmed (Schuldiner et al., 2009) and for statin induced muscle symptoms an association with *SLCO1B1* was found (SEARCH Collaborative Group, 2008) in a GWA study. In a GWA study on acenocoumarol maintenance dose, an additional effect was found for polymorphisms in *CYP4F2* and *CYP2C18* (Teichert et al., 2009b). These GWA studies led to more knowledge about several drug-gene interactions, but the causality of the relationship is not always clear in these studies. Another difficulty with this type of analyses is the need of large patient numbers because of the correction for multiple testing.

5.3 Sequencing

DNA sequencing is the determination of the nucleotide bases in DNA. In contrast to GWA studies, where tag SNPs are used to cover as much of the variation within the gene as possible, this technique will determine the exact order of nucleotides in DNA. Instead of tag SNPs that are usually markers for the causal SNP - and thereby introduce noise because they are not always in complete linkage disequilibrium - the causal SNPs can be identified. Therefore, this technique might provide new insights in associations between drug response and pharmacogenetic parameters that are not observed when performing a candidate-gene study or a GWA study. It is possible to sequence a whole genome or whole exome. In addition, there is an option 'targeted sequencing' which means that a candidate gene is sequenced. This technique is relatively new and gaining interest in the last few years, but the same issues (i.e. causality of the relationship is not always clear and large patient numbers are needed) as with the GWA studies occur with sequencing. This warrants that the functionality of the SNP should be studied (Sadee, 2011).

5.4 Point-of-care testing

As discussed earlier, point-of-care tests can be used as mobile genotyping instruments in different settings, including the pharmacy, anticoagulation clinic and physician's office. It avoids the need to collect multiple samples and the genotyping results are available within 2 hours. This technique might be used to genotype the patient before the start of the therapy. However, the applicability of a point-of-care test may be different from centralized laboratory testing because of different sensitivity and specificity parameters. Also, it is not attractive to use such a test in research where large patient groups are needed to find a pharmacogenetic interaction, since that would be very labor intensive.

6. Conclusion

There is considerable potential for pharmacogenetic based drug dosing in CVD, but at the moment, these are not widely implemented in clinical practice. Convincing evidence was found for several CVD drugs. Carriers of a variant allele of the *SLCO1B1* gene could be treated with a *SLCO1B1* independent statin to increase the safety of the treatment. Clopidogrel is less metabolized into its active form by patients carrying a variant allele of *CYP2C19*, resulting in a less effective therapy. Information about the patient's *VKORC1* and *CYP2C9* genotype could be used when defining the appropriate dose during the anticoagulation therapy with coumarins to enhance the efficacy and increase the safety of the treatment. However, implementation of this knowledge is challenging and depends on multiple factors. First, clinical trials are needed to provide evidence for and enhance the implementation of pharmacogenetic testing. However, it is not feasible to perform a clinical trial for every newly found gene-drug interaction. Therefore it is desirable to develop guidelines to which observational studies should apply before implementing the gene-drug interaction in clinical practice. Secondly, multiple parties are involved, such as patients, health care professionals, regulatory authorities, health insurance companies and researchers. We discussed the different parties involved and their rationales. Thirdly, several facilities should be in place before pharmacogenetic testing can be implemented in clinical practice, such as availability of genotyping results and authority guidelines. Lastly, before it comes to implementation, the cost-effectiveness of the pharmacogenetic approach should be investigated. Health insurance companies may require proof of cost-effectiveness before considering reimbursement and therefore implementation of pharmacogenetic testing.

For the coming years, researchers will continue to develop the different genotyping methods. Larger studies will be performed and meta-analyses will be carried out to investigate less frequent genetic profiles. Analysis of GWA studies and sequencing is challenging due to the enormous amount of data obtained by this technique.

In the field of oncology, pharmacogenetic testing already is part of daily practice. We expect that pharmacogenetic testing will also be implemented in CVD in the near future.

7. References

Anderson, C., Biffi, A., Greenberg, S. & Rosand, J. (2010). Personalized approaches to clopidogrel therapy: are we there yet? *Stroke* 41, 12, (Dec 2010), 2997-3002.

Ansell, J., Hirsh, J., Hylek, E., Jacobson, A., Crowther, M. & Palareti, G. (2008). Pharmacology and management of the vitamin K antagonists: American College of Chest Physicians Evidence-Based Clinical Practice Guidelines (8th Edition). *Chest* 133, 6 suppl, (Jun 2008), 160S-198S.

Arnett, D. & Claas, S. (2009). Pharmacogenetics of antihypertensive treatment: detailing disciplinary dissonance. *Pharmacogenomics* 10, 8, (Aug 2009), 1295-1307.

Collet, J. & O'Connor, S. (2011). Clinical effects and outcomes with new P2Y12 inhibitors in ACS. *Fundam. Clin. Pharmacol.* (Sep 2011).

Crespin, D., Federspiel, J., Biddle, A., Jonas, D. & Rossi, J. (2011). Ticagrelor versus genotype-driven antiplatelet therapy for secondary prevention after acute coronary syndrome: a cost-effectiveness analysis. *Value Health.* 14, 4, (Jun 2011), 483-491 (2011).

Custodio das Dores, S., Booth, S., Martini, L., de Carvalho Gouvea, V., Padovani, C., de Abreu Maffei, F., Campana, A. & Rupp de Paiva, S. (2007). Relationship between diet and anticoagulant response to warfarin: a factor analysis. *Eur J Nutr* 46, 3, (Apr 2007), 147-154.

Daly, A. (2010). Genome-wide association studies in pharmacogenomics. *Nat. Rev. Genet.* 11, 4, (Apr 2010), 241-246.

European Medicines Agency [EMA]. (2006). Guideline on pharmacogenetics briefing meetings.

European Medicines Agency [EMA]. (2007). ICH Topic E15 Definitions for genomic biomarkers, pharmacogenomics, pharmacogenetics, genomic data and sample coding categories.

Food and Drug Administration [FDA]. (2007). Transcript of the FDA press conference on Warfarin held on 16 August.

Food and Drug Administration [FDA]. (2008). Guidance for Industry E15 Definitions for Genomic Biomarkers, Pharmacogenomics, Pharmacogenetics, Genomic Data and Sample Coding Categories

French, B., Joo, J., Geller, N., Kimmel, S., Rosenberg, Y., Anderson, J., Gage, B., Johnson, J., Ellenberg, J. & COAG investigators. (2010). Statistical design of personalized medicine interventions: the Clarification of Optimal Anticoagulation through Genetics (COAG) trial. *Trials* 11, (Nov 2010), 108.

Furuya, H., Fernandez-Salguero, P., Gregory, W., Taber, H., Steward, A,, Gonzalez, F. & Idle, J. (1995) Genetic polymorphism of CYP2C9 and its effect on warfarin maintenance dose requirement in patients undergoing anticoagulation therapy. *Pharmacogenetics*. 5(6), (dec 1995), 389-392.

Goodsaid, F. (2006). 42nd annual meeting; Joint USFDA-EU Pharmacogenomic Initiatives.

Harmsze, A., van Werkum, J., Ten Berg, J., Zwart, B., Bouman, H., Breet, N., van 't Hof, A., Ruven, H., Hackeng, C., Klungel, O., de Boer, A. & Deneer, V. (2010a). CYP2C19*2 and CYP2C9*3 alleles are associated with stent thrombosis: a case-control study. *Eur. Heart J.* 31, 24, (Dec 2010) 3046-3053.

Harmsze, A., van Werkum, J., Bouman, H., Ruven,H., Breet, N., Ten Berg, J., Hackeng, C., Tjoeng, M., Klungel, O., de Boer, A. & Deneer, V. (2010b). Besides CYP2C19*2, the variant allele CYP2C9*3 is associated with higher on-clopidogrel platelet reactivity in patients on dual antiplatelet therapy undergoing elective coronary stent implantation. *Pharmacogenet Genomics* 20, 1, (Jan 2010), 18-25.

Howard, R., Leathart, J., French, D., Krishan, E., Kohnke. H., Wadelius, M., van Schie, R., Verhoef, T., Maitland-van der Zee, A., Daly, A. & Barallon, R. (2011). Genotyping for CYP2C9 and VKORC1 alleles by a novel point of care assay with HyBeacon(R) probes. *Clin. Chim. Acta,* (Jul 2011).

Hoskins, J., Carey, L. & McLeod, H. (2009). CYP2D6 and tamoxifen: DNA matters in breast cancer. *Nature Rev. Cancer,* 9, 576-586.

Huang, S. (2008). Warfarin Pharmacogenetic Testing is Now Ready for Prime Time, AACC Annual Meeting, Washington DC, July 28, 2008.

Hulot, J., Bura, A., Villard, E., Azizi, M., Remones, V., Goyenvalle, C., Aiach, M., Lechat, P. & Gaussem, P. (2006) Cytochrome P450 2C19 loss-of-function polymorphism is a major determinant of clopidogrel responsiveness in healthy subjects. *Blood* 108, 2244-2247

Jakubowski, J., Riesmeyer, J., Close, S., Leishman, A. & Erlinge, D. (2011). TRITON and Beyond: New Insights into the Profile of Prasugrel. *Cardiovasc. Ther.* (Feb 2011).

James, A., Britt, R., Raskino, C. & Thompson, S. (1992). Factors affecting the maintenance dose of warfarin. *J Clin Pathol* 45, 8, (Aug 1992), 704-6.

Law, M. & Rudnicka, A. (2006). Statin safety: a systematic review. *Am. J. Cardiol.* 97, 8A, (Apr 2006), 52C-60C.

Levy, H. & Young, J. (2008). Perspectives from the clinic: will the average physician embrace personalized medicine? *Clin. Pharmacol. Ther.* 83, 3, (Mar 2008), 492-493.

Li, T., Chang, C., Jin, D., Lin, P., Khvorova, A., & Stafford, D. (2004). Identification of the gene for vitamin K epoxide reductase. *Nature,* 427, 541-544.

Nice. (2008). Guide to the methods of technology appraisal.

Niemi, M., Pasanen, M. & Neuvonen, P. (2006). SLCO1B1 polymorphism and sex affect the pharmacokinetics of pravastatin but not fluvastatin. *Clin. Pharmacol. Ther.* 80, 4, (Oct 2006), 356-366.

Niemi, M. (2007). Role of OATP transporters in the disposition of drugs. *Pharmacogenomics* 8, 7, (Jul 2007), 787-802.

Pasanen, M., Neuvonen, M., Neuvonen, P. & Niemi, M. (2006). SLCO1B1 polymorphism markedly affects the pharmacokinetics of simvastatin acid. *Pharmacogenet Genomics* 16, 12 (Dec 2006), 873-879.

Pearson, T., Laurora, I., Chu, H. & Kafonek, S. (2000). The lipid treatment assessment project (L-TAP): a multicenter survey to evaluate the percentages of dyslipidemic patients receiving lipid-lowering therapy and achieving low-density lipoprotein cholesterol goals. *Arch. Intern. Med.* 160, 4, (Feb 2000), 459-467.

Penning-van Beest, F., van Meegen, E., Rosendaal, F. & Stricker, B. (2001). Drug interactions as a cause of overanticoagulation on phenprocoumon or acenocoumarol predominantly concern antibacterial drugs. *Clin Pharmacol Ther* 69, 6, (Jun 2001), 451-457.

Peters, B., Klungel, O., Visseren, F., de Boer, A. & Maitland-van der Zee, A. (2009). Pharmacogenomic insights into treatment and management of statin-induced myopathy. *Genome Med.* 1, 1, (Dec 2009), 120.

Peters, B. (2010). Thesis: "Methodological approaches to the pharmacogenomics of statins"

Rettie A., Korzekwa, K., Kunze, K. , Lawrence, R. Eddy, A., Aoyama, T., Gelboin, J., Gonzalez, F. & Trager, W. (1992) Hydroxylation of warfarin by human cDNA-expressed cytochrome P-450: A role for P-4502C9 in the etiology of (S)-warfarin-drug interactions. *Chem. Res. Toxicol.* 5, 54-59.

Romaine, S., Bailey, K., Hall, A. & Balmforth, A. (2010). The influence of SLCO1B1 (OATP1B1) gene polymorphisms on response to statin therapy. *Pharmacogenomics J.* 10, 1, (Feb 2010), 1-11.

Rost, S., Fregin, A., Ivaskevicius, V., Conzelmann, E., Hörtnagel, K., Pelz, H., Lappegard, K., Seifried, E., Scharrer, E., Tuddenham, E., Müller, C., Strom, T. & Oldenburg, J. (2004). Mutations in VKORC1 cause warfarin resistance and multiple coagulation factor deficiency type 2. *Nature*, 427, 537-541.

Sadee, W., (2011). Pharmacogenomic biomarkers: validation needed for both the molecular genetic mechanism and clinical effect. *Pharmacogenomics*, 12, 5, (May 2011), 675-80.

Schalekamp, T., Oosterhof, M., van Meegen, E., van Der Meer, F., Conemans, J., Hermans, M., Meijerman, I. & de Boer, A. (2004). Effects of cytochrome P450 2C9 polymorphisms on phenprocoumon anticoagulation status. *Clin. Pharmacol. Ther.* 76, 5, (Nov 2004), 409-417.

Schalekamp, T. & de Boer, A. (2010). Pharmacogenetics of oral anticoagulant therapy. *Curr Pharm Des* 16, 2, (2010) 187-203.

van Schie, R., Wadelius, M., Kamali, F., Daly, A., Manolopoulos, V., de Boer, A., Barallon, R., Verhoef, T., Kirchheiner, J., Haschke-Becher, E., Briz, M., Rosendaal, F., Redekop, W., Pirmohamed, M. & van der Zee, A. (2009) Genotype-guided dosing of coumarin derivatives: the European pharmacogenetics of anticoagulant therapy (EU-PACT) trial design. *Pharmacogenomics* 10, 10, (Oct 2009), 1687-1695.

van Schie, R., Wessels, J., le Cessie, S., de Boer, A., Schalekamp, T., van der Meer, F., Verhoef, T., van Meegen, E., Rosendaal, F. & Maitland-van der Zee, A., for the EU-PACT Study Group (2011) Loading and maintenance dose algorithms for phenprocoumon and acenocoumarol using patient characteristics and pharmacogenetic data. *Eur Heart J.* 32,15, (Aug 2011), 1909-1917.

Sculpher, M. & Claxton, K. (2005). Establishing the cost-effectiveness of new pharmaceuticals under conditions of uncertainty--when is there sufficient evidence? *Value Health*, 8, 4, (Jul 2005), 433-446.

SEARCH Collaborative Group. (2008). SLCO1B1 variants and statin-induced myopathy--a genomewide study. *N. Engl. J. Med.* 359, 8, (Aug 2008), 789-799.

Shuldiner, A., O'Connell, J., Bliden, K., Gandhi, A., Ryan, K., Horenstein, R., Damcott, C., Pakyz, R., Tantry, U., Gibson, Q., Pollin, T., Post, W., Parsa, A., Mitchel, B., Faraday, N., Herzog, W. & Gurbel, P. (2009). Association of cytochrome P450 2C19 genotype with the antiplatelet effect and clinical efficacy of clopidogrel therapy. *JAMA*, 302, 8, (Aug 2009), 849-857.

Swen, J., Nijenhuis, M., de Boer, A., Grandia, L., Maitland-van der Zee, A., Mulder, H., Rongen, G., van Schaik, R., Schalekamp, T., Touw, D., van der Weide, J., Wilffert, B., Deneer, V. & Guchelaar, H. (2011). Pharmacogenetics: from bench to byte- an update of guidelines. *Clin. Pharmacol. Ther.* 89, 5, (May 2011), 662-673.

Teichert, M., van Schaik, R., Hofman, A., Uitterlinden, A., de Smet, P., Stricker, B. & Visser, L. (2009a). Genotypes associated with reduced activity of VKORC1 and CYP2C9 and their modification of acenocoumarol anticoagulation during the initial treatment period. *Clin. Pharmacol. Ther.* 85, 4, (Apr 2009), 379-386.

Teichert, M., Eijgelsheim, M., Rivadeneira, F., Uitterlinden, A., van Schaik, R., Hofman, A., De Smet, P., van Gelder, T., Visser, L. & Stricker, B. (2009b). A genome-wide association study of acenocoumarol maintenance dosage. *Hum. Mol. Genet.* 18, 19, (Oct 2009), 3758-86.

Torn, M., Bollen, W., van der Meer, F., van der Wall, E. & Rosendaal, F. (2005). Risks of oral anticoagulant therapy with increasing age. *Arch Intern Med* 165, 13, (Jul 2011) 1527-1532.

U.S. Department of Health and Human Services, Food and Drug Administration, Center for Drug Evaluation and Research (CDER), Center for Biologics Evaluation and Research (CBER) & Center for Devices and Radiological Health (CDRH). (2005). Guidance for Industry, Pharmacogenomic Data Submissions.

Verhoef, T., Redekop, W., Darba, J., Geitona, M., Hughes, D., Siebert, U., de Boer, A., Maitland-van der Zee, A. & EU-PACT group. (2010). A systematic review of cost-effectiveness analyses of pharmacogenetic-guided dosing in treatment with coumarin derivatives. *Pharmacogenomics* 11, 7, (Jul 2010), 989-1002.

Voora, D., Shah, S., Spasojevic, I., Ali, S., Reed, C., Salisbury, B. & Ginsburg, G. (2009). The SLCO1B1*5 genetic variant is associated with statin-induced side effects. *J. Am. Coll. Cardiol.* 54, 17, (Oct 2009), 1609-1616.

van Wieren-de Wijer, D., Maitland-van der Zee, A., de Boer, A., Kroon, A., de Leeuw, P., Schiffers, P., Janssen, R., Psaty, B., van Duijn, C., Stricker, B. & Klungel, O. (2009). Reasons for non-response in observational pharmacogenetic research. *Pharmacoepidemiol. Drug Saf.* 18, 8, (Aug 2009), 665-671.

Wilffert, B., Swen, J., Mulder, H., Touw, D., Maitland-van der Zee, A., Deneer, V. & KNMP working Group Pharmacogenetics (2010). From evidence based medicine to mechanism based medicine. Reviewing the role of pharmacogenetics. *Pharm. World Sci.* (Nov 2010).

Yukhanyan, L., Freynhofer, M., Siller-Matula, J., Schror, K. & Huber, K. (2011). Genetic variability in response to clopidogrel therapy and its clinical implications. *Thromb. Haemost.* 105 Suppl 1, (May 2011), S55-9.

Zabalza, M., Subirana, I., Sala, J., Lluis-Ganella, C., Lucas, G., Tomas, M., Masia, R., Marrugat, J., Brugada, R. & Elosua, R. (2011). Meta-analyses of the association between cytochrome CYP2C19 loss- and gain-of-function polymorphisms and cardiovascular outcomes in patients with coronary artery disease treated with clopidogrel. *Heart*, (Jun 2011).

11

Warfarin Enantiomers Pharmacokinetics by CYP2C19

Yumiko Akamine and Tsukasa Uno
Department of Hospital Pharmacy, Faculty of Medicine,
University of the Ryukyus, Okinawa,
Japan

1. Introduction

Warfarin, a coumarin vitamin K antagonist, is the most widely prescribed anticoagulant agent for the control and prevention of atrial fibrillation-related thrombus formation, stroke, and arterial and venous thrombembolism (Hirsh J et al., 1998). The recommend warfarin therapy consists of the lowest dose required to maintain the target international normalized ratio (INR) because of the drug's narrow therapeutic window. However, there can be a 20-fold difference in the dose required by patients to achieve this target INR. It is well known that cytochrome P450 (CYP), predominantly CYP2C9, activity is an important source of variability (Kaminsky LS and Zhang ZY, 1997) . Additionally, Rieder et al. (2005) have reported that an effect of the vitamin K epooxide reductase complex subunit 1 gene (VKORC1) has an important role on dose requirement. However, Takahashi et al. (2006) shows that Caucasians and African-Americans have high frequencies of VKORC1 and CYP2C9 genotypes, which lead to either reduced metabolic activity or attenuated sensitivity to warfarin, whereas only about 20% of the Japanese population possesses these genotypes. Therefore, further study of sources of variability in warfarin dose requirements among Japanese patients is warranted.

Warfarin is administered clinically as a racemic mixture of the *S*- and *R*-enantiomer (Fig. 1), however *S*-warfarin is 3–5 times more potent than *R*-enantiomer. Both enantiomers are extensively metabolized in the liver (Chan E et al., 1994; Takahashi H and Echizen H, 2001). The more potent *S*-enantiomer is metabolized mainly to *S*-7-hydroxywarfarin by CYP2C9, whereas *R*-enantiomer is metabolized to *R*-6, *R*-7, *R*-8 and *R*-10-hydroxywarfarin by several CYPs involving CYP1A2, CYP3A4 and CYP2C19 (Kaminsky LS and Zhang ZY, 1997). Among these CYPs, it has been shown that both CYP2C9 and CYP2C19 are subject to single nucleotide polymorphisms (SNPs). In Japanese, because the heterozygous frequency of the CYP2C9 Leu359 allele is 3.5% (Takahashi H et al., 1998) and the frequency of the defective CYP2C19 alleles is 18.8% (Kubota T et al., 1996), the latter may be more closely associated with the clinical effect of warfarin. In this chapter, we therefore focus on the effect of CYP2C19 genotypes on the pharmacokinetics and pharmacodynamics of warfarin enantiomers. In addition, we characterize the impact of omeprazole, a CYP2C19 inhibitor, on the stereoselective pharmacokinetics and pharmacodynamics of warfarin between CYP2C19 genotypes.

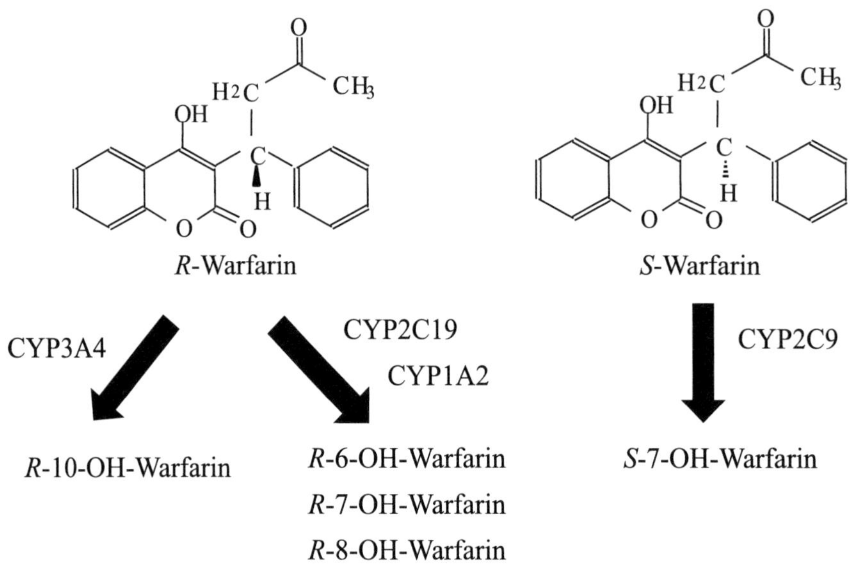

Fig. 1. Metabolic pathways of *R*-warfarin and *S*-warfarin.

2. Analytical methods

2.1 Genotypic identification

17 healthy Japanese volunteers (12 males and 5 females) were enrolled in this study after giving written informed consent. All subjects were enrolled in this study after giving written informed consent. Each Subject underwent a CYP2C19 genotyping test by use of a polymerase chain reaction-restriction fragment length polymorphism (PCR-RFLP) method with allele-specific primer for identifying the *CYP2C19* wild-type (*1) gene and the 2 mutated alleles, *CYP2C19**2 (*2) in exon 5 and *CYP2C19**3 (*3) in exon 4 (De Morais SM et al., 1994), and they were classified into 2 genotype groups as follows: homozygous extensive metabolizers (hmEMs, *1/*1, 10 subjects), poor metabolizers (PMs, *2/*2 or *2/*3, 7 subjects). Similarly, CYP2C9 genotyping test by use of a PCR-RFLP method with allele-specific primer was performed for identifying the *CYP2C9* wild-type (*1) gene and the 2 mutated alleles, *CYP2C9*2* (Arg144Cys) and *CYP2C9*3* (Ile359Leu) (Yasar U et al., 1999). Alleles in which neither *CYP2C9*2* nor *CYP2C9*3* variants were identified were regarded as wild type in all subjects.

2.2 Assay

Plasma concentrations of warfarin enantiomers and *S*-7-hydoxywarfarin were determined using high performance liquid chromatography (HPLC) method developed in our laboratory (Uno T et al., 2007). In brief, warfarin enantiomers, *S*-7-hydroxywarfarin and an internal standard, diclofenac sodium, were extracted from 1 ml of plasma sample using diethyl ether-chloroform (80:20, v/v). The extract was injected onto column I (TSK precolumn BSA-C8, 5 µm, 10 mm x 4.6 mm i.d.) for clean-up and column II (Chiralcel OD-RH analytical column, 150 mm x 4.6 mm i.d.) coupled with a guard column (Chiralcel OD-

RH guard column, 10 mm x 4.6 mm i.d.) for separation. The mobile phase consisted of phosphate buffer-acetonitrile (84:16 v/v, pH 2.0) for clean-up and phosphate buffer-acetonitrile (45:55 v/v, pH 2.0) for separation. The peaks were monitored with an ultraviolet detector set at a wavelength of 312 nm, and total time for chromatographic separation was about 25 minutes. The retention times of *S*-7-hydoxywarfarin, *R*-warfarin, I.S. and *S*-warfarin were 17.6 min, 19.1 min, 20.0 min and 21.2 min, respectively. The validated concentration ranges of this method were 3-1000 ng/ml for *R*- and *S*-warfarin, and 3-200 ng/ml for *R*- and *S*-7-hydroxywarfarin, respectively. Intra- and inter-day coefficients of variation were less than 4.4 and 4.9% for *R*-warfarin and 4.8 and 4.0% for *S*-warfarin, and 5.1 and 4.2% for *R*-7-hydroxywarfarin and 5.8 and 5.0% for *S*-7-hydroxywarfarin at the different concentrations. The limit of quantification was 3 ng/ml for both warfarin and 7-hydroxywarfarin enantiomers. Plasma samples for the pharmacokinetic study were stored at -20 ˚C and analyzed within 3 months after sampling, and then were stable at -70 ˚C for 12 months.

Plasma concentrations of omeprazole and 5-hydroxyomeprazole were quantitated using HPLC method developed in our laboratory (Shimizu M et al., 2006). In brief, after alkalization with 0.1 mL of 0.5 M disodium hydrogen phosphate, 1 mL plasma was extracted with 4 mL of diethyl ether-dichloromethane (55:45, v/v). The organic phase was evaporated at 60 ˚C to dryness. The residue was dissolved with 30 µL of methanol and 100 µL of 50 mM disodium hydrogen phosphate buffer (pH 9.3), and then a 30-µL aliquot was injected to an HPLC system (SHIMADZU CLASS-VP, SHIMADZU Corporation, Kyoto, Japan), with a Inertsil ODS-80A column as an analytical column (particle size 5 µm; GL Science Inc, Tokyo, Japan). The mobile phase consisted of phosphate buffer-acetonitrile-methanol (65:30:5 v/v/v, pH6.5). Flow rate was 0.8 mL/min and wavelength was set at 302 nm. Limit of quantification was 3 ng/mL for omeprazole and 5-hydroxyomeprazole. Intra- and inter-day coefficient variations were less than 5.1 and 6.6% for omeprazole concentrations ranging from 4 to 1600 ng/mL and 4.6 and 5.0% for 5-hydroxyomeprazole concentration ranging from 4 to 400 ng/mL, respectively.

3. Pharmacokinetics of warfarin enantiomers

We examined the pharmacokinetics of warfarin enantiomers by administering 10 mg of racemic warfarin to 17 healthy volunteers (Uno T et al., 2008). Blood samples were obtained before and over the course of 120 hours after dosing for the determination plasma warfarin enantiomer concentrations and prothrombin time-INR (PT-INR). Fig. 2 shows the mean plasma concentration-time curves for *R*- and *S*-warfarin between the CYP2C19 genotypes. The mean pharmacokinetic parameters of these compounds are summarized in Table 1.

In this study, the area under the plasma concentration-time curve ($AUC_{0-\infty}$) and the elimination half-life ($t_{1/2}$) of *R*-warfarin were about 2-fold greater than those of *S*-warfarin in 17 subjects (Table 1). These values of *R*- and *S*-warfarin were in line with a previous report in which the same dose of racemic warfarin was administered (Lilja JJ et al., 1984). Additionally, $AUC_{0-\infty}$ and $t_{1/2}$ of *R*-warfarin in PMs were significantly greater than those in hmEMs ($P < 0.001$ and $P = 0.010$, respectively). Similarly, there is a significant difference ($P = 0.007$) in the apparent oral clearance (CL) in hmEMs compared with that in PMs. The *S/R* ratios of $AUC_{0-\infty}$ of warfarin enantiomers were 0.51 in hmEMs and 0.37 in PMs ($P = 0.005$). Whereas, no difference was found in all pharmacokinetic parameters of *S*-warfarin and *S*-7-hydroxywarfarin in hmEMs compared with PMs of CYP2C19.

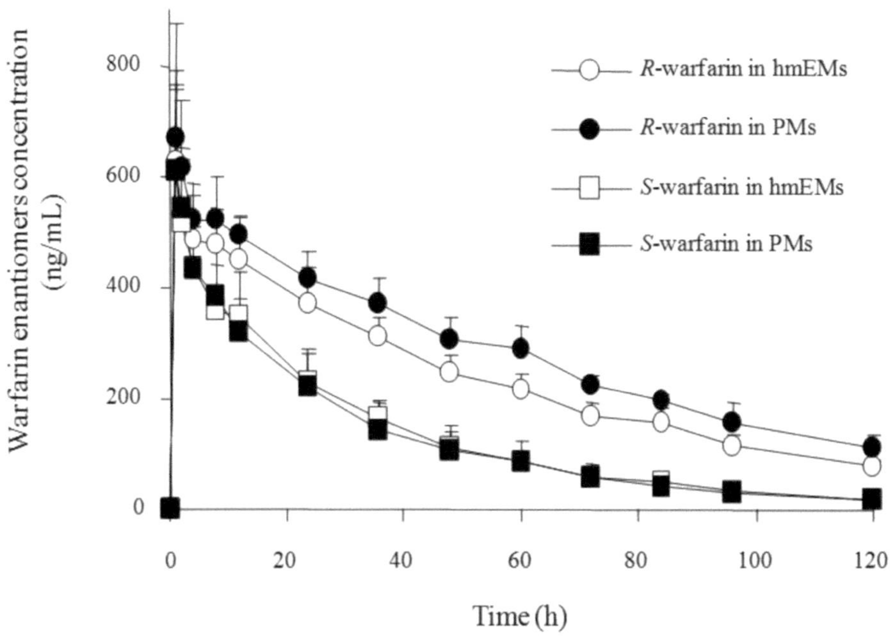

Fig. 2. Plasma concentrations-time curves (mean + S.D.) of *R*-warfarin or *S*-warfarin in hmEMs (*R*-; open circles, *S*-; open square) and PMs (*R*-; closed circles, *S*-; closed square) after a single dose of 10 mg warfarin.

4. Drug interaction between omeprazole and warfarin enantiomers

Omeprazole 20 mg/daily was given orally to 17 healthy volunteers for 11 days, and on day 7, a single dose of racemic warfarin 10 mg was added (Uno T et al., 2008).

The pharmacokinetic parameters are summarized in Table 1. In hmEMs, the omeprazole treatment significantly increased *R*-warfarin $AUC_{0-\infty}$ (P = 0.004), and prolonged its $t_{1/2}$ (P = 0.017) without any effect on *R*-warfarin C_{max} or t_{max}. However, the omeprazole treatment did not alter any pharmacokinetic parameters of *S*-warfarin in both hmEMs and PMs as well as those of *R*-warfarin in hmEMs. Consequently, the omeprazole treatment decreased the *S*/*R* enantiomer ratio of warfarin $AUC_{0-\infty}$ from 0.51 to 0.43 in hmEMs (P = 0.010), but not in PMs.

In addition, significant differences were found in mean C_{max} (P < 0.001), $t_{1/2}$ (P = 0.005), and AUC_{0-24} (P < 0.001) of omeprazole between different CYP2C19 genotypes, though there was no difference in mean C_{max} or AUC_{0-24} of 5-hydroxyomeprazole between hmEMs and PMs.

Variable	hmEMs			PMs		
	Control	Omeprazole	Fold change	Control	Omeprazole	Fold change
***R*-warfarin**						
C_{max} (ng/mL)	692 (616, 768)	629 (556, 702)	0.92 (0.70-1.18)	706 (599, 813)	589 (474, 703)	0.84 (0.55-1.08)
t_{max} (h)	1.4 (0.8, 2.0)	3.3 (1.3, 5.3)	3.02 (0.25-12)	2.6 (0.6, 4.5)	3.6 (0.6, 6.5)	2.79 (0.5-12)
$t_{1/2}$ (h)	40.8 (36.1, 45.6)	46.4 (44.2, 48.7)†	1.12 (0.96-1.27)	49.6 (46.9, 52.3)*	48.8 (42.5, 55.0)	0.97 (0.63-1.18)
$AUC_{0-\infty}$ (ng*h/mL)	34613 (32702, 36524)	41387 (37221, 45552)††	1.19 (1.02-1.39)	42938 (39342, 46533)**	39100 (34802, 43399)	0.92 (0.74-1.08)
CL (mL*kg/h)	2.4 (2.1, 2.5)	2.1 (1.8, 2.2)††	0.87 (0.72-1.09)	1.9 (1.6, 2.3)**	2.1 (1.6, 2.6)	1.12 (0.93-1.36)
***S*-warfarin**						
C_{max} (ng/mL)	659 (570, 748)	600 (528, 673)	0.93 (0.62-1.36)	630 (520, 739)	554 (469, 638)	0.90 (0.69-1.12)
t_{max} (h)	1.3 (0.7, 1.9)	1.7 (1.1, 2.3)	1.63 (0.25-2)	1.1 (0.9, 1.4)	1.1 (0.9, 1.4)	1.07 (0.5-2)
$t_{1/2}$ (h)	25.4 (22.0, 28.9)	27.0 (21.3, 32.8)	1.13 (0.50-1.80)	22.7 (19.7, 25.8)	25.4 (21.7, 29.0)	1.13 (0.82-1.37)
$AUC_{0-\infty}$ (ng*h/mL)	16968 (15233, 18701)	18166 (15705, 20628)	1.07 (0.87-1.54)	15851 (12686, 19016)	14756 (11768, 17745)	0.93 (0.78-1.03)
CL (mL*kg/h)	5.0 (4.6, 5.4)	4.7 (4.1, 5.3)	0.95 (0.65-1.13)	5.6 (4.7, 6.4)	6.0 (4.9, 7.1)	1.08 (0.97-1.28)
The S/R ratios of $AUC_{0-\infty}$	0.51 (0.47, 0.54)	0.43 (0.40, 0.46)††	0.82 (0.76-0.88)	0.37 (0.31, 0.43)***	0.38 (0.31, 0.44)	1.05 (0.98-1.12)
***S*-7-hydroxywarfarin**						
C_{max} (ng/mL)	69.8 (61.7, 77.8)	72.0 (62.8, 81.2)	1.03 (0.91-1.18)	68.1 (63.1, 73.1)	67.6 (63.0, 72.2)	1.00 (0.83-1.08)
t_{max} (h)	18.0 (13.0, 23.0)	26.0 (19.7, 32.3)	2.35 (1.0-12.0)	24.0 (16.7, 27.5)	18.9 (9.1, 28.6)	0.74 (0.3-1.5)
$t_{1/2}$ (h)	28.8 (19.3, 38.2)	25.2 (20.5, 30.0)	1.07 (0.33-2.14)	22.1 (16.7, 27.4)	24.6 (16.3, 33.0)	1.24 (0.39-2.41)
$AUC_{0-\infty}$ (ng*h/mL)	2584 (1997, 3171)	2695 (2101, 3289)	1.06 (0.87-1.21)	2471 (1982, 2959)	2429 (2065, 2792)	1.00 (0.85-1.13)
The metabolic ratio	0.15 (0.12, 0.19)	0.16 (0.12, 0.19)	1.04 (0.89-1.11)	0.17 (0.11, 0.24)	0.18 (0.12, 0.24)	1.03 (0.97-1.22)

AUC, area under plasma concentration-time curve; C_{max}, peak concentration; t_{max}, time to C_{max}; $t_{1/2}$, elimination half-life; CL, apparent oral clearance. The S/R ratios of AUC; $AUC_{0-\infty}$ *S*-warfarin / $AUC_{0-\infty}$ *R*-warfarin. The metabolic ratio; $AUC_{0-\infty}$ of *S*-7-hydroxywarfarin / $AUC_{0-\infty}$ of *S*-warfarin.
$^{*}P<0.05$, $^{**}P<0.01$, $^{***}P<0.001$, between hmEMs and PMs., †$P<0.05$,††$P<0.01$, between control and omeprazole phase. Data are shown as mean and 95% confidence interval ; t_{max} and fold change data are shown as a median wich a range.

Table 1. The summary of pharmacokinetics of warfarin enantiomers

5. Pharmacodynamics of warfarin

No significant difference was found between hmEMs and PMs in either the PT-INR AUC_{0-120} or the PT-INR max during the placebo phase, and the omeprazole treatment did not affect these parameters in both hmEMs and PMs (Uno T et al., 2008).

6. The effect of CYP2C19 genotypes on the pharmacokinetics

Previous studies in patients with different CYP2C19 genotypes reported not to affect plasma *R*-warfarin concentrations at the steady state in clinical studies, in which the concentrations were evaluated at a one sampling point (Obayashi K et al., 2006; Scordo MG et al., 2002; Takahashi et al., 1998). However, two of the reports (Obayashi K et al., 2006; Scordo MG et al., 2002) observed that the *S*/*R* ratio based on steady-state concentrations in PMs was smaller than that in hmEMs. The third study (Takahashi et al., 1998) compared PMs with EMs which included both hmEMs and heterozygous EMs with one mutated CYP2C19 allele. Therefore, the present study was designed to evaluate the elimination phase of warfarin and examine the effect of the CYP2C19 genotype on the pharmacokinetics of warfarin enantiomers. Although the pharmacokinetics was measured after a single administration in this study, our results indicated that the plasma concentrations and $t_{1/2}$ of *R*-warfarin in PMs were markedly higher compared with those of the corresponding *R*-enantiomer in hmEMs. In addition, the $AUC_{0-\infty}$ *S*/*R* ratio in PMs decreased significantly more than that in hmEMs, thereby showing that the pharmacokinetics of *R*-warfarin may be significantly affected by CYP2C19 polymorphism. In contrast, no difference was found in any pharmacokinetic parameters of *S*-warfarin between the hmEMs and the PMs. Consequently, these findings suggest that CYP2C19 activity is an important determinant of *R*-warfarin pharmacokinetics.

We also demonstrated that the reported interaction of *R*-warfarin with omeprazole was found only in the hmEMs of CYP2C19. In previous pharmacokinetic studies (Sutfin T et al., 1989; Unge P et al., 1992), omeprazole has been reported to cause a minor but significant increase in *R*-warfarin plasma concentrations [9.5% (Unge P et al., 1992) and 12% (Sutfin T et al., 1989)]. In our present study, although the pharmacokinetics of warfarin enantiomers of the PMs were not affected by the omeprazole treatment, mean *R*-warfarin $AUC_{0-\infty}$ and $t_{1/2}$ of the hmEMs increased after the omeprazole treatment to the levels comparable to those of the PMs. Mean *R*-warfarin $AUC_{0-\infty}$ of our hmEMs showed an 18 % increase, and the increase was greater than that of the previous studies (Sutfin T et al., 1989; Unge P et al., 1992), probably due to recruiting the same genotype in the present study. Omeprazole is known to be an inhibitor of some CYP enzymes including CYP2C9 and 2C19 (Ko JW et al., 1997; Li XQ et al., 2004). CYP2C9 is known to be responsible for the biotransformation from *S*-warfarin to *S*-7-hydroxywarfarin (Kaminsky LS and Zhang ZY, 1997), and the ratio of *S*-7-hydroxywarfarin AUC to *S*-warfarin AUC would reflect the *in vivo* activity of CYP2C9. Previous report suggested that the clearance of omeprazole is markedly reduced and plasma concentrations of omeprazole in CYP2C19 PMs are much more elevated than those in CYP2C19 EMs (Sohn DR et al., 1992). Increased plasma concentrations of omeprazole in CYP2C19 PMs might affect the pharmacokinetics of warfarin *S*-enantiomer, a substrate of CYP2C9 (Kaminsky LS and Zhang ZY, 1997), as well as its *R*-enantiomer, compared to those in CYP2C19 EMs. In this study, the inhibitory effect of omeprazole was noted only in the hmEMs of CYP2C19 despite higher omeprazole concentrations in the PMs, and the $AUC_{0-\infty}$ ratio of *S*-7-hydroxywarfarin to *S*-warfarin was relatively constant between the placebo and the omeprazole phases, suggesting that the 7-day administration of omeprazole 20 mg once daily would affect the CYP2C19 activity solely.

7. The effect of CYP2C19 genotypes on the pharmacodynamics

Interestingly, no significant difference was found in PT-INR between the hmEMs and PMs in both the control and the omeprazole phases even though the CYP2C19 genotypes affected the *R*-warfarin pharmacokinetic parameters. However, these findings are not surprising because the anticoagulant effect of *S*-enantiomer is 3-5 times more potent than that of *R*-enantiomer (Takahashi H and Echizen H, 2001), and a concentration rises of *R*-enantiomer was seemed to have little influence on the anticoagulant effect of warfarin. These results therefore suggest that altered pharmacokinetics of *R*-warfarin may play a minor role in determining the average clinical doses of warfarin. Moreover, these results also imply that inhibition of the *in vivo* CYP2C19 activity by the co-administration of a CYP2C19 inhibitor, such as omeprazole, lansoprazole or fluvoxamine (Hemeryck A and Belpaire FM, 2002; Ko JW et al., 1997; Li XQ et al., 2004), may scarcely modify the anticoagulant effects of warfarin. Recently, Rieder et al. (2005) have shown that there is an effect of the VKORC1 on dose requirement. Furthermore, Obayashi et al. (2006) reported that the genotyping of the vitamin K epooxide reductase complex subunit 1 gene (VKORC1) may be more predictive of the anticoagulant effect than genotyping of CYPs, which reflects the warfarin plasma concentrations. Therefore, these studies suggest that VKORC1 activity may be an important determinant of the pharmacodynamics of warfarin in Japanese patients.

8. Conclusion

These results indicate that CYP2C19 activity is important in the pharmacokinetics of *R*-warfarin because the pharmacokinetics of warfarin enantiomers were different between the CYP2C19 genotypes and the omeprazole affected the *R*-warfarin pharmacokinetics of CYP2C19 in only hmEMs. However, these affects are not translated into any significant effect in the pharmacodynamics of warfarin.

9. References

Chan E, McLachlan AJ, Pegg M, MacKay AD, Cole RB, Rowland M. (1994). Disposition of warfarin enantiomers and metabolites in patients during multiple dosing with rac-warfarin. *Br J Clin Pharmacol*, Vol. 37, pp. 563-569.

De Morais SM, Wilkinson GR, Blaisdell J, Meyer UA, Nakamura K, Goldstein JA. (1994). Identification of a new genetic defect responsible for the polymorphism of (S)-mephenytoin metabolism in Japanese. *Mol Pharmacol*, Vol. 46, pp. 594-598.

Hemeryck A, Belpaire FM. (2002). Selective serotonin reuptake inhibitors and cytochrome P-450 mediated drug-drug interactions: an update. *Curr Drug Metab*, Vol.3, pp. 13-37.

Hirsh J, Dalen JE, Anderson DR, Poller L, Bussey H, Ansell J, Deykin D, Brandt JT. (1998). Oral anticoagulants: mechanism of action, clinical effectiveness, and optimal therapeutic range. *Chest*, Vol. 114, pp. 445S-469S.

Kaminsky LS, Zhang ZY. (1997). Human P450 metabolism of warfarin. *Pharmacol Ther*, Vol. 73, pp. 67-74.

Ko JW, Sukhova N, Thacker D, Chen P, Flockhart DA. (1997). Evaluation of omeprazole and lansoprazole as inhibitors of cytochrome P450 isoforms. *Drug Metab Dispos*, Vol. 25, pp. 853-62.

Kubota T, Chiba K, Ishizaki T. (1996). Genotyping of S-mephenytoin 4'-hydroxylation in an extended Japanese population. *Clin Pharmacol Ther*, Vol. 60, pp. 661-666.

Lilja JJ, Backman JT, Neuvonen PJ. (2005). Effect of gemfibrozil on the pharmacokinetics and pharmacodynamics of racemic warfarin in healthy subjects. *Br J Clin Pharmacol*, Vol. 59, pp. 433-439.

Li XQ, Andersson TB, Ahlström M, Weidolf L. (2004). Comparison of inhibitory effects of the proton pump-inhibiting drugs omeprazole, esomeprazole, lansoprazole, pantoprazole, and rabeprazole on human cytochrome P450 activities. *Drug Metab Dispos*, Vol. 32, pp. 821-7.

Obayashi K, Nakamura K, Kawana J, Ogata H, Hanada K, Kurabayashi M. (2006). VKORC1 gene variations are the major contributors of variation in warfarin dose in Japanese patients. *Clin Pharmacol Ther*, Vol. 80, pp. 169-178.

Rieder MJ, Reiner AP, Gage BF, Nickerson DA, Eby CS, McLeod HL, Blough DK, Thummel KE, Veenstra DL, Rettie AE. (2005). Effect of VKORC1 haplotypes on transcriptional regulation and warfarin dose. *New England Journal of Med*, Vol. 352, pp. 2285-2293.

Scordo MG, Pengo V, Spina E, Dahl ML, Gusella M, Padrini R. (2002). Influence of CYP2C9 and CYP2C19 genetic polymorphisms on warfarin maintenance dose and metabolic clearance. *Clin Pharmacol Ther*, Vol. 72, pp. 702-710.

Shimizu M, Uno T, Niioka T, Yaui-Furukori N, Takahata T, Sugawara K, Tateishi T. (2006). Sensitive determination of omeprazole and its two main metabolites in human plasma by column-switching high-performance liquid chromatography: application to pharmacokinetic study in relation to CYP2C19 genotypes. *J Chromatogr B*, Vol. 832, pp. 241-248.

Sohn DR, Kobayashi K, Chiba K, Lee KH, Shin SG, Ishizaki T. (1992). Disposition kinetics and metabolism of omeprazole in extensive and poor metabolizers of S-mephenytoin 4'-hydroxylation recruited from an Oriental population. *J Pharmacol Exp Ther*, Vol. 262, pp. 1195-1202.

Sutfin T, Balmer K, Bostrom H, Eriksson S, Hoglund P, Paulsen O. (1989). Stereoselective interaction of omeprazole with warfarin in healthy men. *Ther Drug Monit*, Vol. 11, pp. 176-184.

Takahashi H, Wilkinson GR, Nutescu EA, Morita T, Ritchie MD, Scordo MG, Pengo V, Barban M, Padrini R, Ieiri I, Otsubo K, Kashima T, Kimura S, Kijima S, Echizen H. (2006). Different contributions of polymorphisms in VKORC1 and CYP2C9 to intra- and inter-population differences in maintenance dose of warfarin in Japanese, Caucasians and African-Americans. *Pharmacogenetics and Genomics*, Vol. 16, pp. 101-110.

Takahashi H, Echizen H. Pharmacogenetics of warfarin elimination and its clinical implications. (2001). *Clin Pharmacokinet*, Vol. 40, pp. 587-603.

Takahashi H, Kashima T, Nomizo Y, Muramoto N, Shimizu T, Nasu K, Kubota T, Kimura S, Echizen H. (1998). Metabolism of warfarin enantiomers in Japanese patients with heart disease having different CYP2C9 and CYP2C19 genotypes. *Clin Pharmacol Ther*, Vol. 63, pp. 519-528.

Unge P, Svedberg LE, Nordgren A, Blom H, Andersson T, Lagerstrom PO, Idstrom JP. (1992). A study of the interaction of omeprazole and warfarin in anticoagulated patients. *Br J Clin Pharmacol*, Vol.34, pp. 509-512.

Uno T, Sugimoto K, Sugawara K, Tateishi T. (2008). The role of cytochrome P2C19 in R-warfarin pharmacokinetics and its interaction with omeprazole.*Ther Drug Monit*, Vol. 30, pp.276-281.

Uno T, Niioka T, Hayakari M, Sugawara K, Tateishi T. (2007). Simultaneous determination of warfarin enantiomers and its metabolite in human plasma by column-switching high-performance liquid chromatography with chiral separation. *Ther Drug Monit*, Vol. 29, pp. 333-339.

Yasar U, Eliasson E, Dahl ML, Johansson I, Ingelman-Sundberg M, Sjoqvist F. (1999). Validation of methods for CYP2C9 genotyping: frequencies of mutant alleles in a Swedish population. *Biochem Biophys Res Commun*, Vol. 254, pp. 628-631.

12

Pharmacogenetics – A Treatment Strategy for Alcoholism

Anjana Munshi* and Vandana Sharma
Institute Of Genetics and Hospital for Genetic Diseases, Osmania University, Begumpet, Hyderabad, India

1. Introduction

Alcoholism is a complex relapsing disorder of heterogeneous etiology, affecting people internationally. Alcohol dependence is a cumulative response of inability to stop drinking, craving and developing the symptoms of physical dependence and tolerance. In past two decades, mounting evidence has suggested that alcoholism or alcohol addiction is a host of major psychological, social, financial and health problems (Poznyak et al., 2005). According to World Health Organization, alcoholism is responsible for 4% of global disease burden and is the third major preventable risk factor for premature death and disability in developed nations (World Health Organization, 2002). Although, the exclusive biological mechanisms underlying the development of alcoholism are still uncertain, the major risk factors contributing towards the development of alcoholism are age (adolescents are at higher risk of developing alcoholism), gender (men are more prone to develop alcoholism as compared to women due to depression), personality (experience seeking), and psychiatric or behavioral disorders. The prevalence, age of onset, clinical symptoms and outcome of alcoholism differs from individual to individual and varies according to ethnicity (Kenneth et al., 2011). In addition to this, lower social status and low education have also been found to be associated with alcoholism in cross sectional and longitudinal studies (Fukuda et al., 2005; Poznyak et al., 2005; Subramanian et al., 2005; Wray et al., 2005).

According to World Health Organization report on global alcohol status, it has been found that approximately 2 billion people consume alcoholic beverages and there are about 76.3 million people with diagnosable alcohol disorder (World Health Organization, 2004). In India the prevalence of alcoholism has been found to be 21.4% as recoded by epidemiological surveys (Benegal, 2005).The deleterious effects of alcohol on central nervous system can be observed in the form of changes in mood and personality, anxiety and depression. Although, it affects all the organs in the body, brain neurotransmitters are the main target sites of alcohol (Wertheimer et al., 2003). The specific physiological effects of alcohol depend on dose, concentration in blood, absorption, distribution, metabolism, excretory conditions, prior drinking experience, concurrent use of other drugs, and

* Corresponding Author

comorbid conditions. The body adapts metabolically and neurally to repeated exposure of alcohol so as to develop tolerance (Zaleski et al., 2004).

Recent advances in the field of neurobiology have improved our understanding about associated risk factors and neurochemical mechanisms responsible for the development of alcoholism. Evidences suggest that there is large inter-individual variation in terms of development of alcohol dependence and treatment of alcoholism. People consume alcohol and respond to its effects in a number of ways e.g. some develop no side effects even in moderate to higher levels and some may develop problems even when consumed in smaller doses. This variation is the result of individual's genetic makeup directly influencing the metabolism of alcohol (Strat et al., 2008).

Genetic factors have been found to play a critical role in the etiology of alcoholism (Heath et al., 2001; Sloan et al., 2008; Kenneth et al., 2011). Researchers have suggested that 50-60% of alcohol dependence is determined by genetics (Goldman and Bergen 1998; McGue et al., 1999). Based on results of adoption, twin, and family studies it is now clear that the vulnerability to alcoholism is determined by genetic factors as well as by environmental factors (Moussas et al., 2009). However, it is difficult to determine the individual determinant of alcoholism (Flensborg-Madsen et al., 2007). The candidate gene approach has revealed a number of biomarkers, which are responsible for alcoholism. Certain variants of alcohol dehydrogenase and aldehyde dehydrogenase genes (genes encoding for alcohol metabolizing enzymes) have been found to alter the metabolism of alcohol in a dramatic way (Nurnberger et al., 2004). In addition to this, polymorphisms in neurotransmitter genes (target receptor genes) such as gamma amino butyric acid and opioid receptor genes have also been reported to be associated with marked risk of alcohol dependence (Strat et al., 2008). Current treatment approaches to alcoholism are moderately effective with perhaps as many as half of the patients receiving treatment due to abstinent or significantly reducing episodes of binge drinking (Group, 1997). Pharmacotherapy and behavioral therapy including psychosocial support are two main types of treatment in alcoholism. The pharmacological agents approved by FDA prescribed in the treatment of alcoholism are disulfiran (antabuse), naltrexone (revia), acamprosate (campral) and Vivitrol (Krishnan-Sarin & O'Malley et al., 2008).

The major drawback of ineffectiveness of pharmacotherapy of alcoholism is inter-individual variation in response to medication (Radel and Goldman, 2001). There are individuals, showing lesser/no therapeutic efficacy of a drug prescribed, known as non-responders. Another group of individuals showing high therapeutic efficacy towards the same drug are known as responders (McLeod et al., 2000).

Recent advances in the area of molecular biology have increased our knowledge of understanding the influence of genetic variants on pharmacokinetic and pharmacodynamic profile of alcohol and neurobiology of alcoholism (Ray et al., 2010a). The unavoidable alcohol withdrawl symptoms, depression, unpredicted death, medical complications, socioeconomic repercussions of alcoholism suggest that the treatment strategies should be improved with new and targeted approach of pharmacogenetics.

Pharmacogenetics is a measure of predicting individual's genetic profile responsible for variable drug responses. The genetic analysis along with consideration of other factors of alcoholic patients can lead to the identification of clinical subtypes of patients with specific treatments. This will improve the treatment of alcoholism. Alcohol pharmacogenetics has great potential in improving treatment strategies for alcoholism (Radel and Goldman, 2001; Quickfall and el-Guebaly, 2006). The treatment strategy of combining clinician's views based on genotypic information would individualize and optimize the treatment for alcoholism with best possible outcome of individual's good health free of alcohol dependence. Pharmacogenetics is expected to add new dimensions and would tailor the therapeutic treatment of alcoholism.

The chapter provides an overview of the molecular, pharmacological and neurological aspects of alcoholism with main emphasis on pharmacogenetics of alcoholism treatment.

2. Metabolism of alcohol

Alcohol is generally taken orally, absorbed unchanged through the whole length of digestive tract. Almost 20% absorption takes place rapidly through stomach and 80% through small gut (Caballeria, 2003). The rate of absorption depends on volume, concentration, nature of alcoholic drink, presence and absence of food in stomach, permeability of gastric and intestinal tissues and genetic variation. After absorption into the blood-stream, alcohol is distributed quickly throughout the total body fluid (Pawan, 1972). The distribution of alcohol is accelerated by vascularization and blood flow e.g. organs rich in blood supply such as brain and lungs achieve the higher initial concentrations of alcohol.

Liver is the main site of alcohol metabolism. In hepatocytes three systems are involved in alcohol metabolism located in three different cellular compartments. These are alcohol dehydrogenase (*ADH*) located in cytosol, microsomal ethanol oxidizing system (*MEOS*) situated in endoplasmic reticulum and catalase in peroxisomes (Caballeria, 2003). These are involved in conversion of alcohol to acetaldehyde (Figure 1).

The metabolic pathway involves conversion of alcohol (ethanol) to acetaldehyde via oxidation catalyzed by *ADH* in cytoplasm of hepatocytes, a rate limiting step. The second reaction is catalyzed by aldehyde dehydrogenases (*ALDH*), acetaldehyde is converted to acetic acid and finally to carbon dioxide and water through citric acid cycle into circulation. Acetaldehyde plays central role in the toxicity produced by alcohol consumption as in liver it reaches to saturation point and escapes into blood circulation. Further it impairs mitochondrial functions and reactions leading to damage of hepatocytes. The rate of metabolism of alcohol differs from person to person because it is influenced by genetic variants of metabolizing enzymes mentioned above (Quertemont, 2004).

2.1 Alcohol dehydrogenase system

Alcohol dehydrogenase (ADH) occurs in multiple forms and is encoded by 7 different genes. These are ADH1A, ADH1B, ADH1C, ADH4, ADH5, ADH6 and ADH7. These genes are aligned along a small region of chromosome 4. ADH enzymes encoded by ADH gene function as dimers i.e. the active forms are composed of two subunits. On the basis of their similar amino acid sequences and kinetic properties, these seven ADH types have been divided into five classes. The class I genes ADH1A, ADH1B and ADH1C are closely related. These encode for α, β and γ subunits respectively, which form homodimers or heterodimers and account for most of the alcohol oxidizing capacity in liver (Hurley et al., 2002; Lee et al.,

2006). Further, ADH1A, ADH1B and ADH1C are mainly present in liver and linings of stomach. ADH4 encodes п-ADH which has been reported to contribute significantly to ethanol oxidation at higher concentration. The ADH5 gene encodes for χ-ADH, a ubiquitously expressed formaldehyde dehydrogenase, which has low affinity for ethanol. ADH6 mRNA is found in fetal and adult liver. Since the enzyme has not been isolated from tissues so far, therefore little is known about it. ADH7 encodes for σ-ADH, which oxidizes both ethanol and retinol (Edenberg, 2007).

2.2 Aldehyde dehydrogenase

These enzymes rapidly convert acetaldehyde to acetate using cofactor NAD^+ via oxidation. ALDH is divided into nine major categories. Some of these are significantly involved in acetaldehyde metabolism, and others metabolize a variety of substrates. Two main ALDH enzymes reported to be involved in metabolization of acetaldehyde during the oxidation of ethanol are ALDH1 and ALDH2. ALDH1 encoded by ALDH1A1 gene is found in fluid filling cells (the cytosol) while ALDH2 is found in mitochondria and is encoded by the ALDH2 gene. The two genes are 52 kb and 43 kb in length and are present on chromosome 9 and chromosome 12 respectively. Both genes have a similar structure with 13 exons and the protein encoded by both the genes is 70% similar in sequence and structure (Hurley et al., 2002). ALDH1A1, ALDH1B1 and ALDH2 are mainly involved in acetaldehyde oxidation.

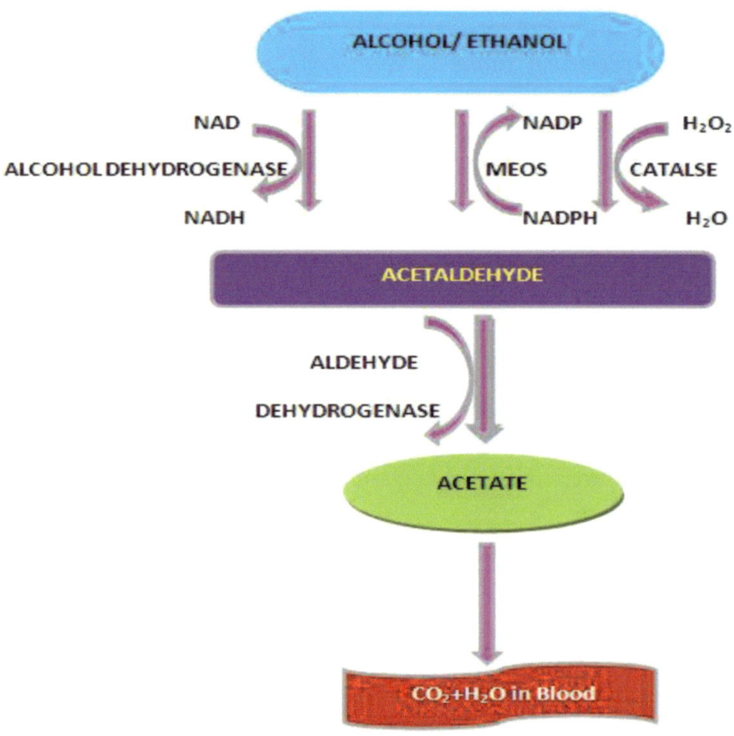

Fig. 1. Metabolism of alcohol in liver hepatocytes using 3 systems, (i) Alcohol dehydrogenase, (ii) Microsomal ethanol oxidizing enzyme (iii) Catalase and finally Aldehyde dehydrogenase converts acetaldehyde into acetate

2.3 Microsomal ethanol oxidizing enzymes

Apart from ADH which accounts for greater part of ethanol oxidation, a quantitatively small portion of alcohol is catalyzed by microsomal ethanol oxidizing system involving CYP2E1 (Edenberg, 2007). Studies have shown that CYP2E1 is induced by high ethanol concentration and by chronic intake of alcohol or ethanol (up to 10 fold) (Quertemont, 2004). It has been found that after chronic ethanol consumption CYP2E1 increases the rate of ethanol clearance and this may result in development of ethanol tolerance (Lieber et al., 1968; 1988; Takahashi et al., 1993; Tsutsumi et al., 1989). CYP2E1 induction may further lead to higher concentrations of acetaldehyde leading to injuries in hepatocytes.

2.4 Catalase

Catalase oxidizes alcohol to acetaldehyde within the peroxisomes (Oshino et al., 1973). This reaction is hydrogen peroxide (H_2O_2) dependent. Under normal conditions catalase plays a minor role in ethanol oxidation. However, the functional activity of catalase is accelerated in the presence of reactive oxygen species and H_2O_2 (Quertemont, 2004). Zimatkin et al. (1997) have suggested that catalase may be one of alternative metabolic pathways for ethanol oxidation in brain where CYP2E1 and ADH appear to be of minor importance. However, the precise role of catalase in brain ethanol oxidation is still not clear.

2.5 Nonoxidative ethanol metabolism

Apart from oxidative metabolism of alcohol, nonoxidative metabolism also takes place in organs lacking oxidative metabolism such as heart (Beckemeier et al., 1998). A minor extent of alcohol is metabolized by nonoxidative pathway using enzyme fatty acid ethyl synthases resulting in the formation of fatty acid ethyl esters (Caballeria 2003). Further, these esters have been found to be involved in alcohol-induced organ injuries (Beckemeier et al., 1998).

3. Genetic variants affecting alcohol metabolism

Genes encoding for alcohol metabolizing enzymes are supposed to have major influence on development of alcoholism. There are multiple ADH and ALDH enzymes encoded by different genes. Some of these genes have been reported to occur in several variants or alleles. The enzymes encoded by different alleles can differ in the rate at which they metabolize ethanol (Edenburg, 2007).

3.1 Genetic variants of alcohol dehydrogenase

Researchers have studied the genetic variants of ADH1B and ADH1C genes that result in the production of enzymes with different kinetic properties and have been implicated in the susceptibility to develop alcoholism. These genetic variants or SNPs and their effects have been widely studied in different populations and three different alleles have been reported which alter the amino acid sequence of the encoded beta subunit. ADH1B*1 allele, (reference allele) encodes for $\beta1$ subunit that has arginine at positions 48 and 370. ADH1B*1 is the predominant allele in most populations. ADH1B*2 encodes for $\beta2$ subunit with histidine at position 48 and is commonly found in Asians. ADH1B*3 encodes for $\beta3$ subunit that has cysteine at position 370 and is prevalent in people of African descent. In $\beta2$ and $\beta3$ subunits, amino acid substitutions occur at an amino acid which contacts with coenzyme nicotineamide dinucleotide (required for ethanol oxidation) (Hurley et al., 2002). The substitution results in enzymes, which have 70- to 80- fold higher turnover rate than the β1 subunit. This is because the coenzyme is released more rapidly at the end of reaction.

For ADH1C gene, there are 3 alleles ADH1C*1 encoding γ1 subunit with arginine at position 272 and isoleucine at position at position 350. ADH1C*2 encodes the γ2 subunit which has glutamine (Gln) at position 272 and a valine (Val) at position 350. These two SNPs occur together (i.e., are in very high linkage disequilibrium). It has been found that the ADH with two γ1 subunits (i.e., the γ1γ1 homodimeric enzyme) has a turnover rate that is about 70 percent higher than that of the γ2γ2 enzyme (Edenberg, 2007). ADH1C*Thr352 encodes for a subunit with threonine at position 352 and has been found in Native Americans (Osier et al., 2002). However, the studies on this protein are still lacking. Researchers have identified the differences in the rate of metabolism of ethanol in liver on the basis of difference in amino acid sequence resulting in difference in kinetic properties of encoded enzyme. If a person carries two copies of reference allele i.e. ADH1B*1 and ADH1C*1 alleles (homozygous for ADH1B*1and ADH1C*1) the enzyme (together α, β, γ subunits) together accounts for liver's 70% ethanol oxidizing capacity, additionally π ADH accounts for 30% (Hurley et al., 2002). ADH1B*1 allele has been reported to reduce the occurrence of alcohol abuse and alcoholism in Asians, in Whites and in Jewish populations where this allele has a relatively high prevalence (Carr et al., 2002; Neumark et al., 1998). ADH1B*2 has been found to occur in a higher frequency in nonalcoholics and in moderate drinkers relative to heavy drinkers. As far as ADH1B*2 is concerned, this allele has been found to be associated with lower rates of heavy drinking and alcohol dependence in Native Americans (Quertemont, 2007).

A meta-analysis conducted by Whitfield has concluded that ADH1B*1 allele is associated with a threefold increase in risk of alcoholism in comparison with ADH1B*2 allele.ADH1B*2 allele encodes for an enzyme with a faster ethanol oxidation rate (Whitfield, 1997). It has been assumed that this allele protects against alcoholism and alcohol abuse because of the unpleasant effects associated with acetaldehyde accumulation (Yin, 1994). The frequency of ADH1C*1 allele has been reported to about 50% in European population and up to 90% in some Asian and African populations (Goedde et al., 1992; Osier et al., 2002). This allele has also been shown to provide a protection against alcohol abuse and alcoholism since a higher frequency of this allele has been found in nonalcoholics especially from Asian population.

Gene-gene interactions have also been found to play an intricate role in development of alcoholism. Oseir et al. (2004) found that there is potential epistatic interaction between ADH1B and ADH7 which leads to protective effect against alcoholism among Han Chinese population (Oseir et al., 2004).

3.2 Genetic variants of aldehyde dehydrogenase (ALDH)

The best known variation of alcohol metabolizing enzymes has been associated with ALDH2 gene. A variant of this gene known as ALDH2*2 allele leads to the substitution of lysine to glutamine at 504 position (Chou et al., 1999). This substitution results in the production of a nearly inactive ALDH2 enzyme which no longer oxidizes acetaldehyde to acetate. Studies have demonstrated that this variant is dominant because people who are heterozygous (ALDH2*1 and ALDH2*2) have almost no detectable activity of ALDH2 enzyme in the liver. People with an ALDH2*2 allele show an alcohol flush reaction even when they consume alcohol in relatively small amounts (Harada et al., 1981). The presence of even a single ALDH2*2 allele has been shown to be strongly protective against alcohol dependence. The protective effect of ALDH2*2 is the most widely reproduced association of a specific gene with alcoholism (Chen et al., 1999; Hurley et al., 2002; Luczak et al., 2006; Thomasson et al., 1991).

3.3 Genetic variants of microsomal ethanol oxidizing system

Another enzyme, microsomal ethanol oxidizing enzyme involved in alcohol metabolism is encoded by CYP2E1 gene. CYP2E1 is induced (increase in activity up to 10 fold) by chronic alcohol drinking and may contribute to development of metabolic tolerance in alcoholics. Studies have revealed that polymorphism in CYP2E1 (CYP2E1*1D) has been found to be significantly associated with alcohol dependence in Canadian native Indians (Howard et al., 2003; Itoga et al., 1999). Another rare mutant named as c2 allele (CYP2E1*5B) in CYP2E1 gene has been found to be associated with higher transcriptional activity leading to elevated level of the enzyme as compared to wild type c1 allele i.e. CYP2E1*5A (Hayashi et al., 1991).

3.4 Genetic variants of catalase

Studies have revealed that subjects with positive family history of alcoholism have a higher mean activity of catalase as compared to control subjects (Koechling and Amit et al., 1992). A significant positive correlation was observed in brain and blood catalase activity in rats (Amit and Aragon., 1988). Koechling and Amit (1992) have reported a significant coorelation between blood catalase activity with alcohol consumption. However, there are no studies on the association of genetic polymorphism of catalase with alcoholism.

4. Neuropharmacological aspects of chronic alcoholism

The neuropharmacological actions of alcohol such as cognitive impairment and other behavioral changes are mediated via their interaction with brain neurotransmitters. Neurotransmitters are the chemicals involved in communication of neurons in brain and may be inhibitory or excitatory depending upon their mechanism of action. Although alcohol does not have any specific target neurotransmitter, it acts on multiple neurotransmitter systems (Deitrich and Erwin, 1996; Tabakoff and Hoffman, 1992).

Chronic alcohol consumption may cause cognitive impairment, tolerance and physical dependence due to changes in neurotransmitter system in brain. The neuropharmacological changes caused by chronic alcoholism involve monoamine oxidase, neurotransmitter amino acids and calcium ion channels and some other pathways leading to neuroadaptations and development of tolerance (Zaleski et al., 2004). The complex mechanism of action involving neurochemical changes explains why even moderate doses of alcohol may lead the subject to develop psychiatric complications and alcohol dependence. The addictive and alcohol seeking behavior can be explained by understanding the neurotransmitter involved in the processes (Vengeliene et al., 2006).

Few of the neurotransmitters involved in alcohol dependence are as follows:

4.1 Alcohol and monoamines

Ethanol affects the release of the main neurotransmitters present in central nervous system, such as dopamine, gamma amino butyric acid (GABA), serotonin, noradrenaline and opioid peptides (Kianmaa &Tabakoff, 1983; Tabakoff, 1977, 1983). Alcohol activates the firing of dopaminergic neurons in the ventral tegmental area and nucleus accumbens structures which together are a part of mesolimbic pathway and play an important role for the rewarding effect of ethanol (Diana et al., 1992). Studies have demonstrated that the stimulation of dopaminergic neurons may indirectly activate serotonergic pathways. The low levels of serotonin have been reported to be a risk factor for development of alcoholism (Lovinger, 1991).

4.2 Alcohol and neurotransmitter amino acids

Several studies have demonstrated the actions of ethanol on neurotransmitter amino acids which consist of glutamate-main excitatory neurotransmitter in the central nervous system. It has N-methyl-D-aspartate (NMDA) and amino-3-hydroxy-5-methyl-4-isoxazoleproprionate (AMPA), and kainate receptors. The NMDA receptors are controlled by several regulatory sites. To open the channel of NMDA receptor, presence of glycine is required. Glycine is an amino acid which has its own site, acting as a coagonist. Alcohol has been reported to act on glycine binding site therefore, inhibiting the function of NMDA receptor (Woodword, 1994). The receptor has been found to play an important role in learning and memory and in development of alcohol tolerance (Longo et al., 2002). Glutamate, a neurotransmitter has been found to play a significant role in the pathogenesis of alcohol dependence by mediating excitatory pathways (Sander et al., 2000). Chronic alcohol use has been found to be associated with upregulation of NMDA receptors. Alcohol shows lower affinity for AMPA and kainate glutamate receptors (Ferreira & Morato, 1997). In case of acute ethanol withdrawal, NMDA receptor releases increased amount of glutamate which is associated with tremors, anxiety, ataxia, and convulsions.

Alcohol produces sedative-hypnotic effects mediated via GABA, an inhibitory neurotransmitter. There are three types of GABA receptors, GABA A, GABA B, and GABA C in brain. GABA A receptors are responsible for the intoxicating effects of alcohol such as motor incoordination, anxiolysis and sedation. The neurobehavioral effects of ethanol mediated via neurotransmitter GABA are directly dose-dependent. The effects of alcohol at GABA A receptors vary across brain regions. This might be due to the differential expression of GABA A receptor subunits (Loh et al., 1999).

Another neurotransmitter, Neuropeptide Y (NPY) is an amino acid peptide which has been associated with reward, appetite and anxiety. The association of NPY has also been reported with alcohol dependence in animal models. NPY-deficient mice have been reported to show higher alcohol consumption as compared with wild type mice (Thiele et al., 1998).

4.3 Alcohol and calcium ion channels

Voltage sensitive calcium channels (VSCCs) play a major role in gating synaptic calcium influx and thereby modulating a range of calcium dependent intracellular processes, membrane potential, and neurotransmitter release (Kennedy & Liu, 2003). The types of

VSCC are of L-type (dihydropyridine-sensitive), N-type (neuronal), P-type (Purkinje), R-type (Resistant), and T type (transient) channels. It has been found that alcohol (ethanol) blocks L-type channels. The L-type VSCC antagonists show some ethanol, like effects in rats. Evidence suggested that chronic administration of alcohol in mice up-regulates the number and function of N-type calcium channels. Ethanol actions at VSCCs may modulate its behavioral effects in humans (Zaleski et al., 2004). It has been reported that there is an increase in the inflow of Calcium ions through these channels, contributing to the development of withdrawal symptoms such as seizures and craving.

4.4 Alcohol and other mechanisms of actions

Studies assessing cognitive functions have associated the chronic ingestion of ethanol with the reduction in concentration of acetylcholine in humans as well as mice, caused by the degeneration of brain tissues which seems to be related to the development of tolerance of alcohol. Chronic consumption of alcohol may affect opioid receptor system thus exerting neurobehavioral effects such as reinforcement. The three major classes of opioid system are μ, δ and κ. Alcohol may stimulate the release of certain opioid peptides such as endorphins and enkephalins, which in turn, could interact with the centers (mesolimbic dopamine pathway) of the brain, associated with reward and positive reinforcement and may lead to further alcohol consumption (Vengeliene et al., 2008). Human and animal studies have suggested that μ opioid receptor is mainly involved in initial sensitivity and response to alcohol. The increased activity of brain opioid peptide systems, in response to ethanol exposure, may be important for initiating and maintaining high alcohol consumption and for mediating the positive reinforcing effects of alcohol (Gianoulakis et al., 1996).

5. Genetic variants of neurotransmitters

Alcohol exerts its effects such as reward and reinforcement by acting on a number of neurotransmitter in the brain. Studies have revealed that polymorphisms in genes encoding for neurotransmitter may increase the risk of developing alcoholism (Radel & Goldman, 2001; Foley et al., 2006). The knowledge of gene variants affecting neurotransmitters is very important as it serves the basis for developing novel and targeted therapeutic agents in treatment of alcoholism. A few of the genetic variants of neurotransmitters associated with alcohol dependence are as:

5.1 Glutamate

Candidate gene studies have shown that individuals bearing G603A polymorphism of glial glutamate transporter gene (EAAT2) are at increased risk of alcoholism (Sander et al., 2000). The individuals with genetic variants of NMDA (subunit NR2A) and glutamate receptor metabotropic gene (mGLUR5) have been studied in a hospital based study in Germany (Schumann et al., 2008). It was found that carriers of the NR2A risk genotypes for rs2072450 CC and rs9924016 Del/Del had higher risk of developing alcohol dependence as compared to the individuals with protective genotypes rs2072450 AC and rs9924016 Del/Ins (Schuman et al., 2008). In the case of mGLUR5 gene, individuals of the risk genotypes rs3824927 C/C and rs 3462 G/G have been found to be at higher risk of developing alcohol dependence when compared with individuals bearing the protective genotypes rs3824927 CA and rs3462 GA.

5.2 Gamma amino butyric acid

Association of genetic variants of GABARA1 and GABAR6 with alcoholism has been reported in Korean population (Park et al., 2006).The GG genotype of GABAA1 receptor has been found to be significantly associated with early onset and severity of alcoholism in Korean population (Park et al., 2006). It has been also been reported that Pro385Ser substitution in GABA A6 is associated with alcohol dependence and with antisocial alcoholism (Sander et al., 1999).

5.3 Norepinephrine

Studies have suggested that alcohol produces biphasic effects on norepinephrine turnover in the brain, with low doses increasing turnover and higher doses depressing turnover. The sensitivity of noradrenergic systems to ethanol effects varies among brain regions. A few studies have been attempted to see the effect of genetic variants of norepinephrine on alcoholism. Huang et al. (2008) reported that norepinephrine transporter polymorphisms T-182C and G1287A are not associated with alcohol dependence and its clinical subgroups in Han Chinese population.

5.4 Dopamine

Research studies have revealed that there is a positive association between polymorphism in Dopamine receptor gene (DRD) with alcoholism. Ponce et al. (2008) reported that the two SNPs (-141C Ins/Del) and TaqI A, present on DRD2 gene locus were associated with alcoholism in North Indian population. Studies from South Indian population have reported no association between TaqI A polymorphism and alcoholism.

The -141 Ins/Del polymorphism in DRD2 gene has been found to be associated with alcoholism in several studies across different populations, but with inconsistent results. This promoter polymorphism plays a significant role in D2 receptor expression via altering the transcriptional activity. Johann et al. (2005) studied the association of -141I Del variant (-141C) SNP in German alcoholics. It was found that -141 Del C variant of DRD2 gene might be a protective factor against development of alcoholism. On the other hand the -141 Ins allele has been found to be a genetic risk factor for alcoholism in Mexican-Americans. This can be correlated with decreased DRD2 receptor density in alcoholic patients which in turn stimulates craving-reward pathway- thereby promoting alcoholism.

Another polymorphism in DRD2 gene Taq I A in Ankyrin repeat and Kinase Domain containing (ANKK1)(rs 1800497) is one of the most frequently studied mutations. The DRD2 gene is actually not located on DRD2 but rather within the protein coding region exon 8 of the adjacent ANKK1gene (Neville et al., 2004). TaqI A SNP causes an amino acid substitution within the 11th ankyrin repeat of the putative protein and has been found to affect the substrate binding specificity (Ponce et al., 2008). In a meta-analysis, the single nucleotide variant TaqIA (rs 1800497) of the DRD2 gene has been found as a vulnerability gene for alcoholism in more than 40 studies, but with conflicting results.

5.5 Serotonin

The genetic variants of serotonin receptor gene for example rs1042173 may influence alcohol dependence (Jhonsan et al., 2011). The presence of genetic variation may lead to manipulation of serotonergic transmission therefore affecting the rate of development of tolerance and alcohol dependence (Yoshimoto et al., 1996).

5.6 Cholinergic and nicotinic receptor gene

Evidence from genetic studies suggested that alcohol dependence as well as cigarette smoking in families share the genetic vulnerability. Research studies have identified a missense mutation (rs16969968) in exon 5 of the nicotinic receptor (CHRNA5) gene and a variant in the 3'-UTR of the CHRNA3 gene in association with alcoholism and nicotine dependence (Wang et al., 2009). Cholinergic muscarinic 2 receptor (CHRM2) SNP (rs1824024) has been significantly associated with the pathogenesis of depression and alcohol dependence disorders (Jung et al., 2011; Luo et al., 2005).

5.7 Opioids

Bart et al. (2005) have identified positive association between A118G polymorphism and increased risk of alcohol dependence in individuals from Sweden. The single nucleotide polymorphism A118G in exon 1 of opioid receptor gene (OPRM1) results in increase in 3 fold binding capacity of beta endorphin. However, the results of a number of research studies are contradictory. Few studies have failed to find the association between the A118 G allele and alcoholism (Bergen et al., 1997; Franke et al., 2001; Gelernter et al., 1999; Kim et al., 2004; Kranzler et al., 1998; Schinka et al., 2002), while few others have found positive association between the A118 allele and alcoholism (Town et al., 1999). The explanations for these conflicting reports may be small sample size of the populations under study and the ethnic variation.

5.8 Other neurotransmitters (Neuropeptide Y)

In Humans, Leu7Pro polymorphism in NPY gene has been established to affect the release of mature NPY. Individuals with Pro7/Leu7 allele have 42% higher plasma concentration of NPY as compared with Leu7/Leu7 variant. Kauhanen et al. (2000) reported that Pro7allele is associated with more (34% higher) alcohol consumption in a cohort of Finnish middle aged men. Lappalainnen and others have reported that NPYPro7 allele significantly contributes towards the heritability of alcohol dependence in European American population (Lappalainnen et al., 2002).

6. Pharmacotherapy of alcoholism

The first step in the treatment of alcoholism is detoxification assisted by medical treatment (Wertheimer and Chaney 2003). Detoxification is required to manage the clinical and psychological symptoms of alcoholism. After detoxification there is need for counseling or psychotherapy and rehabilitation (Williams, 2001). The pharmacological agents or medicines in use for alcoholism treatment act on specific neurotransmitter systems. The treatment is aimed at normalizing the alcohol specific neuroadaptations (Krishnan-Sarin et al., 2008). The selection criteria for treatment of alcoholism is based on the length of illness and additional amount of alcohol related problems (Wertheimer &Chaney, 2003).

6.1 FDA approved drugs for treatment of alcoholism

Some of the drugs approved by FDA for treatment of alcoholism are as follows (Krishnan-Sarin et al., 2008).

6.1.1 Disulfiram

Disulfiram has been in use to treat alcoholism since 1940. Disulfiram produces an aversive effect by disrupting alcohol metabolism. The proposed mechanism of action of disulfiram on alcohol use has been found to be primarily related to the inhibition of liver aldehyde dehydrogenase (metabolizing enzyme of alcohol) and secondarily related to central nervous system actions, via modulation of catecholamine neurotransmission. It blocks ALDH activity by forming intermolecular disulfide bridges resulting in acetaldehyde accumulation. Excessive buildup of acetaldehyde results in many unpleasant effects including lowered blood pressure, palpitation, nausea, vomiting, headache and difficulty in breathing.

In clinical doses, disulfiram inhibits the enzyme dopamine-β-hydroxylase, which converts dopamine to norepinephrine, leading to increase in dopamine levels in brain (Goldstein & Nakajima, 1967; Goldstein et al., 1964). It has been found in clinical trials of disulfiram that there are lower rates of relapse to drinking in those who are compliant with the medication (Fuller et al., 1986). However, due to aversive nature of this drug, noncompliance is one of the biggest problems encountered with its use. The use of disulfiram is supervised in many clinical settings.

6.1.2 Naltrexone

Naltrexone is a drug used mainly for the treatment of alcohol dependence, and is available as oral medication and in injectable form. The drug is well tolerated with primary gastrointestinal side effects (O'Malley et al., 1992; Volpicelli et al., 1992). The efficacy of naltrexone in reducing alcohol drinking is mediated via interactions between the endogenous opioid system and dopamine systems, specifically through antagonism of the μ-opioid receptors. The studies on animal models suggested that alcohol increases release of β-endorphins in certain portions of the brain known to be involved in alcohol reward (Marinelli et al., 2003; Zalewska-Kaszubska et al., 2006). Nalotrexane blocks the release of these endorphins. Naltrexone has also been shown to reduce drinking in animal models (Froehlich et al. 2003; Swift, 2000).

A number of clinical trials indicate that alcoholics receiving naltrexone treatment in combination with behavioral intervention have lower levels of relapse and reduced levels of alcohol craving (O'Malley et al., 1992). Recent reports (Bouza et al., 2004; Srisurapanont & Jarusuraisin, 2002) suggest that naltrexone has modest efficacy in preventing relapse to drinking. Although, naltrexone is well tolerated, the potential risk of toxicity of liver at high doses is the major cause of concern in patients with liver disease.

6.1.3 Acamprosate

Acamprosate is available in an oral, delayed release formula, Camprel. The mechanism of action is through antagonizing of the N-methyl D-aspartate (NMDA) glutamate receptor site or via modulation of glutamate neurotransmission (DeWitte et al., 2005; Harris et al., 2002).

It has been found that acamprosate reduces neuronal hyperexcitability during alcohol withdrawal, due to reductions in glutamate levels, so as to normalize the balance between excitatory and inhibitory neurotransmitters produced in chronic alcohol consumption (Spanagel et al., 1996; Dahchour et al., 1998; Littleton & Zieglgansberger, 2003).

6.2 Other promising medicines

In addition to the drugs approved by FDA for treating alcoholism there are other medications which are in use because of some clinical evidence of efficacy.

6.2.1 Ondansetron

Ondansetron is a 5HT3 receptor antagonist used mainly as antinausea medicine after postoperative nausea and as anticraving medicine in alcoholism. Human laboratory studies have demonstrated that ondansetron decreases alcohol preference and desire to drink (Johnson et al., 1993). The efficacy of ondansetron in reducing drinking behavior has also been reported in Clinical trials, especially in drinkers with early onset alcoholism (Kranzler et al., 2003).

6.2.2 Baclofen

Baclofen, a GABA B receptor antagonist is used clinically for the treatment of muscle spasticity. The preclinical trials have shown the effectiveness of baclofen in reducing chronic alcoholism (Colombo et al., 2004). In a recent clinical trial, it was found that the drug is well tolerated in alcohol dependent patients with liver cirrhosis and has some efficacy in improving abstinence rates. However, more clinical research is needed to establish its efficacy and tolerability in alcoholic patients.

6.2.3 Topiramate

Topiramate is an antiseizure medication which has been shown to be effective in reducing alcohol use in recent clinical trials. Its action is mediated via antagonizing α amino-3-hydroxy 5-methylisoxazole 4-propionic acid (AMPA) and kainate glutamate receptors as well as inhibition of GABA A receptors, L type calcium channels, and voltage dependent sodium channels (SCN). Topiramate has been shown to reduce alcohol use in animal models (Farook et al., 2007). It also helps in reducing alcohol withdrawl induced convulsions. It has some side effects such as numbness, anorexia, cognitive difficulty, and taste distortion, as well as some rare incidents of visual side effects including myopia, glaucoma, and increased intraocular pressure. The clinical trials used a slow titration over several weeks to the desired dose to reduce the incidence of side effects.

6.2.4 Selective serotonin reuptake inhibitors (SSRI)

Selective serotonin reuptake inhibitors such as fluoxetine, citalopram, and sertraline are used in the treatment of alcoholism because existing evidence has shown that lowering brain serotonin levels decrease preference for alcohol and SSRI. SSRI's are basically used in the treatment of depression, therefore the effectiveness has been found in depressed alcoholics in some clinical trials.

7. Pharmacogenetics of alcoholism

The sequencing of the human genome has become the foundation for one of the most significant scientific contribution, the idea that although all human individuals are genetically similar, each retains a unique genetic identity. The publication of the human blueprint has triggered an explosion in pharmaceutical research to utilize this knowledge in the prescription of drugs for various ailments including alcoholism to be tailored according to the genetic makeup of susceptible individuals or in other words personalized medicine.

Just before half a century ago the Human Genome Project, scientists had realized that inheritance was an important factor which accounts for individual variation in drug response (Kalow, 1962; Venter et al., 2001). This led to the birth of the term Pharmacogenetics. Pharmacogenetics is the study of the role of inter-individual genetic variation in drug response. Although human beings are 99.9% similar in their genetic makeup, 0.1% variability in terms of single-nucleotide polymorphisms is significantly accountable for an individual's susceptibility to diseases and inter- and intra-individual variation of drug response (Brooks, 1999).

On the basis of our current understanding of neurobiology numerous candidate genes have been implicated in the etiology and response to treatments for different addictions including alcoholism. The focus is on functional genetic variants of proteins involved in the neural response to alcohol including alcohol sensitivity, reward and tolerance and variants of the enzyme involved in metabolism of alcohol.

8. Genetic predictors of medication response

The inter-individual variation in drug response results in categorization of alcoholic patients into responders and nonresponders. The responders experience therapeutic efficacy with a particular drug given in therapeutic range without any toxicity or adverse effects. The nonresponders do not show any therapeutic effect, even when the administered drug reaches to peak level in blood, leading to ineffective treatment, known as poor as poor metabolizers. Therefore the traditional approach of one dose fits for all is no longer helpful in predicting the therapeutic efficacy of a drug. The pharmacogenetics focuses on identifying genetic factors that is with are responsible responsible for variability in pharmacotherapeutic effect both in terms of pharmacodynamics and efficacy (Evans &Johnson, 2001). The field has greatly benefitted from advances in molecular genetic tools, developments in bioinformatics and functional genomics for identifying genetic variants.

Genetic factors can account for interindividual differences in drug toxicity and efficacy in many ways e.g. the variability in genes may lead to differences in drug metabolism and disposition through functional differences in activity of enzymes or drug transporters (Ray et al., 2010a). Alternatively genetic variation may impact a drug's target such as particular receptor. Genetic variants that may modulate the effects of naltrexane have been identified in the gene coding for μ OPRM1, which is the primary target of naltrexaone (Oslin et al., 2003). One of the most widely studied SNPs in OPRM1 is +118A/G (rs 1799971) located in the +118 position of exon1 one which encodes for Asn40Asp substitution (Bond et al., 1998). This A/G substitution has been reported to affect the receptor affinity for endogenous ligands, β-endorphin leading to gain in function such that the G variant was thought to bind β-endorphin with greater affinity than A allele. However, some recent studies have shown that G allele has a loss of function rather than a gain. Further, the results of the study testing the relationship between this SNP of the OPRM1 gene and alcoholism have shown inconsistent results, some support the association of this SNP and alcohol dependence while others have failed to replicate this association (Schinka et al., 2002; Kranzler et al., 1998; Town et al., 1999). Further, this SNP of OPRM1 gene has also been associated with a differential response in clinical trials of naltrexone. Oslin et al. (2003) has reported that this SNP is associated with clinical response to naltrexaone among alcohol dependent patients such that individuals with at least one copy of the G allele, coding for more potent OPRM1 receptor reported lower relapse rates and longer time to return to heavy drinking after treatment with naltrexone, in comparison with individuals who were homozygous for the A allele.

It has been reported that persons of Asian descent possess an ALDH2*2 genetic variant (Quertemont et al., 2004). ALDH2*2 genetic variant of the ALDH enzyme metabolizes slowly and leads to accumulation of acetaldehyde (Edenberg, 2007). When the individuals bearing this variant drink alcohol they develop high acetaldehyde blood concentration and experience of flushing reaction similar to that seen in combination of ethanol and disulfiram. ALDH2*2 variation is the best characterized genetic factor protecting against the development of alcohol dependence. Pharmacogenomic studies suggest that it is highly unlikely that disulfiram will be helpful in treating the patients who have genetically compromised ALDH.

In addition disulfiram chelates copper and thus inhibits copper containing enzyme dopamine beta hydroxylase which further inhibits norepinephrine and dopamine in brain (Haile et al., 2009). The individuals harboring TT allele of dopamine beta hydroxylase (DβH) gene with C1021T polymorphism respond better to disulfiram treatment and need less dose whereas carriers (CT) would need intermediate dose and those with CC allele need maximum concentration to reach the efficacy level.

Acamprosate, is a drug used for abstinence and maintenance as it reduces craving in alcoholic patients who have undergone detoxification (De Witte et al., 2005). The effective acamprosate response in alcohol dependent subjects may be influenced by genetically controlled variation of NMDA receptor and the type of glutaminergic mGLU5 receptor. Confirmation of this hypothesis could lead to development of effective individualized treatment and recommendation for alcohol dependent patients based on pharmacogenetically relevant genetic variant.

Ondansetron, an antagonist of serotonin is important in the treatment of alcoholism. Serotonin transporter gene is an important regulator of neuronal 5-HT's function. The genetic difference in this gene may modulate the severity of alcohol consumption and predict the therapeutic response to 5-HT3 receptor antagonist ondansetron. A variable tandem repeat polymorphism (5-HTT LPR) is common in the promoter region of 5-HTT gene which alters the transcriptional activity. Two important variants are long (insertion LL) and short (SS) version. It has been reported in a randomized clinical trial that individuals with LL genotype (Homozygous for the long version) of 5-HTT gene showed significant results in improvements of alcoholism with treatment of ondansetron as compared to LS and SS genotype (Johnson et al., 2011).

Another functional T/G polymorphism (rs1042173) as in the 3/ untranslated region of the 5-HTT gene may alter the therapeutic response in alcoholism treatment with ondansetron in alcohol addiction treatment (Jhonsan et al., 2011). The effect of ondensateron will be higher in individuals possessing the combination of LL genotype and TT genotype of 5-HTT gene.

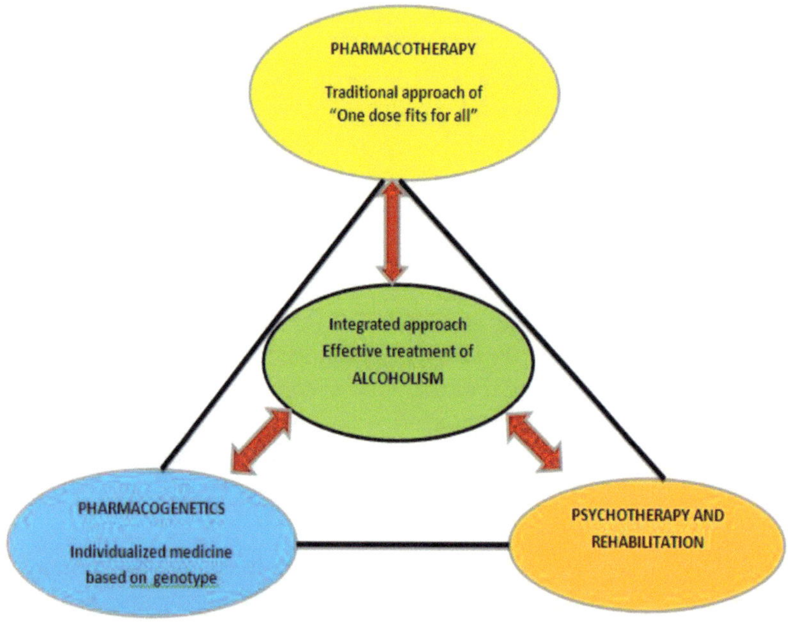

Fig. 2. Alcoholism Treatment: A Treatment approach to use a trio of Pharmacotherapy using pharmacological agents, where a traditional approach of "One dose for all" is used and Psychotherapy - an important part of treatment in alcoholism and Pharmacogenetics based on Genetic makeup of the Individual for better and effective treatment in alcoholism

9. Conclusion

Lot of work still needs work still needs to be done in order to improve our understanding of the genetic and environmental factors underlying alcohol dependence and also utilizing the genetic information in prescribing the drugs as per the genetic architecture of the individuals. The integrated approach of incorporating a trio of pharmacogenetic, pharmacotherapy and psychotherapy would be more promising in treatment of alcoholism (Fig 2). As the genetic testing becomes more common in the practice of medicine variety of ethical and practical challenges unique to alcohol addiction, will also need to be addressed.

10. References

Amit, Z. Aragon, C.M. (1988). Catalase activity measured in rats naive to ethanol correlates with later voluntary ethanol consumption: possible evidence for a biological marker system of ethanol intake. *Psychopharmacology*, Vol. 95. pp. 512–515

Bart, G. Kreek, M.J. Ott, J. LaForge, K.S. Proudnikov, D. Pollak, L. Heilig, M. (2005). Increased attributable risk related to a functional mu-opioid receptor gene polymorphism in association with alcohol dependence in central Sweden. *Neuropsychopharmacology*, Vol. 30, No. 2, pp. 417-422

Beckemeier, M.E. Bora, P.S. (1998). Fatty acid ethyl esters: potentially toxic products of myocardial ethanol metabolism. *J Mol Cell Cardiol,* Vol. 30, pp. 2487–2494

Benegal, V. (2005). India alcohol and public health.*Addiction* August vol.100 No. 8, pp. 1051-1056

Bergen, A.W. Kokoszka, J. Peterson, R. Long, J.C. Virkkunen, M. Linnoila, M. Goldman, D. (1997). Mu-opioid receptor gene variants: lack of association with alcohol dependence. *Mol Psychiatry,* Vol. 2, pp. 490–494

Bond, C. LaForge, K.S. Tian, M. Melia, D. Zhang, S. Borg, L. Gong, J. Schluger, J. Strong, J.A. Leal, S.M. Tischfield, J.A. Kreek, M.J. Yu, L. (1998). Single-nucleotide polymorphism in the human mu opioid receptor gene alters beta-endorphin binding and activity: possible implications for opiate addiction. *ProcNatlAcadSci,* Vol. 95, pp. 9608-9613

Bouza, C. Angeles, M. Muñoz, A. Amate, J.M. (2004). Efficacy and safety of naltrexone and acamprosate in the treatment of alcohol dependence: A systematic review. *Addiction,* Vol. 99, No.7, pp. 811– 828

Brooks, A.J. (1999). The essence of SNPs. *Gene,* Vol. 234, pp. 177–186

Caballeria, J. (2003). Current concepts in Alcoholmetabolism.*Annals of Hepatology,* Vol. 2, No. 2, pp. 60-68

Carr, L.G. Foroud, T. Stewart, T. Castellucio, P. Edenberg, H.J. Li, T. (2002). Influence of ADH1B polymorphism on alcohol use and its subjective effects in a Jewish population.*Am J Med Genet,* Vol. 112, pp. 138–143

Chen, C.C. Lu, R.B. Chen, Y.C. Wang, M.F. Chang, Y.C. Li, T.K. Yin, S.J. (1999). Interaction between the functional polymorphisms of the alcohol-metabolism genes in protection against alcoholism.*American Journal of Human Genetics,* Vol. 65, No. 3, pp. 795–807

Chou, W.Y. Stewart, M.J. Carr, L.G. Zheng, D. Stewart, T.R. Williams, A. Pinaire, J. Crabb, D.W. (1999). AnA/G polymorphism in the promoter of mitochondrial aldehyde dehydrogenase (ALDH2): Effects of the sequence variant on transcription factor binding and promoter strength. *Alcohol Clin and Experimental Res,* Vol. 23, No. 6, pp. 963–968

Colombo G, Addolorato G, Agabio R, Carai MA, Pibiri F, Serra S, Vacca G, Gessa GL. (2004). Role of GABA(B) receptor in alcohol dependence: Reducing effect of baclofen on alcohol intake and alcohol motivational properties in rats and amelioration of alcohol withdrawal syndrome and alcohol craving in human alcoholics. *Neurotoxicity Research,* Vol. 6, No. 5, pp. 403–414

Dahchour, A. De Witte, P. Bolo, N. Nedelec, J.F. Muzet, M. Durbin, P. Macher, J.P. (1998). Central effects of acamprosate: Part 1. Acamprosate blocks the glutamate increase in the nucleus accumbens microdialysate in ethanol withdrawn rats. *Psychiatry Research,* Vol. 82, No. 2, pp. 107–114

De Witte, P. Littleton, J. Parot, P. Koob, G. (2005). Neuroprotective and abstinence-promoting effects of acamprosate: elucidating the mechanism of action. *CNS drugs,* Vol. 19, No. 6, pp. 517–537

Deitrich, R.A.&Erwin, V.G. E. (1996).Pharmacological Effects of Ethanol on the Nervous System.*Hand book of Pharmacology and toxicology,* CRC Press, ISBN: 9780849383892

Diana, M. Gessa, G.L. Rossetti, Z.L. (1992). Lack of tolerance to ethanol-induced stimulation of dopamine mesolimbic system. *Alcohol,* Vol. 2, No. 4, pp. 329-333

Edenberg, H.J. (2007). The Genetics of Alcohol Metabolism.Role of Alcohol Dehydrogenase and Aldehyde dehydrogenase variants.*Alcohol Research and Health,* Vol. 30, No.1, pp. 5-13

Evans, W.E. Johnson, J.A. (2001). Pharmacogenomics the inherited basis for inter-individual differences in drug response. *Annu Rev Genomics Hum Genet.* Vol. 2, pp. 9-39

Farook, J.M. Morrell, D.J. Lewis, B. Littleton, J.M. Barron, S. (2007). Topiramate (Topamax) reduces conditioned abstinence behaviors and handling-induced convulsions (HIC) after chronic administration of alcohol in Swiss-Webster mice. *Alcohol and Alcoholism,* Vol. 42, No. 4, pp. 296–300

Ferreira, V.M.M. Morato, G.S. (1997). D-Cycloserine blocks the effects of ethanol and HA-906 in rats tested in the elevated plus-maze. *Alcohol Clin Exp Res,* Vol. 21, No. 9, pp. 1638-1642

Flensborg-Madsen, T. Knop, J. Mortensen, E. L. Becker, U.&Gronbek, M. (2007). Amount of Alcohol consumption and risk of developing alcoholism in men and women. *Alcohol and Alcoholism,* Vol. 42, No.5 pp. 442-447

Foley, P.F.Loh, E.W. Innes, D.J. Williams, S.M. Tannenberg, A.E. Harper, C.G. Dodd, P.R. (2004).Association studies of neurotransmitter gene polymorphisms in alcoholic Caucasians.*Ann N Y AcadSci,* Vol 1025pp39-46.

Franke, P. Wang, T. Nothen, M.M. Knapp, M. Neidt, H. Albrecht, S. Jahnes, E. Propping, P. Maier, W. (2001). Nonreplication of association between μ-opioid-receptor gene (OPRM1) A118G polymorphism and substance dependence.*Am J Med Genet,* Vol. 105, pp. 114 -119

Froehlich J, O'Malley S, Hyytia P, Davidson D, Farren C. (2003). Preclinical and clinical studies on naltrexone: What have they taught each other? Alcoholism: *Clinical and Experimental Research,* Vol. 27, No. 3, pp. 533–539

Fukuda, Y. Nakamura, K. Takano, T. (2005). Accumulation of health risk behaviours is associated with lower socioeconomic status and women's urban residence: a multilevel analysis inJapan. *BMC Public Health,* Vol.5, No. 53.doi:10.1186/1471-2458-5-53,ISSN 1755-7682

Fuller, R.K. Branchey, L. Brightwell, D.R. (1986). Disulfiram treatment of alcoholism: A Veterans Administration cooperative study. *Journal of the American Medical Association,* Vol. 256, No. 11,pp. 1449–1455

Gelernter, J. Kranzler, H. Cubells, J. (1999). Genetics of two μ-opioid receptor gene (OPRM1) exon I polymorphisms: population studies, and allele frequencies in alcohol- and drug-dependent subjects. *Mol Psychiatry,* Vol. 4, pp. 476–483

Gianoulakis,C. (1996). Implications of endogenous opioids and dopaminein alcoholism: human and basic science studies. *Alcohol AlcoholSuppl,* Vol. 1, pp. 33–42

Goedde, H.W. Agarwal, D.P. Fritze, G. Meier-Tackmann, D. Singh, S. Beckmann, G. Bhatia, K, Chen, L.Z. Fang, B. Lisker, R. (1992). Distribution of Adh2 and Aldh2 Genotypes in Different Populations.*Hum Genet,* Vol. 88, pp. 344–346

Goldman, D. & Bergen, A. (1998).General and specific inheritance of substance abuse and alcoholism.*Archives of General Psychiatry,* Vol.55, pp. 964–965

Goldstein, M. &Nakajima, K. (1967). The effect of disulfiram on catecholamine levels in the brain. *Journal of Pharmacol and Exp Therap,* Vol. 157, No. 1, pp. 96–102

Goldstein, M. Anagnoste, B. Lauber, E. &Mckeregham, M.R. (1964).Inhibition of dopamine-beta-hydroxylase by disulfiram.*Life Sciences,* Vol. 3, pp. 763–767

Group, P.M.R. (1997).Matching Alcoholism Treatments to Client heterogeity: Project MATCH posttreatment drinking outcomes.*J Stud Alcohol,* Vol.58, No.1, pp. 7-29

Haile, C.N. Kosten, T.R. Kosten, T.A. (2009). Pharmacogenetic treatments for drug addiction: cocaine, amphetamine and methamphetamine. *Am J Drug Alcohol Abuse,* Vol. 35, No. 3, pp.161-77

Harris, B.R. Prendergast, M.A. Gibson, D.A. Rogers, D.T. Blanchard, J.A. Holley, R.C. Fu, M.C. Hart, S.R. Pedigo, N.W. Littleton, J.M. (2002). Acamprosate inhibits the binding and neurotoxic effects of trans-ACPD, suggesting a novel site of action at metabotropic glutamate receptors. *Alcohol Clin Exp Res,* Vol. 26, No.12, pp. 1779–1793

Hayashi, S. Watanabe, J. Kawajiri, K. (1991). Genetic polymorphisms in the 5'-flanking region change transcriptional regulation of the human cytochrome P450IIE1 gene. *J Biochem,* Vol. 110, pp. 559–565

Heath, A.C. Madden, P.A.F. Bucholz, K.K. Bierut, L.J. Whitefild, J.B. Dinwiddie, W.S. Slutske, D.B. Statham, D.B.&Martin, N.G. (2001). Towards a molecular epidemiology of alcohol dependence: analyzing the interplay of genetic and environmental risk factors. *British Journal of Psychiatry,* Vol. 178, No.40, pp. s33-s40

Hoerner, M. Behrens, U. Worner, T. Lieber, C.S. (1986). Humoralimmuneresponses to acetaldehyde adducts in alcoholic patients. *Res CommunChemPathol Pharmacol,* Vol. 54, pp. 3-12

Howard, L.A. Ahluwalia, J.S. Lin, S.K. Sellers, E.M. Tyndale, R.F. (2003). CYP2E1*1D regulatory polymorphism: association with alcohol and nicotine dependence. *Pharmacogenetics,* Vol. 13, No. 7, pp. 441-442

Huang, S.Y. Lu, R.B. Ma, K.H. Shy, M.J. Lin, W.W. (2008). Norepinephrine transporter polymorphisms T-182C and G1287A are not associated with alcohol dependence and its clinical subgroups. *Drug Alcohol Depend,* Vol. 92, No. 1-3, pp. 20-26

Hurley, T.D. Edenberg, H.J. Li, T.K. (2002). The pharmacogenomics of alcoholism. In: *Pharmacogenomics: The Search for Individualized Therapies.*Weinheim, Germany: Wiley-VCH, pp. 417–441

Itoga, S. Nomura, F. Harada, S. Tsutsumi, M. Takase, S. Nakai, T. (1999).Mutations in the exons and exon–intron junction regions of human cytochrome P-4502E1 gene and alcoholism.*Alcohol Clin Exp Res,* Vol. 23, pp. 13s–16s

Jessica, E. Sturgess, J.E. George, T.P. Kennedy J.L. Heinz, A.& Müller, D.J.(2011). Pharmacogenetics of alcohol, nicotine and drug addiction treatments.*Addiction Biology,* Vol. 16, No.3, pp. 357-376

Johann, M. Putzhammer, A. Eichhammer, P. Wodarz, N. (2005). Association of the -141C Del variant of the dopamine D2 receptor (DRD2) with positive family history and suicidality in German alcoholics.*Am J Med Genet B Neuropsychiatr Genet,* Vol. 132, No.1, pp. 46-49

Johnson, B.A. Ait-Daoud, N. Seneviratne, C. Roache, J.D. Javors, M.A. Wang, X.Q. Liu, L. Penberthy, J.K. DiClemente, C.C. Li, M.D. (2011). Pharmacogenetic approach at the serotonin transporter gene as a method of reducing the severity of alcohol drinking.*Am J Psychiatry,* Vol. 168, No. 3, pp. 265-275

Johnson, B.A. Campling, G.M. Griffiths, P. Cowen, P.J. (1993). Attenuation of some alcohol-induced mood changes and the desire to drink by 5-HT3 receptor blockade: A preliminary study in healthy male volunteers. *Psychopharmacology*, Vol. 112, No.1, pp.142–144

Jung, M.H. Park, B.L. Lee, B.C. Ro, Y. Park, R. Shin, H.D. Bae, J.S. Kang, T.C. Choi, I.G. (2011).Association of CHRM2 polymorphisms with severity of alcohol dependence.*Genes Brain Behavior,* Vol. 10, No. 2, pp. 253-256

Kalow, W. (1962). Pharmacogenetics: Heredity and the response to drugs. Philadelphia, W.B. Saunders.

Kauhanen, J. Karvonen, M.K. Pesonen, U. Koulu, M. Tuomainen, T.P. Uusitupa, M.I.J. Salonen, J.T. (2000). Neuropeptide Y polymorphism and alcohol consumption in middle-aged men.*Am J Med Genet,* Vol. 93, pp. 117-121

Kennedy, R.H.& Liu, S.J. (2003). Sex differences in L-type calcium current after chronic ethanol consumption in rats.*ToxicolApplParmacol,* Vol. 15, No. 3, pp. 196-203

Kenneth, S. Kendler, M.D. Andrew, C. Heath, D. Michael, C. Neale. Kessler R.D.& Eaves L.J. (2011). A population - based Twin study of Alcoholism in Women. *JAMA,* Vol. 268, No.14, pp. 1877-1882

Kianmaa, K. Tabakoff, B. (1983). Neurochemical correlates of tolerance and strain differences in the neurochemical effects of ethanol. *Pharmacol BiochemBehav,* Vol. 8, pp. 383-388

Kim, S.G. Kim, C.M. Kang, D.H. Kim, Y.J. Byun, W.T. Kim, S.Y. Park, J.M. Kim M.J. Oslin, D.W. (2004). Association of functional opioid receptor genotypes with alcohol dependence in Koreans.*Alcohol Clin Exp Res,* Vol. 28, pp. 986–990

Koechling, U.M. Amit, Z. (1992). Relationship between blood catalase activity and drinking history in a human population, a possible biological marker of the affinity to consume alcohol.*Alcohol,* Vol. 27, pp. 181–188

Kranzler, H.R. Gelernter, J. O'Malley, S. Hernandez-Avila, C.A. Kaufman, D. (1998). Association of alcohol or other drug dependence with allelesofthe μ-opioid receptor gene (OPRM1). *Alcohol Clin Exp Res,* Vol. 22, pp. 1359–1362

Kranzler, H.R. Pierucci-Lagha, A. Feinn, R. Hernandez-Avila, C. (2003). Effects of ondansetron in early- versus late-onset alcoholics: A prospective, open-label study. *Alcoholism: Clinical and Experimental Research,* Vol. 27, No. 7, pp. 1150–1155

Krishnan-Sarin, S. O'Malley, S. &Krystal, J.H. (2008). Treatment Implications: Using Neuroscience to Guide the development of new Pharmacotherapies for Alcoholism. *Alcohol, Res &Health,*pp. 400-407

Lappalainen, J. Kranzler, H.R. Malison, R. Price, L.H. Van Dyck, C. Rosenheck, R.A. Cramer, J. Southwick, S. Charney, D. Krystal, J. Gelernter, J. (2002). A functional neuropeptide Y Leu7Pro polymorphism associated with alcohol dependence in a large population sample from the United States.*Arch Gen Psychiatry,* Vol. 59, No. 9, pp. 825-831

Lee, S.L.Chau, G.Y. Yao, C.T. Wu, C.W. Yin, S.J. (2006). Functional assessment of human alcohol dehydrogenase family in ethanol metabolism: Significance of first-pass metabolism. *Alcoholism: Clinical and Experimental Research,* Vol. 30, No.7 pp.1132–1142

Lieber, C.S. DeCarli, L.M. (1968). Ethanol oxidation by hepatic microsomes: adaptive increase after ethanol feeding. *Science,* Vol.162, pp. 917–918

Lieber, C.S. Lasker, J.M. DeCarli, L.M. Saeli, J. Wojtowicz, T. (1988).Role of acetone, dietary fat, and total energy intake in the induction of the hepatic microsomal ethanol oxidizing system.*J Pharmacol Exp Ther,* Vol. 247, pp. 791–795

Lieber, C.S. (1999). Microsomal ethanol-oxidizing system: the first 30 years (1968–1998) a review. *Alcohol Clin Exp Res,* Vol. 23, pp. 991–1007

Littleton, J. &Zieglgänsberger, W. (2003).Pharmacological mechanisms of naltrexone and acamprosate in the prevention of relapse in alcohol dependence.*American Journal on Addictions,* Vol. 12, No. 1, pp. S3–S11

Loh, E.W. Smith, I. I. Murray, R. McLaughlin, M. McNulty, S. Ball, D. (1999). Association between variants at the GABAAbeta2, GABAAalpha6 and GABAAgamma2 gene cluster and alcohol dependence in a Scottish population.*Mol Psychiatry,* Vol. 4, No.6, pp. 539–544

Longo, L.P. Campbell, T. Hubatch, S. (2002). Divalproex sodium (Depakote) for alcohol withdrawal and relapse prevention.*J Addict Dis,* Vol. 21, No. 2, pp. 55-64

Lovinger, D.M. (1991).Ethanol potentiation of 5HT3 receptor-mediated ion current in NCB-20 neuroblastoma cells.*Neurosci Lett,* Vol. 122, pp. 57-60

Luczak, S.E. Glatt, S.J. & Wall, T.J. (2006).Meta-analyses of ALDH2 and ADH1B with alcohol dependence in Asians. *Psychological Bulletin,* Vol. 132, No. 4, pp. 607–621

Luo, X. Kranzler, H.R. Zuo, L. Wang, S. Blumberg, H.P. Gelernter, J. (2005). CHRM2 gene predisposes to alcohol dependence, drug dependence and affective disorders: results from an extended case-control structured association study. *Human Molecular Genetics,* Vol. 14, No.16, pp. 2421-2434

Marinelli, P.W. Quirion, R. Gianoulakis, C. (2003). A microdialysis profile of beta-endorphin and catecholamines in the rat nucleus accumbens following alcohol administration.*Psychopharmacology,* Vol. 169, No.1, pp. 60–67

McGue, M. (1999).The behavioral genetics of alcoholism.*Current Directions in Psychological Science,* Vol. 8, pp. 109–115

McLeod, H.L.Krynetski, E.Y.Relling, M.V. Evans, W.E. (2000). Genetic polymorphisms of thiopurinemethyltransferase and its clinical relevance for childhood lymphoblastic leukemia.*Leukemia,* Vol. 14, pp. 567–572

Moussas, G. Christodoulou, C.Douzenis, A. (2009). A Short review on the etiology of alcoholism. *Annals of General Psychiatry,* Vol. 8, No.10, doi:10.1186/1744-859X-8-10

Neumark, Y.D. Friedlander, Y. Thomasson, H.R. Li, T.K. (1998). Association of the ADH2*2 allele with reduced ethanol consumption in Jewish men in Israel: a pilot study. *J Stud Alcohol,* Vol. 59, pp. 133–139

Neville, M.J. Johnstone, E.C. Walton, R.T. (2004). Identification and characterization of ANKK1: a novel kinase gene closely linked to DRD2 on chromosome band 11q23.1.*Human Mutation,* Vol. 23, pp. 540-545

Nurnberger, J.I. Wiegand, R. Bucholz, K. O'Connor, S. Meyer, E.T. Reich, T. Rice, J. Schuckit, M. King, L. Petti, T. Bierut, L. Hinrichs, A.L. Kuperman, S. Hesselbrock, V.&Porjesz, B. (2004). A Family Study of Alcohol Dependence - Coaggregation of Multiple Disorders in Relatives of Alcohol- Dependent Probands.*Arch Gen Psychiatry,* Vol. 61, pp. 1246-1256

O'Malley, S.S.Jaffe, A.J. Chang, G. Rode, S.Schottenfeld, R. Meyer, R.E.Rounsaville, B. (1992). Naltrexone and coping skills therapy for alcohol dependence: A controlled study. *Archives of General Psychiatry,* Vol. 49, No.11, pp. 881–887

Oshino, N. Oshino, R. Chance, B. (1973). The characteristics of the peroxidatic reaction in ethanol oxidation.*Biochem J,* Vol. 131, pp. 555–567

Osier, M.V. Pakstis, A.J.Soodyall, H. Comas, D. Goldman, D. Odunsi, A.Okonofua, F.Parnas, J. Schulz, L.O.Bertranpetit, J. Bonne-Tamir, B. Lu, R.B. Kidd, J.R. Kidd, K.K. (2002). Aglobal perspective on genetic variation at the ADH genes reveals unusual patterns of linkage disequilibrium and diversity. *Am J Genet,* Vol. 71, pp. 84–99

Osier, M.V. Lu, R.B. Pakstis, A.J. Kidd, J.R. Huang, S.Y. Kidd, K.K. (2004). Possible epistatic role of ADH7 in the protection against alcoholism.*American Journal of Medical Genetics.* Part B *Neuropsychiatric Genetics,* Vol. 126, pp.19–22

Oslin, D.W. Berrettini, W. Kranzler, H.R. Pettinati, H. Gelernter, J Volpicelli, J.R. O'Brien, C.P. (2003). A functionalpolymorphism of the mu-opioid receptor gene is associated withnaltrexone response in alcohol-dependent patients. *Neuropsychopharmacology,* No. 28, pp.1546-1552

Park, C.S. Park, S.Y. Lee, C.S. Sohn, J.W. Hahn, G.H. Kim, B.J. (2006). Association between Alcoholism and the Genetic polymorphism of the GABA A receptor genes on chromosome 5q33-34 in Korean population.*J Korean Med Sci,* Vol. 21, No. 3, pp. 533-538

Pawan, G.L.S. (1972). Meatbolism of Alcohol (ethanol) in Man. *ProcNutrSoc,* Vol. 3I, pp. 83-89

Ponce, G. Hoenicka, J. Jiménez-Arriero, M.A. Rodríguez-Jiménez, R. Aragüés, M. Martín-Suñé, N. Huertas, E. Palomo, T. (2008). DRD2 andANKK1 genotype in alcohol-dependent patients with psychopathic traits: association and interaction study.*Br J Psychiatry,* Vol. No. 2, pp. 121-125

Poznyak, V. Saraceno, B. Obot, I.S. (2005). Breaking the vicious circle of determinants and consequences of harmful alcohol use.*Bulletin of the World Health Organization.*Vol.83, pp 803

Quertemont, E. (2004). Genetic polymorphism in ethanol metabolism: acetaldehyde contribution to alcohol abuse and alcoholism.*MoleculPsychiat,* Vol. 9, pp. 570-581

Quickfall, J.& el-Guebaly, N. (2006). Genetics and Alcoholism: How close are we to potential clinical applications? *Can Journal of Psychiatry,* Vol. 51, No.7, pp. 461-467

Radel, M. Goldman, D. (2001). Pharmacogenetics of alcohol response and alcoholism: the interplay of genes and environmental factors in thresholds for alcoholism.*DrugMetabDispos,* Vol. 29, No. 4, pp. 489-494

Ray, L.A. Mackillop, J.&Monti, P.M. (2010a). Subjective responses to alcohol consumption as endophenotypes: Advancing behavioral Genetics in etiological and treatment models of Alcoholism. *Substance Use and Misuse,* Vol. 45, pp. 1742-1765

Ray, L.R. Chin, P.F. Miotto, K. (2010b). Naltrexone for the treatment of Action and Pharmacogenetics.*CNS & Neurological Disorders Drug Targets.* Vol. 9, pp. 13-22

Sander, T. Ball, D. Murray, R. Patel, J. Samochowiec, J. Winterer, G.Rommelspacher, H. Schmidt, L.G. Loh, E.W.(1999). Association analysis of sequence variants of GABA(A) alpha 6, beta 2, and gamma 2 gene cluster and alcohol dependence. *Alcohol Clin Exp Res,* Vol.23, No. 3, pp. 427–431

Sander, T. Ostapowicz, A. Samochowiec, J. Smolka, M. Winterer, G. Schmidt, L.G. (2000).Genetic variation of the glutamate transporter EAAT2 gene and vulnerability to alcohol dependence.*Psychiatry Genet,* Vol. 10, No. 3, pp. 103–107

Schinka, J.A. Town, T. Abdullah, L. Crawford, F.C. Ordorica, P.I. Francis, E. (2002).A functional polymorphism within the μ-opioid receptor gene and risk for abuse of alcohol and other substances.*Mol Psychiatry,* Vol. 7, pp. 224 -228

Schumann, G. Johann, M. Frank, J. Preuss, U. Dahmen, N. Laucht, M. Rietschel, M. Rujescu, D. Lourdusamy, A. Toni-Kim, C. Krause, K. Dyer, A. Depner, M. Wellek, S. Treutlein, J. Szegedi, A. Giegling, I. Cichon, S. Blomeyer, D. Heinz, A. Heath, S. Lathrop, M. Wodarz, N. Soyka, M. Spanagel, R. Mann, K. (2008). Systematic analysis of glutaminergic neurotransmission genes in alcohol dependence and adolescent risky drinking behavior.*Arch Gen Psychiatry,* Vol. 65, No.7, pp. 826-838

Sloan, C.D. Sayarath, V.&Moore, J.H. (2008). Systems Genetics of Alcoholism.*Alcohol Research and Health,*Vol. 31,No.1, pp. 14-25

Spanagel, R. Putzke, J. Stefferl, A. Schöbitz, B. Zieglgänsberger, W. (1996). Acamprosate and alcohol: II. Effects on alcohol withdrawal in the rat.*Europ Journal of Pharmacol,* Vol. 305, No. 1-3, pp. 45–50

Srisurapanont, M. &Jarusuraisin, N. (2002).Opioid antagonists for alcohol dependence. *Cochrane Database Syst Rev.* No. 1, CD001867

Strat, Y.L. Ramoz, N. Schumann, G.&Gorwood, P.(2008).Molecular Genetics of Alcohol Dependence and Related endophenotypes. *Current Genomics,* Vol. 9, pp. 444-451.

Subramanian, S.V.Nandy, S. Irving, M. Gordon, D. Davey, Smith, G. (2005) Role of socioeconomic markers and state prohibition policy inpredicting alcohol consumption among men and women in India:a multilevel statistical analysis. *Bulletin of the World Health Organization,* Vol. 83, pp. 829–836

Swift, R.M. (2000). Opioid antagonists and alcoholism treatment.*CNS Spectrums,*Vol. 5, No. 2, pp. 49–57

Tabakoff, B. Hoffman, P.L. Moses, F.(1977). Neurochemical correlates of ethanol withdrawal: alterations in serotonergic function. *J Pharm Pharmacol,* Vol. 29, pp. 471-476

Tabakoff, B. (1983). Current trends in biologic research on alcoholism.*Drug Alcohol Depend,* Vol. 11, No. 1, pp. 33-37

Tabakoff, B.&Hoffman, P.L. (1992). Alcohol: Neurobiology. *Substance Abuse,* 2nd edition, pp. 152–185

Takahashi, T. Lasker, J.M. Rosman, A.S. Lieber, C.S. (1993). Induction of cytochrome P-4502E1 in the human liver by ethanol is caused by a corresponding increase in encoding messenger RNA. *Hepatology,* Vol. 17, pp. 236–245

Thiele, T.E. Marsh, D.J. Ste Marie, L. Bernstein, I.L. Palmiter, R.D. (1998). Ethanol consumption and resistance are inversely related to neuropeptide Y levels. *Nature,* Vol. 396, pp. 366–369

Thomasson, H.R. Edenberg, H.J. Crabb, D.W. Mai, X.L. Jerome, R.E. Li, T. K. Wang, S.P. Lin, Y.T. Lu, R.B. Yin, S.J. (1991).Alcohol and aldehyde dehydrogenase genotypes and alcoholism in Chinese men. *American Journal of Human Genetics,* Vol. 48, No. 4, pp. 677–681

Town, T. Abdullah, L. Crawford, F. Schinka, J. Ordorica, P.I. Francis, E. Hughes, P. Duara, R. Mullan, M. (1999). Association of a functionalμ-opioid receptor allele (+118A) with alcohol dependency.*Am J Med Genet,* Vol. 88, pp. 458–461

Tsutsumi, M. Lasker, J.M. Shimizu, M. Rosman, A.S. Lieber, C.S. (1989). Theintralobular distribution of ethanol-inducible P-450IIE1 in rat and human liver.*Hepatology,* Vol. 10, pp. 437–446

Vengeliene, V. Bilbao, A. Molander, A.&Spanagel, R. (2006). Neuropharmacology of Alcohol addiction.*British Journal of Pharmacology,* Vol. 154, pp. 299-315

Vengeliene, V. Bilbao, A. Molander, A. Spanagel, R. (2008).Neuropharmacology of alcohol addiction. *Br J Pharmacol,* Vol. 154, No. 2, pp. 299-315

Venter, J.C. Adams, M.D. Myers, E.W.Li, P.W. Mural, R.J. Sutton, G.G (2001). The sequence of the human genome.*Science,* Vol. 291, pp. 1304–1351

Volpicelli, J.R. Alterman, A.I. Hayashida, M. O'Brien, C.P. (1992). Naltrexone in the treatment of alcohol dependence. *Archives of General Psychiatry,* Vol. 49, No.11, pp. 876–880

Wang, J.C. Grucza, R. Cruchaga, C. Hinrichs, A.L. Bertelsen, S. Budde, J. P. Fox, L. Goldstein, E. Reyes, O. Saccone, N. Saccone, S. Xuei, X. Bucholz, K. Kuperman, S. Nurnberger, J. Rice, J.P. Schuckit, M.J. Tischfield, J. Hesselbrock, V. Porjesz, B. Edenberg, H.J. Bierut, L.J. Goate, A.M. (2009). Genetic variation in the CHRNA5 gene affects mRNA levels and is associated with risk for alcohol dependence Association of CHRNA5 with alcohol dependence. *Molecul Psychiatry,* Vol.14, pp. 501-510

Wertheimer, A.I.& Chaney, N.M. (2003). The full extent of Alcoholism: A WorldwideEconomic and Social Tragedy. *Malaysian Journal of Pharmacy,* Vol.1, No.3, pp. 54-58

Whitfield, J.B. (1997). Meta-analysis of the effects of alcohol dehydrogenase genotype on alcohol dependence and alcoholic liver disease.*Alcohol,* Vol. 32, pp. 613–619

Williams, S. (2001). Introducing an in-patient treatment for alcohol detoxification into community settings. *J Clin Nursing,* Vol. 10, pp. 635-642

Woodward, J.J. (1994). A comparison of the effects of ethanol and the competitiveglycine agonist 7-chlorokynurenic acid on N-methyl-D-aspartate acid-inducedneurotransmitter release from rat hippocampal slices. *J Neurochem,* Vol. 62, No. 98, pp. 7-91

World Health Organization.(2002). The World Health Report 2002- Reducing risks, Promoting Healthy Life.*World Health Organization, Geneva,* pp. 65-67.

World Health Organization.(2004). *WHO Global Status Report on Alcohol.* pp. 1-68

Yin, S.J. (1994). Alcohol dehydrogenase: enzymology and metabolism. *Alcohol AlcoholSuppl,* Vol. 29, No. 2, pp. 113–119

Wray, L.A. Alwin, D.F. &McCammon, R.J. (2005). Social statusand risky health behaviors: results from the health and retirement study. *Journals of Gerontology Series B-Psychological Sciences and Social Sciences,* Vol.60, No 2, pp. 85–92.

Yoshimoto, K. Yayama, K. Sorimachi, Y. Tani, J. Ogata, M. Nishimura, A. Yoshida, T. Ueda, S. Komura, S. (1996). Possibility of 5-HT3 receptor involvement in alcohol dependence: a microdialysisstudy of nucleus accumbens dopamine and serotonin releasein rats with chronic alcohol consumption. *Alcohol Clin Exp Res,* Vol. 20, No. 9, pp. 311A–319A

Zaleski, M. Morato, G.S. da Silva V.A. Lemos, T. (2004). Neuropharmacological aspects of chronic alcohol use and withdrawl symptoms. *Rev Brain Psiquiater,* Vol. 26, pp. 40-42

Zalewska-Kaszubska, J. Gorska, D. Dyr, W. Czarnecka, E. (2006). Effect of acute administration of ethanol on beta-endorphin plasma level in ethanol preferring and non-preferring rats chronically treated with naltrexone. *Pharmacol, Biochemistry, and Behavior,* Vol. 85, No.1, pp. 155–159

Zimatkin, S.M. Deitrich, R.A. (1997). Ethanol metabolism in the brain.*Addict Biol,* Vol. 2, pp. 387–399

Part 4

Clinical Pharmacology

13

Pharmacological Approaches to Improve Ageing

Pedro J. Camello, Cristina Camello-Almaraz and Maria J. Pozo
Department of Physiology, University of Extremadura, Cáceres, Spain

1. Introduction

Aging is generally considered as a progressive and irreversible set of structural and functional changes, due both to the genetic background of the individual and the oxidative damage and modifications of intracellular signaling mechanisms. Although the anatomical and physiological alterations associated to aging (e.g. sarcopenia, cognitive and sensorial decline, functional loss in cardiovascular system…) are not a disease, they reduce the functional reserve of the organism, ultimately leading to pathological alterations and death.

Improvements of nutrition, hygiene and public health, and medical diagnosis and treatments have dramatically extended life expectancy in the last decades. However, the rate of human aging is to the moment an elusive target in biomedical interventions. The achievement of a slowing of human age is not necessarily linked to an increase of morbid, unhealthy population, but is likely to postpone the onset of age-related pathologies (Blagosklonny, 2010). Pharmacological intervention to decelerate aging and age-related diseases is highly attractive because it would target all the population during many years. If successful, antiaging therapy will be more efficient in reducing mortality than to fight separately each age-related disease (Olshansky *et al.*, 2007). Research on anti-aging interventions has evolved along the main theories of aging. We describe here the available explanations for aging before presenting the updated status of each approach.

2. Oxidative stress, aging and antioxidant treatments

2.1 Mitochondrial free radicals theory of aging

After formulation of the "rate of living" hypothesis at the beginning of the last century, proposing that longevity is determined by the metabolic rate (Pearl, 1928), the main explanation for aging has been oxidative damage due to free radicals, especially when comparative studies made clear that metabolic rate alone could not explain longevity (see Speakman & Selman, 2011). The oxidative theory of aging (Harman, 1956) proposes that aging is driven by the damage inflicted to cellular components by reactive oxygen species (ROS) produced by mitochondria in the course of respiration, and has evolved into the mitochondrial free radicals theory of aging pointing to this organelle as a key factor in aging (Harman, 1972;Miquel *et al.*, 1980), including some refinement (de Grey, 2004). Briefly, endogenous ROS (and some nitrogen reactive species derived from them) modify lipids, DNA and proteins, leading to functional and structural alterations of the cell, both directly and by modifications of the nuclear and mitochondrial genomic material (Pak *et al.*, 2003), the later especially exposed to ROS due to proximity and to the lack of histones (Yakes & Van, 1997).

ROS are formed in the inner mitochondrial membrane by transfer of electrons to molecular oxygen from complex I and III of the electron transport system (ETS) during the flow of electrons from reduced NADH and FADH generated by metabolism. At resting, about 0.1% of consumed oxygen (in spite of the erroneous figure of about 2%) (Fridovich, 2004) produces the highly reactive superoxide anion, enzymatically mutated to H_2O_2 and then to H_2O. It is important to note that the rate of ROS formation is not determined by the level of O_2 consumption, but by electrochemical potential of the inner membrane (generated by the H^+ gradient created by the ETS) and by the amount, efficiency and reduction level of complex I and III (Skulachev, 2004). This led to the "uncoupling to survive" theory of aging: H^+-permeating proteins at the inner mitochondrial membrane inhibit ROS production and are correspondingly enhanced in more long-lived species and in some life-extending manipulations (Brand, 2000).

To limit oxidative damage cells have developed enzymatic (superoxide dismutase, catalase,…) and non-enzymatic (glutathione) antioxidants to scavenge and metabolize radicals and have reduced the most ROS-sensitive components of proteins and lipids, i.e. methionine and cysteine contents of mitochondrial proteins and the number of double bonds of unsaturated fatty acids (lipid oxidation forms long lasting reactive carbonyl species which attack lipids, proteins and DNA) (Pamplona & Barja, 2011).

Although a causal link for mitochondrial radical production in aging has been generally accepted in the last three decades, the actual status is rather controversial. This view was supported by correlative studies between longevity and mitochondrial ROS production (Ku *et al.*, 1993;Sohal *et al.*, 1990). These reports did not controlled for phylogeny, body mass and metabolic rate level (Speakman, 2005), but posterior controlled studies confirmed the correlation and extended it to mitochondrial DNA oxidation (see Pamplona & Barja, 2011). On the other hand, initial studies with transgenic mice showed that inhibition or enhancement of endogenous antioxidant enzymes respectively shortens (Yamamoto *et al.*, 2005) or extends (Hu *et al.*, 2007;Schriner *et al.*, 2005) lifespan, but more recent studies did not reproduce this (Lapointe & Hekimi, 2010;Page *et al.*, 2010) or were ambiguous (Perez *et al.*, 2009). In addition, although mice with defective mitochondrial DNA repair enzymes show normal ROS production they age faster (Trifunovic *et al.*, 2005), supporting the idea that mitochondria alterations drive senescence even with normal oxidative damage.

The conflicting results of genetic experiments and the poor effects of antioxidants therapy in longevity (see 2.2) have been used to refute the free radical theory of aging (e.g., Lapointe & Hekimi, 2010;Perez *et al.*, 2009). However, it is likely that ROS production and not antioxidant defenses is the main factor determining longevity, as indicated by comparative and phylogenic studies on the correlation between longevity and antioxidants (Pamplona & Barja, 2011). This is supported by the finding that caloric restriction (CR) (the most successful life-extending manipulation) decreases mitochondrial ROS output and DNA oxidation (Migliaccio *et al.*, 1999), and by life extension in mice with genetic ablation of the protein p66shc (which produces mitochondrial ROS in response to insulin/IGF-1 signaling and stress factors) (e.g. Vendelbo & Nair, 2011).

It is clear that even if mitochondrial ROS were not the only cause of aging, is unlikely that oxidative stress and mitochondria do not participate in the aging process. Several modifications of the theory have focused on the mitochondrial DNA alterations induced by radicals (de Grey, 2004;Pamplona, 2011). Other authors have proposed that although high ROS concentration are detrimental, physiological levels protect from aging by increasing stress defense systems, so that non physiological increases of antioxidant activity can paradoxically accelerate aging (mitochondrial hormesis or mitohormesis, Tapia, 2006).

2.2 Antioxidative therapies

Given the large evidence linking oxidative stress with aging, the use of antioxidants has been a repeated approach in anti-aging research for decades. Even if aging itself is not due to oxidative damage, this approach could extend average life by reducing the mortality of a number of pathological conditions associated to oxidation.

The most frequently assayed antioxidants are present in vegetables and fruits, not only vitamins E (tocopherols), A (carotenes) and C, but also flavonoids (from tea and *Ginkgo biloba),* phenolic compounds (e.g. resveratrol in grapes), catechins and others. A number of artificial antioxidants have also been assayed (deprenyl, NDGA, PBN, thioproline,...). It must be noted that efficiency not only depends on their oxidant scavenging activity, but also in humans bioavailability factors (absorption, lifetime,...) so that animal studies are a requisite even for initial evaluation of the potential utility of an antioxidant.

Part of the initial studies in rodent models showed that some antioxidants could extend average and/or maximum lifespan (see Meydani *et al.*, 1998;Spindler, 2011). Unfortunately no measurements of the oxidative stress were performed in the initial reports, a requisite to confirm that a treatment lowers oxidative stress (Knasmuller *et al.*, 2008). Also, the effects could be due to a decrease in caloric intake of the animals and not by direct antioxidant effects, but when other authors controlled this variable still found an increase in mice lifespan (Bezlepkin *et al.*, 1996;Miquel & Economos, 1979). Recently, an extensive meta-analysis of the rodent lifespan studies reveals that a range of antioxidants (from chemicals such as deprenyl to naturally occurring compounds such as polyphenols) extend lifespan independently of the CR effect observed in other studies (Spindler, 2011).

In human, the available information is epidemiological or observational, including transversal studies about alimentary habits. Vitamins C, E and A operate synergistically against lipid peroxidation (see a review in Fusco *et al.*, 2007), and vitamin C can also regenerate vitamin E levels (Niki *et al.*, 1995). There is a negative correlation between plasmatic levels of antioxidants, mainly vitamin E, and incidence of cardiovascular diseases and some types of cancer (see Fusco *et al.*, 2007 and Hercberg *et al.*, 2009). This correlation is also present for fruits and vegetables intake (Genkinger *et al.*, 2004) and flavonoids and polyphenols (Manach *et al.*, 2005) and for other age-related diseases such as Alzheimer disease (Viña *et al.*, 2004) or diabetes (Czernichow *et al.*, 2006).

The life-extending effects of antioxidants in humans must be inferred from trials assessing the mortality of age-related pathologies. Contrary to the observational studies, randomized trials have not confirmed the expected decrease of mortality after long-term antioxidant treatment. In the trial SUVIMAX, with low doses of antioxidants, a reduction in mortality after 7.5 years of treatment was observed only in men (Hercberg *et al.*, 2004), which could be explained by a possible lower level of endogenous antioxidants compared to women, similar to a trial in a Chinese population with poor nutritive status (Blot *et al.*, 1993). Other large scale trials have not found beneficial effects of vitamin E supplementation (alone or with other antioxidants) on the incidence of cardiovascular and cancer mortality (Jacobs *et al.*, 2003;Lee *et al.*, 2005;Lonn *et al.*, 2005). It has been suggested that only individuals with low levels of antioxidant would benefice from these treatments, as found in lung cancer rates and selenium supplement (Reid *et al.*, 2002).

A concerning outcome of the controlled trials is the finding that supplementation can have detrimental effects in some groups (Hercberg *et al.*, 2009;Pham & Plakogiannis, 2005). Therefore, the official recommendation is an adequate intake of antioxidant-enriched aliments until more evidence makes clear if supplementation is safe (Fusco et al., 2007).

The discrepancy between the epidemiological and interventional studies could be due to limitations in the design of the studies. As pointed above, the "shotgun" approach of "flooding" the tissues with an antioxidant is likely inefficient or even detrimental *per se* (see 2.1) and it depends critically on the dosage (supplementation does not guarantee redox normalization (Knasmuller et al., 2008)) and the moment of application (in rodent models lifespan effects require initiation at late (PBN) or early age (vitamins mixture, NDGA) (Bezlepkin *et al.*, 1996;Spindler, 2011)). Also, it is likely that only certain combinations of antioxidants can block the redox network of multiple endogenous radicals (as shown in experimental models, (Rebrin *et al.*, 2005)). Last, the plasma measurements commonly used in human studies are not an unequivocal account of systemic redox (Knasmuller et al., 2008). On the other hand, the epidemiological results could be due to differences in lifestyles and genetic and environmental influences, all of them factors cancelled in randomized controlled trials.

A great interest has been raised by resveratrol, a polyphenol found in grapes and red wine. Resveratrol extends longevity in mice fed a high calorie diet (Baur *et al.*, 2006), but not under normal diet (Pearson *et al.*, 2008) and, relevant for human studies, improves in rodent models several markers for senescence and oxidative stress, mimicking caloric restriction (see Minor *et al.*, 2010a). Moreover, resveratrol also improves endothelial function in human patients with coronary heart disease (Lekakis *et al.*, 2005) (see also section 4).

The mechanism of action of resveratrol is however different to other antioxidants. Its main targets seem to be activation of sirtuins, deacetylases that activate transcription of antioxidant enzymes and promote mitogenesis (Vendelbo & Nair, 2011), although recent data indicate that its action on Sirt1 is indirect. It is noteworthy that Sirt1 and Sirt3 interact with metabolic pathways related to aging (see 4), working as sensors of energy availability (Guarente, 2000): upon low energy levels, increased NAD+ concentration activates Sirt1, which in turn operates on FOXO3, a transcription factor correlated with longevity in humans (Willcox *et al.*, 2008) that increases transcription of antioxidants in response to caloric restriction. Sirt3 is genetically linked to longevity in humans (Rose *et al.*, 2003), declines with age (Lanza *et al.*, 2008) and also activates FOXO3 (Sundaresan *et al.*, 2009).

A special mention is deserved by melatonin, the hormone released during the night by the pineal gland (see section 3). In addition to its chronobiological function it is one of the most potent antioxidants known. Melatonin not only acts as a direct antioxidant and inductor of the antioxidant enzymes, but it also generates, after oxidative cleavage, a series of derivatives with potent antioxidant activity (see Hardeland *et al.*, 2009). Melatonin accumulates in nuclei and mitochondria, protecting against oxidation of genetic material and it has been repeatedly shown to be an excellent antioxidant in conditions of oxidative stress, both in animals and humans (for recent reviews see Anisimov *et al.*, 2006 or Pozo *et al.*, 2010). Melatonin has also been shown in animal models to slow functional changes associated to aging in a number of systems (Camello-Almaraz *et al.*, 2008;Gomez-Pinilla *et al.*, 2008;Pascua *et al.*, 2011). More important, melatonin extends lifespan in more than 50% of rodent studies and has well established anticarcinogenic properties for mammary and colon cancer in animal models (Anisimov et al., 2006). Although to date there are no human mortality data in healthy individuals treated with melatonin, the results from clinical assays are promising. For example, a meta-analysis shows in human patients of solid tumors a decrease in risk of death at 1 year (Mills *et al.*, 2005), and numerous animal and human (clinical) studies support the potential of this hormone to limit cancer development (see a review in Karasek, 2004). Additionally, controlled trials in humans have shown the absence of toxicity and significant side effects (Singer *et al.*, 2003).

3. Hormonal replacement as antiaging therapy

The observation that several endocrine secretions decay with aging (sexual hormones, growth hormone (GH), melatonin and others (Pandi-Perumal *et al.*, 2008), laid the basis for attempts for hormonal replacement as antiaging therapy.

3.1 Melatonin

Melatonin, discovered 50 years ago, is a hormone synthesized by the pineal gland, retina, gastrointestinal tract and immune cells. Melatonin plasma levels follow a circadian rhythm: it is secreted by the pineal gland during the dark phase of the day, because light input into retinal cells activates nerve impulses to the suprachiasmatic nuclei of hypothalamus (SCN), which in turn suppresses the excitatory sympathetic input to the pineal gland and the release of melatonin. Thus, melatonin monitors the onset and duration of the dark phase, synchronizing the central circadian oscillator (SCN) and the peripheral organs with the environmental light-dark cycle, but is also involved in vasomotor control, sleep initiation,... (Pandi-Perumal et al., 2008). In humans the rhythmic secretion starts around the 6th month of age, peak levels are achieved at 4 - 7th years, melatonin concentration drops at puberty and diminishes gradually in old people (Karasek, 1999). Melatonin acts through plasma membrane and nuclear receptors and by interaction with intracellular signalling proteins and it has potent antioxidant properties (this aspect has been treated above).

The decline in melatonin secretion with age is accompanied by a progressive deterioration of the central circadian oscillator (Hofman & Swaab, 1994) and by sleep disruption, a feature of aging in humans (Neubauer, 1999). Although a meta-analysis did not find conclusive evidence that melatonin was effective to improve sleep parameters in patients with insomnia due to great discrepancies in pharmacological preparation, dose and time of treatment and measurements of melatonin and circadian parameters (Buscemi *et al.*, 2005), a more recent meta-analysis supports the effectiveness of exogenous melatonin in patients with delayed sleep phase disorder (van Geijlswijk *et al.*, 2010). The study found three requisites for optimal melatonin therapy: adequate dose (too low is inefficient, too high is hypnotic), administration 3-6 hours before the so-called dim light melatonin onset and choice of appropriate patients (with a delayed biological timing).

A recent improvement is a formulation that releases melatonin slowly in the gut after oral administration and increases its plasma concentration over the following 8-10 h (Circadin®, Neurim Pharmaceuticals, Israel), which has been approved by the European Medicines Evaluation Agency in June 2007 for the short-term treatment of primary insomnia. Several studies have shown its efficiency and safety for short-term treatment (3 weeks) of adults and old people (Luthringer *et al.*, 2009), including a double-blind, placebo-controlled randomized trial evaluating the short and long-term effects of Circadin (Wade *et al.*, 2010). Circadin also seems to improve blood pressure rhythms (Grossman *et al.*, 2006).

The effects of melatonin on sleep rhythm are due to its plasma membrane receptors (MT1 and MT2) in the suprachiasmatic nucleus. MT1 receptors inhibit firing of suprachiasmatic neurons and MT2 receptors entrain circadian rhythms and have phase-shifting effects (Hunt *et al.*, 2001). This finding lead to the design of specific agonists ramelteon (Rozerem®, Takeda Pharmaceuticals, Japan) and agomelatine (Valdoxan®, Servier and Novartis). Ramelteon, approved by the FDA (July 2005) for the treatment of insomnia, has been assayed for the treatment of primary insomnia in humans (Erman *et al.*, 2006). Although these studies found it effective and safe, the European Medicines Evaluation Agentcy found the efficacy of ramelteon insufficient for marketing authorization. Agomelatine binds to melatonin receptors but is also an antagonist of serotonin 5-HT2C receptors used to decrease anxiety and promote sleep (Lemoine *et al.*, 2007). Its efficacy, tolerability and safety have been assessed by several randomized, placebo and active-controlled studies (Kennedy & Emsley, 2006) and improves the disrupted sleep of depressed patients (Lemoine et al., 2007).

3.2 GH

The growth hormone (GH) and its key mediator insulin-like growth factor-I (IGF-I) regulate somatic growth and development, metabolism and body composition, but seems to be also related to aging. The pulsatile GH secretion shows an age-related decay after the high amplitude pulses of the postnatal and puberty stages (Finkelstein *et al.*, 1972), and correlates to aging-related changes in body composition (sarcopenia, osteopenia, increase in fat content,...) (Veldhuis *et al.*, 1995). This correlation, together with the fact that replacement therapy in GH deficient adults and elderly improves body composition, lipoprotein profile, exercise capacity and bone density (Rudman, 1985), elicited interest in the possible use of GH as antiaging therapy. However, a higher mortality has been found in patients critically ill treated with GH (Takala *et al.*, 1999) and in rodents and humans suffering high levels of GH (acromegaly) (Sheppard, 2005). This is in keeping with the increased lifespan of mutant mice with defects in GH/IGF-1 secretion/pathways (Bartke, 2003) and by some data on human lifespan (Suh *et al.*, 2008). Therefore, the clinical use of GH is only approved in US for treatment of GH deficiency, idiopathic short stature and HIV/AIDS.

3.3 Vitamin D

In addition to its key role in calcium homeostasis, there are evidences that vitamin D can influence longevity by decreasing the morbidity of age-related diseases, such as cancer or cardiovascular diseases, in addition to osteoporosis (not treated in this review). The active form of vitamin D3 (1,25(OH)2-cholecalciferol or calcitriol) binds to nuclear receptors (VDRs) to modulate the transcription of genes involved in systemic and intracellular Ca^{2+}

homeostasis and in cellular proliferation. The later are also due to fast, non genomic effects mediated by plasma membrane VDRs (Dusso *et al.*, 2005).

The main actions of vitamin D of interest as antiaging therapy are its anti-inflammatory and anti-cytokine effects in humans (shown in controlled trials (Schleithoff *et al.*, 2006)), and its ability to promote neuronal survival in different experimental models (Regulska *et al.*, 2006). In fact, human observational studies show a negative correlation of levels of vitamin D3 with cardiovascular disease (Zittermann *et al.*, 2005) (an inflammatory process), and with cognitive performance in elderly (Llewellyn *et al.*, 2009;Oudshoorn *et al.*, 2008). Additional support for vitamin D3 as antiaging treatment comes up from evidences that serum concentration of vitamin D decreases with age (Utiger, 1998) and its role in the control of cell cycle and apoptosis, which are altered in aging: calcitriol reduces proliferation of normal and cancer cells (Ylikomi *et al.*, 2002) and up-regulates apoptosis of cells damaged by redox stress and DNA alteration (Higami & Shimokawa, 2000).

The beneficial effects of vitamin D in age-associated diseases is expected to result in a prolongation of average lifespan. A study showed that vitamin D deprivation decreased the lifespan of male, but not female, rats (Thomas *et al.*, 1984). In humans, a recent meta-analysis of randomized trial showed a clear reduction in all-cause mortality in old individuals under vitamin D supplementation (Autier & Gandini, 2007). However, some reports have raised concerns with the safety of calcitriol supplementation (Stolzenberg-Solomon, 2009), although limitations in the design of the studies avoid definitive conclusions.

4. Caloric restriction

CR is the most robust non-genetic nutritional experimental intervention for slowing aging, and maintaining health and vitality in organisms ranging from budding yeast (*Sacharomyces cerevisiae*) to humans (Fontana *et al.*, 2010b). It is defined as a reduction of total macronutrient intake without causing malnutrition, with food intake reduced by 30-40% compared to *ad libitum* levels. Experiments involving CR in rodents in 1935 provided the first promise for modulation of lifespan (McCay *et al.*, 1935). Since then CR has been repeatedly proved to be effective in extending average and maximum lifespan and delaying the onset of age-associated pathologies in diverse species (for review see (Minor *et al.*, 2010a;Omodei & Fontana, 2011)). It was not until the 1990s that CR became widely viewed as a scientific model that could provide insights into the underlying mechanisms of aging and lifespan extension. The fact that CR significantly increased the average and maximum lifespan in many simpler eukaryotes, including the common model organisms used in aging research, *Drosophila melanogaster*, *Caenorhabditis elegans* and *Saccharomyces cerevisiae* pointed out that CR represents an evolutionarily conserved mechanism for modulating longevity and opened the possibility of using genetic tools in these models that helped to unveil intracellular pathways related to pro-longevity.

Alternative approaches to CR are a controlled reduction of a particular macronutrient of the diet (dietary restriction, DR) or temporal variations of food intake (intermittent fasting, IF). Particularly, protein restriction, PR, where a percentage of calories derived from protein is replaced by fat or carbohydrate, has been investigated in rodents and decreases in mitochondrial reactive oxygen species production and DNA and protein oxidative modifications have been reported (Ayala *et al.*, 2007), which could explain the increase in lifespan previously reported for PR (Leto *et al.*, 1976). Similar effects were obtained with reduction of the amino acid methionine (Naudi *et al.*, 2007), but they could not be replicated by restricting lipid intake alone (Sanz *et al.*, 2006a) or carbohydrate intake alone (Sanz *et al.*, 2006b). IF, a regimen of either alternate day fasting or fasting for a day after 2 days of feeding, both increases lifespan and delays or prevents some age-related diseases (reviewed in Mattson & Wan, 2005). However, CR is by now the most powerful nutritional intervention to prolong life.

4.1 Effects of caloric restriction

It is totally accepted that the effects of CR on lifespan and mortality in rodents increase linearly with the extent of the restriction until reaching approximately a 50-60% of restriction at which lifespan is negatively affected. In addition, the effect of CR on lifespan is stronger when initiated at weaning and weaker later in life (reviewed in (Fontana, 2009b;Speakman & Hambly, 2007;Speakman & Mitchell, 2011)). In fact, CR increases rather than decreases mortality if initiated in advanced age (Forster *et al.*, 2003). CR inhibits growth and body size after maturation and reduces body weight, as consequence of changes in the endocrine profile as discussed below. CR also inhibits fertility, especially in females, but there is an increase in their reproductive performance when they are subsequently returned to *ad libitum* feeding (Selesniemi *et al.*, 2008)

CR induces transcriptional alterations that are indicative of metabolic reprogramming, a change in how energy is generated and how fuel is utilized. A key metabolic change during CR is a shift from fat storage to fat utilization impacting stress signaling pathways and ROS production (Anderson & Weindruch, 2010). Immediately following food intake there was a period of endogenous fatty acid synthesis that was then followed by a period of prolonged fatty acid oxidation, which induces large changes in the respiratory quotient (RQ) (Speakman & Mitchell, 2011). In addition, during CR there is an increase in the AMP/ATP ratio which leads to the activation of the AMP-activated protein kinase (AMPK) that promotes fat oxidation increasing the transport of fatty acids into the mitochondrion. In fact, marked phosphorylation of AMPK has been found after long term CR (Edwards *et al.*, 2010). Because fatty acid substrates enter the electron transport chain predominantly via complex II rather than complex I, the main ROS generator is bypassed when the metabolism is switched predominantly to fatty acid oxidation. This might represent a mechanism minimizing oxidative stress under CR.

The hormonal profile of long-term CR is characterized by a suppression of the gonadal, thyroid and GH-insulin-like growth factor I (GH-IGF-I) axes, an increase in the insulin sensitivity and an increase in the daily peak levels of plasma corticosterone that takes part in successfully coping with stressors (Xiang & He, 2011). CR also results in decreased levels of leptin and increased blood concentration of ghrelin and adiponectin, a modulator of a number of metabolic processes appearing to have anti-inflammatory, anti-diabetic, and anti-atherogenic properties that seem to play an important role in life extension effect of CR (Chiba *et al.*, 2002;Lago *et al.*, 2007).

The reductions in IGF-I and insulin signaling that occur under CR have been suggested to be causally linked to the lifespan enhancing effects of CR. This is in part based on the observation that several rodent models that present mutations that modified insulin/GH/IGF-I signals, live longer than controls and there is considerable phenotypic overlap between long-lived mutant mice and normal mice on chronic CR. These models include, amongst others, *Prop-1* (Ames mice) and *pit-1* (Snell mice) mutant dwarf mice, GH receptor/binding protein homozygous knockout mice (*GHR/BP*$^{-/-}$ or GHRKO), insulin receptor substrate 1 knockout mice (*Irs1*$^{-/-}$)... Most of these mice have a body weight smaller than their normal siblings and present decreased levels of IGF-I , and increased sensibility to insulin (Chiba *et al.*, 2007), except *Irs1*$^{-/-}$ mice whose IGF-I levels are unchanged and show a mild but lifelong insulin resistance having increased lifespan and reduced markers of aging (Selman *et al.*, 2008). In GHRKO mice CR increased lifespan only in females and failed to further enhance the remarkable insulin sensitivity and the insulin signaling cascade in GHRKO mutants (Bonkowski *et al.*, 2006;Bonkowski *et al.*, 2009). These data imply that somatotropic signaling is critically important in mediating the effects of CR on lifespan and also support the notion that enhanced sensitivity to insulin plays a prominent role in the actions of CR and GH resistance on longevity. It was originally reported that long-term severe CR did not reduce serum IGF-I concentration or the IGF-I/IGF binding protein ratio in humans but total and free IGF-I concentrations were significantly lower in moderately protein-restricted individuals (Fontana *et al.*, 2008). In addition, it has been recently shown that CR for 4 years leads to reduced IGF-I serum levels in formerly obese women relative to normal-weight women eating *ad libitum* (Mitterberger *et al.*, 2011), which suggests that growth hormone/IGF-I axis is also important in the effects of CR in humans.

4.2 Caloric restriction in non-human primates

Most CR research on longevity in mammals has been performed in rodents, mainly in mice. However, studies designed to evaluate the effects of CR on species closer to humans are of great interest in order to translate the knowledge to humans. Two prospective investigations of the effects of CR on long-lived nonhuman primate species began nearly 25 years ago and are still under way. These studies (randomized controlled trials) revealed beneficial effects of CR on physiological functions and the retardation of disease. In the study conducted in the Wisconsin National Primate Research Center a recent report showed that animals on 30% of CR appeared subjectively younger than controls, the body weight was reduced and the age-related sarcopenia attenuated. Improvements in metabolic function (improved insulin sensitivity and glucose tolerance) and preservation of grey matter volume in subcortical regions were reported. In addition, there was a lower incidence of neoplasia, cardiovascular disease and type 2 diabetes mellitus. Survival analysis considering only age-related deaths revealed a significant effect of CR in increasing survival, but when assessing "all-cause" mortality CR did not provide a statistically significant lifespan increase (Colman *et al.*, 2009). In any case, the reduction of age-related diseases and the potential increase in longevity are promising. Data regarding CR-induced longevity from the National Institute of Aging's are not yet available, although a decrease in age-related diseases and beneficial effects on other physiological parameters have been provided (Mattison *et al.*, 2007).

4.3 Caloric restriction in humans

The studies about human responses to CR have some limitations that should be taken into account when interpreting the results. An important amount of data come from members of the CR Society International (www.calorierestriction.org) which has the mission to promote the use of CR in humans. In agreement with the research results from animal studies, voluntary CR in humans results in sustained beneficial effects on the major atherosclerosis risk factors, and has protective effect against obesity and insulin resistance. In addition, the CR society members have reduced circulating levels of insulin, PDGF, TGF-β and pro-inflammatory cytokines (reviewed in Fontana, 2009a). Nonetheless, despite high serum adiponectin and low inflammation, approximately 40% of CR individuals exhibited an exaggerated hyperglycemic response to a glucose load. This impaired glucose tolerance is associated with lower circulating levels of IGF-1, total testosterone, and triiodothyronine, which are typical adaptations to life-extending CR in rodents (Fontana *et al.*, 2010a). Assuming the importance of these findings, it should be noted that these volunteers are clearly a self selected population and this is not a randomized controlled trial.

There is a randomized controlled trial for the effects of CR on humans, and that is the CALERIE (Comprehensive Assessment of the Long term Effects of Reducing Intake of Energy) trial sponsored by the NIA in the USA. In the phase 1 of the trial all the studies have been performed in non-obese healthy but overweight subjects, therefore it is difficult to separate beneficial effects due to the weight loss or to CR. The most relevant findings of phase 1 trials were the reduced body weight and total fat mass, the reduced fasting levels of insulin, leptin and T3 and the increased insulin sensitivity. Activity energy expenditure and core body temperature were decreased in response to the CR. In addition, CR decreased cardiovascular risk, increased some antioxidant defenses and reduced markers of inflammation (reviewed in (Speakman & Hambly, 2007)). Interestingly, "in vitro" studies utilizing CR human serum to examine effects on markers of health and longevity in cultured cells resulted in increased stress resistance and an up-regulation of genes (sirt1 and PGC1α) proposed to be indicators of increased longevity (Allard *et al.*, 2008). In the phase 2 trial of the study, a two-year CR period was selected to attempt to provide for a sustained period of weight stability following weight loss that would more accurately unveil the effects of CR in humans (Rickman *et al.*, 2011). Whether CR extends life in humans and the magnitude of this potential effect also remain unclear and far for been resolved

4.4 Intracellular pathways mediating CR effects

For many individuals, the hardships of maintaining a CR lifestyle are too great to justify the improved health profile and potential life-extension benefits. Nevertheless, identifying the genetic and physiological mediators of CR could aid in the discovery of compounds/treatments that would act on those pathways, thereby mimicking the positive aspects of CR without imposed food restriction.

TOR, a serine/threonine protein kinase that belongs to the family of phosphoinositide-3-kinase (PI3K)-related kinases (PIKK), is the primary candidate involved in the regulation of lifespan in animals under CR. Its name, Target Of Rapamycin, indicates that it mediates the effects of rapamycin, an antifungal and immunosuppressant agent that inhibits TOR. In mammalian cells, TOR participates in the mammalian complex 1 (mTORC1) that is sensitive to rapamycin and controls cell size, proliferation and lifespan via a variety of downstream pathways. mTORC1 is a homodimer that has four components in addition to the Serine/Threonine kinase mTOR: Raptor, mLST8, PRAS40 and Deptor. Raptor binds mTOR and recruits the downstream kinase substrates (S6K and 4E-BP) in a manner that enables their phosphorylation by the mTOR catalytic domain. Other proteins that participate in TORC1 regulation are Tuberous Sclerosis Complex proteins TSC1 and TSC2, with a GTPase-activating (GAP) domain, and the Ras-like small GTPase RHEb, the preferred substrate of the TSC2 GAP activity. TSC complex inhibits TOR signaling as the result of its ability to deactivate Rheb (reduced GTP/GDP) (reviewed in Kapahi *et al.*, 2010).

TORC1 integrates responses to growth factor stimulation, changes in energy status, nutrients, oxygen levels and various types of stress. Thus growth factors like IGF and insulin, via Akt, directly phosphorylate several sites on TSC2, which decrease the inhibitory activity of TSC and the increase TORC1 activity. A drop in the cell energy content, as that induced by glucose deprivation, is reflected in the rise of the AMP/ATP ratio that triggers AMP-dependent activation of AMPK. In turn, AMPK reduces the activity of TORC1 by direct phosphorylation and stimulation of Tsc2 activity and inhibition of Raptor. Amino-acid regulation is exerted predominantly through Rag GTPases (RagA, RagB, RagC, and RagD) that sense amino acid levels. In the presence of amino acids the complex interacts with raptor and promotes TORC1 through relocalization to RHEB rich cellular compartments. Conversely, deprivation of amino acid inhibits mTORC1 with leucine or arginine withdrawal mimicking total amino acid deprivation. Amongst the environmental stresses to which cells are exposed, TORC1 also senses hypoxia. Low levels of oxygen, through stabilization of HIF1α induce the transcription of hypoxic response genes, mostly REDD1 that inhibits TORC1 activity by a TSC2-dependent mechanism. In addition, hypoxia reduces ATP levels, and then it controls TORC1 through AMPK. Genotoxic stress represses TORC1 activity through p53-mediated increased expression of PTEN, TSC2 and REDD1 (reviewed in Kapahi *et al.*, 2010;Ma & Blenis, 2009;Speakman & Mitchell, 2011).

TORC1 controls cell growth maintaining the adequate balance between anabolic processes such as protein synthesis and catabolic processes like autophagy. As commented before, S6K and 4E-BP1 are the best-known substrates of TORC1 and through them TORC1 regulates protein synthesis by regulating the activity of the translational machinery and also specifically controlling the translation of subset of mRNAs that are thought to promote cell growth and proliferation (Ma & Blenis, 2009). The limiting step of protein synthesis is translation initiation. The recruitment of the small ribosomal subunit to mRNA requires the participation of the translation initiation factor 4F (eIF4F) complex. 4E-BP binds eIF4E, a component of this complex, and prevents translation initiation. When hyperphosphorylated by mTORC1, 4E-BP1 dissociates from eIF4E, allowing the initiation of translation. Evidence suggests that S6Ks modulate the functions of translation initiation factors during protein synthesis and also coordinate the regulation of ribosome biogenesis, which in turn drives efficient translation (see for review (Ma & Blenis, 2009)). S6K1 interacts back with the insulin signaling pathway by phosphorylating the insulin receptor substrates IRS1 and IRS2, which seems related to insulin resistance. Consistent with the important role of S6K on mediating mTOR induced lifespan extension, $S6K1^{-}/^{-}$ mice have gene expression profiles similar to those of CR mice, and females have extended longevity with evidence of fewer age-related diseases (Selman *et al.*, 2009).

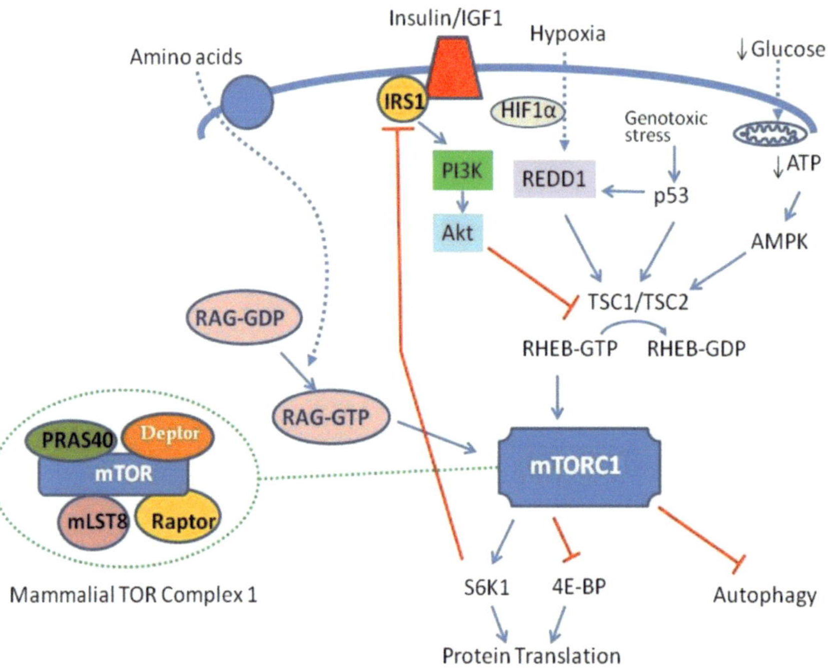

In mammalial cells mTORC1 receives positive inputs from RHEB-GTP, but it is inhibited when RHEB is bound mainly to GDP. TSC1/TSC2 complex, through its GTPase-activating domain favors GDP-bound RHEB and then it mediates mTORC1 inhibition. Several extracellular and intracellular pathways activate (by phosphorylation) TSC complex, such as the ATP sensor AMPK that is stimulated when cellular energy decreases, the hypoxic response gene REDD1 that senses hypoxia, and p53 that senses genotoxic stress. TSC complex is inhibited by Akt-mediated phosphorylation, which results in mTORC1 activation. An important pathway for Akt activation is the insulin/IGF signaling. The amino acid level in the cell controls the state of Rag GTPases. The presence of amino acids enhances Rag-GTP and activates mTORC1 through relocalization to RHEB rich cellular compartments. Activation of mTORC1 increases mRNA translation and protein synthesis through phosphorylation of S6K1 and 4E-BP and inhibits autophagy, which results in cell growth and also in senescence. Inhibition of mTORC1 increases autophagy, reduces protein synthesis and cell grothw/differentiation decreasing senescence and extending lifespan.

Fig. 1. mTORC1 and insulin/IGF1 signalling and lifespan.

Accumulating evidence demonstrates that longevity pathways, including mTOR, interact with the macroautophagic process. Autophagy is a lysosome-mediated degradative process of eukaryotic cells to digest their own constituents during development or starvation. Macroautophagy (hereafter referred as autophagy) is a type of autophagy that involves the formation of subcellular double membrane-bound structures called autophagosomes to sequester cytoplasmatic materials and deliver them into lysosomes for breakdown by acid hydrolases. According to the current knowledge, the first signalling component downstream of mTOR in the autophagy pathway in mammals is ULK1, a serine/threonine kinase. ULK1 plays a key role at the nucleation (the early event when membrane structures are initiated) and formation of the preautophagosome structures. mTOR-induced ULK1 phosphorylation avoids the recruitment of proteins to the autophagosome membranes inhibiting downstream events essential for autophagy (reviewed in (Jung *et al.*, 2010)).

Sirtuins are a family of NAD+-dependent protein deacetylases that exert multiple cellular functions by interacting with, and deacetylating a wide range of signaling molecules, transcription factors, histones and enzymes (Yamamoto *et al.*, 2007). In mammals, the family is represented by seven members (SIRT1-7) with different cellular locations. Several studies have demonstrated that CR regulates sirtuin system and that a functional sirtuin system is required for lifespan extension to occur (Bamps *et al.*, 2009;Cohen *et al.*, 2004). Thus, CR does not have any effects of lifespan extension in SIRT1 deficient mice (Boily *et al.*, 2008). By contrast, elevation of SIRT1 expression results in a phenotype resembling that of caloric restriction (Bordone *et al.*, 2007). In humans SIRT1 gene expression also appears to be responsive to caloric restriction (reviewed in (Kelly, 2010)). SIRT1 elicits anti-senescence activity by targeting a wide range of protein substrates that are critically involved in regulating key cellular processes, such as oxidative stress, DNA damage, mitochondrial biogenesis and autophagy. Targets for SIRT1-mediated deacetylation include p53, NFkB, PGC-1a (peroxisome proliferator-activated receptor-c coactivator 1a], eNOS, mTOR and FoxOs. It is also of great importance the interaction of SIRT1 with LKB/AMPK. While acute activation of the LKB1/AMPK pathway confers adaption to stress, sustained stimulation of this pathway leads to irreversible senescence. SIRT1-mediated deacetilation of LKB, and consequent ubiquintination and degradation serves to prevent persistent AMPK signaling, reinforcing the anti-age effects of SIRT1 (reviewed in (Wang *et al.*, 2011)).

4.5 Therapies based on caloric restriction

The knowledge of the intracellular pathways related to aging led to the development of drugs, named generically caloric restriction mimetics (CRM) that replicate the effects of CR. These drugs targets the main pathways affected by CR: insulin/IGF1, mTOR, and sirtuins.

4.5.1 Insulin/IGF1 pathway

The firts CRM used was 2-deoxy-D-glucose (2DG), a compound that inhibits glycolisis. In keeping with the effects of CR, 2DG in rodents reduced body temperature, body weight and circulating glucose and insulin and increased glucocorticoids and heat-shock proteins. In addition, reduced tumors and increased stress resistance to neurotoxins and cold shock (Le Couteur *et al.*, 2011;Minor *et al.*, 2010a). Despite of these findings, long-term administration of 0.4% 2DG did not enhanced lifespan but increased mortality due to cardiac toxicity and adrenal tumors (Minor *et al.*, 2010b), which indicates that this drug could have therapeutic value for short-term treatment but it would not be indicated for aging interventions.

The biguanide antidiabetic drug metformin has been shown to molecularly recapitulate most of the pro-longevity effects occurring upon CR (Dhahbi *et al.*, 2005) and to suppress S6K1 activity in cultured proliferating epithelial cells (Vazquez-Martin *et al.*, 2009). In keeping with these effects, it has been reported that chronic metformin treatment of mice from different strains predisposed to high incidence of mammary tumors decreased body temperature, increased mean and maximal lifespan and postponed tumors and age-related switch-off of estrous function. These effects were dependent on the gender and the strain of mice (reviewed in (Anisimov, 2010)). In humans a retrospective study has reported an impressive 56% decrease in breast cancer risk among diabetic receiving metformin (Bodmer *et al.*, 2010), which together with the animal studies suggest that metformin could increase lifespan in humans. Metformin treatment phenocopies the effects of amino acid-deprivation on mTORC1, suggesting that this drug may inhibit mTORC1 via modulation of Rag signaling (Kalender *et al.*, 2010). The effects of metformin on mTOR and its effector S6K1 can also be due to the well recognized activation of AMPK by the drug (Hardie, 2011), which as described above, inhibits mTORC1. Other bioguanides such as buformin and phenformin have shown promising results in rodent tumor suppression, but they have to be withdrawn from the clinical practice due to association with lactic acidosis (Minor *et al.*, 2010a).

4.5.2 mTOR pathway

Rapamycin, a macrolide antibiotic with antitumor and immunosuppressant actions, selectively and effectively inhibits mTORC1 as CR does, as discussed above. The inhibitory action of rapamycin on TOR signaling requires the formation of the rapamycin/FKBP12 complex, which interferes with the proper interaction between raptor and mTOR, rather than or in addition to a more direct inhibition of mTOR catalytic activity. Many roles of mTORC1 on cell growth and survival have been unveiled by the use of rapamycin. Rapamycin is, by now, the pharmacological treatment that more resembles CR-induced lifespan extension. One of the most important contributions to this field has been the report of the National Institute on Aging Intervention Testing Program (ITP) showing that rapamycin supplementation late in life (20 months of age) induced a significant mean lifespan extension in both male and female mice fed a standard diet. This study was conducted in three different sites in the USA and used genetically heterogenous mice to avoid genotype-specific effects on disease susceptibility. According to this study, rapamycin may extend lifespan by postponing death from cancer, by retarding mechanisms of ageing, or both (Harrison *et al.*, 2009). Rapamycin treatment increases autophagy, reduces cell senescence and have anti-inflammatory as well as antitumor effects. In addition rapamycin and rapamycin analogs (rapalogs) ameliorate age-related diseases such as cancer, metabolic syndrome, neurodegenerative and cardiovascular diseases (reviewed in (Sharp & Richardson, 2011)).

4.5.3 Sirtuin pathway

Resveratrol, in addition to its antioxidant properties, has been reported to mediate yeast lifespan extension through the activation of the sirtuin family of deacetylases (Howitz *et al.*, 2003). This led to the idea that resveratrol might act as a CRM, and was supported by results on rodents showing impressive protection against age-related diseases including neurodegeneration, cancer, cardiovascular diseases and obesity (Markus & Morris, 2008). Regarding the targets of resveratrol, biochemical studies indicate that resveratrol may not activate sirtuins directly but thorugh activation of AMPK (Hwang *et al.*, 2009). Although in mice fed with a high fat diet resveratrol induces lifespan extension and its commonly associated features (increased insulin sensitivity and AMPK activity, reduced IGF-I levels, ...) (Baur *et al.*, 2006), there are no reports of increased lifespan in healthy mammals. This may indicate that resveratrol induces effects by targeting intracellular pathways activated by CR without slowing aging. The effects of resveratrol have led to development of more potent SIRT1 activators. These newly synthesized compounds (by a pharmaceutical biotechnology company called Sirtris Pharmaceuticals) are potent small-molecule activators of SIRT1 that are structurally unrelated to natural polyphenols. There are promising data regarding the effects of these compounds in mouse models and some of them are in phase II clinical trials for type 2 diabetes, opening an approach for other age-related diseases (reviewed in Camins *et al.*, 2010).

5. Conclusion

The evolution of our understanding of the biological basis of aging has focused antiaging research on antioxidant, metabolic and hormonal replacement therapies. Although beneficial effects of antioxidant therapies are not in doubt, controlled trials have revealed poor efficiency for hormonal and antioxidant treatments. Thus, more controlled and properly designed trials are needed to determine the potential of these approaches. The recent advances in knowledge about metabolic signalling pathways involved in the aging process especially in mTOR/Insulin/IGF-1 pathway that mediate the beneficial effects of CR, have opened new venues for the development of effective antiaging or CRM treatments. The results reported for rapamycin treatment starting later in life are of great interest in terms of the potential use of this inhibitor of mTORC1 for slowing aging and probably its combination with resveratrol, an stimulator of Sirt1 that improves age-related diseases without increasing lifespan in mammals, will render a more potent and efficient treatment. In addition, future research in how the different pathways integrate and interact to mediate CR effects will provide us with new pharmacological interventions that can slow the process of aging. An important issue in the prescription of these drugs to healthy humans is that aging is not recognized as a condition to be treated. Thus, the anti-aging drugs should be introduced in human if they affect disease, and later on, when showed effective the day will come when they become anti-aging drugs.

6. Acknowledgments

Financial support from BFU2011-24365, RETICEF (RD06/0013/1012), Junta de Extremadura (GR10009) and FEDER.

7. References

Allard, J.S., Heilbronn, L.K., Smith, C., Hunt, N.D., Ingram, D.K., Ravussin, E. & de, C.R. (2008). In vitro cellular adaptations of indicators of longevity in response to treatment with serum collected from humans on calorie restricted diets. *PLoS One* Vol.3, No.9, (2008), pp. e3211

Anderson, R.M. & Weindruch, R. (2010). Metabolic reprogramming, caloric restriction and aging. *Trends Endocrinol Metab* Vol.21, No.3, (March 2010), pp. 134-141

Anisimov, V.N. (2010). Metformin for aging and cancer prevention. *Aging (Albany NY)* Vol.2, No.11, (November 2010), pp. 760-774

Anisimov, V.N., Popovich, I.G., Zabezhinski, M.A., Anisimov, S.V., Vesnushkin, G.M. & Vinogradova, I.A. (May 2006). Melatonin as antioxidant, geroprotector and anticarcinogen. *Biochim Biophys Acta* Vol.1757, No.5-6, (May 2006), pp. 573-589

Autier, P. & Gandini, S. (2007). Vitamin D supplementation and total mortality: a meta-analysis of randomized controlled trials. *Arch Intern Med* Vol.167, No.16, (September 2007), pp. 1730-1737

Ayala, V., Naudi, A., Sanz, A., Caro, P., Portero-Otin, M., Barja, G. & Pamplona, R. (2007). Dietary protein restriction decreases oxidative protein damage, peroxidizability index, and mitochondrial complex I content in rat liver. *J Gerontol A Biol Sci Med Sci* Vol.62, No.4, (April 2007), pp. 352-360

Bamps, S., Wirtz, J., Savory, F.R., Lake, D. & Hope, I.A. (2009). The Caenorhabditis elegans sirtuin gene, sir-2.1, is widely expressed and induced upon caloric restriction. *Mech Ageing Dev* Vol.130, No.11-12, (November 2009), pp. 762-770

Bartke, A. (2003). Can growth hormone (GH) accelerate aging? Evidence from GH-transgenic mice. *Neuroendocrinology* Vol.78, No.4, (October 2003), pp. 210-216

Baur, J.A., Pearson, K.J., Price, N.L., Jamieson, H.A., Lerin, C., Kalra, A., Prabhu, V.V., Allard, J.S., Lopez-Lluch, G., Lewis, K., Pistell, P.J., Poosala, S., Becker, K.G., Boss, O., Gwinn, D., Wang, M., Ramaswamy, S., Fishbein, K.W., Spencer, R.G., Lakatta, E.G., Le, C.D., Shaw, R.J., Navas, P., Puigserver, P., Ingram, D.K., de, C.R. & Sinclair, D.A. (2006). Resveratrol improves health and survival of mice on a high-calorie diet. *Nature* Vol.444, No.7117, (November 2006), pp. 337-342

Bezlepkin, V.G., Sirota, N.P. & Gaziev, A.I. (1996). The prolongation of survival in mice by dietary antioxidants depends on their age by the start of feeding this diet. *Mech Ageing Dev* Vol.92, No.2-3, (December 1996), pp. 227-234

Blagosklonny, M.V. (2010). Why human lifespan is rapidly increasing: solving "longevity riddle" with "revealed-slow-aging" hypothesis. *Aging (Albany NY)* Vol.2, No.4, (April 2010), pp. 177-182

Blot, W.J., Li, J.Y., Taylor, P.R., Guo, W., Dawsey, S., Wang, G.Q., Yang, C.S., Zheng, S.F., Gail, M., Li, G.Y. & . (1993). Nutrition intervention trials in Linxian, China: supplementation with specific vitamin/mineral combinations, cancer incidence, and disease-specific mortality in the general population. *J Natl Cancer Inst* Vol.85, No.18, (September 1993), pp. 1483-1492

Bodmer, M., Meier, C., Krahenbuhl, S., Jick, S.S. & Meier, C.R. (2010). Long-term metformin use is associated with decreased risk of breast cancer. *Diabetes Care* Vol.33, No.6, (June 2010), pp. 1304-1308

Boily, G., Seifert, E.L., Bevilacqua, L., He, X.H., Sabourin, G., Estey, C., Moffat, C., Crawford, S., Saliba, S., Jardine, K., Xuan, J., Evans, M., Harper, M.E. & McBurney, M.W. (2008). SirT1 regulates energy metabolism and response to caloric restriction in mice. *PLoS One* Vol.3, No.3, (2008), pp. e1759

Bonkowski, M.S., Dominici, F.P., Arum, O., Rocha, J.S., Al Regaiey, K.A., Westbrook, R., Spong, A., Panici, J., Masternak, M.M., Kopchick, J.J. & Bartke, A. (2009). Disruption of growth hormone receptor prevents calorie restriction from improving insulin action and longevity. *PLoS One* Vol.4, No.2, (2009), pp. e4567

Bonkowski, M.S., Rocha, J.S., Masternak, M.M., Al Regaiey, K.A. & Bartke, A. (2006). Targeted disruption of growth hormone receptor interferes with the beneficial actions of calorie restriction. *Proc Natl Acad Sci U S A* Vol.103, No.20, (May 2006), pp. 7901-7905

Bordone, L., Cohen, D., Robinson, A., Motta, M.C., van, V.E., Czopik, A., Steele, A.D., Crowe, H., Marmor, S., Luo, J., Gu, W. & Guarente, L. (2007). SIRT1 transgenic mice show phenotypes resembling calorie restriction. *Aging Cell* Vol.6, No.6, (Dec. 2007), pp. 759-767

Brand, M.D. (2000). Uncoupling to survive? The role of mitochondrial inefficiency in ageing. *Exp Gerontol* Vol.35, No.6-7, (September 2000), pp. 811-820

Buscemi, N., Vandermeer, B., Hooton, N., Pandya, R., Tjosvold, L., Hartling, L., Baker, G., Klassen, T.P. & Vohra, S. (2005). The efficacy and safety of exogenous melatonin for primary sleep disorders. A meta-analysis. *J Gen Intern Med* Vol.20, No.12, (December 2005), pp. 1151-1158

Camello-Almaraz, C., Gomez-Pinilla, P.J., Pozo, M.J. & Camello, P.J. (2008). Age-related alterations in Ca2+ signals and mitochondrial membrane potential in exocrine cells are prevented by melatonin. *J Pineal Res* Vol.45, No.2, (September 2008), pp. 191-198

Camins, A., Sureda, F.X., Junyent, F., Verdaguer, E., Folch, J., Pelegri, C., Vilaplana, J., Beas-Zarate, C. & Pallas, M. (2010). Sirtuin activators: designing molecules to extend life span. *Biochim Biophys Acta* Vol.1799, No.10-12, (October 2010), pp. 740-749

Chiba, T., Yamaza, H., Higami, Y. & Shimokawa, I. (2002). Anti-aging effects of caloric restriction: Involvement of neuroendocrine adaptation by peripheral signaling. *Microsc Res Tech* Vol.59, No.4, (November 2002), pp. 317-324

Chiba, T., Yamaza, H. & Shimokawa, I. (2007). Role of insulin and growth hormone/insulin-like growth factor-I signaling in lifespan extension: rodent longevity models for studying aging and calorie restriction. *Curr Genomics* Vol.8, No.7, (Nov. 2007), pp. 423-428

Cohen, H.Y., Miller, C., Bitterman, K.J., Wall, N.R., Hekking, B., Kessler, B., Howitz, K.T., Gorospe, M., de, C.R. & Sinclair, D.A. (2004). Calorie restriction promotes mammalian cell survival by inducing the SIRT1 deacetylase. *Science* Vol.305, No.5682, (July 2004), pp. 390-392

Colman, R.J., Anderson, R.M., Johnson, S.C., Kastman, E.K., Kosmatka, K.J., Beasley, T.M., Allison, D.B., Cruzen, C., Simmons, H.A., Kemnitz, J.W. & Weindruch, R. (2009). Caloric restriction delays disease onset and mortality in rhesus monkeys. *Science* Vol.325, No.5937, (July 2009), pp. 201-204

Czernichow, S., Couthouis, A., Bertrais, S., Vergnaud, A.C., Dauchet, L., Galan, P. & Hercberg, S. (2006). Antioxidant supplementation does not affect fasting plasma glucose in the Supplementation with Antioxidant Vitamins and Minerals (SU.VI.MAX) study in France: association with dietary intake and plasma concentrations. *Am J Clin Nutr* Vol.84, No.2, (August 2006), pp. 395-399

de Grey, A.D. (2004). Mitochondria in homeotherm aging: will detailed mechanisms consistent with the evidence now receive attention? *Aging Cell* Vol.3, No.2, (April 2004), pp. 77

Dhahbi, J.M., Mote, P.L., Fahy, G.M. & Spindler, S.R. (2005). Identification of potential caloric restriction mimetics by microarray profiling. *Physiol Genomics* Vol.23, No.3, (November 2005), pp. 343-350

Dusso, A.S., Brown, A.J. & Slatopolsky, E. (2005). Vitamin D. *Am J Physiol Renal Physiol* Vol.289, No.1, (July 2005), pp. F8-28

Edwards, A.G., Donato, A.J., Lesniewski, L.A., Gioscia, R.A., Seals, D.R. & Moore, R.L. (2010). Life-long caloric restriction elicits pronounced protection of the aged myocardium: a role for AMPK. *Mech Ageing Dev* Vol.131, No.11-12, (Nov. 2010), pp. 739-742

Erman, M., Seiden, D., Zammit, G., Sainati, S. & Zhang, J. (2006). An efficacy, safety, and dose-response study of Ramelteon in patients with chronic primary insomnia. *Sleep Med* Vol.7, No.1, (January 2006), pp. 17-24

Finkelstein, J.W., Roffwarg, H.P., Boyar, R.M., Kream, J. & Hellman, L. (1972). Age-related change in the twenty-four-hour spontaneous secretion of growth hormone. *J Clin Endocrinol Metab* Vol.35, No.5, (November 1972), pp. 665-670

Fontana, L. (2009b). The scientific basis of caloric restriction leading to longer life. *Curr Opin Gastroenterol* Vol.25, No.2, (March 2009b), pp. 144-150

Fontana, L. (2009a). The scientific basis of caloric restriction leading to longer life. *Curr Opin Gastroenterol* Vol.25, No.2, (March 2009a), pp. 144-150

Fontana, L., Klein, S. & Holloszy, J.O. (2010a). Effects of long-term calorie restriction and endurance exercise on glucose tolerance, insulin action, and adipokine production. *Age (Dordr)* Vol.32, No.1, (March 2010a), pp. 97-108

Fontana, L., Partridge, L. & Longo, V.D. (2010b). Extending healthy life span--from yeast to humans. *Science* Vol.328, No.5976, (April 2010b), pp. 321-326

Fontana, L., Weiss, E.P., Villareal, D.T., Klein, S. & Holloszy, J.O. (2008). Long-term effects of calorie or protein restriction on serum IGF-1 and IGFBP-3 concentration in humans. *Aging Cell* Vol.7, No.5, (October 2008), pp. 681-687

Forster, M.J., Morris, P. & Sohal, R.S. (2003). Genotype and age influence the effect of caloric intake on mortality in mice. *FASEB J* Vol.17, No.6, (April 2003), pp. 690-692

Fridovich, I. (2004). Mitochondria: are they the seat of senescence? *Aging Cell* Vol.3, No.1, (February 2004), pp. 13-16

Fusco, D., Colloca, G., Lo Monaco, M.R. & Cesari, M. (2007). Effects of antioxidant supplementation on the aging process. *Clin Interv Aging* Vol.2, No.3, (2007),377-387

Genkinger, J.M., Platz, E.A., Hoffman, S.C., Comstock, G.W. & Helzlsouer, K.J. (2004). Fruit, vegetable, and antioxidant intake and all-cause, cancer, and cardiovascular disease mortality in a community-dwelling population in Washington County, Maryland. *Am J Epidemiol* Vol.160, No.12, (December 2004), pp. 1223-1233

Gomez-Pinilla, P.J., Gomez, M.F., Sward, K., Hedlund, P., Hellstrand, P., Camello, P.J., Andersson, K.E. & Pozo, M.J. (2008). Melatonin restores impaired contractility in aged guinea pig urinary bladder. *J Pineal Res* Vol.44, No.4, (May 2008), pp. 416-425

Grossman, E., Laudon, M., Yalcin, R., Zengil, H., Peleg, E., Sharabi, Y., Kamari, Y., Shen-Orr, Z. & Zisapel, N. (2006). Melatonin reduces night blood pressure in patients with nocturnal hypertension. *Am J Med* Vol.119, No.10, (October 2006), pp. 898-902

Guarente, L. (2000). Sir2 links chromatin silencing, metabolism, and aging. *Genes Dev* Vol.14, No.9, (May 2000), pp. 1021-1026

Hardeland, R., Tan, D.X. & Reiter, R.J. (2009). Kynuramines, metabolites of melatonin and other indoles: the resurrection of an almost forgotten class of biogenic amines. *J Pineal Res* Vol.47, No.2, (September 2009), pp. 109-126

Hardie, D.G. (2011). Sensing of energy and nutrients by AMP-activated protein kinase. *Am J Clin Nutr* Vol.93, No.4, (April 2011), pp. 891S-6

Harman, D. (1956). Aging: a theory based on free radical and radiation chemistry. *J Gerontol* Vol.11, No.3, (July 1956), pp. 298-300

Harman, D. (1972). The biologic clock: the mitochondria? *J Am Geriatr Soc* Vol.20, No.4, (April 1972), pp. 145-147

Harrison, D.E., Strong, R., Sharp, Z.D., Nelson, J.F., Astle, C.M., Flurkey, K., Nadon, N.L., Wilkinson, J.E., Frenkel, K., Carter, C.S., Pahor, M., Javors, M.A., Fernandez, E. & Miller, R.A. (2009). Rapamycin fed late in life extends lifespan in genetically heterogeneous mice. *Nature* Vol.460, No.7253, (July 2009), pp. 392-395

Hercberg, S., Czernichow, S. & Galan, P. (2009). Tell me what your blood beta-carotene level is, I will tell you what your health risk is! The viewpoint of the SUVIMAX researchers. *Ann Nutr Metab* Vol.54, No.4, (2009), pp. 310-312

Hercberg, S., Galan, P., Preziosi, P., Bertrais, S., Mennen, L., Malvy, D., Roussel, A.M., Favier, A. & Briancon, S. (2004). The SU.VI.MAX Study: a randomized, placebo-controlled trial of the health effects of antioxidant vitamins and minerals. *Arch Intern Med* Vol.164, No.21, (November 2004), pp. 2335-2342

Higami, Y. & Shimokawa, I. (2000). Apoptosis in the aging process. *Cell Tissue Res* Vol.301, No.1, (July 2000), pp. 125-132

Hofman, M.A. & Swaab, D.F. (1994). Alterations in circadian rhythmicity of the vasopressin-producing neurons of the human suprachiasmatic nucleus (SCN) with aging. *Brain Res* Vol.651, No.1-2, (July 1994), pp. 134-142

Howitz, K.T., Bitterman, K.J., Cohen, H.Y., Lamming, D.W., Lavu, S., Wood, J.G., Zipkin, R.E., Chung, P., Kisielewski, A., Zhang, L.L., Scherer, B. & Sinclair, D.A. (2003). Small molecule activators of sirtuins extend Saccharomyces cerevisiae lifespan. *Nature* Vol.425, No.6954, (September 2003), pp. 191-196

Hu, D., Cao, P., Thiels, E., Chu, C.T., Wu, G.Y., Oury, T.D. & Klann, E. (2007). Hippocampal long-term potentiation, memory, and longevity in mice that overexpress mitochondrial superoxide dismutase. *Neurobiol Learn Mem* Vol.87, No.3, (March 2007), pp. 372-384

Hunt, A.E., Al-Ghoul, W.M., Gillette, M.U. & Dubocovich, M.L. (2001). Activation of MT(2) melatonin receptors in rat suprachiasmatic nucleus phase advances the circadian clock. *Am J Physiol Cell Physiol* Vol.280, No.1, (January 2001), pp. C110-C118

Hwang, J.T., Kwon, D.Y. & Yoon, S.H. (2009). AMP-activated protein kinase: a potential target for the diseases prevention by natural occurring polyphenols. *N Biotechnol* Vol.26, No.1-2, (October 2009), pp. 17-22

Jacobs, E.J., Connell, C.J., Chao, A., McCullough, M.L., Rodriguez, C., Thun, M.J. & Calle, E.E. (2003). Multivitamin use and colorectal cancer incidence in a US cohort: does timing matter? *Am J Epidemiol* Vol.158, No.7, (October 2003), pp. 621-628

Jung, C.H., Ro, S.H., Cao, J., Otto, N.M. & Kim, D.H. (2010). mTOR regulation of autophagy. *FEBS Lett* Vol.584, No.7, (April 2010), pp. 1287-1295

Kalender, A., Selvaraj, A., Kim, S.Y., Gulati, P., Brule, S., Viollet, B., Kemp, B.E., Bardeesy, N., Dennis, P., Schlager, J.J., Marette, A., Kozma, S.C. & Thomas, G. (2010). Metformin, independent of AMPK, inhibits mTORC1 in a rag GTPase-dependent manner. *Cell Metab* Vol.11, No.5, (May 2010), pp. 390-401

Kapahi, P., Chen, D., Rogers, A.N., Katewa, S.D., Li, P.W., Thomas, E.L. & Kockel, L. (2010). With TOR, less is more: a key role for the conserved nutrient-sensing TOR pathway in aging. *Cell Metab* Vol.11, No.6, (June 2010), pp. 453-465

Karasek, M. (1999). Melatonin in humans-where we are 40 years after its discovery. *Neuro Endocrinol Lett* Vol.20, No.3-4, (1999), pp. 179-188

Karasek, M. (2004). Melatonin, human aging, and age-related diseases. *Exp Gerontol* Vol.39, No.11-12, (November 2004), pp. 1723-1729

Kelly, G. (2010). A review of the sirtuin system, its clinical implications, and the potential role of dietary activators like resveratrol: part 1. *Altern Med Rev* Vol.15, No.3, (September 2010), pp. 245-263

Kennedy, S.H. & Emsley, R. (2006). Placebo-controlled trial of agomelatine in the treatment of major depressive disorder. *Eur Neuropsychopharmacol* Vol.16, No.2, (Feb.2006), pp. 93-100

Knasmuller, S., Nersesyan, A., Misik, M., Gerner, C., Mikulits, W., Ehrlich, V., Hoelzl, C., Szakmary, A. & Wagner, K.H. (2008). Use of conventional and -omics based methods for health claims of dietary antioxidants: a critical overview. *Br J Nutr* Vol.99 E Suppl 1, (May 2008), pp. ES3-52

Ku, H.H., Brunk, U.T. & Sohal, R.S. (1993). Relationship between mitochondrial superoxide and hydrogen peroxide production and longevity of mammalian species. *Free Radic Biol Med* Vol.15, No.6, (December 1993), pp. 621-627

Lago, F., Dieguez, C., Gomez-Reino, J. & Gualillo, O. (2007). The emerging role of adipokines as mediators of inflammation and immune responses. *Cytokine Growth Factor Rev* Vol.18, No.3-4, (June 2007), pp. 313-325

Lanza, I.R., Short, D.K., Short, K.R., Raghavakaimal, S., Basu, R., Joyner, M.J., McConnell, J.P. & Nair, K.S. (2008). Endurance exercise as a countermeasure for aging. *Diabetes* Vol.57, No.11, (November 2008), pp. 2933-2942

Lapointe, J. & Hekimi, S. (2010). When a theory of aging ages badly. *Cell Mol Life Sci* Vol.67, No.1, (January 2010), pp. 1-8

Le Couteur, D.G., McLachlan, A.J., Quinn, R.J., Simpson, S.J. & de, C.R. (2011). Aging Biology and Novel Targets for Drug Discovery. *J Gerontol A Biol Sci Med Sci* (August 2011)

Lee, I.M., Cook, N.R., Gaziano, J.M., Gordon, D., Ridker, P.M., Manson, J.E., Hennekens, C.H. & Buring, J.E. (2005). Vitamin E in the primary prevention of cardiovascular disease and cancer: the Women's Health Study: a randomized controlled trial. *JAMA* Vol.294, No.1, (July 2005), pp. 56-65

Lekakis, J., Rallidis, L.S., Andreadou, I., Vamvakou, G., Kazantzoglou, G., Magiatis, P., Skaltsounis, A.L. & Kremastinos, D.T. (2005). Polyphenolic compounds from red grapes acutely improve endothelial function in patients with coronary heart disease. *Eur J Cardiovasc Prev Rehabil* Vol.12, No.6, (December 2005), pp. 596-600

Lemoine, P., Guilleminault, C. & Alvarez, E. (2007). Improvement in subjective sleep in major depressive disorder with a novel antidepressant, agomelatine: randomized, double-blind comparison with venlafaxine. *J Clin Psychiatry* Vol.68, No.11, (November 2007), pp. 1723-1732

Leto, S., Kokkonen, G.C. & Barrows, C.H. (1976). Dietary protein life-span, and physiological variables in female mice. *J Gerontol* Vol.31, No.2, (March 1976), pp. 149-154

Llewellyn, D.J., Langa, K.M. & Lang, I.A. (2009). Serum 25-hydroxyvitamin D concentration and cognitive impairment. *J Geriatr Psychiatry Neurol* Vol.22, No.3, (September 2009), pp. 188-195

Lonn, E., Bosch, J., Yusuf, S., Sheridan, P., Pogue, J., Arnold, J.M., Ross, C., Arnold, A., Sleight, P., Probstfield, J. & Dagenais, G.R. (2005). Effects of long-term vitamin E supplementation on cardiovascular events and cancer: a randomized controlled trial. *JAMA* Vol.293, No.11, (March 2005), pp. 1338-1347

Luthringer, R., Muzet, M., Zisapel, N. & Staner, L. (2009). The effect of prolonged-release melatonin on sleep measures and psychomotor performance in elderly patients with insomnia. *Int Clin Psychopharmacol* Vol.24, No.5, (September 2009), pp. 239-249

Ma, X.M. & Blenis, J. (May 2009). Molecular mechanisms of mTOR-mediated translational control. *Nat Rev Mol Cell Biol* Vol.10, No.5, (May 2009), pp. 307-318

Manach, C., Mazur, A. & Scalbert, A. (2005). Polyphenols and prevention of cardiovascular diseases. *Curr Opin Lipidol* Vol.16, No.1, (February 2005), pp. 77-84

Markus, M.A. & Morris, B.J. (2008). Resveratrol in prevention and treatment of common clinical conditions of aging. *Clin Interv Aging* Vol.3, No.2, (2008), pp. 331-339

Mattison, J.A., Roth, G.S., Lane, M.A. & Ingram, D.K. (2007). Dietary restriction in aging nonhuman primates. *Interdiscip Top Gerontol* Vol.35, (2007), pp. 137-158

Mattson, M.P. & Wan, R. (2005). Beneficial effects of intermittent fasting and caloric restriction on the cardiovascular and cerebrovascular systems. *J Nutr Biochem* Vol.16, No.3, (March 2005), pp. 129-137

McCay, C.M., Crowell, M.F. & Maynard, L.A. (1935). The effect of retarded growth upon the length of life span and upon the ultimate body size. *J Nutr* Vol.10, (May 1935), pp. 63-79

Meydani, M., Lipman, R.D., Han, S.N., Wu, D., Beharka, A., Martin, K.R., Bronson, R., Cao, G., Smith, D. & Meydani, S.N. (1998). The effect of long-term dietary supplementation with antioxidants. *Ann N Y Acad Sci* Vol.854, (Nov. 1998), pp. 352-360

Migliaccio, E., Giorgio, M., Mele, S., Pelicci, G., Reboldi, P., Pandolfi, P.P., Lanfrancone, L. & Pelicci, P.G. (1999). The p66shc adaptor protein controls oxidative stress response and life span in mammals. *Nature* Vol.402, No.6759, (November 1999), pp. 309-313

Mills, E., Wu, P., Seely, D. & Guyatt, G. (2005). Melatonin in the treatment of cancer: a systematic review of randomized controlled trials and meta-analysis. *J Pineal Res* Vol.39, No.4, (November 2005), pp. 360-366

Minor, R.K., Allard, J.S., Younts, C.M., Ward, T.M. & de, C.R. (2010a). Dietary interventions to extend life span and health span based on calorie restriction. *J Gerontol A Biol Sci Med Sci* Vol.65, No.7, (July 2010a), pp. 695-703

Minor, R.K., Smith, D.L., Jr., Sossong, A.M., Kaushik, S., Poosala, S., Spangler, E.L., Roth, G.S., Lane, M., Allison, D.B., de, C.R., Ingram, D.K. & Mattison, J.A. (2010b). Chronic ingestion of 2-deoxy-D-glucose induces cardiac vacuolization and increases mortality in rats. *Toxicol Appl Pharmacol* Vol.243, No.3, (March 2010b), pp. 332-339

Miquel, J. & Economos, A.C. (1979). Favorable effects of the antioxidants sodium and magnesium thiazolidine carboxylate on the vitality and life span of Drosophila and mice. *Exp Gerontol* Vol.14, No.5, (1979), pp. 279-285

Miquel, J., Economos, A.C., Fleming, J. & Johnson, J.E., Jr. (1980). Mitochondrial role in cell aging. *Exp Gerontol* Vol.15, No.6, (1980), pp. 575-591

Mitterberger, M.C., Mattesich, M., Klaver, E., Piza-Katzer, H. & Zwerschke, W. (2011). Reduced Insulin-Like Growth Factor-I Serum Levels in Formerly Obese Women Subjected to Laparoscopic-Adjustable Gastric Banding or Diet-Induced Long-term Caloric Restriction. *J Gerontol A Biol Sci Med Sci* (August 2011)

Naudi, A., Caro, P., Jove, M., Gomez, J., Boada, J., Ayala, V., Portero-Otin, M., Barja, G. & Pamplona, R. (2007). Methionine restriction decreases endogenous oxidative molecular damage and increases mitochondrial biogenesis and uncoupling protein 4 in rat brain. *Rejuvenation Res* Vol.10, No.4, (December 2007), pp. 473-484

Neubauer, D.N. (1999). Sleep problems in the elderly. *Am Fam Physician* Vol.59, No.9, (May 1999), pp. 2551-2560

Niki, E., Noguchi, N., Tsuchihashi, H. & Gotoh, N. (1995). Interaction among vitamin C, vitamin E, and beta-carotene. *Am J Clin Nutr* Vol.62, No.6 Suppl, (December 1995), pp. 1322S-1326S

Olshansky, S.J., Perry, D., Miller, R.A. & Butler, R.N. (2007). Pursuing the longevity dividend: scientific goals for an aging world. *Ann N Y Acad Sci* Vol.1114, (October 2007), pp. 11-13

Omodei, D. & Fontana, L. (2011). Calorie restriction and prevention of age-associated chronic disease. *FEBS Lett* Vol.585, No.11, (June 2011), pp. 1537-1542

Oudshoorn, C., Mattace-Raso, F.U., van, d., V, Colin, E.M. & van der Cammen, T.J. (2008). Higher serum vitamin D3 levels are associated with better cognitive test performance in patients with Alzheimer's disease. *Dement Geriatr Cogn Disord* Vol.25, No.6, (2008), pp. 539-543

Page, M.M., Richardson, J., Wiens, B.E., Tiedtke, E., Peters, C.W., Faure, P.A., Burness, G. & Stuart, J.A. (2010). Antioxidant enzyme activities are not broadly correlated with longevity in 14 vertebrate endotherm species. *Age (Dordr)* Vol.32, No.2, (June 2010), pp. 255-270

Pak, J.W., Herbst, A., Bua, E., Gokey, N., McKenzie, D. & Aiken, J.M. (2003). Mitochondrial DNA mutations as a fundamental mechanism in physiological declines associated with aging. *Aging Cell* Vol.2, No.1, (February 2003), pp. 1-7

Pamplona, R. (2011). Mitochondrial DNA damage and animal longevity: insights from comparative studies. *J Aging Res* Vol.2011, (2011), pp. 807108

Pamplona, R. & Barja, G. (2011). An evolutionary comparative scan for longevity-related oxidative stress resistance mechanisms in homeotherms. *Biogerontology* (July 2011)

Pandi-Perumal, S.R., Trakht, I., Srinivasan, V., Spence, D.W., Maestroni, G.J., Zisapel, N. & Cardinali, D.P. (2008). Physiological effects of melatonin: role of melatonin receptors and signal transduction pathways. *Prog Neurobiol* Vol.85, No.3, (July 2008), pp. 335-353

Pascua, P., Camello-Almaraz, C., Camello, P.J., Martin-Cano, F., Vara, E., Tresguerres, J. & Pozo, M.J. (2011). Melatonin, and to a lesser extent growth hormone, restores colonic smooth muscle physiology in old rats. *J Pineal Res* (May 2011)

Pearl R (1928). *The rate of living* Alfred A Knopf, Inc., New York.

Pearson, K.J., Baur, J.A., Lewis, K.N., Peshkin, L., Price, N.L., Labinskyy, N., Swindell, W.R., Kamara, D., Minor, R.K., Perez, E., Jamieson, H.A., Zhang, Y., Dunn, S.R., Sharma, K., Pleshko, N., Woollett, L.A., Csiszar, A., Ikeno, Y., Le, C.D., Elliott, P.J., Becker, K.G., Navas, P., Ingram, D.K., Wolf, N.S., Ungvari, Z., Sinclair, D.A. & de, C.R. (2008). Resveratrol delays age-related deterioration and mimics transcriptional aspects of dietary restriction without extending life span. *Cell Metab* Vol.8, No.2, (August 2008), pp. 157-168

Perez, V.I., Bokov, A., Van, R.H., Mele, J., Ran, Q., Ikeno, Y. & Richardson, A. (2009). Is the oxidative stress theory of aging dead? *Biochim Biophys Acta* Vol.1790, No.10, (October 2009), pp. 1005-1014

Pham, D.Q. & Plakogiannis, R. (2005). Vitamin E supplementation in cardiovascular disease and cancer prevention: Part 1. *Ann Pharmacother* Vol.39, No.11, (November 2005), pp. 1870-1878

Pozo, M.J., Gomez-Pinilla, P.J., Camello-Almaraz, C., Martin-Cano, F.E., Pascua, P., Rol, M.A., cuna-Castroviejo, D. & Camello, P.J. (2010). Melatonin, a potential therapeutic agent for smooth muscle-related pathological conditions and aging. *Curr Med Chem* Vol.17, No.34, (2010), pp. 4150-4165

Rebrin, I., Zicker, S., Wedekind, K.J., Paetau-Robinson, I., Packer, L. & Sohal, R.S. (2005). Effect of antioxidant-enriched diets on glutathione redox status in tissue homogenates and mitochondria of the senescence-accelerated mouse. *Free Radic Biol Med* Vol.39, No.4, (August 2005), pp. 549-557

Regulska, M., Leskiewicz, M., Budziszewska, B., Kutner, A., Basta-Kaim, A., Kubera, M., Jaworska-Feil, L. & Lason, W. (2006). Involvement of PI3-K in neuroprotective effects of the 1,25-dihydroxyvitamin D3 analogue - PRI-2191. *Pharmacol Rep* Vol.58, No.6, (November 2006), pp. 900-907

Reid, M.E., Duffield-Lillico, A.J., Garland, L., Turnbull, B.W., Clark, L.C. & Marshall, J.R. (2002). Selenium supplementation and lung cancer incidence: an update of the nutritional prevention of cancer trial. *Cancer Epidemiol Biomarkers Prev* Vol.11, No.11, (November 2002), pp. 1285-1291

Rickman, A.D., Williamson, D.A., Martin, C.K., Gilhooly, C.H., Stein, R.I., Bales, C.W., Roberts, S. & Das, S.K. (2011). The CALERIE Study: Design and methods of an innovative 25% caloric restriction intervention. *Contemp Clin Trials* (July 2011)

Rose, G., Dato, S., Altomare, K., Bellizzi, D., Garasto, S., Greco, V., Passarino, G., Feraco, E., Mari, V., Barbi, C., BonaFe, M., Franceschi, C., Tan, Q., Boiko, S., Yashin, A.I. & De, B.G. (2003). Variability of the SIRT3 gene, human silent information regulator Sir2 homologue, and survivorship in the elderly. *Exp Gerontol* Vol.38, No.10, (October 2003), pp. 1065-1070

Rudman, D. (1985). Growth hormone, body composition, and aging. *J Am Geriatr Soc* Vol.33, No.11, (November 1985), pp. 800-807

Sanz, A., Caro, P., Sanchez, J.G. & Barja, G. (2006a). Effect of lipid restriction on mitochondrial free radical production and oxidative DNA damage. *Ann N Y Acad Sci* Vol.1067, (May 2006a), pp. 200-209

Sanz, A., Gomez, J., Caro, P. & Barja, G. (2006b). Carbohydrate restriction does not change mitochondrial free radical generation and oxidative DNA damage. *J Bioenerg Biomembr* Vol.38, No.5-6, (December 2006b), pp. 327-333

Schleithoff, S.S., Zittermann, A., Tenderich, G., Berthold, H.K., Stehle, P. & Koerfer, R. (2006). Vitamin D supplementation improves cytokine profiles in patients with congestive heart failure: a double-blind, randomized, placebo-controlled trial. *Am J Clin Nutr* Vol.83, No.4, (April 2006), pp. 754-759

Schriner, S.E., Linford, N.J., Martin, G.M., Treuting, P., Ogburn, C.E., Emond, M., Coskun, P.E., Ladiges, W., Wolf, N., Van, R.H., Wallace, D.C. & Rabinovitch, P.S. (2005). Extension of murine life span by overexpression of catalase targeted to mitochondria. *Science* Vol.308, No.5730, (June 2005), pp. 1909-1911

Selesniemi, K., Lee, H.J. & Tilly, J.L. (2008). Moderate caloric restriction initiated in rodents during adulthood sustains function of the female reproductive axis into advanced chronological age. *Aging Cell* Vol.7, No.5, (October 2008), pp. 622-629

Selman, C., Lingard, S., Choudhury, A.I., Batterham, R.L., Claret, M., Clements, M., Ramadani, F., Okkenhaug, K., Schuster, E., Blanc, E., Piper, M.D., Al-Qassab, H., Speakman, J.R., Carmignac, D., Robinson, I.C., Thornton, J.M., Gems, D., Partridge, L. & Withers, D.J. (2008). Evidence for lifespan extension and delayed age-related biomarkers in insulin receptor substrate 1 null mice. *FASEB J* Vol.22, No.3, (March 2008), pp. 807-818

Selman, C., Tullet, J.M., Wieser, D., Irvine, E., Lingard, S.J., Choudhury, A.I., Claret, M., Al-Qassab, H., Carmignac, D., Ramadani, F., Woods, A., Robinson, I.C., Schuster, E., Batterham, R.L., Kozma, S.C., Thomas, G., Carling, D., Okkenhaug, K., Thornton, J.M., Partridge, L., Gems, D. & Withers, D.J. (2009). Ribosomal protein S6 kinase 1 signaling regulates mammalian life span. *Science* Vol.326, No.5949, (October 2009), pp. 140-144

Sharp, Z.D. & Richardson, A. (2011). Aging and cancer: can mTOR inhibitors kill two birds with one drug? *Target Oncol* Vol.6, No.1, (March 2011), pp. 41-51

Sheppard, M.C. (2005). GH and mortality in acromegaly. *J Endocrinol Invest* Vol.28, No.11 Suppl International, (2005), pp. 75-77

Singer, C., Tractenberg, R.E., Kaye, J., Schafer, K., Gamst, A., Grundman, M., Thomas, R. & Thal, L.J. (2003). A multicenter, placebo-controlled trial of melatonin for sleep disturbance in Alzheimer's disease. *Sleep* Vol.26, No.7, (Nov. 2003), pp. 893-901

Skulachev, V.P. (2004). Mitochondria, reactive oxygen species and longevity: some lessons from the Barja group. *Aging Cell* Vol.3, No.1, (February 2004), pp. 17-19

Sohal, R.S., Svensson, I. & Brunk, U.T. (1990). Hydrogen peroxide production by liver mitochondria in different species. *Mech Ageing Dev* Vol.53, No.3, (April 1990), pp. 209-215

Speakman, J.R. (2005). Correlations between physiology and lifespan:two widely ignored problems with comparative studies. *Aging Cell* Vol.4, No.4, (Aug.2005), pp. 167-175

Speakman, J.R. & Hambly, C. (2007). Starving for life: what animal studies can and cannot tell us about the use of caloric restriction to prolong human lifespan. *J Nutr* Vol.137, No.4, (April 2007), pp. 1078-1086

Speakman, J.R. & Mitchell, S.E. (2011). Caloric restriction. *Mol Aspects Med* (August 2011)

Speakman, J.R. & Selman, C. (2011). The free-radical damage theory: Accumulating evidence against a simple link of oxidative stress to ageing and lifespan. *Bioessays* Vol.33, No.4, (April 2011), pp. 255-259

Spindler, S.R. (2011). Review of the literature and suggestions for the design of rodent survival studies for the identification of compounds that increase health and life span. *Age (Dordr)* (March 2011)

Stolzenberg-Solomon, R.Z. (2009). Vitamin D and pancreatic cancer. *Ann Epidemiol* Vol.19, No.2, (February 2009), pp. 89-95

Suh, Y., Atzmon, G., Cho, M.O., Hwang, D., Liu, B., Leahy, D.J., Barzilai, N. & Cohen, P. (2008). Functionally significant insulin-like growth factor I receptor mutations in centenarians. *Proc Natl Acad Sci U S A* Vol.105, No.9, (March 2008), pp. 3438-3442

Sundaresan, N.R., Gupta, M., Kim, G., Rajamohan, S.B., Isbatan, A. & Gupta, M.P. (2009). Sirt3 blocks the cardiac hypertrophic response by augmenting Foxo3a-dependent antioxidant defense mechanisms in mice. *J Clin Invest* Vol.119, No.9, (September 2009), pp. 2758-2771

Takala, J., Ruokonen, E., Webster, N.R., Nielsen, M.S., Zandstra, D.F., Vundelinckx, G. & Hinds, C.J. (1999). Increased mortality associated with growth hormone treatment in critically ill adults. *N Engl J Med* Vol.341, No.11, (September 1999), pp. 785-792

Tapia, P.C. (2006). Sublethal mitochondrial stress with an attendant stoichiometric augmentation of reactive oxygen species may precipitate many of the beneficial alterations in cellular physiology produced by caloric restriction, intermittent fasting, exercise and dietary phytonutrients: "Mitohormesis" for health and vitality. *Med Hypotheses* Vol.66, No.4, (2006), pp. 832-843

Thomas, M.L., Armbrecht, H.J. & Forte, L.R. (1984). Effects of long-term vitamin D deficiency and response to vitamin D repletion in the mature and aging male and female rat. *Mech Ageing Dev* Vol.25, No.1-2, (April 1984), pp. 161-175

Trifunovic, A., Hansson, A., Wredenberg, A., Rovio, A.T., Dufour, E., Khvorostov, I., Spelbrink, J.N., Wibom, R., Jacobs, H.T. & Larsson, N.G. (2005). Somatic mtDNA mutations cause aging phenotypes without affecting reactive oxygen species production. *Proc Natl Acad Sci U S A* Vol.102, No.50, (Dec.2005), pp. 17993-17998

Utiger, R.D. (1998). The need for more vitamin D. *N Engl J Med* Vol.338, No.12, (March 1998), pp. 828-829

van Geijlswijk, I.M., Korzilius, H.P. & Smits, M.G. (2010). The use of exogenous melatonin in delayed sleep phase disorder: a meta-analysis. *Sleep* Vol.33, No.12, (December 2010), pp. 1605-1614

Vazquez-Martin, A., Oliveras-Ferraros, C. & Menendez, J.A. (2009). The antidiabetic drug metformin suppresses HER2 (erbB-2) oncoprotein overexpression via inhibition of the mTOR effector p70S6K1 in human breast carcinoma cells. *Cell Cycle* Vol.8, No.1, (January 2009), pp. 88-96

Veldhuis, J.D., Liem, A.Y., South, S., Weltman, A., Weltman, J., Clemmons, D.A., Abbott, R., Mulligan, T., Johnson, M.L., Pincus, S. & . (1995). Differential impact of age, sex steroid hormones, and obesity on basal versus pulsatile growth hormone secretion in men as assessed in an ultrasensitive chemiluminescence assay. *J Clin Endocrinol Metab* Vol.80, No.11, (November 1995), pp. 3209-3222

Vendelbo, M.H. & Nair, K.S. (2011). Mitochondrial longevity pathways. *Biochim Biophys Acta* Vol.1813, No.4, (April 2011), pp. 634-644

Viña, J., Lloret, A., Orti, R. & Alonso, D. (2004). Molecular bases of the treatment of Alzheimer's disease with antioxidants: prevention of oxidative stress. *Mol Aspects Med* Vol.25, No.1-2, (February 2004), pp. 117-123

Wade, A.G., Ford, I., Crawford, G., McConnachie, A., Nir, T., Laudon, M. & Zisapel, N. (2010). Nightly treatment of primary insomnia with prolonged release melatonin for 6 months: a randomized placebo controlled trial on age and endogenous melatonin as predictors of efficacy and safety. *BMC Med* Vol.8, (2010), pp. 51

Wang, Y., Liang, Y. & Vanhoutte, P.M. (2011). SIRT1 and AMPK in regulating mammalian senescence: a critical review and a working model. *FEBS Lett* Vol.585, No.7, (April 2011), pp. 986-994

Willcox, B.J., Donlon, T.A., He, Q., Chen, R., Grove, J.S., Yano, K., Masaki, K.H., Willcox, D.C., Rodriguez, B. & Curb, J.D. (2008). FOXO3A genotype is strongly associated with human longevity. *Proc Natl Acad Sci U S A* Vol.105, No.37, (September 2008), pp. 13987-13992

Xiang, L. & He, G. (2011). Caloric restriction and antiaging effects. *Ann Nutr Metab* Vol.58, No.1, (2011), pp. 42-48

Yakes, F.M. & Van, H.B. (1997). Mitochondrial DNA damage is more extensive and persists longer than nuclear DNA damage in human cells following oxidative stress. *Proc Natl Acad Sci U S A* Vol.94, No.2, (January 1997), pp. 514-519

Yamamoto, H., Schoonjans, K. & Auwerx, J. (2007). Sirtuin functions in health and disease. *Mol Endocrinol* Vol.21, No.8, (August 2007), pp. 1745-1755

Yamamoto, M., Clark, J.D., Pastor, J.V., Gurnani, P., Nandi, A., Kurosu, H., Miyoshi, M., Ogawa, Y., Castrillon, D.H., Rosenblatt, K.P. & Kuro-o M (2005). Regulation of oxidative stress by the anti-aging hormone klotho. *J Biol Chem* Vol.280, No.45, (November 2005), pp. 38029-38034

Ylikomi, T., Laaksi, I., Lou, Y.R., Martikainen, P., Miettinen, S., Pennanen, P., Purmonen, S., Syvala, H., Vienonen, A. & Tuohimaa, P. (2002). Antiproliferative action of vitamin D. *Vitam Horm* Vol.64, (2002), pp. 357-406

Zittermann, A., Schleithoff, S. & Koerfer, R.(2005). Putting cardiovascular disease and vitamin D insufficiency into perspective.*Br J Nutr* Vol.94,No.4,(Oct.2005), pp.483-492

14

Pharmacological Neuromodulation in Autism Spectrum Disorders

Bill J. Duke
Child Psychopharmacology Institute
USA

1. Introduction

This chapter will examine pharmacological approaches to neuromodulation in Autism Spectrum Disorders (ASD), pharmacological clinical trials and pharmacological strategies on the horizon.

Drugs used in autism target neuromodulation at different neuronal sites. Those utilizing anti-convulsant, neurolepic, anti-depressant, stimulant, cholinesterase inhibitors, anxiolytics, mood stabilizers and other pharmacological interventions in autism do so for a variety of purposes. Each of these classes of drugs will be examined relative to their proposed neuromodulatory actions as they relate to the Autism Spectrum Disorder population.

Children with ASD demonstrate deficits in 1) social interaction, 2) verbal and nonverbal communication, and 3) repetitive behaviors or interests. Many have unusual sensory responses. Symptoms range from mild to severe and present with individual uniqueness and complexity. Some aspects of learning may seem exceptional while others may lag. These children reflect a mix of communication, social, and behavioral patterns that are individual but fit into the overall diagnosis of ASD. Aggression, irritability and/or self-injury in children with autistic spectrum disorders often meet the threshold indicating pharmacological intervention.

Autism Spectrum Disorders have been shown to be related to complex combinations of environmental, neurological, immunological, and genetic factors. In addition to strong genetic links, environmental factors such as infection and drug exposure during pregnancy, perinatal hypoxia, postnatal infections and metabolic disorders have each been implicated in autistic populations. Summarizing an earlier Centers for Disease Control and Prevention Study (CDC) with subsequent major studies on autism prevalence, the CDC estimates 2-6 per 1,000 (from 1 in 500 to 1 in 150) children have an ASD. The risk is 3-4 times higher in males than females (Rice 2006)(CDC 2011).

The pathogenetic components and biological endophenotypes in autism spectrum disorders were described by Sacco and colleagues as: Circadian & Sensory Dysfunction; Immune Dysfunction; Neurodevelopmental Delay; and Stereotypic Behavior (Sacco R, et al 2010).

The heterogeneity of Autism Spectrum Disorders has resulted in many genes being studied that are thought to have an impact on the development of the pathological characteristics associated with Autism Spectrum Disorder (Greer PL, et al 2010). The developmental neurobiology of ASD is incrementally illuminated at the cutting edges of science. The permutations of mutations and epigenetic effects in ASD are both daunting yet increasingly identifiable targets for pharmacologic intervention. Clinical necessity and clincial trials drive discoveries for therapeutic interventions until stem cell or genetic solutions arrive.

Some states or effects seen in ASD may be responsive to developmental interventions while others may not. As we know, prompt thyroid replacement in a hypothyroid infant will generally allow normative intellectual development and prevent developmental disability. An example of variation of developmental impact is a mutation in MECP2, which encodes the epigenetic regulator methyl-CpG-binding protein 2 and is associated with Rett Syndrome. A recent study asked the question whether providing MeCP2 function exclusively during early post-natal life might prevent or mitigate disease in adult animals. Re-expression of MeCP2 in symptomatic mice rescued several features of the disease. The investigators argue "...the temporal association of disease with the postnatal period of development may be unrelated to any 'developmental' or stage restricted function of MeCP2, at least in mouse models." They concluded that "...therapies for RTT, like MeCP2 function must be continuously maintained" (McGraw, et al 2011).

Genetic-environment interactions in ASD that continue to be investigated include: parental age; maternal genotype; maternal-fetal immunoreactivity; in vitro fertilization; maternal ingestion of drugs; toxic chemicals in the environment during pregnancy; and maternal illnesses during pregnancy such as maternal diabetes or infections (Hallmayer J, 2011) . Recent studies are consistent with a fetal programming hypothesis of ASD that considers environmental risk factors that affect the fetal environment and interact with genetic variants (Szatmari 2011). The pathogenic potential of dysregulated states may further stress developmentally vulnerable neurodevelopment (Duke, B. , 2008).

As these genes and interacting effects become better characterized therapeutic strategies can be developed (Buxbaum 2009) (Levy et al, 2011)(Sanders et al, 2011)(Gilman et al, 2011). These genes include those involved in the patterning of the central nervous system; those that govern biochemical pathways; those responsible for the development of dendrites and synapses; and, genes associated with the immune system and autoimmune disorders (Ashwood et al, 2006) (Careaga M et al, 2010).

Neuroimaging studies further enlighten our theoretical models and techniques such as diffusion tensor imaging (DTI) have gained prominence as a means of assessing brain development (Isaacson & Provenzale, 2011). Studies of emotional perception demonstrated that while listening to either happy or sad music, individuals with ASD activated cortical and subcortical brain regions known to be involved in emotion processing and reward. The investigators, using functional magnetic resonance imaging compared ASD participants with neurotypical individuals and found ASD individuals had decreased brain activity in the premotor area and in the left anterior insula, especially in response to happy music excerpts. Their findings illuminate our understanding of the neurobiological correlates of preserved and altered emotional processing in ASD (Caria A, et al 2011).

Other imaging studies have found: diminished gray matter within the hypothalamus in autism disorder and suggest this is a potential link to hormonal effects (Kurth F, et al 2011); elevated repetitive and stereotyped behavior (RSB) associated with decreased volumes in several brain regions: left thalamus, right globus pallidus, left and right putamen, right striatum and a trend for left globus pallidus and left striatum within the ASD group (Estes A, et al 2011); alterations in frontal lobe tracts and corpus callosum in young children with autism spectrum disorder (Kumar A, et al 2010); and, revealed pervasive microstructural abnormalities (Groen WB, et al 2011).

As our theoretical constructs are tested and enriched clinical scientists are poised to learn exponentially as treatment response databases and measurement methods and systems are further developed. We are ready to experience an evolution and fusion of medical arts strengthened by scientific methods and information technology.

Psychopharmacological treatment guidelines for very young children suggest that children with persistent moderate to severe symptoms and impairment, despite psychotherapeutic interventions, may be better served by carefully monitored medication trials than by continuing ineffective treatments (Gleason MM, et al 2007).

The treatment of children with ASD has challenges that are also present in the treatment of many mood disorders and in schizophrenia. In Stephen Stahl's text, Essential Psychopharmacology (Stahl 2010), he deconstructs the syndrome of schizophrenia into five symptom dimensions: Positive and Negative symptoms, aggression, affect and cognition. These symptom dimensions are also relevant to children with ASD and many children with mood disorders. Individual presentations and variability of treatment response can be managed by enlisting the parents to be observers utilizing defined measurements.

Multiple medications have utility in ASD treatment and are sometimes used in combination. Thoughtful utilization and management of medications can offer children with autism spectrum disorders significiant reductions of impairment. Each of the medications used, as true with any medication, has varying degrees and potential related to benefits, risk and limitations. Although the antipsychotic risperidone has been demonstrated as effective in reducing serious behavioral problems, it shares adverse neurological and metabolic risks with other typical and atypical antipsychotic agents. Nevertheless, risperidone has demonstrated efficacy at relatively low doses and treatment monitoring can assist in managing risks when substantial benefit is possible.

Antidepressants have been reported as helpful for some with ASD, particularly related to repetitive or obsessive compulsive behaviors, however, studies reviewing off-label uses of anti-depressants have also reported adverse effects of increased agitation, behavioral activation and sleep disturbance. If we consider these findings as evidence suggesting antidepressants, in some, perturb inhibitory- excitatory neuronal balance or, in a broad sense, contribute to central nervous system hyperarousal, it follows that such effects could contribute to pathogenesis rather than decrease the allostatic load. This does not suggest that anti-depressant medications can't be helpful. It is recognized that in many cases antidepressants are helpful; however, vigilance for signs of disinhibition or other dysregulation is prudent.

Known stimulant benefits include increased ability to sustain attention, reduced motoric hyperactivity and reduced impulsivity. Adverse effects associated with stimulants include dysphoric responses, sleep disturbances and appetite supression.

Anticonvulsants have demonstrated their place in the treatment regimen of many children with ASD and approximately twenty percent of those with ASD are thought to have a seizure disorder (Tuchman & Cuccaro, 2011). Benefits can include seizure control and mood stabilization while adverse effects can include cognitive dulling. When anticonvulsants are useful, cognitive dulling can often be managed by anticonvulsant selection and dosing.

Current pharmacological interventions in autism spectrum disorders are essentially directed at reducing cognitive and behavioral impairments. Treatment studies have demonstrated little observable benefit to core deficits of ASD, however, the argument is made that, in addition to the practical benefits of reducing behavioral and cognitive impairments, symptom reduction is a reflection of more efficient neural processing and development.

Effective impairment reduction often allows children to remain in a family home, function in a school setting, optimize reponsiveness to behavioral and educational methods and, generally, function more normally than would otherwise be possible. Those of us who treat children who will otherwise be excluded from normal environments appreciate the importance and complexity of these interventions. The greater promise of pharmacological interventions is their potential, through early intervention, to inhibit or reduce the development of pathological and pathogenic endophenotypes.

2. Conceptualization of clinical hypotheses, treatment strategies and measurement of treatment response

Physicians and clinician- scientists are humbled distinguishing among nosological categories in the context of the diverse and complex treatment circumstances presented by those significantly impaired within the spectrum of autism disorders.

Treatment decisions are based on symptom profiles, types and severity of impairment, risk-benefit calculations, potential treatments available and clinical hypotheses related to the nature of the disorder. Unlike elegantly designed experiments with exquisitely defined variables and thoughtful control of confounding variables, those suffering functional and qualitative impairment present with inherent experimental limitations. Despite these limitations, the application of scientific principles related to individual measurement and monitoring of treatment response provides a platform from which to assess treatment response and dynamically test clinical hypotheses.

The deconstruction of psychiatric syndromes into symptoms is described as a way to establish a diagnosis, deconstruct the condition into its symptoms, match the symptoms to a hypothetically malfunctioning circuit and consider the collection of neurotransmitters and neuromodulators known to regulate the circuit. "Next, one can match each symptom to a hypothetically malfunctioning circuit and - with knowledge of the neurotransmitters regulating that circuit and drugs acting on those neurotransmitters - choose a therapeutic agent to reduce that symptom. If such a strategy proves unsuccessful, it is possible that adding or switching to another agent acting on another neurotransmitter in that circuit can be effective. Repeating this strategy for each symptom can result in remission of all symptoms in many patients." (Stahl, 2010)

Knowledge gained in the study of abnormal circuitry in mood disorders, schizophrenia and other neuropsychiatric and neurological conditions provide models by which treatment responses and clinical hypotheses can be tested. Whether the symptoms are hyperkinetic movement disorders or hyperactive mesolimbic systems, pharmacological strategies can inform and interact with the rapidly developing basic and translational sciences. Dysregulation of neuronal inhibition and excitability appears as a common theme among many disorders.

Consideration of the pathological developmental aspects of autism spectrum disorders provokes the possibility that altering disease progression may rescue or support improved functional neurodevelopmental outcomes. In a broad statement regarding psychiatric disorders that supports that potential, Stephen Stahl remarks, "It may also be possible to prevent disease recurrence and progression to treatment resistance by treating not only symptoms but also inefficient brain circuits that are asymptomatic. Failing to do so may allow 'diabolical learning' where circuits run amok, become more efficient in learning how to mediate symptoms, and are therefore more difficult to treat." (Stahl, 2010, p. 274)

The lessons and theoretical models related to pharmacological interventions in other neurological and psychiatric syndromes can be applied to treatment conceptualizations with the autistic spectrum disordered as well. For example, constructs investigated with antiepileptic drugs (AED) can also be considered within the neural circuitry issues involved in Autism Spectrum Disorders.

"Several pathophysiological mechanisms inducing a neuronal excitability seems to be involved in an imbalance of both GABAergic and glutamatergic neurotransmissions and therefore could be similar in epilepsy and hyperkinetic movement disorders. The main targets for the action of the AEDs include enhancement of GABAergic inhibition, decreased glutamatergic excitation, modulation of voltage-gated sodium and calcium channels, and effects on intracellular signaling pathways. All of these mechanisms are of importance in controlling neuronal excitability in different ways." (Siniscalchi, Gallelli & De Sarro, 2010)

When pharmacological interventions are applied, secondary to their clinical intent, they serve as probes of endophenotypic neural functioning and circuitry states revealing response to particular pharmacodynamic and pharmacokinetic profiles. The classes of antipsychotic drugs considered to be atypical are described by Schwartz with such considerations in mind.

"The second generation antipsychotics are clearly delineated in the treatment of psychosis and mania and share similar mechanisms of action to achieve these results: dopamine-2 receptor antagonism for efficacy and serotonin-2a receptor antagonism for EPS tolerability. From here, each agent has a unique pharmacodynamic and pharmacokinetic profile where some agents carry more, or less antidepressant, anxiolytic, or hypnotic profiles. Choosing an agent and dosing it in low, middle, or high ranges may result in differential effectiveness and tolerability" (Schwartz & Stahl, 2011).

We are further humbled by the incomplete pharmacodynamic and pharmacokinetic profiles of the drugs we employ. Many of the drugs and compounds used have poorly understood neuromodulary effects in addition to known receptor specific actions. Nevertheless, contributions to our knowledge continue to further characterize and define drugs as well as continue to discover relationships of enviromental effects and immunological response. Researchers, for example, have recently shown the inhibitory effects of some antidepressants as well as some typical/atypical antipsychotics on the release of inflammatory cytokines and free radicals from activated microglia, which the investigators state have been discovered to cause synaptic pathology, a decrease in neurogenesis, and white matter abnormalities found in the brains of patients with psychiatric disorders. (Monji A, 2011). We operate with limited visibility that is increased by clinical experience and science.

Despite the complexity and challenges of ASD, potential for early interventions are supported by animal research. An example is the recent demonstration that autism risk genes differentially impact cortical development (Eagleson K, et al 2011). The demonstrations of these risk genes and their interaction with various states, illustrate animal models that may further elucidate pathogenic developmental processes. The role of glutamate (Hamberger A, et al 1992), serotonin (Levitt P, 2011) and sigma 1 ligands (Yagasaki Y, et al 2006) have each demonstrated potential importance in modulating glutamatergic and other developmentally critical signaling processes.

In autism spectrum disorders as well as in other neurological and neurodegenerative disorders, discoveries in developmental neurobiology and genetics will continue to provide increasingly sophisticated models in which interventions of developmentally specific neuropathogenic processes can be assessed and clinical hypotheses considered and tested. Coinciding are increasingly sophisticated objective measures that will allow greater definition of treatment response characteristics and endophenotypic response profiles. Applications related to treatment response measurement and management utilizing on-line observational and other measurements related to eye, facial, voice, reaction time consistency, sleep and activity are currently being studied and developed at the Child Psychopharmacolgy Institute.

3. Registered clinical trials (NIH- USA) in autism spectrum disorders

We can learn a great deal from the current foci of pharmacological interventions in ASD by reviewing clinical trials that have been conducted and those that are current.

	Frequency	Percent
Drug Studies	151	53.5
Behavioral Studies	43	15.2
Dietary Studies	18	6.4
Device or Procedure Studies	5	1.8
Obervational and Other Studies	65	23.0
Total	282	100.0

Table 1. ASD Study Types- NIH Registrations of Record July 2011

Drug Classes Used In Autism Spectrum Disorder Clinical Trials
Antidepressant
Stimulant
Anticonvulsant
Antipsychotic
NMDA Antagonists And Glutamatergic
Antibacterial Anti-Infective
Immunomodulator
Hyperbaric Oxygen
Hormone Or Enzyme Factors
Adrenergic
Anti-Hypertensive
Diruretic
Opioid Antagonist
Anti-Oxidants
Hypoglycemic Agents
Supplements
GABA B Recepter Agonist
Trichuris Suis Ova
Antidote Heavy Metal
Ampa Receptor Modulator
Anxioytic

Table 2. Drug Classes Used in Autism Spectrum Disorder July 2011 NIH

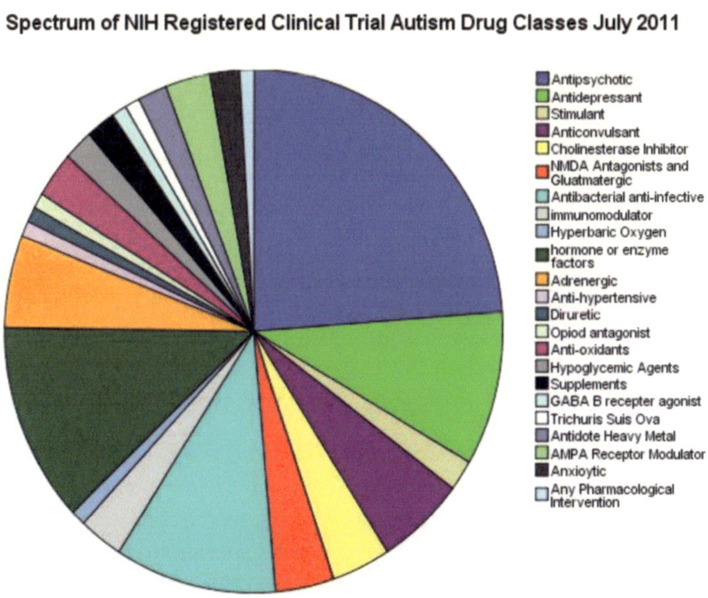

Fig. 1. Spectrum of Drug Classes in Autism Spectrum Disorders

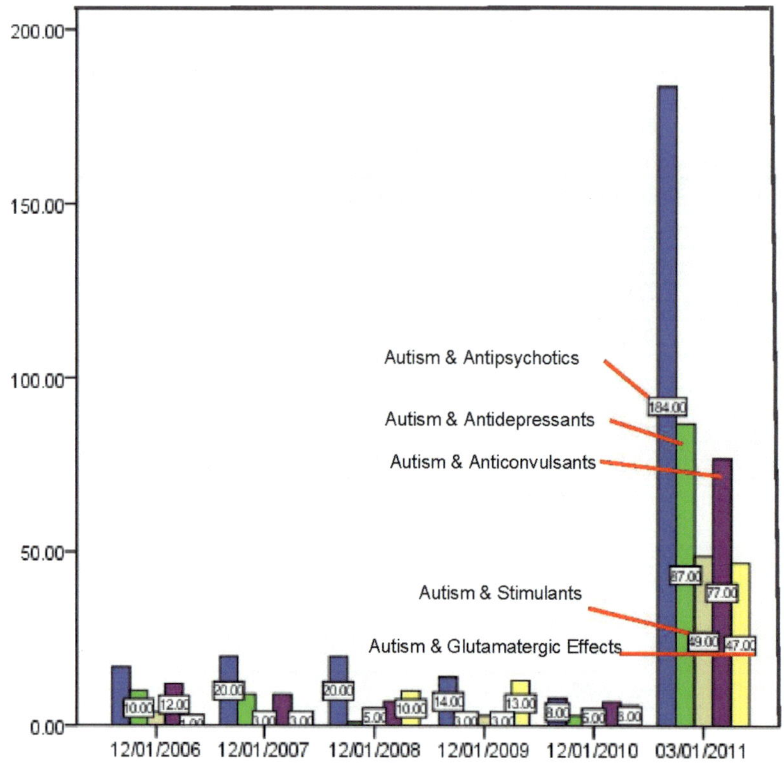

Fig. 2. NLM Clinical Trial Reviews 2006 to 2011

Table 3 displays a sampling of drugs in clinical trials and their generally proposed actions.

Antipsychotic Drugs
Risperidone is a selective blocker of dopamine d2 receptors and serotonin 5-ht2 receptors that acts as an atypical antipsychotic agent.
Aripiprazole has both presynaptic dopamine autoreceptor agonistic activity and postsynaptic D2 receptor antagonistic activity; use associated with hyperglycemia. It can also be described as a Dopamine Partial Agonist.
Ziprasidone -antipsychotic-A benzisothiazoylpiperazine derivative; has combined dopamine and serotonin receptor antagonist activity; structurally related to tiospirone.
Zyprexa (olanzapine) has combined dopamine and serotonin receptor antagonist activity.
Antidepressant Drugs
Fluoxetine: serotonin specific uptake inhibitor
Citalopram serotonin specific uptake inhibitor. The drug is also effective in reducing ethanol uptake in alcoholics and is used in depressed patients who also suffer from tardive dyskinesia
The SSRI fluvoxamine is not only an inhibitor of SERT, but also acts at sigma receptors, perhaps as a sigma-1 agonist, with some preclinical evidence that fluvoxamine can improve PCP-induced cognitive deficits
Atomoxetine: norepinephrine selective reuptake inhibitor.

Anticonvulsant Drugs
Divalproex sodium: A fatty acid with anticonvulsant properties used in the treatment of epilepsy. The mechanisms of its therapeutic actions are not well understood. It may act by increasing gamma-aminobutyric acid levels in the brain.
Riluzole: A glutamate antagonist (receptors, glutamate) used as an anticonvulsant (anticonvulsants) and to prolong the survival of patients with amyotrophic lateral sclerosis.
Lamotrigine,Sodium Valproate, or Carbamazepine: Anticonvulsants
Stimulant Drugs
Methylphenidate is a racemic mixture comprised of the d- and l-threo enantiomers. The d-threo enantiomer is more pharmacologically active than the l-threo enantiomer. Methylphenidate HCl is a central nervous system (CNS) stimulant.
Methylphenidate transdermal system: Methylphenidate HCl is a central nervous system (CNS) stimulant.
Choline and Cholinesterase Inhibitors
Choline: Precursor to Acetylcholine
Donepezil: Current theories on the pathogenesis attribute some symptoms to a deficiency of cholinergic neurotransmission. Donepezil hydrochloride is postulated to exert its therapeutic effect by inhibiting AChe boosting the availability of ACh.
Drugs with Glutaminergic Effects, AMPA Modulators and NMDA Antagonists
Acamprosate is a derivative of the amino acid taurine and, like alcohol, reduces excitatory glutamate neurotransmission and enhances inhibitory GABA neurotransmission
Memantine: a weak NMDA antagonist. Persistent activation of central nervous system N-methyl-D-aspartate (NMDA) receptors by the excitatory amino acid glutamate has been hypothesized to contribute to the symptomatology of Alzheimer's disease.
Dextromethorphan and quinidine sulfate (Nuedexta): NMDA antagonist; Sigma 1 agonist; binds to SERT; proposed neuromodulator.
Hormones
Oxytocin: A nonapeptide hormone released from the neurohypophysis (pituitary gland, posterior). it differs from vasopressin by two amino acids at residues 3 and 8.
Vasopressin
Anti-infective-Anti-bacterial-Immunomodulators
N Acetylcysteine N-acetyl derivative of cysteine. It is used as a mucolytic agent to reduce the viscosity of mucous secretions. It has also been shown to have antiviral effects in patients with HIV due to inhibition of viral stimulation by reactive oxygen.
Cycloserine Antibiotic substance produced by Streptomyces garyphalus.
Sapropterin: reduces blood phenylalanine (Phe) levels in patients with hyperphenylalaninemia (HPA) due to tetrahydrobiopterin- (BH4-) responsive Phenylketonuria (PKU). Proposed Neuroprotective and neurotransmitter effects.
Mecobalamin: a study (PMID: 20406575) demonstrated a progressive decrease of sciatic nerve IGF-1 mRNA and peptide contents, and peripheral nerve dysfunction in the saline-treated diabetics over 12 weeks in contrast to the normal control non-diabetics.

Table 3. Sampling of Drugs in ASD Clinical Trials and Their Generally Proposed Actions

Study of Aripiprazole to Treat Children and Adolescents With Autism	Phase II	The Clinical Global impression (CGI) Improvement Scale.; The Irritability subscale of the Aberrant Behavior Checklist (ABC); The Clinical Global Impression Severity Scale.
A Study of Aripiprazole in Children and Adolescents With Aspergers and Pervasive Developmental Disorder.	Phase II	The Clinical Global impression(CGI) Improvement Scale.; The Irritability subscale of the Aberrant Behavior Checklist (ABC); The Clinical Global Impression Severity Scale.;CY-BOCS (Children's Yale-Brown Obsessive Compulsive Scale)
Study of Aripiprazole in the Treatment of Serious Behavioral Problems in Children and Adolescents With Autistic Disorder (AD)	Phase III	Number of Participants With Serious Adverse Events (SAEs), Treatment-Emergent Adverse Events (AEs), Deaths, AEs Leading to Discontinuation, Extra Pyramidal Syndrome (EPS)-Related AEs; Mean Change From Baseline in Total Simpson-Angus Scale (SAS)
Aripiprazole in Children With Autism: A Pilot Study	Phase II	Clinical Global Impressions; Children's Psychiatric Rating Scale
An Open-Label Trial of Aripiprazole in Autism Spectrum Disorders	Phase II	Clinical Global Impressions-Improvement; Aberrant Behavior Checklist-Irritability subscale
Pilot Study of the Effect of Aripiprazole Treatment in Autism Spectrum Disorders on Functional Magnetic Resonance Imaging (fMRI) Activation Patterns and Symptoms	Phase IV	RBS-R (Repetitive Behavior Scale - Revised); CY-BOCS (Children's Yale-Brown Obsessive Compulsive Scale)
OPT - Phase IV Long Term Maintenance Study of Aripiprazole for the Treatment of Irritability Associated With Autistic Disorder	Phase IV	Time from randomization to relapse; Mean change from end of Phase 1 to Week 16 endpoint (LOCF) on the Aberrant Behavior Checklist - Irritability Subscale; Mean Clinical Global Impression - Improvement scale score at Week 16 endpoint (LOCF)
Study of Aripiprazole in the Treatment of Children and Adolescents With Autistic Disorder (AD)	Phase III	Mean Change (Week 8 - Baseline) in the Autistic Behavior Checklist (ABC) Irritability Subscale Score; Mean Clinical Global Impressions Improvement Scale (CGI-I) Score; Number of Participants With Response at Week 8; Mean Change (Week 8 - Baseline)
Study of Aripiprazole in the Treatment of Children and Adolescents With Autistic Disorder (AD)	Phase III	Mean Change (Week 8 - Baseline) in the Autistic Behavior Checklist (ABC) Irritability Subscale Score; Mean Clinical Global Impressions Improvement Scale (CGI-I) Score; Number of Participants With Response at Week 8; Mean Change (Week 8 - Baseline)

Evaluating the Effectiveness of Aripiprazole and D-Cycloserine to Treat Symptoms Associated With Autism	Phase III	Aberrant Behavior Checklist (ABC) Irritability Subscale; Clinical Global Impression (CGI) Scale; ABC Subscales; Vineland Maladaptive Behavior Subscales; A modified version of the Compulsion Subscale of the Children's Yale-Brown Obsessive Compulsive Scale.
Efficacy of Aripiprazole Versus Placebo in the Reduction of Aggressive and Aberrant Behavior in Autistic Children	Phase I	Clinical Global Impression Improvement (CGI-AD); Aberrant Behavior Checklist; Abnormal Involuntary Movement Scale (AIMS)
Long-Term Olanzapine Treatment in Children With Autism	Phase II Phase III	Children's Psychiatric Rating Scale; Aberrant Behavior Checklist; Clinical Global Impressions; Treatment Emergent Symptoms Scale; Olanzapine Untoward Effects Checklist; Abnormal Involuntary Movement Scale; Neurological Rating Scale

Table 4. Antipsychotic Clinical Trials, Trial Phase and Outcome Measures (Continued on table 5)

A Controlled Study of Olanzapine in Children With Autism	Phase II	Children's Psychiatric Rating Scale; Clinical Global Impressions; Abberant Behavior Checklist; Treatment Emergent Symptoms Scale; Olanzapine Untoward Effects Checklist; Abnormal Involuntary Movement Scale; Neurological Rating Scale
Study of Paliperidone ER in Adolescents and Young Adults With Autism	Phase III	The IrritabIrritibility subscale of the Aberrant Behavior Checklist (ABC) will be used as the caregiver-rated primary outcome measure. The Clinical Global Impression- Improvement(CGI-I) will be included as a primary outcome measure
A Study of the Effectiveness and Safety of Two Doses of Risperidone in the Treatment of Children and Adolescents With Autistic Disorder	Phase IV	Allocation: Randomized; Endpoint Classification: Safety/Efficacy Study; Intervention Model: Parallel Assignment; Masking: Double Blind (Subject, Caregiver, Investigator); Primary Purpose: Treatment
A Study of the Effectiveness and Safety of Risperidone Versus Placebo in the Treatment of Children With Autistic Disorder and Other Pervasive Developmental Disorders (PDD)	Phase III	Change in the Irritability Subscale of the Aberrant Behavior Checklist (ABC) and other ABC subscales at end of treatment compared with baseline; Change from baseline to end of treatment in Nisonger Child Behavior Rating Form (N-CBRF), Visual Analogue Scale

Pharmacogenomics in Autism Treatment	Phase II Phase III	ABC and CGI; ABC
Treatment of Autism in Children and Adolescents	Phase III	
Risperidone Pharmacokinetics in Children With Pervasive Developmental Disorder (PDD)	Phase I	Quantify tVariability of clearance and volume of distribution among AE rating, weight gain and ABC responder status; Exploratory analysis will be performed to examine the relationship of other factors to risperidone and metabolite concentrations.
Pharmacogenetics of Risperidone in Children With Pervasive Developmental Disorder (PDD)	Phase I	
Comparison of Applied Behavioral Analysis (ABA) Versus ABA and Risperidone		
RUPP PI PDD: Drug and Behavioral Therapy for Children With Pervasive Developmental Disorders		Home Situations Questionnaire; Vineland Daily Living Skills Scale; Irritability subscale-Aberrant Behavioral Checklist; Clinical Global Impressions-Improvement (CGI-I)
Risperidone Treatment In Children With Autism Spectrum Disorder And High Levels Of Repetitive Behavior	Phase II	Aberrant Behavior Checklist
Ziprasidone in Children With Autism: A Pilot Study	Phase II	Clinical Global Impressions; Children's Psychiatric Rating Scale
An Observational Study to Evaluate the Safety and the Effects of Risperidone Compared With Other Atypical Antipsychotic Drugs on the Growth and Sexual Maturation in Children		To comparZ-scores for height, age at current Tanner stage, and prolactin-related adverse events between patients exposed to risperidone and patients exposed to other atypical antipsychotic drugs.; Assess the prolactin value and risk of hyperprolactine

Table 5. Antipsychotic Clinical Trials, Trial Phase and Outcome Measures (Continued)

Citalopram for Children With Autism and Repetitive Behavior (STAART Study 1)	Phase II	Clinical Global Improvement; Safety Monitoring Uniform Research Form (SMURF); Children's Yale-Brown Obsessive-Compulsive Scale (CYBOCS); Repetitive Behavior Scale-Revised (RBS-R); Parent Chief Complaint; Aberrant Behavior Checklist;
Functional MRI Evaluation of the Effect of Citalopram in Autism Spectrum Disorders	PhaseI	Functional Magnetic Resonance Imaging; Clinicians Global Improvement Scale; Childrens Yale- Brown Obsessive Compulsive Scale
Randomized Study of Fluoxetine in Children and Adolescents With Autism	Phase I	
Study of Fluoxetine in Adults With Autistic Disorder	PhaseI	
Extended Management and Measurement of Autism	Phase III	Safety Outcomes: Laboratory determinations, Urine drugs of abuse tests,Vital Signs,Physical Examinations, Adverse Events/Serious Adverse Events, Clinical Global Impression of Severity (CGI-S AD)
Fluoxetine Essay in Children With Autism	Phase II	Subscores of Autism Diagnostic Interview (ADI-R)at each visit of the protocol (LECOUTER et RUTTER, 1989); Sides effect scale (FSEC); Aberrant Behavior Checklist (Aman et al., 1985); Clinical Global Impressions (CGI) severity and improvement.
Study of Fluoxetine in Autism	Phase III	The percentage change from baseline to the endpoint visit for the CYBOCS-PDD score; The time and dose related course of therapeutic effects; The inter-relationship between these effects in the context of global clinical changes; The indirect effect.
Effectiveness of Early Intervention With Fluoxetine in Enhancing Developmental Processes in Children With Autism (STAART Study 2)	Phase III	Feasibility and safety of conducting placebo control trial of fluoxetine; Side effect and drop out evaluation
Fluvoxamine and Sertraline in Childhood Autism - Does SSRI Therapy Improve Behaviour and/or Mood?	Phase III	The severity of the autistic child's behaviour or condition (assessed by parents); Weight and vital signs; Blood count and liver function studies
Mirtazapine Treatment of Anxiety in Children and Adolescents With Pervasive Developmental Disorders	Phase III	Pediatric Anxiety Rating Scale (PARS); Clinical Global Impressions (CGI)

Table 6. Antidepressant Clinical Trials, Trial Phase and Outcome Measures

Methylphenidate for Attention Deficit Hyperactivity Disorder and Autism in Children	Phase III	Conners' Teacher Rating Scale-Revised (CTRS-R); Continuous Performance Test (CPT); Matching Familiar Figures Test (MFFT); Speeded Classification Task (SCT); Delay of Gratification Task (DOG); Conners' Parent Rating Scale (CPRS)-Short Form;
A Pilot Study of Daytrana TM in Children With Autism Co-Morbid for Attention Deficit Hyperactivity Disorder (ADHD) Symptoms	Phase III	Determine if Daytrana is safe and well-tolerated by children with Autism co-morbid for ADHD; Determine if Daytrana is effective in both school and home

Table 7. Stimulant Clinical Trials, Trial Phase and Outcome Measures

Divalproex Sodium ER vs Placebo in Childhood/Adolescent Autism valproex Sodium vs. Placebo in Childhood/Adolescent Autism	Phase II	Clinical Global Impression-Improvement; Aberrant Behavior Checklist Clinical Global Impression-Improvement; Aberrant Behavior Checklist; Clinical Global Impression-Improvement; Aberrant Behavior Checklist
Divalproex Sodium ER in Adult Autism	Phase IV	
A Study of Divalproex Sodium in Children With ASD and Epileptiform EEG	Phase II	epileptiform EEG discharges; Improvement in behavior
Oxcarbazepine Versus Placebo in Childhood Autism	1	Vineland Adaptive Behavior Scales; Aberrant Behavior Checklist; Clinical Global Impression Improvement Scale; Autism Diagnostic Observation Schedule
Riluzole to Treat Child and Adolescent Obsessive-Compulsive Disorder With or Without Autism Spectrum Disorders	Phase II	Reduction of 30% or more in Children's Yale-Brown Obsessive-Compulsive Scale (CY-BOCS) and Repetitive Behavior Scale; Much/Very much improved on Clinical Global Impressions - Improvement score (CGI-I)
Valproate Response in Aggressive Autistic Adolescents	Phase III	

Table 8. Anticonvulsant Clinical Trials, Trial Phase and Outcome Measures

Treatment With Acetyl-Choline Esterase Inhibitors in Children With Autism Spectrum Disorders	Phase IV	Core autistic symptoms (ATEC); Side effects and adverse events questionnaire; Linguistic performance (CELF-4); Adaptive functioning (Vineland-II); Co-morbid behaviors (CSI-4 questionnaire); Executive functions (BRIEF) questionnaire
Drug Treatment for Autism	Phase II	Cognitive Assessment
The Effect of Donepezil on REM Sleep in Children With Autism	Phase II	The primary outcome measure of this protocol is to determine if donepezil can increase the percentage of time that subjects with autism spend in REM sleep.; A secondary aim of this protocol is to examine changes in functional outcome, including cognitive.
Galantamine Versus Placebo in Childhood Autism	Phase III	Autism Diagnostic Observation Schedule-Generic (ADOS-G)- Change from Baseline to Final Visit; Clinical Global Impression Improvement (CGI)- Change from Baseline to Final Visit; Aberrant Behavior Checklist (ABC) (hyperactivity/irritability sections).

Table 9. AcetylCholine Esterase Inhibitors Clinical Trials, Trial Phase and Outcome Measures

An Open Label Extension Study of STX209 in Subjects With Autism Spectrum Disorders	Phase II	Irritability subscale of the Aberrant Behavior Checklist
Study of Arbaclofen for the Treatment of Social Withdrawal in Subjects With Autism Spectrum Disorders	Phase II	Aberrant Behavior Checklist-Social Withdrawal Subscale
Open-Label Study of the Safety and Tolerability of STX209 in Subjects With Autism Spectrum Disorders	Phase II	Adverse events; Irritability Subscale of the Aberrant Behavior Checklist, Community Version

Table 10. Immunomodulator Clinical Trials, Trial Phase and Outcome Measures

Open-Label Extension Study of Kuvan for Autism	Phase II Phase III	Clinical Global Impressions Scale; Vineland Adaptive Behavior Scale; Clinical Global Impression: Severity; Children's Yale Brown Obsessive Compulsive Scale; Parental Global Assessment; Preschool Language Scale; Connor's Preschool ADHD question
Intranasal Oxytocin for the Treatment of Autism Spectrum Disorders	Phase II	Change from Baseline to week 12 on the Diagnostic Analysis of Nonverbal Accuracy (DANVA2); Change from Baseline to week 12 on the Social Responsivity Scale (SRS); Change from Baseline to week 12 on the Clinical Global Impressions Scale - Improvement
Intranasal Oxytocin in the Treatment of Autism	Phase II	Clinical Global Impressions Scale (CGI); Diagnostic Analysis of Nonverbal Accuracy, Adult Paralanguage Test (DANVA2-AP); Repetitive Behavior Scale (RBS); Event Contingent Reporting; Yale-Brown Obsessive-Compulsive Scale (YBOCS); Social Responsiveness.
An fMRI Study of the Effect of Intravenous Oxytocin vs. Placebo on Response Inhibition and Face Processing in Autism	Phase I	
A Study of Oxytocin in Children and Adolescents With Autistic Disorder	Phase II	Tolerability of Oxytocin Nasal Spray; Biomarkers; Feasibility; Acceptability of Oxytocin Nasal Spray
Brain Imaging Study of Adults With Autism Spectrum Disorders	Phase I	Changes in brain activations; Performance scores and reaction time on behavioral tasks.
Study of Glutathione, Vitamin C and Cysteine in Children With Autism and Severe Behavior Problems	Phase I	Improvement in both developmental skills and behavior with either glutathione or glutathione, Vitamin C and N-acetylcysteine therapy as compared to placebo therapy. Subjects will also be monitored using clinical and laboratory safety parameters.
Synthetic Human Secretin in Children With Autism	Phase III	
Synthetic Human Secretin in Children With Autism and Gastrointestinal Dysfunction	Phase III	

Sapropterin as a Treatment for Autistic Disorder	Phase II	Clinical Global Impression -- Improvement (CGI-I) Scale; Preschool Language Scale (PLS); Vineland Adaptive Behavior Scale-II; Children's Yale Brown Obsessive Compulsive Scale (C-YBOCS); Connor's Preschool ADHD questionnaire; Adverse Events Scale
Secretin for the Treatment of Autism	Phase III	
The Effects of Oxytocin on Complex Social Cognition in Autism Spectrum Disorders	Phase I	Empathic accuracy performance; fmri BOLD response during empathic accuracy task
Cholesterol in ASD: Characterization and Treatment	Phase I Phase II	Behavioral Changes

Table 11. Hormone or Related Clinical Trials, Trial Phase and Outcome Measures

A Study of Atomoxetine for Attention Deficit and Hyperactive/Impulsive Behaviour Problems in Children With ASD
Atomoxetine and Parent Management Training in Treating Children With Autism and Symptoms of Attention Deficit Disorder With Hyperactivity
Effectiveness of Atomoxetine in Treating ADHD Symptoms in Children and Adolescents With Autism
Atomoxetine Versus Placebo for Symptoms of Attention-Deficit/Hyperactivity Disorder (ADHD) in Children and Adolescents With Autism Spectrum Disorder
Atomoxetine, Placebo and Parent Management Training in Autism
Efficiency of Bumetanide in Autistic Children
Early Pharmacotherapy Aimed at Neuroplasticity in Autism : Safety and Efficacy
Buspirone in the Treatment of 2-6 Year Old Children With Autistic Disorder
A Trial of CM-AT in Children With Autism- Open Label Extension Study
A Trial of CM-AT in Children With Autism
Effects of CX516 on Functioning in Fragile X Syndrome and Autism
Mercury Chelation to Treat Autism
Dimercaptosuccinic Acid (DMSA) Treatment of Children With Autism and Heavy Metal Toxicity
Trial of Low-Dose Naltrexone for Children With Pervasive Developmental Disorder (PDD)
A Pilot Trial of Mecamylamine for the Treatment of Autism
Treatment of Sleep Problems in Children With Autism Spectrum Disorder With Melatonin

An Open-label Trial of Metformin for Weight Control of Pediatric Patients on Antipsychotic Medications.
Efficacy Study of Subcutaneous Methyl-B12 in Children With Autism
Methylphenidate in Children and Adolescents With Pervasive Developmental Disorders
Omega-3 Fatty Acids Monotherapy in Children and Adolescents With Autism Spectrum Disorders
Evaluation and Treatment of Copper/Zinc Imbalance in Children With Autism
Dose Finding Study of Pioglitazone in Children With Autism Spectrum Disorders (ASD)
Transcranial Magnetic Stimulation (TMS) Measures of Plasticity and Excitatory/Inhibitory Ratio as Biomarkers: R-baclofen Effects in Normal Volunteers
Melatonin for Sleep in Children With Autism
Trichuris Suis Ova Adult Autism Symptom Domains
Multidimensional Measurement of Psychopharmacological Treatment Response * CPI

Table 12. Other Clinical Trials

4. Pharmacological strategies in autism spectrum disorders

Treatment monitoring and treatment response measurement provide methods by which treatment strategies may be assessed, tested and dynamically applied to the treatment process. Two examples are presented. The first illustrates the longitudinal measurement of risperidone response and the second illustrates a treatment review and re-conceptualization of treatment strategy.

The first case is an actigraphic, psychometric and observational study of risperidone response in a six year old autism spectrum disordered child with Kabuki Syndrome. It provides an illustration of circadian and behavioral disturbances in a child, and the utility of single subject repeated actigraphic, psychometric and observational measurements of treatment response (Duke, 2010).

Actigraphic measurements, such as those used in the following case, are not necessary to obtain meaningful treatment response data, although additional measurements, such as actigraphic data, are helpful.

The non-invasive nature of watch-like actigraphy devices (Rispironics Actiwatch) is particularly attractive for use in pediatric populations. Meaningful treatment response measurements are obtained when actigraphic data is combined with psychometric and observational repeated measurements.

This case study includes baseline and repeated psychological, observational and actigraphic measurements that were initiated prior to treatment with risperidone and repeated throughout the treatment process.

Actigraphic measurements provide a basis by which to measure sleep and sleep onset latency as well as periods of mobility and immobility. In this case the actigraphic device was programmed to record activity every thirty seconds.

Actigraphic measurements were made utilizing a watch-like actigraphic device with an 11 day baseline actigraphic measurement period and continued measurements that included the initiation of a pharmacological intervention for 6 days, followed by a planned adjustment to b.i.d. dosing that was measured for an additional 4 days. This initial actigraphic study resulted in over 65,000 measurements of activity. Repeated observations continued throughout the treatment period and actigraphic studies were repeated after 23 months of risperidone treatment.

The measurement methods included the Personality Inventory for Children (PIC) an objective multidimensional measurement of affect, behavior, ability and family function. The PIC was administered prior to treatment with risperidone and repeated after 23 months of treatment. The PIC serves as both an actuarial pre-treatment diagnostic tool as well as a post-treatment repeated measurement indicating treatment and developmentally associated change (Duke, B., 1991).

Observational methods were employed throughout the treatment process. A primary observer (The Child's Mother) was trained to report symptom percentages present since previous observations utilizing the operationally defined and observer defined items of the Systematic Observation Scale™ (Duke, B., 1990) throughout the treatment process. The Systematic Observation Scale™ utilizes single-subject repeated measurements. Symptoms and issues of interest are defined and a variety of frequency and sampling methods can be applied. The Systematic Observation Scale was designed so Primary Observers (parents, guardians, self observers or others) can make pre-treatment and subsequent observations to track, document and evaluate symptom variation over the course of an illness. The measurement utilized is the percentage of time the symptom is observed by the primary observer since the previous observation.

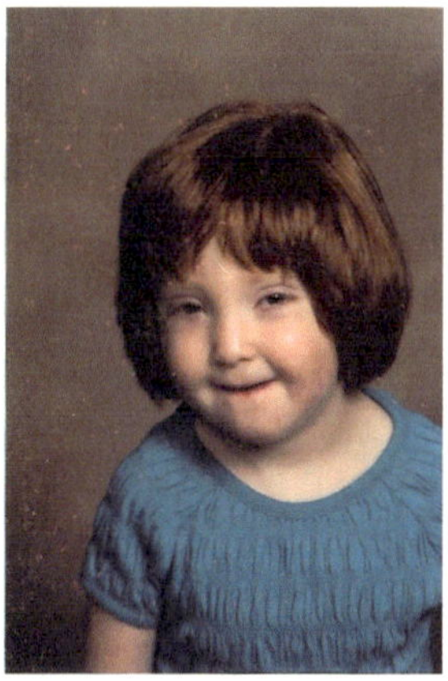

Fig. 3. The child's parents kindly consented to the use of this photograph.

The actigraphic study was designed to select a child anticipating a psychopharmacological intervention.

The study was reviewed and approved by the Child Psychopharmacology Institute Institutional Review Board and was registered with the National Institutes of Health Protocol Registration System (NCT00723580) as a non-randomized, single subject, case study clinical trial.

The Study Investigator's DSM-IV diagnoses were:

- Axis I
- 299.80 Pervasive Developmental Disorder Not Otherwise Specified
- 314.01 Attention-Deficit Hyperactivity Disorder
- 327.30 Circadian Rhythm Sleep Disorder (unspecified type)
- Axis II
- 317 Mild Mental Retardation
- Axis III
- Kabuki Syndrome*
- Hearing Impairment

The child's impulsivity and inability to sleep represented a significant symptom and risk factors. She frequently moved about restlessly until 5:00 AM and would often sleep (or partially sleep) with her eyes open. She had frequent infections and had been previously stimulated by diphenylhydramine, over-sedated on clonidine and had mood destabilization when tried on mirtazapine. The child's diagnosis of Kabuki Syndrome had been previously established by a geneticist at the Mayo Clinic. The child presented with severe impulsivity, psychomotor acceleration, severe insomnia and obsessive compulsive behaviors that included touching objects to the whites of her eyes (these behaviors occurred multiple times an hour). An MLL2 mutation has been verified in this child. It has recently been reported that Kabuki Syndrome is caused by mutations in MLL2, a gene that encodes a Trithorax-group histone methyltransferase, a protein important in the epigenetic control of active chromatin states (Hannibal et, al, 2011).

Dr. Niikawa and Dr. Kuroki described Kabuki Syndrome in 1981. The term was used because of the affected children's facial resemblance to the famous Kabuki actors that perform in traditional Japanese theater.

Kabuki Syndrome is rare and diagnosis is complicated by the diverse spectrum of characteristics. Arched eyebrows, thick eyelashes, eversion of the lateral lower lid and long palpebral fissures contribute to the resemblance. Skeletal and dermatological abnormalities are common along with short stature, behavioral and pervasive developmental disorders and mild to moderate intellectual disability. Congenital heart defects and hearing impairment are often associated with the syndrome. The proportion of male to female occurrence is equal and no correlation with birth order has been found (Adam & Hudgins, 2005).

The assessment and treatment plan included a baseline biopsychosocial history, a baseline cognitive and personality assessment and the initiation of actigraphy measurements. The initial 21 day study of actigraphic measurements included an eleven day baseline prior to pharmacological interventions. The pharmacological Intervention following the medication free baseline utilized risperidone .25 mg q.h.s. initiated for seven days and then increased to twice daily dosing. Subsequent actigraphic measurements reflected the subsequent risperdal dose of .5 mg three times daily. Systematic observations continued throughout the treatment period and the personality assessment was repeated at the study end point. The established treatment goals were to: improve sleep; reduce general impairment; reduce hyperactivity; reduce impulsivity; reduce irritability and improve social functioning.

Hypotheses and Outcome Measures:

H1: Reduced percentages of primary symptoms will be associated with increased sleep during sleep periods (activity and sleep measurements). Actiwatch Communication and Sleep Analysis Instruction Manual (Respironics).

H2: Sleep quality will be reflected by reduced standard deviations of activity during sleep periods.

H3: Positive treatment response as reflected by reduced percentages of primary symptoms will be associated with decreased activity during activity periods.

H4: Reduced impulsivity will be associated with reduced standard deviations of activity during activity periods.

Outcome Measures

a. Actigraphic Measurement of Treatment Conditions:
b. Baseline May 12, 2008 and two additional 21 day periods between May 12, 2008 to July 14, 2010
c. Systematic Observation Scale™ Measurements: May 7, 2008 to July 14th, 2010
d. Personality Inventory for Children-Revised: pre-test May 2008 and post-test April 2010

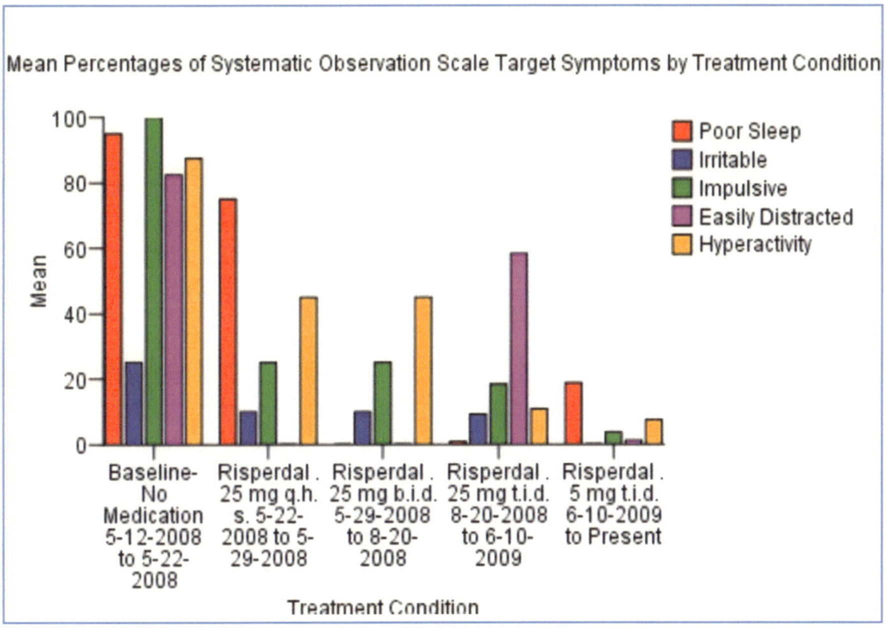

Fig. 4. Target Symptoms by Treatment Condition (BL- .25 mg - .5 mg t.i.d)

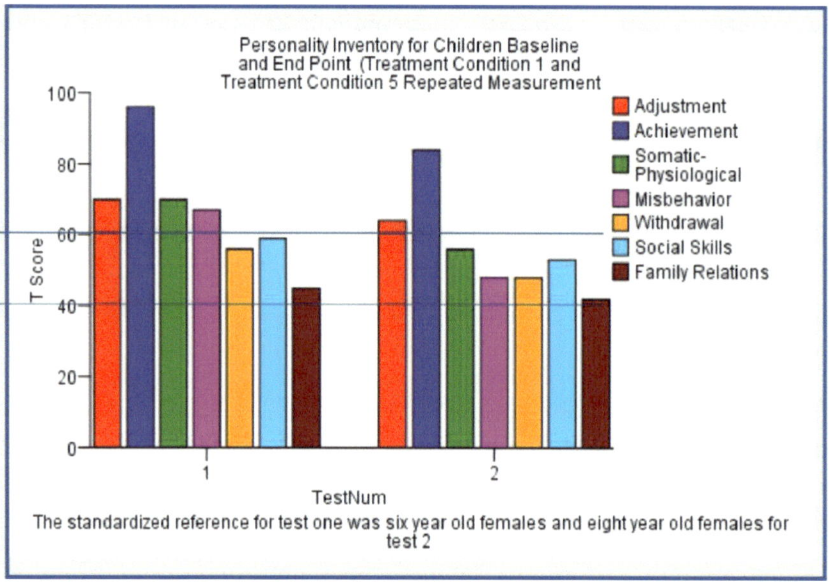

Fig. 5. Personality Inventory Pre-Test and Post-Test

Study conclusions: Sleep quantity was increased; Sleep quality was improved; Hyperactivity was reduced; Impulsivity was reduced; Significance between treatment conditions, activity and target symptoms was demonstrated.

The second case is a ten year old male who had received numerous medications over the past several years. Despite these treatments, and optimal family environment and commitment, the primary symptoms of mood instability and cognitive impairment continued. The child was receiving aripiprazole 5 mg q.a.m. and Concerta 36 mg q.a.m. Prior to the treatment review, the child had become disinhibited and severely impulsive in response to treatment with an SSRI, which was discontinued. He had also demonstrated a dose related worsening when tried on quetiapine. The quetiapine was discontinued due to associated insomnia and worsened mood and behavioral states.

At the time of the review the child presented with neurological immaturity, delayed fine motor integration, jerky saccadic eye movements and possible symptoms of partial complex seizures. The child's episodic emotional dyscontrol, attention and cognitive functioning did not appear to be, pharmacologically, optimally addressed.

DSM IV Diagnoses: Axis I:

299.80 Pervasive Developmental Disorder NOS

296.90 Mood Disorder NOS

314.01 Attention Deficit/Hyperactivity Disorder, Combined Type

307.7 Encopresis

		Sum of Squares	df	Mean Square	F	Sig.
Activity	Between Groups	4.476E8	3	1.492E8	1057.569	.000
	Within Groups	2.698E10	191235	141065.613		
	Total	2.742E10	191238			
Poor Sleep	Between Groups	16583.631	4	4145.908	10.542	.002
	Within Groups	3539.583	9	393.287		
	Total	20123.214	13			
Impulsive	Between Groups	13278.274	4	3319.568	15.707	.000
	Within Groups	1902.083	9	211.343		
	Total	15180.357	13			
Hyperactivit y	Between Groups	11034.524	4	2758.631	10.994	.002
	Within Groups	2258.333	9	250.926		
	Total	13292.857	13			
Irritable	Between Groups	838.095	4	209.524	4.481	.029
	Within Groups	420.833	9	46.759		
	Total	1258.929	13			
Easily Distracted	Between Groups	14721.131	4	3680.283	4.379	.031
	Within Groups	7564.583	9	840.509		
	Total	22285.714	13			

Fig. 6. Treatment Response: Analysis of Variance

Following the treatment review the initial strategy was to add carbamazepine 200 mg ER q.p.m. x 7 days then b.i.d. Subsequent to improved emotional stability and broadly reduced symptoms the contribution of aripiprazole was assessed by a dose reduction to 2.5 mg q.a.m. for four days and subsequently replaced with risperidone .5 mg b.i.d. Plans were made to subsequently assess his stimulant treatment response as the monitoring continued. Figure 7 displays symptom percentage averages over the treatment transition.

Printable observation forms and item defintions are available and free for non-commercial use on the Child Psychopharmacology Institute website (www. ChildPsychopharmacologyInstitute.org).

5. Pharmacological protection and prevention strategies on the horizon: Glutamatergic modulation and neuroprotection

Although pharmacological interventions utilized in Autistic Spectrum Disorders are generally associated with targeting behavioral or emotional impairments, little attention has been given to the important potential of glutamatergic regulation and neuroprotection in this vulnerable population.

While a single drug has not triumphed in the treatment of autism spectrum disorders, many drugs have proven helpful to varying degrees and for various purposes. The dearth of children's pharmacological studies stand in stark contrast to wide use of pharmacological interventions in ASD children.

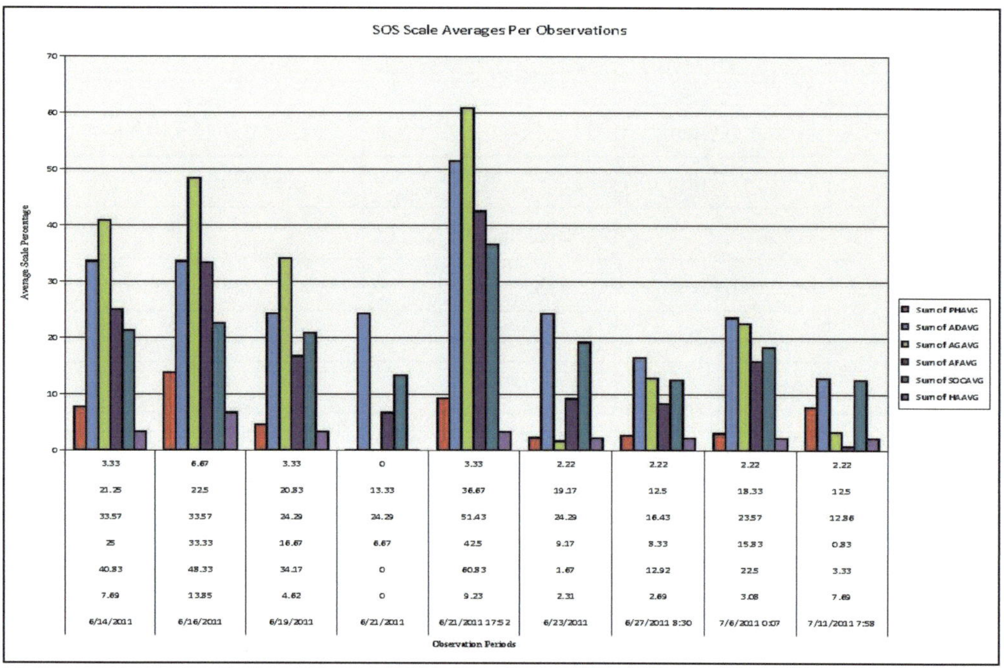

Fig. 7. Symptom Percentage Observation Scale Averages

Alternative pathways of ASD pathology being explored include the study of tetrahydrobiopterin (BH_4) as a novel therapeutic intervention and point to ASD children as having low levels of BH_4. Early studies suggest low BH_4 levels during development have devastating consequences on the central nervous system leading to or potentiating the neuropathology of ASD (Frye, et al, 2010). These studies are promising and may suggest a role for BH_4 treatment or treatment augmentation in the ASD population.

It is proposed that pharmacological approaches with neuroprotective characteristics have potential to reduce the dynamic pathogenic states that are likely occurring in highly symptomatic young children who are in developmentally critical stages of neural patterning and maturation. In a manner similar to the example provided regarding atypical antipsychotics, drugs will increasingly be chosen based on their particular characteristics or used together for separate or synergistic effects.

Arriving at a full understanding of these approaches will take further studies that consider the potential for unwanted effects. The Frye study, for example, noted that based on seven studies in which 451 patients with autism were treated with sapropterin (synthetic BH_4) that ninety-seven (21.5%) experienced adverse effects for which a causal relationship with the study drug could not be ruled out. The most frequently reported adverse effects were sleep disorders, excitement, hyperkinesia, enuresis and diarrhea. It will be important to learn if sapropterin's benefits are primarily from developmentally critical neuroprotective effects and/or effects on neurotransmitters. It will also be important to determine if indiscriminate neurotransmitter potentiation in dysregulated neurons and circuits are being reflected in the adverse effect profile that some demonstrate.

Synaptic molecules are important targets for protective treatments, to slow disease progression and preserve cognitive and functional abilities by preserving synaptic structure and function. Glutamate receptors and post synaptic density proteins play a central role in excitatory synaptic plasticity. Synaptic dysregulation may contribute to brain disorders present in those with Autism Spectrum Disorders by preventing appropriate synaptic signaling and plasticity.

The NMDA receptor is fundamental to excitatory synaptic plasticity and neurological diseases. Synaptic loss is a pathologic correlate of cognitive decline. Synaptic dysfunction is evident long before synapses and neurons are lost. The synapse constitutes an important target for treatments to slow progression and preserve cognitive and functional abilities in these diseases. (van Spronsen & Hoogenraad, 2010)

5.1 Excitotoxity and glutamatergic activity

Current hypotheses propose excessive glutamate activity can lead to excitotoxicity interfering with normal neurodevelopment in schizophrenia. Similarly, these effects may be involved in the neurodevelopment in ASD. The excitotoxicity is hypothesized to continue and is linked to disease progression in schizophrenia ultimately resulting in pathologically functioning NMDA glutamate receptors. These hypotheses are consistent with those that identify the final common pathway of many neuropsychiatric diseases as synaptic pathology.

While the future promises biomarkers, RNAi strategies, stem cell transplantation and other genetic treatments, arresting and/or reducing developmental pathogenic potential by discovering and developing methods of effecting glutamatergic regulation by NMDA antagonism or other methods is a worthy, if not urgent, treatment goal for Autism Spectrum Disordered children. Blocking or moderating excessive glutamate neurotransmission with NMDA antagonists may prevent or mitigate damage, maladaptive neurodevelopment or neurodegenerative processes.

Some NMDA antagonists appear to be neuromodulators that reduce the excitotoxicity effects of dysregulated circuits and support dendritic health, long term potentiation and neural plasticity. Such treatments may one day provide preventative pharmacological interventions as well as those that can reduce impairment and improve functioning.

Two NMDA antagonists are particuilarly interesting candidates for therapeutic potential in the ASD population, memantine and dextromethorphan/quinidine (Duke & Kaye, 2010).

Memantine, as an augmenting agent, demonstrated significant improvements in open-label use for language function, social behavior, and self-stimulatory behaviors, although self-stimulatory behaviors comparatively improved to a lesser degree. Chronic use so far appears to have no serious side effects (Chez MG, et al 2007).

Dextromethorphan/quinidine (DM/Q) shares the attributes of being an uncompetitive NMDA antagonist with memantine, however, importantly; DM/Q is a sigma 1 agonist and binds to SERT. Binding data comparing memantine with DM/Q demonstrate the presence of Sigma 1 and SERT binding in DM/Q but not in memantine (Werling, et al 2007).

One of the characteristics that suggests DM/Q might have therapeutic potential in ASD is its efficacy in pseudobulbar affect (PBA). The efficacy and safety of dextromethorphan and quinidine was demonstrated in clinical trials of late stage neurological conditions (amyotrophic lateral Sclerosis and Multiple Sclerosis) demonstrating reductions of emotional lability and improvements in sleep. These findings suggest that the pharmacological characteristics of DM/Q may, at some level rescue synaptic signaling and may have the potential to affect neurodevelopmental trajectory in dysregulated developing nervous systems such as those with Autism Spectrum Disorders.

AVP-923 was approved by the FDA in 2010 as Nuedexta™ the first and only treatment for Pseudobulbar Affect (PBA). This is an important therapeutic for those suffering the debilitating effects of pseudobulbar affect. The efficacy in reducing dysregulated and involuntary congruent and incongruent emotional expressions is a significant achievement. Why is DM/Q (Nuedexta) effective in PBA? That, of course, is unknown, but PBA is often considered the result of connectivity and neural circuitry failures and ASD is known to have signaling and connectivity pathologies. Emotional lability is often associated with behavioral dyscontrol, irritibility, assaultive and raging behaviors that prompt pharmacological intervention in children with ASD.

NMDA antagonists may offer a therapeutic pathway through modulation or regulation of dysregulated glutamatergic processes. The potential of DM/Q (Nuedexta) in ASD, particularly in the early developmental stages of the illness, to rescue and support synaptic function is worthy of further study.

Although the mechanism of action of DM/Q is not fully characterized, its unique properties as an NMDA receptor antagonist and as a Sigma 1 receptor agonist appear to convey effects of both neuroprotection and neuromodulation. Future studies will help us determine if these unique characteristics will lead to improved outcomes for those with autism spectrum disorders.

6. Conclusion

The distress, irritability and emotional lability often seen in Autism Spectrum Disorders may be a reflection of pathological glutamatergic functioning or otherwise dysregulated circuits relative to inhibitory-excitatory balance. When sustained, these symptoms demonstrate potential for pathological development of abnormal neural circuits capable of dysregulation through neural synchronicity and state dependent effects on genetic expression. Within the framework of this hypothesis the neural plasticity and critical periods, present in developing brains, place them at particular risk.

We currently have drugs and compounds that have the ability to reduce impairment and improve functioning in many with ASD when used, monitored and managed thoughtfully. Early pharmacological intervention related to severe emotional lability, irritability and dysregulated circuits may also reduce the pathogenic potential and reduce or prevent the development or maintenance of pathological processes.

7. Acknowledgement

As a faculty member of the Child Psychopharmacology Institute and as a consultant for Avanir Pharmaceuticals I wish to express my gratitude to my colleagues Randall Kaye, M.D., MPH, R. Dennis Staton, Ph.D., M.D. and Scott Siegert, Pharm.D. for their collegial support and expertise.

8. References

Adam, MP & Hudgins, L. "Kabuki Syndrome: A Review." Clin Genet, 2005: Mar;67(3):209-19.

Ashwood, P., Wills S., and Van de Water, J. "The immune response in autism: a new frontier for autism research." *Journal of Leukocyte Biology*, 2006 : Volume 80, July.

Buxbaum, JD. "Multiple rare variants in the etiology of autism spectrum disorders." *Dialogues Clin Neurosci.*, 2009: 11(1)35-43.

Careaga M, Van de Water J, Ashwood P. "Immune dysfunction in autism: a pathway to treatment." *Neurotherapeutics*, 2010 : Jul;7(3) 283-92.

Caria A, Venuti P, & de Falco S. "Functional and Dysfunctional Brain Circuits Underlying Emotional Processing of Music in Autism Spectrum Disorders." *Cereb Cortex*, 2011: May 6. CDC. *Autism Spectrum Disorders.* August 1, 2011. http://www.cdc.gov/ncbddd/autism/research.html (accessed August 1, 2011).

Chez MG, Burton Q, Dowling T, Chang M, Khanna P, Kramer C. "Memantine as adjunctive therapy in children diagnosed with autistic spectrum disorders: an observation of initial clinical response and maintenance tolerability." *J Child Neurol.* , 2007: May;22(5):574-9.

Duke, B. & Kaye, R. "Breaking Pharmacological Barriers to Innovation: The Case for Assessing Dextromethorphan/Quinidine in Autistic Spectrum Disorders." *Journal of Brain Research Meeting: Emerging Neuroscience of Autism Spectrum Disorders.* San Diego: Elsevier, 2010.

Duke, B. "A 23 Month Longitudinal Actigraphic, Psychometric and Observational Study." *Journal of Brain Research Meeting: Emerging Neuroscience of Autism Spectrum Disorders.* San Diego: Elsevier, 2010. Poster.

Duke, B. "Measuring Response to Psychopharmacologic Interventions." *Proceedings of the American Psychological Association symposium, the Personality Inventory for Children: Assessment Linking Families and Schools.* San Francisco: American Psychological Association, 1991. D. Lachar, Chair.

Duke, B. "Pathogenic Effects of Central Nervous System Hyperarousal." *Medical Hypothesis,* 2008: 71: 212-217.

Duke, B.J. "Child Psychotherapy and the Scientific Method: The Systematic Observation Scale." *Proceedings of the Pacific Division, American Association For The Advancement of Science,* 1990: (9)1:21. .

Eagleson K., Campbell D., Thompson, B., Bergman, M., and Levitt, P. "The Autism Risk Genes MET and PLAUR Differentially Impact Cortical Development." *Autism Research 4:,* 2011: 68-83.

Estes A, Shaw DW, Sparks BF, Friedman S, Giedd JN, Dawson G, Bryan M, & Dager SR. "Basal ganglia morphometry and repetitive behavior in young children with autism spectrum disorder. ." *Autism Res.* , 2011 : Jun;4(3):212-20. .

Frye, R, Huffman, L, & Elliot, G. Tetrahydrobiopterin as a novel therapeutic intervention for autism. Neurotherapeutics, 2010 July;7(3): 241-249

Gilman, S. R. et al. "Rare de novo variants associated with autism implicate a large functional network of genes involved in formation and function of synapses." *Neuron,* 2011: 70, 898–907 .

Gleason MM, Egger HL, Emslie GJ, Greenhill LL, Kowatch RA, Lieberman AF, Luby JL,. "Psychopharmacological treatment for very young children: contexts and guidelines." *J Am Acad Child Adolesc Psychiatry. 2007 Dec;46(12):1532-72.,* 2007: Dec;46(12):1532-72.

Greer PL, Hanayama R, Bloodgood BL, Mardinly AR, Lipton DM, Flavell W, Kim TK, Griffith EC, Waldon Z, Maehr R, Ploegh HL, Chowdhury S, Worley PF, Steen J, Greenberg ME. "The Angelman Syndrome protein Ube3A regulates synapse development by ubiquitinating arc. ." *Cell,* 2010: Mar 5;140(5):704-16.

Groen WB, Buitelaar JK, van der Gaag RJ & Zwiers MP. "Pervasive microstructural abnormalities in autism: a DTI study." *J Psychiatry Neurosci.,* 2011: Jan;36(1): 32-40.

Hallmayer J, Cleveland S, Torres A, Phillips J, Cohen B, Torigoe T, Miller J, Fedele A, Collins J, Smith K, Lotspeich L, Croen LA, Ozonoff S, Lajonchere C, Grether JK, Risch N. "Genetic heritability and shared environmental factors among twin pairs with autism." *Archives of General Psychiatry,* 2011: July.

Hamberger A, Gillberg C, Palm A, Hagberg B. "Elevated CSF glutamate in Rett syndrome." *Neuropediatrics,* 1992 : Aug;23(4) 212-3.

Hannibal, MC et al. "Spectrum of MLL2 (ALR) mutations in 110 cases of Kabuki syndrome." Am J Med Genet A. 2011 Jul;155A(7):1511-6.

Isaacson, J. & Provenzale, J. "Diffusion tensor imaging for evaluation of the childhood brain and pediatric white matter disorders." *Neuroimaging Clin N Am.*, 2011: Feb;21(1):179-89, ix.

Kumar A, Sundaram SK, Sivaswamy L, Behen ME, Makki MI, Ager J, Janisse J, Chugani HT, & Chugani DC. "Alterations in frontal lobe tracts and corpus callosum in young children with autism spectrum disorder." *Cereb Cortex*, 2010: Sep;20(9):2103-13.

Kurth F, Narr KL, Woods RP, O'Neill J, Alger JR, Caplan R, McCracken JT, & Toga AW. "Diminished gray matter within the hypothalamus in autism disorder: a potential link to hormonal effects?" *Biol Psychiatry*, 2011: Aug 1;70(3):278-82.

Levitt, P. "Serotonin and the Autisms." *Arch Gen Psychiatry*, 2011: Commentary.

Levy, D. et al. "Rare de novo and transmitted copy-number variation in autistic spectrum disorders." *Neuron*, 2011: 70, 886–897 .

McGraw, C., Samaco, R. & Zoghbi, H. "Adult Neural Function Requires MeCP2." *Science*, 2011: July Vol333 p186.

Monji, A. "The microglia hypothesis of psychiatric disorders." *Nihon Shinkei Seishin Yakurigaku Zasshi*, 2011 : Feb;31(1):1-8.

Rice, C. "Prevalence of Autism Spectrum Disorders --- Autism and Developmental Disabilities Monitoring Network." (CDC United States) 2006.

Sacco R, Curatolo P, Manzi B, Militerni R, Bravaccio C, Frolli A, Lenti C,Saccani M, Elia M, Reichelt KL, Pascucci T, Puglisi-Allegra S. "Principal pathogenetic components and biological endophenotypes in autism spectrum disorders." *Autism Res.*, 2010: Sep 27.

Sanders, S. J. et al. "Multiple recurrent de novo CNVs, including duplications of the 7q11.23 Williams syndrome region, are strongly associated with autism." *Neuron*, 2011: 70:863–885 .

Schwartz, T and Stahl S. "Treatment strategies for dosing the second generation antipsychotics." *CNS Neurosci Ther.*, 2011 : Apr;17(2):110-7.

Siniscalchi, A. Gallelli, L. and De Sarro, G. "Use of Antiepileptic Drugs for Hyperkinetic Movement Disorders." *Current Neuropharmacology*, 2010: 8, 359-366.

Stahl, Stephen. *Stahl's Essential Psychopharmacology Online: Neuroscientific Basis and Practical Applications.* New York: Cambridge University Press, 2010 p. 274.

Szatmari, P. "Is Autism, at Least in Part, a Disorder of Fetal Programming?" *Arch Gen Psychiatry*, 2011: July 5, 2011.

Tuchman, R. & Cuccaro, M. "Epilepsy and Autism: Neurodevlopmental Perspective." *Curr Neurol Neurosci Rep.*, 2011: Aug;11(4):428-34.

van Spronsen M, Hoogenraad CC. "Synapse pathology in psychiatric and neurologic disease." *Curr Neurol Neurosci Rep.*, 2010 : May;10(3) 207-14.

Werling, L., Keller, A., Frank, J., & Nuwayhid, S. "A comparison of the binding profiles of dextromethorphan, memantine,fluoxetine and amitriptyline: Treatment of involuntary emotional expression disorder." *Experimental Neurology*, 2007: 248–257.

Yagasaki Y, Numakawa T, Kumamaru E, Hayashi T, Su TP, Kunugi H. "Chronic antidepressants potentiate via sigma-1 receptors the brain-derived neurotrophic factor-induced signaling for glutamate release." *J Biol Chem.*, 2006: May 5;281(18):12941-9.

15

Pharmacology of Hormone Replacement Therapy in Menopause

Adela Voican et al.*
[1]*Universitatea de Medicina din Craiova (AV,LN),*
[2]*Univ Paris-Sud, Faculté de Médecine Paris-Sud UMR-S693, Le Kremlin Bicêtre,*
[1]*Romania*
[2]*France*

1. Introduction

Menopause represents the final stage of the continuous process of reproductive aging in a woman's life, marking the end of her fertility. According to the World Health Organization (WHO), the natural menopause is defined *as the permanent cessation of menstruation resulting from the loss of ovarian follicular activity* (WHO Report, 1996). Preceded by endocrine and menstrual cycle changes described as "menopausal transition", natural menopause occurs at an average age of approximately 51 years, although a high inter-individual variability is supported by results from epidemiological studies. However, occurrence of menopause outside the estimated normal age interval (45-55 years) is associated with increased morbidity, either when a late or on the contrary, a premature cessation of menstruation appears. A late menopause implies a longer exposure to estrogens and a possible increased risk for breast (Colditz, 1993; Kelsey & Bernstein, 1996) and endometrial cancer (Dossus et al., 2010; McPherson et al., 1996) or for venous thromboembolism (Simon et al., 2006). On the other hand, women entering menopause earlier are facing a hypo-estrogenic state for a longer period compared to women undergoing normal menopause. That is the case for about 1% of women, which are confronted with the diagnosis of primary ovarian insufficiency (POI). POI is defined by the presence of amenorrhea associated with elevated follicle-stimulating hormone (FSH) levels in the menopausal range in women younger than 40 years (Bachelot et al., 2009). Women facing a premature cessation of the ovarian function were shown to be at increased risk for premature death, cardiovascular disease, neurologic disease, mood disorders, osteoporosis or psychosexual dysfunction (Shuster et al., 2010). As the main rationale for these disorders was linked to hormonal changes, maintaining a certain level of ovarian steroids for a given period of time arose as an essential condition for conserving life quality in women (Wilson, [1966]). Accentuated by the increasing life span, researches related to menopause and its treatment have provided scientific community with an increased body of data during the last decades. However, different aspects regarding the benefit/risk balance or the ideal doses and routes of administration of hormone replacement therapy (HRT) in menopausal women remain uncertain (Grodstein et al., 1997; Rossouw et al., 2002).

---

* Bruno Francou, Liliana Novac, Nathalie Chabbert-Buffet, Marianne Canonico, Geri Meduri, Marc Lombes, Pierre-Yves Scarabin, Jacques Young, Anne Guiochon-Mantel and Jérôme Bouligand
Univ Paris-Sud, France

In this context, our paper addresses various issues related to steroid hormone substitution, ranging from the basic pharmacology of sex steroids to their clinical use in HRT and subsequent benefits and risks.

2. Sex steroids

2.1 Natural oestrogens and progestogens

During a woman's reproductive lifetime, sex steroids (Oestrogens and Progestogens - the two main classes of female steroids) result mainly from the process of ovarian steroidogenesis and only small amounts are being secreted by the peripheral compartments (e.g. adrenals, adipose tissue). This characteristic is maintained until menopause, when subsequent to a decline in ovarian synthesis, sex steroid plasmatic levels rely only to the less significant amounts produced peripherally. In the particular case of pregnant women, the pivotal role for steroid secretion shifts from ovaries to placenta.

Ovarian secretion of sex steroids during reproductive age follows a monthly cyclic evolution under the control of pituitary gonadotropins (Figure 1A). This precise central control of the ovarian function depends on the coordinated pulsatile secretions of the hypothalamic GnRH (Bouligand et al., 2009) and of pituitary gonadotropins. The decrease in sex steroids levels in menopause abolishes the normal negative feedback at the hypothalamus and pituitary glands, resulting in an over-secretion of gonadotropins, especially FSH (Figure 1B). The pharmacological basis of hormone replacement therapy is to compensate the decrease of estradiol production by ovaries in order to limit the adverse events due to sex steroids deficiency.

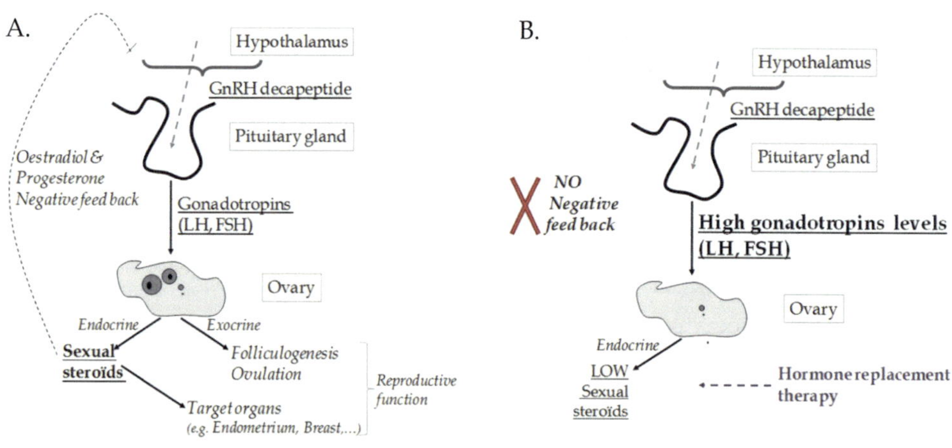

Fig. 1. The Hypothalamic-Pituitary-Gonadal (HPG) axis in women. A. Characteristics of HPG axis during the reproductive age. B. Changes in HPG axis following menopause.

Among the three forms of **natural circulating oestrogens** (i.e. estradiol, estriol and estrone, Figure 2), the main biological effect is exerted by estradiol, with a potency of approximately ten times that of estrone (Coldham et al., 1997; Van den Belt et al., 2004), while estriol exhibits the weakest estrogenic activity. In the second class of female sex steroids, **progesterone** represents the most important component, with significantly higher secreted levels than 17-hydroxyprogesterone, the other naturally occurring progestogen (Figure 2).

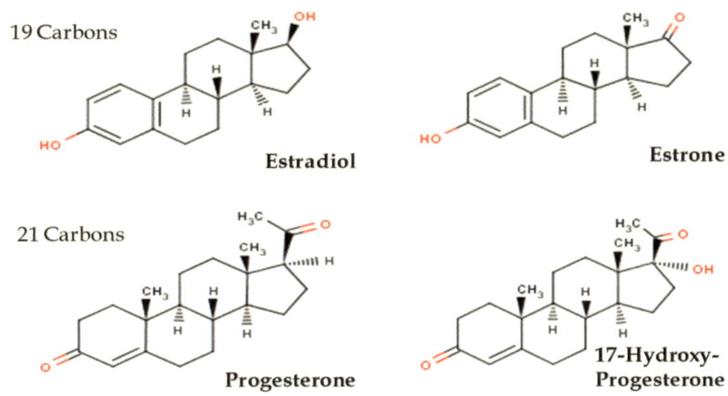

Fig. 2. Chemical Structure of Natural Sex Steroids

2.2 Mechanisms of action of sex steroids

The mechanisms by which oestrogen and progesterone exert their effects are complex (Figure 3A), and involve both classic pathways of hormone gene transcription through their cognate receptors, as well as "non-genomic" actions, the latter being characterized by significantly faster response rates (e.g. seconds, minutes).

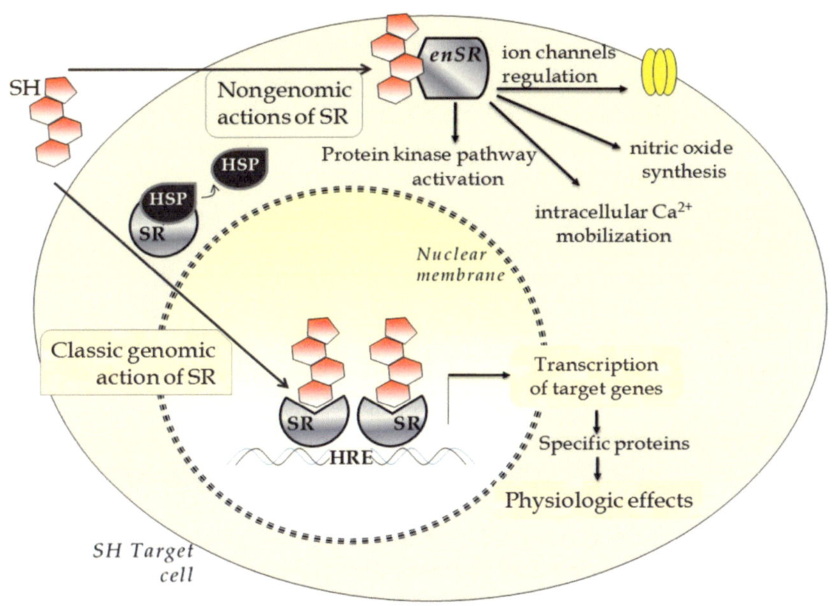

SH: steroid hormones (oestrogen, progesterone) ; SR: steroid receptor (ER, PR) ; enSR: extranuclear steroid receptors ; HSP: heat shock proteins ; HRE: hormone response elements.

Fig. 3.a. Sex steroids mechanism of action

Oestradiol and progesterone receptors (ERs and PRs respectively) belong to the large family of nuclear receptors (NRs), sharing several structural features (Loosfelt et al., 1986) and acting as transcriptional factors in a ligand dependent manner (For review, (Edwards, 2005).

Two major forms have been identified for each of the two types of ovarian steroid receptor, namely ERα and ERβ (Kuiper et al., 1996; Walter et al., 1985), and PR-A and PR-B respectively (Conneely et al., 1989; Huckaby et al., 1987; Kastner et al., 1990; Khan et al., 2011) (Figure 3B).

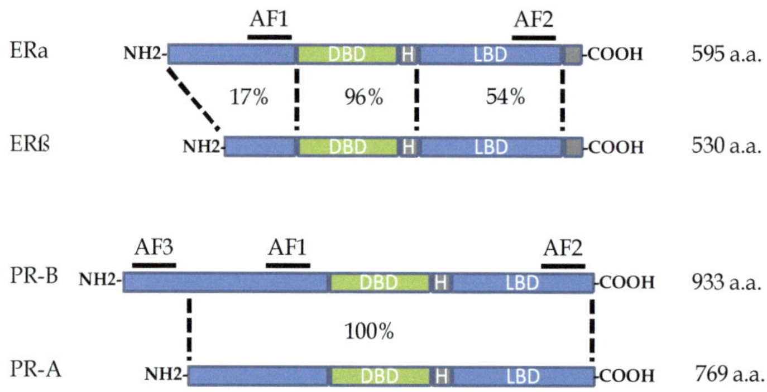

LBD: ligand binding domain; DBD: DNA binding domain; AF: transcription activation domain (AF-1, AF-2, AF-3); H: Hinge region, a.a. : amino-acids. The percentages indicate the amino acid identity between domains of ERa and ERβ and between A and B forms of PR.

Fig. 3.b. Domain structures of estrogen (ER) and progesterone (PR) receptors.

Most of ERs and PRs are constitutively localized in the nucleus in the absence of their ligands (Welshons et al., 1985), and nuclear localization signals have been described in the hinge region (Guiochon-Mantel et al., 1989; Picard et al., 1990). Due to their lipophilic nature, steroids will easily cross the cell membrane and bind to specific receptors, resulting in hormone-receptor complexes. Prior to ligand binding, receptors are inactive and associate protein complexes, among which the heat shock proteins (hsp) play important roles (e.g. hsp 90, hsp 70)(Pratt & Toft, 1997). But in the presence of their ligands, receptors undergo conformational changes with subsequent release of the associated protein complexes and bind to specific DNA sequences (hormone-response elements) from the promoter regions of target genes. The expression of target genes is thus modulated after interaction with various coregulators (Rosenfeld & Glass, 2001; Amazit et al., 2011). ERs and PRs bind DNA as dimers and have the ability to form both homodimers and heterodimers ($ER_{\alpha/\beta}$, $PR_{A/B}$ respectively)(Cowley et al., 1997; Leonhardt et al., 1998). Furthermore, the complexity of oestrogen and progesterone actions is enhanced by the growing body of evidence supporting the non-genomic mechanisms of steroid hormones action (Hammes & Levin, 2007; Levin, 2011; Losel & Wehling, 2003). These rapid effects may not be explained by the classic pathway and involve a variety of signalling events, such as the activation of various kinases, ion channels regulation and intracellular calcium mobilization or nitric oxide synthesis (Edwards, 2005; Madak-Erdogan et al., 2008). Responsible for generating these effects may be either membrane forms of classically ERs and PRs or alternative unrelated molecules (Wendler et al., 2010).

2.3 Physiological effects

Oestrogens and progestogens main effects concern the **reproductive organs**, initiating and supporting their development and functionality. Secondary sex characteristics are under the close control of gonadal steroids. During the reproductive lifetime of a woman, oestrogens dictate the proliferation of the uterine endometrium and the development of endometrial glands, while progesterone promotes secretory changes of the endometrium, in a process of preparation of the ideal milieu for implantation of the fertilized ovum. In the **breast,** oestrogens promote the development of the stromal and ductal systems together with fat deposition at this level, and progesterone induces the development of the secretory units of the breast, causing alveolar cells to proliferate.

Although the reproductive system represents the principal target for sex steroids, their effects are far from being limited only to this system. **Bone health,** for instance, is greatly influenced by oestrogens levels, as they play an important role in the process of bone remodelling. Under their action, skeletal resorption is diminished due to a decreased osteoclastic activity and by consequence, bone formation is promoted. Furthermore, a **cardioprotective** role exerted by ovarian steroids was inferred due to the significantly lower rates of cardiovascular diseases manifested by women prior to menopause compared to men and the cancelation of these gender differences following menopause. Several **metabolic effects** are also described, oestrogens slightly increasing the metabolic rate, promoting deposition of the fat in subcutaneous tissue and changing lipoprotein profiles by increasing HDL and decreasing LDL cholesterol (Edwards, 2005; Guyton & Hall, c2006).

3. Menopause principal consequences

Given the multitude of physiological effects exerted by sex steroids in women, it is not surprising that the hormonal changes related to menopause have been linked to a wide spectrum of symptoms and disorders. The most frequent menopausal symptoms include vasomotor disorders (e.g. hot flashes, night sweets), urogenital atrophy (e.g. vaginal dryness, urinary symptoms), or psychological disturbances (e.g. sleep disturbances, forgetfulness, mood changes or depression), all of which may seriously impact on women's quality of life. Decreased oestrogen levels in menopause result in an altered bone structure with reduced bone mineral density (BMD) and increased risk for subsequent fractures. Postmenopausal women, compared to the premenopausal period, are also more prone to develop cardiovascular disease (CVD), which represents the leading cause of death in women. Furthermore, the increased risk of dementia and Alzheimer disease in postmenopausal women was also partially attributed to endogenous oestradiol depletion (Yaffe et al., 2007).

If the aforementioned effects are present in women undergoing natural menopause, the magnitude of these consequences is even higher in POI women and the dimension of each long-term effect may vary in relation to the exact cause of POI and to the rapidity of apparition of the oestrogen deficit (e.g. women undergoing surgical oophorectomy will face a sudden decrease in steroids levels compared to women experiencing a spontaneous POI) (Maclaran et al., 2010). All-cause mortality rates in women appear to be associated with age at menopause, women entering menopause before 40 years having mortality rates twice as the ones seen in the 50-54 years group (Snowdon et al., 1989). Studies on the cardiovascular risk in POI demonstrated that several risk factors for CVD are influenced by a premature occurence of menopause (e.g. alteration of lipid profiles (Knauff et al., 2008), decreased insulin sensitivity(Corrigan et al., 2006) or the presence of metabolic syndrome (Eshtiaghi et al., 2010)). Moreover, the impaired endothelial function found in women with POI, precursor of more severe vascular abnormalities, was improved by hormonal replacement, further supporting the role of steroids in normal cardiovascular function (Kalantaridou et al., 2004). POI patients present with low BMD, which seems to be greatly influenced by the accelerated bone loss during the first 4-5 years of menopause (Amarante et al., 2011; Anasti et al., 1998; Gallagher, 2007; Uygur et al., 2005; van Der Voort et al., 2003), and hence having an increased risk of fractures compared to their peers who underwent a physiological menopause. Finally, an increased risk for cognitive impairment, dementia and Parkinson disease, inversely proportional with age at menopause, was reported in premature menopausal women following oophorectomy (Rocca et al., 2007, 2008).

4. Hormone replacement therapy

4.1 Basis for the hormone replacement therapy in menopause

When an installed hormonal deficiency generates symptoms in an individual, disturbing its well-being, it is expected that by adjusting the deficit, an improvement or even an offset of the symptoms should be reached (Wilson, [1966]). That was the hypothesis guiding clinicians decisions about substitution of ovarian steroids in menopause. Hormone replacement therapy (HRT) has been a common practice during the last decades, being initially used for both treatment of symptoms and prevention of chronic medical conditions related to menopause (e.g. heart and bone diseases). But 2002, the year when the first results from a large randomized and placebo-controlled trial (the Women Health Initiative - WHI) were published, marked a major change in both clinicians and patients perception towards the use of HRT(Rossouw et al., 2002). Conducted with the aim of evaluating HRT major benefits and risks, WHI results contradicted previous observational studies and showed an increased risk for cardiovascular events together with that of breast cancer rates in the studied population. Even if this resulted in a significant reduction in the use of HRT worldwide (Hersh et al., 2004; Lagro-Janssen et al., 2010; MacLennan et al., 2004), it represented also the subject to some major controversies. One major debate is the legitimacy of applying these conclusions to all women, when most of the women concerned by HRT prescription belong to the 50-54 years age group while participants in the WHI study had an average age of 63 years and a high body mass index. Thus, following the release of the first WHI report, various studies intended to better evaluate the real risks and benefits associated with HRT were conducted. The resulting body of evidence has led to the necessity of periodic revision of the existing recommendations and statements in this field (North American Menopause Society (NAMS) position statement, 2010; Santen et al., 2010; Sturdee et al., 2011).

4.2 Current recommendations

Current recommendations specify that HRT use should be restricted mainly to moderate or severe menopausal symptoms alleviation. It should not be used as a mean of chronic disease prevention and it is advisable to restrict treatment administration to the shortest period and the lowest dosage possible to control symptoms effectively. Nevertheless, in selected cases, HRT may be used to treat or to reduce the risk of diseases (e.g. osteoporosis). This involves HRT use *in prevention of further bone loss and/or reduction of osteoporotic fracture in menopausal women when alternate therapies are not appropriate or cause side effects* (NAMS position statement, 2010) or for *women younger than 60 years, with an increased risk of fracture* (Sturdee et al., 2011). In the particular case of women diagnosed with POI, HRT is recommended at least until the median age of natural menopause is reached (NAMS position statement, 2010).

4.3 Hormone replacement therapy regimens

4.3.1 Oestrogens and progestins in HRT

HRT comprises a variety of regimens, compounds, dosages and routes of administration. In most women, excepting hysterectomized patients, menopausal treatment requires preparations combining oestrogens with a progestin, the latter being used mainly to balance oestrogen's effects on the endometrium and to avoid endometrial hyperplasia and an increased risk of secondary carcinoma. This combination therapy may be administrated either in a sequential cyclic regimen or in a continuous one. The sequential regimen involves the alternation of a pure oestrogenic period to an oestro-progestative one, leading to withdrawal bleeding when the progestin administration is discontinued. This regimen is commonly administrated with a monthly cyclicity including at least 10 days of progestin treatment. Quarterly regimens are also available, involving progestin administration every 3 months, although in this case the risk for endometrial hyperplasia needs further evaluation. The continuous combined treatment implies the administration of both compounds on a daily basis and uses lower doses of progestin compared to the sequential regimen. This constitutes an option especially in older women not desiring a monthly withdrawal bleeding, even if uterine bleeding with unpredictable onset may not be excluded particularly during the first administrations (Doren, 2000; Ylikorkala & Rozenberg, 2000). Available formulations for the estrogens and progestins in HRT and their commonly used doses are listed in Table 1.

4.3.2 Other therapeutic options

Androgens are thought to play a role in maintaining a normal libido and sexual function in postmenopausal women and to potentially prevent the decline of bone quality, muscular force and cognitive function. Thus, after exclusion of other possible causes, androgen therapy represents an option for menopausal women with hypoactive sexual desire disorder undergoing concomitant oestrogen treatment, especially in those who have suffered a surgical menopause (Davis et al., 2008).

Tibolone is a synthetic compound with mixed oestrogenic, progestogenic and androgenic activities, representing an alternative to conventional HRT (Lazovic et al., 2008). It represents an efficient option for vasomotor symptoms alleviation or prevention of BMD loss in menopausal women (Gallagher et al., 2001; Swanson et al., 2006).

Another possible option in menopausal therapy refers to the **selective oestrogen receptor modulators (SERMs)**. These are pharmacologic agents characterised by variable oestrogen activity, acting as oestrogen agonists in some tissues while in other tissues they exert oestrogen antagonist effects. Examples of SERMs of interest in menopause treatment include raloxifene together with novel molecules like bazedoxifene, lasofoxifene or ospemifene.

Route	Oestrogens	Dosage
Oral	Conjugated estrogens (conjugated equine oestrogens)	0.625 mg
	Micronized 17 beta oestradiol	1, 2 mg
	Oestradiol valerate	1, 2 mg
	Estropipate (piperazine estrone sulphate)	0.75, 1.5, 3 mg
Transdermal	17 beta oestradiol (patch)	25, 37.5, 50, 75, 100 μg/day
	Oestradiol (gel)	1 mg/ 1g
Subcutaneous	Oestradiol (implant)	20, 50, 100 mg
Vaginal	Estriol (gel)	1mg/g
	Estradiol (tabs)	25μg
	Progestins	
Oral	Norethisterone acetate	0.5, 1 mg
	Medroxyprogesterone acetate	2.5, 5 mg
	Chlormadinone acetate	2, 5, 10 mg
	Drospirenone	2 mg
	Dydrogesterone	5, 10 mg
	Nomogestrol acetate	3.75, 5 mg
	Promegestone	0.125, 0.25, 0.5 mg
	Micronized progesterone	100, 200 mg
Transdermal	Levonorgestrel	7, 10μg/24h
Intrauterine	Levonorgestrel intrauterine device	20 μg/24h

Table 1. Commonly used oestrogens and progestins

4.4 Primary ovarian insufficiency: Particular requirements

Current publications highlight the lack of specifically designed HRT regimens for women with POI and the fact that existing observations from studies conducted on older women undergoing natural menopause should not be extrapolated to the much younger category of POI women. In the absence of a consensus regarding the ideal hormonal replacement regimen for women facing a premature cessation of the ovarian function, the oestro-progestative substitution commonly involves either HRT or combined oral contraceptive pills (COCP) prescription. Even if the use of the latter may be associated with a lower emotional impact for these patients, being perceived less as a treatment, it must be underlined that COCP standard preparations contain synthetic steroids in higher doses than the ones required for physiologic hormonal replacement in POI (Nelson et al., 2005). There is an urgent need to develop evidence-based guidelines relying on solid research in order to optimize the care of this group of women (Panay & Kalu, 2009).

4.5 Benefit versus risk of hormonal replacement therapy based 1 on the reviews of clinical studies

Despite the wide agreement that hormonal substitution remains the most effective option for the alleviation of menopausal symptoms, a careful evaluation of the benefit-risk balance is however essential prior to prescribing a HRT regimen because of its associated risks (Santen et al., 2010). The principal benefits and risks related to HRT in the light of recent evidences are further discussed in this paragraph.

The **cardiovascular events** represent the first cause of mortality in postmenopausal women and constituted a major subject of controversy regarding the use of HRT, an uncertainty accentuated by the discrepant results between randomised controlled trials (RCTs) (Hulley et al., 1998; Rossouw et al., 2002; Vickers et al., 2007) and observational studies (Bush et al., 1987; Grodstein et al., 1997; Stampfer et al., 1991). Initially, as expected from the physiological functions of oestrogens, several observational studies suggested a protective role of HRT on the cardiovascular system. Contrary to these observations, the WHI, a randomised, placebo-controlled trial, failed to validate the cardioprotective effect of HRT. The primary outcome of this study was related to the effects of menopausal substitution on the cardiovascular function and breast cancer risk, participants receiving either conjugated equine estrogens (CEE) alone (0.625mg/day) if hysterectomised (Anderson et al., 2004) or 0.625mg/day CEE in combination with 2.5mg/day medroxyprogesterone acetate (MPA) if they presented with an intact uterus (Rossouw et al., 2002). In an attempt to explain the disparity between these results the "timing hypothesis" arose as a possible answer, supported by differences between women enrolled in this study and those participating in observational studies (Grodstein et al., 2003). Thus, while the former included women more than a decade away from the onset of menopause, in the latter HRT was usually initiated shortly after menopause. Animal studies supported this hypothesis and demonstrated that the positive cardiovascular effects of hormonal substitution are inversely correlated with the delay of initiating the treatment (Clarkson, 2007). Several analysis, including some of the WHI subgroup data, tested the timing hypothesis and showed a trends towards a decreased risk in women younger and closer to menopause (Rossouw et al., 2007; Salpeter et al., 2006). Trials addressing specifically the effects of HRT in younger women (e.g. Kronos EarlyEstrogen Prevention Study (KEEPS) (Harman et al., 2005), Early Versus Late Intervention Trial With Estradiol (ELITE, *NCT00114517*) are currently under way and their results will probably shed a better light on these controversial facts.

Venous thromboembolism (VTE) is one of the major harmful effects of hormone therapy use among postmenopausal women (Olie et al., 2010). A recent meta-analysis on the risk of VTE in women using HRT indicated an increased risk by twofold to threefold when oral oestrogens were administrated (the combined relative risk (RR) from both trials and observational studies of 1.9 and confidence interval (CI) of 1.3 to 2.3, with a higher risk within the first year of treatment (Canonico, Plu-Bureau et al., 2008). When VTE risk was analysed in women receiving transdermal oestrogen, there was a combined RR of 1.0 (CI, 0.9 - 1.1). The impact of the route of administration on VTE risk and the recent pharmacogenetic studies providing support for the implication of the first pass effect in these different outcomes are detailed in chapter 5.

Musculoskeletal effects. Both observational studies (Cauley et al., 1995; Grodstein, Stampfer et al., 1999; Kiel et al., 1987) and RCTs (Cauley et al., 2003; Jackson et al., 2006; Lindsay et al., 2005) have proven HRT efficacy in reducing bone loss in menopausal women. Additionally, this positive effect appears to be present even when lower doses of oestrogen are used (Lindsay et al., 2005). However, rapidly after its discontinuation the protective effect on BMD is no longer evident. A recent study, evaluating hip fracture incidence after HRT cessation in a large cohort of 80.955 postmenopausal women, reported a significantly increased risk of hip fracture within only two years following HRT cessation compared to women who continued using HRT (Karim et al., 2011).

HRT and cancer risks. There is a large body of studies investigating the association between HRT and the risk for various types of cancer, primarily those hormone-dependent and particularly **breast cancer**. Breast cancer was one of the reasons for the premature discontinuation after 5.2 years of follow-up of the arm receiving combined HRT in the WHI trial, as the increased risk in breast cancer exceeded the stopping boundary for this adverse effect (RR 1.26; 95% CI 1.00-1.59) (Rossouw et al., 2002). Contrary to these findings, in the oestrogen-only group the relative risk was inferior compared to the control group (RR 0.77, 95% CI 0.57–1.06) (Anderson et al., 2004), suggesting that in addition to oestrogen, progestins have also a role in breast cancer pathophysiology. The risk of developing breast cancer increases with longer duration of HRT use (Beral, 2003; Fournier et al., 2008). One meta-analysis assessing the impact of HRT on the risk of invasive breast cancer in epidemiological studies and RCTs reported an increased annual risk for breast cancer varying between 0–9% in the case of E+P regimens and 0–3% in oestrogen-only administration (Greiser et al., 2005).

Although the risk of CHD was reported to increase when HRT is started a long time after the onset of menopause, the reverse situation seems to apply in the case of breast cancer. Data from the WHI trial supported this so called "gap time hypothesis" and reported an increased risk for breast cancer when HRT is started less than 5 years after the onset of menopause in both E (with a RR of 1.12 versus 0.58 when HRT was initiated less than 5 and respectively more than 5 years from menopause in women without a prior HRT use, or a relative risk (RR) of 1.00 versus 0.77 in women with prior HRT use) and E+P arms (with a RR of 1.77 versus 0.99 when HRT was initiated less than 5 and respectively more than 5 years from menopause in women without a prior HRT use, or a RR of 2.06 versus 1.30 in women with prior HRT use)(Prentice et al., 2009). The fact that ER positive breast tumours in postmenopausal women, but not in premenopausal ones, respond to treatment with high-dose oestrogen further supports this hypothesis and suggests that the decline in oestrogen levels associated with menopause may sensitize breast cancer cells to the proapoptotic effects of estrogen (Taylor & Manson, 2011).

Endometrial cancer (EC) constitutes another adverse effect linked to HRT use. The most common form of EC, the endometrioid (type I) variant, is generally hormonally responsive and women with an unbalanced oestrogen exposure are at increased risk for this form of EC. No risk increase was reported in women using a continuous combined HRT regimen, while the use of sequential HRT resulted in different risk profiles according to the duration of treatment (Jaakkola et al., 2011). Thus, when used for less than 5 years, the sequential E+P regimen showed a decreased risk for EC (RR 0.67, 95% CI 0.52-0.86), while continuing treatment after 5 years resulted in an increased risk for EC (RR 1.11,

95%CI 0.87-1.41 for the 5-10 years interval and RR 1.38, 95%CI 1.15-1.66 for an use exceeding 10 years).

Several studies reported an increased risk for **ovarian cancer** in women using HRT (Beral et al., 2007; Morch et al., 2009), with a stronger association in the case of unopposed oestrogen administration (Hildebrand et al., 2010). However, due to the small excess risk, the overall benefit-risk balance in HRT appears not to be significantly influenced by these results (Taylor & Manson, 2011).

Colorectal cancer. Observational studies have suggested an association between the use of HRT and a reduced incidence in colorectal cancer (Grodstein, Newcomb et al., 1999), an observation also validated by data from the E+P arm from the WHI trial (Chlebowski et al., 2004). However, despite a reduced overall rate, poor prognosis forms of colon cancer were diagnosed more frequently in women receiving HRT than in the placebo group. In contrast to the group receiving E+P, the reduced incidence of colorectal cancer was not found in the oestrogen-alone arm of WHI (Ritenbaugh et al., 2008). The relation between colorectal cancer and hormone exposure is further complicated by recent evidences suggesting that a greater endogenous estrogen exposure may increase the risk of colorectal cancer in postmenopausal women (Clendenen et al., 2009; Zervoudakis et al., 2011).

Finally, results from several studies comprising those of WHI (Chlebowski et al., 2009) have led to the inclusion of **lung cancer** on the list of potential adverse effects of HRT, although a neutral effect of HRT on lung cancer risk (Ayeni & Robinson, 2009) or even lower risks (Rodriguez et al., 2008) have been reported by others. Post-hoc analysis of WHI showed than even if the incidence of lung cancer in women using HRT did not increase, the number of death from lung cancer was significantly higher (in particular deaths from non-small-cell lung cancer) in women receiving combined HRT (Chlebowski et al., 2009), contrary to the use of oestrogen alone where the death rates were similar to the control group (Chlebowski et al., 2010).

The effect of HRT on a variety of conditions (e.g. mood disturbances, neurocognitive impairment, gallbladder disease, immune disorders, etc) have also been investigated. However, as either current evidences are insufficient or their impact on the overall benefit-risk balance is not significant, we will not detail them.

Particularities of the HRT benefit-risk balance in POI patients. Available results from studies evaluating HRT effects, especially its risks, do not address particularly the population of POI patients, but rather there is a tendency to apply to this group an extrapolation of findings from natural menopause, although there are evident differences in the HRT benefit-risk ratio between the two populations.

Cardiovascular and breast cancer risks, the two main adverse effects related to HRT use, need a special consideration in the context of women diagnosed with POI. First, the "timing hypothesis" for cardiovascular effects of HRT suggest a clear trend towards cardiovascular benefits in young women using HRT and hence, it is possible that the benefits in the younger POI patients might be even greater (Panay & Fenton, 2008). Secondly, the breast cancer risk profile differs in women undergoing a premature menopause compared to the general population. A younger age at menopause is protective against breast cancer regardless of whether the menopause was natural or surgical (Hulka & Moorman, 2008).

Thus, POI patients should be informed that results from reports on HRT associated breast cancer do not necessarily apply to their case, in which treatment is intended to provide the hormones that should be physiologically present at their age (Maclaran & Panay, 2011).

These particularities of the HRT risk profile in women facing a premature cessation of the ovarian function, together with the beneficial bone effects (Farquhar et al., 2009), support the current recommendations regarding the need for HRT substitution until the average age of natural menopause (Vujovic et al., 2010).

5. Pharmacology of hormone replacement therapy

The pharmacology of hormone replacement therapy is of a particular interest given the complex benefit/risk balance and the importance of this treatment for women health. As illustrated in previous paragraphs, there is a wide diversity of drugs and protocols proposed for HRT. Our analysis will be limited to the pharmacology of the natural sex steroid 17β-estradiol.

5.1 The route of oestradiol administration (oral versus transdermal) highlights the hepatic first pass effect

Oral oestradiol is commonly used by women receiving HRT, being seen as a convenient and inexpensive option. In turn, following oral administration, oestradiol is subject to the first-pass effect, a term that encompasses the metabolic changes underwent by a drug before it reaches systemic circulation. This results in the use of higher doses of oestradiol (~ 1,5 mg/day) compared to parenteral routes (patch ~ 50μg/24h). Moreover, subsequent to the various metabolic changes suffered by oestrogens once absorbed in the intestinal tract, a specific profile of oestradiol metabolites and oestrogen-dependent serum parameters with particular pathophysiological implications will appear, widely different from what is observed after the use of transdermal oestradiol where the first-pass effect is avoided.

The oestradiol metabolism pathway (Raftogianis et al., 2000) is outlined in Figure 4. Rapidly after the intestinal absorption, part of oral oestradiol is converted to oestrone, a reversible reaction catalysed by 17β-hydroxysteroid-dehydrogenase (HSD), and the conversion may continue towards their inactive conjugates (i.e. sulfates and glucuronides). Subsequent to this process, the oestrone/ oestradiol ratio resulting from oral administration is significantly higher (approximately 5:1) than the one observed following transdermal administration (approximately 1:1, which is similar to the physiologic ratio found in premenopausal women)(Kuhl, 2005). Contrary to the aforementioned transformations, further phase I reactions (oxidation reactions catalysed by cytochrome P450 (CYP) enzymes) are no more reversible. The final steps in oestrogen metabolism involve the process of detoxification under the action of phase II enzymes.

The first pass effect of oestradiol results in various biological consequences (De Lignieres et al., 1986). For instance, a well known effect attributed to hepatic first pass is the decrease of IGF-1 after oral oestradiol, whereas no significant change was observed with transdermal oestrogens (Sonnet et al., 2007). Furthermore, an increased synthesis of blood coagulation factors (Caine et al., 1992) and resistance to activated protein C (Oger et al., 2003) constitute another important consequences which are directly implicated in VTE pathophysiology, one of the major adverse events of oral oestrogens.

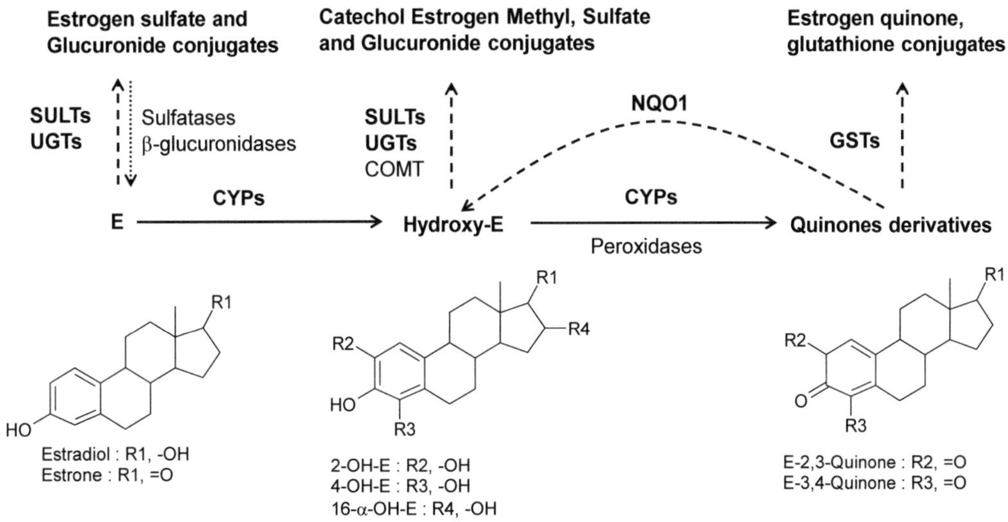

Various isoforms of cytochromes P450s (CYP3A, CYP1A and CYP1B families) activate estrogens during phase-1 metabolism. Oxidative metabolites, such as hydroxyestradiol and quinone derivatives, are conjugated by various phase-2 enzymes. The expression of several of these enzymes (SULTs, UGTs, GSTs and NQO1) is regulated by Nrf2. E: estradiol or estrone; CYPs: cytochrome P450s; UGTs: UDP-glucuronosyltransferase; COMT: catechol-o-methyltransferase; GSTs: glutathione S-transferases; NQO1: NAD(P)H dehydrogenase, quinone 1. Phase-1 metabolism is represented by horizontal arrows. Phase-2 metabolism is represented by vertical arrows (dashed).

Fig. 4. Oestrogens hepatic metabolism

5.2 Pharmacokinetic of oral *versus* transdermal oestrogens

The pharmacokinetics of exogenous estrogens is complex and most efficacy studies of transdermal *versus* oral oestrogens have not included the measurement of oestrogens concentrations. The oral route of oestradiol administration is easy and convenient, however the hormone is extensively metabolized in the gut and the liver leading to first-pass effect and, as previously mentioned, to a high estrone/oestradiol ratio (Kuhl, 2005). On the other hand, transdermal 17β-oestradiol is well absorbed through the epidermis and produces higher parent oestrogens serum concentrations and lower metabolites ratios because it bypasses the liver. Moreover, owing to a very low bioavailability [0.1 - 12%] of oral micronized 17β-oestradiol (O'Connell, 1995), higher doses are needed for the oral route compared to transdermal administration (O'Connell, 1995; Powers et al., 1985).

Pharmacokinetic profiles of transdermal and oral oestradiol are very different with oral administration producing fluctuant concentrations compared to the more constant levels achieved with transdermal formulations (Kopper et al., 2009). Interestingly, there is no pharmacokinetic/pharmacodynamic relationship between serum levels and positive effects of oestradiol treatment. It has been clearly shown that serum level after transdermal oestradiol does not predict the outcome when treating hot flushes (Steingold et al., 1985). The precise oestradiol and oestrone concentrations required to prevent bone loss and cardiovascular disease after either oral or transdermal oestrogen administration are also unknown (O'Connell, 1995).

5.3 Venous thromboembolism risk and HRT

As previously mentioned, VTE represents one of the main adverse effects of HRT in postmenopausal women (Canonico, Plu-Bureau et al., 2008; Cushman et al., 2004). Yet, while oral oestrogen was associated with a significantly increased risk for VTE, this was not observed in women treated with transdermal oestrogen (Canonico et al., 2010; Canonico et al., 2007; Olie et al., 2010; Scarabin et al., 2003; Straczek et al., 2005). An explanation for the distinct VTE risk profile following the two routes of administration involves the first-pass effect of oestrogen. This was shown to affect the synthesis of various oestrogen-dependent hepatic serum factors (Kuhl, 2005), including coagulation and fibrinolysis factors, resulting in blood coagulation activation (Scarabin et al., 1997; Vehkavaara et al., 2001), increased thrombin generation (Scarabin et al., 2011) or induction of resistance to activated protein C (Hemelaar et al., 2006; Oger et al., 2003). However, the precise mechanisms by which these changes occur are still unclear.

5.4 Pharmacogenetics: Genetics factors predisposing to venous thromboembolism (VTE) after oral oestradiol

Straczek et al. investigated the impact of the route of oestrogen administration on the association between a prothrombotic mutation (factor V Leiden or prothrombin G20210A mutation) and VTE risk. This study confirms the increase risk of VTE due to oral 17β-oestradiol in women presenting a genetic predisposition to VTE (Straczek et al., 2005). On the other hand, we have recently suggested that the hepatic metabolism of oestrogen may modulate the risk of VTE either through an increased phase I metabolism or through a decreased phase II metabolism. To address this important question, we have tested genetic polymorphisms capable to modulate oestradiol phase I or phase II liver metabolism. These polymorphisms do not increase the risk of VTE in the absence of HRT. First, we have demonstrated that increased expression of CYP3A5, a phase I enzyme of particular interest in oestrogen liver metabolism, in women carrying the CYP3A5*1 allele, is associated with a higher risk of VTE during oral oestrogen administration (RR 14.5; CI 2.8 - 73.9), without observing the same interaction in women receiving transdermal oestrogen (Canonico, Bouaziz et al., 2008). Further, we have investigated the association between VTE and nuclear factor (erythroid-derived 2)-like 2 (NFE2L2) polymorphisms (Bouligand et al., 2011). NFE2L2 gene encodes for a transcription factor also known as Nrf2 (NF-E2 related factor 2), essential for both maintenance and induction of phase II metabolism (Thimmulappa et al., 2002). One functional polymorphism (rs6721961) from the promoter region of NFE2L2 was described to be associated with an impaired auto-induction of this transcription factor (Marzec et al., 2007). The presence of this polymorphism may subsequently alter the expression of phase II genes, including those essential for the detoxification of oestrogen metabolites (see Figure 5) (Raftogianis et al., 2000). Our post-hoc analysis of the ESTHER Study (Canonico et al., 2007; Scarabin et al., 2003; Straczek et al., 2005) demonstrated the association between VTE risk and the NFE2L2 polymorphism (i.e. rs672196) in oral oestrogen users (RR 17.9; CI 3.7 – 85.7).

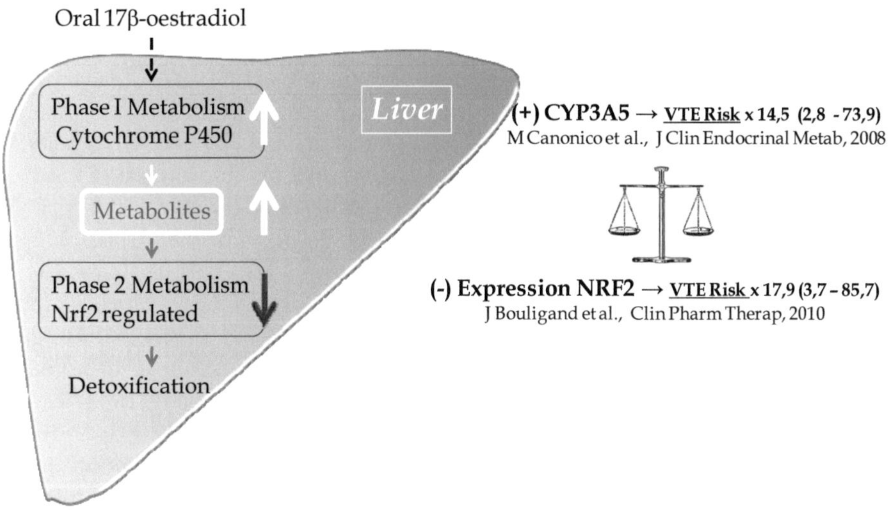

Fig. 5. Genetic polymorphisms modulating liver metabolism and first pass effect of oestrogens.

These pharmacogenetic studies provide new insights suggesting that liver metabolism of oestrogens may be implicated in the pathophysiology of VTE among women using HRT with oral oestrogen therapy. This original finding deserves further investigations in largest and independent series of women receiving oral 17β-oestradiol as well as other oestrogens with different metabolic pathways, not only to treat postmenopausal symptoms but also for contraception. Taking into account the proportion of women using exogenous hormone therapy, these new results may have important clinical implications to improve the stratification of thrombotic risk and identify new groups at high risk.

6. Conclusion

The increasing life expectancy observed during the last century, without an equivalent change in the average age of menopause, resulted in an increased number of women facing the effects of low ovarian steroids for a longer period of time. Thus, the high interest towards therapeutic options capable to alleviate menopausal symptoms and the extensive research in this field are not surprisingly. Despite the current controversies summarised here which encompass HRT use, further researches will likely improve therapeutic outcomes. In this context, pharmacogenetics studies play a key role in fulfilling the aim of providing patients with an individualised therapy which will reduce risks and improve benefits related to HRT.

7. References

Amarante, F., Vilodre, L. C., Maturana, M. A.& Spritzer, P. M. (2011). Women with primary ovarian insufficiency have lower bone mineral density. *Braz J Med Biol Res,* Vol. 44, No. 1, (Jan 2011), pp. 78-83.

Amazit, L., Roseau, A., Khan, J. A., Chauchereau, A., Tyagi, R. K., Loosfelt, H., Leclerc, P., Lombes, M.& Guiochon-Mantel, A. (2011). Ligand-dependent degradation of SRC-1 is pivotal for progesterone receptor transcriptional activity. *Mol Endocrinol,* Vol. 25, No. 3, (Mar 2011), pp. 394-408.

Anasti, J. N., Kalantaridou, S. N., Kimzey, L. M., Defensor, R. A.& Nelson, L. M. (1998). Bone loss in young women with karyotypically normal spontaneous premature ovarian failure. *Obstet Gynecol,* Vol. 91, No. 1, (Jan 1998), pp. 12-15.

Anderson, G. L., Limacher, M., Assaf, A. R., Bassford, T., Beresford, S. A., Black, H., Bonds, D., Brunner, R., Brzyski, R., Caan, B., Chlebowski, R., Curb, D., Gass, M., Hays, J., Heiss, G., Hendrix, S., Howard, B. V., Hsia, J., Hubbell, A., Jackson, R., Johnson, K. C., Judd, H., Kotchen, J. M., Kuller, L., LaCroix, A. Z., Lane, D., Langer, R. D., Lasser, N., Lewis, C. E., Manson, J., Margolis, K., Ockene, J., O'Sullivan, M. J., Phillips, L., Prentice, R. L., Ritenbaugh, C., Robbins, J., Rossouw, J. E., Sarto, G., Stefanick, M. L., Van Horn, L., Wactawski-Wende, J., Wallace, R.& Wassertheil-Smoller, S. (2004). Effects of conjugated equine estrogen in postmenopausal women with hysterectomy: the Women's Health Initiative randomized controlled trial. *JAMA,* Vol. 291, No. 14, (Apr 2004), pp. 1701-1712.

Ayeni, O.& Robinson, A. (2009). Hormone replacement therapy and outcomes for women with non-small-cell lung cancer: can an association be confirmed? *Curr Oncol,* Vol. 16, No. 3, (May 2009), pp. 21-25.

Bachelot, A., Rouxel, A., Massin, N., Dulon, J., Courtillot, C., Matuchansky, C., Badachi, Y., Fortin, A., Paniel, B., Lecuru, F., Lefrere-Belda, M. A., Constancis, E., Thibault, E., Meduri, G., Guiochon-Mantel, A., Misrahi, M., Kuttenn, F.& Touraine, P. (2009). Phenotyping and genetic studies of 357 consecutive patients presenting with premature ovarian failure. *Eur J Endocrinol,* Vol. 161, No. 1, (Jul 2009), pp. 179-187.

Beral, V. (2003). Breast cancer and hormone-replacement therapy in the Million Women Study. *Lancet,* Vol. 362, No. 9382, (Aug 2003), pp. 419-427.

Beral, V., Bull, D., Green, J.& Reeves, G. (2007). Ovarian cancer and hormone replacement therapy in the Million Women Study. *Lancet,* Vol. 369, No. 9574, (May 2007), pp. 1703-1710.

Bouligand, J., Cabaret, O., Canonico, M., Verstuyft, C., Dubert, L., Becquemont, L., Guiochon-Mantel, A.& Scarabin, P. Y. (2011). Effect of NFE2L2 genetic polymorphism on the association between oral estrogen therapy and the risk of venous thromboembolism in postmenopausal women. *Clin Pharmacol Ther,* Vol. 89, No. 1, (Jan 2011), pp. 60-64.

Bouligand, J., Ghervan, C., Tello, J. A., Brailly-Tabard, S., Salenave, S., Chanson, P., Lombes, M., Millar, R. P., Guiochon-Mantel, A.& Young, J. (2009). Isolated familial hypogonadotropic hypogonadism and a GNRH1 mutation. *N Engl J Med,* Vol. 360, No. 26, (Jun 2009), pp. 2742-2748.

Bush, T. L., Barrett-Connor, E., Cowan, L. D., Criqui, M. H., Wallace, R. B., Suchindran, C. M., Tyroler, H. A.& Rifkind, B. M. (1987). Cardiovascular mortality and noncontraceptive use of estrogen in women: results from the Lipid Research Clinics Program Follow-up Study. *Circulation,* Vol. 75, No. 6, (Jun 1987), pp. 1102-1109.

Caine, Y. G., Bauer, K. A., Barzegar, S., ten Cate, H., Sacks, F. M., Walsh, B. W., Schiff, I.& Rosenberg, R. D. (1992). Coagulation activation following estrogen administration to postmenopausal women. *Thromb Haemost,* Vol. 68, No. 4, (Oct 1992), pp. 392-395.

Canonico, M., Bouaziz, E., Carcaillon, L., Verstuyft, C., Guiochon-Mantel, A., Becquemont, L.& Scarabin, P. Y. (2008). Synergism between oral estrogen therapy and cytochrome P450 3A5*1 allele on the risk of venous thromboembolism among postmenopausal women. *J Clin Endocrinol Metab,* Vol. 93, No. 8, (Aug 2008), pp. 3082-3087.

Canonico, M., Fournier, A., Carcaillon, L., Olie, V., Plu-Bureau, G., Oger, E., Mesrine, S., Boutron-Ruault, M. C., Clavel-Chapelon, F.& Scarabin, P. Y. (2010). Postmenopausal hormone therapy and risk of idiopathic venous thromboembolism: results from the E3N cohort study. *Arterioscler Thromb Vasc Biol,* Vol. 30, No. 2, (Feb 2010), pp. 340-345.

Canonico, M., Oger, E., Plu-Bureau, G., Conard, J., Meyer, G., Levesque, H., Trillot, N., Barrellier, M. T., Wahl, D., Emmerich, J.& Scarabin, P. Y. (2007). Hormone therapy and venous thromboembolism among postmenopausal women: impact of the route of estrogen administration and progestogens: the ESTHER study. *Circulation,* Vol. 115, No. 7, (Feb 2007), pp. 840-845.

Canonico, M., Plu-Bureau, G., Lowe, G. D.& Scarabin, P. Y. (2008). Hormone replacement therapy and risk of venous thromboembolism in postmenopausal women: systematic review and meta-analysis. *BMJ,* Vol. 336, No. 7655, (May 2008), pp. 1227-1231.

Cauley, J. A., Robbins, J., Chen, Z., Cummings, S. R., Jackson, R. D., LaCroix, A. Z., LeBoff, M., Lewis, C. E., McGowan, J., Neuner, J., Pettinger, M., Stefanick, M. L., Wactawski-Wende, J.& Watts, N. B. (2003). Effects of estrogen plus progestin on risk of fracture and bone mineral density: the Women's Health Initiative randomized trial. *JAMA,* Vol. 290, No. 13, (Oct 2003), pp. 1729-1738.

Cauley, J. A., Seeley, D. G., Ensrud, K., Ettinger, B., Black, D.& Cummings, S. R. (1995). Estrogen replacement therapy and fractures in older women. Study of Osteoporotic Fractures Research Group. *Ann Intern Med,* Vol. 122, No. 1, (Jan 1995), pp. 9-16.

Chlebowski, R. T., Anderson, G. L., Manson, J. E., Schwartz, A. G., Wakelee, H., Gass, M., Rodabough, R. J., Johnson, K. C., Wactawski-Wende, J., Kotchen, J. M., Ockene, J. K., O'Sullivan, M. J., Hubbell, F. A., Chien, J. W., Chen, C.& Stefanick, M. L. (2010). Lung cancer among postmenopausal women treated with estrogen alone in the women's health initiative randomized trial. *J Natl Cancer Inst,* Vol. 102, No. 18, (Sep 2010), pp. 1413-1421.

Chlebowski, R. T., Schwartz, A. G., Wakelee, H., Anderson, G. L., Stefanick, M. L., Manson, J. E., Rodabough, R. J., Chien, J. W., Wactawski-Wende, J., Gass, M., Kotchen, J. M., Johnson, K. C., O'Sullivan, M. J., Ockene, J. K., Chen, C.& Hubbell, F. A. (2009). Oestrogen plus progestin and lung cancer in postmenopausal women (Women's Health Initiative trial): a post-hoc analysis of a randomised controlled trial. *Lancet,* Vol. 374, No. 9697, (Oct 2009), pp. 1243-1251.

Chlebowski, R. T., Wactawski-Wende, J., Ritenbaugh, C., Hubbell, F. A., Ascensao, J., Rodabough, R. J., Rosenberg, C. A., Taylor, V. M., Harris, R., Chen, C., Adams-Campbell, L. L.& White, E. (2004). Estrogen plus progestin and colorectal cancer in postmenopausal women. *N Engl J Med,* Vol. 350, No. 10, (Mar 2004), pp. 991-1004.

Clarkson, T. B. (2007). Estrogen effects on arteries vary with stage of reproductive life and extent of subclinical atherosclerosis progression. *Menopause,* Vol. 14, No. 3 Pt 1, (May-Jun 2007), pp. 373-384.

Clendenen, T. V., Koenig, K. L., Shore, R. E., Levitz, M., Arslan, A. A.& Zeleniuch-Jacquotte, A. (2009). Postmenopausal levels of endogenous sex hormones and risk of colorectal cancer. *Cancer Epidemiol Biomarkers Prev,* Vol. 18, No. 1, (Jan 2009), pp. 275-281.

Coldham, N. G., Dave, M., Sivapathasundaram, S., McDonnell, D. P., Connor, C.& Sauer, M. J. (1997). Evaluation of a recombinant yeast cell estrogen screening assay. *Environ Health Perspect,* Vol. 105, No. 7, (Jul 1997), pp. 734-742.

Colditz, G. A. (1993). Epidemiology of breast cancer. Findings from the nurses' health study. *Cancer,* Vol. 71, No. 4 Suppl, (Feb 1993), pp. 1480-1489.

Conneely, O. M., Kettelberger, D. M., Tsai, M. J., Schrader, W. T.& O'Malley, B. W. (1989). The chicken progesterone receptor A and B isoforms are products of an alternate translation initiation event. *J Biol Chem,* Vol. 264, No. 24, (Aug 1989), pp. 14062-14064.

Corrigan, E. C., Nelson, L. M., Bakalov, V. K., Yanovski, J. A., Vanderhoof, V. H., Yanoff, L. B.& Bondy, C. A. (2006). Effects of ovarian failure and X-chromosome deletion on body composition and insulin sensitivity in young women. *Menopause,* Vol. 13, No. 6, (Nov-Dec 2006), pp. 911-916.

Cowley, S. M., Hoare, S., Mosselman, S.& Parker, M. G. (1997). Estrogen receptors alpha and beta form heterodimers on DNA. *J Biol Chem,* Vol. 272, No. 32, (Aug 1997), pp. 19858-19862.

Cushman, M., Kuller, L. H., Prentice, R., Rodabough, R. J., Psaty, B. M., Stafford, R. S., Sidney, S.& Rosendaal, F. R. (2004). Estrogen plus progestin and risk of venous thrombosis. *JAMA,* Vol. 292, No. 13, (Oct 2004), pp. 1573-1580.

Davis, S. R., Moreau, M., Kroll, R., Bouchard, C., Panay, N., Gass, M., Braunstein, G. D., Hirschberg, A. L., Rodenberg, C., Pack, S., Koch, H., Moufarege, A.& Studd, J. (2008). Testosterone for low libido in postmenopausal women not taking estrogen. *N Engl J Med,* Vol. 359, No. 19, (Nov 2008), pp. 2005-2017.

De Lignieres, B., Basdevant, A., Thomas, G., Thalabard, J. C., Mercier-Bodard, C., Conard, J., Guyene, T. T., Mairon, N., Corvol, P., Guy-Grand, B.& et al. (1986). Biological effects of estradiol-17 beta in postmenopausal women: oral versus percutaneous administration. *J Clin Endocrinol Metab,* Vol. 62, No. 3, (Mar 1986), pp. 536-541.

Doren, M. (2000). Hormonal replacement regimens and bleeding. *Maturitas,* Vol. 34 Suppl 1, (Jan 2000), pp. S17-23.

Dossus, L., Allen, N., Kaaks, R., Bakken, K., Lund, E., Tjonneland, A., Olsen, A., Overvad, K., Clavel-Chapelon, F., Fournier, A., Chabbert-Buffet, N., Boeing, H., Schutze, M., Trichopoulou, A., Trichopoulos, D., Lagiou, P., Palli, D., Krogh, V., Tumino, R., Vineis, P., Mattiello, A., Bueno-de-Mesquita, H. B., Onland-Moret, N. C., Peeters, P. H., Dumeaux, V., Redondo, M. L., Duell, E., Sanchez-Cantalejo, E., Arriola, L., Chirlaque, M. D., Ardanaz, E., Manjer, J., Borgquist, S., Lukanova, A., Lundin, E., Khaw, K. T., Wareham, N., Key, T., Chajes, V., Rinaldi, S., Slimani, N., Mouw, T., Gallo, V.& Riboli, E. (2010). Reproductive risk factors and endometrial cancer: the European Prospective Investigation into Cancer and Nutrition. *Int J Cancer,* Vol. 127, No. 2, (Jul 2010), pp. 442-451.

Edwards, D. P. (2005). Regulation of signal transduction pathways by estrogen and progesterone. *Annu Rev Physiol,* Vol. 67, pp. 335-376.

Eshtiaghi, R., Esteghamati, A.& Nakhjavani, M. (2010). Menopause is an independent predictor of metabolic syndrome in Iranian women. *Maturitas,* Vol. 65, No. 3, (Mar 2010), pp. 262-266.

Farquhar, C., Marjoribanks, J., Lethaby, A., Suckling, J. A.& Lamberts, Q. (2009). Long term hormone therapy for perimenopausal and postmenopausal women. *Cochrane Database Syst Rev,* No. 2, pp. CD004143.

Fournier, A., Fabre, A., Mesrine, S., Boutron-Ruault, M. C., Berrino, F.& Clavel-Chapelon, F. (2008). Use of different postmenopausal hormone therapies and risk of histology- and hormone receptor-defined invasive breast cancer. *J Clin Oncol,* Vol. 26, No. 8, (Mar 2008), pp. 1260-1268.

Gallagher, J. C. (2007). Effect of early menopause on bone mineral density and fractures. *Menopause,* Vol. 14, No. 3 Pt 2, (May-Jun 2007), pp. 567-571.

Gallagher, J. C., Baylink, D. J., Freeman, R.& McClung, M. (2001). Prevention of bone loss with tibolone in postmenopausal women: results of two randomized, double-blind, placebo-controlled, dose-finding studies. *J Clin Endocrinol Metab,* Vol. 86, No. 10, (Oct 2001), pp. 4717-4726.

Greiser, C. M., Greiser, E. M.& Doren, M. (2005). Menopausal hormone therapy and risk of breast cancer: a meta-analysis of epidemiological studies and randomized controlled trials. *Hum Reprod Update,* Vol. 11, No. 6, (Nov-Dec 2005), pp. 561-573.

Grodstein, F., Clarkson, T. B.& Manson, J. E. (2003). Understanding the divergent data on postmenopausal hormone therapy. *N Engl J Med,* Vol. 348, No. 7, (Feb 2003), pp. 645-650.

Grodstein, F., Newcomb, P. A.& Stampfer, M. J. (1999). Postmenopausal hormone therapy and the risk of colorectal cancer: a review and meta-analysis. *Am J Med,* Vol. 106, No. 5, (May 1999), pp. 574-582.

Grodstein, F., Stampfer, M. J., Colditz, G. A., Willett, W. C., Manson, J. E., Joffe, M., Rosner, B., Fuchs, C., Hankinson, S. E., Hunter, D. J., Hennekens, C. H.& Speizer, F. E. (1997). Postmenopausal hormone therapy and mortality. *N Engl J Med,* Vol. 336, No. 25, (Jun 1997), pp. 1769-1775.

Grodstein, F., Stampfer, M. J., Falkeborn, M., Naessen, T.& Persson, I. (1999). Postmenopausal hormone therapy and risk of cardiovascular disease and hip fracture in a cohort of Swedish women. *Epidemiology,* Vol. 10, No. 5, (Sep 1999), pp. 476-480.

Guiochon-Mantel, A., Loosfelt, H., Lescop, P., Sar, S., Atger, M., Perrot-Applanat, M.& Milgrom, E. (1989). Mechanisms of nuclear localization of the progesterone receptor: evidence for interaction between monomers. *Cell,* Vol. 57, No. 7, (Jun 1989), pp. 1147-1154.

Guyton, A. C.& Hall, J. E. (c2006). *Textbook of medical physiology,* Elsevier Saunders, 0721602401, Philadelphia.

Hammes, S. R.& Levin, E. R. (2007). Extranuclear steroid receptors: nature and actions. *Endocr Rev,* Vol. 28, No. 7, (Dec 2007), pp. 726-741.

Harman, S. M., Brinton, E. A., Cedars, M., Lobo, R., Manson, J. E., Merriam, G. R., Miller, V. M., Naftolin, F.& Santoro, N. (2005). KEEPS: The Kronos Early Estrogen Prevention Study. *Climacteric,* Vol. 8, No. 1, (Mar 2005), pp. 3-12.

Hemelaar, M., Rosing, J., Kenemans, P., Thomassen, M. C., Braat, D. D.& van der Mooren, M. J. (2006). Less effect of intranasal than oral hormone therapy on factors associated with venous thrombosis risk in healthy postmenopausal women. *Arterioscler Thromb Vasc Biol,* Vol. 26, No. 7, (Jul 2006), pp. 1660-1666.

Hersh, A. L., Stefanick, M. L.& Stafford, R. S. (2004). National use of postmenopausal hormone therapy: annual trends and response to recent evidence. *JAMA,* Vol. 291, No. 1, (Jan 2004), pp. 47-53.

Hildebrand, J. S., Gapstur, S. M., Feigelson, H. S., Teras, L. R., Thun, M. J.& Patel, A. V. (2010). Postmenopausal hormone use and incident ovarian cancer: Associations differ by regimen. *Int J Cancer,* Vol. 127, No. 12, (Dec 2010), pp. 2928-2935.

Huckaby, C. S., Conneely, O. M., Beattie, W. G., Dobson, A. D., Tsai, M. J.& O'Malley, B. W. (1987). Structure of the chromosomal chicken progesterone receptor gene. *Proc Natl Acad Sci U S A,* Vol. 84, No. 23, (Dec 1987), pp. 8380-8384.

Hulka, B. S.& Moorman, P. G. (2008). Breast cancer: hormones and other risk factors. *Maturitas,* Vol. 61, No. 1-2, (Sep-Oct 2008), pp. 203-213; discussion 213.

Hulley, S., Grady, D., Bush, T., Furberg, C., Herrington, D., Riggs, B.& Vittinghoff, E. (1998). Randomized trial of estrogen plus progestin for secondary prevention of coronary heart disease in postmenopausal women. Heart and Estrogen/progestin Replacement Study (HERS) Research Group. *JAMA,* Vol. 280, No. 7, (Aug 1998), pp. 605-613.

Jaakkola, S., Lyytinen, H. K., Dyba, T., Ylikorkala, O.& Pukkala, E. (2011). Endometrial cancer associated with various forms of postmenopausal hormone therapy: a case control study. *Int J Cancer,* Vol. 128, No. 7, (Apr 2011), pp. 1644-1651.

Jackson, R. D., Wactawski-Wende, J., LaCroix, A. Z., Pettinger, M., Yood, R. A., Watts, N. B., Robbins, J. A., Lewis, C. E., Beresford, S. A., Ko, M. G., Naughton, M. J., Satterfield, S.& Bassford, T. (2006). Effects of conjugated equine estrogen on risk of fractures and BMD in postmenopausal women with hysterectomy: results from the women's health initiative randomized trial. *J Bone Miner Res,* Vol. 21, No. 6, (Jun 2006), pp. 817-828.

Kalantaridou, S. N., Naka, K. K., Papanikolaou, E., Kazakos, N., Kravariti, M., Calis, K. A., Paraskevaidis, E. A., Sideris, D. A., Tsatsoulis, A., Chrousos, G. P.& Michalis, L. K. (2004). Impaired endothelial function in young women with premature ovarian failure: normalization with hormone therapy. *J Clin Endocrinol Metab,* Vol. 89, No. 8, (Aug 2004), pp. 3907-3913.

Karim, R., Dell, R. M., Greene, D. F., Mack, W. J., Gallagher, J. C.& Hodis, H. N. (2011). Hip fracture in postmenopausal women after cessation of hormone therapy: results from a prospective study in a large health management organization. *Menopause,* (Jul 2011).

Kastner, P., Krust, A., Turcotte, B., Stropp, U., Tora, L., Gronemeyer, H.& Chambon, P. (1990). Two distinct estrogen-regulated promoters generate transcripts encoding the two functionally different human progesterone receptor forms A and B. *EMBO J,* Vol. 9, No. 5, (May 1990), pp. 1603-1614.

Kelsey, J. L.& Bernstein, L. (1996). Epidemiology and prevention of breast cancer. *Annu Rev Public Health,* Vol. 17, pp. 47-67.

Khan, J. A., Amazit, L., Bellance, C., Guiochon-Mantel, A., Lombes, M.& Loosfelt, H. (2011). p38 and p42/44 MAPKs Differentially Regulate Progesterone Receptor A and B Isoform Stabilization. *Mol Endocrinol*, (Aug 2011).doi:10.1210/me.2011-1042

Kiel, D. P., Felson, D. T., Anderson, J. J., Wilson, P. W.& Moskowitz, M. A. (1987). Hip fracture and the use of estrogens in postmenopausal women. The Framingham Study. *N Engl J Med,* Vol. 317, No. 19, (Nov 1987), pp. 1169-1174.

Knauff, E. A., Westerveld, H. E., Goverde, A. J., Eijkemans, M. J., Valkenburg, O., van Santbrink, E. J., Fauser, B. C.& van der Schouw, Y. T. (2008). Lipid profile of women with premature ovarian failure. *Menopause,* Vol. 15, No. 5, (Sep-Oct 2008), pp. 919-923.

Kopper, N. W., Gudeman, J.& Thompson, D. J. (2009). Transdermal hormone therapy in postmenopausal women: a review of metabolic effects and drug delivery technologies. *Drug Des Devel Ther,* Vol. 2, pp. 193-202.

Kuhl, H. (2005). Pharmacology of estrogens and progestogens: influence of different routes of administration. *Climacteric,* Vol. 8 Suppl 1, (Aug 2005), pp. 3-63.

Kuiper, G. G., Enmark, E., Pelto-Huikko, M., Nilsson, S.& Gustafsson, J. A. (1996). Cloning of a novel receptor expressed in rat prostate and ovary. *Proc Natl Acad Sci U S A,* Vol. 93, No. 12, (Jun 1996), pp. 5925-5930.

Lagro-Janssen, A., Knufing, M. W., Schreurs, L.& van Weel, C. (2010). Significant fall in hormone replacement therapy prescription in general practice. *Fam Pract,* Vol. 27, No. 4, (Aug 2010), pp. 424-429.

Lazovic, G., Radivojevic, U.& Marinkovic, J. (2008). Tibolone: the way to beat many a postmenopausal ailments. *Expert Opin Pharmacother,* Vol. 9, No. 6, (Apr 2008), pp. 1039-1047.

Leonhardt, S. A., Altmann, M.& Edwards, D. P. (1998). Agonist and antagonists induce homodimerization and mixed ligand heterodimerization of human progesterone receptors in vivo by a mammalian two-hybrid assay. *Mol Endocrinol,* Vol. 12, No. 12, (Dec 1998), pp. 1914-1930.

Levin, E. R. (2011). Minireview: Extranuclear steroid receptors: roles in modulation of cell functions. *Mol Endocrinol,* Vol. 25, No. 3, (Mar 2011), pp. 377-384.

Lindsay, R., Gallagher, J. C., Kleerekoper, M.& Pickar, J. H. (2005). Bone response to treatment with lower doses of conjugated estrogens with and without medroxyprogesterone acetate in early postmenopausal women. *Osteoporos Int,* Vol. 16, No. 4, (Apr 2005), pp. 372-379.

Loosfelt, H., Atger, M., Misrahi, M., Guiochon-Mantel, A., Meriel, C., Logeat, F., Benarous, R.& Milgrom, E. (1986). Cloning and sequence analysis of rabbit progesterone-receptor complementary DNA. *Proc Natl Acad Sci U S A,* Vol. 83, No. 23, (Dec 1986), pp. 9045-9049.

Losel, R.& Wehling, M. (2003). Nongenomic actions of steroid hormones. *Nat Rev Mol Cell Biol,* Vol. 4, No. 1, (Jan 2003), pp. 46-56.

Maclaran, K., Horner, E.& Panay, N. (2010). Premature ovarian failure: long-term sequelae. *Menopause Int,* Vol. 16, No. 1, (Mar 2010), pp. 38-41.

Maclaran, K.& Panay, N. (2011). Premature ovarian failure. *J Fam Plann Reprod Health Care,* Vol. 37, No. 1, (Jan 2011), pp. 35-42.

MacLennan, A. H., Taylor, A. W.& Wilson, D. H. (2004). Hormone therapy use after the Women's Health Initiative. *Climacteric,* Vol. 7, No. 2, (Jun 2004), pp. 138-142.

Madak-Erdogan, Z., Kieser, K. J., Kim, S. H., Komm, B., Katzenellenbogen, J. A.& Katzenellenbogen, B. S. (2008). Nuclear and extranuclear pathway inputs in the regulation of global gene expression by estrogen receptors. *Mol Endocrinol,* Vol. 22, No. 9, (Sep 2008), pp. 2116-2127.

Marzec, J. M., Christie, J. D., Reddy, S. P., Jedlicka, A. E., Vuong, H., Lanken, P. N., Aplenc, R., Yamamoto, T., Yamamoto, M., Cho, H. Y.& Kleeberger, S. R. (2007). Functional polymorphisms in the transcription factor NRF2 in humans increase the risk of acute lung injury. *FASEB J,* Vol. 21, No. 9, (Jul 2007), pp. 2237-2246.

McPherson, C. P., Sellers, T. A., Potter, J. D., Bostick, R. M.& Folsom, A. R. (1996). Reproductive factors and risk of endometrial cancer. The Iowa Women's Health Study. *Am J Epidemiol,* Vol. 143, No. 12, (Jun 1996), pp. 1195-1202.

Morch, L. S., Lokkegaard, E., Andreasen, A. H., Kruger-Kjaer, S.& Lidegaard, O. (2009). Hormone therapy and ovarian cancer. *JAMA,* Vol. 302, No. 3, (Jul 2009), pp. 298-305.

Nelson, L. M., Covington, S. N.& Rebar, R. W. (2005). An update: spontaneous premature ovarian failure is not an early menopause. *Fertil Steril,* Vol. 83, No. 5, (May 2005), pp. 1327-1332.

North American Menopause Society. Estrogen and progestogen use in postmenopausal women: 2010 position statement of The North American Menopause Society. (2010). *Menopause,* Vol. 17, No. 2, (Mar 2010), pp. 242-255.

O'Connell, M. B. (1995). Pharmacokinetic and pharmacologic variation between different estrogen products. *J Clin Pharmacol,* Vol. 35, No. 9 Suppl, (Sep 1995), pp. 18S-24S.

Oger, E., Alhenc-Gelas, M., Lacut, K., Blouch, M. T., Roudaut, N., Kerlan, V., Collet, M., Abgrall, J. F., Aiach, M., Scarabin, P. Y.& Mottier, D. (2003). Differential effects of oral and transdermal estrogen/progesterone regimens on sensitivity to activated protein C among postmenopausal women: a randomized trial. *Arterioscler Thromb Vasc Biol,* Vol. 23, No. 9, (Sep 2003), pp. 1671-1676.

Olie, V., Canonico, M.& Scarabin, P. Y. (2010). Risk of venous thrombosis with oral versus transdermal estrogen therapy among postmenopausal women. *Curr Opin Hematol,* Vol. 17, No. 5, (Sep 2010), pp. 457-463.

Panay, N.& Fenton, A. (2008). Premature ovarian failure: a growing concern. *Climacteric,* Vol. 11, No. 1, (Feb 2008), pp. 1-3.

Panay, N.& Kalu, E. (2009). Management of premature ovarian failure. *Best Pract Res Clin Obstet Gynaecol,* Vol. 23, No. 1, (Feb 2009), pp. 129-140.

Picard, D., Kumar, V., Chambon, P.& Yamamoto, K. R. (1990). Signal transduction by steroid hormones: nuclear localization is differentially regulated in estrogen and glucocorticoid receptors. *Cell Regul,* Vol. 1, No. 3, (Feb 1990), pp. 291-299.

Powers, M. S., Schenkel, L., Darley, P. E., Good, W. R., Balestra, J. C.& Place, V. A. (1985). Pharmacokinetics and pharmacodynamics of transdermal dosage forms of 17 beta-estradiol: comparison with conventional oral estrogens used for hormone replacement. *Am J Obstet Gynecol,* Vol. 152, No. 8, (Aug 1985), pp. 1099-1106.

Pratt, W. B.& Toft, D. O. (1997). Steroid receptor interactions with heat shock protein and immunophilin chaperones. *Endocr Rev,* Vol. 18, No. 3, (Jun 1997), pp. 306-360.

Prentice, R. L., Manson, J. E., Langer, R. D., Anderson, G. L., Pettinger, M., Jackson, R. D., Johnson, K. C., Kuller, L. H., Lane, D. S., Wactawski-Wende, J., Brzyski, R., Allison, M., Ockene, J., Sarto, G.& Rossouw, J. E. (2009). Benefits and risks of postmenopausal hormone therapy when it is initiated soon after menopause. *Am J Epidemiol,* Vol. 170, No. 1, (Jul 2009), pp. 12-23.

Raftogianis, R., Creveling, C., Weinshilboum, R.& Weisz, J. (2000). Estrogen metabolism by conjugation. *J Natl Cancer Inst Monogr*, No. 27, pp. 113-124.

Ritenbaugh, C., Stanford, J. L., Wu, L., Shikany, J. M., Schoen, R. E., Stefanick, M. L., Taylor, V., Garland, C., Frank, G., Lane, D., Mason, E., McNeeley, S. G., Ascensao, J.& Chlebowski, R. T. (2008). Conjugated equine estrogens and colorectal cancer incidence and survival: the Women's Health Initiative randomized clinical trial. *Cancer Epidemiol Biomarkers Prev,* Vol. 17, No. 10, (Oct 2008), pp. 2609-2618.

Rocca, W. A., Bower, J. H., Maraganore, D. M., Ahlskog, J. E., Grossardt, B. R., de Andrade, M.& Melton, L. J., 3rd. (2007). Increased risk of cognitive impairment or dementia in women who underwent oophorectomy before menopause. *Neurology,* Vol. 69, No. 11, (Sep 2007), pp. 1074-1083.

Rocca, W. A., Bower, J. H., Maraganore, D. M., Ahlskog, J. E., Grossardt, B. R., de Andrade, M.& Melton, L. J., 3rd. (2008). Increased risk of parkinsonism in women who underwent oophorectomy before menopause. *Neurology,* Vol. 70, No. 3, (Jan 2008), pp. 200-209.

Rodriguez, C., Spencer Feigelson, H., Deka, A., Patel, A. V., Jacobs, E. J., Thun, M. J.& Calle, E. E. (2008). Postmenopausal hormone therapy and lung cancer risk in the cancer prevention study II nutrition cohort. *Cancer Epidemiol Biomarkers Prev,* Vol. 17, No. 3, (Mar 2008), pp. 655-660.

Rosenfeld, M. G.& Glass, C. K. (2001). Coregulator codes of transcriptional regulation by nuclear receptors. *J Biol Chem,* Vol. 276, No. 40, (Oct 2001), pp. 36865-36868.

Rossouw, J. E., Anderson, G. L., Prentice, R. L., LaCroix, A. Z., Kooperberg, C., Stefanick, M. L., Jackson, R. D., Beresford, S. A., Howard, B. V., Johnson, K. C., Kotchen, J. M.& Ockene, J. (2002). Risks and benefits of estrogen plus progestin in healthy postmenopausal women: principal results From the Women's Health Initiative randomized controlled trial. *JAMA,* Vol. 288, No. 3, (Jul 2002), pp. 321-333.

Rossouw, J. E., Prentice, R. L., Manson, J. E., Wu, L., Barad, D., Barnabei, V. M., Ko, M., LaCroix, A. Z., Margolis, K. L.& Stefanick, M. L. (2007). Postmenopausal hormone therapy and risk of cardiovascular disease by age and years since menopause. *JAMA,* Vol. 297, No. 13, (Apr 2007), pp. 1465-1477.

Salpeter, S. R., Walsh, J. M., Greyber, E.& Salpeter, E. E. (2006). Brief report: Coronary heart disease events associated with hormone therapy in younger and older women. A meta-analysis. *J Gen Intern Med,* Vol. 21, No. 4, (Apr 2006), pp. 363-366.

Santen, R. J., Allred, D. C., Ardoin, S. P., Archer, D. F., Boyd, N., Braunstein, G. D., Burger, H. G., Colditz, G. A., Davis, S. R., Gambacciani, M., Gower, B. A., Henderson, V. W., Jarjour, W. N., Karas, R. H., Kleerekoper, M., Lobo, R. A., Manson, J. E., Marsden, J., Martin, K. A., Martin, L., Pinkerton, J. V., Rubinow, D. R., Teede, H., Thiboutot, D. M.& Utian, W. H. (2010). Postmenopausal hormone therapy: an Endocrine Society scientific statement. *J Clin Endocrinol Metab,* Vol. 95, No. 7 Suppl 1, (Jul 2010), pp. s1-s66.

Scarabin, P. Y., Alhenc-Gelas, M., Plu-Bureau, G., Taisne, P., Agher, R.& Aiach, M. (1997). Effects of oral and transdermal estrogen/progesterone regimens on blood coagulation and fibrinolysis in postmenopausal women. A randomized controlled trial. *Arterioscler Thromb Vasc Biol,* Vol. 17, No. 11, (Nov 1997), pp. 3071-3078.

Scarabin, P. Y., Hemker, H. C., Clement, C., Soisson, V.& Alhenc-Gelas, M. (2011). Increased thrombin generation among postmenopausal women using hormone therapy:

importance of the route of estrogen administration and progestogens. *Menopause,* Vol. 18, No. 8, (Aug 2011), pp. 873-879.

Scarabin, P. Y., Oger, E.& Plu-Bureau, G. (2003). Differential association of oral and transdermal oestrogen-replacement therapy with venous thromboembolism risk. *Lancet,* Vol. 362, No. 9382, (Aug 2003), pp. 428-432.

Shuster, L. T., Rhodes, D. J., Gostout, B. S., Grossardt, B. R.& Rocca, W. A. (2010). Premature menopause or early menopause: long-term health consequences. *Maturitas,* Vol. 65, No. 2, (Feb 2010), pp. 161-166.

Simon, T., Beau Yon de Jonage-Canonico, M., Oger, E., Wahl, D., Conard, J., Meyer, G., Emmerich, J., Barrellier, M. T., Guiraud, A.& Scarabin, P. Y. (2006). Indicators of lifetime endogenous estrogen exposure and risk of venous thromboembolism. *J Thromb Haemost,* Vol. 4, No. 1, (Jan 2006), pp. 71-76.

Snowdon, D. A., Kane, R. L., Beeson, W. L., Burke, G. L., Sprafka, J. M., Potter, J., Iso, H., Jacobs, D. R., Jr.& Phillips, R. L. (1989). Is early natural menopause a biologic marker of health and aging? *Am J Public Health,* Vol. 79, No. 6, (Jun 1989), pp. 709-714.

Sonnet, E., Lacut, K., Roudaut, N., Mottier, D., Kerlan, V.& Oger, E. (2007). Effects of the route of oestrogen administration on IGF-1 and IGFBP-3 in healthy postmenopausal women: results from a randomized placebo-controlled study. *Clin Endocrinol (Oxf),* Vol. 66, No. 5, (May 2007), pp. 626-631.

Stampfer, M. J., Colditz, G. A., Willett, W. C., Manson, J. E., Rosner, B., Speizer, F. E.& Hennekens, C. H. (1991). Postmenopausal estrogen therapy and cardiovascular disease. Ten-year follow-up from the nurses' health study. *N Engl J Med,* Vol. 325, No. 11, (Sep 1991), pp. 756-762.

Steingold, K. A., Laufer, L., Chetkowski, R. J., DeFazio, J. D., Matt, D. W., Meldrum, D. R.& Judd, H. L. (1985). Treatment of hot flashes with transdermal estradiol administration. *J Clin Endocrinol Metab,* Vol. 61, No. 4, (Oct 1985), pp. 627-632.

Straczek, C., Oger, E., Yon de Jonage-Canonico, M. B., Plu-Bureau, G., Conard, J., Meyer, G., Alhenc-Gelas, M., Levesque, H., Trillot, N., Barrellier, M. T., Wahl, D., Emmerich, J.& Scarabin, P. Y. (2005). Prothrombotic mutations, hormone therapy, and venous thromboembolism among postmenopausal women: impact of the route of estrogen administration. *Circulation,* Vol. 112, No. 22, (Nov 2005), pp. 3495-3500.

Sturdee, D. W., Pines, A., Archer, D. F., Baber, R. J., Barlow, D., Birkhauser, M. H., Brincat, M., Cardozo, L., de Villiers, T. J., Gambacciani, M., Gompel, A. A., Henderson, V. W., Kluft, C., Lobo, R. A., MacLennan, A. H., Marsden, J., Nappi, R. E., Panay, N., Pickar, J. H., Robinson, D., Simon, J., Sitruk-Ware, R. L.& Stevenson, J. C. (2011). Updated IMS recommendations on postmenopausal hormone therapy and preventive strategies for midlife health. *Climacteric,* Vol. 14, No. 3, (Jun 2011), pp. 302-320.

Swanson, S. G., Drosman, S., Helmond, F. A.& Stathopoulos, V. M. (2006). Tibolone for the treatment of moderate to severe vasomotor symptoms and genital atrophy in postmenopausal women: a multicenter, randomized, double-blind, placebo-controlled study. *Menopause,* Vol. 13, No. 6, (Nov-Dec 2006), pp. 917-925.

Taylor, H. S.& Manson, J. E. (2011). Update in hormone therapy use in menopause. *J Clin Endocrinol Metab,* Vol. 96, No. 2, (Feb 2011), pp. 255-264.

Thimmulappa, R. K., Mai, K. H., Srisuma, S., Kensler, T. W., Yamamoto, M.& Biswal, S. (2002). Identification of Nrf2-regulated genes induced by the chemopreventive agent sulforaphane by oligonucleotide microarray. *Cancer Res,* Vol. 62, No. 18, (Sep 2002), pp. 5196-5203.

Uygur, D., Sengul, O., Bayar, D., Erdinc, S., Batioglu, S.& Mollamahmutoglu, L. (2005). Bone loss in young women with premature ovarian failure. *Arch Gynecol Obstet,* Vol. 273, No. 1, (Nov 2005), pp. 17-19.

Van den Belt, K., Berckmans, P., Vangenechten, C., Verheyen, R.& Witters, H. (2004). Comparative study on the in vitro/in vivo estrogenic potencies of 17beta-estradiol, estrone, 17alpha-ethynylestradiol and nonylphenol. *Aquat Toxicol,* Vol. 66, No. 2, (Feb 2004), pp. 183-195.

van Der Voort, D. J., van Der Weijer, P. H.& Barentsen, R. (2003). Early menopause: increased fracture risk at older age. *Osteoporos Int,* Vol. 14, No. 6, (Jul 2003), pp. 525-530.

Vehkavaara, S., Silveira, A., Hakala-Ala-Pietila, T., Virkamaki, A., Hovatta, O., Hamsten, A., Taskinen, M. R.& Yki-Jarvinen, H. (2001). Effects of oral and transdermal estrogen replacement therapy on markers of coagulation, fibrinolysis, inflammation and serum lipids and lipoproteins in postmenopausal women. *Thromb Haemost,* Vol. 85, No. 4, (Apr 2001), pp. 619-625.

Vickers, M. R., MacLennan, A. H., Lawton, B., Ford, D., Martin, J., Meredith, S. K., DeStavola, B. L., Rose, S., Dowell, A., Wilkes, H. C., Darbyshire, J. H.& Meade, T. W. (2007). Main morbidities recorded in the women's international study of long duration oestrogen after menopause (WISDOM): a randomised controlled trial of hormone replacement therapy in postmenopausal women. *BMJ,* Vol. 335, No. 7613, (Aug 2007), pp. 239.

Vujovic, S., Brincat, M., Erel, T., Gambacciani, M., Lambrinoudaki, I., Moen, M. H., Schenck-Gustafsson, K., Tremollieres, F., Rozenberg, S.& Rees, M. (2010). EMAS position statement: Managing women with premature ovarian failure. *Maturitas,* Vol. 67, No. 1, (Sep 2010), pp. 91-93.

Walter, P., Green, S., Greene, G., Krust, A., Bornert, J. M., Jeltsch, J. M., Staub, A., Jensen, E., Scrace, G., Waterfield, M.& et al. (1985). Cloning of the human estrogen receptor cDNA. *Proc Natl Acad Sci U S A,* Vol. 82, No. 23, (Dec 1985), pp. 7889-7893.

Welshons, W. V., Krummel, B. M.& Gorski, J. (1985). Nuclear localization of unoccupied receptors for glucocorticoids, estrogens, and progesterone in GH3 cells. *Endocrinology,* Vol. 117, No. 5, (Nov 1985), pp. 2140-2147.

Wendler, A., Baldi, E., Harvey, B. J., Nadal, A., Norman, A.& Wehling, M. (2010). Position paper: Rapid responses to steroids: current status and future prospects. *Eur J Endocrinol,* Vol. 162, No. 5, (May 2010), pp. 825-830.

WHO Report. Research on the menopause in the 1990s. Report of a WHO Scientific Group. (1996). *World Health Organ Tech Rep Ser,* Vol. 866, pp. 1-107.

Wilson, R. A. ([1966]). *Feminine forever,* M. Evans; distributed in association with Lippincott, New York.

Yaffe, K., Barnes, D., Lindquist, K., Cauley, J., Simonsick, E. M., Penninx, B., Satterfield, S., Harris, T.& Cummings, S. R. (2007). Endogenous sex hormone levels and risk of cognitive decline in an older biracial cohort. *Neurobiol Aging,* Vol. 28, No. 2, (Feb 2007), pp. 171-178.

Ylikorkala, O.& Rozenberg, S. (2000). Efficacy and tolerability of fully transdermal hormone replacement in sequential or continuous therapy at two doses of progestogen in postmenopausal women. *Maturitas,* Vol. 37, No. 2, (Dec 2000), pp. 83-93.

Zervoudakis, A., Strickler, H. D., Park, Y., Xue, X., Hollenbeck, A., Schatzkin, A.& Gunter, M. J. (2011). Reproductive history and risk of colorectal cancer in postmenopausal women. *J Natl Cancer Inst,* Vol. 103, No. 10, (May 2011), pp. 826-834.

16

A Multi-Level Analysis of World Scientific Output in Pharmacology

Carlos Olmeda-Gómez, Ma-Antonia Ovalle-Perandones and Antonio Perianes-Rodríguez
Carlos III University of Madrid
Spain

1. Introduction

Over the last few decades and particularly in the present economic context, the distribution of economic resources has been a concern addressed by governmental and corporate scientific policy, which has either benefitted only part of the scientific and technological community or furthered certain lines of research. The pharmaceutical industry in particular has had to confront not only this situation, but also ongoing internationalisation, supported by the relentless advances in communication technologies.

Until the nineteen eighties, industry internationalisation, in terms of R&D, was a marginal matter, not only for economics theory and business in general, but also for governments and the other organisations involved. Globalisation began to acquire importance after the mid nineteen nineties, although not all manufacturing industries have experienced the same degree of R&D internationalisation. The pharmaceutical industry, for one, pioneered this more universal approach to research and development (Noisi, 1999).

Contrary to the widely held opinion according to which R&D internatianlisation is the fruit of domestic innovation in many industries, pharmaceutical constitutes an exception. Indeed, international innovation intensifies the industry's R&D (Patel and Pavitt, 2000), whereas in other lines of business domestic innovation is the driver. In addition to internationalising its R&D, the pharmaceuticals industry has increased its research spending exponentially in recent years (Congressional Budget Office, 2006).

A number of earlier papers studied the bibilometric characteristics of the pharmacological publications generated as a result of the R&D effort in places such as the United States (Narin and Rozek, 1988), India (Kaur and Gupta, 2009; Gupta and Kaur, 2009) or the Middle East (Biglu and Omidi, 2010). Others stressed the contribution of pharmaceutical firms to scientific knowledge (Koening, 1983; McMillan and Hamilton, 2000; Rafols, et al. 2010; Perianes-Rodríguez, et al. 2011). The assessment of the international impact of scientific papers is a present, but not a new concern: it has been a frequent object of study since the nineteen eighties. The use of scientific indicators for several decades to characterise research by subject area, country or institution has confirmed that, although they have their limitations, they are the only suitable tool for scientific assessment (Braun T et al., 1985).

The purpose of this chapter is to analyse international research in "pharmacology, toxicology and pharmaceutics" (hereafter pharmacology) on the basis of the scientific papers listed in the Scopus multidisciplinary database. This primary objective is reached by answering the following questions (in the section on results). What weight does the subject area "pharmacology, toxicology and pharmaceutics" carry in world-wide science? What is the percentage contribution made by the various regions of the world to the subject area "pharmacology, toxicology and pharmaceutics"? Can certain regions be identified as leaders on that basis, as in other scientific contexts? Are emerging countries present in the field? Do the most productive countries also publish the largest number of journals? What features characterise the scientific output of companies that publish pharmacological papers?

2. Methodology

2.1 Database

The possible sources of information for scientometric research include multi-disciplinary databases such as Thomson Reuters' Web of Science, Elsevier's Scopus and resources such as Google Scholar, as well as specialised services such as Medline. These sources analyse research results in the form of scientific papers published in international journals and their subsequent citation by the rest of the scientific community.

Scopus, the Elsevier database created in 2004, lists over 18 000 journals edited by over 5 000 publishers[1]. When it first appeared, it was analysed by many authors and compared to other resources in a whole stream of papers (Fingerman, 2005; LaGuardia, 2005). It was chosen for the present study because of its broad subject area and linguistic coverage; in the understanding that world-wide scientific production is more fully represented in Scopus than in other databases (Sciverse Scopus, 2011). In addition, as a resource suitable for research conducted after 1996, it is particularly apt for a subject area such as pharmacology (Gorraiz and Schloegl, 2008).

Scopus' strong points as a source of information are reinforced by an open access, on-line tool known as SCImago Journal and Country Rank (SJR, 2007). As its name infers, this system of scientific information, drawing from Scopus contents from 1996 to 2010, ranks journals and countries using data intended for world-wide scientific assessment. The tool provides open access to both data and indicators by region or country, with international coverage. It proved to be particularly useful for the aims pursued in the present study.

2.2 Indicators

Two sets of bibliometric indicators were used in this study: one to determine the quantitative characteristics of scientific output and the other to analyse its quality, i.e., the qualitative characteristics of citations and journals (Rehn, 2007). The indicators included in each group are described below.

This study calculated the number of scientific papers published by the units analysed (world, region, country or industry) over the time span defined. All of the various possible types of papers (such as articles, reviews and notes to the editor,) were included in the *output* indicator.

[1] Available from http://www.info.sciverse.com/scopus/scopus-in-detail/facts/. 20/08/2011

When papers were co-authored by researchers from institutions in different countries, a complete computational approach was adopted. The growth rate, when provided, indicates the rise or decline in world-wide output in 2009 with respect to the baseline year, 1996.

A number of indicators were used to obtain an approximate view of the quality of world scientific output in the field of pharmacology. The number of *citations* received refers to the total number of times papers published by the unit analysed were cited during the period studied. This indicator provides an overview of the scientific impact of the articles published by the unit in question. The number of *citations per paper* was calculated as the mean number of citations received by all the papers published by the unit analysed in the period studied.

The *domestic citations* were separated from the total to determine the proportion of the output that was used as a reference in the same geographic area (region or country) and consequently, by simple subtraction, the proportion involving knowledge transfer to other areas. The results are shown as the percentage of the citations used for research conducted in the same geographic area. The *normalised citation* indicator is the relative number of times papers produced by a specific unit were cited, compared to the world-wide mean for papers of the same type, age and subject area.

While citations denote the subsequent use of papers once published, the *references* list the literature cited in papers published by a journal at any given time. The number of *references per paper* was found by dividing the total number of references by the number of papers published by the unit.

A country's *H index*, in turn, specifies the number of papers (h) produced in that country and receiving at least h citation. It relates a country's scientific productivity (output) to its scientific impact (citations). The *international collaboration* indicator is the percentage of papers with author affiliations in more than one country. This indicator measures institutions' international networking capacity. In this chapter a journal's *% output in Q1* is the percentage of scientific papers published by an institution in what are classified as the most influential journals in the respective category, i.e., the periodicals in the first quartile or Q1, the upper 25 %, based on their SJR value.

Another qualitative indicator used, homonymous with the aforementioned scientific information system (SCImago Journal and Country Rank), was the *Scimago Journal Rank (SJR)*, used as an alternative to the traditional impact factor (I.F.). This indicator, which measures the visibility of the journals in the Scopus® database, is established by the SCImago[2] research team on the grounds of the well-known Google PageRank™ algorithm. It differs from the I.F. in two ways: citations are computed over 3 rather than 2 years; and article citations are weighted, with citations in more visible or prominent journals carrying greater weight than citations in lower-ranking journals (González-Pereira et al., 2009).

3. Results

3.1 World-wide science and pharmacology

World-wide scientific output, as listed in the Scopus database for the period running from 1996 to 2009, came to 21 100 138 papers. The total citations received by those papers during the

[2] http://www.scimago.es/. 20.08.2011

same period amounted to 217 388 448, for a mean of 10.03 citations per paper. The absolute numbers for pharmacology, as one of the 27 subject areas established by Scopus, were logically much smaller. The totals were 564 914 papers and 6 266 408 citations. The mean number of citations in pharmacology was therefore higher than the world average, at 11.09. The growth rate for this subject area was 4.76 %, reflecting the growth in its scientific output.

Figure 1 shows the percentage contribution of the Scopus subject areas to world-wide scientific output during the period studied. Medicine played a predominant role in the international scientific scenario, with a mean yearly contribution of over 20 %. Decision science and dentistry stood at the other extreme, with a mean yearly output of 0.35 %, shown on the figure as very thin lines. The mean yearly contribution of pharmacology to international scientific output in the period was 2.7 %, shown in red on the right half of the graph. When pooled, all the subject areas with relative outputs of under 4 %, which include pharmacology, earth and planet sciences, immunology and microbiology, accounted for 34.83 % of the scientific papers published world-wide.

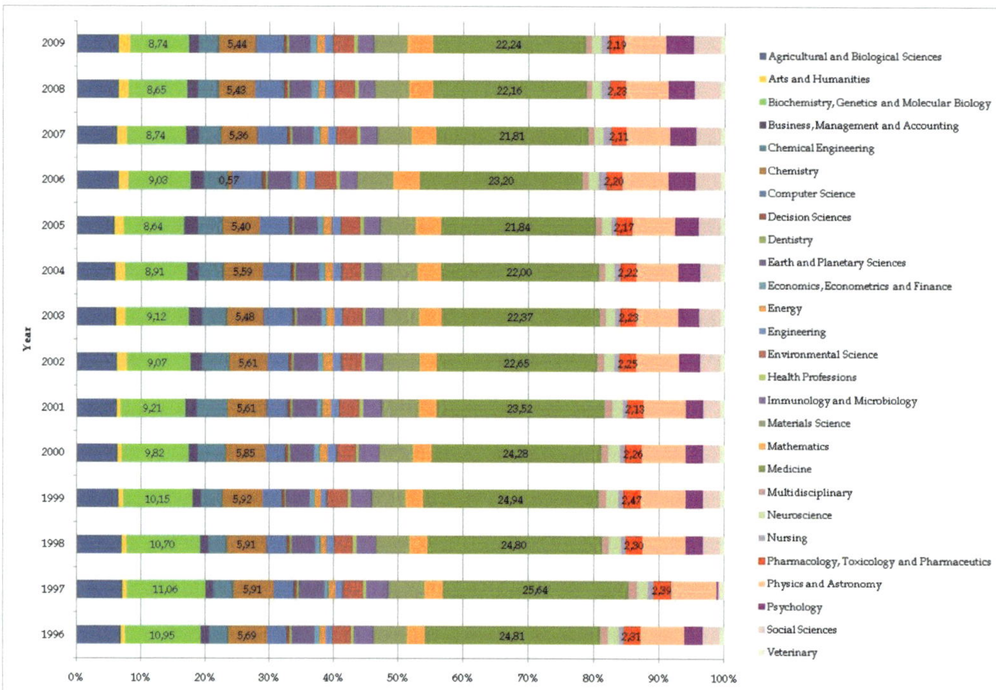

Fig. 1. World output by subject areas (%) (Scopus, 1996-2009)

3.2 Pharmacology by region

While scientific output by region is an important indicator to determine regional contributions to pharmacology, quantitative information alone is incomplete and must be supplemented with data on the impact of these papers on the scientific community. Table 1 gives the vales of some of the indicators described earlier for a number of regions, along with colour bar graphs for readier interpretation.

Region	Output	Citations	Domestic citations	%Domestic citations	Citations per paper
North America	155373	2714951	2209503	81.38	17.47
Western Europe	159512	2383236	1671534	70.14	14.94
Asia	113741	1095409	626665	57.21	9.63
Eastern Europe	21951	178157	57830	32.46	8.12
Latin America	18122	164264	78623	47.86	9.06
Pacific Region	11802	161126	45651	28.33	13.65
Middle East	10256	105817	27329	25.83	10.32
Southern Africa	2167	23987	7406	30.88	11.07
Central Africa	2035	11101	4650	41.89	5.46
Northen Africa	827	7559	1808	23.92	9.14

Table 1. Pharmacological scientific output, citations and domestic citations by region (Scopus, 1996-2009)

The behaviour of the domestic citations indicator merits comment. In North America, these citations accounted for over 80 % percent of the total. The number of domestic citations was likewise very high in Western Europe; in both regions most of the citations were found in articles published in the same country as the paper cited. Consequently, in these two regions, the large number of domestic citations led to an inordinately large number of total citations.

The regions with smaller numbers of citations also had a smaller proportion of domestic citations. In other words, their output was acknowledged primarily by other regions, while domestic citations were less frequent. The region that best illustrates this observation is Northern Africa, where only 23.92 % of the citations received were domestic.

The number of citations per paper was also highest in North America and Western Europe, with the Pacific Region ranking a close third. Central Africa's low scientific output in pharmacology was only scantly acknowledged, with only 5.46 citations per paper on average. Asia, Eastern Europe, Latin America and Northern Africa had similar citations per paper values, which ranged from 8 to 9.

The pharmacological output by regions over the period 1996 to 2009 is shown in Figure 2. The three most productive regions in that period were Western Europe (red), North America (blue) and Asia (green). Asia had a higher growth rate in the latter years of the period and was the most productive region in 2009. This rise may have been the result of greater participation in the pharmacology, particularly in countries that in those years began to adopt a very active role in the field.

3.3 Countries and pharmacology

The basic unit for the regions listed above was defined as the individual country. A total of 194 countries published pharmacological research in the period studied. The analysis conducted of their output provided greater insight into the values found for the regional indicators.

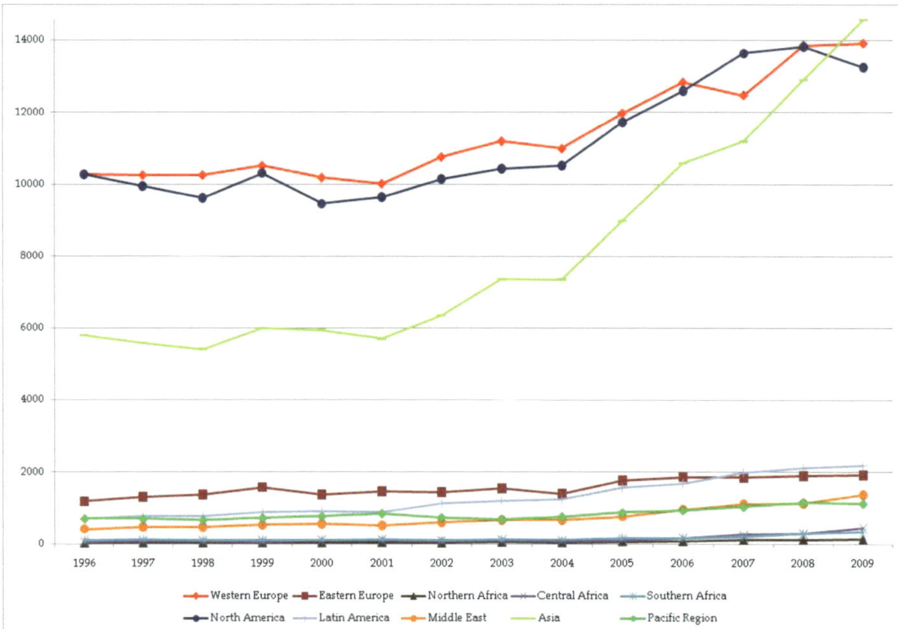

Fig. 2. Pharmacological scientific output by region (Scopus, 1996-2009)

The ten most productive countries accounted for around 71 % of world-wide pharmacological output in the period studied. These ten countries are listed in Table 2, which shows their total output in the period, the number of total and domestic citations received, the citations per paper and the H index. The list is headed by the United States, which had the largest output and number of citations, although the number per paper should be interpreted bearing in mind the impact of the large number of domestic citations identified. At 293, its H index was likewise high, indicating that 293 papers were cited in 293 other articles.

Table 3 ranks the countries whose overall data for the entire period are given in Table 2, year by year across the period. Grey shading indicates that the country changed its position from the preceding year and maroon shading that the country joined the top ten in the year in question.

The regional study showed the enormous progress in Asia in the latter years of the period. That growth was the result of greater participation in the subject area by Asian countries. Although until 2005 Japan was the second largest producer in pharmacology, from 2006 onward it was overtaken by an emerging neighbour: China. In the three earliest years China ranked tenth; in the intermediate years it gradually climbed to higher positions and finally reached second place in 2006. While still among the most productive countries, Japan's position slid, denoting its tendency to contribute less and less to pharmacological output. In the last year of the series, 2009, four of the ten most productive countries were Asian (China, India, Japan and South Korea).

The United States maintained its lead throughout the period. That leadership and Canada's contribution, from lower but still productive positions, made North America the sole region with an output comparable to Asia's in the latter years. All the other most productive countries in pharmacology were from Western Europe: United Kingdom, Germany, Italy and France, and the Netherlands and Spain in some years. Only one Latin American country was among the most productive during the period: Brazil, in 2007.

Country	Output	Citations	Domestic citations	Citations per paper	H Index
United States	154941	2516137	1221126	17.38	293
Japan	47322	543692	164265	11.38	139
United Kingdom	40531	644728	143933	16.9	195
China	36079	178269	80870	6.34	84
Germany	34443	442517	106046	13.49	157
India	23323	144862	59885	9.22	91
Italy	22593	304775	75527	14.88	128
France	21925	320578	64831	15.28	148
Canada	18667	297798	61608	17.18	143
Spain	14232	165910	41389	12.66	101

Table 2. Pharmacological scientific output, domestic citations, citations per document and H index for the 10 most productive countries (Scopus, 1996-2009)

1996	1997	1998	1999	2000	2001	2002	2003	2004	2005	2006	2007	2008	2009
USA	USA	USA	USA	USA	USA	USA	USA	USA	USA	USA	USA	USA	USA
Japan	Japan	Japan	Japan	Japan	Japan	Japan	Japan	Japan	Japan	China	China	China	China
U.K.	U.K.	U.K.	U.K.	U.K.	U.K.	U.K.	U.K.	U.K.	China	Japan	Japan	U.K.	India
Germany	Germany	Germany	Germany	Germany	Germany	Germany	Germany	Germany	U.K.	U.K.	U.K.	Japan	U.K.
France	France	France	France	France	France	Italy	China	China	Germany	Germany	Germany	India	Japan
Italy	Italy	Italy	Italy	Italy	Italy	France	France	Italy	Italy	India	India	Germany	Germany
Canada	Canada	Canada	Canada	China	China	China	Italy	France	India	Italy	Italy	Italy	Italy
Spain	Spain	Netherlands	China	Canada	Canada	Canada	Canada	Canada	France	France	France	France	France
Netherlands	Netherlands	Spain	Netherlands	Spain	Netherlands	India	India	India	Canada	Canada	Canada	Canada	Canada
China	China	China	Spain	India	Spain	Netherlands	Spain	Netherlands	Spain	Spain	Brazil	South Korea	South Korea

Table 3. Country position by output (Scopus, 1996-2009)

Figures 3 and 4 show the relationship between international collaboration and citations per paper in countries publishing at least 1 000 papers. The position occupied by the countries in each region is shown in both figures, but only Western European and North American countries are depicted in Figure 3. All the Asian, Eastern European and Latin American countries are shown in Figure 4, although only the BRIC countries (Brazil, Russia, India, China) are labelled.

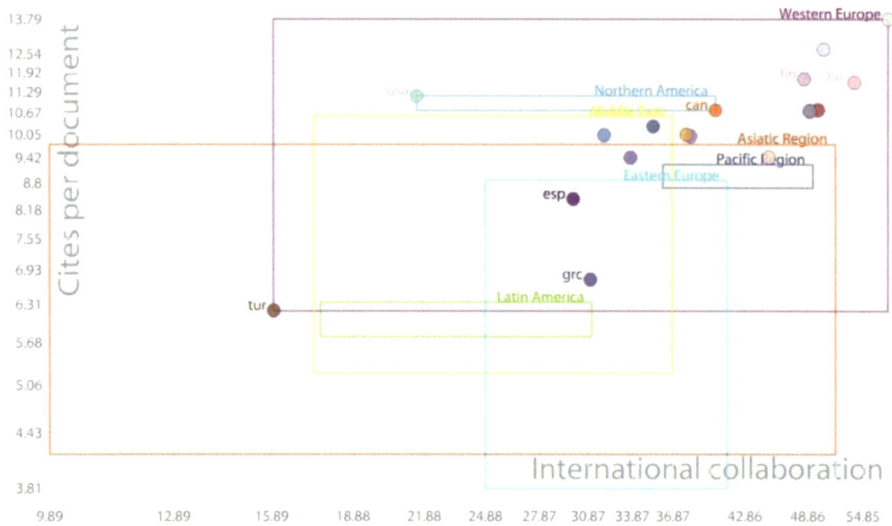

Fig. 3. International collaboration and citations per paper in North American and Western European countries (www.scimagoir.com), 2003-2009.

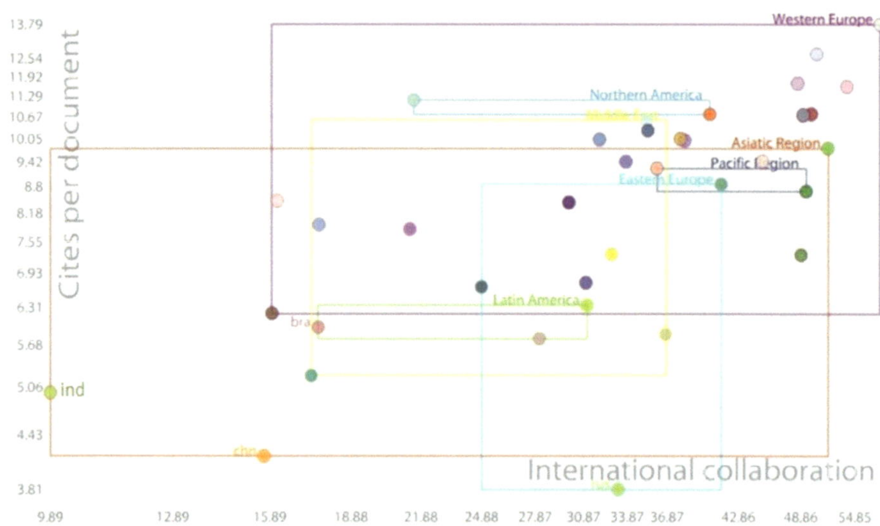

Fig. 4. International collaboration and citations per paper in BRIC countries (www.scimagoir.com), 2003-2009.

The country in Figure 3 with the smallest number of citations per paper and least intense international collaboration was Turkey. With 6.18 citations per paper and an international co-authorship percentage of 16.12, it stood at the low end of its region, Western Europe, and had lower citation values than Latin America or Eastern Europe. In Western Europe, Sweden and Belgium were the two countries both in that region and the world with the highest international collaboration indices and a mean of 12 citations per paper. Both, as well as other countries, also had higher values than the USA (in terms of international collaboration) and Canada.

Measuring their scientific status in terms of citations per paper and international collaboration values, the BRIC countries still have room for improvement. Three of those four countries were positioned very close to the origin on the graph. Of the four, only Brazil showed values close to the results recorded for Turkey.

3.4 Pharmacology in journals

The analysis of the journals that published pharmacological papers included the data for the periodicals that published at least one such paper in 2009. Under that criterion, a total of 482 journals were identified, 61 of which had been recently added to the database and consequently lacked the data needed to calculate their SJR.

Of the remaining 421 (that had published more than one paper and had an SJR index), 110 were edited in the United States, although a fair number were also published in other countries: Netherlands (87), United Kingdom (75), Germany (25), China (12), India (12), Japan (11), Spain (11), France (8), Switzerland (7) and New Zealand (6).

The remaining journals were published in a total of 33 countries, each with less than six journals.

10 top journals by SJR value	SJR	Ouput (2009)	Citations (3years)	Citations per paper (2years)	Refs	Ref per doc	Country
Annual Review of Pharmacology and Toxicology	3.56	19	1429	22.94	2367	124.58	United States
Pharmacological Reviews	3.3	19	1433	17.16	6531	343.74	United States
Nature Reviews Drug Discovery	2.68	202	5827	15.67	7865	38.94	United Kingdom
Trends in Pharmacological Sciences	1.64	84	2588	9.56	5718	68.07	Netherlands
Drug Resistance Updates	1.52	16	530	11.79	1836	114.75	United States
DNA Repair	1.44	169	2237	4.15	10528	62.3	Netherlands
Pharmacology and Therapeutics	1.22	104	3367	9.23	20152	193.77	United States
Current Opinion in Pharmacology	1.14	117	2138	7.57	6206	53.04	Netherlands
Advanced Drug Delivery Reviews	1.1	143	4030	12.34	15219	106.43	Netherlands
10 top journals by total documents in 2009	**SJR**	**Ouput (2009)**	**Citations (3years)**	**Citations per paper (2years)**	**Refs**	**Ref per doc**	**Country**
Bioorganic and Medicinal Chemistry Letters	0.21	1546	10591	2.72	39742	25.71	Netherlands
Pharmaceutical Journal	0.03	1058	124	0.1	972	0.92	United Kingdom
Deutsche Apotheker Zeitung	0.02	967	11	0.02	1440	1.49	Germany
Bioorganic and Medicinal Chemistry	0.2	910	7859	2.88	34194	37.58	Netherlands
Chemosphere	0.15	905	11704	3.41	32003	35.36	Netherlands
European Journal of Pharmacology	0.27	619	6875	2.76	26762	43.23	Netherlands
British Journal of Pharmacology	0.6	616	6819	5.29	28480	46.23	United Kingdom
Medical Hypotheses	0.12	612	1835	1.55	16902	27.62	United States
Japanese Journal of Cancer and Chemotherapy	0.03	611	163	0.09	889	1.45	Japan
International Journal of Pharmaceutics	0.19	528	5930	3.33	17075	32.34	Netherlands

Table 4. Pharmacology journals: SJR, output, citations, citations per paper, references, references per paper and country of publication (Scopus), 2009

The large and unwieldy original table was abbreviated to build Table 4, which gives the values for only the journals with the 10 highest SJR and the 10 scientific journals that published the largest number of pharmacological articles in the last year of the series. Note that none of these journals appears on both lists.

Of the scientific journals with the highest SJR, two were published in the US, *Annual Review of Pharmacology and Toxicology* and *Pharmacological Review*, and one in the United Kingdom, *Nature Reviews and Drug Discovery*. These three journals had SJR scores of 3.56, 3.3 and 2.68, respectively. That means that they received large numbers of citations, but also that since they are weighted by journal prestige to calculate the indicator, those citations appeared in other high quality journals. Neither of the US journals was very productive, with only 19 papers each in 2009, compared to a much larger output by the English periodical, which published a total of 202 articles.

The scientific journals with the highest output in pharmacology were The Netherlands' *Bioorganic and Medicinal Chemistry Letters*, with 1 546 papers, followed by the UK's *Pharmaceutical Journal*, with 1 058 and Germany's *Deutsche Apotheker Zeitung*, with 967. Their SJR indices were lower than for the journals mentioned in the preceding paragraph, however, with scores of 0.21, 0.03 and 0.02, respectively. In other words, in the period calculated for the SJR index (three years), either the absolute number of citations received by this group of more productive journals was very low or the citations were published in lower quality journals.

Each country's contribution to pharmacological scientific output can be analysed from two perspectives: as specified earlier, by the contribution made by its scientists through their published papers, or by the journals edited in the country. These two factors are compared in Figure 5. Each country's scientific output is shown in red and its publishing activity in blue. Many countries, such as the United States, show similar percentages for both types of contribution, while in others the values vary widely. A case in point is The Netherlands, whose scientific output was a mere 2 % while its journals published over 20 % of the pharmacological articles.

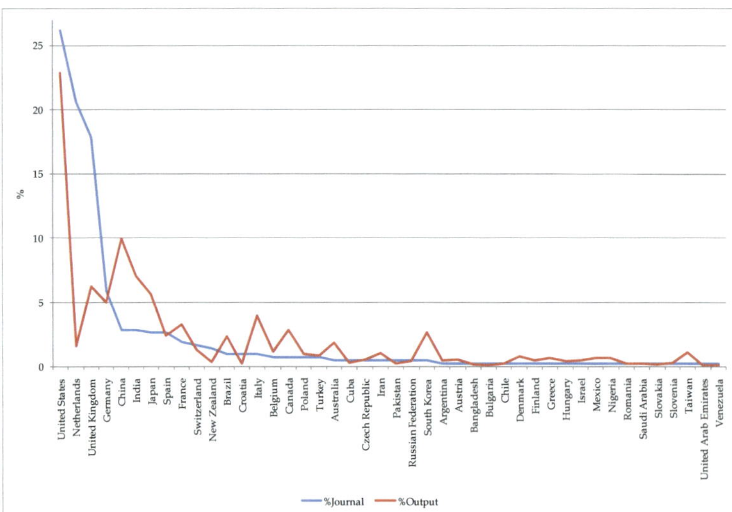

Fig. 5. Percentage of pharmacology-related journals and papers published by country (Scopus, 2009)

3.5 Scientometric indicators for pharmaceutical companies

The pharmaceutical industry, in addition to being one of the most profitable, is also one of the most globalised and fastest growing lines of business. Moreover, its large investment in research makes it an innovation-intensive activity. This innovation is the result of the direct or indirect interaction of a large number of actors: different types of companies, research institutes, financial institutions, public bodies and authorities, public and private universities, research centres, regulating bodies, governments, health systems, consumers and physicians, to name a few.

The industry comprises three categories of companies. The first covers (primarily North American and European) multinational companies that operate globally and invest huge sums in R&D, which is centralised in some cases and decentralised with laboratories in many countries and on many continents in others. The second category consists of small companies that supply their domestic markets with drugs that require no substantial R&D investment. The third includes firms that specialise in biotechnology and invest considerable sums in research despite their small size.

In 2010, biopharmaceutical companies invested an estimated 67.4 **billion** dollars in pursuit of new drugs (Figure 6). The total R&D spending by Pharmaceutical Research and Manufacturers of America (PhRMA) members, including industry majors such as AstraZeneca, Bayer, Boehringer, Ingelheim, Bristol-Myers, Squibb, Eli Lilly, Genzyme, GlaxoSmithKline, Hoffmann-La Roche, Merck, Novartis, Pfizer, and Sanofi-Aventis, as well as non-members, are shown in the figure.

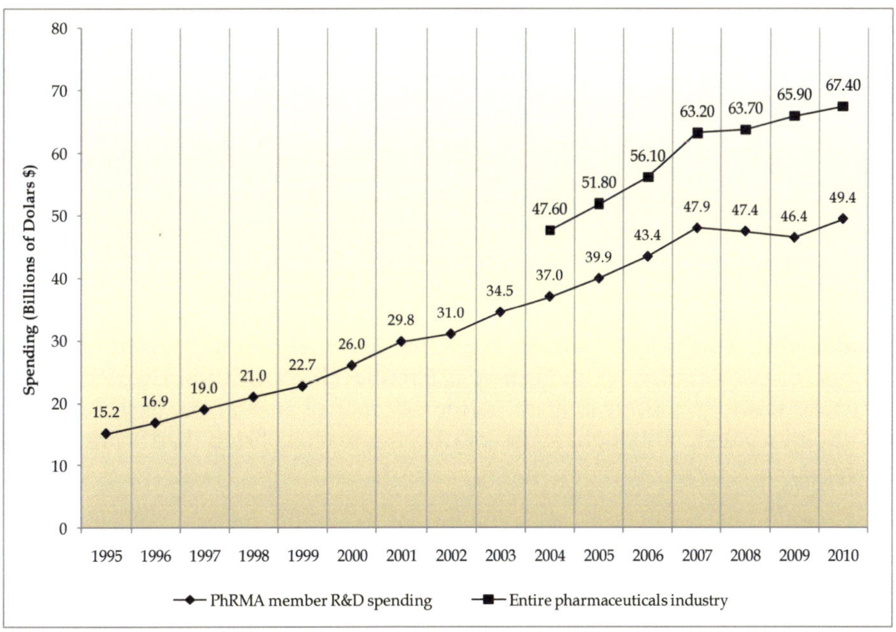

Fig. 6. Biopharmaceutical company R&D and PhRMA member R&D: 1995-2010 (Sources: Burrill and Company, analysis for PhRMA, 2005-2011 (Includes PhRMA research associates and non-members); PhRMA, PhRMA Annual Member Survey, 1996-2010)

Figure 7 shows the R&D spending by PhRMA members in and outside the United States. The total R&D investment by pharmaceutical companies has continued to rise. In 2010 PhRMA members invested 49.4 **billion** dollars, up 6 % from 2009 and 90 % since 2009.

PhRMA members spent most of their R&D budgets (76.1 %) in the United States, Western Europe (16.6 %) and Japan (1.5 %), while spreading the rest across other countries around the world (PhRMA, 2011).

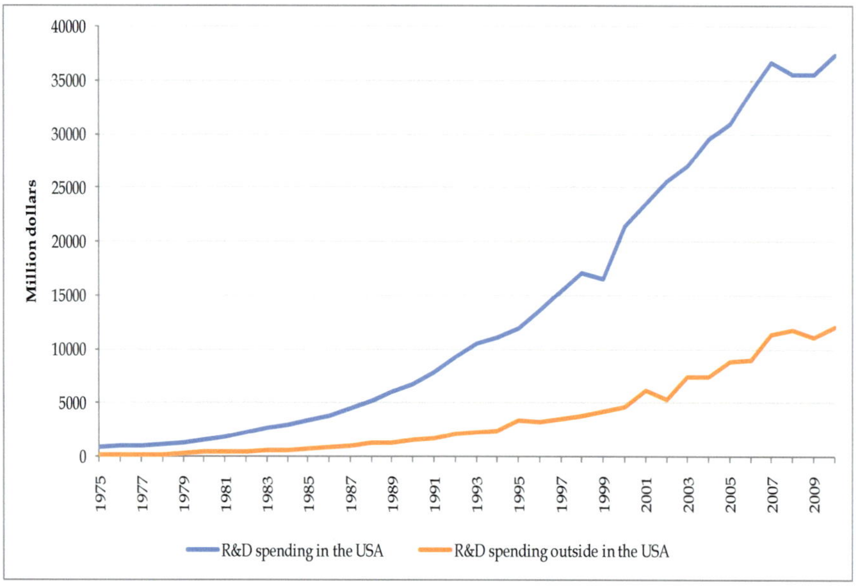

Fig. 7. R&D spending by Pharmaceutical Research and Manufacturers of America (PhRMA) members, 1975-2010 (PhRMA, 2011)

Bibliometric indicators can be constructed for the pharmaceutical industry on the grounds of the research results made public by the authors. As noted earlier, the industry has been gradually internationalising its high research and innovation potential since the mid nineteen seventies (McMillan and Hamilton, 2000).

The values of the bibliometric parameters for the pharmaceutical majors are given in Table 5. The data, which cover a seven-year period and are based on these companies' research publications, reveal a number of interesting differential characteristics. The ranking criterion followed was scientific output defined as the number of papers published in 2003-2009, initially disaggregated, although some of the companies listed had parent-subsidiary relationships.

The first significant result was the volume of scientific papers published by these companies. These elite, all of whose members published at least 125 papers in the period considered, was headed by the Pfizer headquarters site, which averaged 353 papers yearly throughout the period, followed by Merck with a yearly mean of 251.

The second statistic of interest was the citations per paper, which ranged from fairly low (7.86 for Dow Chemical Co., 8.47 for the Indian firm Dr Reddy´s and 9.26 for Sanofi-Aventis GmbH in Germany) to very high values (18.47 for Astra Zeneca in the United Kingdom and

18.21 for Hoffmann-La Roche in Switzerland). These findings suggest substantial differences in the visibility or quality of firms' scientific knowledge.

Organisation	Country	Output	Citations per paper	International collaboration	Normalised Citation	% Output in Q1
Pfizer Inc.	USA	2476	12.4	18.54	1.55	79.36
Merck & Co., Inc.	USA	1759	14.34	18.08	1.74	83.63
Eli Lilly and Company	USA	820	16.13	25.24	1.68	81.1
GlaxoSmithKline. United States	USA	788	15.17	29.7	1.77	86.68
GlaxoSmithKline. United Kigdom	GBR	781	13.76	42.77	1.74	85.66
Bristol-Myers Squibb Company	USA	677	12.97	13	1.58	87.59
Novartis	CHE	595	16.82	66.72	1.8	77.98
Abbott Laboratories United States	USA	571	14.75	12.61	1.65	88.27
Amgen	USA	497	12.27	16.9	1.59	77.46
F. Hoffmann-La Roche. Ltd.	USA	452	14.81	21.46	1.84	83.19
Pfizer Ltd	GBR	379	14.8	43.54	1.73	79.16
Bayer AG	DEU	362	10.46	36.74	1.34	64.36
Johnson & Johnson Pharmaceutical Research	USA	356	13.45	18.54	1.68	87.64
AstraZeneca R&D	SWE	294	14.64	57.82	1.8	87.07
F. Hoffmann-La Roche. Ltd.	CHE	272	18.21	55.15	1.86	83.09
Sanofi-Aventis. S.A.	FRA	224	15.64	43.75	1.55	66.52
Laboratoires SERVIER	FRA	200	17.16	37.5	1.71	91.5
Novartis Pharma SA. East Hanover	USA	192	16.2	34.9	1.89	73.96
AstraZeneca Pharmaceuticals. LP	USA	188	15.77	30.85	1.69	75
Sanofi-Aventis Deutschland GmbH	DEU	167	9.26	26.35	0.95	57.49
Schering-Plough Research Institute	USA	165	12.8	12.73	1.46	86.67
AstraZeneca	GBR	161	18.47	40.37	1.81	77.64
Novartis Institutes for Biomedical Research	USA	161	12.93	60.87	1.77	84.47
Laboratoires Pierre Fabre. S.A.	FRA	155	10.18	23.23	1.17	81.94
Novo Nordisk A/S	DNK	153	12.77	46.41	1.32	77.12
Dr. Reddy's Laboratories Ltd.	IND	150	8.47	7.33	0.88	59.33
H. Lundbeck A/S	DNK	150	18.11	45.33	1.73	91.33
GlaxoSmithKline. Italy	ITA	127	11.52	66.14	1.57	81.89
Dow Chemical Company	USA	125	7.86	34.4	0.9	66.4

Table 5. Bibliometric performance indicators for pharmaceutical firms, 2003-2009 (www.scimagoir.com)

Pharmaceuticals is generally agreed to be one of the industries whose research is most intensely internationalised, defining that to mean the proportion of the research conducted outside the headquarters country. The industry's business has become more international since the nineteen nineties as a result of the convergence of a number of processes. New industrial activities have cropped up around biotechnological research, primarily in the US;

market dynamics with a view to capitalising on research incentives has favoured the location of new laboratories in different countries; global excellence centres with research responsibilities have been created; and inter- and intra-firm networking has been intensified.

When companies were ranked in descending order of the percentage of their papers involving international collaboration, two different patterns emerged, one for European and the other for North American companies. The percentages were higher in the former than in the latter. Several explanations can be given for this difference between countries on the two sides of the Atlantic. The United States is the critical location for pharmaceutical alliances as a result of the quality of the research conducted there, but especially of the size of its research base, i.e., the number and size of universities, companies and research departments. Other factors that distinguish the European and US include the latter's easy financing and marketing terms and fairly large number of start-up incubators and venture capitalists.

The result is that companies based in the US have lower percentages of internationally co-authored papers than European companies: Abbott Laboratories 12.67 %, Schering-Plough Research Institute, 12.73 %, Bristol-Myers Squibb Company, 13 %.

Switzerland's Novartis, by contrast, co-authored 66.72 % of its papers with other countries. Its US subsidiary had a collaboration rate of 69.87 %, while the figure for the French firm Sanofi-Aventis was 43.75 %.

The final indicator analysed was normalised citation, which measures a company's impact on the scientific community as a whole and compares the quality of the research conducted by organisations of different sizes. The highest score was obtained by Swiss Novartis' North American subsidiary, with a mean citation value 89 % higher than the world-wide mean (1.89). It was followed by its parent company, which had a mean citation value 86 % higher than the world-wide mean, and the Swiss subsidiary of North America's F. Hoffman La Roche, with a score of 84 %. The lowest values were recorded for Dow Chemical's pharmaceuticals division (US) and the Dr. Reddy laboratories in India, whose citation values were below the international average.

4. Conclusions

This chapter reports on a multi-level analysis of scientific results in pharmacology. The findings confirmed that despite its scant weight in world-wide science, pharmacological scientific output is characterised by high quality and has citation per paper values higher than the mean for international scientific output as a whole.

Two regions of the world have traditionally occupied the leading positions in terms of pharmacological scientific output, North America and Western Europe. Moreover, the impact of this output is high, measured in terms of citations in other papers. When only citations outside the home region are considered, however, other regions, such as Northern Africa, prove to have higher values. The regions with the largest absolute number of citations also have the highest percentage of domestic citations. By contrast, since the regions with smaller numbers of citations in absolute terms receive fewer domestic citations, the acknowledgement coming primarily from countries outside their own region carries much heavier weight.

During the period studied, certain emerging countries such as Brazil or India joined the list of top ten producers, while China, which was already on the list, climbed almost to the summit. As might be expected, the countries in the most productive regions occupied the highest positions throughout the period analysed, but the appearance of these BRIC countries should prompt reflection on their scientific potential in the field of pharmacology.

The most productive journals, i.e., the ones that publish the largest number of pharmacological articles, do not generally earn high SJR impact values. These values are attained by journals publishing smaller numbers of papers. Consequently, journal quality and the number of papers published are inversely related. An analysis relating papers published and journals edited in each country showed that intense pharmacological publishing is not necessarily attendant upon the presence of numerous researchers working in the field (The Netherlands). US publishing in pharmacology, by contrast, is as predominant in the area as its research community.

Companies carry specific weight in pharmacology. Their investment and innovative capacity are mirrored by the scientific results attained, primarily by US and European pharmaceutical laboratories.

5. Acknowledgement

The authors wish to thank Scimago Lab for its generous assistance in compiling the data used.

6. References

Biglu, M.H. and Omidi, Y. (2010). Scientific profile of Pharmacology, Toxicology and Pharmaceutics fields in Middle East Countries: Impacts of Iranian Scientists. *International Journal of Advances in Pharmaceutical Sciences*, Vol. 1, pp. 122-127, ISSN 0976-1055

Braun, T.; Glänzel, W. and Schubert, A. Scientometric indicators: a 32-country comparative evaluation of *publishing performance and citation impact*. Singapore, Philadelphia: World Scientific, 1985, 425 p.

Congressional Budget Office. (2006). *A CBO Study: Research and Development in hte Pharmaceutical Industry*. Congress of the United States. 20/08/2011. Available from http://www.cbo.gov/ftpdocs/76xx/doc7615/10-02-DrugR-D.pdf

Fingerman, S. (2006). Web of Science and Scopus: current features and capabilities. Issues in *Science and Technology Librarianship*, Fall, ISSN 1092-1206, 20/08/2011, Available from http://www.istl.org/06-fall/electronic2.html

Gambardella, A. (1995). *Science and innovation: the US pharmaceutical industry during the 1980s*. Cambridge: Cambridge University Press. ISBN: 0521451183

González-Pereira, B.; Guerrero-Bote, V. and Moya-Anegón, F. (2009). The SJR indicator: A new indicator of journals' scientific prestige. *Arxiv Preprint* arXiv:0912.4141, 02/08/2011, Available from http://arxiv.org/ftp/arxiv/papers/0912/0912.4141.pdf

Gorraiz, J. and Schloegl, C. (2008). A bibliometric analysis of pharmacology and pharmacy journals: Scopus versus Web of Science. *Journal of Information Science*, Vol. 34, No. 5, pp. 715-725, ISSN 0165-5515

Gupta, B.M. and Kaur, H. (2009). Status of India in science and technology as reflected in its publication output in the Scopus international database, 1996-2006. *Scientometrics*, Vol. 80, No. 2, pp. 473-490, ISSN 0138-9130

Kaur, H. and Gupta, B.M. (2009). Indian Contribution in Pharmacology, Toxicology and Pharmaceutics during 1998-2007: A Scientometric Analysis. *Collnet Journal of Scientometrics and Information Management*, Vol. 3, No. 1, pp. 1-9, ISSN 0973-7766

Koening, M. (1983). Bibliometric analysis of pharmaceutical research. Research Policy, Vol. 12, No. 1, pp. 15-36, ISSN 0048-7333

LaGuardia, C. (2005). E-views and reviews: Scopus vs Web of Science. Library Journal, (January 2005), eISSN 0000-0027, 20.08.2011, Available from http://www.libraryjournal.com/article/CA491154.html

McMillan, G.S. and Hamilton, R.D. (2000). Using Bibliometrics to Measure Firm Knowledge: An Analysis of the US Pharmaceutical Industry. Technology *Analysis and Strategic Management*. Vol. 12, No. 4, pp. 465-475. ISSN 0953-7325

Noisi, J. (1999). The internationalization of industrial R&D from technology transfer to the learing organization. *Research Policy*, Vol. 28, pp. 107-117, ISSN 0048-7333

Narin, F. and Rozek, R.P. (1988). Bibliometric analysis of United States pharmaceutical industry research performance. *Research Policy*, Vol. 17, No. 3, pp. 139-154, ISSN 0048-7333

Patel, P. and Pavitt, K. (2000). National systems of innovation under strain: The internationalization of coporate R&D. In: Barrel, R.; Mason, G.; Mahony, M. (eds). *Productivity, Innovation and Economic Performance*. Cambridge: Cambridge University Press, pp. 217-235. ISBN 0521780314

Perianes-Rodríguez, A.; Rafols, I.; O'Hare, A.; Hopkins, M.M. and Nightingale, P. (2011). Benchmarking and visualizing the knowledge base of pharmaceutical firms (1995-2009). *Proceedings of the 13th ISSI Conference*. Durban: International Society for Scientometrics and Informetrics, Vol. 2, pp. 656-661, ISBN 9789081752701

Pharmaceutical Research and Manufacturers of America. *Pharmaceutical Industry Profile 2011*. Washington, DC: PhRMA, April 2011

Rafols, I.; O'Hare, A.; Perianes-Rodríguez, A.; Hopkins, M.M. and Nightingale, P. (2010). *Collaborative practices and technological trajectories in large pharmaceutical firms. Tentative Governance in Emerging Science and Technology*. Enschede: University of Twente, pp. 93-95.

Rehn, C. (2007). Bibliometric indicators: definitions and usage at Karolinska Institutet. 20/08/2011, Available from http://ki.se/content/1/c6/01/79/31/Bibliometric%20indicators%20-%20definitions_1.0.pdf

Sciverse Scopus (2011). What dos it Cover?. 2.08.2011. Available from http://www.info.sciverse.com/scopus/scopus-in-detail/facts

SJR. SCImago Research Group. *SCImago Journal and Country Rank*. 2007. 20/08/2011. Available from: http://www.scimagojr.com

17

Mephedrone-Related Fatalities in the United Kingdom: Contextual, Clinical and Practical Issues

John M. Corkery, Fabrizio Schifano and A. Hamid Ghodse
University of Hertfordshire & St George's, University of London
United Kingdom

1. Introduction

The misuse of mephedrone (4-methylmethcathinone) has been increasing greatly in Western countries over the last two years or so, especially in the club and dance scenes. This period has also been marked by claims that the substance has been implicated in a rising number of deaths in the USA and Western Europe, especially the United Kingdom (UK).

This chapter explores the context(s) and evolution of mephedrone use in the UK, and the circumstances in which these fatalities occurred. Particular attention is paid to the settings in which these incidents took place, their symptomatology and physical characteristics; intervention/treatment opportunities; and toxicological and pathological findings. These results are related to the known pharmacological facts regarding mephedrone, its possible interactions with alcohol and other psychoactive drugs, and suggested clinical interventions and treatment(s).

The relationship between mephedrone, other methcathinones, and other emerging novel psychoactive substances, as well as established stimulants is also examined. These developments are important as novel substances used for recreational use become more globally accessible through the use of the Internet.

2. Recreational use

Mephedrone (4-methylmethcathinone; 'Plant Food', 'Meow Meow', 'Miaow', 'Drone', 'Meph', 'Bubbles', 'Spice E', 'Charge', 'M-Cat', 'Rush', 'Ronzio', 'Fiskrens' and 'MMC Hammer') (Schifano et al, 2011) is the most popular of the cathinone derivatives, which also include butylone, flephedrone, MDPV, methedrone, methylone, pentylone, and other compounds (ACMD, 2010; Morris, 2010). It has been readily available for purchase both online and in head shops as a 'legal high', and more recently as a 'research chemical'; its circulation has been promoted by aggressive web-based marketing (Deluca et al., 2009). Mephedrone elicits stimulant and empathogenic effects similar to amphetamine, methylamphetamine, cocaine and MDMA (Winstock et al., 2010). However, as we write, relatively few formal related papers and experimental/clinical data have been published (Dargan et al., 2010; Winstock et al., 2010; Winstock et al., 2011).

The synthesis of mephedrone was first described over 80 years ago (Saem de Burnaga Sanchez, 1929). However, the first Internet reference to it occurred reportedly in May 2003 (Power, 2009), but both its availability for purchase online (Camilleri et al., 2010; Roussel et al., 2009) and its related popularity only started in 2007 (Deluca et al., 2009). Data collected by the European Monitoring Centre for Drugs and Drug Addiction (EMCDDA) indicate that during the first quarter of 2010, there were detections in some 20 EU Member States, with most of them reporting small- to medium-sized seizures (Europol-EMCDDA, 2010). During the second quarter of 2009, the UK Forensic Science Service received submissions of three times as many samples of mephedrone for analysis than it had in the previous 12-month period (ACMD, 2010; Ghodse et al., 2010). Since mephedrone appeared comparatively recently on the market, it does not feature in most drug use household surveys, and it is uncertain how many people present with a history of mephedrone misuse. Most available data originate from self-reported surveys and small focus group research.

The main settings for mephedrone use appear to be nightclubs, parties and people's homes (Newcombe, 2009). A survey of readers of the dance magazine 'Mixmag' found that 41.7% of respondents had ever tried mephedrone and 33.2% had used it during the previous month (Winstock et al., 2011). Dargan et al. (2010) assessed both the prevalence and frequency of use of mephedrone by students in Tayside (Scotland) in February 2010. Some 20.3% reported previous use of mephedrone; 23.4% reported using only using mephedrone on one occasion previously and 4.4% reported daily use. A total of 48.8% of users had sourced mephedrone from street-level dealers and 10.7% from the Internet. Heightened awareness and interest in mephedrone was reflected by a rise in the number of both telephone inquiries and visits to both the TOXBASE and FRANK web sites (ACMD, 2010; James et al., 2010). The 2011 sweep of the British Crime Survey, which covers households in England and Wales, found that 4.4% of adults aged 16 to 24 years had used mephedrone in the last year, compared to only 0.6% of those aged 25 to 59 years (Smith & Flatley, 2011). The rate for the younger age-group is similar to that for cocaine. The majority of respondents who had taken mephedrone in the last year had also taken another drug. It is, therefore, likely that it is existing users of drugs that are taking mephedrone rather than new users drawn to drug taking.

The emergence of mephedrone on the UK recreational drug scene may be linked to decreasing purity in the UK of both MDMA (ecstasy) and cocaine (Mulchandani et al., 2010; Fleming, 2010; Measham et al., 2010; NTA, 2010). As a consequence, drug users may have switched to mephedrone, as it was seen as cheaper and more powerful than the currently available 'traditional' stimulants (Deluca et al., 2009). Its availability over the Internet and its status as a 'legal high' (and therefore presumed not to be harmful) may have boosted its appeal (Daly, 2010; Ramsey et al., 2010).

3. Legal status

Mephedrone is not scheduled under the 1971 United Nations Convention on Psychotropic Substances. In Australia, New Zealand, and the USA mephedrone is considered as an analogue of other illegal substances already and can be controlled by laws similar to the Federal Analog Act. In March 2010, the EMCDDA and Europol submitted a joint report on mephedrone to the Council of the European Union, the European Commission and the European Medicines Agency (EMA), presenting the case for a formal risk assessment of the drug (Europol-EMCDDA, 2010). The risk assessment report, which was submitted to the European Commission and the Council of the European Union on 26 May 2010, examined the health and social risks of the drug, as well as information on international trafficking and the involvement of organised crime. Furthermore, the report considers the potential implications for placing the drug under control in the EU. On the basis of this report – and on the initiative of the European Commission – on 2 December 2010, the Council decided that mephedrone is to be subject to control measures (EMCDDA, 2011).

In the UK, where mephedrone had been attracting great attention from both the mass media and the Government, the Advisory Council on the Misuse of Drugs (ACMD) submitted a report to the Home Office on the cathinone derivatives, recommending their inclusion in the Misuse of Drugs Act 1971 as a Class B drug (ACMD, 2010). The Home Office announced on 30 March 2010 that this recommendation would be enforced from 16 April 2010 (Home Office, 2010).

4. Chemistry

Mephedrone is a semi-synthetic compound belonging to the chemical class of cathinone derivatives (or substituted cathinones). Cathinone is a natural amphetamine-like alkaloid found in the fresh leaves and stems of the African shrub Khat (Catha edulis) (Kalix, 1992). The systematic name of mephedrone is 2-(methylamino)-1-(p-tolyl)propan-1-one(2S)-2-(methylamino)-1-(4-methylphenyl)propan-1-one, in accordance with the International Union of Pure and Applied Chemistry. The structure of mephedrone differs from cathinone by methylation of the amino group and the benzene ring present (Gustaffsson and Escher, 2009; Osorio-Olivares et al., 2003). The cathinones are beta-keto derivatives of phenethylamines, and hence analogues of amphetamines (Chemspider, 2010). Since they are mainly synthetic in origin, beta-keto amphetamines are also known as 'bk designer drugs'. It is relatively easy to produce mephedrone in nonprofessional laboratories via bromination of 4-methylpropiophenone followed by reaction with methylamine or by oxidation of 4-methylephedrine (Archer, 2009; Europol-EMCDDA, 2010).

Although mainly sold in powder and crystal forms, mephedrone may be commercially available in tablets and included within vegetable-based capsules. It has been reported that mephedrone is sometimes sold in some countries as either ecstasy or 'synthetic' cocaine (Deluca et al., 2009; Schifano et al., 2011). Furthermore, it may be found mixed with adulterants, such as caffeine, paracetamol and even cocaine, amphetamine and ketamine (Camilleri et al., 2010), as well as with other methcathinones (as revealed by information supplied to the National Programme on Substance Abuse Deaths by coroners - see below).

5. Pharmacology

Given the affiliation of cathinone derivatives to beta-keto amphetamines, mephedrone would be expected to act as a Central Nervous System stimulant. In vitro studies on the effects of the cathinone derivatives methcathinone and methylone confirm that the main mechanism of action is very similar to that of amphetamine, being characterised by a predominant action on plasma membrane catecholamine transporters (Cozzi et al., 1999). The presence of the ring substituent on the phenethylamine core modifies the pharmacological properties by giving the compound some MDMA-like effects (Europol-EMCDDA, 2010). Cathinones' potencies are mostly lower than those of amphetamines as beta-keto amphetamines show a reduced ability to cross the blood–brain barrier due to the presence of the beta group (Nagai et al., 2007; Gygi et al., 1996).

N-demethylation to the primary amine, reduction of the keto moiety to the respective alcohol, and oxidation of the tolyl moiety to the corresponding alcohols and carboxylic acid is the major metabolic pathway for mephedrone, followed by N-dealkylation.

6. Routes of administration, dosage, use in combination with other drugs, effects

The most common routes for recreational use include insufflation (snorting) and oral ingestion. Because of its solubility in water, mephedrone is reportedly used by rectal administration or injected intravenously. Other typical methods of intake include oral ingestion as capsules or tablets; swallowing mephedrone powder wrapped up in cigarette paper (bombing); or mixed with water. Insufflation is likely to be the most common modality as, when snorted, mephedrone elicits its effects within a few minutes, with the peak being reached in less than 30 min followed by a rapid comedown. According to online users, the mephedrone dosage for snorting may range between 25 and 75 mg, with a lower threshold at 5-15 mg and levels in excess of 90 mg considered a high dosage (Sumnall and Wooding, 2009). Dosing is more frequent when taken intranasally; this route is allegedly associated with greater abuse liability than the oral route (Winstock et al., 2010, 2011). On average, the most common oral dosages are higher than the snorting ones (Sumnall & Wooding, 2009), in the range 150 to 250 mg.

Time of onset may be from 45 min to 2 h and may vary in association with the amount of food in the stomach. Because of this, users suggest taking mephedrone on an empty stomach. Psychoactive effects may last longer (up to 2–4 h) with oral ingestion; side-effects might be milder and the need to re-dose less urgent. Some users employ both insufflation and oral ingestion in combination to obtain faster onset and long-lasting effects (Deluca et al., 2009). Users report that rectal administration is characterised by faster onset of the effects and requires lower doses, e.g. 100 mg on average than oral ingestion (Deluca et al., 2009). Although not typically advised, because this may increase the drug's addictive liability levels (Deluca et al., 2009), mephedrone may also be injected either intramuscularly (Wood et al., 2010a) or intravenously, at one half or two-thirds of the oral dose (Deluca et al., 2009). According to online user fora, mephedrone may be taken in combination with a number of stimulants, sedatives and psychedelics (Deluca et al., 2009; Schifano et al., 2011).

As mephedrone has the capacity to induce tolerance on repeated dosing, an increasing number of user reports have stated a quick progression to either regular drug use and/or uncontrolled bingeing behaviour (known as 'fiending'), with 1–4 g of mephedrone consumed in a session to prolong the duration of its effects (Deluca et al., 2009; Europol-EMCDDA, 2010; Dargan et al., 2010). A recent survey carried out by a drug-related web site has unveiled an average monthly use of 11.16 g for each mephedrone consumer (Drugs-forum, 2010). Although withdrawal symptoms are not commonly reported, users often display strong cravings for mephedrone (Newcombe, 2009).

The effects of mephedrone have been compared by users variously to those of cocaine, amphetamine and MDMA. Self-reported subjective effects may include (Winstock et al., 2011; Deluca et al., 2009): intense stimulation and alertness, euphoria; empathy/feelings of closeness, sociability and talkativeness; intensification of sensory experiences; moderate sexual arousal; and perceptual distortions (reported with higher dosages only).

7. Adverse effects

Dargan et al. (2010) report that some 56% of those who had used mephedrone may complain of at least one unwanted effect associated with mephedrone use. These may include (ACMD, 2010; Deluca et al., 2009; James et al., 2010; Wood et al., 2009, 2010b): loss of appetite, nausea, vomiting and stomach discomfort; tremors, headache (very common), dizziness/light-headedness, seizures, nystagmus, pupil dilation, blurred vision, numbness of tactile sensitivity (reported at higher dosages); anxiety, confusion, dysphoria, aggression, depression, long-lasting hallucinations, paranoid delusions, short-term psychosis, short-term mania, insomnia and nightmares, impaired short-term memory, poor concentration, tachycardia, elevated blood pressure, respiratory difficulties, chest pain. Possibly due to vasoconstriction, users have anecdotally described cold/blue fingers. Of particular interest are recent reports of clinical significance: severe refractory left ventricular failure (Chhabra et al., 2010); and acute myocarditis (Nicholson et al., 2010). Further unwanted effects may include: difficulties in urination, possible nephrotoxicity, anorgasmia; changes in body temperature regulation, with hot flushes and sweating; immunological toxicity (vasculitis, infections and ulcerations); posterior reversible encephalopathy syndrome (Omer & Doherty, 2010); and finally serotonin syndrome (Garrett & Sweeney, 2011).

Most of the above untoward effects seem to be similar to those already documented for amphetamine, methylamphetamine and MDMA (Schifano et al., 2010), implicitly supporting a sympathomimetic activity of mephedrone. Conversely, symptoms of depression and anhedonia could be tentatively associated to a putative depletion of serotonin and dopamine as a consequence of drug use (ACMD, 2010), similarly to what may occur with other stimulants (Schifano, 1996). It is impossible to determine a 'safe' dose for mephedrone since negative side-effects may present in association with any dosage taken. Furthermore, similar dosages may have dramatically different consequences in different individuals (Dickson et al., 2010).

8. Fatalities

During the last few months of 2009 and the first few months of 2010, the UK media were constantly reporting fatalities allegedly related to mephedrone consumption, but only a proportion of them had by that time been formally confirmed. A report on a mephedrone-related fatality first appeared in Sweden, referring to an 18-year-old female death which occurred in December 2008. No other drugs, apart from mephedrone, were identified by the toxicological screenings (Gustaffson & Escher, 2009). Previously, a Danish teenager found in possession of mephedrone died in May 2008, although toxicology reports were inconclusive (Campbell, 2009). The first mephedrone-related death in the USA involved the combined use of mephedrone and heroin (Dickson et al., 2010). More recently, the first cases from the Netherlands (Lusthof et al., 2011) and the Republic of Ireland (EMCDDA, 2011:85) have been reported.

Given the potentially large numbers of consumers involved in the use of mephedrone across both the EU and the UK (EMCDDA, 2011), the main aims of this study were to report and analyse information relating to the socio-demographics and clinical circumstances of all recorded mepherone-related deaths for the whole of the UK, both when the index drug was taken on its own and when in combination with other drugs. The rationale for doing this is to make accessible a corpus of material which will help inform treatments and interventions so as to reduce deaths associated with the use of this drug and other methcathinones.

9. Methodology for identifying potential mephedrone-related fatalities

In the UK and Islands all sudden, unexpected or violent deaths - as well as deaths in custody - are formally investigated by Coroners (or their equivalent in the Islands), or Procurators Fiscal in the case of Scotland. Most drug-related deaths are subject to these processes, typically by way of a coronial inquest (Corkery, 2002).

Since its establishment in 1997, the National Programme on Substance Abuse Deaths (np-SAD) has been regularly receiving coroners' information on drug-related deaths amongst both addicts and non-addicts in the UK, the Channel Islands and the Isle of Man. The average annual response rate from coroners in England and Wales to np-SAD has been between 89% and 95% (Ghodse et al., 2010). Since 2004, information has also been received from the Scottish Crime &Drug Enforcement Agency and the General Register Office for Northern Ireland. To date, details of some 25,000 deaths have been received. The information reported here on deaths associated with mephedrone consumption are based on all relevant cases recorded in the Special Mortality Register of the np-SAD based at St George's Hospital Medical School, University of London.

To be recorded in the np-SAD database as a drug-related death, at least one of the following criteria must be met: (a) presence of one or more psychoactive substances directly implicated in death; (b) history of dependence or abuse of drugs; and (c) presence of controlled drugs at post-mortem. Full details of the np-SAD data collection form and its surveillance work can be found in the Programme's annual report (Ghodse et al., 2010). Ethical approval is not required in the UK for studies whose subjects are deceased. However, confidentiality arrangements are in place with each of the respective data providers.

A range of documents are contained in coronial inquest files, although the variety differs from case to case. Typically, the coroner has access to: statements from witnesses, family and friends; General Practitioner records (if the deceased is registered with one); reports from ambulance, police or other emergency services; hospital Emergency Department and clinical ward reports; psychiatric and substance abuse team reports; as well as post mortem and toxicology reports. Internet searches of toxicological as well as newspaper and other media websites revealed information on further cases. The media reports available for some cases were used to supplement the information provided on the np-SAD data collection form, especially where access to the full coronial files was not possible.

In addition to its routine surveillance activities, the Programme also provides real-time information on the emergence of novel substances or new ways of taking existing substances to the UK Early Warning System and the Advisory Council on the Misuse of

Drugs (ACMD). This information comes both from notifications of deaths and from 'alerts' or other information provided by the various agencies and networks, national and international, with which the Programme maintains contacts. Regular searches of media reports are also undertaken.

Through these channels (including coroners, forensic toxicologists - principally the London Toxicology Group, Drug & Alcohol Action Teams, and the Scottish Crime & Drug Enforcement Agency) the Programme became aware of the emerging issue of the use of methcathinones, especially mephedrone, and similar substances (including chemicals), and of their potential adverse health consequences. It was decided to take a pro-active approach to monitor the situation especially in respect of the potential role of these new substances in causing or contributing to death. For those cases not formally reported to the Programme, contact was made with the relevant coroners to request the submission of an np-SD form so as to obtain the appropriate information. Information on these cases was added to the database when forms were received by the Programme team.

The np-SAD database was searched using the terms 'mephedrone' and '4-methylmethcathinone' to identify potentially relevant cases. The database fields searched were those holding data on: drugs present at post-mortem; drugs implicated; cause(s) of death; accident details; and 'other relevant information'. The data presented here relate to all concluded cases for which forms had been submitted to the Programme by 31 August 2011. Details of some of these cases have previously been published (Torrance & Cooper, 2010; Wood et al., 2010b; Maskell et al., 2011; EMCDDA, 2011:78-85).

Analyses were performed using IBM® SPSS® Statistics, version 18 for Windows™. Demographic details, risk factors, and categorical data were expressed as frequencies and percentages within groups; ages were compared using Levene's Test for Equality of Variances (two-tailed). The results for statistical tests were regarded as significant at or below the 5% probability level.

10. Results

A total of 125 alleged or suspected mephedrone-associated fatalities have been identified by the np-SAD team (Fig. 1). However, in 25 cases (20.0%) mephedrone was not found at post mortem and for 13 cases (10.4%) the toxicology results are still pending. For those 87 cases (69.6%) where mephedrone was identified at post mortem, inquests have been concluded in 60 cases. These were considered as confirmed fatalities meeting the above inclusion criteria, and on which the present analysis will focus.

10.1 Demographics

The mean age of the sample was 28.7 years (SD 11.3), range 14-64 years old. The mean age for males was 28.9 years compared to 28.0 years for females; this difference was not statistically significant ($t = 0.27$ (two-tailed for equality of means) $p = 0.79$ (95% CI = -5.87 to +7.72). Where known, most victims were described as 'White' (Table 1). Where place of birth was given, 39 were born in the UK and Islands and 8 overseas. Many were in employment ($n = 25$), but one-quarter ($n = 16$) were unemployed, and 11 were students.

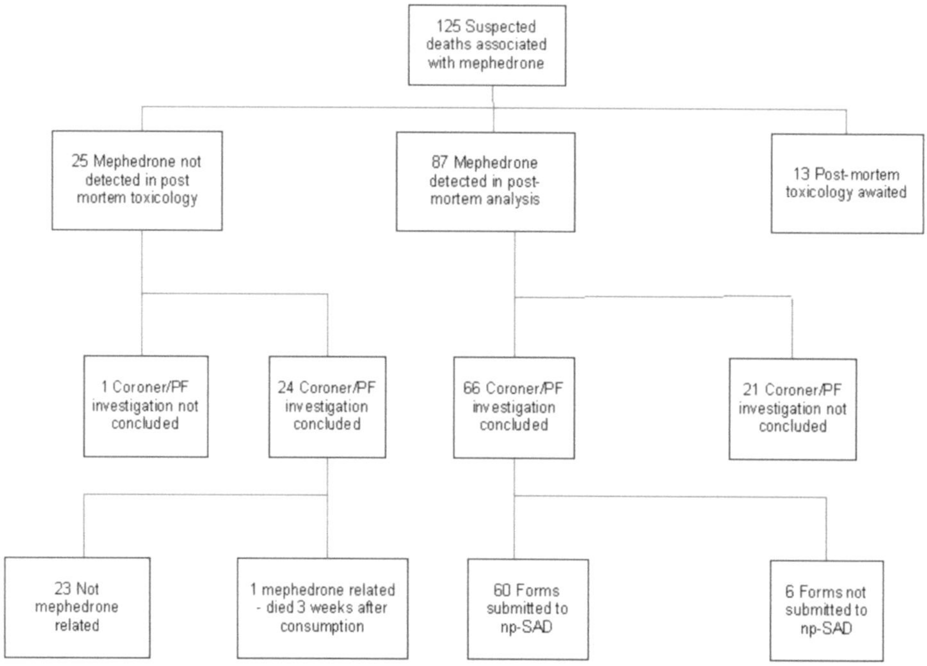

Fig. 1. Flow-chart of UK deaths associated with mephedrone

Demographic variable	Characteristics
Age (years):	
male (n=45)	mean = 28.9, median = 24.9, minimum = 17.1, maximum = 63.8, range = 46.8, SD = 11.1.
female (n=15)	mean = 28.0, median = 24.9, minimum = 14.8, maximum = 55.1, range = 40.3, SD = 12.2.
all (n=60)	mean = 28.7, median = 24.9, minimum = 14.8, maximum = 63.8, range = 49.0, SD = 11.3.
Age-group (years)	< 15 = 1; 15-24 = 30; 25-34 = 16; 35-44 = 6; 45-54 = 5; 55-64 = 2; >64 = 0.
Ethnicity	White = 50; Black = 0; Asian = 1; Other (Filipina) = 1; Not known = 8.
Country of birth	England = 32, Wales = 2, Scotland = 1, Northern Ireland = 2, Guernsey = 2; overseas = 8; unknown/unavailable = 13.
Employment status	non-manual = 9; manual = 14; unemployed = 16; self-employed = 2; invalidity/sickness = 1; student = 11; housewife = 0; unknown = 7.
Living arrangements	alone = 11; with parents = 20; with partner = 14; with partner and children = 2; with friends = 4; no fixed abode = 2; self & children = 1; Other = 1; unknown = 5.
Addict status	non-addict = 10; addict/drug abuser = 27; unknown = 23.

Table 1. Socio-demographics of 60 UK deaths associated with mephedrone reported to np-SAD

Just over half (33) died in their home or that of a friend and 12 in hospital (Table 2). The verdict/conclusion returned by the coroners or procurators fiscal in 35 instances was accidental death or misadventure; (non-dependent) abuse of drugs in 5 cases, suicide in 10 cases, homicide in one case, natural causes in one case, and an open verdict in 8 cases. Forty-four of these deaths occurred in England; nine in Scotland, four in Northern Ireland, two on Guernsey, and one in Wales.

Twenty-seven were known to be as 'addicts' (either dependent on or misusing drugs), and 10 were not addicts; for 23 cases the information was not known. Only 11 of the deceased were known to have been prescribed psychoactive drugs: these included diazepam, antidepressants, antipsychotics, antiepileptics, methadone, and opioid analgesics, often in combination.

Demographic variable	Characteristics
Place of death	at home = 28; friend's home = 5; hospital = 12; open space/woodland/river = 7; other = 7; unknown = 1.
Country of death	England = 44; Wales = 1; Scotland = 9; Northern Ireland = 4; Guernsey = 2; Jersey = 0; Isle of Man = 0.
Day of week of death (this is not necessarily day of consumption)	Sunday = 13; Monday = 12; Tuesday = 10; Wednesday = 8; Thursday = 2; Friday = 5; Saturday = 10.
Month of death	Sep 2009 = 1; Oct 2009 = 1; Nov 2009 = 1; Dec 2009 = 5; Jan 2010 = 7; Feb 2010 = 7; Mar 2010 = 9; Apr 2010 = 6; May 2010 = 3; Jun 2010 = 1; Jul 2010 = 7; Aug 2010 = 2; Sep 2010 = 0; Oct 2010 = 2; Nov 2010 = 2; Dec 2010 = 0; Jan 2011 = 0; Feb 2011 = 2; Mar 2011 = 0; Apr 2011 = 2; May 2011 = 2; Jun 2011 = 0; Jul 2011 = 0; Aug 2011 = 0.
Verdict (legal conclusion)	accident/misadventure = 35; (non-dependent) abuse of drugs = 5; open/undetermined = 8; suicide = 10; killed unlawfully = 1; other = 1.
Manner of death (intentionality)	natural = 1; accidental = 41; suicidal = 11; homicidal = 1; undetermined = 6.

Table 2. Circumstances of 60 deaths associated with mephedrone reported to np-SAD

The first known death in the UK occurred in September 2009. The number steadily rose to 7 both in January and February 2010, peaked at 9 in March, falling to 6 in April, and declining in the next couple of months to one in June. However, there was a further peak of 7 cases in July, followed by two deaths in August and another 2 in both October and November. There then followed a period of a few months without any reported fatalities, but the most recent deaths occurred in April and May 2011 (Fig. 2). There were twice as many deaths on Saturdays, Sundays, Mondays and Tuesdays (n = 45, average 11.2 per day) compared to the other days of the week (n = 15; average of 5.0 per day). It should be noted that the day of death was not necessarily the day that mephedrone was consumed, as in a few cases death occurred several days later in hospital - in one case three weeks after the event.

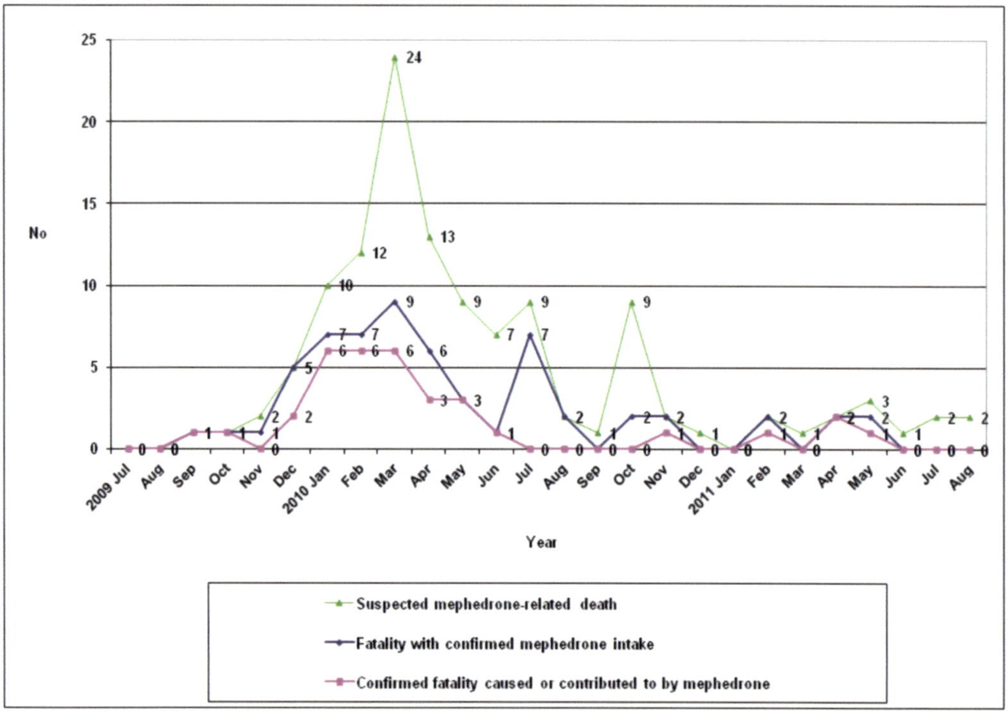

Fig. 2. Evolution of suspected deaths (n = 125) and cases with confirmed positive toxicology for mephedrone submitted to np-SAD as at 31 August 2011 (n = 60)

10.2 Events leading to death

As might be expected given the typical purpose of using mephedrone to experience its psychoactive effects, many deaths occurred following recreational consumption of the drug (Table 3), often in the deceased's or another's home. However, some deaths (road traffic collisions, drowning, hypothermia, etc.) occurred as the result of accidents through impaired judgement due to mephedrone use. In two cases, the deceased had been engaged in sexual activity.

There was a significant number (n = 18) of deaths involving violent means, and especially hanging (13 cases). In several of these cases, mephedrone was considered by the pathologist/coroner/Procurator Fiscal to have played a role although it was not being specifically mentioned in the cause of death field. Mephedrone withdrawal was considered a contributory factor in one suicide by hanging. There were also three fatal road traffic accidents following consumption of mephedrone (and other drugs), and one homicide when the deceased was killed for his supply of mephedrone (about 500 g).

10.3 Cause(s) of death

The effects ('adverse', poisoning, intoxication, toxicity) of mephedrone, including other substances, were recorded in the cause of death for 24 cases (Table 4). Consumption of mephedrone led to a seizure in one case, and cardiac arrest in another. In a further case, cardiac arrest was caused by multiple drug toxicity (including mephedrone) and/or excited delirium. In two cases the ingestion of mephedrone with other drugs led to hypoxic brain injury (one with cerebral oedema). Health issues were present in a number of cases. These, along with mephedrone (and other substances) contributed to death; for example, cardiovascular conditions - 4, bronchopneumonia - 3.

Found unresponsive/dead after taking mephedrone (and other substance) - 14
Found hanging after paranoiac/suicidal behaviour - 6
Found hanging following depression relationship broke up – 1
Found hanging following row with girlfriend over his drug misuse - 1
Self-suspension when intoxicated with alcohol and cocaine – 1
Found hanging after no apparent untoward behaviour – 1
Found dead after cutting own throat – 1
Suicide by gun-shot following consumption of mephedrone, other methcathinone(s) and cocaine – 1
Had consumed mephedrone and other substances, jumped from bridge where relative had previously committed suicide – 1
Committed suicide by drug overdose, including mephedrone – 2
Following family argument, took fatal levels of amitriptyline and methadone, consumed mephedrone – 1
Reported missing after argument with partner, found dead next day on running track with suicide note, had consumed prescribed medications and mephedrone - 1
Had taken mephedrone, but was stabbed and his large supply of mephedrone was stolen, bled to death – 1
Took drugs (including mephedrone and cocaine), started behaving bizarrely, aggressively and abusively; police tried unsuccessfully to calm him down and had to arrest him; collapsed whilst under restraint and suffered cardiac arrest - 1
Attended party, collapsed with cardiac arrest, died in hospital – 1
Attended party, collapsed with breathing difficulties, died in hospital – 1
Attended party, took mephedrone 'bomb', collapsed with very high temperature which prevented blood from clotting, causing abdominal haemorrhages, never regained consciousness - 1
Took mephedrone and other substances, collapsed with chest pains – 2
Took mephedrone and other methcathinones, together with cocaine, which caused fatal heart attack – 1
Took cocaine and mephedrone at party, collapsed and died following day - 1
Had consumed mephedrone but died from heroin and alcohol toxicity – 1
Found dead after consuming Datura, dihydrocodeine, alcohol and mephedrone - 1
Had consumed mephedrone and other stimulants, attempted to swim across river but drowned - 1
Had taken mephedrone and other drugs, driving vehicle involved in fatal road traffic accident – 3
Following consumption of alcohol and mephedrone, felt sick, collapsed, died in hospital – 1

Took alcohol and mephedrone, collapsed and unrouseable, died in hospital - 1
Collapsed after taking mephedrone, died in hospital 3 weeks later from acute liver failure – 1
Attended party where took mephedrone and heroin, collapsed died in hospital 3 weeks later – 1
Died in hospital after taking mephedrone – 1
Indulged in sexual activity, self-injected mephedrone, had seizure and collapsed – 1
Had taken large amounts of methcathinones, engaged in auto-erotic asphyxiation with plastic bag over head, but accidentally suffocated - 1
Consumed amphetamine & mephedrone, vomited, felt cold & sleepy; taken to hospital where, despite treatment, suffered liver problems & multi-organ failure – 1
Found unresponsive in bed, death certified at scene; had been feeling unwell, on medication for chronic abdominal & back pain – 1
Admitted to Emergency Department previous day with drug overdose, had been partying but later found hanging – 1
Aspirated blood following mixed drug (including mephedrone) intoxication - 1
Had consumed GHB and mephedrone; found dead beside bed at home by a friend – 1
Not known – 2

Table 3. Events leading to death

1a Hanging - 10
1a Hanging; 2 Mephedrone withdrawal – 1
1a Hanging; 2 alcohol and mephedrone use – 1
1a Hanging; 2 using mephedrone - 1
1a Shotgun wound to head; 2 Use of mephedrone, methylone and cocaine – 1
1a Blood loss following fatal stabbing to thigh [inflicted by third party] – 1
1a Exsanguination; 1b Neck laceration cutting left jugular vein [self-inflicted] - 1
1a Multiple injuries; 1b Blunt force trauma; 1c Vehicular collision (driver) – 1
1a Ruptured inferior vena cava with haemorrhage in abdominal cavity & cervical spine fracture; 1b Road traffic accident; 2 Cirrhosis of liver & misuse of drugs – 1
1a Multiple injuries [road traffic accident] – 1
1a Multiple injuries [fall from height] – 1
1a Drowning; 2 Multiple drug overdose – 1
1a Hypothermia; 1b Drug overdose [quetiapine, lorazepam, venlafaxine, mephedrone] - 1
1a Adverse effects of mephedrone - 1
1a Poisoning by mephedrone – 1
1a Mephedrone toxicity - 1
1a Mephedrone poisoning; 2 Coronary artery disease – 1
1a Adverse effects of mephedrone; 2 Atherosclerotic coronary artery disease; myocardial fibrosis – 1
1a Mephedrone intoxication – 2
1a Cardiac arrest following ingestion of mephedrone – 1

1a Seizure; 1b Effect of mephedrone - 1
1a Cardiac arrest, cause unascertained between multiple drug toxicity [mephedrone, MDPV, fluoromethcathinone] and/or Excited Delirium - 1
1a Aspiration of blood; 1b Mixed drug intoxication [inc. mephedrone] - 1
1a Adverse effects of methadone and mephedrone - 1
1a Overdosage of mephedrone (meow meow) compounded by cocaine; 2 Cocaine abuse - 1
1a Mixed MDMA and mephedrone toxicity - 1
1a Combined toxic effects of amphetamine and mephedrone - 1
1a Patchy bronchopneumonia & pulmonary oedema; 1b Cardiac ischaemia, contributed to by mephedrone, citalopram and diazepam - 1
1a Ischaemic heart disease; 1b Illicit use of cathinones - 1
1a Toxic effects of drugs [inc. mephedrone] - 1
1a Fatal drug intoxication [inc. mephedrone] - 1
1a Mixed drug toxicity [inc. mephedrone] - 1
1a Hypoxic brain injury; 1b Mixed drug overdose [inc. mephedrone] - 1
1a Hypoxic brain injury; 1b Cerebral oedema; 1c Ingestion of psychoactive drug [inc. mephedrone] - 1
1a Toxic effects of alcohol and cocaine - 1
1a Heroin and alcohol toxicity - 1
1a GHB intoxication - 2
1a Acute alcohol poisoning - 1
1a Morphine (heroin) toxicity - 1
1a Morphine toxicity (on balance of probability) - 1
1a BZP and TFMPP toxicity - 1
1a Illicit methadone misuse - 1
1a Combined effects of alcohol and GBL intoxication - 1
1a Combined toxic effects of alcohol, dihydrocodeine and atropine/hyoscine (from Datura Stramonium) together with postural asphyxia - 1
1a Systemic sepsis, resulting in cardiac arrest; 1b Bronchopneumonia; 1c Beta haemolytic Streptococcal Group A infection - 1
1a Medication toxicity; 2 Acute & chronic debilitating back pain, early stage bronchopneumonia - 1
1a Combined methadone and alcohol overdose - 1
1a Amitriptyline/Methadone overdose - 1
1a Asphyxia [plastic bag suffocation] - 1
(Where cause of death sections of the death certificate specifically mentioned mephedrone or where it was included in verdict. Mephedrone was implicated on its own in 18 cases, with other substances in 18 cases. In many of the hanging causes, mephedrone was considered to have played a contributory role although not recorded in the cause of death.)

Table 4. Cause of deaths associated with mephedrone reported to np-SAD

10.4 Drugs implicated

Mephedrone was specifically mentioned as being present at post-mortem in 59 cases. The drug was formally included in the cause of death in 18 cases and implicitly (e.g. polydrug toxicity given in the cause of death without specifying particular drugs, but mephedrone was found in post-mortem analysis or mentioned by the pathologist as contributing to death) in 10 further cases. In a further case, the drug was not mentioned either as being present at post-mortem (death occurred 3 weeks after mephedrone consumption) or in the cause of death although stated by witnesses to have been consumed.

Where details of the drugs present at post-mortem (or ante-mortem) were given, mephedrone alone was used on eight occasions, solely with alcohol in four cases, and in combination with further substances in 18 cases (Table 5). In 15 cases mephedrone was ingested with stimulants, and with diazepam in 13 cases. It is noteworthy that other newly emerging psychoactive substances were also here identified, including: GBL/GHB, ketamine, and piperazines, as well as other methcathinones (n = 8), especially MDPV. Prescribed medications were also present: opioids including methadone; hypnotics/sedatives; antidepressants; antipsychotics; and antiepileptics.

(Mephedrone was present in 59 cases, including 2 ante-mortem. It had been consumed in all cases in the period leading up the incident causing death.)
Mephedrone sole mention – 8
Mephedrone with alcohol – 4
Mephedrone and alcohol and other drugs - 18
Mephedrone with cannabis – 4
Mephedrone with stimulants – 15
Mephedrone with diazepam - 13
Mephedrone with opiates – 12
Mephedrone with piperazines – 7
Mephedrone with GBL/GHB – 5
Mephedrone with ketamine – 2
Mephedrone with other methcathinones – 8
Mephedrone with antidepressants – 5
Mephedrone with antipsychotics - 2
Mephedrone with antiepileptics - 1
Mephedrone with hypnotics/sedatives (exc. Diazepam) – 3

Table 5. Summary of drug combinations and positive toxicological findings for deaths associated with mephedrone reported to np-SAD

10.5 Toxicology

Full details of mephedrone levels are given in Table 6; actual levels were quantified in 36 cases (Table 6). Overall: (n = 36) mean = 1.586mg/l, range = <0.01 - 22.0mg/l; mono-mephedrone cases (n = 10) mean = 1.996mg/l range = <0.01 - 12.15mg/l; combined mephedrone cases (n = 26): mean = 1.429mg/l; range = 0.03 - 22.0mg/l. These figures exclude one combined mephedrone case with a level of >2000mg/l.

Case No.	Mephedrone present	Mephedrone levels	Second drug present	Third drug present	Fourth drug present	Fifth drug present	Sixth drug present
1	Yes	bl 0.04mg/l	methadone	diazepam	olanzapine	chlorpromazine	
2	Yes	bl <0.01mg/l ur +					
3	Yes	bl 0.76mg/l	alcohol	GBL	diazepam & metabolites		
4	Yes	bl 1.3mg/l ur +					
5	Yes	bl 0.07mg/l, 0.15mg/l ur 16mg/l	alcohol	diazepam			
6	Yes	bl 0.41mg/l, 0.42mg/l	diazepam	citalopram			
7	Yes	bl +	alcohol	cocaine & metabolite	lignocaine		
8	Yes	bl 16ug/l	alcohol				
9	Yes	bl detected	alcohol	cocaine	cocaethylene	levamisole	lignocaine
10	Yes	bl 2.1ug/ml	alcohol				
11	Yes	bl 0.21ug/ml ur +	GBL	TFMPP	ketamine	methylamph etamine	diazepam
12	Yes	bl 2.24mg/l, ur +	TFMPP	alcohol			
13	Yes	bl 1.0mg/l	MDMA				
14	Yes	bl 0.32mg/l					
15	Yes	bl 0.88mg/l , ur +, stomach +	paracetamol				
16	Yes	bl 22mg/l	alcohol	amphetamine	diazepam		
17	Yes	bl 0.04mg/l, 0.19mg/l, ur 64.8mg/l, stomach 2.65mg/l					
18	Yes	bl 0.108mg/l, 0.08mg/l	alcohol	diazepam			
19	Yes	bl 3.3mg/l, stomach +, hair 4.2ng/mg, 4.7ng/mg					
20	Yes	bl > 2.0mg/ml	amphetamine	BZP	TFMPP	chlorpheniramine	
21	Yes	bl 9.01ug/ml, ur 0.01ug/ml, stomach +	morphine	cannabis			

Case No.	Mephedrone present	Mephedrone levels	Second drug present	Third drug present	Fourth drug present	Fifth drug present	Sixth drug present
22	No	-	morphine				
23	Yes	AM serum 0.042mg/l, ur +					
24	Yes	bl 12.15mg/l, ur +					
25	Yes	ur +	cocaine	methylone			
26	Yes	ur +	alcohol	pyrovalerone	BZP	FTMPP	
27	Yes	bl 0.31ug/ml	cannabis				
28	Yes	bl trace	morphine	quetiapine			
29	Yes	bl 0.07mg/l	alcohol				
30	Yes	bl +	alcohol	BZP	TFMPP	paracetamol	citalopram
31	Yes	bl +	alcohol	paracetamol	citalopram	zopiclone	
32	Yes	AM bl +					
33	Yes	bl 0.08ug/ml	methylone	MDPV	GBL		
34	Yes	bl +	methadone	alcohol	cocaine		
35	Yes	bl + recent use	alcohol	benzocaine			
36	Yes	bl + recent use	alcohol	benzocaine			
37	Yes	bl 0.03ug/ml	cannabis				
38	Yes	bl + ur +	diazepam				
39	Yes	bl low level	diazepam	cannabis			
40	Yes	bl +	ampheta-mine				
41	Yes	ur +	alcohol	cocaine & metabolites			
42	Yes	bl 6.2mg/l	diazepam & metabolites	gabapentin	oxycodone		
43	Yes	bl +	alcohol	cannabis	diazepam		
44	Yes	bl 0.05mg/l	GHB	alcohol	ampheta-mine	cocaine & metabolites	methadon e
45	Yes	bl 0.033ug/ml, bile 0.05ug/ml, ur 0.24ug/ml					
46	Yes	bl 1.7mg/l	BZP	TFMPP	codeine	diazepam	
47	Yes	bl <0.05mg/l, ur 11.67mg/l	alcohol	venlafaxine	quetiapine	halperidol	lorazepam
48	Yes	bl 0.51mg/l	alcohol				
49	Yes	bl <0.3125, ur +	alcohol	MDPV	cocaine	levamisole	quinine

Case No.	Mephedrone present	Mephedrone levels	Second drug present	Third drug present	Fourth drug present	Fifth drug present	Sixth drug present
50	Yes	bl 0.17mg/l	MDPV	MDMA	MDA	cocaine	diazepam
51	Yes	ur +	methylam-phetamine	amphetamine	GHB	ketamine	
52	Yes	n/k	alcohol	morphine	cocaine	fluoxetine	
53	Yes	bl 0.04mg/l, ur +	alcohol	dihydroco-deine	atropine	hyoscine butylbromide	diazepam
54	Yes	bl <0.005mg/l	morphine	nitrazepam	buprenor-phine	mirtazapine	
55	Yes	bl 0.21mg/l	cocaine	levamisole	alcohol		
56	Yes	n/k	methadone	amitriptyline	nitrazepam		
57	Yes	ur <0.005mg/l	flephedrone	MDPV	ibuprofen	unidentified compounds	
58	Yes	n/k	MDPV	MDPBP	pentylone	cocaine metabolites	
59	Yes	bl 0.05mg/l, ur 0.05mg/l	MDPV	fluoromethcat hinone	diazepam		
60	Yes	bl 1.94mg/l	BZP	TFMPP	diazepam		

Table 6. Combinations of post mortem drugs in deaths associated with mephedrone (levels) reported to np-SAD

11. Discussion

The existence of the Special Mortality Register maintained by the National Programme on Substance Abuse Deaths fulfills several major roles: it provides a unique UK-wide historic repository of unparalleled detailed information on drug-related deaths and deaths of drug addicts since 1997; the provision of a nation-wide surveillance capability for monitoring substance-related deaths; and the provision of information on the epidemiology of such events.

This paper contributes to the knowledge-base on mephedrone by providing supplementary/complementary information on the epidemiology of its use in the UK through the provision of centralised collation of post mortem toxicological results. Furthermore, this report has provided an analysis of the only UK-wide, mephedrone-specific mortality dataset. Although not all cases have yet been fully investigated, to the best of our knowledge this is the most comprehensive and detailed study of deaths associated with mephedrone in the literature.

11.1 User profile

One in five of 'mephedrone fatalities' turned out here not to be actually related to mephedrone, since the drug was actually not identified at post mortem. This might be understood in the context of the high levels of both media attention and public concerns surrounding the unprecedented rapidity of the appearance of mephedrone in the UK recreational drug market (Davey et al., 2010). However, some of these cases turned out to involve other methcathinones such as MDPV.

Typical mephedrone victims in this study were young (78% under 35 years of age); male (75%); White (96% where ethnicity was known); either in full time employment, unemployed or students; and with a previous history of drug misuse (73% where known). With an average age of 29 years and nearly four-fifths under the age of 35, the age profile of this dataset is much younger than cases typically reported to np-SAD (Ghodse et al., 2010).

Mephedrone misuse in the UK is likely to have started as early as 2007 (Davey et al., 2010), and the first mephedrone-related fatality recorded on the np-SAD database occurred in September 2009. Although further studies are needed to confirm present observations, it seems from the information presented here that reports of mephedrone fatalities dropped in the months following the announcement by the Home Office on 30 March 2010 that the chemical, together with other related substances, was going to become a Controlled Drug. However, there was a further peak in July 2010, as well as additional deaths occurring in February, April and May 2011. This suggests that mephedrone, as well as other illegal methcathinones, are still being consumed in the UK.

The excess number (doubling) of observed mephedrone-associated fatalities between Saturdays and Tuesdays, compared to other days of the week, might be explained by its more frequent intake over the weekend, confirming once again its recreational drug profile.

An issue of particular concern and, to the best of our knowledge, something previously unreported is that 16 victims (about 1 in 3 cases of the current sample) either hanged themselves (13 cases), or used particularly violent means to terminate their own lives. In 10 cases, the coroner gave a verdict of suicide and in 8 further cases an open verdict was returned. In most of these cases, mephedrone was considered to have played a contributory role. Although a full psychiatric history is not typically made available to np-SAD, it is worth emphasizing that, out of the whole sample, antipsychotics were here identified at post mortem in 2 cases and antidepressants in 5 cases. Therefore, it can be postulated that mephedrone (either on its own, or in a polydrug misuse combination) has the potential to cause and/or exacerbate psychosis and/or depression, thus facilitating the occurrence of bizarre behaviour/self harm with particularly violent means. In one instance, the possibility of Excited Delirium was recorded. Although the present report comments on only 60 cases, the suicide rates in our other UK studies of stimulant-related fatalities were quantitatively less significant, being in the range of 3-6%: amphetamine-type drugs (Schifano et al., 2010); MDMA/ecstasy (Schifano et al., 2010; Schifano et al., 2003b); cocaine (Schifano & Corkery, 2008). The rate for khat-related fatalities was about 31% (sample size = 13) (Corkery et al., 2010).

Contributory clinical (e.g. sepsis; bronchopneumonia; pre-existing atherosclerotic cardiovascular conditions) and environmental (e.g. involvement in traffic accidents, drowning, hypothermia) factors were here identified at post mortem in respectively 5 and 5 mephedrone fatalities. These observations are overall consistent with the existing literature on stimulant misuse and may reflect the sympathomimetic actions of mephedrone and the accident-proneness or risk-taking behaviour of stimulant, including mephedrone, misusers (Schifano et al., 2011).

Mean mephedrone blood levels at post mortem were of either about 1.43mg/l (in polydrug cases) or 2.00mg/l (mono-intoxication fatalities), which is broadly in line with previous, small scale, anecdotal observations (Dickson et al., 2010; Lusthof et al., 2011).

11.2 Mephedrone use with other substances

Although mephedrone was here identified on its own in the cause of death in only one-third of cases (n = 18, 30%), this finding confirms some of the concerns recently expressed regarding the acute toxicity potential of the drug itself (James et al., 2011; Maskell et al., 2011; Schifano et al., 2011; Torrance & Cooper, 2010; Wood et al., 2010; Regan et al., 2010). It could be argued that the fact there are such a relatively large number of deaths in a comparatively short period (two years) underlines the need to inform consumers of its potential to cause death on its own.

Conversely, most mephedrone victims died of polydrug, and especially alcohol, consumption. Anecdotally, it appears that alcohol is taken in association with stimulants to get a stronger/better 'high'. Similarly, other stimulants such as MDMA/ecstasy, whilst in the presence of alcohol, show more significant physiopathological effects (Pacifici et al., 2002; Schifano et al., 2003a). In 15 cases mephedrone was ingested with stimulants. Cocaine, amphetamines, other methcathinones and/or ecstasy tablets may be taken to maintain arousal and a state of alertness, since the stimulant desired effects of mephedrone fade away in a few hours (Schifano et al., 2011). However, co-ingestion of two stimulants could increase, in a synergic way, both the dopaminergic and serotonergic stimulation, and this is likely to increase mephedrone toxicity effects and harm potential (Schifano et al., 2011). In other cases, arguably to modulate its stimulant effects, mephedrone was associated in this study with opiates (12 cases) and/or diazepam (13 cases). This is likely to be consistent with the observation made here that, where known, about 3 out of 4 victims had a history of drug misuse. It is noteworthy that other newly emerging psychoactive substances (including: GBL/GHB, ketamine, piperazines, as well as other methcathinones) were also found in several cases in conjunction with mephedrone; this is in line with the literature (Deluca et al., 2009; Schifano et al., 2011). In all of these polydrug abuse cases, the precise role of mephedrone in causing fatality was due to simultaneous drug use and remains unclear. Conversely, the use of stimulants might afford some protective effects to those who overdosed with sedatives.

11.3 Treatment and prevention of fatalities

The patterns of drug use evidenced by post mortem toxicology results are similar to those reported by surveys and online users' fora; polysubstance use is common, especially the co-ingestion of alcohol, stimulants and other 'legal highs'. The pathologies (including psychopathologies) exhibited in many of these cases exhibit close similarities to those previous noted for amphetamine, cocaine, MDMA and khat. The implication of these findings is that similar advice to that already given for adverse events caused by other stimulants should be provided to clinicians, the emergency services and first-aiders. It is suggested that the treatment for more life-threatening conditions might be broadly similar to that for amphetamine poisoning. Individuals with less severe symptoms should be assessed and managed as for any psychoactive drug user; they may simply need reassurance, support and observation. People with underlying cardiac, neurological and psychiatric conditions, especially those on medication, are likely to be at greatest risk of serious adverse events (Winstock et al., 2010).

Although our knowledge of mephedrone's potential neurotoxicity or long-term consequences of its use is still very limited, it is sensible to offer the following advice: avoiding regular use to avoid developing tolerance; not using the drug in combination with other stimulants or large amounts of alcohol and other depressants; not injecting the drug; remaining well hydrated when using the drug; and avoiding becoming overheated. Brief motivational interventions and appropriately adapted psychosocial intervention may be employed to treat mephedrone addiction (Winstock et al., 2010).

11.4 Limitations

A number of limitations need to be borne in mind in respect of this study: (a) not all suspected cases may have been identified; (b) remaining 'positive' cases are awaiting further inquiries or inquest; (c) the fact that mephedrone may have been involved in death cannot be confirmed until the relevant Coroner or Procurator Fiscal has concluded her/his inquest or other formal inquiry; (d) the presence of mephedrone in post mortem toxicology does not necessarily imply that it caused or contributed to a death; (e) not all completed cases have been formally notified to the Programme for recording. Hence, the number of identified cases reported here is likely to be an underestimation.

It is thought unlikely that the changes in fatality rates over time observed here are related to parallel changes in coroner methods, which would in turn affect surveillance. Data collection methods have remained unchanged. However, greater awareness of the phenomenon, improved case identification methods, and the devopment of new approaches in forensic toxicology and the range of substances now routinely screened for may have led to more potential cases being notified and registered.

Further limitations of the present report may include: lack of analytical attention to the role of the possible triggering environmental factors (i.e. overcrowding; hot settings etc); lack of total geographical coverage of coroner's jurisdictions; possible incomplete information relating to the prescription of psychoactive medications; and lack of information for some fatalities on the concentration of mephedrone detected in body fluids, so that some victims might have had only traces of the substance. Finally, since mortality rates (e.g. number of deaths out of number of mephedrone intake occasions) were not here calculated, it may be difficult to determine the true extent of risks associated with mephedrone consumption. However, in at least one case death occurred on the first use of mephedrone (albeit in combination with amphetamine).

12. Conclusions

This chapter has highlighted the dangers associated with mephedrone consumption, especially with regard to recreational use. This study represents the most detailed analysis to date of the largest number of mephedrone-related fatalities world-wide. It is hoped that it will thereby make a major contribution to the evidence-base being built up on this drug, and therefore, to reducing drug-related deaths.

Although identified on its own in only a minority of cases, present data confirm concerns regarding the acute toxicity potential of the drug. It is of concern that about 1 in 3 cases of the current sample used particularly violent means to terminate their own lives.

The number of mephedrone intake occasions was not calculated here, and so it may be difficult to determine the true extent of risks associated with mephedrone consumption. It may be possible to compare the lethality of mephedrone with other substances building on methods developed by King and Corkery (2010).

Further studies of a similar nature should be conducted in other countries, to see if the clinical and toxicity patterns associated with mephedrone use described here are confirmed. Notwithstanding the possible biases outlined above, the number of cases reported here may however suggest a significant level of caution when ingesting mephedrone for recreational purposes.

The limited information yet available on mephedrone underlines the need for basic pre-clinical and in-vitro research (and the necessary funding to carry it out) on the pharmacology, metabolism, etc. of methcathinones so as to provide evidence-based interventions and treatments.

13. Acknowledgements

The authors wish to thank coroners and their staff in England & Wales, Northern Ireland, and the Islands; Procurators Fiscal in Scotland; and the Scottish Crime & Drug Enforcement Agency for their assistance in providing data to the National Programme on Substance Abuse Deaths. Thanks are also due to colleagues in UK forensic toxicology agencies for assistance in identifying and confirming suspected deaths in which mephedrone consumption was positive. The np-SAD regularly received support from the Department of Health in the time frame 2004-2010.

This publication arises as well from the activities of the ReDNet Research Project, for which FS has received funding from the European Commission, in the framework of the Public Health Programme (2009 12 16).

14. Conflicts of interest

No conflicts of interest are declared here which may have influenced the interpretation of present data. Please note the following: JC has been the UK Focal Point expert on Drug-Related Deaths for the European Monitoring Centre for Drugs and Drugs Addiction since 2000; FS is a full member of the UK Advisory Council on the Misuse of Drugs (ACMD); JC and FS are members of the ACMD Working Group on Novel Psychoactive Substances, the UK Early Warning System. All authors are members of the International Centre for Drug Policy (ICDP). AHG is current President of the International Narcotics Control Board (INCB). The views expressed here reflect only those of authors and not necessarily those of the Department of Health, Home Office, the ACMD, the ICDP, the EMCDDA, or the INCB.

15. References

ACMD. (2010). *ACMD letter to Home Secretary - Mephedrone (and related cathinones)*. 13 January. Advisory Council on the Misuse of Drugs, London, Available from: http://www.homeoffice.gov.uk/publications/alcohol-drugs/drugs/acmd1/acmdmephedrone?view=Binary

Archer, R.P. (2009). Fluoromethcathinone, a new substance of abuse, *Forensic Science International*, Vol.185:10–20.

Camilleri, A., Johnston, M.R., Brennan, M., Davis, S. & Caldicott, D.G. (2010). Chemical analysis of four capsules containing the controlled substance analogues 4-

methylmethcathinone, 2-fluoromethamphetamine, alpha-phthalimidopropiophenone and N-ethylcathinone, *Forensic Science International*, Vol.197:59–66.

Campbell, D. (2009). Online sales of legal alternatives to class A drugs raise safety fears. *The Guardian*, 12.03.09, Available from: http://www.guardian.co.uk/society/2009/mar/12/online-legal-drugs-stimulants

Chhabra, J.S., Nandalan, S. & Saad, R. (2010). Mephedrone poisoning - a case of severe refractory left ventricular failure, Poster Presentation 33, *The State of the Art Meeting*, London, 13-14 December 2010, pp. 74-75.

Chemspider. (2010). Mephedrone, Available from: http://www.chemspider.com/Chemical-Structure.21485694.html

Corkery, J.M. (2002). Drug-related mortality in the United Kingdom, in Ghodse, H., Oyefeso, A., Corkery, J. & Baldacchino, A. (eds.), *Drug-related Mortality: Perspectives across Europe*, European Collaborating Centres for Addiction Studies, London, Monograph Series No. 2, pp. 155-184.

Corkery, J.M., Schifano, F., Oyefeso, A., Ghodse, A.H., Tonia, T., Naidoo, V. & Button, J. (2011). 'Bundle of fun' or 'bunch of problems'? Case series of khat-related deaths in the UK, *Drugs Education, Prevention and Policy*, Vol.18(6):408-425.

Cozzi, N.V., Sievert, M.K., Shulgin, A.T., Jacobill, P. & Ruoho, A.E. (1999). Inhibition of plasma membrane monoamine transporters by betaketoamphetamines, *European Journal of Pharmacology*, Vol. 381:63–69.

Daly, M. (2010). Teenage kicks, *Druglink*, Vol.25(No.1) (Jan/Feb):8-10, Available at: http://www.drugscope.org.uk/OneStopCMS/Core/CrawlerResourceServer.aspx?resource=359F1F2D-3D94-4061-AB88-25AFFF1C801C&mode=link&guid=677eca484c614bf995ba90f8f81449d7

Dargan, P.I., Albert, S. & Wood, D.M. (2010). Mephedrone use and associated adverse effects in school and college/university students before the UK legislation change, *Quarterly Journal of* Medicine, Vol.103(No.11):875-9.

Davey, Z., Corazza, O., Schifano, F., Deluca, P. & the Psychonaut Web Mapping Group. (2010). Mass-information: Mephedrone, myths, and the new generation of legal highs, *Drugs and Alcohol Today*, Vol.10:24-28.

Deluca, P., Schifano, F., Davey, Z., Corazza, O., Di Furia, L. & the Psychonaut Web Mapping Research Group. (2009). *Mephedrone Report*, Institute of Psychiatry, King's College London, London (UK), Available from: http://www.psychonautproject.eu

Dickson, A.J., Vorce, S.P., Levine, B. & Past, M.R. (2010). Multiple-Drug Toxicity Caused by the Coadministration of 4-Methylmethcathinone (Mephedrone) and Heroin, *Journal of Analytical Toxicology*, Vol.34:162-168.

Drugsforum. (2010). Mephedrone (4-methylmethcathinone, 4-MMC) Experiences, www.drugs-forum.com, Available at: http://www.drugs-forum.com/forum/showthread.php?t=43273

EMCDDA. (2011). *Report on the risk assessment of mephedrone in the framework of the Council Decision on new psychoactive substances*, May 2011, European Monitoring Centre for Drugs and Drug Addiction, Lisbon, Available from: http://www.emcdda.europa.eu/html.cfm/index116639EN.html

Europol-EMCDDA. (2010). *Europol–EMCDDA Joint Report on a new psychoactive substance: 4-methylmethcathinone (mephedrone)*, March 2010, European Monitoring Centre for Drugs and Drug Addictions, Lisbon, Available from:

http://www.emcdda.europa.eu/html.cfm/index132196EN.html

Feyissa, A.M. & Kelly, J.P. (2008). A review of the neuropharmacological properties of khat, *Progress in Neuro-Psychopharmacology and Biological Psychiatry*, Vol.32:1147-1166.

Fleming, N. (2010). Miaow-miaow on trial: truth or trumped-up charges?, *New Scientist*, 29 March, Available at: http://www.newscientist.com/article/dn18712-miaowmiaow-on-trial-truth-or-trumpedup-charges.html

Garret, G. & Sweeney, M. (2010). The serotonin syndrome as a result of mephedrone toxicity, *BMJ Case Reports*, Doi:10.1136/bcr.04.2010.2925.

Gibbons, S. & Zloh, M. (2010). An analysis of the 'legal high' mephedrone, *Bioorganic & Medicinal Chemistry Letters*, Vol.20:4135–4139

Ghodse, A.H., Corkery, J., Oyefeso, A., Schifano, F., Ahmed, K. & Naidoo, V. (2010). *Drug-related deaths in the UK. Annual Report 2010.* International Centre for Drug Policy, St George's, University of London (UK). Available from: http://www.sgul.ac.uk/research/projects/icdp/pdf/np-SAD%2011th%20annual%20report%20Final.pdf

Gustaffsson, D. & Escher, C. (2009). Mefedron. Internetdrog som tycks ha kommit för att stanna [Mephedrone-Internet drug that seems to have come to stay], *Läkartidningen*, Vol.106:2769-2771.

Gygi, M.P., Gibb, J.W. & Hanson, G.R. (1996). Methcathinone: an initial study of its effects on monoaminergic systems, *Journal of Pharmacology and Experimental Therapeutics*, Vol.276:1066–1072.

Home Office. (2010). A change to the Misuse of Drugs Act 1971: Control of mephedrone and other cathinone derivatives, Home Office Circular 010/2010, 14 April 2010, Home Office, London, Available at: http://www.homeoffice.gov.uk/about-us/corporate-publications-strategy/home-office-circulars/circulars-2010/010-2010/

James, D., Adams, R.D., Spears, R., Cooper, G., Lupton, D.J., Thompson, J.P. & Thomas, S.H.; on behalf of the National Poisons Information Service. (2011). Clinical characteristics of mephedrone toxicity reported to the UK National Poisons Information Service, *Emergency Medical Journal*, Aug, Vol.28(No.8):686-689.

Kalix, P. (1990). Pharmacological properties of the stimulant khat, *Pharmacology and Therapeutics*, Vol.48:397-416.

Kalix, P. (1992). Cathinone, a natural amphetamine, *Pharmacology & Toxicology*, Vol.70:77–86.

King, L.A. & Corkery, J.M. (2010). An index of fatal toxicity for drugs of misuse, *Human Psychopharmacology*, Vol.25(No.2):162-166.

Lee, W.S., Chan, M.F., Tam, W.M. & Hung, M.Y. (2007). The application of capillary electrophoresis for enantiomeric separation of N,Ndimethylamphetamine and its related analogs: intelligence study on N,N-dimethylamphetamine samples in crystalline and tablet forms, *Forensic Science International*, Vol.165:71–77.

Lusthof, K.J., Oosting, R., Maes, A., Verschraagen, M., Dijkhuizen, A. & Sprong, A.G.A. (2011). A case of extreme agitation and death after the use of mephedrone in The Netherlands, *Forensic Science International*, Vol. 206:e93–e95

Mackay, K., Taylor, M. & Bajaj, N. (2011). The adverse consequences of mephedrone use: a case series, *The Psychiatrist*, Vol.35: 203-205.

Maskell, P.D., De Paoli, G., Seneviratne, C. & Pounder, D.F. (2011). Mephedrone (4-Methylmethcathinone)-related deaths, *Journal of Analytical Toxicology*, Vol. 35:188-191.

Measham, F., Moore, K., Newcombe, R. & Welch, Z. (2010). Tweaking, bombing, dabbing and stockpiling: the emergence of mephedrone and the perversity of prohibition, *Drugs and Alcohol Today*, Vol.10:14–21.

Morris, K. (2010). UK places generic ban on mephedrone drug family, *The Lancet*, Vol.9723:1333-1334.

Mulchandani, R., Hand, T. & Panesar, L.K. (2010). *Seizures of drugs in England and Wales, 2009/10*, Home Office Statistical Bulletin 17/10, 28 October 2010, Home Office Research Development and Statistics Directorate, London, Available from: http://webarchive.nationalarchives.gov.uk/20110218135832/rds.homeoffice.gov.uk/rds/pdfs10/hosb1710.pdf

Nagai, F., Nonaka, R. & Kamimura, K.S.H. (2007). The effects of nonmedically used drugs on monoamine neurotransmission in rat brain, *European Journal of Pharmacology*, Vol.559:132–137.

National Treatment Agency. (2010). *Drug treatment in 2009–2010*, National Treatment Agency, London, Available from: http://www.nta.nhs.uk/uploads/nta_annualreport_0910.pdf

Newcombe, R. (2009). *Mephedrone: the use of mephedrone (M-cat, meow) in Middlesbrough*, Lifeline Publications, Manchester

Nicholson, P.J., Quinn, M.J. & Dodd, J.D. (2010). Headshop heartache: acute mephedrone 'meow' myocarditis, *Heart*, Vol.96:2051-2052.

Odenwald, M., Neuner, F., Schauer, M., Elbert, T., Catani, C., Lingenfelder, B., Hinkel, H., Häfner, H. & Rockstroh, B. (2005). Khat use as risk factor for psychotic disorders: a cross-sectional and case–control study in Somalia, *BMC Medicine*, Vol.12:3–5.

Odenwald, M., Hinkel, H., Schauer, E., Schauer, M., Elbert, T., Neuner, F. & Rockstroh, B. (2009). Use of khat and posttraumatic stress disorder as risk factors for psychotic symptoms: a study of Somali combatants, *Social Science & Medicine*, Vol.69:1040–1048

Omer, T.A. & Doherty, C. (2011). Posterior reversible encephalopathy syndrome (PRES) complicating the 'legal high' mephedrone, *BMJ Case Reports*, Doi:10.1136/bcr.02.2011.3904

Osorio-Olivares, M., Caroli Rezende, S., Sepulveda-Boza, B.K., Cassels, R.F. et al. (2003). A two-step method for the preparation of homochiral cathinones, *Tetrahedron: Asymmetry*, Vol.14:1473–1477.

Pacifici, R., Zuccaro, P., Farre, M., Pichini, S., Di Carlo, S., Roset, P.N., Palmi, I., Ortuno, J., Menoyo, E., Segura, J. & de la Torre, R. (2002). Cell-mediated immune response in MDMA users after repeated dose administration: studies in controlled versus noncontrolled settings, *Annals of the New York Academy of Sciences*, Vol.965:421-433.

Power, M. (2009). Mephedrone: the future of drug dealing, *Druglink*, Vol.24.(No.2) (Mar/Apr):6,7,9. Available from: http://www.drugscope.org.uk/Resources/Drugscope/Documents/PDF/Good%20Practice/Druglink_March_09_mephedrone.pdf

Ramsey, J., Dargan, P.I., Smyllie, S., Davies, S., Button, J., Holt, D.W. & Wood, D.M. (2010). Buying 'legal' recreational drugs does not mean that you are not breaking the law, *Quarterly Journal of Medicine*, Vol.103:777–783.

Roussel, O., Perrin, M., Herard, P., Chevance, M. Arpino, P. (2009). La 4-méthyléphédrone sera-t-elle une "Ecstasy" du XXIème siècle?, *Annales de toxicologie analytique*, Vol. 21:169–177.

Regan, L., Mitchelson, M. & Macdonald, C. (2010). Mephedrone toxicity in a Scottish emergency department, *Emergency Medicine Journal*, Dec 23. [Epub ahead of print]

Saem de Burnaga Sanchez, J. (1929). Sur un homologue de l'ephedrine, *Bulletin de la Société Chimique de France*, Vol.45:284–286.

Schifano, F. (1996). Cocaine misuse and dependence, *Current Opinion in Psychiatry*, Vol.9:225–230

Schifano, F., Corkery, J., Naidoo, V., Oyefeso, A. & Ghodse, A.H. (2010). Comparison between amphetamine/ methylamphetamine and ecstasy (MDMA, MDEA, MDA, 4-MTA) mortality data in the UK (1997-2007), *Neuropsychobiology*, Vol.61:122-130.

Schifano, F., Oyefeso, A., Corkery, J., Cobain, K., Jambert-Gray, R., Martinotti, G. & Ghodse, A.H. (2003a). Death rates from ecstasy (MDMA, MDA) and polydrug use in England and Wales 1996-2002, *Human Psychopharmacology Clinical and Experimental*, Vol. 18:519-524.

Schifano, F., Oyefeso, A., Webb, L., Pollard, M., Corkery, J. & Ghodse, A.H. (2003b). Review of deaths related to taking ecstasy, England and Wales, 1997-2000, *British Medical Journal*, Vol. 326:80-81.

Schifano, F. & Corkery, J. (2008). Cocaine/crack cocaine consumption, treatment demand, seizures, related offences, prices, average purity levels and deaths in the UK (1990-2004), *Journal of Psychopharmacology*, Vol. 22:71-79.

Schifano, F., Albanese, A., Fergus, S., Stair, J.L., Deluca, P., Corazza, O., Davey, Z., Corkery, J., Siemann, H., Scherbaum, N., Farre', M., Torrens, M., Demetrovics, Z., Ghodse, A.H., Psychonaut Web Mapping & ReDNet Research Groups. (2011). Mephedrone (4-methylmethcathinone; 'meow meow'): chemical, pharmacological and clinical issues, *Psychopharmacology (Berlin)*, Vol. 214:593-602.

Smith, K. & Flatley, J. (Eds.). (2011). *Drug Misuse Declared: Findings from the 2010/11 British Crime Survey England and Wales*, Home Office Statistical Bulletin 12/11, 28 July 2011, Home Office Research, Development and Statistics Directorate, London, Available from: http://www.homeoffice.gov.uk/publications/science-research-statistics/research-statistics/crime-research/hosb1211/hosb1211?view=Binary

Sumnall, H. & Wooding, O. (2009). *Mephedrone: an update on current knowledge*. Centre for Public Health, Liverpool John Moores University, Liverpool, Available from: http://www.cph.org.uk/showPublication.aspx?pubid=614

Torrance, H. & Cooper, G. (2010) The detection of mephedrone (4-methylmethcathinone) in 4 fatalities in Scotland, *Forensic Sciences International*, Vol.202(No.1-3):e62-3.

Winstock, A.R., Marsden, J. & Mitcheson, L. (2010). What should be done about mephedrone? *British Medical Journal*, Vol.340:c1605.

Winstock, A., Mitcheson, L., Deluca, P., Davey, Z., Corazza, O. & Schifano, F. (2011). Mephedrone; new kid for the chop, *Addiction*, Vol.106(No.1):154-61.

Wood, D.M., Davies, S., Puchnarewicz, M., Button, J., Archer, R., Ovaska, H., Ramsey, J., Lee, T., Holt, D.W. & Dargan, P.I. (2010a). Recreational use of mephedrone (4-

methylmethcathinone, 4-MMC) with associated sympathomimetic toxicity, *Journal of Medical Toxicology*, Vol.6:327–330.

Wood, D.M., Davies, S., Puchnarewicz, M., Button, J., Archer, R. et al. (2009). Recreational use of 4-methylmethcathinone (4-MMC) presenting with sympathomimetic toxicity and confirmed by toxicological screening, *Clinical Toxicology*, Vol.47:7331.

Wood, D.M., Greene, S.L. & Dargan, P.I. (2010b). Clinical pattern of toxicity associated with the novel synthetic cathinone mephedrone, *Emergency Medical Journal*, doi:10.1136/emj.2010.092288

18

Novel Strategies in Drug-Induced Acute Kidney Injury

Alberto Lázaro, Sonia Camaño, Blanca Humanes and Alberto Tejedor
Renal Physiopathology Laboratory, Department of Nephrology, Hospital General Universitario Gregorio Marañón, Madrid, Spain

1. Introduction

1.1 Renal toxicity

Renal toxicity associated with commonly prescribed drugs lengthens hospital stay, worsens prognosis, and limits the potential benefits obtained from therapy (Peracella, 2011; Servais et al., 2008).

Proximal tubule preservation is a clue in strategies aimed to prevent nephrotoxicity. The proximal tubule is a target for filtered drugs that are reabsorbed by solvent drag or pinocytosis, but also for drugs that are secreted into the luminal side.

Proximal tubules recover more than 60% of total filtered load, i.e., a single molecule of toxin that is filtered and reabsorbed will pass through the proximal tubule cell more than 50 times per day. Such a high degree of exposure implies a risk of cell damage causing a variety of clinical syndromes, from proximal acidosis and acquired Fanconi syndrome to tubular cell necrosis (Oh, 2010). This spectrum of diseases is known as acute kidney injury (AKI), which also includes cell death by apoptosis, anoikis, necrosis, or cell dysfunction (Lorz et al., 2006).

Nephrotoxicity can often be expected with certain drugs, such as vancomycin, gentamicin, foscarnet, cisplatin, cyclosporine A (CsA), and tacrolimus. Less often, the toxic effect is unexpected and not predictable, as is the case with iodinated contrast agents and paracetamol.

1.2 Cell death mediation

Intrinsic pathway-mediated apoptosis and extrinsic pathway-mediated apoptosis are both involved in toxic proximal tubule cell death (Pabla & Dong, 2008; Servais et al., 2008; Xiao et al., 2011). With most of toxins, cell death is followed by detachment and anoikis. Paracetamol is a notable exception to this behavior. Caspases activation, mitochondrial depolarization, release of cytochrome C from mitochondria, cell membrane modification, and nucleosome formation are all hallmarks of apoptosis that are regularly observed in toxin-damaged proximal tubules (Camano et al., 2010). Nitric oxide, soluble oxygen radicals, and proinflammatory cytokines are released by damaged proximal tubules, thus amplifying the lesion.

1.3 Nephrotoxicity prevention strategies

Overhydration is the most common maneuver to prevent toxic concentrations in urine and, consequently, inside the cell. However, nephrotoxicity usually requires dose adjustment or drug withdrawal, thus limiting effectiveness.

Other strategies aimed at inhibiting cell drug transport or interfering with mediation of apoptosis also tend to interfere with the therapeutic targets and, consequently, limit the effectiveness of therapy (Pabla & Dong, 2008; Servais et al., 2008).

During the last 5 years, our work on nephrotoxicity has enabled us to better understand the role of proximal tubule behavior in the adaptation of the kidney to toxic aggressions (Camano et al., 2010; Camaño-Paez et al., 2008; Neria et al., 2009; Perez et al., 2004; Tejedor et al., 2007).

Therefore, not surprisingly, the search for alternative protective strategies against toxic damage to the proximal tubule is an important area of investigation today.

1.4 Ability of cilastatin to prevent drug toxicity targeting the proximal tubule

Cilastatin is an inhibitor of brush border dehydropeptidase I (DHP-I), which is present in renal proximal tubular epithelial cells (RPTECs). It was initially designed to inhibit hydrolysis and uptake of the carbapenem antibiotic imipenem, thus enabling it to be more easily recovered from urine (Birnbaum et al., 1985; Norbby et al., 1983). However, cilastatin is also able to inhibit uptake of CsA and cisplatin by RPTECs by decreasing in a dose-dependent way the toxic effect of CsA and cisplatin on RPTECs (Camano et al., 2010; Perez et al., 2004). Clinical studies also support this protective role of cilastatin against CsA-induced nephrotoxicity (Carmellini et al., 1997, 1998; Gruss et al., 1996; Markewitz et al., 1994; Mraz et al., 1987, 1992; Tejedor et al., 2007). Experimental evidence suggests that cilastatin binding to brush border DHP-I could interact with apical cholesterol lipid rafts (Camano et al., 2010; Perez et al., 2004; Tejedor et al., 2007).

The aim of this brief report is to determine whether cilastatin is able to interfere with the direct toxic effect of several known nephrotoxic drugs on cultured RPTECs. We investigated the effect of cilastatin on the toxicity of gentamicin, vancomycin, iodinated contrast agent, amphotericin B, foscarnet, cisplatin, mannitol, chloroform, paracetamol, CsA and tacrolimus.

We describe for the first time the effects of a drug that specifically targets the renal proximal tubule brush border and seems to be able to reduce accumulation and toxicity of the main nephrotoxic drugs by inhibiting internalization of brush border-bound lipid rafts.

2. Methods

2.1 Drugs

We used commercially available parenteral formulations of gentamicin (powder, Guinama, Alboraya, Spain), vancomycin (powder, Combino Pharm, Barcelona, Spain), iodinate contrast agent (iopamidol, Laboratorios Farmacéuticos Rovi, Madrid, Spain), amphotericin B (Bristol Myers Squibb, Madrid, Spain), foscarnet (Foscavir, AstraZeneca, Madrid, Spain), cisplatin (Pharmacia, Barcelona, Spain), mannitol 20%, (Osmofundin®, Braun Medical S.A., Barcelona, Spain), chloroform (Scharlau, Barcelona, Spain), CsA (Sandimmun Neoral®,

Novartis Farmaceutica S.A., Spain), tacrolimus (Prograf®, Fujisawa S.A., Spain), and paracetamol (Perfalgan, Bristol Myers Squibb). The concentrations used were similar to the pharmacologically active recommended plasma level.

Crystalline cilastatin was provided by Merck Sharp & Dohme S.A. (Madrid, Spain). A dose of 200 µg/ml was chosen, because it is cytoprotective and falls within the reference range for clinical use (Camano et al., 2010; Perez et al., 2004).

All drug dilutions were performed with sterile culture medium and cilastatin, and the tested drugs were added simultaneously.

2.2 Primary cultures of renal proximal tubule epithelial cells

Porcine RPTECs were obtained as previously described (Camano et al., 2010; Perez et al., 2004). Briefly, the cortex was sliced and incubated for 30 minutes at 37°C with 0.6 mg/ml of collagenase A (Boehringer Mannheim, Germany) in Ham's F-12 medium. Digested tissue was then filtered through a metal mesh (250 µm), washed 3 times with Ham's F-12 medium, and centrifuged using an isotonic Percoll gradient (45% [v/v]) at 20,000*g* for 30 minutes. Proximal tubules were recovered from the deepest fraction, washed, and resuspended in supplemented DMEM/Ham's F-12 at a 1:1 ratio (with 25 mM HEPES, 3.7 mg/ml sodium bicarbonate, 2.5 mM glutamine, 1% non-essential amino acids, 100 U/ml penicillin, 100 mg/ml streptomycin, 5 x 10^{-8} M hydrocortisone, 5 mg/ml insulin-transferrin-sodium selenite media supplement, and 2% fetal bovine serum). Proximal tubules were seeded at a density of 0.66 mg/ml and incubated at 37°C in a 95% air/5% CO_2 atmosphere. Culture medium was renewed every 2 days. RPTECs were used after they had reached confluence (80%).

2.3 Cell death studies

2.3.1 Nuclear morphology

Cell nuclei were visualized following DNA staining with the fluorescent dye DAPI (Sigma-Aldrich, Missouri, USA). Briefly, cells were seeded on cover slips in a 24-well plate, fixed in 4% formaldehyde for 10 minutes, and permeabilized with 0.5% Triton X-100. They were then rinsed with PBS and incubated with DAPI (12.5 µg/ml) for 15 minutes. Excess dye was removed. Cells imaging was performed with the 40X PL-APO 1.25 NA oil objective of a Leica-SP2 confocal microscope (Leica Microsystems, Heidelberg, Germany). DAPI was excited with a 405 nm laser-diode. Emission between 420 nm and 490 nm was collected following the manufacturer's recommendations. Six fields with ~200 cells per field were examined in each condition to estimate the percentage of nuclei with an apoptosis-like appearance.

2.3.2 Nucleosomal quantification

To evaluate DNA fragmentation in the context of apoptosis, RPTECs were incubated for 48 hours under specific conditions with the nephrotoxic compounds selected. At the end of this period RPTECs were lysed and centrifuged at 200*g* for 10 minutes to remove cell debris. DNA and histones present in the soluble fraction were quantified using an enzyme-linked immunosorbent assay (*Cell Death Detection ELISA^PLUS^* kit, Boehringer Mannheim, Germany), as previously described (Camano et al., 2010; Perez et al., 2004).

2.3.3 Cell viability assay

The cell survival assay relies on the capacity of cells to reduce 3-(4, 5- dimethylthiazol-2-yl)-2, 5-diphenyltetrazolium bromide (MTT) (Calbiochem, California, USA) to colored formazan in metabolically active cells. RPTECs were seeded onto 96-well plates and incubated with toxins alone or in combination with cilastatin. Twenty-four hours later, 0.5 mg/ml of MTT was added, plates were incubated for 3 hours in the dark at 37°C, and 100 µL of 50% dimethylformamide in 20% SDS (pH 4.7) was added. Plates were incubated at 37°C overnight, and absorbance was measured at 595 nm. All assays were performed in triplicate.

Alternatively, MTT assays were performed in real time, following MTT reduction on single cells, with an Olympus IX70 inverted microscope fitted to a spectrofluorometer SLM AMINCO 2000. MTT was measured by reading cell absorbance at 570 nm.

2.4 Cell viability: Quantification of colony-forming units

RPTECs were treated for 24 hours with CsA, tacrolimus or paracetamol in the presence or absence of cilastatin (200 µg/ml). Adherent cells were washed in saline serum, harvested with trypsin-EDTA, seeded in Petri dishes (100 mm), and cultured for 7 days in drug-free complete medium. Surviving adherent cells were fixed for 5 minutes with 5% paraformaldehyde/PBS and stained with 0.5% crystal violet/20% methanol for 2 minutes. Excess dye was rinsed with PBS. Finally, the intracellular dye was eluted with 50% ethanol/50% sodium citrate 0.1 M (pH 4.2) and quantified by spectrometry at 595 nm.

2.5 Cellular drug transport and accumulation

RPTECs incubated for 24 hours with increasing concentrations of CsA, tacrolimus or paracetamol in the presence or absence of cilastatin (200 µg/ml), were scraped and lysed in 400 µL of lysis buffer at 70°C (2.22% [w/v] SDS; 19.33 % [v/v] glycerol [87% v/v]; 790 mM Tris HCl pH 6.8 in dH_2O, phenylmethylsulfonyl fluoride, and protease inhibitors). Cell lysates were heated at 100°C for 5 minutes, homogenized in ice, and centrifuged at 12,000*g* for 5 minutes at 4°C. The supernatant was analyzed for total protein content and the presence of nephrotoxins. The concentrations of CsA, tacrolimus and paracetamol were measured using fluorescence polarization immunoassay technology on a TDX Chemistry Analyzer (Abbot Laboratories, USA) in accordance with the instructions provided by the manufacturer. The calibrators and controls supplied with each kit were applied, and the results were expressed as ng drug/µg protein.

2.6 Localization of lipids rafts by immunofluorescence

To study the interaction of cilastatin with cholesterol lipid rafts, we used FITC-conjugated cholera toxin B (Molecular Probes, Oregon, USA), as its internalization is mediated by lipid rafts.

RPTECs cultured on glass coverslips were preincubated with culture medium alone or cilastatin 200 µg/ml for 15 minutes. The cells were then incubated with 10 µg/ml FITC-labelled cholera toxin B for 1 and 2.5 hours. Cells were washed with PBS and fixed in 4%

formaldehyde in PBS for 10 minutes before being rinsed with PBS. The nuclei were counterstained with DAPI. After washing, cells were mounted in fluorescent mounting medium (Dako North America, Inc., Carpinteria, California). Images of the distribution of cholera toxin immunolocalization across membranes were obtained with the 20X PL-APO 0.7-numerical aperture objective of a Leica-SP2 confocal microscope (Leica Microsystems).

2.7 Dehydropeptidase I and IV activity assays

RPTECs were incubated overnight with Gly-Phe-*p*-nitroanilide (DHP-I substrate; Sigma-Aldrich) 1mM in PBS for DHP-I activity determination or with Gly-Pro-*p*-nitroanilide (DHP-IV substrate; Sigma-Aldrich) 1 mM for DHP-IV activity determination. Both activities were measured in the presence or absence of cilastatin (200 µg/ml). *P*-Nitroanilide was quantified in aliquots from supernatants by measuring at 410 nm absorbance.

2.8 Statistical analysis

Quantitative variables were expressed as the mean ± standard error of the mean (SEM). Differences were considered statistically significant for bilateral alpha values less than 0.05. Factorial ANOVA was used when more than 1 factor was considered. When a single factor presented more than 2 levels and the model showed significant differences between factors, a post-hoc analysis (least significant difference) was performed. When results are shown, they represent a minimum of at least 3 repeats. When possible, a quantification technique (e.g. dye recovery) was used to illustrate reproducibility. When figures illustrated an effect, paracetamol was chosen as the example.

3. Results

3.1 Cilastatin as a broad nephroprotective drug: reduction of toxin-induced proximal tubular cell death

After 48 hours of exposure to the drugs tested, apoptosis of RPTECs measured as nucleosomal DNA fragmentation and migration from nuclei to cytosol was quantified and compared with apoptosis under the same conditions, although in the presence of cilastatin (Fig. 1). RPTECs exposed to toxins present different increases in the number of nucleosomes recovered from cytosol. Cilastatin significantly partially or totally prevented these changes in most of the selected drugs (Fig. 1).

When the magnitude of cilastatin protection was plotted against the magnitude of basal cell death under every treatment tested, a clear linear trend was observed ($r=0.839$, $p<0.0005$). None of the drugs tested differed significantly from this trend (Fig. 2).

We made a detailed study of the effect of 3 of these drugs: CsA, tacrolimus and paracetamol. A more selective qualitative estimation of apoptotic cell death was also obtained in adherent cells treated with CsA, tacrolimus, and paracetamol and stained with DAPI (Fig. 3). Incubation with toxins led to cell shrinkage with significant nuclear condensation, fragmentation, and formation of apoptosis-like bodies (see arrows). Cilastatin was able to reduce nuclear damage in all cases. Apoptosis-like nuclei are quantified in Fig. 3B, C, and D.

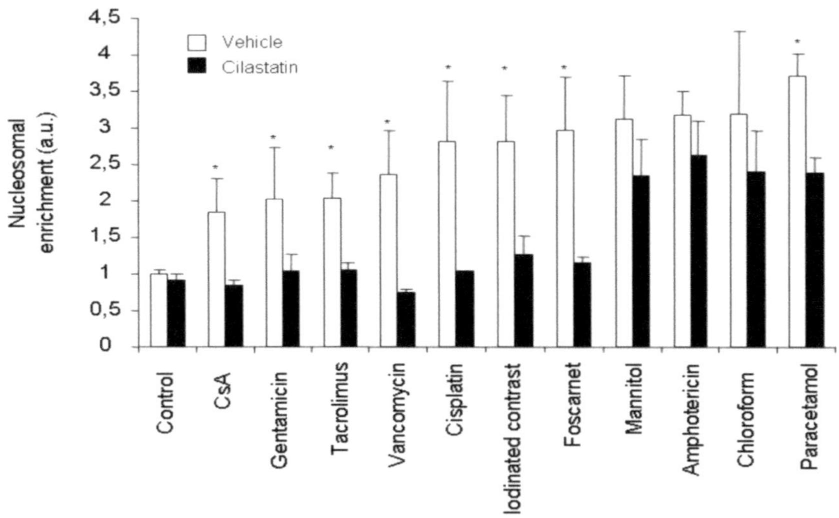

Fig. 1. Effect of cilastatin on nephrotoxin-induced apoptosis. Renal proximal tubular epithelial cells were exposed to CsA (1 µg/ml), gentamicin (20 mg/ml), tacrolimus (50 ng/ml), vancomycin (600 µg/ml), cisplatin (10 µM), iodinated contrast (1 mg/ml), foscarnet (1 mM), mannitol (100 mosm/l), amphotericin B (10 µg/ml), chloroform (100 µg/ml), and paracetamol (300 µg/ml) with and without cilastatin (200 µg/ml) for 48 hours. Oligonucleosomal DNA fragmentation was detected by ELISA. Data are represented as the mean ± SEM of at least 3 separate experiments. ANOVA model: $p<0.0001$. *$p<0.05$ vs. same data with cilastatin.

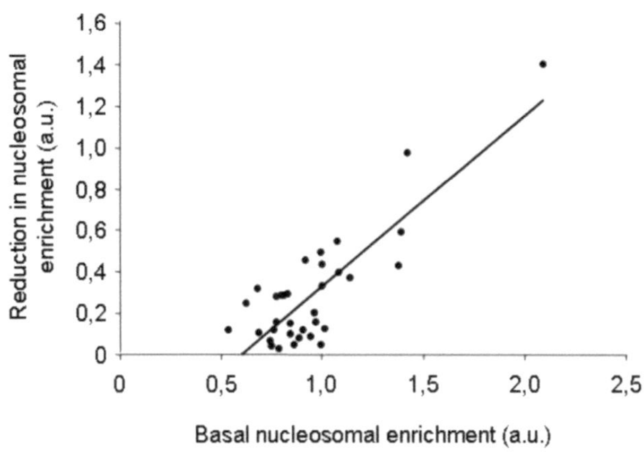

Fig. 2. Reduction in nucleosomal enrichment induced by cilastatin over basal nucleosomal enrichment induced by each toxin. Individual experimental data are provided. There is a common trend for all the data, suggesting a common behavior, with cilastatin protection being proportional to basal damage. Linear regression of "cilastatin-induced reduction" vs. "basal nucleosomal enrichment", slope=0.82, r=0.839, adjusted $r^2=0.695$, $p<0.0005$.

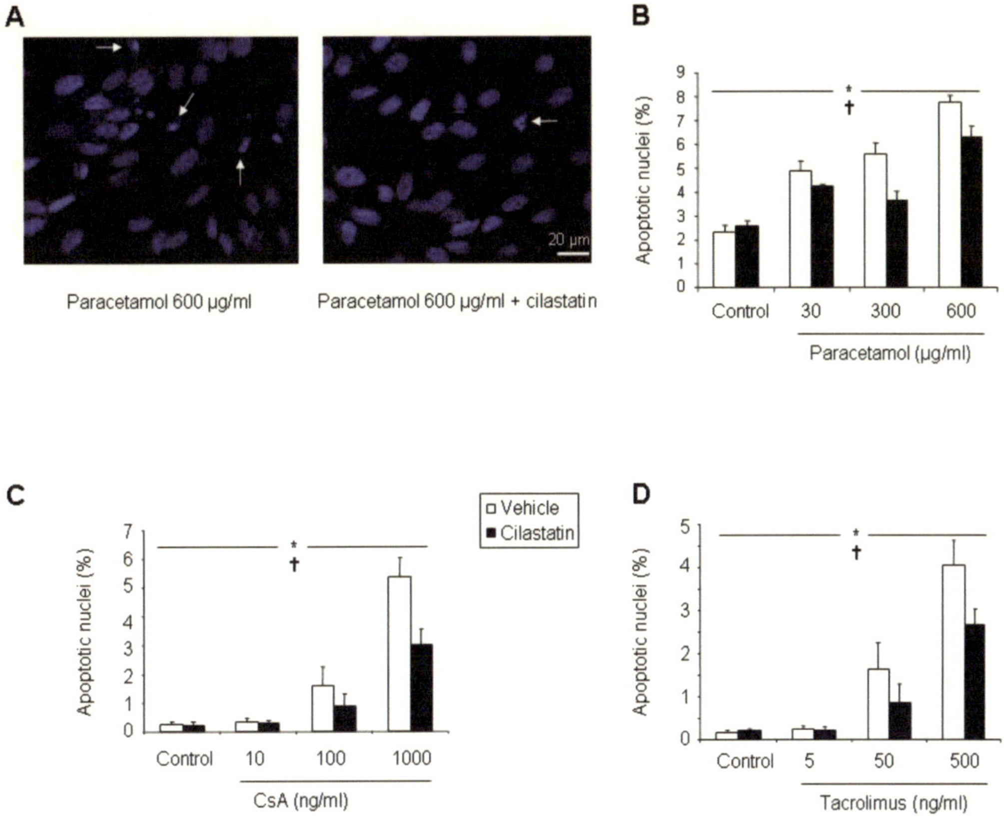

Fig. 3. Effects of cilastatin on the nuclear morphology of renal proximal tubular epithelial cells (RPTECs) during treatment with toxins. RPTECs were cultured in the presence of paracetamol (30, 300 and 600 µg/ml), cyclosporine (CsA, 10, 100, and 1000 ng/ml) and tacrolimus (5, 50, and 500 ng/ml) with or without cilastatin (200 µg/ml) for 24 hours. A, Example of nuclear staining with DAPI to determine whether an apoptotic-like nuclear morphology was present. Arrows point to fragmented, apoptotic nuclei. B, C and D, Quantitative approach to staining for paracetamol, CsA and tacrolimus, respectively. Data are represented as the mean ± SEM of at least 3 separate experiments. ANOVA models $p<0.0001$. * cilastatin effect, $p<0.05$; †dose effect, $p<0.05$.

We quantified the functional impact of CsA, tacrolimus and paracetamol treatments on cell survival by measuring the percentage of adherent cells still able to reduce MTT to formazan after exposure to increasing doses of toxins. After 24 hours of incubation with toxins, the amount of surviving cells able to reduce MTT decreases progressively as the concentrations of CsA, tacrolimus, and paracetamol increase. However, in the presence of cilastatin, all surviving cells keep their capacity to reduce MTT (Fig. 4). Cilastatin is able to counteract both the structural and functional damage induced by toxins.

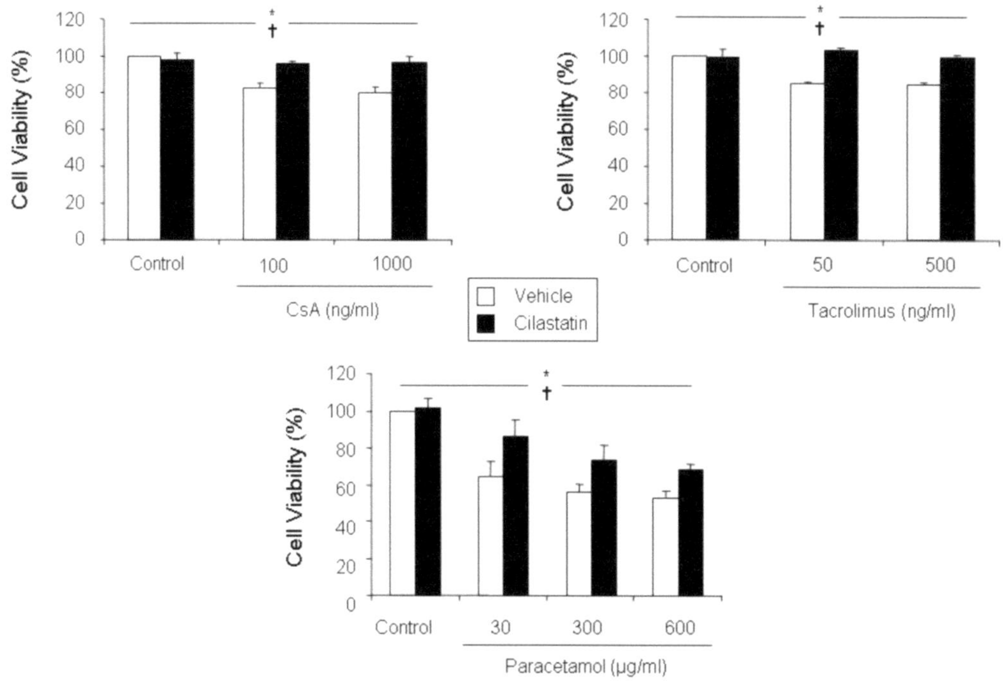

Fig. 4. Effect of cilastatin on toxin-induced loss of cell viability determined by the ability to reduce MTT (see Methods). Renal proximal tubular epithelial cells were exposed to toxins and toxins + cilastatin (200 µg/ml) for 24 hours. Results are expressed as the percentage of the value obtained relative to control (without toxins and cilastatin) of at least 3 separate experiments. ANOVA: for CsA, *dose effect, $p \leq 0.05$; †cilastatin effect, $p < 0.05$; for tacrolimus, *dose effect, $p < 0.05$; †cilastatin effect, $p \leq 0.04$; for paracetamol, *dose effect, $p \leq 0.05$; †cilastatin effect, $p \leq 0.05$.

3.2 Cilastatin prevents toxin-induced mitochondrial damage

The effect of cilastatin on mitochondria may be observed very early after CsA, tacrolimus, or paracetamol is added to cell culture plates. In Fig. 5, an inverted IX-80 microscope was fitted with a black chamber, a photomultiplier, and a spectrofluorimeter (SML Aminco) to obtain absorbance readings at specific wavelengths on single (or small groups of) cells in culture. This set-up allows real time follow-up of colorimetric in vivo reactions.

Recording the first seconds after MTT addition shows the initial kinetics of MTT reduction and formazan precipitation, thus offering a first approach to the activity of the mitochondrial chain in intact cells. Although not suitable for detailed kinetic studies, this method allows a quick check of mitochondrial oxidative activity.

RPTECs exposed to toxins showed a quick and deep depression in the reduction of MTT activity compared with controls (Fig. 5). Coincubation with cilastatin partially recovers this effect, although the effect was less visible for paracetamol. Differences are observed even during the first 5 minutes of drug additions.

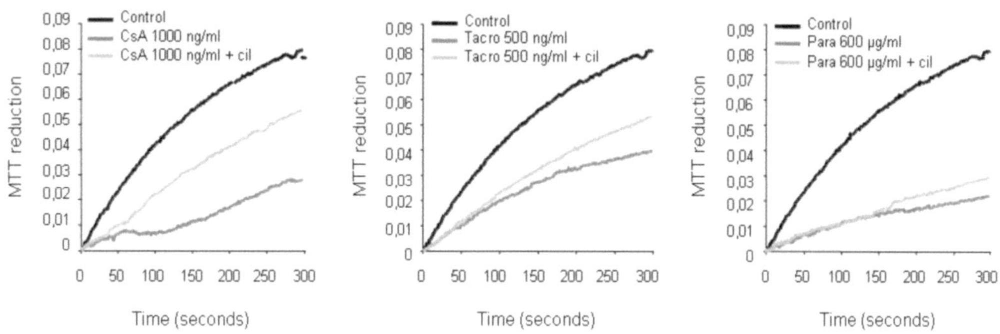

Fig. 5. Effect of cilastatin on toxin-induced mitochondrial damage. Changes in the mitochondrial oxidative capacity of RPTECs were assessed by MTT reduction at 570 nm. The graphs show formation of formazan as detected in isolated cells in real time with no treatment (control) and CsA (cyclosporin, 1000 ng/ml), tacro (tacrolimus, 500 ng/ml) and para (paracetamol, 600 µg/ml) with or without 200 µg/ml cilastatin, after the incubation times on the X-axis.

3.3 Cilastatin improves long-term recovery and viability of RPTECs after exposure to CsA, tacrolimus, and paracetamol

To know the long-term viability of surviving RPTECs after 24 hours of exposure to CsA, tacrolimus, or paracetamol, we tested the ability of those cells to proliferate into new cell colonies. Colony-forming units (CFUs) were quantified as specified in Methods. The CFUs count decreased after 24 hours of treatment with CsA, tacrolimus, and paracetamol, and this decrease was clearly dose-dependent (Fig. 6). If the cells were exposed to toxins in the presence of cilastatin, the number of CFUs was significantly greater after 7 days of recovery for every CsA, tacrolimus, and paracetamol concentration studied. The intracellular dye was extracted, and absorbance was quantified al 595 nm (Fig. 6B, C and D).

3.4 Cilastatin reduces intracellular accumulation of CsA, tacrolimus, and paracetamol

In many cases, nephrotoxicity is largely dependent on the intracellular concentration of drug reached. As cilastatin is a ligand of the brush border membrane, we investigated whether it affected toxin uptake by RPTECs. To test this hypothesis, we measured the intracellular content of CsA, tacrolimus, and paracetamol by TDX analysis, as described in Methods. Cellular CsA, tacrolimus and paracetamol content increased progressively in a dose-dependent manner when RPTECs were incubated for 24 hours in the presence of different concentrations of toxins (Fig. 7). Coincubation with cilastatin consistently reduced accumulation of CsA, tacrolimus and paracetamol in the cells for every concentration studied (Fig. 7). These results confirm that adding cilastatin to primary cultures of proximal cells decreases cellular toxin accumulation. This effect may be involved in the reduced impact of CsA, tacrolimus, and paracetamol on damage to and survival and death of RPTECs.

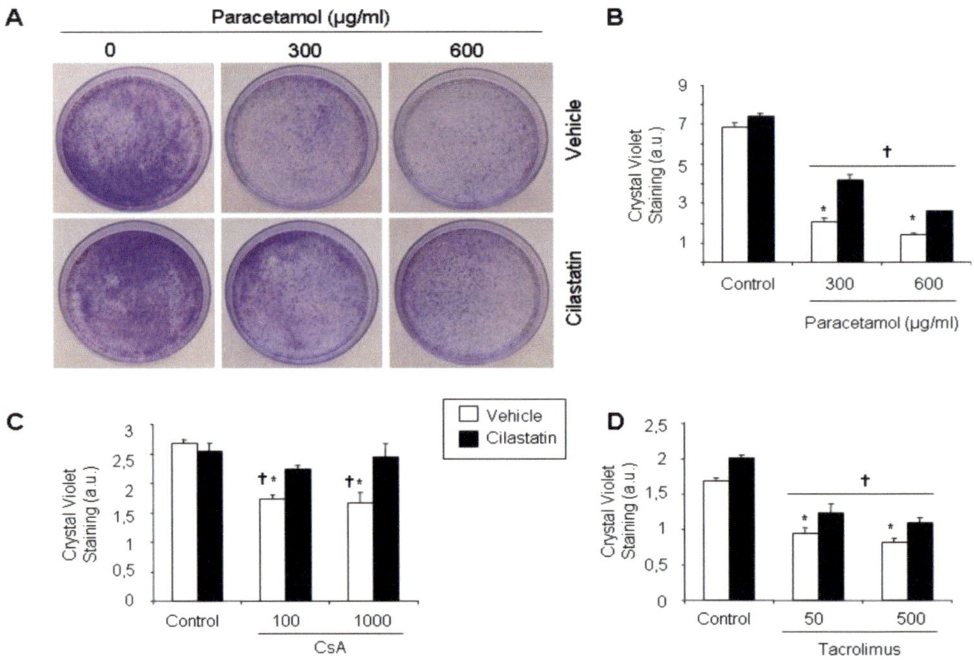

Fig. 6. Cilastatin preserves long-term recovery of toxin-treated RPTECs. A, RPTECs were incubated with paracetamol, CsA (cyclosporin), or tacrolimus in the presence or absence of 200 µg/ml cilastatin for 24 hours. The number of colony-forming units was determined by staining with crystal violet after 7 days (the figure shows the experiment with paracetamol). B, C, and D, Quantification of crystal violet staining for paracetamol, CsA and tacrolimus, respectively. Data are expressed as mean ± SEM; of 3 separate experiments. ANOVA model, $p<0.0001$. †$p<0.05$ vs. control; *$p\leq0.05$ vs. same data with cilastatin.

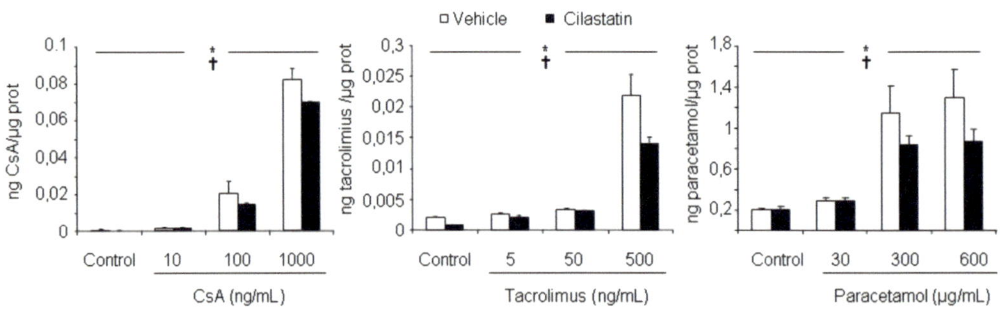

Fig. 7. Effects of cilastatin on accumulation of toxins by RPTECs. Intracellular accumulation was measured in the lysates of RPTECs treated with nephrotoxins for 24 hours, in the presence or absence of cilastatin (200 µg/ml), using a specific fluorescence polarization immunoassay (TDX). Cilastatin was shown to prevent entry of all nephrotoxins into RPTECs. Values were expressed as means ± SEM of drug concentrations (n=4 different experiments). ANOVA model, $p<0.0001$; *, cilastatin effect $p<0.05$; †, dose effect $p<0.05$.

3.5 Effect of cilastatin on lipid rafts distribution

According to these results, which suggest that cilastatin interferes with intracellular administration of the nephrotoxins tested, cilastatin appears to be able to inhibit an intracellular nephrotoxin accumulation pathway as a result of its binding to renal DHP-I. We explored the possibility that cilastatin, through its interaction with DHP-I and when anchored to cholesterol lipid rafts by a glycosyl-phosphate-inositol (GPI) group (Adachi et al., 1990; Parkin et al., 2001), could block transport through lipid rafts or interfere with the cholesterol lipid raft-dependent endocytic pathway. The expression and cell membrane localization of cholera toxin, which specifically binds to its ganglioside GM1 receptor present in cholesterol lipid rafts, were assessed using confocal microscopy in RPTECs treated for very short periods. In Fig. 8, cholera toxin is identified on the cell surface after 15 minutes incubation, but it disappeared from the membrane after 1 hour (top) and accumulated in a perinuclear position. In the presence of 200 μg/ml cilastatin and after 1 hour of treatment, cholera toxin was still attached to the membrane, suggesting interference with the cholera toxin internalization site. No significant changes in FITC-cholera toxin staining patterns were observed at 2.5 hours in the presence of cilastatin.

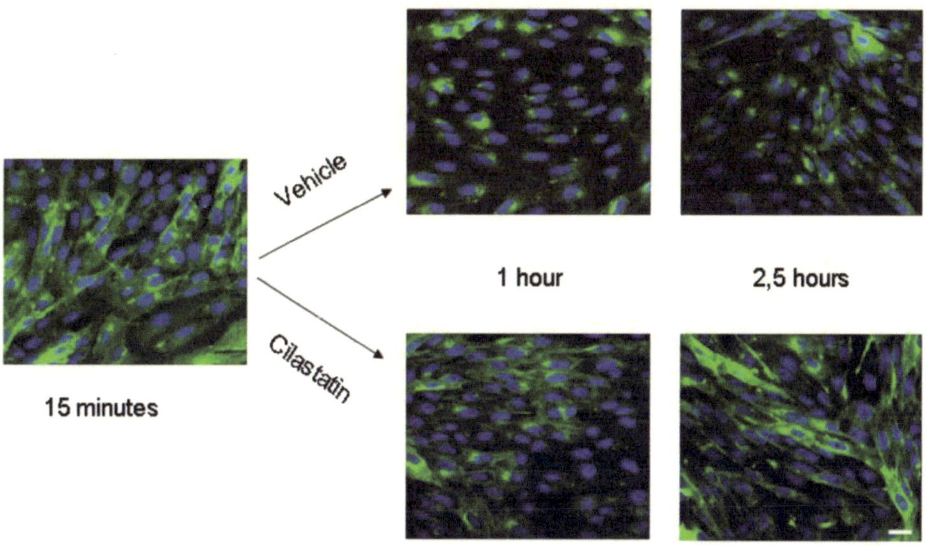

Fig. 8. Blockade of circulation of cholesterol rafts by cilastatin. This picture shows the change in cholera toxin fluorescence internalization over time in control cells and cells incubated in the presence of cilastatin (200 μg/ml). Bar, 20 μm.

4. Conclusion

We report that cilastatin, a powerful and specific inhibitor of DPH-I, is able to reduce both intracellular accumulation and induction of apoptosis by antibiotic, cytotoxic, anti-inflammatory, antiretroviral, anesthetic, and immunosuppressive drugs. These findings expand our previous results with cisplatin (Camano et al., 2010) and CsA (Perez et al., 2004; Tejedor et al., 2007).

Cilastatin inhibits the activity of DPH-I, but not of DPH-4, in the brush border of renal RPTECs (Fig. 9).

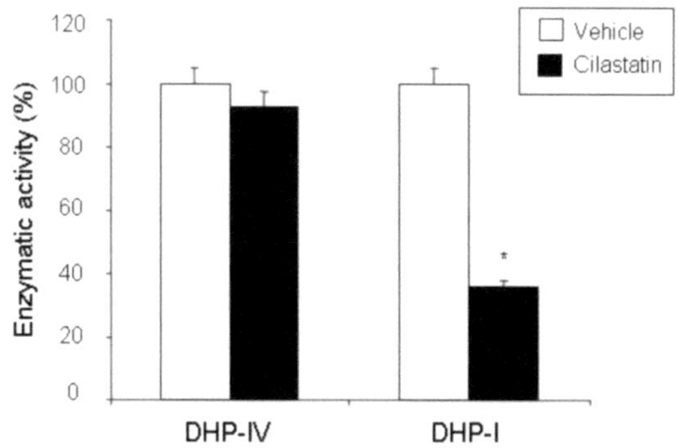

Fig. 9. Effect of cilastatin on the activity of dehydropeptidase I and IV. Activities were determined by the hydrolysis of specific substrates. Results are expressed as a percentage of enzyme activity compared to untreated controls (100% activity) and as the mean ± SEM of 3 experiments. ANOVA model, $p<0.0001$. * $p<0.01$ vs. the same data without cilastatin.

Although this inhibition is probably irrelevant in the degree of nephroprotection observed—none of the nephrotoxins studied have a chemical structure that could potentially be affected by dipeptidase activity—binding to DPH-I may partially explain this protection.

DPH-I is anchored to brush border lipid rafts (Pang et al., 2004; Parkin et al., 2001). Binding of FITC-labelled B-cholera toxin to lipid rafts leads to their rapid internalization. However, internalization does not occur in the presence of cilastatin.

This mechanism is probably behind the reduction observed in the intracellular concentration of the different drugs analyzed.

We previously showed that cilastatin modifies brush border membrane fluidity by interfering with membrane-bound cholesterol (Perez et al., 2004).

The drugs tested in Fig. 1 have many different chemical structures, and their mechanisms of cell permeation are not well established in some cases. However, for all those drugs, intracellular concentrations were measured and cilastatin always reduced intracellular accumulation. By inhibiting lipid raft–dependent vesicle circulation, cilastatin seems able to reduce luminal entry of drugs, even if they are not substrates for DPH-I activity.

This interference with drug entry may explain the almost instantaneous protection observed in the real-time experiments of MTT reduction. MTT reduction relies on mitochondrial oxidative chain integrity. When single cell oxidative capacity is recorded in real time, addition of the toxin inhibits MTT reduction activity relative to the single control cell, and this is evident from the first seconds. Cilastatin partially protects against this effect. The quick time course of the effect strongly suggests that a mechanism of cilastatin inhibits drug intake by the cell.

However, other mechanisms may be implicated in the broad renal protection observed. We recently published that, when exposed to toxic concentrations of cisplatin, RPTECs increase expression of Fas and Fas L. Fas targets brush border lipid rafts (Dimanche-Boitrel et al., 2005), binds its ligand, and triggers the extrinsic pathway of apoptosis. Internalization of Fas/Fas L seems a necessary step (Camano et al., 2010).

Cilastatin reduced cisplatin-induced cell apoptosis but not cell necrosis (Camano et al., 2010). When the extrinsic apoptosis pathway was checked, the initial step blocked by cilastatin was Fas L/Fas internalization (Camano et al., 2010).

Cilastatin reduces apoptosis (nuclear damage, nucleosome formation, MTT reduction capacity) and ameliorates surviving cell recovery. Both reductions in drug intake by proximal cells and blockade of lipid raft internalization are probably involved in these protective actions (Fig. 10).

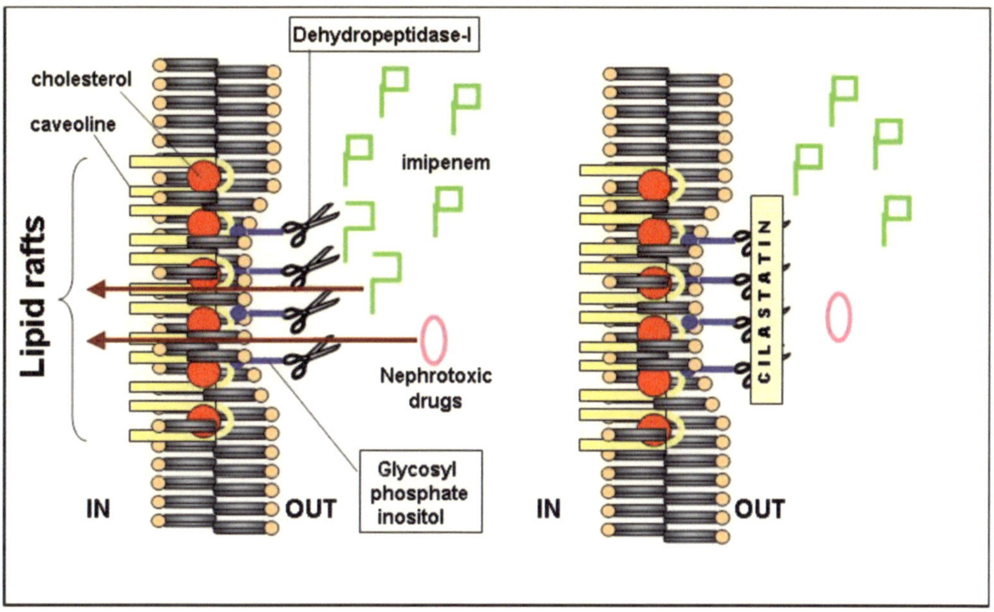

Fig. 10. Diagram of the possible protective mechanism of cilastatin. Cilastatin is a dehydropeptidase-I inhibitor used in human clinical practice combined with imipenem. Dehydropeptidase inhibition affects the structure of lipid rafts by preventing hydrolysis of the lactam ring and inhibits the absorption of imipenem and other nephrotoxic drugs, thus reducing their renal toxicity.

Protection by cilastatin depends on its interaction with DPH-I, an enzyme that is found almost exclusively in proximal tubules. Therefore, cilastatin-induced nephroprotection is specific for tissue and cell type, but not for the drug tested.

More research is necessary to confirm the mechanism of protection, the ability to protect in animal models of acute renal failure, and the absence of an effect on the pharmacological targets of tested drugs. Nevertheless, cilastatin offers a new protective strategy, as it is a tissue-specific designed drug, with unexpected tissue-specific antiapoptotic actions.

5. Acknowledgments

This work was partially supported by the Fondo de Investigaciones Sanitarias [Grants FIS-PI05/2259, FIS-PI 08/1481], Comunidad de Madrid [Grant BIO-S-0283/2006], and Fundacion Mutua Madrileña. AL holds a "Sara Borrell" post-doctoral research contract from the ISCIII.

The authors are grateful to Dr. Rafael Samaniego for help with confocal microscopy, Dr. Miguel L.F. Ruano for technical assistance with the TDX assays, and Merck Sharp & Dohme for providing cilastatin.

6. References

Adachi, H.; Tawaragi, Y.; Inuzuka, C.; Kubota, I.; Tsujimoto, M.; Nishihara, T. & Nakazato, H. (1990). Primary structure of human microsomal dipeptidase deduced from molecular cloning. *The Journal of Biological Chemistry*, Vol.265, No.7, (March 1990), pp. 3392-5, ISSN 0021-9258

Birnbaum, J.; Kahan, F.M.; Kropp, H. & MacDonald, .JS. (1985). Carbapenems, a new class of beta-lactam antibiotics. Discovery and development of imipenem/cilastatin. *The American Journal of Medicine*, Vol.78, No.6A, (June 1985), pp. 3-21, ISSN 0002-9343

Camano, S.; Lazaro, A.; Moreno-Gordaliza, E.; Torres, A.M.; de Lucas, C.; Humanes, B.; Lazaro, J.A.; Gomez-Gomez, M.; Bosca, L. & Tejedor, A. (2010). Cilastatin attenuates cisplatin-induced proximal tubular cell damage. *The Journal of Pharmacology and Experimental Therapeutics*, Vol.334, No.2, (April 2010), pp. 419-29, ISSN 0022-3565

Camaño-Páez, S.; Lázaro-Fernández, A.; Callejas-Martínez, R.; Lázaro-Manero, J.A.; Castilla-Barba, M.; Martín-Vasallo, P.; Martínez-Escandel, A: & Tejedor-Jorge A. (2008). Study on the role of the tubule in renal vasoconstriction induced by cyclosporine. *Actas Urológicas Españolas*, Vol.32, No.1, (January 2008), pp. 128-39, ISSN 0210-4806

Carmellini. M.; Frosini, F.; Filipponi, F.; Boggi, U. & Mosca, F. (1997). Effect of cilastatin on cyclosporine-induced acute nephrotoxicity in kidney transplant recipients. *Transplantation*, Vol.64, No.1, (July 1997), pp. 164-6, ISSN 0041-1337

Carmellini, M.; Matteucci, E.; Boggi, U.; Cecconi, S.; Giampietro, O. & Mosca, F. (1998). Imipenem/cilastatin reduces cyclosporin-induced tubular damage in kidney transplant recipients. *Transplantation Proceedings*, Vol.30, No.5, (August 1998), pp. 2034-5, ISSN 0041-1345

Dimanche-Boitrel, M.T.; Meurette, O.; Rebillard, A. & Lacour, S. (2005) Role of early plasma membrane events in chemotherapy-induced cell death. *Drug Resistance Update: reviews and commentaries in antimicrobial and anticancer chemotherapy*, Vol.8, No.1-2, (April 2005), pp. 5-14, ISSN 1368-7646

Gruss. E.; Tomas, J.F.; Bernis, C.; Rodriguez, F.; Traver, J.A. & Fernandez-Ranada, J.M. (1996). Nephroprotective effect of cilastatin in allogeneic bone marrow transplantation. Results from a retrospective analysis. *Bone Marrow Transplantation*, Vol.18, No.4, (October 1996), pp. 761-5, ISSN 0268-3369

Lorz, C.; Benito-Martin, A.; Justo, P.; Sanz, A.B.; Sanchez-Niño, M.D.; Santamaria, B.; Egido, J. & Ortiz, A. (2006). Modulation of renal tubular cell survival: where is the evidence?. *Current Medicinal Chemistry*, Vol.13, No.4, pp. 449-54, ISSN 0929-8673

Markewitz, A.; Hammer, C.; Pfeiffer, M.; Zahn, S.; Drechsel, J.; Reichenspurner, H. & Reichart, B. (1994). Reduction of cyclosporine-induced nephrotoxicity by cilastatin following clinical heart transplantation. *Transplantation*, Vol.57, No.6, (March 1994), pp. 865-70, ISSN 0041-1337

Mraz, W.; Modic, P.K. & Hammer, C. (1992). Impact of imipenem/cilastatin on cyclosporine metabolism and excretion. *Transplantation Proceedings*, Vol.24, No.5, (October 1992), pp. 1704-8, ISSN 0041-1345.

Mraz. W.; Sido, B.; Knedel, M. & Hammer, C. (1987). Concomitant immunosuppressive and antibiotic therapy--reduction of cyclosporine A blood levels due to treatment with imipenem/cilastatin. *Transplantation Proceedings*, Vol.19, No.5, (October 1987), pp. 4017-20, ISSN 0041-1345

Neria, F.; Castilla, M.A.; Sanchez, R.F.; Gonzalez-Pacheco, F.R.; Deudero, J.J.; Calabia, O.; Tejedor, A.; Manzarbeitia, F.; Ortiz, A. & Caramelo, C. (2009). Inhibition of JAK2 protects renal endothelial and epithelial cells from oxidative stress and cyclosporin A toxicity. *Kidney International*, Vol.75, No.2, (September 2008), pp. 227-34, ISSN 0085-2538

Norrby, S.R.; Alestig, K.; Björnegård, B.; Burman, L.A.; Ferber, F.; Huber, J.L.; Jones, K.H.; Kahan, F.M.; Kahan, .J.; Kropp, H.; Meisinger, M.A. & Sundelof, J.G. (1983). Urinary recovery of N-formimidoyl thienamycin (MK0787) as affected by coadministration of N-formimidoyl thienamycin dehydropeptidase inhibitors. *Antimicrobial Agents and Chemotherapy*, Vol.23, No.2, (February 1983), pp. 300-7, ISSN 0066-4804

Oh, M.S. (2010). Unconventional views on certain aspects of toxin-induced metabolic acidosis. *Electrolyte & Blood Pressure*, Vol.8, No.1, (June 2010), pp.32-7, ISSN 17385997

Pabla, N. & Dong, Z. (2008) Cisplatin nephrotoxicity: mechanisms and renoprotective strategies. *Kidney International*, Vol.73, No.9, (May 2008), pp. 994-1007, ISSN 0085-2538

Pang, S.; Urquhart, P. & Hooper, N.M. (2004). N-glycans, not the GPI anchor, mediate the apical targeting of a naturally glycosylated, GPI-anchored protein in polarised epithelial cells. *Journal of Cell Science*, Vol.117, No.Pt21, (October 2004), pp. 5079-86, ISSN 0021-9533

Parkin, E.T.; Turner, A.J. & Hooper, N.M. (2001). Differential effects of glycosphingolipids on the detergent-insolubility of the glycosylphosphatidylinositol-anchored membrane dipeptidase. *The Biochemical Journal*, Vol.358, No.Pt1, (August 2005), pp. 209-16, ISSN 0264-6021

Perazella, M.A. (2009). Renal vulnerability to drug toxicity. *Clinical Journal of the American Society of Nephrology*, Vol.4, No.7, (July 2009), pp. 1275-83, ISSN 1555-9041

Perez, M.; Castilla, M.; Torres, A.M.; Lázaro, J.A.; Sarmiento, E. & Tejedor, A. (2004) Inhibition of brush border dipeptidase with cilastatin reduces toxic accumulation of cyclosporin A in kidney proximal tubule epithelial cells. *Nephrology, dialysis, transplantation*, Vol.19, No.10, (July 2004), pp. 2445-55, ISSN 0931-0509

Servais, H.; Ortiz, A.; Devuyst, O.; Denamur, S.; Tulkens, P.M. & Mingeot-Leclercq, M.P. (2008). Renal cell apoptosis induced by nephrotoxic drugs: cellular and molecular mechanisms and potential approaches to modulation. *Apoptosis*, Vol. 13, No.1, (January 2008), pp. 11-32, ISSN 1360-8185

Tejedor, A.; Torres, A.M.; Castilla, M.; Lazaro, J.A.; de Lucas, C. & Caramelo, C. (2007). Cilastatin protection against cyclosporin A-induced nephrotoxicity: clinical evidence. *Current Medical Research Opinion*, Vol.19, No.10, (March 2007), pp. 505-13, ISSN 0300-7995

Xiao, Z.; Li, C.; Shan, J.; Luo, L.; Feng, L.; Lu, J.; Li, S.; Long, D. & Li, Y. (2011). Mechanisms of renal cell apoptosis induced by cyclosporine A: a systematic review of in vitro studies. *American Journal of Nephrology*, Vol.33, No.69, (May 2011), pp. 558-66, ISSN 0250-8095

19

Chemical and Physical Enhancers for Transdermal Drug Delivery

José Juan Escobar-Chávez[1,*], Isabel Marlen Rodríguez-Cruz[2]
and Clara Luisa Domínguez-Delgado[2]
[1]*Unidad de Investigación Multidisciplinaria, Laboratorio 12: Materiales Nanoestructurados y Sistemas Transdérmicos, Facultad de Estudios Superiores Cuautitlán-Universidad Nacional Autónoma de México, Carretera Cuautitlán–Teoloyucan, San Sebastián Xhala, Cuautitlán Izcalli, Estado de México,*
[2]*Departamento de Ingeniería y Tecnología, Sección de Tecnología Farmacéutica, Facultad de Estudios Superiores Cuautitlán-Universidad Nacional Autónoma de México, Cuautitlán Izcalli, Estado de México, México*

1. Introduction

The application of preparations to the skin for medical purposes is as old as the history of medicine itself, with references to the use of ointments and salves found in the records of Babylonian and Egyptian medicine.(López-Castellano & Merino, 2010) The historical development of permeation research is well described by Hadgraft & Lane, 2005. Over time, the skin has become an important route for drug delivery in which topical, regional or systemic effects are desired (Domínguez-Delgado, et al., 2010). Nevertheless, skin constitutes an excellent barrier and presents difficulties for the transdermal delivery of therapeutic agents, since few drugs possess the characteristics required to permeate across the stratum corneum in sufficient quantities to reach a therapeutic concentration in the blood. In order to enhance drug transdermal absorption different methodologies have been investigated developed and patented (Rizwan et al., 2009). To date many chemical and physical approaches have been applied to increase the efficacy of the material transfer across the intact skin. These are termed 'Novel' due to recent development with satisfactory results in the field of drug delivery (Patel et al., 2010). Improvement in physical permeation-enhancement technologies has led to renewed interest in transdermal drug delivery. Some of these novel advanced transdermal permeation enhancement technologies include: iontophoresis, electroporation, ultrasound, microneedles to open up the skin and the use of transdermal nanocarriers (Díaz-Torres, 2010; Escobar-Chávez & Merino, 2010a).

---

* Corresponding Author

2. Chemical enhancers

Chemical percutaneous enhancers have long been used to increase the range of drugs that can be effectively delivered through the skin (López-Castellano & Merino, 2010). To date, a plethora of chemicals have been evaluated as enhancers, but their inclusion in topical or transdermal formulations is limited due to fact that the underlying mechanisms of action of these agents remain unclear. Although different chemicals are employed by the industry as percutaneous enhancers, some of which have several desirable properties, to date none has proved to be ideal. An ideal chemical penetration enhancer should have the following attributes (Barry, 1983; López- Castellano & Merino, 2010): a) It should be non-toxic, non-irritating and non-allergenic, b) It should work rapidly, and its activity and duration of effect should be both predictable and reproducible, c) It should exert no pharmacological activity within the body, d) It should work unidirectionally, e) When removed, the skin's barrier properties should return both rapidly and fully, f) It should be compatible with both excipients and drugs, and g) It should be cosmetically acceptable and, ideally, odourless and colourless.

2.1 Percutaneous penetration routes of drugs

There are three major potential routes of percutaneous penetration: appendageal, transcellular (through the stratum corneum), and intercellular (through the stratum corneum) (Figure 1). There is a weight of evidence that suggests that passage through the intact stratum corneum constititutes the predominant route by which most molecules penetrate the skin, as the appendageal route is characterized by a limited available fractional

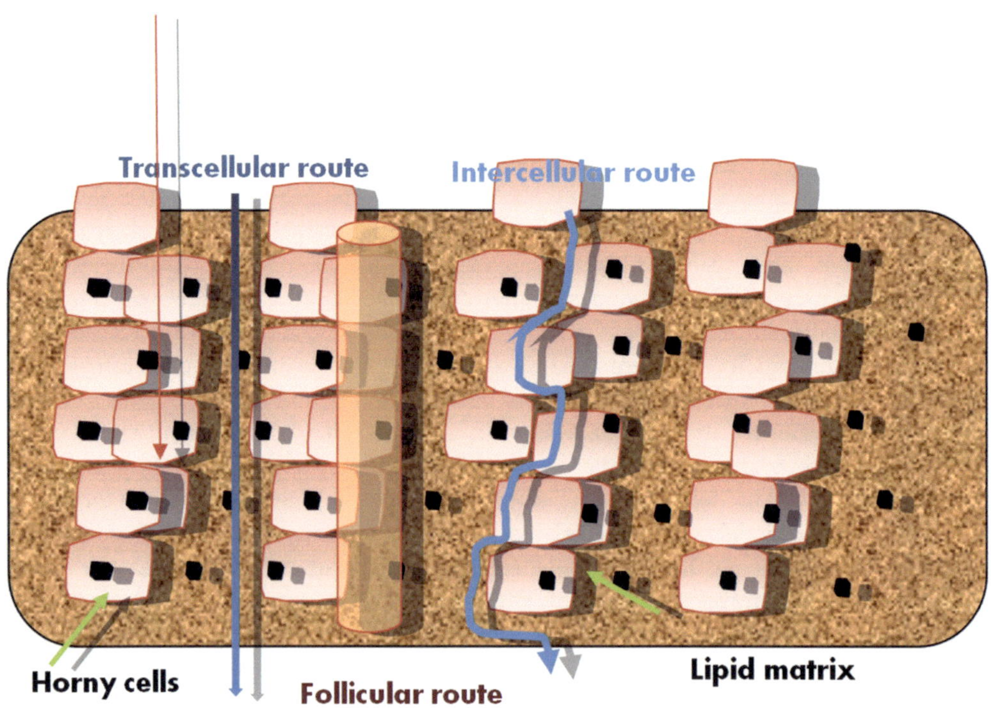

Fig. 1. Processes of percutaneous absorption

area of 0.1%. In this way, diffusion through the skin is controlled by the particular characteristics of the stratum corneum. In order to obtain a sufficient drug flux and, in turn, the therapeutical objectives in question, an alternative is to use chemical percutaneous enhancers. These substances alter some of the properties of the stratum corneum. (López-Castellano & Merino, 2010)

2.2 Direct effects on the skin due to the use of transdermal penetration enhancers

The lipid-protein-partititioning theory sets out the mechanisms by which enhancers alter skin lipids, proteins and/or partitioning behaviour (Barry, 1991): i) They act on the stratum corneum intracellular keratin by denaturing it or modifying its conformation, causing subsequent swelling and increased hydration; ii) They affect the desmosomes that maintain cohesion among corneocytes; iii) They modify the intercellular lipid domains to reduce the barrier-like resistance of the bilayer lipids. Disruption to the lipid bilayers can be homogeneous when the enhancer is distributed evenly within the complex bilayer lipids, but the accelerant is more likely to be heterogeneously concentrated within the domains of the bilayer lipids and iv) They alter the solvent nature of the stratum corneum, thus aiding the partitioning of the drug or a co-solvent into the tissue.(López-Castellano & Merino, 2010)

2.3 Indirect effects on the skin due to the use of transdermal penetration enhancers

Chemical enhancers can produce: *a)* Modification of the thermodynamic activity of the vehicle. The permeation of a good solvent from the formulation, such as ethanol, can increase the thermodynamic activity of a drug; *b)* It has been suggested that, by permeating through the membrane, a solvent can 'drag' the permeant with it, though this concept is somewhat controversial and requires confirmation; *c)* Solubilising the permeant within the donor, especially when solubility is very low, as in the case of aqueous donor solutions, can reduce depletion effects and prolong drug permeation.(López-Castellano & Merino, 2010)

2.4 Classification of percutaneous chemical enhancers

The classification of percutaneous enhancers is frequently based on the chemical class to which the compounds belong. Table 1 shows the principal classes of percutaneous enhancers.

CHEMICAL CLASS	COMPOUNDS
Water	Water
Sulfoxides and similar chemicals	Dimethyl sulfoxide, Dodecyl methyl sulfoxide
Ureas	Urea
Alcohols	Ethanol, Caprylic alcohol, Propylene glycol
Pyrrolidones and derivatives	N-methyl-2-pyrrolidone, 2-pyrrolidone
Azone and derivatives	Azone® (1-dodecylazacycloheptan-2-one)
Dioxolane derivatives	SEPA®
Surfactants (Anionic, Cationic, Nonionic, Zwitterionic)	Sodium lauryl sulfate, Cetyltrimethyl amonium bromide, Sorbitan monolaurate, Polisorbate 80, Dodecyl dimethyl ammoniopropane sulfate
Terpenes	Menthol, Limonene
Fatty acids	Oleic acid, Undecanoic acid

Table 1. Principal classes of percutaneous enhancers.

2.5 Determination of permeation enhancement

The great majority of studies of the effects of enhancers on skin permeability have been carried out by means of *in vitro* diffusion experiments in which various kinds of diffusion cells have been used. The most well-known of these cells are the Franz diffusion systems. These cells have two receptor compartments - donor and receptor (donor positioned above receptor) - between which the skin is placed. In general, the skin is pretreated with a solution of the chemical enhancer to be evaluated. The transdermal flux (J) of drugs can be estimated from the slope of the linear region (steady-state portion) of the accumulated amount of drug in the receptor compartment versus time plot. Permeation enhancing activity, expressed as enhancement ratio of flux (ER_{flux}), is determined as the ratio between the flux value obtained with the chemical enhancer and that obtained with the control. A number of variables can strongly influence the permeation enhancement of drugs. The most important are the skin used in the experiments, temperature, humidity, enhancer concentration, vehicle employed and degree of saturation of the drug in the donor and receptor compartments. (López-Castellano & Merino, 2010)

2.6 Uses in topical/transdermal formulations

Some examples of drugs delivered throughout the skin using chemical enhancer are shown in Table 2.

Drug	*Chemical enhancer*
Sodium salicylate (Hadgraft et al., 1985; Smith & Irwin, 2000); *Sodium naproxen* (Escobar-Chavez et al., 2005); *Ibuprofen* (Philips & Michniak,1995; Shen et al., 2007); *Nonivamide acetate* (Fang et al., 1997); *Meloxicam* (Zhang et al., 2009); *Flurbiprofen* (Ma et al., 2010); *Naloxone* (Xu et al., 2007); *Furosemide* (Agyralides et al., 2004); *Methotrexate* (Allan, 1995); *Sumatriptan succinate* (Balaguer-Fernandez et al., 2010).	Azone®
Sodium naproxen (Escobar-Chavez et al., 2005); *Sodium diclofenac* (Escribano et al., 2003); *Lidocaine* (Cazares-Delgadillo et al., 2005); *Testosterone* (Hathout et al., 2010); *Mometasone furoate* (Senyiğit et al., 2009); *Ketorolac* (Amrish et al., 2009).	Transcutol ®
Haloperidol (Vaddi et al., 2009); *Indomethacin* (Ogiso et al., 1995); *Leuprolide* (Lu et al., 1992).	Urea
Tizanidine hydrochloride (Mutalik et al., 2009); *Minoxidil* (Mura et al., 2009); *Metopimazine* (Bounoure et al., 2008); *Nortriptyline hydrochloride* (Merino et al., 2008; Escobar-Chavez et al., 2011).	Alcohols
Lidocaine (Lee et al., 2006); *Bupranolol* (Babu et al., 2008); *Propanolol* (Amnuaikit et al., 2005); *Acyclovir* (Montenegro et al., 2003).	Pyrrolidones
Tizanidine hydrochloride (Mutalik et al., 2009); *Daphnetin* (Wen et al., 2009); *Nitrendipin* (Mittal et al., 2008).	Fatty acids
Diclofenac (Kigasawa et al., 2009); *Nortiptyline hydrochloride* (Merino et al., 2008); *Verapamil hydrochloride* (Güngör et al., 2008); *Minoxidil* (Mura et al., 2009)	Terpenes
Retinol (Mélot et al., 2009); *Morphine* (Monti et al., 2001); *Arginine vasopressin* (Nair&Pachangula, 2003); *Insulin* (Pillai & Pachangula, 2003); *Enoxacin* (Fang et al., 1998).	Surfactants

Table 2. Examples of drugs delivered throughout the skin using chemical penetration enhancers.

3. Sonophoresis

Absorption of ultrasonic energy leads to tissue heating, and this has been used with therapeutic intent in many conditions. More recently it has been realized that benefit may also be obtained from the non-thermal effects that occur as ULTS travels through tissue. ULTS therapies can broadly be divided into "high" power and "low" power therapies where high power applications include high intensity focused ULTS and lithotripsy, and low power encompasses sonophoresis, sonoporation, gene therapy and bone healing. There are three distinct sets of ULTS conditions based on frequency range and applications: 1) High frequency (3–10 MHz) or diagnostic ULTS, 2) Medium frequency (0.7–3 MHz) or therapeutic ULTS, and 3) Low frequency (18 to 100 KHz) or power ULTS.

3.1 The ultrasound

The term ultrasonic refers to sound waves whose frequency is >20 KHz. The intensity (I, expressed in W/cm^2), or concentration of power within a specific area in an ULTS beam, is proportional to the square of the amplitude, p, which is the maximum increase or decrease in the pressure relative to ambient conditions in the absence of the sound wave. The complete relationship is: $I= p^2/2\rho c$, where ρ is the density of the medium and c is the speed of the sound (in human soft tissue, this velocity is 1540 m/s). The intensity is progressively lost when a sound wave passes through the body or is deviated from its initial direction, a phenomenon referred to as attenuation. In homogeneous tissue, the attenuation occurs as a result of absorption, in which case the sound energy is transformed into heat and scattered. The sound waves are produced in response to an electrical impulse in the piezoelectric crystal, allowing the conversion of electrical into mechanical or vibrational energy; this transformation requires a molecular medium (solid, liquid, or gas) to be effective. The ULTS beam is composed of two fields, the "near field," in the region closest to the transducer face, and the "far field," corresponding to the conical diverging portion of the beam (Figure 2). The parameters controlling this configuration of the ULTS beam are principally the frequency and the size of transducer.

3.2 Mechanisms of action

3.2.1 Cavitation effects

Cavitation is the formation of gaseous cavities in a medium upon ULTS exposure. The primary cause of cavitation is ULTS-induced pressure variation in the medium. Cavitation involves both the rapid growth and collapse of a bubble (inertial cavitation), or the slow oscillatory motion of a bubble in an ULTS field (stable cavitation). Collapse of cavitation bubbles releases a shock wave that can cause structural alteration in the surrounding tissue (Clarke et al., 2004) ULTS can generate violent microstreams, which increase the bioavailability of the drugs (Tachibana & Tachibana, 1999). Tissues contain air pockets that are trapped in the fibrous structures that act as nuclei for cavitation upon ultrasound exposure. The cavitational effects vary inversely with ULTS frequency and directly with ULTS intensity. Cavitation might be important when low-frequency ULTS is used, gassy fluids are exposed or when small gas-filled spaces are exposed. Cavitation occurs due to the nucleation of small gaseous cavities during the negative pressure cycles of ULTS, followed by the growth of these bubbles throughout subsequent pressure cycles (Tang et al., 2001).

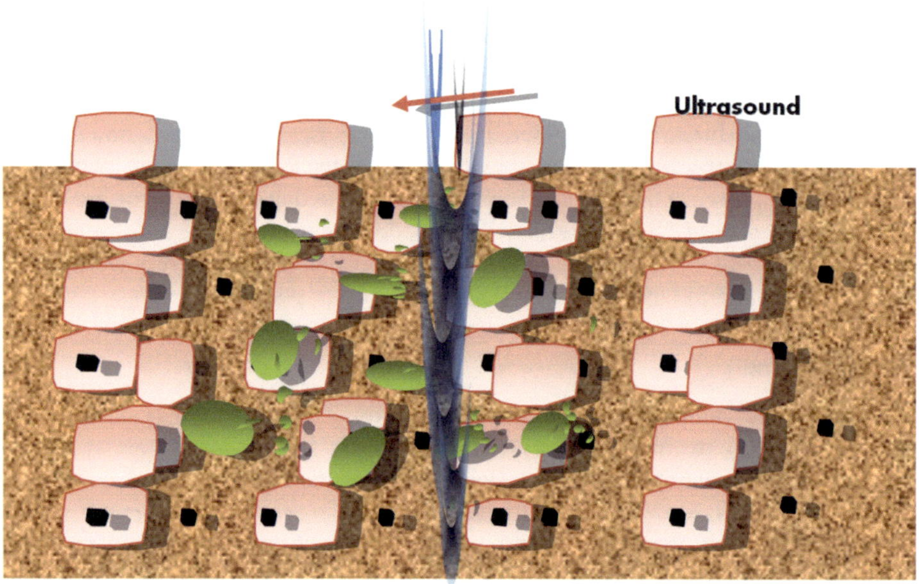

Fig. 2. Enhanced permeation by disruption of lipid barrier and cavitation by use of ULTS.

3.2.2 Thermal effects

Absorption of ULTS increases temperature of the medium. Materials that possess higher ULTS absorption coefficients, such as bone, experience severe thermal effects compared with muscle tissue, which has a lower absorption coefficient (Lubbers et al., 2003). The increase in the temperature of the medium upon ULTS exposure at a given frequency varies directly with the ULTS intensity and exposure time. The absorption coefficient of a medium increases directly with ULTS frequency resulting in temperature increase.

3.2.3 Convective transport

Fluid velocities are generated in porous medium exposed to ultrasound due to interference of the incident and reflected ULTS waves in the diffusion cell and oscillations of the cavitation bubbles. Fluid velocities generated in this way may affect transdermal transport by inducing convective transport of the permeant across the skin, especially through hair follicles and sweat ducts.

3.2.4 Mechanical effects

ULTS is a longitudinal pressure wave inducing sinusoidal pressure variations in the skin, which, in turn, induce sinusoidal density variation. At frequencies greater than 1 MHz, the density variations occur so rapidly that a small gaseous nucleus cannot grow and cavitational effects cease. But other effects due to density variations, such as generation of cyclic stresses because of density changes that ultimately lead to fatigue of the medium, may continue to occur. Lipid bilayers, being self-assembled structures, can easily be disordered by these stresses, which result in an increase in the bilayer permeability. This increase is, however, non-significant and hence mechanical effects do not play an important role in therapeutic sonophoresis. Thus cavitation induced lipid bilayer disordering is found to be the most important cause for ultrasonic enhancement of transdermal transport.

3.3 Advantages and disadvantages of sonophoresis

Sonophoresis is capable of expanding the range of compounds that can be delivered transdermally. In addition to the benefits of avoiding the hepatic first-pass effect, and higher patient compliance, the additional advantages and disadvantages that the sonophoretic technique offers can be summarized as follows in Table 3.

Advantages	Disadvantages
Enhanced drug penetration (of selected drugs) over passive transport.	Can be time-consuming to administer.
Allows strict control of transdermal penetration rates. Permits rapid termination of drug delivery through termination of ULTS. Skin remains intact, therefore low risk of introducing infection. Less anxiety provoking or painful than injection	Minor tingling, irritation, and burning have been reported (these effects can often be minimized or eradicated with proper ULTS adjustment (Maloney et al., 1992). SC must be intact for effective drug penetration.
In many cases, greater patient satisfaction.	
Not immunologically sensitizing.	
Less risk of systemic absorption than injection.	

Table 3. Advantages and disadvantages of using sonophoresis as a physical penetration enhancer.

3.4 Applications of ultrasound

Table 4 summarizes the research on sonophoresis uses in the transdermal administration of drugs.

Anesthetics		
Research	**Outcome**	**References**
Topical skin penetration of lidocaine	Increase in the concentration of lidocaine transmitted into rabbit subdermal tissues when topical application was followed by use of ULTS	Wells et al., 1977.
Double blind, vehicle-controlled, crossover trial in healthy volunteers for lidocaine cream	No increase in absorption of lidocaine cream by using ULTS	McEnlay et al., 1985.
Trial in healthy volunteers for lidocaine oil	Other variables include differences in ULTS frequencies and drug concentrations.	Novak et al., 1964.

Skin lidocaine penetration	250 kHz induced the highest penetration of lidocaine.	Griffin & Touchstone, 1972.
Anesthetic effect of lidocaine in legs of hairless mice	ULTS in conjunction with a topical aqueous lidocaine solution was rapidly effective in inducing an anesthetic effect in the legs of hairless mice	Tachibana et al., 1993
Sonophoresis of topical benzocaine and dibucaine	No detectable increase in the rate of anesthetic penetration	Williams et al., 1990.
Administration of lidocaine hydrochloride trandermally on healthy volunteers applying 0.5 MHz ULTS.	0.5 MHz ULTS in sonophoresis for conduction anesthesia using lidocaine hydrochloride for a nerve block, it is more effective than the 1 Mhz that is widely used in clinical situations	Kim et al., 2007.
Permeation of procaine hydrochloride through cell monolayers applying therapeutical ULTS.	Extent and velocity of the permeation of procaine hydrochloride through MDCK monolayer can be controlled by sonophoresis	Hehn et al., 1996.
Analgesic and anti-inflammatory drugs		
Effect of intensity, mode, and duration of ULTS application on the transport of three non steroidal anti-inflammatory drugs (NSAIDs) across cellulose membrane and hairless rabbit-skin	Demonstrated the synergistic effect of temperature and ULTS operation parameters on drug transport of NSAIDs	Meshali et al., 2008.
Effect of an ULTS (1 MHz) on transdermal absorption of indomethacin from an ointment in rats	Intensity and duration of application play an important role in the transdermal sonophoretic delivery; intensity of 0.75 W/cm^2 for 10 min was most effective for delivering indomethacin	Miyazaki et al., 1992.
Study of the influence of ultrasound on percutaneous absorption of ketorolac tromethamine *in vitro* across hairless rat skin	A significant increase in permeation of ketorolac through rat skin was observed with the applied sonication at 3 W/cm^2 when compared with permeation at 1 and 2 W/cm^2.	Tiwari et al., 2004.
To determine if a ketorolac tromethamine (KT) gel solution could be administered *in vivo* via phonophoretic transdermal delivery using pulsed ULTS by examining its anti-inflammatory effects in a rat carrageenan inflammation model.	The transdermal application of KT gel using sonophoresis had significant anti-hyperalgesic and anti-inflammatory effects. These findings suggest that the transdermal administration of a KT gel using sonophoresis with pulsed ULTS might be useful for treating acute inflammation and pain.	Yang et al., 2008.
Application of ultraphonophoresis of 5% ibuprofen nurofen gel to affected joints of 20 patients.	Analgesic efficacy of transcutaneous 5% gel nurofen in osteoarthrosis.	Serikov et al., 2007.

Examination of therapeutic effects of sonophoresis with ketoprofen in gel form in patients with enthesopathy of the elbow.	Positive effects of sonophoresis using a pharmacologically active gel with ketoprofen were shown to be highly significant in assessments, objective (clinical examination) and subjective (interview). The pain symptoms in the elbow resolved in most of the patients.	Cabak et al., 2005.
Quantitative study of sodium diclofenac (Voltaren Emulgel, Novartis) phonophoresis in humans	Previously applied therapeutic ULTS irradiation enhances the percutaneous penetration of the topical diclofenac gel, although the mechanism remains unclear	Rosim et al., 2005.
Investigation of *in vitro* penetration and the *in vivo* transport of flufenamic acid in dependence of ULTS.	Using this *in vitro* model it is possible to compare the transdermal delivery of commercial flufenamic ointment in volunteers.	Hippius et al., 1998.
Antibiotics		
Effect of ULTS on the delivery of topically applied amphotericin B ointment in guinea pigs.	Amphotericin B content in the skin and subcutaneous fatty tissues was much higher when the drug was delivered in the presence of ULTS.	Rornanenko & Araviiskii, 1991.
Administration of tetracycline in healthy rabbits using electrophoresis and sonophoresis	It was found that the tissue levels of tetracycline administered with the modified methods of electro and sonophoresis increased with an increase in the current density or ULTS intensity, the procedure time and antibiotic concentration.	Ragelis et al., 1981.
Immunosuppressives		
Investigated the topical transport of Cyclosporin A using low-frequency US throughout rat skin	The enhanced skin accumulation of Cyclosporin A by the combination of low-frequency ULTS and chemical enhancers could help significantly to optimize the targeting of the drug without of a concomitant increase of the systemic side effects.	Liu et al., 2006.
Evaluation of the efficacy of low frequency sonophoresis (LFS) at 25KHz produced by a sonicator apparatus for treatment of alopecia areata, melasma and solar lentigo.	The study showed that LFS, a not aggressive technique, enhanced penetration of topic agents obtaining effects at the level of the epidermis, dermis and appendages (intradermal delivery), giving better results in the treatment of some cosmetic skin disorders.	Santoianni et al., 2004.

Anticancer drugs		
Application of a method using ULTS and nano/microbubbles to cancer gene therapy using prodrug activation therapy.	Dramatic reductions of the tumor size by a factor of four.	Aoi et al., 2007.
Investigation of competitive transport across skin of 5-fluorouracil into coupling gel under the influence of ULTS, heat-alone and Azone® enhancement.	Ultrasonication produced a decrease in percutaneous drug penetration. This effect was due to the diffusive loss of the hydrophilic substance 5-fluorouracil from the skin surface.	Meidan et al., 1999.
Insulin		
To determine if the 3x1 rectangular cymbal array perform significantly better than the 3x3 circular array for glucose reduction in hyperglycemic rabbits.	Using the rectangular cymbal array, the glucose decreased faster and to a level of -200.8±5.9 mg/dL after 90 min.	Luis et al., 2007.
To demonstrate ultrasonic transdermal delivery of insulin *in vivo* using rabbits with a novel, low-profile two-by-two ULTS array.	For the ULTS-insulin group, the glucose level was found to decrease to -132.6 ± 35.7 mg/dL from the initial baseline in 60 min	Lee et al., 2004.
The purpose of this study was to demonstrate the feasibility of ULTS-mediated transdermal delivery of insulin *in vivo* using rats with a novel, low profile two-by-two US array based on the "cymbal" transducer.	For the 60-min ULTS exposure group, the glucose level was found to decrease from the baseline to -267.5 ± 61.9 mg/dL in 1 h. Moreover, to study the effects of ULTS exposure time on insulin delivery, the 20-min group had essentially the same result as the 60-min exposure at a similar intensity.	Smith et al., 2003.
Corticosteroids		
Determination of the effect of ULTS on the transcutaneous absorption of dexamethasone.	A sonophoretic effect occurred with dexamethasone when its application saturated the skin.	Saliba et al., 2007.
To determine if ULTS enhances the diffusion of transdermally applied corticosteroids.	The effects of sonophoresed dexamethasone can be measured in terms of reduced collagen deposition as far down as the subcutaneous tissue but not in the submuscular or subtendinous tissue	Byl et al., 1993.
Comparison of effectiveness of 0.4% Dexamethasone sodium phosphate (DEX-P) sonophoresis (PH) with 0.4% DEX-P iontophoresis (ION) therapy in the management of patients with knee joint osteoarthritis	Significant improvement in total WOMAC scores was observed in 15 (60%) and 16 (64%) patients in the PH and ION groups respectively, indicating no significant difference in the improvement rate.	Akinbo et al., 2007.

Designing a sonophoretic drug delivery system to enhance the triamcinolone acetonide (TA) permeability.	The highest permeation of TA was observed under the ULTS treatment conditions of low frequency, high intensity, and in continuous mode.	Yang et al., 2006.
Cardiotonics		
The sonophoresis of digoxin *in vitro* through human and hairless mouse skin.	There was no enhancement of digoxin absorption across human skin by ULTS.	Machet et al., 1996.
Vasodilators		
Skin penetration enhancement effect of ULTS on methyl nicotinate in 10 healthy human volunteers.	ULTS treatment applied prior to methyl nicotinate led to enhanced percutaneous absorption of the drug	McEnlay et al., 1993.
Hormones		
Effect of permeation enhancers and application of low frequency (LUS) and high frequency ultrasound (HUS) on testosterone (TS) transdermal permeation after application of testosterone solid lipid microparticles (SLM).	Skin exposure to HUS or LUS before application of 1% dodecylamine for 30 min had no superior enhancement effect over application of either LUS or HUS alone. Application of drug loaded SLM offered skin protection against the irritation effect produced by TS and 1% DA.	El-Kamel et al., 2008.
Cicatrizants		
The effectiveness of sonophoresis on the delivery of high molecular weight (MW) hyaluronan (HA) into synovial membrane using an animal model of osteoarthritis (OA).	Synovial fluid analysis revealed increased absorption and fluorescence microscopy showed deeper penetration of both HA1000 and HA3000.	Park et al., 2005.
Calcein		
The skin permeation clearance of model hydrophilic solutes, calcein (MW 623) and-labeled dextrans [MW 4400 (FD-4) and MW 38000 (FD-40)], across the skin under the influence of ULTS.	Good correlations were observed between the $3H_2O$ flux and solute clearances and, unexpectedly, the slope values obtained from linear regression of the plots were consistent for all solutes examined.	Morimoto et al., 2005.
Oligonucleotids		
Assessment of the potential of low frequency ULTS (20 kHz, 2.4 W/cm^2) in delivering therapeutically significant quantities of anti-sense oligonucleotides into skin.	Microscopic evaluations using revealed heterogeneous penetration into the skin. Heterogeneous penetration led to the formation of localized transport pathways, which occupied about 5% of the total exposed skin area.	Tezel et al., 2004.
Stimulants		
The effect of low-frequency sonophoresis on fentanyl and caffeine permeation through human and hairless rat skin.	Discontinuous ULTS mode was found to be more effective in increasing transdermal penetration of fentanyl while transdermal transport of caffeine was enhanced by both continuous and pulsed mode.	Boucaud et al., 2001.

Calcium		
Manipulation of the Ca^{2+} content of the upper epidermis by sonophoresis across hairless mouse SC.	Sonophoresis at 15 MHz did not alter barrier function.	Menon et al., 1994.
Panax notoginseng		
Effect of a therapeutic US coupled with a Panax notoginseng gel for medial collateral ligament repair in rats.	This study reveals a positive ultrasonic effect of Panax notoginseng extract for improving the strength of ligament repair.	Ng et al., 2008.
Other applications *i)To study the mechanisms of penetration due to US throughout the skin*		
To demonstrate the calcein permeability through the localized transport regions (LTRs) from the exposure to the ULTS/ Sodium lauryl sulphate (SLS) system.	LTRs and the non-LTRs exhibit significant decreases in skin electrical resistivity relative to untreated skin, suggesting the existence of two levels of significant skin structural perturbation due to ULTS exposure in the presence of SLS.	Kushner IV et al., 2004.
To shed light on the mechanism(s) by which low-frequency ULTS (20 KHz) enhances the permeability of the skin.	Significant fractions (30%) of the intercellular lipids of SC were removed during the application of low frequency sonophoresis.	Alvarez-Roman et al., 2003.
Investigation of short time sonication effects of human skin at variable intensities and on the dynamics of fluorescein transport across the skin.	A short application of ULTS enhanced the transport of fluorescein across human skin by a factor in the range of 2–9 for full thickness skin samples and by a factor in the range of 2–28 000 for heat-stripped SC samples	Cancel et al., 2004.
Use of quantum dots as a tracer and confocal microscopy and transmission electron microscopy (TEM) as visualization methods, on low frequency sonophoresis.	ULTS significantly increased the frequency of occurrence of the otherwise scattered and separated lacunar spaces in the SC. A significant increase in lacunar dimensions was observed when 1% w/v sodium lauryl sulfate was added to the coupling medium.	Paliwal et al., 2006.
ii)Kelloids		
ULTS therapy with a water-based gel alone	"Complete flattening" of keloids in two young men when 1 MHz at 0.8 W/cm 2 was applied for approximately 4 minutes.	Walker, 1983.
iii) Tumours		
Optimization of ULTS parameters for *in vivo* bleomycin delivery	An effective antitumor effect was demonstrated in solid tumors of both murine and human cell lines.	Larkin et al., 2008.

Investigation of high-intensity focused ULTS (HIFU) exposure of (111) In-MX-B3.	The HIFU exposure shortened the peak tumor uptake time (24 vs. 48 h for the control) and increased the peak tumor uptake value (38 vs. 25 %ID/g for the control). The HIFU effect on enhancing tumor uptake was greater at earlier times up to 24 h.	Khaibullina et al., 2008.
Supurative wounds		
Treatment of suppurative wounds with ULTS.	sonophoresis of ethylenediaminetetra acetic acid with the quinoxaline antibiotic dioxidine was effective in accelerating wound purification an delimination of necrotic issues	Levenets et al., 1989.
Treatment of suppurative wounds with ULTS.	Sonophoresis of a 1% papain solution together with dimethyl sulfoxide was an effective method for treating purulent wounds and inflammatory infiltrates.	Matinian et al., 1990.

Table 4. Research on uses of sonophoresis to administer different drugs through the skin

4. Iontophoresis

Transdermal iontophoresis consists of the application of a low density current and low voltage (typically 0.5 A/cm^2) via an electrical circuit constituted by two drug reservoirs (anode and cathode) deposited on skin surface. During application of the current, the drug is repelled by the corresponding electrode and pushed through the stratum corneum. A substance can pass through the skin by electromigration, electroosmosis or passive diffusion. The latter of the three mechanisms is a result of changes caused by the electric field to the permeability of the skin, and its effects are negligible compared with those of the other two mechanisms. When ions are repelled by the electrode of the same charge and attracted by the electrode of the opposite charge is electromigration. When neutral substances are transported with the solvent flow is electroosmosis, which at physiological pH favours the movement from the anode to the skin.

The advantages and disadvantages that the iontophoretic technique offers are summarized in Table 5.

4.1 Mechanisms of action

Skin is a complex membrane and controls the movement of molecules across it in the presence of an electric field. Skin has an isoelectric point (pI) of 4–4.5. Above this pH, the carboxylic acid groups are ionized. Therefore, at higher pH values, the skin behaves as a permselective membrane which especially attracts cations that have been repelled by the anode, thus favouring the passage of molecules by electromigration (Merino et al., 1999). The movement of small sized cations (mainly Na+) generates a solvent flow that promotes the passage of non-charged molecules through the skin. This process is identified as electroosmosis (Delgado-Charro and Guy, 1994). Electrical mobility decreases with molecular weight, and, as a consequence, the electroosmotic contribution becomes increasingly important for larger molecules (Guy et al., 2000). The dependence of iontophoretic flux on the intensity of the current applied has been clearly demonstrated by Faraday's law (Sage et al., 1992): where Ja is the flux (in moles per unit time), ta is the transport number, Za is the valence of ion a, I is the current applied (Amperes), and F is Faraday's constant (Coulombs/mol). The transport number, ta, is the fraction of the total current transported by a specific ion, and is a measure of its efficiency as a charge carrier: ta=Ia / I. It follows that knowledge of a compound's transport number allows the feasibility of its iontophoretic delivery or extraction to be predicted. The sum of the transport numbers of all the ions present during iontophoresis equals 1 ($\Sigma ti=1$), illustrating the competitive nature of electrotransport.

Advantages	Disadvantages
Enhance penetration of ionized and unionized molecules. Moreover, improving the delivery of polar molecules as well as high molecular weight compounds (e. g. peptides and oligonucleotides). Enabling continuous or pulsatile delivery of drug (depending on the current applied). Permitting easier termination of drug delivery. Offering better control over the amount of drug delivered since the amount of compound delivered depends on applied current, duration of applied current, and area of skin exposed to the current. Restoration of the skin barrier functions without producing severe skin irritation. Ability to be used for systemic delivery or local (topical) delivery of drugs. Reducing considerably the inter and intraindividual variability, since the rate of drug delivery is more dependent on applied current than on stratum corneum characteristics.	Can be time-consuming to administer. The actual current density in the follicle maybe high enough to damage growing hair. SC must be intact for effective drug penetration.

Table 5. Advantages and disadvantages of using iontophoresis as a physical penetration enhancer.

4.2 Types of iontophresis

4.2.1 Direct iontophoresis

Direct iontophoresis can be anodal if the drug is neutral or positively charged and cathodal if the drug is negatively charged. Although cations have better properties for iontophoresis, anions can also increase their transdermal drug flux with respect to passive diffusion.

4.2.2 Reverse iontophoresis

Reverse iontophoresis across the skin is a potentially useful alternative for non-invasive clinical and therapeutic drug monitoring. During current application, reverse iontophoresis allows the movement of neutral and positively charged entities into the cathode while negatively charged entities move into the anode. The main problem with this is that skin contains some of the entities to be analyzed, which implies that there is a period of time within which it is necessary to withdraw skin reserves and after which it is possible to correlate extracted levels of the analytes with levels in the blood (Leboulanger et al., 2004).

4.3 Applications of iontophoresis

The most extended uses of iontophoresis are the treatment of palmoplantar hyperhidrosis and the diagnosis of cystic fibrosis. However, iontophoresis is also used for the topical delivery of others drugs such as lidocaine, acyclovir and dexamethasone. The only system commercially available at present is the fentanyl iontophoretic transdermal system. It is indicated for the shortterm management of acute postoperative pain in adult patients requiring opioid analgesia during hospitalization. Currently, the iontophoretic delivery of apomorphine for the treatment of idiopathic Parkinson's disease is being evaluated in human subjects. Peptide drugs including various series of amino acid derivatives and tripeptides, thyrotropin release hormones, LHRH and analogues, vasopressin and calcitonin can also be administered by means of this technique. One peptide that has focused the attention of researchers in the field of iontophoresis is insulin.

5. Electroporation

Electroporation is the phenomenon in which cell membrane permeability to ions and macromolecules is increased by exposing the cell to short high electric field pulses. The increase in permeability is attributed to the electric field induced "breakdown" of the cell membrane and the formation of nano- scale defects or "pores" in the membrane - and hence electro-"poration". Electroporation can be of two types - reversible and irreversible. In irreversible electroporation the electric field is such that the membrane permeabilization leads to cell death. This may be caused by either permanent permeabilization of the membrane and cell lysis (necrosis) or by temporary permeabilization of a magnitude which can cause a severe disruption of the cell homeostasis that can finally results in cell death, either necrotic or apoptotic. In reversible electroporation the electric pulse causes only a temporary increase in permeability and the cell survives. The reversible electroporation mode has numerous applications in biotechnology and medicine both, *in vitro* and *in vivo*. Irreversible electroporation has applications in the food industry, for sterilization and in medicine for tissue ablation (Ball et al., 2010).

5.1 Mechanisms of transdermal electroporation

The theory postulates two paths for electroporation induced transdermal transport, through pores formed in the multiple lipid bilayers connecting corneocytes and through appendage cells. Small lipid-soluble molecules can partition into the SC, and then diffuse across the lipid bilayer membranes, but water soluble molecules, particularly charged molecules, cannot penetrate significantly by this route. High voltage pulsing (> 50V) creates aqueous pathways ("pore") through stratum corneum (SC) lipid bilayer membranes, and short pathway segments are formed across 5--6 lipid bilayer membranes which connect adjacent corneocyte interiors forming transcellular straight-through pathways. Moderate voltage (= 5 to 50V) pulses appear to electroporate cell linings of the appendages. Temperature is considered to play a role in the permeabilization.

5.2 Advantages and disadvantages of electroporation for transdermal drug delivery

The advantages and disadvantages that the electroporation technique offers are summarized in Table 6.

Advantages	Disadvantages
Enhanced drug penetration (of selected drugs) over passive transport. Allows strict control of transdermal penetration rates. Versatility: electroporation is effective nearly with all cells and species types (Sung et al., 2003). Efficiency: a large majority of cells take in the target DNA or molecule (Huang et al., 2005). Permits rapid termination of drug delivery through termination of electroporation. The procedure may be performed with intact tissue (Heller et al., 1996). Less anxiety provoking or painful than injection. In many cases, greater patient satisfaction.	Cell damage: If the pulses are of the wrong length or intensity, some pores may become too large or fail to close after membrane discharge causing cell damage or rupture (Murthy et al., 2004). The transport of material into and out of the cell during the time of electropermeability is relatively nonspecific (Murthy et al., 2004).
Not immunologically sensitizing.	

Table 6. Advantages and disadvantages of using electroporation as a physical penetration enhancer.

5.3 Applications of electroporation

The field of skin electroporation is made of two aspects. The first deal with electroporation in a conventional sense in relation to the cells of the skin and the second is unique and relates to transdermal effects. The concept of transdermal electroporation may be traced to fundamental research on the breakdown of flat lipid bilayer membranes. Prausnitz et al., (1993) addresses the fact that transdermal transport normally occurs primarily through the intracellular lipids organized in bilayers. Small molecular weight lipophilic drugs can be effectively delivered by passive transdermal delivery. However, the stratum corneum does not permit passage of polar/hydrophilic molecules and macromolecules. The paper suggests that microsecond to millisecond electroporation type pulsed electric fields applied across the skin produce, in a manner similar to that found in studies on flat lipid bilayers, trans bilayer aqueous pores. It reports that electroporation produces transient structural changes in the skin resulting in an up to four orders of magnitude increase in transdermal mass transfer flux of polar molecules in human skin *in vitro* and animal skin *in vivo*.

6. Microneedles

The use of microneedles is another method for bypassing the stratum corneum barrier, which have been introduced as a form of transdermal drug delivery. They can penetrate the upper layer of the skin without reaching the dermis, to be an efficient method to deliver drugs transdermally in an almost painless method. The drug diffuses across the rest of the epidermis into the dermis where it is absorbed into the blood circulation. Nowadays different types of microneedles have been designed by other researchers as well, varying in their materials of fabrication, shapes, dimensions, modes of application, etc. (Chabri et al., 2009).

6.1 Microneedle types and their methods of transdermal delivery

Microneedles are available as both solid and hollow microneedles made of various materials (Figure 3). Till date, five methods of transdermal delivery mediated by microneedles have been attempted (Gill & Prausnitz, 2007): *Poke with patch approach*: It can be inserted into the skin to pierce the stratum corneum and create micro conduits through which drug can enter into the lower layers of the epidermis (Henry et al., 1998). *Coat and poke approach:* It involves coating the drug to be delivered around the surface of the microneedle. By inserting the microneedles through the skin, the drug coating dissolves off in the skin fluid and the dissolved drug diffuses through the skin into the blood microcirculation. The coating methods are used to roll coating, spray coating and dip coating (Gill & Prausnitz, 2006). *Dip and scrape:* The dip and scrape method involves placing the array in contact with the drug solution and then scraping multiple times across the skin to create microabbrassions (Mikszta et al., 2002). *Dissolving microneedles:* It is referred to microneedles made from a biodegradable polymeric material with the drugs encapsulated inside them. In this method, the drug is released in a controlled manner as the microneedle dissolves off when inserted into the skin (Lee W. J et al., 2007). *Injection through hollow microneedles:* This occurs where the microneedles are designed with holes at the centre or with side openings through which drugs are microinjected into the lower layers of the skin and then diffuses across the viable skin until it reaches the blood vessels in the dermis (Griss & Stemme, 2003).

Solid microneedles: These are easier to fabricate, have better mechanical strength and sharper tips as compared to hollow microneedles (Rhoxed et al., 2008a). Solid silicon microneedles have been widely used for the transdermal drug delivery studies (Donnelly et al., 2009; Haq et al., 2009). However, silicon is expensive, not biocompatible and brittle. Therefore it breaks easily during the penetration across skin (Chen et al., 2008). Polymer has been used as an alternative material because it is a cheaper and stronger material which could reduce tissue damage (Fernandez et al., 2009). Polymer increases the bluntness of the microneedle tip due to the low modulus and yield strength of polymer. Polymer microneedles have a main limitation with its mechanical properties which could cause needle failure during the penetration across skin (Park et al., 2007). Bevelled tip microneedles have been fabricated using biodegradable polymers (Park, 2004). Metal is the third material used to manufacture microneedles. It is mechanically strong and relatively cheap to produce.

Hollow microneedles: The purpose of this type of microneedles is to deliver drugs through the bore at the needle tip. This reduces the sharpness of needle tip which affect the penetration of this needle into skin. These issues have been resolved recently including openings at the side in the microneedles rather than at the bottom (Roxhed et al., 2008). These microneedles have their tip closed initially; however they can be opened on insertion into the skin where the tip dissolves in the high saline solution in the interstitial fluid. The tips can also be opened as a result of applied pressure. It has been proposed the use of rotary drilling and mechanical vibration as methods to enhance insertion of hollow microneedles and the fluid infusion flow rate (Wang et al., 2006).

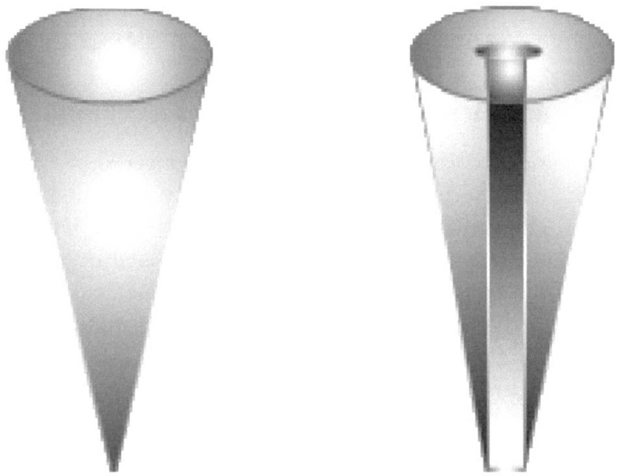

Fig. 3. Two dimensional view of hollow and solid microneedle.

6.2 Microneedles manufacturing

The methods that have been adopted for microneedle fabrication include wet etching, deep reactive ion etching (DRIE) (Teo et al., 2005), microinjection moulding (Sammoura et al., 2007), isotropic etching, isotropic etching in combination with deep etching and wet etching respectively, dry etching, isotropic and anisotropic, photolithography, thin film deposition (Moon & Lee, 2003), laser cutting (Martanto et al., 2004), and inclined LIGA process (Perennes et al., 2006). Studies have shown that factors such as microneedle geometry, coating depth on solid microneedle and skin thickness affect the drug delivery efficiency using microneedles (Al-Qallaf et al., 2009a; 2009b). To ensure that both the insertion and delivery occur at the right location, they should be sharp enough and at least 100μm in length (Stoeber & Liepmann, 2000).

6.3 Microneedles applications

Vaccination against virus: Researchers have recently presented microneedle patches as a better alternative for immunization. The vaccine can be coated unto microneedle array and presented as a simple patch which can allow patients to immunize themselves without the necessity for intense medical training (Stoeber & Liepmann, 2005). *Cutaneous fluid extraction and glucose monitoring:* A prototype of a disposable microneedle based glucose monitoring devices has been designed in which, the fluid extraction chamber attached to the microneedle can be connected to a sensing device which measures and indicates the glucose concentration in the body (Zimmermann et al., 2003). *Acne treatment:* The treatment is limited by the low rate of penetration of drugs through the stratum corneum. So, experiments have been carried out by applying the TheraJectMAT™ dissolving microneedles containing API in a GRAS matrix to the surface of human skin with acne (Kwon, 2006). *Delivery of nanoparticles:* It was showed that the delivery of particles of 1μm in diameter is enhanced when the skin is pre-treated with microneedles by adopting the poke with patch approach. Therefore, it seems to us that the delivery of micro and nano-particles is important in order to facilitate controlled/ delayed delivery after the drug is inserted into the skin (McAllister et al., 2003). *Insulin delivery:* Microneedles have been shown to deliver insulin with a significant biological effect as the blood glucose concentration was reduced by substantial amount using microneedles.

7. Nanocarriers

Nanocarriers are so small to be detected by immune system and they can deliver the drug in the target organ using lower drug doses in order to reduce side effects. Nanocarriers can be administrated into the organisms by all the routes; one of them is the dermal route. The nanocarriers most used and investigated for topic/transdermal drug delivery in the pharmaceutical field are liposomes, dendrimers, nanoparticles and nanoemulsions (Table 7).

Nanocarrier	Size	Preparation Methods	Characteristics	References
Nanoparticles	10-1000 nm	In situ polymerization, emulsification-evaporation, emulsification-diffusion, emulsification-diffusion by solvent displacement	Solid or hollow particles wich have entraped, binded or encapsulated drugs.	Domínguez-Delgado et al., 2011; oppimath et al., 2001
Solid lipid nanoparticles	50-1000 nm	High-pressure homogenization.	Similar to polymeric nanoparticles but made of solid lipids.	Almeida & Souto, 2007
Inorganic nanoparticles	<50nm	Sol-gel technique	Nanometric particles, made up of inorganic compounds such as silica, titania and alumina.	García-González, 2009
Liposomes	25 nm-100 μm	Sonication, extrusion, mozafari method	Vesicles composed of one or more concentric lipid bilayers, separated by water or aqueous buffer compartments.	El Maghraby et al., 2008
Dendrimers	3–10 nm	Polymerization	Macromolecular high branched structures.	Menjoge et al., 2010
Quantum dots	2-10nm	Colloidal assembly, viral assembly, electrochemical assembly.	Made up of organic surfactants, precursors and solvents.	Rzigalinski & Strobl, 2009
Lipid globules	1-100 nm	Emulsification espontaneous systems.	Multicomponent fluid made of water, a hydrophobic liquid, and one or several surfactants resulting in a stable system.	Dan et al., 2010

Nanocarrier	Size	Preparation Methods	Characteristics	References
Lipid microcylinders	<1 µm	Self emulsification	Self organizing system in which surfactants crystallize into tightly packed bilayers that spontaneously form cylinders	Dodla & Bellamkonda, 2008
Lipid microbubbles	<2 µm	Sonication	Gas filled microspheres stabilized by phospholipids, polymers or low density proteins.	Tartis et al., 2008
Lipospheres	0.2-100 µm	Melt method, multiple microemulsion, cosolvent method	Solid lipid core stabilized by a monolayer of phospholipids molecules embedded in the particle surface.	Fang et al., 2007
Ethosomes	<400 nm	Cold method, hot method	Non invasive delivery carriers that enable drugs to reach the deep skin layers and/or the systemic circulation.	Elsayed et al., 2006
Aquasomes	60-300 nm	Self-assembling of hydroxyapatite by co-precipitation method	The particle core is composed of noncrystalline calcium phosphate or ceramic diamond, and it is covered by a polyhydroxyl oligomeric film.	Rojas-Oviedo et al., 2007
Pharmacosomes	<200 nm	Hand-shaking method, Ether-injection method	Pure drug vesicles formed by amphiphilic drugs	Jin et al., 2006
Colloidosomes	200 nm – 1.5 µm	Self-assembly of colloidal particles at the interface of emulsion droplets	Hollow capsules with elastic shells.	Rossier-Miranda et al., 2009
Niosomes	10-1000 nm	Self-assembly of nonionic surfactant	Bilayered structures made of non-ionic surfactant vesicles.	Hong et al., 2009
Nanoemulsions	20-200 nm	High-pressure, homogenization, microfluidization, phase inversion Temperature.	Submicron emulsions o/w or w/o	Elnaggar et al., 2009

Table 7. Examples of Nanocarriers used for transdermal drug delivery

7.1 Liposomes

Liposomes are hollow lipid bilayer structures that can transport hydrophilic drugs inside the core and hydrophobic drugs between the bilayer (Bangham, 1993). They are structures made of cholesterol and phospholipids. They can have different properties depending on the excipients included and the process of their elaboration. The nature of liposomes makes them one of the best alternatives for drug delivery because they are non-toxic and remain inside the bloodstream for a long time. Liposomes can be surface-charged as neutral, negative or positive, depending on the functional groups and pH medium. Liposomes can encapsulate both lipophilic and hydrophilic drugs in a stable manner, depending on the polymer added to the surface (Rodriguez-Justo & Morae et al., 2011). There are small unilamellar vesicles (25 nm to 100nm), medium-sized unilamellar vesicles (100 nm and 500nm), large unilamellar vesicles, giant unilamellar vesicles, oligolamellar vesicles, large multilamellar vesicles and multivesicular vesicles (500 nm to microns). The thickness of the membrane measures approximately 5 to 6 nm. These shapes and sizes depend of the preparation technique, the lipids used and process variables. Depending on these parameters, the behavior both *in vivo* and *in vitro* can change and opsonization processes, leakage profiles, disposition in the body and shelf life are different due to the type of liposome (Rodriguez-Justo & Morae et al., 2011).

Liposomes preparation techniques follow three basic steps with particular features depending on safety, potential scale up and simplicity: 1) Lipid must be hydrated, 2) Liposomes have to be sized and 3) Nonencapsulated drug has to be removed. The degree of transdermal drug penetration is affected by the lamellarity, lipid composition, charge on the liposomal surface, mode of application and the total lipid concentrations (Cevc & Blume, 1992). Some examples of drugs delivered throughout the skin by using liposomes are melatonin (Dubey et al., 2007b), indinavir (Dubey et al., 2010), amphotericin B (Manosroi et al., 2004), methotrexate (Dubey et al., 2007a), ketoprofen (Maestrelli et al., 2005), estradiol (Essa et al., 2004), clindamicyn hydrochloride and lignocaine (Sharma et al., 1994).

7.2 Dendrimers

Dendrimers are monodisperse populations that are structurally and chemically uniform. They allow conjugation with numerous functional groups due to the nature of their branches. The amount of branches increases exponentially and dendrimers growth is typically about 1 nm per generation (Svenson & Tomalia, 2005). The dendrimers classification is based on the number of generations. After the creation of a core, the stepwise synthesis is called first generation; after that, every stepwise addition of monomers creates the next generation. This approach allows an iterative synthesis, providing the ability to control both molecular weight and architecture.

The kind of polymer chosen to construct the dendrimer by polimerization is very important with regard to the final architecture and features. In addition, the use of branched monomers has the peculiarity of providing tailored loci for site-specific molecular recognition and encapsulation. Notably, 3D and fractal architecture, as well as the peripheral functional groups, provide dendrimers with important characteristic physical and chemical properties. In comparison with linear polymers, dendritic structures have "dendritic voids" that give these molecules important and useful features. These spaces inside dendrimers can mimic the molecular recognition performed by natural proteins. Furthermore, dendrimers have a high surface-charge density due to ionizable groups that help them to attach drugs by electrostatic forces, regardless of the stoichimetry. This dendrimer-drug association provides drugs with better solubility, increasing their transport through biological membranes and sometimes increasing drug stability. The number of molecules that can be incorporated into dendrimers is related to the number of surface functional groups; therefore, later-generation dendrimers are more easily incorporated into dendritic structure. However, not all the functional groups are available for interaction due to steric volume, molecule rotation or stereochemistry effects. Dendrimers can have positive and negative charges, which allows them to complex different types of drugs (Kabanov et al., 1998). The main problems with this kind of transdermal carrier are poor biodegradation and inherent cytotoxicity (Parekh, 2007). In order to reduce their toxicity, dendrimers have been linked to peptides and which are formed from amino acids linked via peptide-amide bonds to the branches of dendrimers in the core or on the surface. When they are bio-transformed, dendrimer-peptide systems produce amino-acid derivatives. Finally, the synthesis of these structures is less expensive and purification does not present any difficulty (Niederhafner et al., 2005). Due to their form and size, these molecules can carry drugs, imaging agents, etc. Dendrimers interact with lipids present in membranes, and they show better permeation in cell cultures and intestinal membranes (Cheng et al., 2008). Dendrimers also act like solubility enhancers, increasing the permeation of lipophilic drugs; nevertheless, they are not good carriers for and hydrophilic drugs.

7.3 Nanoparticles

Nanoparticles are smaller than 1,000 nm. Nowadays, it is possible to insert many types of materials such as drugs, proteins, peptides, DNA, etc. into the nanoparticles. They are constructed from materials designed to resist pH, temperature, enzymatic attack, or other problems (Huang L. et al., 2010; Wei et al., 2010). The nanoparticle technology can be divided into three stages: first generation (involves those nanoparticles that had only one component in their structure and these delivery systems are able to transport drugs in the blood until they reach the target), second generation (implies nanoparticles made of one main component and additional substances and these complexes are able to cross barriers and reach difficult targets such as the brain) and third generation is represented by nanoparticles that can be made of nanoparticles with one main component combined with a second component to reach a specific target (Cui et al., 2005; Herffernan & Murthy, 2005). Moreover, nanoparticles can be classified as nanospheres or nanocapsules (Figure 4). Nanospheres are solid-core structures and nanocapsules are hollow-core structures (Yoo et al., 2005). Nanoparticles can be composed of polymers, lipids, polysaccharides and proteins (Goswami et al., 2010; Li et al., 2009). Nanoparticles preparation techniques are based on their physicochemical properties. They are made by emulsification-diffusion by solvent displacement, emulsification-polymerization, in situ-polymerization, gelation, nanoprecipitation, solvent evaporation/extraction, inverse salting out, dispersion polymerization and other derived from these one.

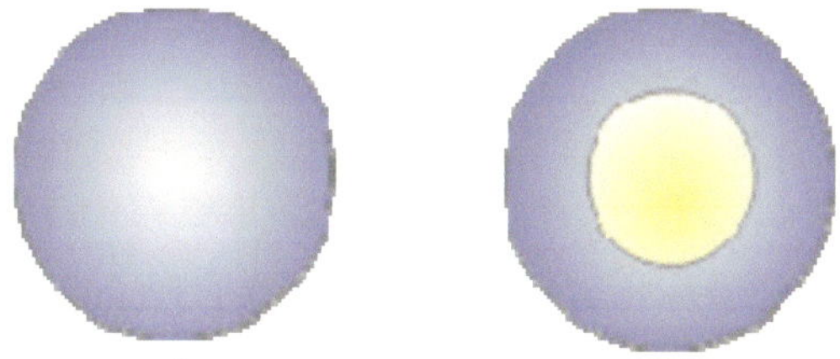

Fig. 4. a) Nanospheres and b) nanocapsules.

7.4 Nanoemulsions

Nanoemulsion are isotropic dispersed systems of two non miscible liquids, normally consisting of an oily system dispersed in an aqueous system (o/w nanoemulsion), or an aqueous system dispersed in an oily system but forming droplets or other oily phases of nanometric sizes (100 nm). They can be stable (methastable) for long times due to the extremely small sizes and the use of adequate surfactants. Nanoemulsions can use hydrophobic and hydrophilic drugs because it is possible to make both w/o or o/w nanoemulsions (Sonneville-Aubrun, et al. 2004). They are non-toxic and non-irritant systems and they can be used for skin or mucous membranes, parenteral and non parenteral administration in general and they have been used in the cosmetic field. Nanoemulsions can be prepared by three methods mainly: high-pressure homogenization, microfluidization and phase inversion temperature. Transdermal delivery using nanoemulsions has been reduced due to the stability problems inherent to this dosage form. Some examples of drugs using nanoemulsions to transdermal drug delivery are gamma tocopherol, caffeine, plasmid DNA, aspirin, methyl salicylate, insulin and nimesulide (Shakeel & Ramadan, 2010).

8. Conclusions

Transdermal drug delivery has several potential advantages over other parenteral delivery methods. Apart from the convenience and noninvasiveness, the skin also provides a "reservoir" that sustains delivery over a period of days. Furthermore, it offers multiple sites to avoid local irritation and toxicity, yet it can also offer the option to concentrate drugs at local areas to avoid undesirable systemic effects. However, at present, the clinical use of transdermal delivery is limited by the fact that very few drugs can be delivered transdermally at a viable rate. This difficulty is because the skin forms an efficient barrier for most molecules, and few noninvasive methods are known to significantly enhance the penetration of this barrier.

In order to increase the range of drugs available for transdermal delivery the use of chemical and physical enhancement techniques have been developed in an attempt to compromise skin barrier function in a reversible manner without concomitant skin irritation. Recently, several alternative physical methods have emerged to transiently break the stratum corneum barrier and also the use of chemical enhancers continues expanding. The projectile methods use propelled microparticles and nanoparticles to penetrate the skin barrier. Microneedle arrays are inserted through the skin to create pores. "Microporation" creates arrays of pores in the skin by heat and radio frequency ablation. Also, ultrasound has been employed to disrupt the skin barrier. All these methods have their own advantages and drawbacks, but a reality is that new developments are expected in the future to make these methods even more versatile.

9. Acknowledgments

José Juan Escobar-Chávez wishes to acknowledge PAPIIT TA 200312 y PAPIIT IN 209709-3. The authors report no conflict of interests.

10. References

Aditya NP, Patankar S, Madhusudhan B, Murthy RSR & Souto EB. (2010). Arthemeter-loaded lipid nanoparticles produced by modified thin-film hydration: Pharmacokinetics, toxicological and *in vivo* anti-malarial activity. *European Journal of Pharmaceutical Sciences*, Vol. 40, pp.448-455, ISSN 0928-0987.

Agyralides, GG.; Dallas PP.; Rekkas, DM. (2004). Development and *in vitro* evaluation of furosemide transdermal formulations using experimental design techniques. *International Journal of Pharmaceutics*, Vol. 281, No.1-2, (August 2004), pp. 35-43, *ISSN 0378-5173*.

Akinbo, SR.; Aiyejusunle, CB.; Akinyemi, OA.; Adesegun, SA, & Danesi MA. (2007). Comparison of the therapeutic efficacy of phonophoresis and iontophoresis using dexamethasone sodium phosphate in the management of patients with knee ostheoarthritis. *Nigerian Postgraduate Medical Journal*; Vol. 14, No. 3, (September 2007), pp.190-94, ISSN 1117-1936.

Allan, G. Azone®. (1995). In: *Percutaneous Penetration Enhancers*, Smith EW, Maibach HI, Eds, pp. 129-3, Florida, Boca Raton.

Almeida AJ, Souto E. (2007). Solid lipid nanoparticles as a drug delivery system for peptides and proteins. *Advanced Drug Delivery Reviews*, vol. 59 pp.478-490, ISSN 0169-409X.

Al-Qallaf B, Das DB & Davidson A. (2009a). Transdermal drug delivery by coated microneedles: Geometry effects on drug concentration in blood. *Asia-Pacific Journal of Chemical Engineering*. Vol. 4, No. 6, (November/December 2009), pp. 845-857, ISSN 1932-2143.

Al-Qallaf B, Das DB. (2009b). Optimizing microneedle arrays to increase skin permeability for transdermal drug delivery. *Annals of the New York Academy of Sciences*. 1161: 83-94.

Alvarez-Roman R, Naik A, Kalia YN, Guy RH & Fessi H. (2004). Skin penetration and distribution of polymeric nanoparticles. *Journal of Controlled Release*, Vol. 99, pp.53-62, ISSN 0168-3659.

Alvarez-Román, R.; Merino, G.; Kalia, YN.; Naik, A, Guy & RH. (2003). Skin permeability enhancement by low frequency sonophoresis: Lipid extraction and transport pathways. *Journal of Pharmaceutical Sciences*, Vol. 92, No. 6, (June 2003), pp. 1138-46, ISSN 0022-3549.

Amnuaikit, C.; Ikeuchi, I.; Ogawara, K.; Higaki, K. & Kimura, T. (2005). Skin permeation of propranolol from polymeric film containing terpene enhancers for transdermal use. *International Journal of Pharmaceutics*, Vol. 289, No. 1-2, (January 2005), pp.167-78, ISSN 0378-5173.

Amrish, C. & Kumar SP. (2009). Transdermal delivery of ketorolac. *Yakugaku Zasshi*, Vol.129, No.3, (March 2009), pp. 373-9, ISSN *1347-5231*.

Aoi, A.; Watanabe, Y, Mori S, et al. (2007). Herpes simplex virus thymidine kinase mediated suicide gene therapy using nano/microbubbles and ultrasound. *Ultrasound In Medicine & Biology*, Vol. 34, No. 39, (March 2008) pp. 425-434, ISSN *0301-5629*.

Arias JL, López-Viota M, López-Viota J & Delgado AV. (2009). Development of iron/ethylcellulose (core/shell) nanoparticles loaded with diclofenac sodium for arthritis treatment. *International Journal of Pharmaceutics*. Vol.382, pp.270-276, ISSN: 0378-5173.

Babu, RJ.; Dhanasekaran, M.; Vaithiyalingam, SR.; Singh, PN. & Pandit, JK. (2008). Cardiovascular effects of transdermally delivered bupranolol in rabbits: effect of chemical penetration enhancers. *Life Science*, Vol. 82, No. 5-6, (January 2008), pp. 273-8, ISSN 0024-3205.

Balaguer-Fernández, C.; Padula, C.; Femenía-Font, A.; Merino, V.; Santi, P. & López-Castellano A. (2010). Development and evaluation of occlusive systems employing polyvinyl alcohol for transdermal delivery of sumatriptan succinate. *Drug Delivery*, Vol. 17, No. 2, (February 2010), pp. 83-91, ISSN *1521-0464*.

Ball C, Thomson KR, Kavnoudias H. Irreversible Electroporation: A New Challenge in "Out of Operating Theater" Anesthesia. Anesthesia Analgesia, Vol. 110, No. 5, (May 2010), pp. 1305-9, ISSN 1526-7598.

Banga AK, Bose S & Ghosh TK. (1999). Iontophoresis and electroporation: comparisons and contrasts. *International Journal of Pharmaceutics*. Vol.179 pp. 1–19, ISSN: 0378-5173.

Bangham AD. (1993). Liposomes: the Babraham connection. *Chemistry and Physics of Lipids*. Vol. 64, pp.275-285, ISSN 0009-3084.

Barry, BW & Williams, AC. (1991). Terpenes and the lipid-protein-partititioning theory of skin penetration enhancement. *Pharmaceutical Research*, Vol. 8, No. 1, (January 1991), pp. 17–24, ISSN 1573-904X.

Barry, BW. (1983). *Dermatological Formulations: Percutaneous Absorption*, Marcel Dekker, ISBN 0824717295, New York.

Barry, BW. (2001). Novel mechanisms and devices to enable successful transdermal drug delivery. *European Journal of Pharmaceutical Sciences*, Vol. 14, No. 2, (September 2001), pp. 101–4, ISSN 0928-0987.

Becker SM, Kuznetsov AV. (2007). Numerical assessment of thermal response associated with *in vivo* skin electroporation: the importance of the composite skin model. Journal of Biomechanical Engineering, Vol. 129, No. 3, (June 2007), pp.330-40, ISSN 0148-0731.

Boucaud, A.; Machet, L.; Arbeille, B.; et al. (2001). In vitro study of low-frequency ultrasound-enhanced transdermal transport of fentanyl and caffeine across human and hairless rat skin. *International Journal of Pharmaceutics*, Vol. 228, No. 1-2, (October 2001), pp. 69-77, ISSN 0378-5173.

Bounoure, F.; Lahiani-Skiba, M.; Besnard, M.; Arnaud, P.; Mallet, E. & Skiba M. (2008). Effect of iontophoresis and penetration enhancers on transdermal absorption of metopimazine. *Journal of Dermatological Science*, Vol. 52, No. 3, (December 2008), pp. 170-7, ISSN *0923-1811*.

Byl, NN.; McKenzie, A.; Halliday, B.; Wong, T.& O'Connell J. (1993) The effects of phonophoresis with corticosteroids controlled pilots study. *Journal of Orthopaedic Sports Physical Therapy*, Vol. 18, No. 5, (November 1993), pp. 590-600, ISSN 0190-6011.

Cabak, A.; Maczewska, M.; Lyp, M.; Dobosz, J. & Gasiorowska U. (2005). The effectiveness of phonophoresis with ketoprofen in the treatment of epocondylopathy. *Ortopedia, Traumatologia, Rehabilitacja*; Vol. 37, No. 6, (December 2005), pp. 660-65. ISSN 1509-3492.

Cancel, LM.; Tarbell, JM. & Ben-Jebria A. (2004). Fluorescein permeability and electrical resistance of human skin during low frequency ultrasound application. *Journal of Pharmacuy and Pharmacology*, Vol. 56, No. 9, (September 2004), pp. 1109-18, ISSN 0022-3573.

Cázares-Delgadillo, J.; Naik, A.; Kalia, YN.; Quintanar-Guerrero, D. & Ganem-Quintanar A. (2005) Skin permeation enhancement by sucrose esters: A pH-dpendent phenomenon. *International Journal of Pharmaceutics*, Vol. 297, No. 1-2, (June 2005), pp. 204-212, ISSN 0378-5173.

Cevc G, Blume G. (1992). Lipid vesicles penetrate into intact skin owing to the transdermal osmotic gradients and hydration force. Biochimica et Biophysica Acta. *Vol.* 1104, pp. 226-232.

Chabri F, Bouris K, Jones T, Barrow D, Hann A, Allender C, Brain K & Birchall J. (2009). Microfabricated silicon microneedles for nonviral cutaneous gene delivery. *The British Journal of Dermatology*, Vol. 150, No. 5, pp. 869–77, ISSN: 0007-0963.

Chen B, Wei J, Tay FE, Wong YT & Iliescu C. (2008). Silicon microneedle array with biodegradable tips for transdermal drug delivery. *Microsystem Technologies*. Vol. 14, No. 7, pp. 1015-19, ISSN: 0946-7076.

Chen T, D'Addio SM, Kennedy MT, Swietlow A, Kevrekidis IG & Panagiotopoulos AZ. (2009). Protected Peptide Nanoparticles: Experiments and Brownian Dynamics Simulations of the Energetics of Assembly. Nano Letters, Vol. 9, pp. 2218-2222, ISSN: 1530-6984.

Cheng Y, Xu Z, Ma M & Xu T. (2008). Dendrimers as drug carriers: Applications in different routes of drug administration. *Journal of Pharmaceutical Sciences*, Vol. 97, pp.123-143, ISSN 0022-3549.

Clarke, L.; Edwards, A.; Graham, E. (2004) Acoustic streaming: an in vitro study. *Ultrasound In Medicine & Biol*ogy, Vol. 30, No. 4, (April 2004), pp. 559–62, ISSN 0301-5629.

Cui Z, Han S, Padinjarae D & Huang L. (2005). Immunsotimulation mechanism of LPD nanoparticles as a vaccine carrier. Molecular Pharmacology, Vol. 2, pp. 22-28, ISSN: 0026-895X.

Dan Y, Liu H, Gao W & Chen S. (2010). Activities of essential oils from Asarum heterotropoides var. mandshuricum against five phytopathogens. *Crop Protection*. Vol. 29, No. 295-299. ISSN: 0261-2194.

Davis SP, Martanto W, Allen MG & Prausnitz MR. (2005). Hollow metal microneedles for insulin delivery to diabetic rats. IEEE T. *BioMedical Engineering*, Vol. 52, No 5, pp. 909-15, ISSN: 0018-9294.

Delgado-Charro MB, Guy RH. (1994). Characterization of convective solvent flow during iontophoresis. Pharmaceutical Research, Vol. 11, No. 7, (July 1994), pp. 29-35, ISSN 0724-8741.

Díaz-Torres, R. (2010). Transdermal nanocarriers. In: *Current Technologies to Increase the Transdermal Delivery of Drugs*, José Juan Escobar-Chávez/Virginia Merino (Eds.), pp., 120-40, Bentham Science Publishers, ISBN 978-1-60805-191-5, The Netherlands.

Dodla MC, Bellamkonda RV. (2008). Differences between the effect of anisotropic and isotropic laminin and nerve growth factor presenting scaffolds on nerve regeneration across long peripheral nerve gaps. *Biomaterials.* Vol. 29, pp.33-46, ISSN: 0142-9612.

Domínguez-Delgado C. L., Rodríguez-Cruz I. M. & López-Cervantes M. (2010). Chapter 1: The skin a valuable route for administration of drugs. In: José Juan Escobar-Chávez (Ed), *Current Technologies To Increase The Transdermal Delivery Of Drugs*. Bentham Science Publishers Ltd. ISBN: 978-1-60805-191-5, Bussum, The Netherlands.

Domínguez-Delgado C. L., Rodríguez-Cruz I. M., Escobar-Chávez J. J., Calderón-Lojero I. O., Quintanar-Guerrero David & Ganem-Quintanar Adriana. (2011). Triclosan nanoparticles as a novel option for acne treatment. *European Journal of Pharmaceutics and Biopharmaceutics.* IN PRESS, ISSN: 0928-0987.

Donnelly RF, Morrow DI, McCarron PA, Woolfson AD, Morrissey A, Juzenas P, Juzeniene A, Lani, V, McCarthy HO & Moan J. (2009). Microneedle arrays permit enhanced intradermal delivery of a preformed photosensitizer. *Photochemistry and Photobiology.* Vol. 85, pp. 195-204, ISSN 1751-1097.

Dubey V, Mishra D & Jain NK. (2007b). Melatonin loaded ethanolic liposomes: Physicochemical characterization and enhanced transdermal delivery. *European Journal of Pharmaceutics and Biopharmaceutics.* Vol. 67, pp. 398-405, ISSN: 0928-0987.

Dubey V, Mishra D, Dutta T, Nahar M, Saraf DK & Jain NK. (2007a). Dermal and transdermal delivery of an anti-psoriatic agent via ethanolic liposomes. *Journal of Controlled Release,* Vol. 123, pp.148-154, ISSN 0168-3659.

Dubey V, Mishra D, Nahar M, Jain V & Jain NK. (2010). Enhanced transdermal delivery of an anti-HIV agent via ethanolic liposomes. *Nanomedicine: Nanotechnology, Biology and Medicine.* Vol. 6. No. 4, (2010 August), pp. 590-6, ISSN: 1549-9634.

El Maghraby GM, Barry BW & Williams AC. (2008). Liposomes and skin: From drug delivery to model membranes. *European Journal of Pharmaceutical Sciences,* Vol. 34, pp.203-222, ISSN 0928-0987.

El-Kamel, AH.; Al-Fagih, IM. & Alsarra IA. (2008). Effect of sonophoresis and chemical enhancers on testosterone transdermal delivery from solid lipid microparticles:an in vitro study, *Current Drug Delivery,* Vol. 5, No. 1, (January 2008), pp. 20-26, ISSN 1567-2018.

Elnaggar YSR, El-Massik MA & Abdallah OY. (2009). Self-nanoemulsifying drug delivery systems of tamoxifen citrate: Design and optimization. *International Journal of Pharmaceutics.* Vol.380, pp.133-141, ISSN: 0378-5173.

Elsayed MMA, Abdallah OY, Naggar VF & Khalafallah NM. (2006). Deformable liposomes and ethosomes: Mechanism of enhanced skin delivery. *International Journal of Pharmaceutics.* Vol. 322, pp. 60-66, ISSN: 0378-5173.

Escobar-Chávez JJ, Bonilla-Martínez D, Villegas-González M.A. (2010b). Sonophoresis: A valuable physical enhancer to increase transdermal drug delivery. In: *Current Technologies to Increase the Transdermal Delivery of Drugs,* José Juan Escobar-Chávez/Virginia Merino (Eds.), pp. 53-76, Bentham Science Publishers, ISBN 978-1-60805-191-5, The Netherlands.

Escobar-Chávez JJ, Melgoza-Contreras LM, López-Cervantes M, et al. (2009c). The tape stripping technique as a valuable tool for evaluating topical applied compounds. In: *Frontiers in Drug Design & Discovery,* Gary W. Caldwell /Atta-ur-Rahman / Z.

Yan / M. Iqbal Choudhary (Eds.) Vol. 4, pp. 189-227, Bentham Science Publishers, eISBN 978-1-60805-202-8.

Escobar-Chávez JJ, Merino-Sanjuán V, López-Cervantes M, et al. (2009d). The use of iontophoresis in the administration of nicotine and new non nicotine drugs through the skin for smoking cessation. *Current Drug Discovery Technologies*, Vol. 6, No. 3, (September 2009), 171-185, ISSN 1570-1638.

Escobar-Chávez JJ, Quintanar-Guerrero D, and Ganem-Quintanar A. (2005). *In vivo* skin permeation of sodium naproxen formulated in PF-127 gels: Effect of Azone® and Transcutol®. *Drug Development and Industrial Pharmacy*; Vol. 31 No. 4-5, (May 2005), pp.447-54, ISSN 0363-9045.

Escobar-Chávez, JJ. & Merino, V. 2010a. *Current Technologies to increase the Transdermal Delivery of Drugs*, Bentham Science Publishers, ISBN: 978-1-60805-191-5, Bussum, The Netherlands.

Escobar-Chávez, JJ.; Bonilla-Martínez, D.; Villegas-González, A.; Rodríguez-Cruz, IM.; Domínguez-Delgado, CL. (2009a). The use of sonophoresis in the administration of drugs through the skin. *Journal of Pharmacy and Pharmaceutical Sci*ences, Vol. 12, No. 1, (April 2009), pp. 88-115, ISSN: 1482-1826.

Escobar-Chávez, JJ.; Bonilla-Martínez, D.; Villegas-González, A.; Revilla-Vazquez, AL. (2009b). The electroporation as an efficient physical enhancer for transdermal drug delivery. *Journal of Clinical Pharmaco*logy, Vol. 49, No. 11, (August 2008), pp. 1262-83, ISSN: 0091-2700.

Escobar-Chávez, JJ.; López-Cervantes, M.; Naïk, A.; et al. (2006). Applications of the thermoreversible Pluronic F-127 gels in pharmaceutical formulations. *Journal of Pharmacy and Pharmceutical Sciences*; Vol. 9, No. 3, (November 2006), pp. 339-58, ISSN 1482-1826.

Escobar-Chávez, JJ.; Merino, V.; Díez-Sales, O.; Nácher-Alonso, A.; Ganem-Quintanar, A.; Herráez, M.; Merino-Sanjuán, M. (2008). The tape-stripping technique as a method for drug quntification in the skin. *Journal of Pharmacy and Pharmaceutical Sci*ences, Vol. 11, No. 1, (March 2008):104-30, ISSN 1482-1826.

Escobar-Chávez, JJ.; Merino, V.; Díez-Sales, O.; Nácher-Alonso, A.; Ganem-Quintanar, A.; Herráez, M.; Merino-Sanjuán, M. (2011). Transdermal nortriptyline hydrocloride patch formulated within a chitosan matrix intended to be used for smoking cessation. *Pharmaceutical Development Technology*, Vol. 16, No. 2, (February 2010), pp. 162-9, ISSN *1083-7450*

Escribano, E.; Calpena, AC.; Queralt, J.; Obach, R.; Doménech J. (2003). Assessment of diclofenac permeation with different formulations: anti-inflammatory study of a selected formula, *European Journal of Pharmaceutical Sciences*, Vol. 19, No. 4, (July 2003), pp. 203-210, ISSN 0928-0987.

Essa EA, Bonner MC & Barry BW. (2004). Electrically assisted skin delivery of liposomal estradiol; phospholipid as damage retardant. *Journal of Controlled Release*, Vol. 95, pp.535-546, ISSN 0168-3659.

Fang J, Hung C, Liao M & Chien C. (2007). A study of the formulation design of acoustically active lipospheres as carriers for drug delivery. *European Journal of Pharmaceutics and Biopharmaceutics*. Vol. 67, pp. 67-75.

Fang JY, Lin HH, Chen HI, Tsai YH. (1998). Development and evaluation on transdermal delivery of enoxacin via chemical enhancers and physical iontophoresis. *Journal of Controlled Release*, Vol. 54, No. (August 1998), pp. 293-304, ISSN *0168-3659.*

Fang, JY.; Fang, CL.; Huang, YB.; Tsai, YH. (2002). Transdermal iontophoresis of sodium nonivamide acetate. V. Combined effect of pre-treatment by penetration enhancers. *International Journal of Pharm*aceutics, Vol. 235, No. 1-2, (March 2002), 95-105, ISSN 0378-5173.

Fang, JY.; Leu, YL.; Wang, YY.; Tsai, YH. (2002). *In vitro* topical application and *in vivo* pharmacodynamic evaluation of nonivamide hydrogels using Wistar rat as an animal model. *European Journal of Pharmaceutical Sciences*, Vol. 15, No. 5, (June 2002), pp. 417-23, ISSN 0928-0987.

García-González CA, Sampaio da Sousa AR, Argemí A, López Periago A, Saurina J, Duarte CM & Domingo C. (2009). Production of hybrid lipid-based particles loaded with inorganic nanoparticles and active compounds for prolonged topical release. *International Journal of Pharmaceutics.* Vol.382 No.1-2 (December 2009), pp.296-304. ISSN: 0378-5173.

Gardeniers HJ, Luttge R, Berenschot EJ, de Boer MJ, Yeshurun SY, Hefetz M, van't Oever R & van den Berg A. (2003). Silicon micromachined hollow microneedles for transdermal liquid transport. Journal of Medieval and Early Modern Studies. Vol. 12, pp 855-62.

Gill SH, Prausnitz RM. (2006). Coated microneedles for transdermal drug delivery. *Journal of Controlled Release,* Vol. 117, pp.227-37, ISSN 0168-3659.

Goswami S, Bajpai J & Bajpai AK. (2010). Designing Gelatin Nanocarriers as a Swellable System for Controlled Release of Insulin: An *In-Vitro* Kinetic Study. Journal of Macromolecular Science. Vol. 47, pp.119-130, ISSN 1060-1325.

Griffin, JE. & Touchstone, JC. (1972). Effects of ultrasound frequency on cortisone into swine tissue. *American Journal of Physcal Medicine,* Vol. 51, No. 2, (April 1972), pp. 62-78, ISSN 0002-9491.

Güngör, S.; Bektaş, A.; Alp, FI.; Uydeş-Doğan, BS.; Ozdemir, O.; Araman, A.; Ozsoy, Y. (2008). Matrix-type transdermal patches of verapamil hydrochloride: in vitro permeation studies through excised rat skin and pharmacodynamic evaluation in rats. *Pharmaceutical Development Technology,* Vol. 13, No. 4, pp. 283-9, ISSN *1083-7450.*

Guy RH, Kalia YN, Delgado-Charro MB, Merino V, Lopez A, Marro D. (2000). Iontophoresis: electrorepulsion and electroosmosis. Journal of Controlled Release, Vol. 64, No. 1-3, (February 2000), pp. 129-32, ISSN 0168-3659.

Hadgraft, J. & Lane, ME. (2005). Skin permeation: The years of enlightenment. *International Journal of Pharmaceutics,* Vol. 305, No. 1-2, (November 2005), pp. 2–12, ISSN 0378-5173.

Hadgraft, J.; Walters, KA. & Wotton, PK. (1985). Facilitated transport of sodium salicylate across an artificial lipid membrane by azone. *Journal of Pharmacy and Pharmacology,* Vol. 37, No. 10, (October 1985), pp. 725-727, ISSN 0022-3573.

Haq MI, Smith E, John DN, Kalavala M, Edwards C, Anstey A, Morrissey A & Birchall JC. (2009). Clinical administration of microneedles: skin puncture, pain and sensation. Biomedical Microdevices. Vol. 11, pp 35–47, ISSN: 1387-2176.

Hathout, RM.; Woodman, TJ.; Mansour, S.; Mortada, ND.; Geneidi, AS.; Guy, RH. (2010). Microemulsion formulations for the transdermal delivery of testosterone. *European Journal of Pharmaceutical Sciences*, Vol. 40, No. 3, (June 2010), pp. 188-96, ISSN *0928-0987*.

Hehn, B. & Moll, F. (1996). Phonophoretic permeation of procaine hydrochloride through and MDCK cell monolayer. *Pharmazie*; Vol. 51, No. 5, (May 1996), pp. 341-5, ISSN 0031-7144.

Heller, R.; Jaroszeski, R.; Glass, LF.; et al. (1996). Phase I / II Trial for the treatment of cutaneous and subcutaneous tumor using electrochemotherapy, *Cancer*, Vol. 77, No. 5, (March 1996), pp. 964–971, ISNN 1097-0142.

Henry S, McAllister V D, Mark GA & Prausnitz RM. (1998). Microfabricated microneedles: A novel approach to transdermal drug delivery. *Journal of Pharmaceutical Sciences*, Vol. 87, pp.922-25, ISSN 0022-3549.

Herffernan M, Murthy N. (2005). Polyketal nanoparticles: A new pH-sensitive biodegradable drug delivery vehicle. *Bioconjugate Chemistry*. Vol. 16, pp.1340-1342,

Hippius, M.; Uhlemann, C.; Smolenski, U.; et al. (1998). In vitro investigations of drug release and penetration enhancing effect of ultrasound on transmembrane transport of flufenamic acid. *International Journal of Clinical Pharmacoloy & Therapeutics*, Vol. 36, No. 2, (September 1998), pp. 107 11, ISSN 0946-1965.

Hong M, Zhu S, Jiang Y, Tang G & Pei Y. (2009). Efficient tumor targeting of hydroxycamptothecin loaded PEGylated niosomes modified with transferrin. *Journal of Controlled Release*, Vol. 133, pp.96-102, ISSN 0168-3659.

Huang X, Du Y, Yuan H & Hu F. (2009). Preparation and pharmacodynamics of low-molecular-weight chitosan nanoparticles containing insulin. Carbohydrate Polymers. Vol. 76, pp. 368-373, ISSN: 0144-8617

Huang, JF.; Sung, KC.; Wang, JJ.; Lin, YH.; Fang, JY. (2005). The effects of electrically assisted methods on transdermal delivery of nalbuphine benzoate and sebacoyl dinalbuphine ester from solutions and hydrogels. *International Journal of Pharmaceutics*,Vol. 297, No. 1-2, (April 2005), pp. 162–171, ISSN 0378-5173.

Jin Y, Tong L, Ai P, Li M & Hou X. (2006). Self-assembled drug delivery systems: 1. Properties and *in vitro/in vivo* behavior of acyclovir self-assembled nanoparticles (SAN). *International Journal of Pharmaceutics*. Vol.309, pp.199-207, ISSN: 0378-5173.

Johnson S, Trejo J, Veisi M, Willhite GP, Liang JT & Berkland C. (2010). Effects of Divalent Cations, Seawater, and Formation Brine on Positively Charged Polyethylenimine/Dextran Sulfate/ Chromium(III) Polyelectrolyte Complexes and Partially Hydrolyzed Polyacrylamide/Chromium(III) Gelation. Journal of Applied Polymer Science. Vol. 115, pp.1008-1014, ISSN 1097-4628.

Joshi M, Patravale V. (2008). Nanostructured lipid carrier (NLC) based gel of celecoxib. *International Journal of Pharmaceutics*. Vol.346, pp.124-132, ISSN: 0378-5173.

Kabanov, V.A.; Zezin, A.B.; Rogacheva, V.B.; Gulyaeva, Z.G.; Zansochova, M.F.; Joosten, J.G.H. & Brackman, J. (1998). Polyelectrolyte behavior of astramol poly(propyleneimine) dendrimers. *Macromolecules*. Vol 31, pp.142-5144, ISSN 0024-9297.

Khaibullina, A.; Jang, BS.; Sun, H.; et al. (2008). Pulsed high intensity focused ultrasound enhances uptake of radiolabeled monoclonal antibody to human epidermoid tumor in nude mice. *Journal of Nuclear Medicine*, Vol. 49, No. 2, (February 2008), pp. 295-302, ISSN 0161-5505.

Kigasawa, K.; Kajimoto, K.; Watanabe, M.; Kanamura, K.; Saito, A.; Kogure, K. (2009). In vivo transdermal delivery of diclofenac by ion-exchange iontophoresis with geraniol. *Biological & Pharmaceutical Bullettin*, Vol. 32, No. 4, (April 2009), pp. 684-7, ISSN *0918-6158.*

Kim, TY.; Jung, DI.; Kim, YI.; Yang, JH.; Shin, SC. (2007). Anesthetic effects of lidocaine hydrochloride gel using low frequency ultrasound of 0.5MHz. *Journal of Pharmacy & Pharmaceutical Sciences*, Vol, 10, No. 1, (February 2007), pp. 1-8, ISSN 1482-1826.

Kushner IV, J.; Blankschtein, D. & Langer, R. (2008). Heterogeneity in skin treated with low-frequency ultrasound. *Journal of Pharmaceutical Sciences*, Vol. 97, No. 10, (October 2008), pp. 4119–28, ISSN 0022-3549.

Kwon S.-Y., (2006). Acne Treatment by a Dissolvable Microneedle Patch, *Proceedings of Controlled Release Society 33st Annual Meeting*; #115.

Larkin, JO.; Casey, GD.; Tangney, M.; et al. (2008). Effective tumor treatment using optimized ultrasound mediated delivery of bleomycin. *Ultrasound In Medicine & Biology*, Vol.34, No. 3, (March 2008), pp. 406-13, ISSN 0301-5629.

Lboutounne H, Chaulet J, Ploton C, Falson F & Pirot F. (2002). Sustained ex vivo skin antiseptic activity of chlorhexidine in poly(ε-caprolactone) nanocapsule encapsulated form and as a digluconate. *Journal of Controlled Release,* Vol. 82, pp.319-334, ISSN 0168-3659.

Leboulanger B, Aubry JM, Bondolfi G, Guy RH, Delgado-Charro MB. (2004). Lithium monitoring by reverse iontophoresis*invivo.* Clinical Chemistry, Vol. 50, No. 11, (November 2004), pp. 2091-100, ISSN 1530-8561.

Lee P, Peng S, Su C, Mi F, Chen H, Wei M, Lin, H & Sung H. (2008). The use of biodegradable polymeric nanoparticles in combination with a low-pressure gene gun for transdermal DNA delivery. *Biomaterials.* Vol.29, No. 6, (February 2008) pp. 742-751, ISSN: 0142-9612.

Lee WJ, Park J & Prausnitz RM. (2007). Dissolving microneedles for transdermal drug delivery. *Biomaterials.* Vol. 29, pp. 2113-24, ISSN: 0142-9612.

Lee, PJ.; Ahmad, N.; Langer, R.; Mitragotri, S.; Prasad Shastri, V. (2006). Evaluation of chemical enhancers in the transdermal delivery of lidocaine. *International Journal of Pharmaceutics,* Vol. 308, No. 1-2, (February 2006), pp. 33-9, ISSN *0378-5173.*

Lee, S.; Snyder, B.; Newnham, RE.; Smith, NB. (2004). Noninvasive ultrasonic transdermal insulin delivery in rabbits using the light weight cymbal array. *Diabetes Technology & Therapeutics;* Vol. 6, No. 6, (December 2004), pp. 808-15, ISSN 1520-9156.

Levenets, AA.; Shuvalov, SM.; Poliakov, AV. (1989). The effect of the disodium salt of ethylenediaminetetraacetate on the healing of experimental suppurative wounds. *Stomatologiia (Mosk);* Vol. 68, No. 5, (September-October 1989), pp. 14-16, ISSN 0039-1735.

Li GP, Liu ZG, Liao B & Zhong NS. (2009). Induction of Th1-Type Immune Response by Chitosan Nanoparticles Containing Plasmid DNA Encoding House Dust Mite Allergen Der p 2 for Oral Vaccination in Mice. Cellular and Molecular Immunology. Vol. 6, pp.45-50, ISSN: 1672-7681.

Liu W, Hu M, Liu W, Xue C, Xu H & Yang X. (2008). Investigation of the carbopol gel of solid lipid nanoparticles for the transdermal iontophoretic delivery of triamcinolone acetonide acetate. *International Journal of Pharmaceutics.* Vol.364, pp.135-141, ISSN: 0378-5173.

Liu, H.; Li, S.; Pan, W.; et al. (2006). Investigation into the potential of low-frequency ultrasound facilitated topical delivery of Cyclosporin A. *International Journal of Pharmaceutics*, Vol. 326, No. 1-2, (December 2006), pp. 32-38, ISSN 0378-5173.

Lopez-Castellano, A & Merino V.(2010). Chapter 2: Chemical enhancers. In: José Juan Escobar-Chávez (Ed), *Current Technologies To Increase The Transdermal Delivery Of Drugs*. Bentham Science Publishers Ltd. ISBN: 978-1-60805-191-5, Bussum, The Netherlands.

Lu, MY.; Lee, D. & Rao, GS. (1992). Percutaneous absorption enhancement of leuprolide. *Pharmaceutical Research*, Vol. 9, No. 12, (December 1992), pp. 1575-9, ISSN *0724-8741.*

Lubbers, J.; Hekkenberg, RT. & Bezemer, RA. (2003). Time to threshold (TT), a safety parameter for heating by diagnostic ultrasound. *Ultrasound In Medicine & Biology*, Vol. 29, No. 5, (May 2003), pp. 755-64, ISSN 0301-5629.

Luis, J.; Park, EJ.; Meyer, RJ.; Smith, NB. (2007). Rectangular cymbal arrays for improved ultrasonic transdermal insulin delivery. *Journal of the Acoustical Society of America*, Vol. 122, No. 4, (October 2007), pp. 2022-30, ISSN 0001-4966.

Ma, X.; Fang, L.; Guo, J.; Zhao, N.; He, Z. (2010). Effect of counter-ions and penetration enhancers on the skin permeation of flurbiprofen. *Journal of Pharmaceutical Sciences*, Vol. 99, No. 4, (April 2010), pp. 1826-37, ISSN 0022-3549.

Machet, L.; Pinton, J.; Patat, F.; Arbeille, B.; Pourcelot, L.; Vaillant, L. (1996). In vitro phonophoresis of digoxin across hairless mice and human skin: thermal effect of ultrasound. *International Journal of Pharmaceutics*, Vol. 133, No. 1-2, (May 1996), pp. 39-45, ISSN 0378-5173.

Maestrelli F, González-Rodríguez ML, Rabasco AM & Mura P. (2005). Preparation and characterisation of liposomes encapsulating ketoprofen–cyclodextrin complexes for transdermal drug delivery. *International Journal of Pharmaceutics.* Vol. 298, pp.55-67, ISSN: 0378-5173.

Maloney M, Bezzant JL, Stephen RL. (1992). Iontophoreric administration of lidocaine anesthesia in office practice. *Journal of Dermatologic Surgery & Oncol*ogy, Vol. 18, No. , (November 1992), 937-40, ISSN 0148-0812.

Manosroi A, Kongkaneramit L & Manosroi J. (2004). Stability and transdermal absorption of topical amphotericin B liposome formulations. *International Journal of Pharmaceutics.* Vol. 270, pp.279-286, ISSN: 0378-5173.

Matinian, AL.; Nagapetian, KH.; Amirian, SS.; et al. (1990). Papain phonophoresis in the treatment of suppurative wounds and inflammatory processes. *Khirurgiia (Mosk)*, Vol. 9, (September 1990), pp. 74-6, ISSN 0023-1207.

McCarron PA, Hall M. (2008). Incorporation of novel 1-alkylcarbonyloxymethyl prodrugs of 5-fluorouracil into poly(lactide-co-glycolide) nanoparticles. *International Journal of Pharmaceutics.* Vol. 348, pp. 115-124, ISSN: 0378-5173.

McElnay, JC.; Benson, HA.; Harland, R.; Hadgraft, J. (1993). Phonophoresis of methyl nicotinate. A preliminary study to elucidate the mechanism of action. *Pharmaceutical Research*, Vol. 10, No. 12, (December 1993), pp. 1726-31, ISSN *0724-8741.*

Mei Z, Chen H, Weng T, Yang Y & Yang X. (2003). Solid lipid nanoparticle and microemulsion for topical delivery of triptolide. *European Journal of Pharmaceutics and Biopharmaceutics*. Vol. 56, No. 189-196, ISSN: 0928-0987.

Meidan, VM.; Walmsley, AD.; Docker, MF.; Irwin, WJ. (1999). Ultrasound enhanced diffusion into coupling gel during phonophoresis of 5-fluorouracil. *International Journal of Pharmaceutics*, Vol. 185, No. 2, (August 1999), pp. 205-13, ISSN 0378-5173.

Mélot, M.; Pudney, PD.; Williamson, AM.; Caspers, PJ.; Van Der Pol, A.; Puppels, GJ. (2009). Studying the effectiveness of penetration enhancers to deliver retinol through the stratum cornum by in vivo confocal Raman spectroscopy. *Journal of Controlled Release*, Vol. 138, No. 1, (August 2009), pp. 32-9, ISSN 0168-3659.

Menjoge AR, Kannan RM & Tomalia DA. (2010). Dendrimer-based drug and imaging conjugates: design considerations for nanomedical applications. Drug Discovery Today. Vol. 15, pp. 171-185, ISSN: 1359-6446.

Menon, GK.; Price, LF.; Bommannan, B.; et al. (1994). Selective obliteration of the epidermal calcium gradient leads to enhanced lamellar body secretion. *Journal of Investigative Dermatology*, Vol. 102, No. 5, (May 1994), pp. 789-95, ISSN 0022-202X.

Merino V, Kalia, YN, Guy RH. (1997). Transdermal therapy and diagnosis by iontophoresis. *Trends in Biotechnology*, Vol. 15, No. 8, (August 1997), pp. 288-90. ISSN 0167-7799.

Merino V, Lopez A, Kalia YN, Guy RH. (1999). Electrorepulsion versus electroosmosis: effect of pH on the iontophoretic flux of 5-fluorouracil. Pharmaceutical Research, Vol. 16, No. 5, (May 1999), pp. 758-61, ISSN 0724-8741.

Merino, G.; Kalia, YN. & Guy, RH. (2003). Ultrasound-Enhanced Transdermal Transport. *Journal of Pharmaceutical Sciences*, Vol. 92, No. 6, (June 2003), pp. 1125-37, ISSN 0022-3549.

Merino, V.; Micó-Albiñana, T.; Nácher, A.; Díez-Sales, O.; Herráez, M.; Merino-Sanjuán, M. (2008). Enhancement of nortriptyline penetration through human epidermis: influence of chemical enhancers and iontophoresis. *Journal of Pharmacy & Pharmacology*, Vol. 60, No. 4, (April 2008), pp. 415-20, ISSN 0022-3573.

Meshali, MM.; Abdel-Aleem, HM.; Sakr, FM.; et al. (2008). In vitro phonophoresis: effect of ultrasound intensity and mode at high frequency on NSAIDs transport across cellulose and rabbit skin membranes. *Pharmazie*; Vol. 63, No. 1, (January 2008), pp. 49-53, ISSN 0031-7144.

Mittal A, Sara UV, Ali A, Aqil M. (2008). The effect of penetration enhancers on permeation kinetics of nitrendipine in two different skin models. *Biology & Pharmaceutical Bulletin*, Vol. 31, No. 9, (September 2008), pp. 1766-72, ISSN 0918-6158.

Miyazaki, S.; Mizuoka, H.; Kohata, Y.; Takada, M. (1992). External control of drug release and penetration. Enhancing effect of ultrasound on the transdermal absorption of indomethacin from an oinment in rats. *Chemical & Pharmaceutical Bulletin (Tokyo)*; Vol. 40, No. 10, (October 1992), pp. 2826-2830, ISSN 0009-2363.

Montenegro, L.; Bucolo, C. & Puglisi, G. (2003). Enhancer effects on in vitro corneal permeation of timolol and acyclovir. *Pharmazie*, Vol. 58, No. 7, (July 2003), pp. 497-501, ISSN 0031-7144.

Monti, D.; Giannelli, R.; Chetoni, P.; Burgalassi, S. (2001). Comparison of the effect of ultrasound and of chemical enhancers on transdermal permeation of caffeine and morphine through hairless mouse skin in vitro. *International Journal of Pharm*aceutics, Vol. 229, No. 1-2, (October 2001), pp. 131-7, ISSN 0378-5173.

Morimoto, Y.; Mutoh, TM.; Ueda, H.; et al. (2005). Elucidation of the transport pathway in hairless rat skin enhanced by low-frequency sonophoresis based on the solute-water transport relationship and confocal microscopy. *Journal of Controlled Release*, Vol. 103, (April 2005), pp. 587–97, ISSN 0168-3659.

Mura, S.; Manconi, M.; Sinico, C.; Valenti, D.; Fadda, AM. (2009). Penetration enhancer-containing vesicles (PEVs) as carriers for cutaneous delivery of minoxidil. *International Journal of Pharmaceutics*, Vol. 380, No. 1-2, (October 2009), pp. 72-9, ISSN 0378-5173.

Murthy SN, Sen A, Zhao YL, Hui SW. (2004). Temperature influences the postelectroporation permeability state of the skin. Journal of Pharmaceutical Sciences, Vol. 93, No. 4, (April 2004), pp.908-15, ISSN 0928-0987.

Mutalik S, Parekh HS, Davies NM, Udupa N. (2009). A combined approach of chemical enhancers and sonophoresis for the transdermal delivery of tizanidine hydrochloride. *Drug Delivery*, Vol. 16, No. 2, (February 2009), pp. 82-91, ISSN 1071-7544.

Nair, V. & Panchagnula, R. (2003). Poloxamer gel as vehicle for transdermal iontophoretic delivery of arginine vasopressin: evaluation of in vivo performance in rats. *Pharmacology Research*, Vol. 47, No. 6, (June 2003), pp. 555-62, ISSN 1043-6618.

Ng, GY. & Wong, RY. (2008). Ultrasound phonophoresis of panax notoginseng improves the strength of repairing ligament: a rat model. *Ultrasound In Medicine & Biology*, Vol. 34, No. 12, (December 2008), pp. 1919-23, ISSN 0301-5629.

Niederhafner P, Šebestík J & Ježek J. (2005). Peptide dendrimers. *Journal of Peptide Science*. Vol. 11, pp. 757-788, ISSN: 1099-1387.

Novak, FJ. (1964). Experirnental wansmission of lidocalne through intact skin by ultrasound. *Archives of Physical Medicine & Rehabilitation*, Vol. 64, (May 1996), pp. 231-2, ISSN 0003-9993.

Ogiso T, Iwaki M & Paku T. (1995). Effect of various enhancers on transdermal penetration of indomethacin and urea, and relationship between penetration parameters and enhancement factors. *Journal of Pharmaceutical Sciences*, Vol. 84, pp.482–88, ISSN: 1520-6017.

Okino M, Mohri H. (1987). Effects of a high-voltage electrical impulse and an anticancer drug on *in vivo* growing tumors. Japanese Journal of Cancer Research, Vol. 78, (December 1987), pp. 1319-1321, ISSN 0910-5050.

Orlowskim S, Belehradek JJ, Paoletti C, Mir LM. (1988). Transient electropermeabilization of cells in culture. Increase of the cytotoxicity of anticancer drugs. Biochemical Pharmacology, Vol. 34, (December 1988), pp. 4727-4733, ISSN 0006- 2952.

Paliwal, S.; Menon, GK.; Mitragotri, S. (2006). Low-frequency sonophoresis: ultrastructural basis for stratum corneum permeability assessed using quantum dots. *Journal of Investigative Dermatology*, Vol. 126, No. 5, (May 2006), pp. 1095–1101, ISSN 0022-202X.

Parekh HS. (2007). The Advance of Dendrimers - A Versatile Targeting Platform for Gene/Drug Delivery. Current Pharmaceutical Design. Vol. 13, pp. 2837-2850, ISSN 1381-6128.

Park JH, Allen MG & Prausnitz MR. (2005). Biodegradable polymer microneedles: fabrication, mechanics and transdermal drug delivery. *Journal of Controlled Release*, Vol. 104, pp.51-66, ISSN 0168-3659.

Park JH. (2004). *Polymeric microneedles for transdermal drug delivery*. PhD Thesis. Georgia Institute of Technology.

Perennes F, Marmiroli B, Matteucci M, Tormen M, Vaccari L & Fabrizio ED. (2006). Sharp beveled tip hollow microneedle arrays fabricated by LIGA and 3D soft lithography with polyvinyl alcohol. Journal of Micromechanics and Microengineering. Vol. 16, pp. 473-79, ISSN 1361-6439.

Phillips, CA. & Michniak, BB. (1995). Transdermal delivery of drugs with differing lipophilicities using Azone analogs as dermal penetration enhancers. *Journal of Pharmaceutical Sciences*, Vol. 84, No. 12, (December 1995), pp. 1427-33, ISSN 0022-3549.

Pliquett U, Gallo S, Hui SW, GusbethCh, Neumann E. (2005). Local and transient structural changes in stratum corneum at high electric fields: contribution of Joule heating. Biolectrochemistry, Vol. 67, No.1, (September 2005), pp. 37-46, ISSN1567-5394.

Pliquett U, GusbethCh, Nuccitelli R. (2008). A propagating heat wave model of skin electroporation. Journal of Theoretical Biology, Vol. 251, No. 2, (March 2008), pp. 195-201, ISSN 0022-5193.

Prausnitz MR, Bose VG, Langer R, Weaver JC. (1993). Electroporation of mammalian skin: a mechanism to enhance transdermal drug delivery. Proceeding of the National Academy of Sciences of the united states of American, Vol. 90, No. 22, (November 1993), pp. 10504-8, ISSN 0027-8424.

Ragelis, Siu. (1981). Tetracycline penetration into tissue by modified electro and phonophoretic methods. *Antibiotiki,* Vol. 26, No. 9, (September 1981), pp. 699-703, ISSN 0003-5637.

Rizwan, M.; Aqil, M.; Talegaonkar, S.; Azeem, A.; Sultana, Y:, Ali, A. (2009). Enhanced transdermal drug delivery techniques: an extensive review of patents. Recent Patents on Drug Delivery & Formul*ations,* Vol. 3, No. 2, pp. 105-24, ISSN1872-2113.

Rodriguez-Justo O. & Moraes Â. M..(2011). Analysis of process parameters on the characteristics of liposomes prepared by ethanol injection with a view to process scale-up: Effect of temperature and batch volume. *Chemical Engineering Research and Design*. Vol. 89, No. 6, (June 2011), pp. 785-792, ISSN: 0263-8762.

Rojas-Oviedo I, Salazar-López RA, Reyes-Gasga J & Quirino-Barreda CT. (2007). Elaboration and structural analysis of aquasomes loaded with Indomethacin. *European Journal of Pharmaceutical Sciences*, Vol. 32, pp. 223-230, ISSN 0928-0987.

Rornanenko, IM. & Araviiskii, RA. (1991). Comparative levels of amphoteficin B in the skin and subcutaneous fatty tissue after cutaneous application of amphotericin ointment by phonophoresis and with preliminary treatment by dimethyl sulfoxide. *Antibiotiki i Khimioterapiia*; Vol. 36, No. 9, (September 1991), pp. 29-31, ISSN 0235-2990.

Rosim, GC.; Barbieri, CH.; Lanças, FM.; Mazzer, N. (2005). Diclofenac phonphoresis in human volunteers. *Ultrasound in Medicine & Biology*, Vol. 31, No. 3, (March 2005), pp. 337-43, ISSN 0301-5629.

Rossier-Miranda FJ, Schroën CGPH & Boom RM. (2009). Colloidosomes: Versatile microcapsules in perspective. Colloids and Surfaces A: Physicochemical and Engineering Aspects. Vol. 343, pp. 43-49, ISSN: 0927-7757.

Roxhed N, Samel B, Nordquist L, Griss P & Stemme G. (2008). Painless drug delivery through microneedle-based transdermal patches featuring active infusion. *IEEE Transactions in Biomedical Engineering*. Vol. 55 No.3, pp. 1063-71. ISSN: 0018-9294

Rzigalinski BA, Strobl JS. (2009). Cadmium-containing nanoparticles: Perspectives on pharmacology and toxicology of quantum dots. Toxicology and Applied Pharmacology. Vol. 238, pp. 280-288, ISSN: 0041-008X.

Saliba, S.; Mistry, DJ.; Perrin, DH.; Gieck, J.; Weltman, A. (2007). Phonophoresis and the absorption of dexamethasone in the presence of an occlusive dressing. *Journal of Athletic Training*, Vol. 42, No. 3, (July-September 2007), pp. 349-54, ISSN 1062-6050.

Sammoura F, Kang JJ, Heo YM, Jung TS & Lin L. (2007). Polymeric microneedle fabrication using a microinjection molding technique. *Microsystem Technologies.* Vol. 13, pp. 517-22, ISSN: 1432-1858.

Sanna V, Caria G & Mariani A. (2010). Effect of lipid nanoparticles containing fatty alcohols having different chain length on the ex vivo skin permeability of Econazole nitrate. *Powder Technology.* Vol. 201, pp. 32-36, ISSN: 0032-5910.

Santander-Ortega MJ, Stauner T, Loretz B, Ortega-Vinuesa JL, Bastos-González D, Wenz G, Schaefer UF, Lehr CM. (2010). Nanoparticles made from novel starch derivatives for transdermal drug delivery. *Journal of Controlled Release,* Vol. 141, pp.85-92, ISSN 0168-3659.

Santoianni, P.; Nino, M. & Calabro, G. (2004). Intradermal drug delivery by low frequency sonophoresis (25KHz). *Dermatol Online Journal*, Vol. 10, No. 2, (October 2004), pp. 24-33, ISSN 10872108.

Senyiğit, T.; Padula, C.; Ozer, O.; Santi, P. (2009). Different approaches for improving skin accumulation of topical corticosteroids. *International Journal of Pharmaceutics*, Vol. 380, No. 1-2, (October 2009), pp. 155-60, ISSN 0378-5173.

Serikov, NP. (2007). Efficacy of ibuprofen (nurofen gel) ultraphonophoresis for pain in ostheoarthritis. *Terapevticheskii arkhiv*, Vol. 79, No. 5, pp. 79-81, ISSN 0040-3660.

Shakeel F, Ramadan W. (2010). Transdermal delivery of anticancer drug caffeine from water-in-oil nanoemulsions. Colloids and Surfaces B: Biointerfaces. Vol. 75, pp. 356-362, ISSN: 0927-7765.

Sharma BB, Jain SK & Vyas SP. (1994). Topical liposome system bearing local anaesthetic lignocaine: preparation and evaluation. *Journal of Microencapsulation.* Vol. 11, pp. 279-286, ISSN 0265-2048.

Shelley WB, McConahy JC, Hesbacher EN. (1950). Effectiveness of antihistaminic compounds introduced into normal skin by iontophoresis. The Journal of Investigative Dermatology, Vol. 15, No. 5, (November 1950), pp. 343-4, ISSN 0022-202X.

Shen, Q.; Li, W. & Li, W. (2007). The effect of clove oil on the transdermal delivery of ibuprofen in the rabbit by in vitro and in vivo methods. *Drug Development & Industrial Pharmacy*; Vol. 33, No. 12, (December 2007), pp. 1369-74, ISSN 0363-9045.

Shim J, Seok Kang H, Park W, Han S, Kim J & Chang I. (2004). Transdermal delivery of mixnoxidil with block copolymer nanoparticles. *Journal of Controlled Release,* Vol. 97, pp.477-484, ISSN 0168-3659.

Skauen, DM. (1974). Heat production by ultrasonic equipment. *Journal of Pharmaceutical Sciences*, Vol. 163, No. 1, (January 1974), pp. 114-6, ISSN 0022-3549.

Smith, JC & Irwin, WJ. (2000). Ionisation and the effect of absorption enhancers on transport of salicylic acid through silastic rubber and human skin. *International Journal of Pharmaceutics*, Vol. 210, No. 1-2, (December 2000), pp. 69-82, ISSN 0378-5173.

Smith, NB.; Lee, S. & Shung, KK. (2003). Ultrasound-mediated transdermal in vivo transport of insulin with low profile cymbal arrays. *Ultrasound in Medicine & Biology*, Vol. 29, No. 8, (August 2003), pp. 1205-10, ISSN 0301-5629.

Sonneville-Aubrun O., Simonnet J. -T. & Alloret F. L. (2004). Nanoemulsions: a new vehicle for skincare products. Advances in Colloid and Interface Science. Vols. 108-109, (20 May 2004), pp. 145-149, ISSN 0001-8686.

Soppimath KS, Aminabhavi TM, Kulkarni AR & Rudzinski WE. (2001). Biodegradable polymeric nanoparticles as drug delivery devices. *Journal of Controlled Release*, Vol. 70, pp.1-20, ISSN 0168-3659.

Stoeber B, Liepmann D. (2005). Arrays of hollow out-of-plane microneedles for drug delivery. *Journal of* Microelectronic systems. Vol. 14, No. 3, pp. 472-79, ISSN 0026-2692.

Sung, KC.; Fang, J-Y.; Wang, JJ.; Hu O, Y-P.(2003).Transdermal delivery of nalbuphine and its prodrugs by electroporation. *European Journal of Pharmaceutical Sciences*, Vol. 18, No. 1, (January 2003), pp. 63–70, ISNN 0928-0987.

Svenson S, Tomalia DA. (2005). Dendrimers in biomedical applications - reflections on the field. *Advanced Drug Delivery Reviews*, vol. 57, pp. 2106-2129, ISSN 0169-409X.

Tachibana, K. & Tachibana, S. (1993). Use of ultrasound to enhance the local anesthetic effect of topically applied aqueous Lidocaine. *Anesthesiology*, Vol. 78, No. 6, (June 1993), pp. 1091-6, ISSN 0003-3022.

Tachibana, K. & Tachibana, S. (1999). Application of ultrasound energy as a new drug delivery system. *Nihon Yakurigaku Zasshi*; Vol. 114, No. 1, (October 1999), pp. 138P-141P, ISSN 1340-2544.

Tang, H.; Mitragotri, S.; Blankschtein, D.; Langer, R. (2001). Theoretical description of transdermal transport of hydrophilic permeants: application to low frequency sonophoresis. *Journal of Pharmaceutical Sciences*, Vol. 90, No. 5, (May 2001), pp. 543–66, ISSN 0022-3549.

Tartis MS, Kruse DE, Zheng H, Zhang H, Kheirolomoom A, Marik J & Ferrara KW. (2008). Dynamic microPET imaging of ultrasound contrast agents and lipid delivery. *Journal of Controlled Release.* Vol. 131: No. 3, (November, 2008) pp.160-166, ISSN 0168-3659.

Teeranachaideekul V, Souto EB, Junyaprasert VB & Müller RH. (2007). Cetyl palmitate-based NLC for topical delivery of Coenzyme Q10 - Development, physicochemical characterization and *in vitro* release studies. *European Journal of Pharmaceutical Sciences*, Vol. 67, pp. 141-148, ISSN 0928-0987.

Teo A L, Shearwood C, Kian C N, Jai L & Shabbiir M. (2005). Transdermal Microneedles for Drug Delivery Application. Materials Science and Engineering: B. Vol. 132, pp. 151-54. ISSN 0921-5093.

Tezel H, Dokka S, Kelly S, Hardee GE, Mitragotri S. (2004). Topical delivery of anti-sense oligonucleotides using low-frequency sonophoresis. *Pharmaceutical Research*, Vol. 21, No. 12, (December 2004), pp. 2219-25, ISSN 0724-8741.

Thote AJ, Gupta RB. (2005). Formation of nanoparticles of a hydrophilic drug using supercritical carbon dioxide and microencapsulation for sustained release. Nanomedicine: Nanotechnology, Biology and Medicine. Vol. 1, pp. 85-90, ISSN: 1549-9634.

Tiwari, SB.; Pai, RM.; Udupa, N. (2004). Influence of ultrasound on the percutaneous absorption of ketorolac tromethamine in vitro across rat skin. *Drug Delivery*, Vol. 11, No. 1, (January-February 2004), pp. 47-51, ISSN 1071-7544.

Ugazio E, Cavalli R & Gasco MR. (2002). Incorporation of cyclosporin A in solid lipid nanoparticles (SLN). *International Journal of Pharmaceutics.* Vol. 241, pp.341-344, ISSN: 0378-5173.

Vaddi, HK.; Wang, LZ.; Ho, PC.; Chan, SY. (2001) Effect of some enhancers on the permeation of haloperidol through rat skin in vitro. *International Journal of Pharmaceutics*, Vol. 212, No. 2, (January 2001), pp. 247-55, ISSN 0378-5173.

Walker, JJ. (1983). Ultrasound therapy for keloids. *South African Medical Journal*, Vol. 64, No. 8, (August 1983), pp. 270, ISSN 0256-9574.

Wang, YY.; Hong, CT.; Chiu, WT.; Fang, JY. (2001). In vitro and in vivo evaluations of topically applied capsaicin and nonivamide from hydrogels. *International Journal of Pharmaceutics*, Vol. 224, No. 1-2, (August 2001), pp. 89-104, ISSN 0378-5173.

Wells, PN. (1977). *Biomedical ultrasonics*. Academic Press, pp. 421-30, New York.

Wen Z, Fang L, He Z. (2009). Effect of chemical enhancers on percutaneous absorption of daphnetin in isopropyl myristate vehicle across rat skin in vitro. *Drug Delivery*, Vol. 16, No. 4, (May 2009), pp. 214-23, ISSN 1071-7544.

Williams, AC. & Barry, BW. (2004). Penetration enhancers. *Advance Drug Delivery Reviews*, Vol. 56, No. 5, (March 2004), 603–18, ISSN 0169-409X.

Williams, AR. (1990). Phonophoresis: an in vivo evaluation using three topical anaesthetic preparations. *Ultrasonics*; Vol. 28, No. 3, (May 1990), pp. 137-41, ISSN 0041-624X.

Xu DH, Zhang Q, Feng X, Xu X, Liang WQ. (2007). Synergistic effects of ethosomes and chemical enhancers on enhancement of naloxone permeation through human skin. *Pharmazie*, Vol. 62, No. 4, (April 2007), pp. 316-8, ISSN 0031-7144.

Yang, JH.; Kim, DK.; Yun, MY.; Kim, TY.; Shin, SC. (2006). Transdermal delivery system of triamcinolone acetonide from a gel using phonophoresis. *Archives of Pharmacal Research*, Vol. 29, No. 5, (May 2006), pp. 412-27, ISSN 0253-6269.

Yang, JH.; Kim, TY.; Lee, JH.; et al. (2008). Anti-hyperalgesic and anti-inflammatory effects of ketorolac tromethamine gel using pulsed ultrasound in inflamed rats. *Archives of Pharmacal Research*, Vol. 31, No. 4, (April 2008), pp. 511-17, ISSN 0253-6269.

Yoo HS, Lee JE, Chung H, Kwon IC & Jeong SY. (2005). Self-assembled nanoparticles containing hydrophobically modified glycol chitosan for gene delivery. *Journal of Controlled Release*, Vol. 103, pp.235-243, ISSN 0168-3659.

Zahn DJ, Trebotich D & Liepmann D. (2005). Microdialysis Microneedles for Continuous Medicla Monitoring. Biomedical Microdevices. Vol. 7, No. 1, pp. 59-69, ISSN 1387-2176.

Zhang, JY.; Fang, L.; Tan, Z.; Wu, J.; He, ZG. (2009). Influence of ion-pairing and chemical enhancers on the transdermal delivery of meloxicam. *Drug Development & Industrial Pharmacy*, Vol. 35, No. 6, (June 2009), pp. 663-70, ISSN 0363-9045.

Zheng J, Zhu R, He Z, Cheng G, Wang H & Yao K. (2010). Synthesis and Characterization of PMMA/SiO_2 Nanocomposites by In Situ Suspension Polymerization. Journal of Applied Polymer Science. Vol. 115, pp. 1975-1981, ISSN 0021-8995.

Zimmermann S, Fienbork D, Stoeber B, Flouriders WA & Liepmann D. A. (2003). Microneedle-Base Glucose Monitor: Fabricated on a Wafer-Level Using In-Devoce Enzyme Immobilization. *Proceedings of 12th International Conference on solid state sensors, actuators and Microsystems.* pp.99-102.

Part 5

Diagnostic

20

Application of Matrix-Assisted Laser Desorption/Ionization Imaging Mass Spectrometry

Nobuhiro Zaima
Department of Applied Biological Chemistry,
Graduate School of Agriculture, Kinki University
Japan

1. Introduction

The clarification of metabolic dynamics in lesion areas is important. Many approaches, such as high performance liquid chromatography mass spectrometry, gas chromatography mass spectrometry, immunohistochemistry, are used to define disease-related abnormalities. Matrix-assisted laser desorption/ionization imaging mass spectrometry (MALDI-IMS) is attracting attention as a new valuable tool. MALDI-IMS is a two-dimensional MALDI mass spectrometric technique used to visualize the spatial distribution of molecules without extraction, purification, separation, or labeling of biological samples (Cornett et al., 2007; Zaima et al., 2010b). MALDI-IMS has revealed the characteristic distribution of several biomolecules, including proteins (Caprioli et al., 1997; Groseclose et al., 2007; Morita et al., 2010), peptides (Chansela et al., 2011; Stoeckli et al., 2002), amino acids (Goto-Inoue et al., 2010b; Zaima et al., 2010a), lipids (Hayasaka et al., 2009; Murphy et al., 2009; Zaima et al., 2011a), and carbohydrates (Goto-Inoue et al., 2010b), in various tissues. The versatility of MALDI-IMS has opened a new frontier in several fields, such as pharmacology, medicine, agriculture, biology, and pathology. In this review, we describe the methodology and applications of MALDI-IMS for biological samples.

2. MALDI-MS

MALDI-MS was developed from laser desorption/ionization mass spectrometry (LDI-MS). The first LDI-MS experiment for high-mass molecules was reported in 1987 (Tanaka et al., 1987). In this experiment, a powder of cobalt metal in glycerol was used for the observation of ions with a mass to charge (*m/z*) ratio of 34,000. Soon afterward, MALDI-MS results of serum albumin (67,000 Da) were reported using nicotinic acid as the matrix (Karas & Hillenkamp, 1988). It was reported that MALDI-MS can detect a wide range of molecules ranging from small (*m/z* <1000) to large molecules (*m/z* >1,000,000) (Yates, 1998). The schema of MALDI-MS is shown in Figure 1.

In routine MALDI-MS analysis (i.e., non-imaging analysis), the analyte can be mixed with an excess of matrix. On the other hand, molecular imaging of tissue sections using MALDI-IMS requires the tissue surface to be homogeneously covered by a matrix. On-tissue application of matrix results in the *in situ* extraction of molecules from biological tissues. The cocrystal of matrix and analyte molecules in tissue is irradiated with a pulsed laser of appropriate energy, leading to desorption and ionization of the matrix and analyte molecules. The fragmentation of analyte molecules is prevented by the incorporation of the analyte molecules into matrix crystals. The role of the optical absorption of the matrix in the transfer of energy from the laser beam to the analyte molecules is governed by Beer's law, as described previously (Karas et al., 1985). However, the mechanisms underlying the formation of charged matrix and analyte molecules in the MALDI process are not fully understood.

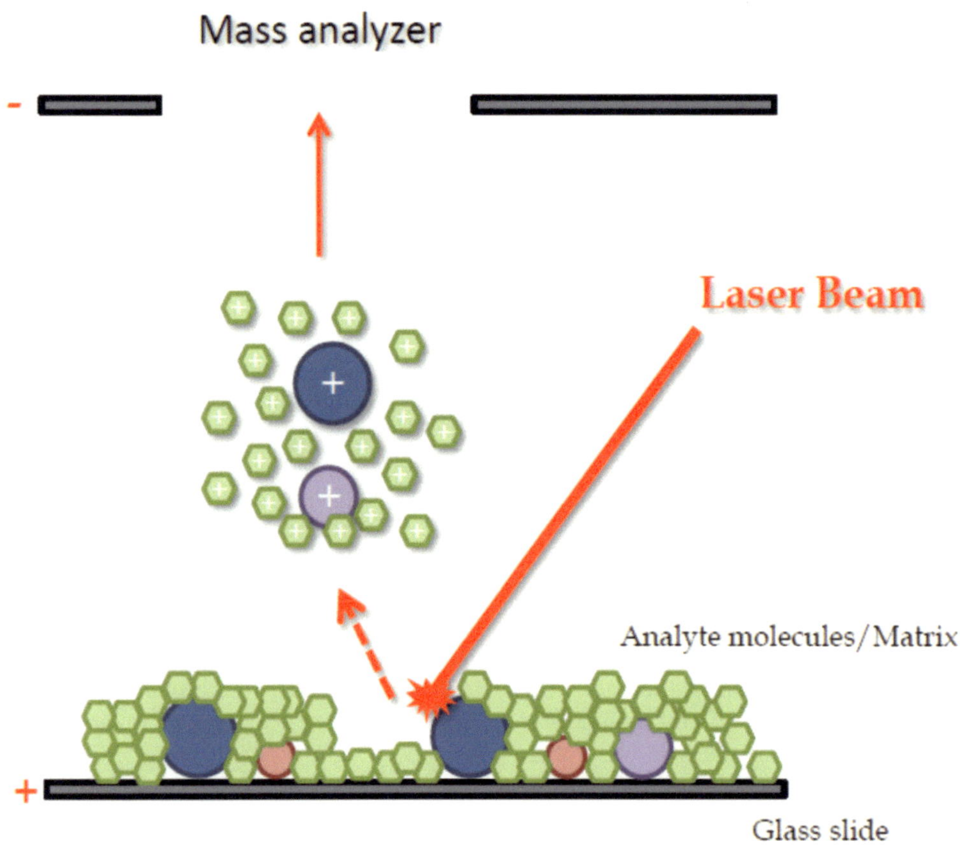

Fig. 1. Schema of MALDI-MS.

The matrix molecules absorb the laser energy and facilitate desorption and ionization of analyte molecules in the tissue. The homogeneous matrix cover is important for MALDI-IMS, because a heterogeneous distribution of matrix results in different ionization efficiencies of analyte molecules based on their location.

3. Methodology of MALDI-IMS

The important experimental steps for visualizing endogenous molecules or administered pharmaceutical agents in tissue using MALDI-IMS are sample preparation (such as fixation, sectioning, and washing), choice of matrix and matrix application, measurement, and data analysis. To obtain meaningful biological images, all steps need to be carefully controlled. In this section, the basic experimental MALDI-IMS procedures are described. The schema of MALDI-IMS is presented in Figure 2.

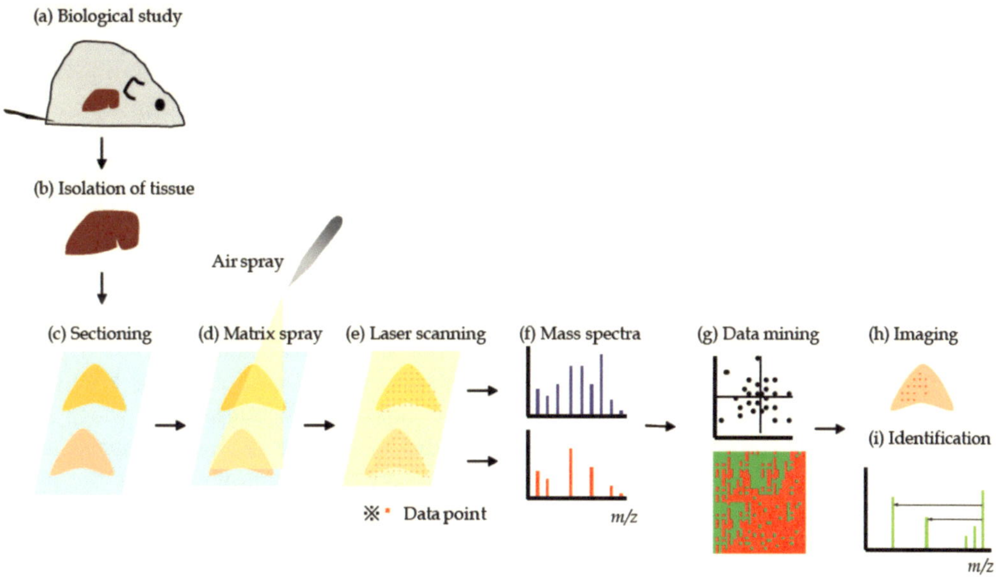

Fig. 2. Schema of MALDI-IMS.

After biological study (a), the tissue of interest should be appropriately isolated (b). A thin section of isolated tissue is mounted on a glass slide (c), coated with matrix (d), and measured by a mass spectrometer (e). The resultant mass spectra (f) can be used for a data mining approach (g). Molecules of interest can be visualized (f) and identified by MS/MS on tissue (f).

3.1 Biological sample preparation

The samples for MALDI-IMS come from a variety of biological sources, including organs, whole animal body dosed with a pharmaceutical compound, or pathological tissues. Optimization of the sample preparation procedure according to the chemical and physical properties of analytes is important. Here, the basic sample preparation steps for MALDI-IMS are described.

3.1.1 Sample condition for MALDI-IMS

Collection and treatment procedures need to be sufficiently fast to prevent rapid tissue degradation, because the sample degradation process starts immediately after the cessation of blood flow. The most preferred sample for MALDI-IMS is a chemically unmodified fresh-frozen one. Fresh-frozen samples can be prepared using dry ice, liquid nitrogen, or liquid nitrogen-chilled isopentane, and can be preserved in a deep freezer until required. The samples should be well sealed to prevent drying during storage, and it is important to ensure that the tissue section morphology is well preserved before MALDI-IMS.

3.1.2 Fixation and embedding

Fixation of samples, such as formalin fixation, is preferably avoided because the protein crosslinking introduced by formalin fixation makes MALDI-IMS analysis difficult. However, many medical samples are routinely formaldehyde-fixed and paraffin-embedded (FFPE) just after dissection. To address this problem, the on-tissue proteolytic digestion method, in which proteins are denatured and digested by enzymes, has been developed (Djidja et al., 2009; Groseclose et al., 2007; Lemaire et al., 2007; Morita et al., 2010). The on-tissue proteolytic digestion method includes a paraffin removal step using xylene and ethanol. In the paraffin removal step, lipophilic molecules are lost; therefore, FFPE samples cannot be used for lipid imaging. When the samples are formaldehyde-fixed without paraffin-embedding, lipid imaging can be performed (Zaima et al., 2011c). However, the detected ion intensities of lipids in formaldehyde-fixed samples are lower than those in fresh-frozen ones are.

Embedding of the tissue samples in supporting material, such as an optimal cutting temperature (OCT) compound, allows the maintenance of tissue morphology and precise sample sectioning. However, supporting materials are often ionized during MALDI-MS analysis and sometimes act as ion suppressors of molecules of interest (Schwartz et al., 2003). Therefore, samples should not be embedded if precise sample sections can be prepared without embedding. When it is difficult to prepare a sample section, the use of carboxymethylcellulose (CMC) or gelatin as embedding material is recommended. Sodium CMC (2%) is reported to be used as an alternative embedding compound that does not interfere with the detection sensitivity of biomolecules in MALDI-IMS analysis (Stoeckli et al., 2006; Zaima et al., 2010a). Chen et al. reported that gelatin provides a cleaner signal background than OCT (Chen et al., 2009). Researchers should ensure compatibility between the supporting material and the biomolecules of interest.

3.1.3 Sectioning

The basic sectioning procedure for MALDI-IMS samples is same as that for pathological examination. Sections for MALDI-IMS can be prepared using a cryostat. The sample stage temperature is typically maintained between -5 and -20°C. To obtain high quality sections from tissues with high fat content (e.g., brain), or atherosclerotic lesions, breast tissue, or lipid storage disease samples lower temperatures are required. In general, 5–20-μm-thick sections are prepared for the analysis of low-molecular-weight molecules. The use of thinner tissue sections (2–5 μm thick) has been recommended for the analysis of high-molecular-weight molecules (range, 3–21 kDa) (Goodwin et al., 2008). Sections are usually thaw-mounted on a stainless steel conductive stage or on commercially available indium-tin oxide (ITO)-coated glass slides. We recommend the use of ITO-coated glass slides because these transparent slides enable microscopic observation of the section after MALDI-IMS. Use of adhesive film is suitable for samples for which thaw-mounted preparation of sections is challenging (e.g., bone or whole-body sections) (Stoeckli et al., 2006; Zaima et al., 2010a). The procedure for sectioning using adhesive film is shown in Figure 3. The prepared section should be immediately dried in a vacuum desiccator to avoid moisture condensation that could cause delocalization of analyte molecules in the tissue. Moisture condensation can be avoided by placing the prepared section in a dry and cold container until return to room temperature.

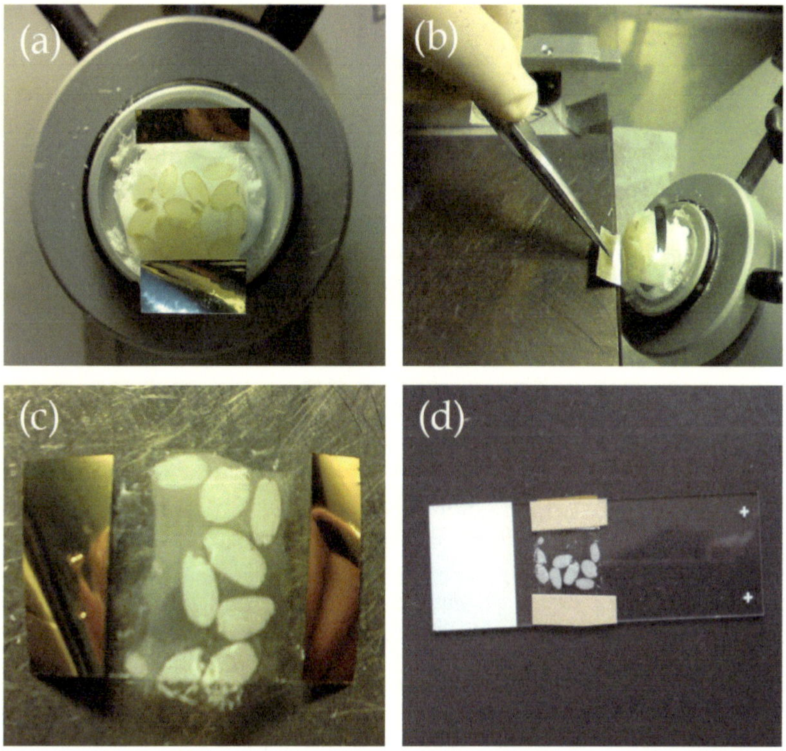

Fig. 3. Procedure for sectioning using adhesive film.

Attachment of adhesive film to the sample block (a). The end of the adhesive film must be anchored with tweezers to prevent adhesion of the film to the sample stage (b). After the sample section is obtained (c), the sample section on the adhesive film is attached to a glass slide (d).

3.1.4 Washing

Washing is required for peptide or protein analysis because their detection is often prevented by large amounts of easily ionized lipid species. Lipid removal simplifies mass spectra in the range of *m/z* 400–1000; thus, lipid removal enables the detection of low-mass peptides that are usually masked by lipid peaks. The washing method should be optimized for the target imaging molecules. Several washing protocols using organic solvents have been reported (Aerni et al., 2006; Andersson et al., 2008; Groseclose et al., 2007; Lemaire et al., 2006; Schwartz et al., 2003).

Washing is also used for removing the matrix from the tissue section after MALDI-IMS analysis. The matrix can be removed using the solvent that is used for preparing the matrix solution. For example, 2,5-dihydroxybenzoic acid (DHB) can be rapidly removed by methanol. Matrix removal enables the microscopic observation of a tissue section followed by pathological staining, such as hematoxylin and eosin (HE) staining, toluidine blue staining etc.

3.2 Matrix application

The matrix plays a central role in MALDI-MS soft ionization (Karas & Hillenkamp, 1988; Karas & Kruger, 2003). Biomolecules are softly ionized in the cocrystal with the matrix, which absorbs the laser beam energy and protects biomolecules from the disruptive energy. Protonated ion ([M + H]+) or deprotonated ion ([M − H]−) molecules are generally detected. Sodium adduct ion ([M + Na]+) and potassium adduct ion ([M + K]+) are often observed by biological sample analysis. It is very important to choose appropriate matrices for obtaining meaningful biomolecular images. An overview of the matrices used for IMS can also be found in other reviews (Chughtai & Heeren, 2010; Kaletas et al., 2009).

3.2.1 Choice of matrix

The choice of matrix used for MALDI-IMS depends on the mass range and chemical properties of the analytes. Among the many kinds of matrices, sinapinic acid (3,5-dimethoxy-4-hydroxycinnamic acid [SA]) is generally used for high-molecular-weight molecules, such as proteins, while α-cyano-4-hydroxycinnamic acid (CHCA) is often used for medium-molecular-weight molecules, such as peptides. 2,6-dihydroxyacetophenone (DHA), DHB, or 9-aminoacridine (9-AA) is generally used for low-molecular-weight molecules, such as pharmaceutical compounds, lipids, or metabolites (Hattori et al., 2010; Hayasaka et al., 2009; Khatib-Shahidi et al., 2006; Sugiura et al., 2009; Woods & Jackson, 2006).

The development of new matrices is still being reported. We and other research groups recently reported the use of nanoparticles as new matrices (Hayasaka et al., 2010; McLean et al., 2005; Moritake et al., 2009; Su & Tseng, 2007; Sugiura & Setou, 2010). For example, iron oxide nanoparticles enable the visualization of sulfatide and phospholipid distribution (Ageta et al., 2009; Taira et al., 2008), silver nanoparticles can be used for the analysis of fatty acids (Hayasaka et al., 2010), and gold nanoparticles are appropriate for the sensitive detection of glycosphingolipids, such as sulfatides and gangliosides (Goto-Inoue et al., 2010a).

3.2.2 Matrix application

There are various methods for applying the matrix onto the section, such as deposition, spraying, and sublimation. The matrix application method also influences analyte extraction efficiency. Compared to other methods, the deposition of matrix solution using automatic depositing robotic devices, such as a chemical inkjet printer (ChIP-1000; Shimadzu Corporation, Kyoto, Japan), increases signal sensitivity, but decreases spatial resolution (Aerni et al., 2006; Chansela et al., 2011; Morita et al., 2010). The other limitation of the inkjet printer is capillary clogging, which occurs when highly concentrated matrix solutions are used. Spraying is the most frequently used method in MALDI-IMS. Using this method, an entire tissue section can be homogeneously coated with relatively small crystals in a short time without special equipment. For its operation, several instruments, including Thin layer chromatography (TLC) sprayers and artistic airbrushes, are available; we use a metal airbrush with a 0.2-mm nozzle because of its simple and easy-to-handle design. This method requires skillful operation because some airbrush parameters are hand-operated. If there is an excess of matrix solution on the tissue, an inhomogeneous crystal can be formed with analytes that have migrated from their original location; on the other hand, if not enough matrix solution is sprayed and it evaporates without sufficiently moisturizing the tissue section, analytes cannot be adequately extracted from the tissue section. The operation should be performed at a constant room temperature and humidity. Beginners are recommended to practice spraying until homogeneous matrix spraying can be reproducibly achieved. Sublimation is a new method for applying matrix to tissue sections (Hankin et al., 2007). Using this technique, a matrix can be applied uniformly over a large sample plate in a few minutes without solvents. Additionally, previous reports demonstrated that this method increases analyte signal and that the fine microcrystals formed from the condensed vapor reduce the image resolution limitation caused by crystal size (Dekker et al., 2009; Vrkoslav et al., 2010).

3.3 Measurement and data analysis

3.3.1 Measurement

MALDI-IMS should be performed as soon as possible after matrix application, regardless of the coating method. The procedure to obtain a good spectrum in MALDI-IMS is almost the same as that for traditional MALDI-MS; mass range, detector gain, and laser power must be optimized. From the mechanical setting perspective, there are 3 differences between MALDI-MS and MALDI-IMS. The first difference is the above-mentioned matrix application. The second difference is the need for focusing of the laser beam. To obtain meaningful biological images by MALDI-IMS, the laser spot size should be reduced to 10–50 µm. The third difference is that a two-dimensional region must be set for analyses. The scan pitch, which signifies the distance between laser irradiation spots, must be fixed. The limitation of the scan pitch, which decides the spatial resolution of the image, depends on the laser spot size and mechanical movement control of the mass spectrometer sample stage. We have developed a new instrument (Mass Microscope) that can move the sample stage by 1 µm, and in which the finest size of the laser diameter is approximately 10 µm (Harada et al., 2009). The measurement time depends on the number of data spots, the frequency of the laser, the number of shots per spot, and the time required to move the sample stage. For example, when researchers select the region of interest as a 1 × 1 mm^2 area with a 10-µm scan pitch (10,000 data points), it takes about 1 h to complete the measurement using a mass microscope equipped with a 1000-Hz laser (100 shots/data point).

MALDI-IMS ionizes numerous compounds in a tissue at the same time. Sometimes, we detect multiple molecules with the same *m/z* value. In such cases, a new imaging technique, "MS/MS imaging," is effective. Using this technique, we can separate each ion derived from their specific fragment ions. Some reports have described the use of MS/MS imaging for IMS of endogenous metabolites and an exogenous drug (Khatib-Shahidi et al., 2006; Porta et al., 2011). Additionally, the combination of ion-mobility separation with MALDI-IMS provides a unique separation dimension to further enhance the capabilities of IMS (Jackson et al., 2007; McLean et al., 2007; Stauber et al., 2010). It can be used to produce images without interference from background ions of similar mass, and this can remove ambiguity from imaging experiments and lead to a more precise localization of the compound of interest.

3.3.2 Data analysis

A large amount of data (a few gigabytes) is obtained from MALDI-IMS; therefore, visualization software packages that can rapidly and efficiently analyze enormous spectra have been developed. BioMap (a free software; Novartis, Basel, Switzerland), FlexImaging

(Bruker Daltonics, Bremen, Germany), and ImageQuest (Thermo Fisher Scientific, CA, USA) are generally used for visualization. For biomarker analysis of the MALDI-IMS dataset, data mining should be used (Hayasaka et al., 2011; Zaima et al., 2011b; Zhang et al., 2004). Data mining software effectively reduce the number of biomarker candidates (Hayasaka et al., 2011; Zhang et al., 2004). We previously reported the use of principal component analysis (PCA) to discover different biomolecules in starvation-induced fatty livers and normal livers (Zaima et al., 2009). Hierarchical clustering was also used to analyze the data obtained from gastric cancer and non-neoplastic mucosa tissue sections (Deininger et al., 2008). Several studies have reported the discovery of biomarkers using MALDI-IMS (Bakry et al., 2011; Ducret et al., 2006; Hong & Zhang, 2011; Solassol et al., 2009; Zaima et al., 2011b).

4. Instruments

The requirement for performing IMS is the availability of an *x-axis-y-axis* moving stage with electronic controls. Most modern MS instruments produced by major MS hardware companies (*i.e.*, Shimadzu, ThermoFisher Scientific, Bruker Daltonics, Applied Biosystems, Waters) can be adapted for MALDI-IMS. Time of flight (TOF) is the most widely used technology. TOF analyzers allow the separation of ionized accelerated molecules according to their *m/z* ratio. TOF-MS offers suitable performance for MALDI-IMS, namely, good transmission ratio (50–100%), sensitivity, mass range, and repetition rate. However, TOF-MS lacks the capability to perform effective tandem MS experiments. This disadvantage of TOF-MS was overcome with the introduction of hybrid analyzers, such as a combination of quadrupole mass analyzer and TOF (so-called qTOF), combination of quadrupole ion trap (QIT) and TOF (so-called QIT-TOF), combination of ion mobility spectrometry (IMS) and TOF (so-called IMS-TOF), or a combination of two TOF mass spectrometers (so-called TOF-TOF). These combination systems revolutionized the application of TOF-MS systems for structural analysis with tandem MS. In general, the first system is used to select a precursor ion for fragmentation, while the second TOF system is employed for fragment analysis. Other mass analyzers (and their combinations), such as linear ion trap (LIT) (Landgraf et al., 2009; Wiseman et al., 2006; Zaima et al., 2010a), triple quadrupole (QqQ) (Hopfgartner et al., 2009; Porta et al., 2011), and Fourier transform ion cyclotron resonance (FTICR) (Taban et al., 2007), are used for MALDI-IMS. The advantages of commercially available LIT instruments are miniaturization, capability of sample analysis on nonconductive glass slides, MALDI performance at intermediate pressure, and superior performance on multistage MS. The QqQ system allows quantitative analysis and single or multiple reaction monitoring (SRM/MRM). The FTICR system offers very high mass resolving power and high mass measurement accuracy.

5. Applications of MALDI-IMS

5.1 Imaging mass spectrometry-based histopathologic examination

Recently, we applied MALDI-IMS for pathologic examination of atherosclerotic aorta (Fig. 4). We named it imaging mass spectrometry-based histopathologic examination (IbHE) (Zaima et al., 2011c). IbHE revealed the characteristic distribution of biomolecules in smooth muscle cells, lipid-rich regions, and calcified regions of an atherosclerotic lesion obtained from aortic roots of apolipoprotein E (ApoE)-deficient mice. We found that phosphatidylcholine (PC), which contains arachidonic acid (20:4) (*m/z* 804.5), was distributed in the smooth muscle cells of the atherosclerotic lesion. Cholesterol linoleate (CE

18:2) (*m/z* 671.6) and cholesterol oleate (CE 18:1) were characteristically distributed in lipid-rich regions, and the ion at *m/z* 566.9 was localized in the calcified region. These biomolecules were hardly detected in the normal aortic roots of ApoE-deficient mice. We applied this method to other vascular diseases, such as varicose veins, arteriovenous fistulae, abdominal aortic aneurysm, and triglyceride deposit cardiomyovasculopathy, and observed the characteristic distribution of biomolecules (Tanaka et al., 2010; Tanaka et al., 2011). In the analysis of several vascular diseases with atherosclerotic lesions, we often observed ectopic TG distribution. Although the role of TG in the evolution of atherosclerosis remains unknown, there is a possibility that TG plays an important role in the evolution of some kinds of atherosclerosis, as we previously found that characteristic atherosclerosis accumulated TG in aortic lesions, while the accumulated cholesterol was normal (Hirano et al., 2008). The reexamination of vascular diseases by IbHE may result in new findings, because IbHE can visualize the localization of low-molecular-weight molecules, which are rarely visualized by other techniques. We believe IbHE is of considerable value as a new histopathological examination because IbHE can visualize metabolic abnormalities in disease.

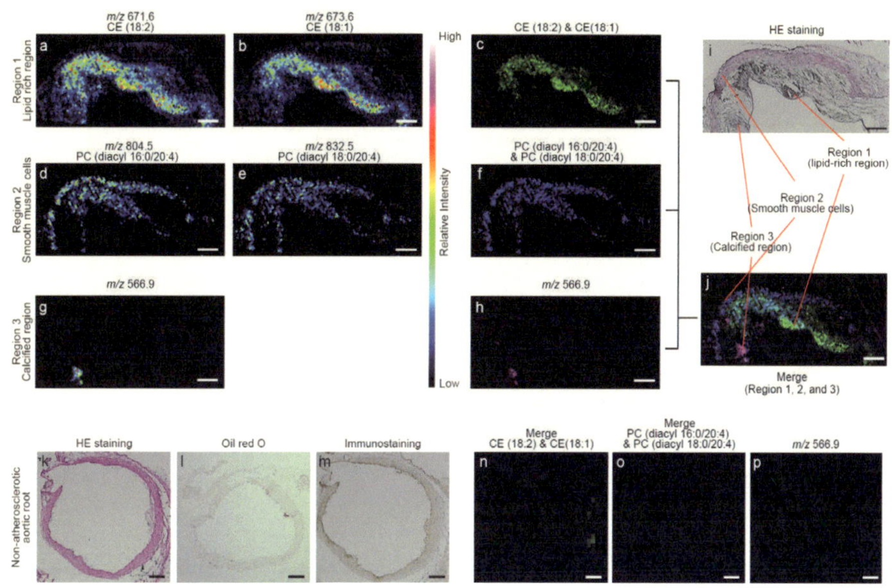

Fig. 4. Representative molecular images of specific ions in a mouse atherosclerotic lesion.

Visualization of biomolecules in atherosclerotic roots (a-j). Scale bar, 100 μm. Specific ion images of region 1 (a and b) and the combined image of *m/z* 671.6 and 673.6 (c). Specific ion images of region 2 (d and e) and the combined image of *m/z* 804.5 and 832.5 (f). Specific ion images of region 3 (g) and the monochrome image of *m/z* 566.9 (h). Comparison of HE staining (i) and the merge images of regions 1, 2, and 3 (j). An image of non-atherosclerotic aortic roots of mice at 12 weeks of age (k-m). Scale bar, 200 μm. HE staining after IMS (k). Oil red O staining (l). Immunostaining of α-actin, which is a marker for smooth muscle cells (m). Merge image of CE (18:2) and CE (18:1) (n). Merge image of PC (diacyl 16:0/20:4) and PC (diacyl 18:0/20:4) (o). Ion image of *m/z* 566.9 (p). "Reprinted from Atherosclerosis, 217. 2, Zaima et al., Imaging mass spectrometry-based histopathologic examination of atherosclerotic lesions, 430., Copyright (2011), with permission from Elsevier."

5.2 IMS for exogenous drugs

MALDI-IMS is a powerful tool for visualizing the distribution of exogenous drugs and their metabolites. Porta et al. reported the visualization of the distribution of cocaine and its metabolites down to a concentration of 5 ng/mg in intact single hair samples from chronic users (Porta et al., 2011) (Fig. 5).

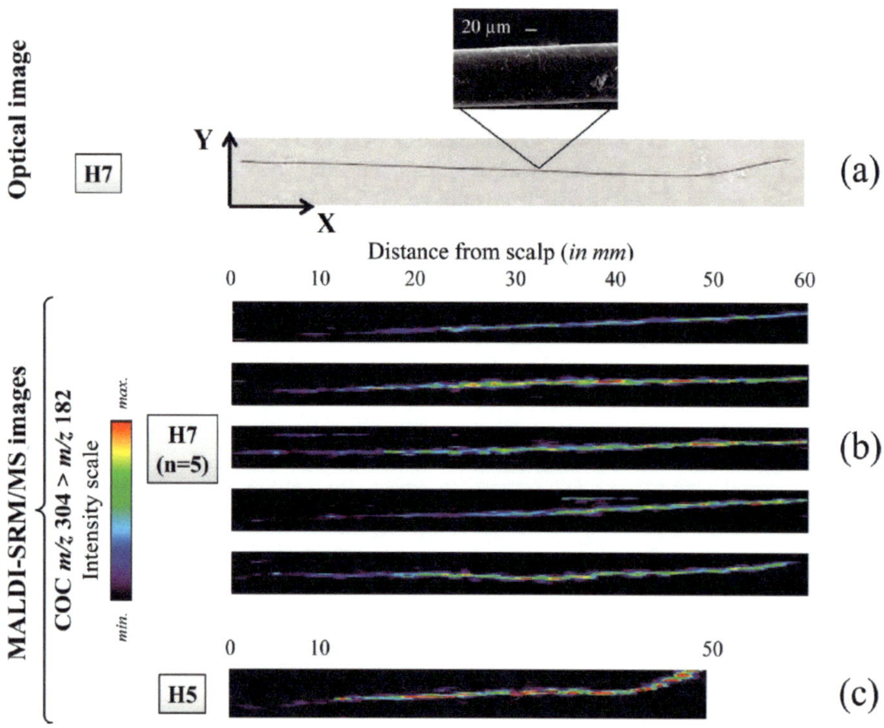

Fig. 5. Imaging of cocaine in hair samples H7 and H5. (H7 and H5 are sample names used in this article)

Optical image of hair sample H7 (a). MALDI-SRM/MS image based on the SRM trace of COC (m/z 305 > m/z 182) for five replicates of single hair samples from individual H7 (b) and single hair analysis from individual H5 (c). The quantitative results from LC-SRM/MS routine analysis were as follows: 130 ng/mg (H7, whole sample); 4.9 ng/mg (H5, segment 0–10 mm), and 8.5 ng/mg (H5, segment 10–50 mm). SRM; selected reaction monitoring. "Reprinted with permission from Porta et al., 2011. Copyright 2011 American Chemical Society."

MALDI-IMS is also applicable to pharmacokinetic analysis. As a Food and Drug Administration (FDA)-mandated pharmacokinetic test, whole-body autoradiography (WBA) is widely performed to determine spatial and quantitative information about a drug compound. Although much information can be acquired by WBA, it has several limitations. First, WBA requires the compound of interest to be radioactively labeled. Furthermore, the detected signal does not distinguish between the original radiolabeled compound and its metabolites that have retained the radiolabel. To complement the disadvantage of WBA, MALDI-IMS and WBA have recently been used together. The combination of MALDI-IMS and

WBA makes it possible to obtain more reliable data for absorption, distribution, metabolism, and excretion of drugs (Atkinson et al., 2007; Caprioli et al., 2008; Clench et al., 2008; Stoeckli et al., 2006). The application of MALDI-IMS to pharmacokinetics in a whole-body mouse section was first reported by Rohner et al. in 2005 (Rohner et al., 2005). In this study, they showed a good correlation between WBA and MALDI-IMS data. Figure 5 shows the simultaneous visualization of drug and metabolites in a whole-rat sagittal tissue section (Khatib-Shahidi et al., 2006). Khatib-Shahidi et al. visualized the temporal distribution of dosed olanzapine (brand name Zyprexa) (8 mg/kg) and its metabolites. In this study, MALDI-IMS was further extended to detect proteins from organs present in a whole-body section.

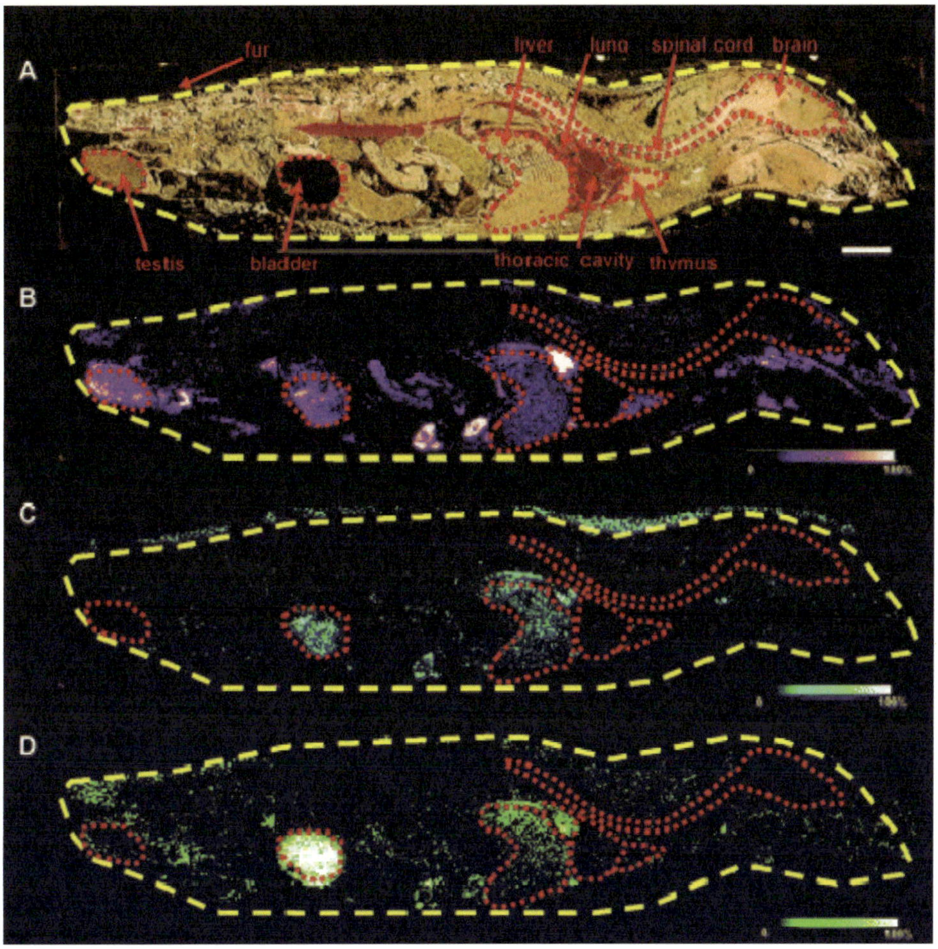

Fig. 6. Detection of drug and metabolite distribution at 6 h post-dose in a whole-rat sagittal tissue section by a single IMS analysis.

Optical images of a 6 h post-olanzapine (OLZ)-dosed rat tissue section across 4 gold MALDI target plates (A). Organs are outlined in red. MS/MS ion image of OLZ (m/z 256) (B). MS/MS ion image of N-desmethyl metabolite (m/z 256) (C). MS/MS ion image of 2-hydroxymethyl metabolite (m/z 272) (D). Scale bar, 1 cm. "Reprinted with permission from Khatib-Shahidi et al., 2006. Copyright 2006 American Chemical Society."

6. Conclusions

MALDI-IMS can be applied to pathological examinations leading to the discovery of potential targets for new drugs, and for the distributional analysis of exogenous drugs in animal and human tissues. We recently used MALDI-IMS in the discovery of metabolites that have pharmacological effects on natural resources. MALDI-IMS will become an essential tool for molecular imaging in pharmacology in the near future.

7. Acknowledgement

This work was supported by the Program for Promotion of Basic and Applied Research for Innovations in Bio-oriented Industry (BRAIN).

8. References

Aerni, H. R., Cornett, D. S., & Caprioli, R. M. (2006). Automated acoustic matrix deposition for MALDI sample preparation. *Anal Chem* 78.3, pp.827-34

Ageta, H., Asai, S., Sugiura, Y., Goto-Inoue, N., Zaima, N., & Setou, M. (2009). Layer-specific sulfatide localization in rat hippocampus middle molecular layer is revealed by nanoparticle-assisted laser desorption/ionization imaging mass spectrometry. *Med Mol Morphol* 42.1, pp.16-23

Andersson, M., Groseclose, M. R., Deutch, A. Y., & Caprioli, R. M. (2008). Imaging mass spectrometry of proteins and peptides: 3D volume reconstruction. *Nat Methods* 5.1, pp.101-108

Atkinson, S. J., Loadman, P. M., Sutton, C., Patterson, L. H., & Clench, M. R. (2007). Examination of the distribution of the bioreductive drug AQ4N and its active metabolite AQ4 in solid tumours by imaging matrix-assisted laser desorption/ionisation mass spectrometry. *Rapid Commun Mass Spectrom* 21.7, pp.1271-6

Bakry, R., Rainer, M., Huck, C. W., & Bonn, G. K. (2011). Protein profiling for cancer biomarker discovery using matrix-assisted laser desorption/ionization time-of-flight mass spectrometry and infrared imaging: A review. *Analytica Chimica Acta* 690.1, pp.26-34

Caprioli, R. M., Cornett, D. S., & Frappier, S. L. (2008). MALDI-FTICR imaging mass spectrometry of drugs and metabolites in tissue. *Analytical Chemistry* 80.14, pp.5648-5653

Caprioli, R. M., Farmer, T. B., & Gile, J. (1997). Molecular imaging of biological samples: localization of peptides and proteins using MALDI-TOF MS. *Anal Chem* 69.23, pp.4751-60

Chansela, P., Goto-Inoue, N., Zaima, N., Sroyraya, M., Sobhon, P., & Setou, M. (2011). Visualization of neuropeptides in paraffin-embedded tissue sections of the central nervous system in the decapod crustacean, Penaeus monodon, by imaging mass spectrometry. *Peptides*

Chen, R., Hui, L., Sturm, R. M., & Li, L. (2009). Three dimensional mapping of neuropeptides and lipids in crustacean brain by mass spectral imaging. *J Am Soc Mass Spectrom* 20.6, pp.1068-77

Chughtai, K., & Heeren, R. M. (2010). Mass spectrometric imaging for biomedical tissue analysis. *Chem Rev* 110.5, pp.3237-77

Clench, M. R., Trim, P. J., Henson, C. M., Avery, J. L., McEwen, A., Snel, M. F., Claude, E., Marshall, P. S., West, A., & Princivalle, A. P. (2008). Matrix-Assisted Laser Desorption/Ionization-Ion Mobility Separation-Mass Spectrometry Imaging of Vinblastine in Whole Body Tissue Sections. *Analytical Chemistry* 80.22, pp.8628-8634

Cornett, D. S., Reyzer, M. L., Chaurand, P., & Caprioli, R. M. (2007). MALDI imaging mass spectrometry: molecular snapshots of biochemical systems. *Nat Methods* 4.10, pp.828-833

Deininger, S. O., Ebert, M. P., Futterer, A., Gerhard, M., & Rocken, C. (2008). MALDI Imaging Combined with Hierarchical Clustering as a New Tool for the Interpretation of Complex Human Cancers. *J Proteome Res* 7.12, pp.5230-5236

Dekker, L. J., van Kampen, J. J., Reedijk, M. L., Burgers, P. C., Gruters, R. A., Osterhaus, A. D., & Luider, T. M. (2009). A mass spectrometry based imaging method developed for the intracellular detection of HIV protease inhibitors. *Rapid Commun Mass Spectrom* 23.8, pp.1183-8

Djidja, M. C., Francese, S., Loadman, P. M., Sutton, C. W., Scriven, P., Claude, E., Snel, M. F., Franck, J., Salzet, M., & Clench, M. R. (2009). Detergent addition to tryptic digests and ion mobility separation prior to MS/MS improves peptide yield and protein identification for in situ proteomic investigation of frozen and formalin-fixed paraffin-embedded adenocarcinoma tissue sections. *Proteomics* 9.10, pp.2750-63

Ducret, A., Meistermann, H., Norris, J. L., Aerni, H. R., Cornett, D. S., Friedlein, A., Erskine, A. R., Augustin, A., Mudry, M. C. D., Ruepp, S., Suter, L., Langen, H., & Caprioli, R. M. (2006). Biomarker discovery by imaging mass spectrometry - Transthyretin is a biomarker for gentamicin-induced nephrotoxicity in rat. *Molecular & Cellular Proteomics* 5.10, pp.1876-1886

Goodwin, R. J., Pennington, S. R., & Pitt, A. R. (2008). Protein and peptides in pictures: imaging with MALDI mass spectrometry. *Proteomics* 8.18, pp.3785-800

Goto-Inoue, N., Hayasaka, T., Zaima, N., Kashiwagi, Y., Yamamoto, M., Nakamoto, M., & Setou, M. (2010a). The detection of glycosphingolipids in brain tissue sections by imaging mass spectrometry using gold nanoparticles. *J Am Soc Mass Spectrom* 21.11, pp.1940-3

Goto-Inoue, N., Setou, M., & Zaima, N. (2010b). Visualization of spatial distribution of gamma-aminobutyric acid in eggplant (Solanum melongena) by matrix-assisted laser desorption/ionization imaging mass spectrometry. *Anal Sci* 26.7, pp.821-5

Groseclose, M. R., Andersson, M., Hardesty, W. M., & Caprioli, R. M. (2007). Identification of proteins directly from tissue: in situ tryptic digestions coupled with imaging mass spectrometry. *J Mass Spectrom* 42.2, pp.254-62

Hankin, J. A., Barkley, R. M., & Murphy, R. C. (2007). Sublimation as a method of matrix application for mass spectrometric imaging. *J Am Soc Mass Spectrom* 18.9, pp.1646-52

Harada, T., Yuba-Kubo, A., Sugiura, Y., Zaima, N., Hayasaka, T., Goto-Inoue, N., Wakui, M., Suematsu, M., Takeshita, K., Ogawa, K., Yoshida, Y., & Setou, M. (2009). Visualization of volatile substances in different organelles with an atmospheric-pressure mass microscope. *Anal Chem* 81.21, pp.9153-7

Hattori, K., Kajimura, M., Hishiki, T., Nakanishi, T., Kubo, A., Nagahata, Y., Ohmura, M., Yachie-Kinoshita, A., Matsuura, T., Morikawa, T., Nakamura, T., Setou, M., & Suematsu, M. (2010). Paradoxical ATP Elevation in Ischemic Penumbra Revealed by Quantitative Imaging Mass Spectrometry. *Antioxid Redox Signal*

Hayasaka, T., Goto-Inoue, N., Ushijima, M., Yao, I., Yuba-Kubo, A., Wakui, M., Kajihara, S., Matsuura, M., & Setou, M. (2011). Development of imaging mass spectrometry (IMS) dataset extractor software, IMS convolution. *Anal Bioanal Chem* 401.1, pp.183-93

Hayasaka, T., Goto-Inoue, N., Zaima, N., Kimura, Y., & Setou, M. (2009). Organ-specific distributions of lysophosphatidylcholine and triacylglycerol in mouse embryo. *Lipids* 44.9, pp.837-48

Hayasaka, T., Goto-Inoue, N., Zaima, N., Shrivas, K., Kashiwagi, Y., Yamamoto, M., Nakamoto, M., & Setou, M. (2010). Imaging mass spectrometry with silver nanoparticles reveals the distribution of fatty acids in mouse retinal sections. *J Am Soc Mass Spectrom* 21.8, pp.1446-54

Hirano, K., Ikeda, Y., Zaima, N., Sakata, Y., & Matsumiya, G. (2008). Triglyceride deposit cardiomyovasculopathy. *N Engl J Med* 359.22, pp.2396-8

Hong, D., & Zhang, F. Q. (2011). Elastic net-based framework for imaging mass spectrometry data biomarker selection and classification. *Statistics in Medicine* 30.7, pp.753-768

Hopfgartner, G., Varesio, E., & Stoeckli, M. (2009). Matrix-assisted laser desorption/ionization mass spectrometric imaging of complete rat sections using a triple quadrupole linear ion trap. *Rapid Commun Mass Spectrom* 23.6, pp.733-6

Jackson, S. N., Ugarov, M., Egan, T., Post, J. D., Langlais, D., Albert Schultz, J., & Woods, A. S. (2007). MALDI-ion mobility-TOFMS imaging of lipids in rat brain tissue. *J Mass Spectrom* 42.8, pp.1093-8

Kaletas, B. K., van der Wiel, I. M., Stauber, J., Guzel, C., Kros, J. M., Luider, T. M., & Heeren, R. M. (2009). Sample preparation issues for tissue imaging by imaging MS. *Proteomics* 9.10, pp.2622-33

Karas, M., Bachmann, D., & Hillenkamp, F. (1985). Influence of the Wavelength in High-Irradiance Ultraviolet-Laser Desorption Mass-Spectrometry of Organic-Molecules. *Analytical Chemistry* 57.14, pp.2935-2939

Karas, M., & Hillenkamp, F. (1988). Laser desorption ionization of proteins with molecular masses exceeding 10,000 daltons. *Anal Chem* 60.20, pp.2299-301

Karas, M., & Kruger, R. (2003). Ion formation in MALDI: the cluster ionization mechanism. *Chem Rev* 103.2, pp.427-40

Khatib-Shahidi, S., Andersson, M., Herman, J. L., Gillespie, T. A., & Caprioli, R. M. (2006). Direct molecular analysis of whole-body animal tissue sections by imaging MALDI mass spectrometry. *Anal Chem* 78.18, pp.6448-56

Landgraf, R. R., Conaway, M. C. P., Garrett, T. J., Stacpoole, P. W., & Yost, R. A. (2009). Imaging of Lipids in Spinal Cord Using Intermediate Pressure Matrix-Assisted Laser Desorption-Linear Ion Trap/Orbitrap MS. *Anal Chem* 81.20, pp.8488-8495

Lemaire, R., Menguellet, S. A., Stauber, J., Marchaudon, V., Lucot, J. P., Collinet, P., Farine, M. O., Vinatier, D., Day, R., Ducoroy, P., Salzet, M., & Fournier, I. (2007). Specific MALDI imaging and profiling for biomarker hunting and validation: fragment of the 11S proteasome activator complex, Reg alpha fragment, is a new potential ovary cancer biomarker. *J Proteome Res* 6.11, pp.4127-34

Lemaire, R., Wisztorski, M., Desmons, A., Tabet, J. C., Day, R., Salzet, M., & Fournier, I. (2006). MALDI-MS direct tissue analysis of proteins: Improving signal sensitivity using organic treatments. *Anal Chem* 78.20, pp.7145-53

McLean, J. A., Ridenour, W. B., & Caprioli, R. M. (2007). Profiling and imaging of tissues by imaging ion mobility-mass spectrometry. *J Mass Spectrom* 42.8, pp.1099-105

McLean, J. A., Stumpo, K. A., & Russell, D. H. (2005). Size-selected (2-10 nm) gold nanoparticles for matrix assisted laser desorption ionization of peptides. *J Am Chem Soc* 127.15, pp.5304-5

Morita, Y., Ikegami, K., Goto-Inoue, N., Hayasaka, T., Zaima, N., Tanaka, H., Uehara, T., Setoguchi, T., Sakaguchi, T., Igarashi, H., Sugimura, H., Setou, M., & Konno, H. (2010). Imaging mass spectrometry of gastric carcinoma in formalin-fixed paraffin-embedded tissue microarray. *Cancer Sci* 101.1, pp.267-73

Moritake, S., Taira, S., Sugiura, Y., Setou, M., & Ichiyanagi, Y. (2009). Magnetic nanoparticle-based mass spectrometry for the detection of biomolecules in cultured cells. *J Nanosci Nanotechnol* 9.1, pp.169-76

Murphy, R. C., Hankin, J. A., & Barkley, R. M. (2009). Imaging of lipid species by MALDI mass spectrometry. *J Lipid Res* 50 Suppl. pp.S317-22

Porta, T., Grivet, C., Kraemer, T., Varesio, E., & Hopfgartner, G. (2011). Single hair cocaine consumption monitoring by mass spectrometric imaging. *Anal Chem* 83.11, pp.4266-72

Rohner, T. C., Staab, D., & Stoeckli, M. (2005). MALDI mass spectrometric imaging of biological tissue sections. *Mech Ageing Dev* 126.1, pp.177-85

Schwartz, S. A., Reyzer, M. L., & Caprioli, R. M. (2003). Direct tissue analysis using matrix-assisted laser desorption/ionization mass spectrometry: practical aspects of sample preparation. *J Mass Spectrom* 38.7, pp.699-708

Solassol, J., Mange, A., Chaurand, P., Perrochia, H., Roger, P., & Caprioli, R. M. (2009). Liquid Chromatography-Tandem and MALDI Imaging Mass Spectrometry Analyses of RCL2/CS100-Fixed, Paraffin-Embedded Tissues: Proteomics Evaluation of an Alternate Fixative for Biomarker Discovery. *Journal of Proteome Research* 8.12, pp.5619-5628

Stauber, J., MacAleese, L., Franck, J., Claude, E., Snel, M., Kaletas, B. K., Wiel, I. M., Wisztorski, M., Fournier, I., & Heeren, R. M. (2010). On-tissue protein identification and imaging by MALDI-ion mobility mass spectrometry. *J Am Soc Mass Spectrom* 21.3, pp.338-47

Stoeckli, M., Staab, D., & Schweitzer, A. (2006). Compound and metabolite distribution measured by MALDI mass spectrometric imaging in whole-body tissue sections. *Int J Mass Spectrom* 260.2-3, pp.195-202

Stoeckli, M., Staab, D., Staufenbiel, M., Wiederhold, K. H., & Signor, L. (2002). Molecular imaging of amyloid beta peptides in mouse brain sections using mass spectrometry. *Anal Biochem* 311.1, pp.33-9

Su, C. L., & Tseng, W. L. (2007). Gold nanoparticles as assisted matrix for determining neutral small carbohydrates through laser desorption/ionization time-of-flight mass spectrometry. *Anal Chem* 79.4, pp.1626-33

Sugiura, Y., Konishi, Y., Zaima, N., Kajihara, S., Nakanishi, H., Taguchi, R., & Setou, M. (2009). Visualization of the cell-selective distribution of PUFA-containing phosphatidylcholines in mouse brain by imaging mass spectrometry. *J Lipid Res* 50.9, pp.1776-88

Sugiura, Y., & Setou, M. (2010). Matrix-assisted laser desorption/ionization and nanoparticle-based imaging mass spectrometry for small metabolites: a practical protocol. *Methods Mol Biol* 656. pp.173-95

Taban, I. M., Altelaar, A. F. M., Van der Burgt, Y. E. M., McDonnell, L. A., Heeren, R. M. A., Fuchser, J., & Baykut, G. (2007). Imaging of peptides in the rat brain using MALDI-FTICR mass spectrometry. *J Am Soc Mass Spectrom* 18.1, pp.145-151

Taira, S., Sugiura, Y., Moritake, S., Shimma, S., Ichiyanagi, Y., & Setou, M. (2008). Nanoparticle-assisted laser desorption/ionization based mass imaging with cellular resolution. *Anal Chem* 80.12, pp.4761-6

Tanaka, H., Zaima, N., Yamamoto, N., Sagara, D., Suzuki, M., Nishiyama, M., Mano, Y., Sano, M., Hayasaka, T., Goto-Inoue, N., Sasaki, T., Konno, H., Unno, N., & Setou, M. (2010). Imaging mass spectrometry reveals unique lipid distribution in primary varicose veins. *Eur J Vasc Endovasc Surg* 40.5, pp.657-63

Tanaka, H., Zaima, N., Yamamoto, N., Suzuki, M., Mano, Y., Konno, H., Unno, N., & Setou, M. (2011). Distribution of phospholipid molecular species in autogenous access grafts for hemodialysis analyzed using imaging mass spectrometry. *Anal Bioanal Chem* 400.7, pp.1873-80

Tanaka, K., Ido, Y., Akita, S., Yoshida, Y., & Yoshida, T. (1987). Detection of High Mass Molecules by Laser Desorption Time-Of-Flight Mass Spectrometry. *Proc. Japan-China Joint Symp. Mass Spectrom.*, pp.185

Vrkoslav, V., Muck, A., Cvacka, J., & Svatos, A. (2010). MALDI imaging of neutral cuticular lipids in insects and plants. *J Am Soc Mass Spectrom* 21.2, pp.220-31

Wiseman, J. M., Ifa, D. R., Song, Q., & Cooks, R. G. (2006). Tissue imaging at atmospheric pressure using desorption electrospray ionization (DESI) mass spectrometry. *Angew Chem Int Ed Engl* 45.43, pp.7188-92

Woods, A. S., & Jackson, S. N. (2006). Brain tissue lipidomics: direct probing using matrix-assisted laser desorption/ionization mass spectrometry. *AAPS J* 8.2, pp.E391-5

Yates, J. R., 3rd (1998). Mass spectrometry and the age of the proteome. *J Mass Spectrom* 33.1, pp.1-19

Zaima, N., Goto-Inoue, N., Adachi, K., & Setou, M. (2011a). Selective analysis of lipids by thin-layer chromatography blot matrix-assisted laser desorption/ionization imaging mass spectrometry. *J Oleo Sci* 60.2, pp.93-8

Zaima, N., Goto-Inoue, N., Hayasaka, T., Enomoto, H., & Setou, M. (2011b). Authenticity assessment of beef origin by principal component analysis of matrix-assisted laser desorption/ionization mass spectrometric data. *Anal Bioanal Chem* 400.7, pp.1865-71

Zaima, N., Goto-Inoue, N., Hayasaka, T., & Setou, M. (2010a). Application of imaging mass spectrometry for the analysis of Oryza sativa rice. *Rapid Commun Mass Spectrom* 24.18, pp.2723-9

Zaima, N., Hayasaka, T., Goto-Inoue, N., & Setou, M. (2010b). Matrix-assisted laser desorption/ionization imaging mass spectrometry. *Int J Mol Sci* 11.12, pp.5040-55

Zaima, N., Matsuyama, Y., & Setou, M. (2009). Principal component analysis of direct matrix-assisted laser desorption/ionization mass spectrometric data related to metabolites of fatty liver. *J Oleo Sci* 58.5, pp.267-73

Zaima, N., Sasaki, T., Tanaka, H., Cheng, X. W., Onoue, K., Hayasaka, T., Goto-Inoue, N., Enomoto, H., Unno, N., Kuzuya, M., & Setou, M. (2011c). Imaging mass spectrometry-based histopathologic examination of atherosclerotic lesions. *Atherosclerosis* 217.2, pp.427-32

Zhang, X., Leung, S. M., Morris, C. R., & Shigenaga, M. K. (2004). Evaluation of a novel, integrated approach using functionalized magnetic beads, bench-top MALDI-TOF-MS with prestructured sample supports, and pattern recognition software for profiling potential biomarkers in human plasma. *J Biomol Tech* 15.3, pp.167-75

21

Closed-Loop Control of Anaesthetic Effect

Santiago Torres, Juan A. Méndez,
Héctor Reboso, José A. Reboso and Ana León
Universidad de La Laguna
Spain

1. Introduction

The interest in automation technologies applied to anaesthesia has been grown exponentially in last decade. The main difference with other fields of automation is that the presence of a human supervisor has been never questioned. In spite of this, the use of automation tools to monitor and control the main variables during surgery notably helps the anaesthetist during surgery. The basic functions of the automation systems in anaesthesia are monitoring and control of the main variables of the process. This leads to two expected benefits. First, the anaesthetist will be freed of some routinary tasks so that he can concentrate more on the state of the patient. On the other hand, using these tools contributes to improve the global performance of the process in terms of safety, costs reduction and patient comfort.

During the surgery operation three main variables have to be regulated: hypnosis, analgesia and muscle relaxation. To achieve this, drugs have to be properly administered to the patient. In recent years many efforts have been made in the development of new drug delivery technologies (Bressan et al., 2009). Most of the difficulties to calculate the proper drug rate to each patient were the inexistence of precise methods to monitor the anaesthetic state of the patient. In the past, patient monitoring was performed just by observing several patient signs (sweat, head lifting, movement, etc.). Nowadays the way that anaesthesia is monitored has changed considerably.

Concerning hypnosis regulation, many efforts have been made to provide the anaesthesiologist with reliable methods for monitoring. In particular, the introduction of the Bispectral Index (BIS) to measure the depth of anaesthesia was one of the key elements in the development of new ways of drug administration (Sigl and Chamoun, 94).

The other main problem in designing control algorithms to regulate hypnosis arises from the complexity of the patient response to drug infusion. This response can be divided in two subsystems. One is the Pharmacokinetics (PK) that refers to the adsorption, distribution, biotransformation and excretion of the drug. And the other is the Pharmacodynamics (PD) that describes the equilibrium relationship between concentration in the body and visible effect produced in the patient. In practice a linear model has been accepted to describe the PK and a nonlinear model for the PD part.

First works involved with anaesthesia control were focused in checking the performance of a fully automated controller compared with the results obtained in a process guided by an anaesthetist. In (Sakai et al., 2000) and (Morley et al., 2000) it is showed that proposed PID controller can assure intraoperative hemodynamic stability and a fast recover of the patient from the hypnosis effects of the drug using closed-loop techniques. In these works and in the works of Absalom (Absalom et al., 2002a, Absalom et al., 2002b, Absalom et al., 2003), it can be shown that the performance of the closed-loop system was as efficient as the observed in the process guided by the specialist, without demonstrating any clinical advantages over the manual techniques.

In the last decade, a lot of research related with automatic control of anaesthesia has been made. Most of them use the intravenous drug propofol as the hypnotic agent. It is important to mention the works that follow a signal-based control, as PID (Liu et al., 2006; Dumont et al., 2009) and fuzzy controllers (Gil, 2004), and the works that follow a model-based control. In this way, many different proposals have been made depending on the controller structure, the controlled variable and the prediction model used. In (Struys. et al., 2001; Sawaguchi et al., 2003; Furutani et al., 2005) the drug concentration in brain is used as controlled variable. In (Ionescu et al., 2008) and (Niño et al., 2009), were EPSAC tecniques are used as controller structure, in (Screenivas et al., 2008), were robust characteristics are added in the design of the controller, and in (S. Syafiie et al., 2009), were nonlinear techinques are used, the authors use predictive control techniques. In (Screenivas et al., 2009) a comparative study between predictive control and PID techniques applied to the control of anaesthetic is done.

The focus of this chapter will be in the regulation of depth of consciousness of patients under general anaesthesia with intravenous propofol.

2. Anaesthetic process: The control problem

The main variables that describe the anaesthetic process are depicted in figure 1. In this figure an input-output description of the system is shown. As can be observed, manipulated variables are anaesthetics, relaxants or serums. Perturbations in the system are signals that can occur at any time (surgical stimulation, blood loss, etc.). The output variables can be measurable and not measurable. The main interest in anaesthesia is focused in non-measurable variables: hypnosis, analgesia and muscular relaxation. Although these variables are not directly measurable, there are methods to estimate them that are used in clinical practice. These methods are based on the use of alternative variables whose behaviour allows the estimation of the non-measurable ones.

Hypnosis is a general term indicating loss of consciousness and absence of the memory of the intervention after awake. Currently, the techniques that have been considered more efficient for this are based in the processing of the patient electroencephalogram (EEG), (Kazama et al., 1999; Struys et al., 2000).

The description of the BIS dynamics has been done mainly with physiological based models. These models consist of a PK part to describe the drug distribution in the internal organs and a PD part to describe the drug effect on the physiological variables of interest.

The drug distribution in the body depends on transport and metabolic processes, which in many cases are not clearly understood. However, dynamical models based on conservation laws that capture the exchange of material between coupled macroscopic subsystems or compartments, are widely used to model these processes.

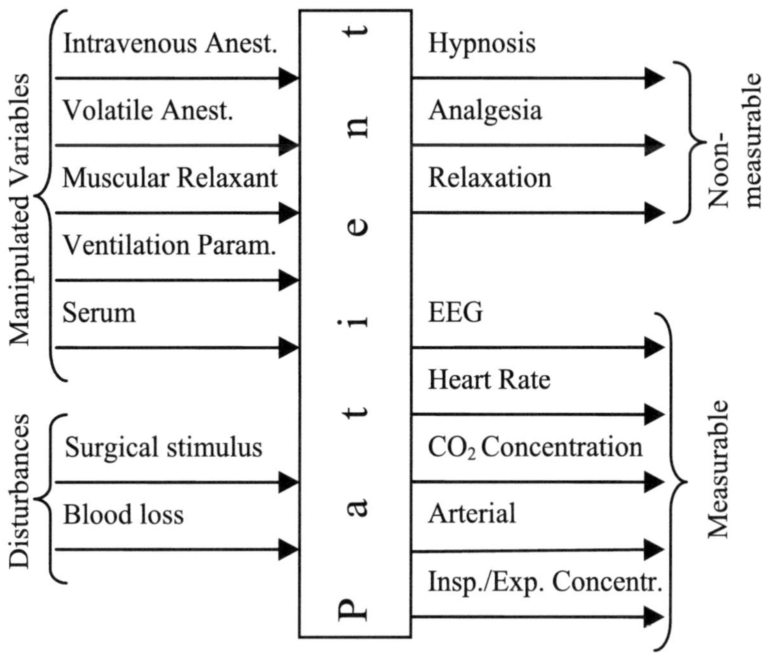

Fig. 1. Input-output description of the anaesthetic process.

2.1 The compartmental model

Figure 2 shows a model based in three compartments: central, fast and slow. The central compartment is the volume in which initial mixing of the drug occurs, and thus can be thought to include the vascular system (blood volume) and for some drugs the interstitial fluid. The fast peripheral compartment represents a compartment of the body that absorbs drug rapidly from the central compartment, and thus can be thought of as comprising tissues of the body that are well-perfused (such as muscles and vital organs). Finally the slow peripheral compartment is used to mathematically represent a compartment into which re-distribution occurs more slowly, and thus can be thought of as including tissues with a poor blood supply (such as adipose tissue).

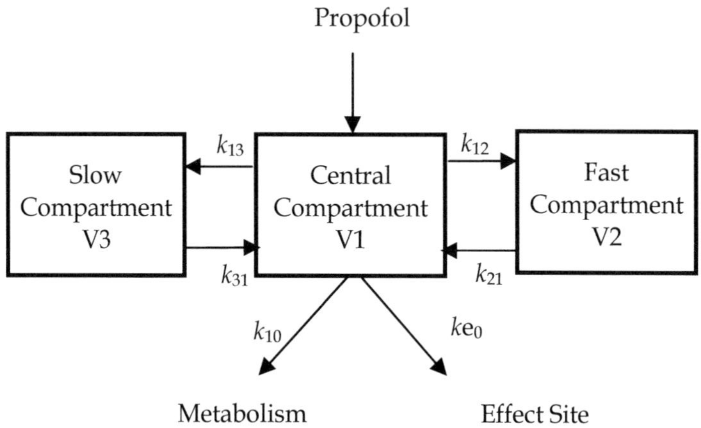

Fig. 2. Compartmental model.

The drug is infused in central compartment and then distributed to the slow and fast compartment and eliminated trough metabolism. Defining the drug concentration variable of the i-th compartment as C_i, the propofol distribution can be described as:

$$V_1 \frac{\partial C_1}{\partial t} = V_2 C_2(t) k_{21} + V_3 C_3(t) k_{31} - V_1 C_1(t)(k_{10} + k_{12} + k_{13}) + u(t) \tag{1}$$

$$V_2 \frac{\partial C_2}{\partial t} = V_1 C_1(t) k_{12} - V_2 C_2(t) k_{21} \tag{2}$$

$$V_3 \frac{\partial C_3}{\partial t} = V_1 C_1(t) k_{13} - V_3 C_3(t) k_{31} \tag{3}$$

$$\frac{\partial C_e}{\partial t} = C_1(t) k_{e0} - C_e(t) k_{e0} \tag{4}$$

where $u(t)$ represents the drug infusion rate in the central compartment and V_i is the volume of the i-th compartment. The dynamics of the compartmental model is defined by the following diffusion constants: k_{10} (rate constant for drug metabolism), k_{12} (rate constant for re-distribution of drug from central to fast peripheral compartment), k_{21} (rate constant for re-distribution of drug from fast to central compartment), k_{13} (rate constant for redistribution of drug from central to slow compartment) and k_{31} (rate constant for redistribution of drug from slow to central compartment). Common PK models for propofol are the Marsh model (Marsh et al., 1991) and the Schnider model (Schnider et al., 1998). Differences between both models can be seen in table 1.

From the point of view of hypnosis control, the variable of interest is not the blood concentration but the concentration in the place where the effect on the controlled variable is produced (effect site concentration). Thus, when there is a simultaneous measure of the drug concentration in blood and its effect on the brain, drug latency can be observed that produces a temporal displacement between the peak of blood concentration and the drug effect.

To include this dynamics in the model a fourth compartment is added. This compartment is known as effect site. It is assumed that this compartment is attached to the central compartment and has negligible volume. The diffusion constant of the effect site is k_{e0}.

	Marsh Model	**Schnider Model**
V_1	0.228 L/Kg	4.27L
k_{10}**(min^{-1})**	0.119	0.0443+0.0107*(BW-77)-0.0159*(LBM-59)+0.0062*(HT-177)
k_{12}**(min^{-1})**	0.112	0.302-0.0056*(Age-53)
k_{13}**(min^{-1})**	0.0419	0.196
k_{21}**(min^{-1})**	0.005	1.29-0.024*(Age-53)
k_{31}**(min^{-1})**	0.0033	0.0035
ke_0**(min^{-1})**	1.21	0.456

Table 1. Comparison of Marsh and Schnider models for PK of propofol. BW stands for Body Weight, LBM is Lean Body Mass and HT is Height.

On the other hand, the drug's pharmacodynamics, that represents the BIS in terms of the effect site concentration, is governed by:

$$BIS = f(C_e) \tag{5}$$

The *f* function is usually taken as an EMAX model whose profile suits the described process:

$$\Delta BIS = \Delta BIS_{\max} \frac{C_e^{\gamma}}{C_e^{\gamma} + EC_{50}^{\gamma}} \tag{6}$$

$$\Delta BIS = BIS - BIS_0 \tag{7}$$

$$\Delta BIS_{\max} = BIS_{\max} - BIS_0 \tag{8}$$

BIS_0 corresponds to the awake state, BIS_{max} represents the minimum achievable BIS and EC_{50} represents the concentration in the effect site for which the effect is half the maximum value, γ represents the sensitivity of the patient to mall concentration variations in the effect site. This parameter can be seen as index that measures the degree of nonlinearity of the model.

2.2 The control problem

From the perspective of the control system three level of complexity can be distinguished. The basic procedure is the open-loop practice in which the anaesthetist, according to the parameters of the patient (age, weight, sex, ASA) directly uses predefined infusion rates of drugs. According to the response observed through his vital signs the drug rates can be modified (the anaesthetist is the controller).

In the next level, it appears the Target Controlled Infusion systems (TCI). In TCI the infusion rate is calculated from models of the pharmacokinetic of the patient, as can be seen in figure

3. Thus, the objective in TCI is to achieve a pre-set target plasma concentration. According to the model of the patient the TCI system (normally implemented in the infusion pump) delivers the adequate drug doses to achieve the objective.

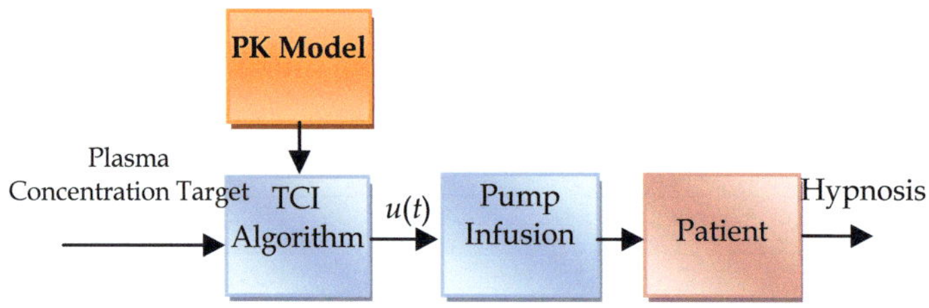

Fig. 3. Hypnosis control with TCI

There is a clear weakness in TCI related to the fact that the real plasma concentration cannot be online measured to compute the infusion rate. That is, TCI is also an open-loop control strategy. Closed-loop strategies appear to solve this problem. The main idea in closed-loop control is to use information of the state of the patient to automatically adjust the drug dosing. Many efforts have been made to provide the anaesthetist with more reliable methods for monitoring this state. In particular, the introduction of the Bispectral Index (BIS) to measure the depth of anaesthesia was one of the key elements in the development of new ways of drug administration (Sigl and Manchoun, 94). BIS has been demonstrated to correlate well with the depth of consciousness of the patient. Thus, it can be used as a feedback system to the controller in order to compute the adequate infusion rate, as can be seen in figure 4.

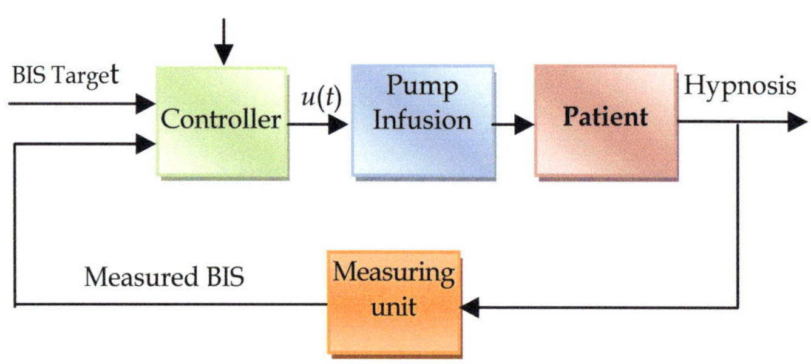

Fig. 4. Hypnosis control with closed-loop controller.

The controller algorithm used for anaesthesia control can be based on signals or in models. Signal based controllers are basically PID algorithms. The key feature of this algorithm is that no model is necessary to compute the infusion rate. Instead, the measured BIS is used to compute an error signal from which the drug dose is calculated. Model based controllers are an alternative to PID controller. The advantage of model-based controller is its ability to predict the behaviour of the patient and anticipate the changes in drug infusion to avoid undesirable responses.

In order to develop an adequate model-based control strategy, it is necessary to obtain a suitable model for the patient behaviour. One common practice is to simplify the model by means of linear approximations around a nominal state (corresponding to BIS target). On the other hand, models are also necessary for offline simulation of the controller structure. The most accepted models for patient representation are those based on compartments to represent the pharmacokinetic together with a nonlinear modelling that describes the PD.

3. Implementation of the closed-loop control of anaesthesia

The main elements that constitute the control system are depicted in figure 5. As can be observed there is a computer that centralizes the monitoring and control task in the system. The BIS monitor is a passive analyser of EEG, that allows monitor the deep of anaesthesia, and has the first objective of adjust in real time the dose of drugs administered to one patient to the actual need. The BIS correlated well with the level of responsiveness and provided an excellent prediction of the level of sedation and loss of consciousness for propofol and midazolam. In this work the Aspect® A-2000 monitor was used. The communication with the computer was implemented via a RS-232 serial interface. Concerning the actuator, the Graseby® infusion pump was used for drug infusion in the patient. The pump is also governed via a RS-232 serial interface.

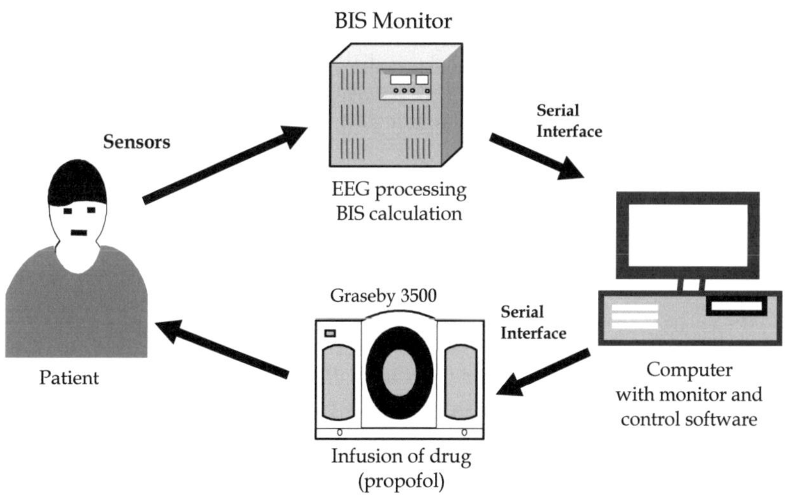

Fig. 5. Main elements of the closed-loop control system.

Apart from sending commands to the pump, the program in the PC reads continuously its state to detect eventual failures of any of the elements in the control loop, like missing BIS signal, excessive infusion rate in the pump syringe changes, etc. The program in the computer has all the routines to monitor and control the system.

The goal is to make a manual induction with propofol and remifentanil and maintain the BIS target during the maintenance of anaesthesia. Remifentanil infusion was adjusted manually and rocuronium was administered in bolus as needs. The operation conditions and the population in which the study was performed are explained in next section.

4. PI control

First control algorithm implemented was a PI controller. This algorithm has been extensively used in several automated closed loop systems. The administration of the drug is made based in the error between the BIS target and the current BIS, and the accumulated error during the operation. Both actions are regulated by gains, which are adjusted in an empirical way trying to get a smooth transitory and a stable response of the patient.

The goal is to make a manual induction with propofol and remifentanil and maintain a BIS target during the maintenance of anaesthesia. Reminfentanil infusion was adjusted manually and rocuronium was administered in bolus as needs. In the real proofs, a BIS target (BIS_r) of 50 is considered while the measurement and actuation period is 5 seconds. Before starting its operation, the software checks that all the security alarms are programmed.

This study was approved by the Ethical and Research Committee of the Hospital Universitario de Canarias and has written informed consent of the patients. The study was performed on a population of 15 patients of 30-60 years. In the real proofs with patients, a BIS target of 50 is considered while the measurement and actuation period is 5 seconds. Before starting its operation, the software checks that all the security alarms are programmed. In the operating room, the patient was connected to the BIS monitor, and the anaesthesia system was started in monitor mode. After the patient had breathed 100% oxygen for 3 min, the system was switched to manual mode, and anaesthesia was induced by means of nearly 2mg/Kg propofol manual bolus. Once the patient achieves a BIS closed to 50, the system is switched to automatic and the interest control algorithm is responsible to regulate the BIS around the objective.

The adjustment of the controller gains was made in an empirical way trying to get a smooth transitory and a stable response. This task was done following standard procedures in online process control engineering. For this, it was necessary the presence of a control expert together with the anaesthesiologist in the operating theatre. Thus, after several trials adequate values for PI controller where found to be Kp=0.67, Ki=0.055. This set of values was tested in the whole population of the study with satisfactory results. Figures 6 and 7 present the evolution of the anaesthesia for two different patients: patient 1 and patient 2. As can be observed, in both cases the system remains stabilised around the reference value with an oscillation of near ±10 units in the worst case (patient 2).

The results obtained with the population submitted to proofs show the patient remains stabilised around the reference value with an oscillation of near ±10 units in the worst case.

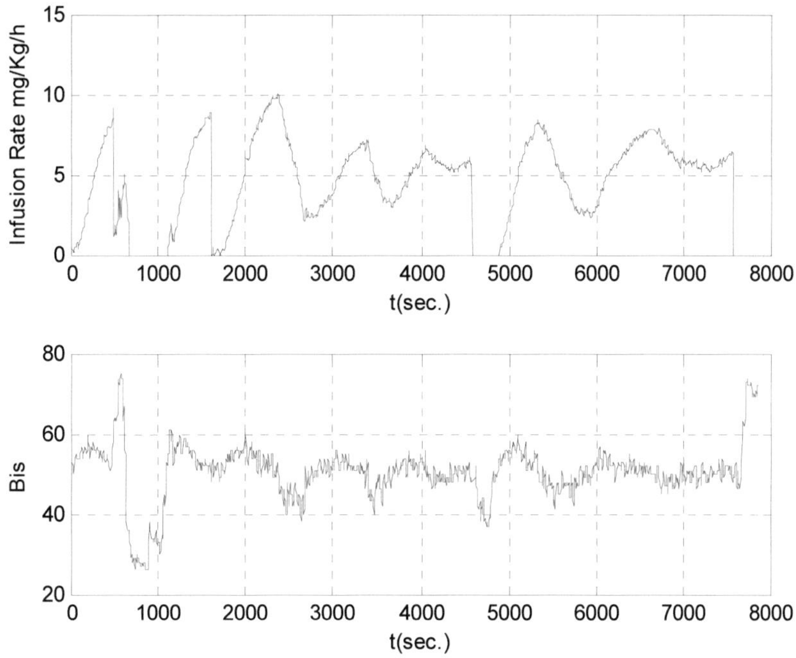

Fig. 6. Results of anaesthesia automatic control on patient 1.

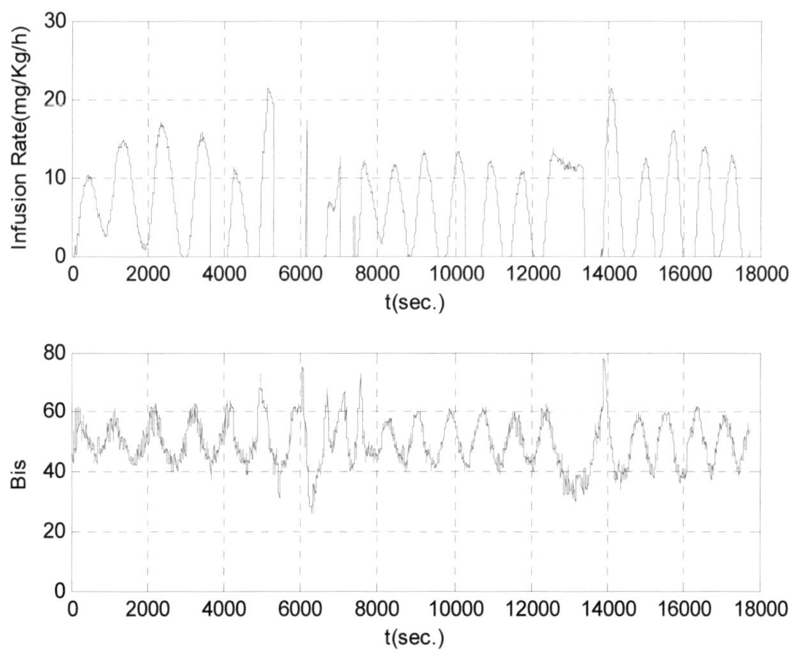

Fig. 7. Results of anaesthesia automatic control on patient 2.

The study revealed that although results are satisfactory, eventually the performance of the controller could decrease. There are two main factors that contribute to this. First of all, the variability between patients implies that the nominal PI parameters chosen are not the best choice for all the patients. Together with this, the dead time present in the system also contributes to reduce the phase margin of the closed loop system. The origin of this time-delay is the period of time since the drug is infused until it causes the adequate effect in the patient. The main effect observed is that the evolution of the BIS is quite oscillatory (see figure 7) around the reference value.

5. Dead-time compensation

In previous section it can be viewed that PI controller usually gives a response with oscillations around the BIS reference value. In this section, the control algorithm is modified in order to compensate these oscillations and get a better transitory. The results shown in this paper are in simulation after having adjusted the patient dynamical model.

The first method implemented to improve the results obtained with the fixed PI controller is to compensate the dead-time present in the system. To do this, a dead-time compensator based on the Smith Predictor theory (Smith, 72) is proposed to act with the PI controller. The basis of the Smith Predictor is to consider the feedback of the controlled variable BIS without delay. As this is variable is not available, the predictor estimates this value and uses this estimation as the feedback signal. To correct the deviations between this estimation and the real value, a correction term, resulting from the error between the estimation and the measured BIS, is added to the feedback signal, as can be seen in the figure 8.

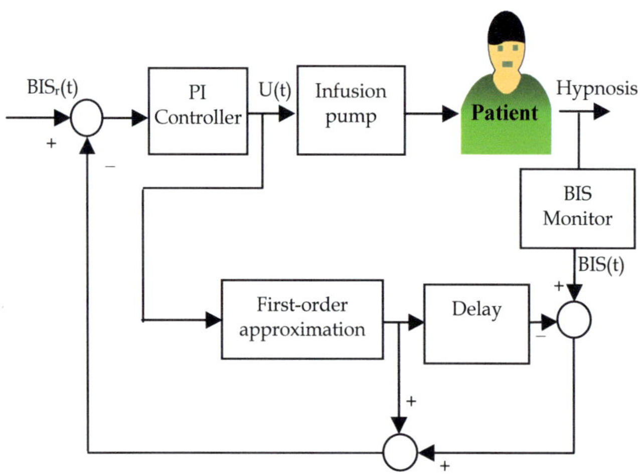

Fig. 8. PI Controller with Smith Predictor for patient hypnosis control.

The basics of this compensation algorithm consider the formulation of the Smith Predictor for linear systems. To apply the Smith Predictor to the nonlinear model of the patient, a first-order plus a time-delay approximation of the patient model is considered. A delay between 90 and 120 seconds is considered.

5.1 Model adjustment

In order to make the simulations proofs of the proposed algorithm, a physiology model of the patient dynamics was designed. As it was told, the model has two parts: pharmacokinetics and pharmacodynamics. The parameters adjustment was made in simulation using the real results obtained from a female, 56 years old patient, 84 Kg. weight, 160 cm. height.

After obtaining a satisfactory manual adjustment, the values for the pharmacokinetics model are k10=0.006, k12=11.0; k21=14.04, k13=10.02, k31=283.50 and ke0=0.0063. The values for the pharmacodynamics model are EC50=610.0, γ=1.5, BIS_0 =100 and BIS_{max}=0.

To validate the model the simulated response is compared with the real one. The obtained results, shown in figure 9a), prove the goodness of the model.

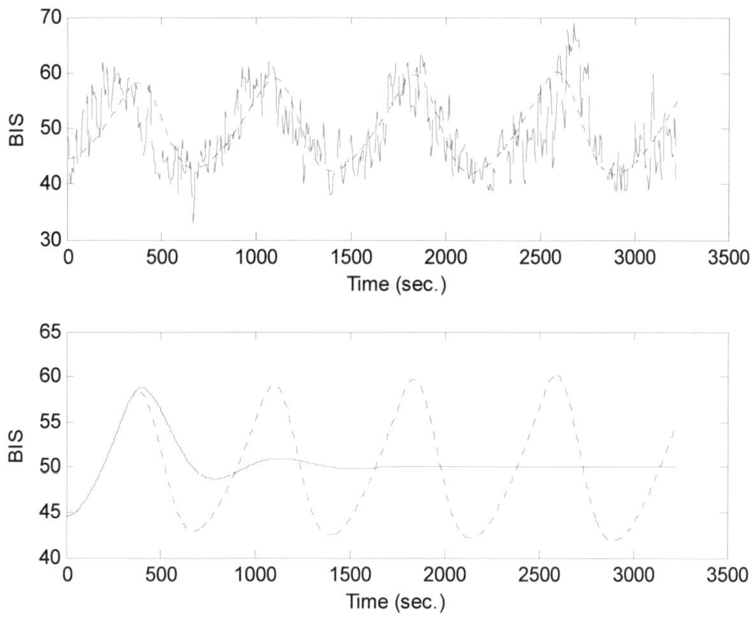

Fig. 9. a) Simulated BIS output (dotted) and real patient BIS output (solid) obtained under the action of a PI controller. b) PI controlled output (dotted) and PI with delay-time compensation output (solid).

5.2 Smith predictor (dead-time compensation)

The proposal here is to improve the performance of the closed-loop system by means of a compensation of the system time-delay. The origin of this time-delay is the period of time between from the infusion pump starts until the drug is distributed along the central compartment. The majority of the works in the literature do not explicitly consider the presence of this time-delay in the proposed models. In fact, in model equations (1)-(4), time-delay is not considered. But in real proofs, some delays between 1 and 2 minutes have to be considered to have a realistic model of the dynamics. Under this hypothesis, a time-delay compensator based on the Smith Predictor theory has been proposed to be added to the PI controller.

5.3 Results with PI controller with dead-time compensation

As it is well known, the basics of this compensation algorithm consider the formulation of the Smith Predictor for linear systems. To apply the Smith Predictor to the nonlinear model of the patient, a first-order plus a time-delay approximation of the patient model is considered. Thus, the configuration employed can be seen in figure 8. A delay between 90 and 120 seconds is considered in the simulations. In figure 9b the results obtained with the patient are shown. The evolution of the BIS signal with the Smith Predictor (in solid line) is much better than with the PI controller (in dotted line), and does not show oscillations around the reference BIS value.

5.4 Self-adaptive dead-time compensation

The main advantage of the time-delay compensation for the PI controller is a better performance in the transitory of the BIS signal. This advantage is conditioned to obtain a good fist-order approximation of the system. However, this model has to be changed in at least two situations. First, when the operation point changes due to a change in the BIS reference for the same patient. Second, when the controller is applied in a different patient, whose physiologic model has to be estimated.

In order to improve the efficiency of that controller, an adaptation of the first-order model patient is added. The aim of this algorithm is to make the time-delay compensator independent of the model assumed for the patient. In order to obtain a simple adaptive algorithm that guarantees the closed-loop stability, model reference adaptive controller - MRAC- (Aström and Wittenmark, 94) is used, as can be seen in figure 10.

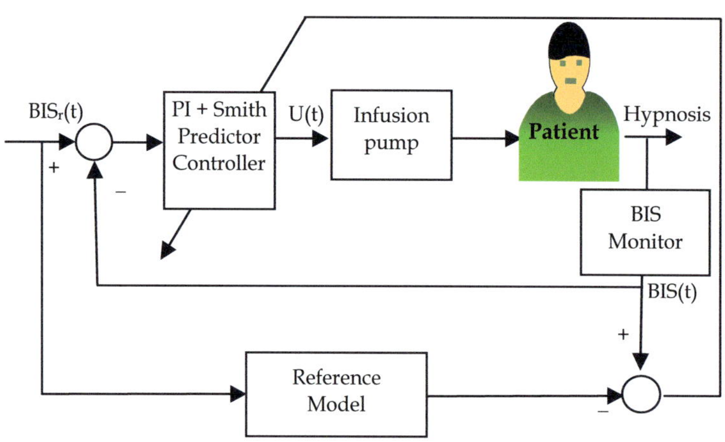

Fig. 10. PI with Smith Predictor controller inserted in the adaptive control scheme MRAC. The error between the system output and the model reference output is used to update the parameters of the PI with Smith Predictor controller.

Following this control scheme, the controller parameters are adjusted by an adaptation law that depends on the error between the system output (BIS) and the model reference output defined for this closed-loop. Minimising a certain cost-function involving this error, an adaptation law of the adjustable controller parameters is obtained. In this case, the adjustable parameters are the static gain and the time constant of the approximated first-order model used in the Smith Predictor.

5.5 Results with the PI controller with self-adaptive dead-time compensation

Several simulation experiments has been made for the patient simulated in previous sections, choosing as the reference model a second-order model with poles, expressed in the z-plane discrete formulation, in z=0.98 and z=-0.75.

The results are shown in figure 11a), where the evolution of the BIS under the self-adaptive compensator algorithm is drawn in solid line and compared with the results obtained in figure 9b) -PI and PI+compensator controllers-. In figure 11b) the evolution of the static gain under this self-adaptive scheme is shown. As it can be observed, some extra oscillations are produced with respect to the previous algorithm, which corresponds to the period of time in that the parameter is adapting.

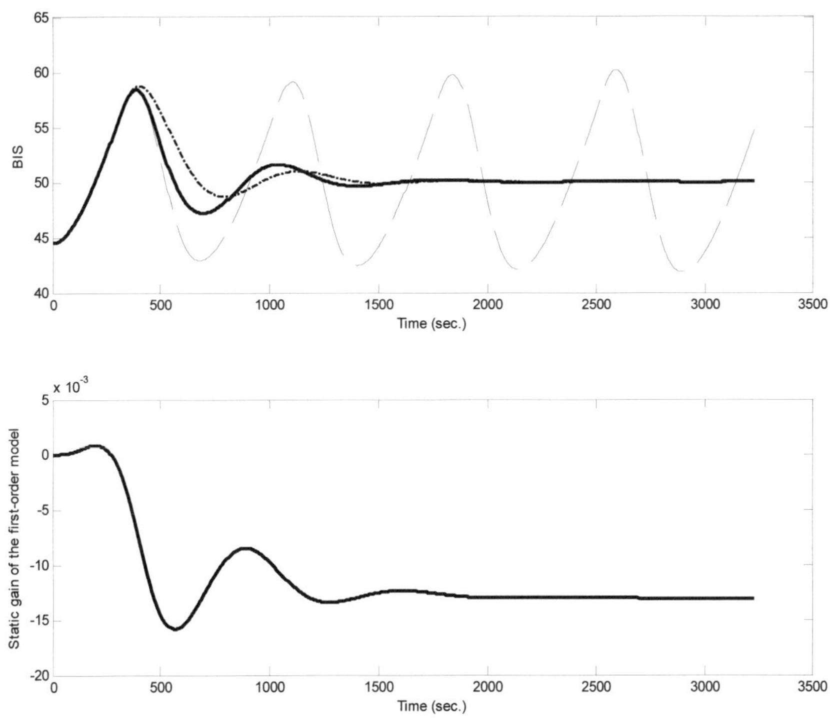

Fig. 11. a) PI controlled system output (dotted), PI with Smith Predictor controlled output (dashed), and self-adaptive time-delay compensation controlled output (solid) compared for the same patient. b) Evolution of the static gain of the first-order approximation model of the time-delay compensation.

Once the optimal values for the parameters are reached, the performance of the system is very similar to the previous controller. In that case, the static gain took a value of -0.037. In this case, the stabilising value for this parameter is near the half. However, the performance is also satisfactory. Moreover, no assumptions over the system had to been made, which is the main advantage of this new algorithm.

Comparing the results obtained with the previous algorithm, some extra oscillations are produced, which corresponds to the period of time in that the parameter is adapting. Once the optimal values for the parameters are reached, the performance of the system is very similar to the previous controller. Moreover, no assumptions over the system had to been made, which is the main advantage of this control algorithm.

6. PI control with self-adaptive gains

Another method to avoid the problem of the oscillations around the BIS reference value occurred with the PI controller is using an adaptive scheme to obtain the gains of the PI controller. The method is based on assuring a desired performance of the closed loop, by emplacing its poles as required, in order to obtain a smooth transition to the BIS reference value.

This method is part of a kind of adaptive controllers, known as self-tuning regulators -STR- (Aström and Wittenmark, 94). They are based on two steps. First, an identification of the system is made in order to get the dynamics in each instant of time. This assures that the controller takes into account the variations in the dynamics of the system. Second step is to compute the control law assuming that the identification results are true. The variety of STR schemes differs in the method used to compute the control law. In this work, an adjustable PI controller is used, which gains are tuned by trying that the closed loop performance of the system be as similar as possible to a desired reference model. This is obtained by emplacing the poles of the reference model into the desired values to get a satisfactory response of the system.

STR controllers have two different parts. The most important part is that they provide an observer in order to identify the dynamics of the system to control. This is an essential point due to the results of the system identification are taken into account to compute the adaptive control law. In this case, a recursive least-squares method based is used to provide the parameters of the dynamics of the observed system.

The second part of the controller is to compute the control law to apply to the system. The results of the identification part are taken to obtain the control action. In this way, the controller takes into account the variations of the dynamics of the system, if they occur. Another advantage of this scheme is its flexibility to be applied to different systems, with the same dynamics but with different parameters, because the identification process adapts the controller to the new situation.

In this case, a pole placement controller is used. Considering the dynamics of the patient as a first order system, and using a PI controller with adaptive gains, the closed loop performance results in a second order system, which dynamics are set by emplacing its poles to the desired values for the closed loop system. Next subsections describe these two parts of the proposed controller.

6.1 Patient dynamics identification

To obtain the dynamics of the patient, a stochastic recursive least-squares method is employed. It consists of an observer of the discrete system that tries to minimize the following cost function:

$$J = \frac{1}{2}\varepsilon^2(k) \tag{9}$$

where $\varepsilon(k)$ is the residual error between the output of the system, $BIS(k)$, and the observed model, being k the instant of time.

Consider the following first order model as an approximation of the patient dynamics, with $u(k)$ being the drug infusion rate of applied to the patient, and $BIS(k)$ the BIS value obtained:

$$BIS(k) + a_1 BIS(k-1) = b_1 u(k-1) \tag{10}$$

It can be expressed by:

$$y(k) = \phi^T(k)\theta \tag{11}$$

$$\varphi(k) = \left[-BIS(k-1) \quad u(k-1)\right]^T \tag{12}$$

$$\theta = \left[a_1 \quad b_1\right]^T \tag{13}$$

In each instant of time, the values of output and input of the system are measured. The iterative process to obtain the best parameters θ that reproduce the performance of the patient is given by the equations:

$$e(k) = y(k) - \phi^T(k)\theta(k-1) \tag{14}$$

$$\theta(k) = \theta(k-1) + W(k)\phi(k)e(k) \tag{15}$$

where:

$$W(k) = \frac{c}{k} \tag{16}$$

being c a constant.

6.2 Pole placement controller

The control law considered for the system is obtained by applying a PI controller. This controller has two gains to adjust: the proportional gain, Kp, and the integer gain, Ki. The discrete version of this controller is given by:

$$G_c(k) = \frac{\alpha + \beta z^{-1}}{1 - z^{-1}} \tag{17}$$

where the relation with the gains is given by:

$$\alpha = K_p + K_i \frac{T}{2} \tag{18}$$

$$\beta = -K_p + K_i \frac{T}{2} \tag{19}$$

being T the sampling time of the system. Considering for the patient the model (10) and for the controller the expression (17), the poles of the closed loop are given by the roots of the following polynomial:

$$D(z^{-1}) = (1 + a_1 z^{-1})(1 - z^{-1}) + b_1 z^{-1}\left(\alpha + \beta z^{-1}\right) \tag{20}$$

Consider the following specification for the closed-loop:

$$Q(z^{-1}) = (1 - q_1 z^{-1})(1 - q_2 z^{-1}) \tag{21}$$

where q_1 and q_2 are the location of the desired poles for the system. It is easy to obtain from (20) and (21) the resulted gains of the PI controller:

$$\alpha = \frac{-1}{b_1}\left(1 + q_1 + q_2 + a_1\right) \tag{22}$$

$$\beta = \frac{1}{b_1}\left(q_1 q_2 + a_1\right) \tag{23}$$

The parameters of the system are obtained in each instant of time form the identification process (15). With the values (22) and (23), the gains of the PI controller are obtained, using (18) and (19), by:

$$K_p = \frac{\alpha - \beta}{2} \tag{24}$$

$$K_i = \frac{\alpha + \beta}{T} \tag{25}$$

6.3 Results with the PI self-adaptive controller

The results shown here correspond to a female of 40 years old, 70 Kg. weight and 170 cm height. The Schnider model presented in section 2 gives an accurate response with the real values obtained for the patient, where the following parameters for (6)-(8) equations are chosen: BIS_0=95, BIS_{max}=8.9, EC_{50}=4.94 μg/ml and γ=2.69. Initially, the patient is infused with a bolus of 1.45 mg/Kg during 2 minutes in order to carry the patient near the desired value for the degree of hypnosis. The reference value is BIS_r=50. After that, the compensated adaptive controller starts controlling the system.

To define the controller, the following assumptions are considered. First, the model for the patient is chosen as:

$$BIS(k) - 0.812BIS(k-1) = -25.389u(k-1) \quad (26)$$

For the second-order reference model, the poles are located in 0.997±0.0027j that correspond to a system with natural frequency 0.05 rad/sec and delta coefficient 0.75. For initiating the identification algorithm (15), the parameters used in (26) are chosen. *c* constant in (16) is set to 0.005.

Figure 12 shows the evolution of the BIS and the parameters of the PI controller in this case. As it can be seen, after the application of the initial bolus, the PI controller varies its gains and the patient remains its degree of freedom around the desired value of 50, but with oscillations.

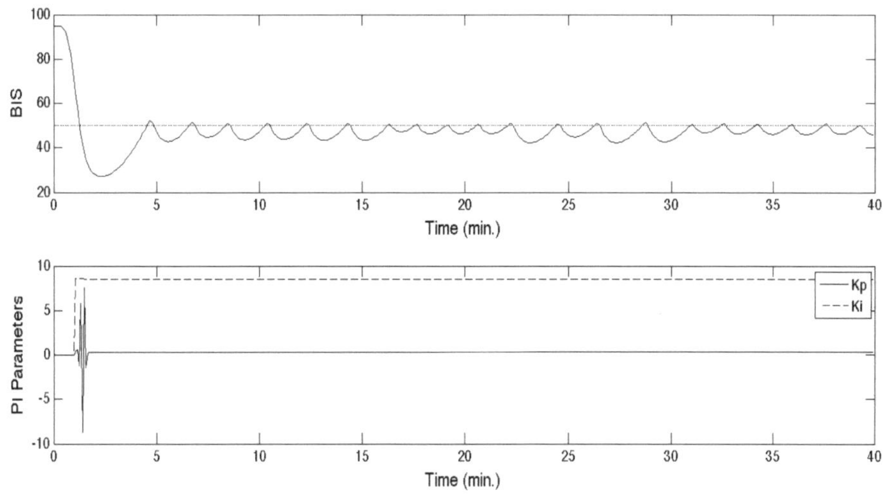

Fig. 12. Results of the PI self-adaptive controller. First graph shows the BIS evolution with respect to BIS_r and second graph are the gains evolution of the PI controller.

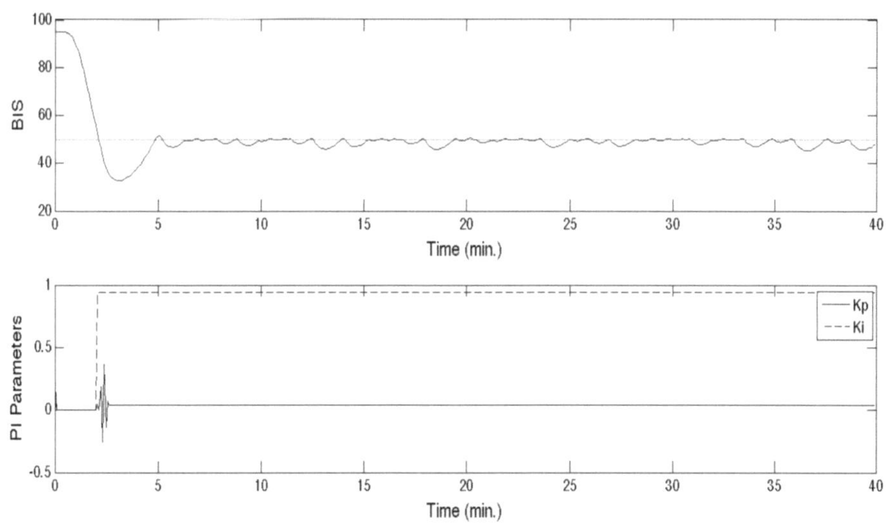

Fig. 13. Results of the compensated self-adaptive PI controller. First graph shows the BIS evolution with respect to BIS_r and second graph are the gains evolution of the PI controller.

To avoid these oscillations in the stationary, the compensation of the time delay by means of a Smith predictor is done in this case. To do that, the time delay considered is 1 minute. Figure 13 shows the results obtained in this case. The oscillations around the objective value are considerably reduced and the performance of the closed loop systems results better than in previous case.

7. Model Predictive Control (MPC)

As an alternative to signal based controllers proposed before, it is shown an algorithm that uses explicitly the model of the patient to compute the drug infusion rate. The objective is to improve the performance of other techniques as those based in PI controllers. Figure 14 shows the structure of the proposed controller. As can be observed, the drug infusion rate is computed as a sum of two terms:

$$u(t) = u_n + \delta u \tag{27}$$

The first term (u_n) is obtained by inverting the model of the patient and is computed to take the BIS variable to the nominal value (BIS_r=50, x_n). That is, from the target BIS (BIS_r) and using the model of the patient (PK+PD) it can be obtained the infusion rate that leads the BIS signal to the desired value. To do this, the inverse dynamics of the system model is evaluated, assuming that the system is approximated by (1)-(5). Taking matrix notation for this model, it can be expressed by:

$$\dot{x} = Ax + Bu \tag{28}$$

where $x = [C_1 \quad C_2 \quad C_3 \quad C_e]^T$.

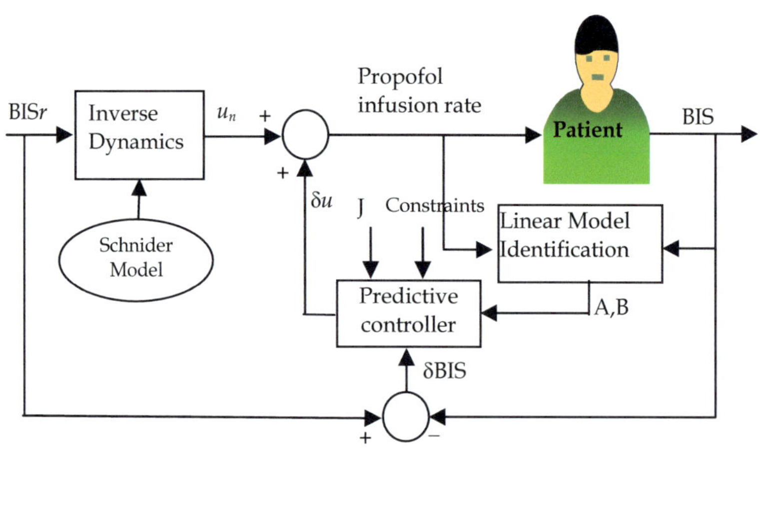

Fig. 14. Structure of the proposed model-based predictive controller.

Assuming that the target state is an equilibrium state $x_n = \begin{bmatrix} C_{1n} & C_{2n} & C_{3n} & C_{en} \end{bmatrix}^T$, the nominal input can be obtained by solving:

$$Ax_n + Bu_n = 0 \tag{29}$$

C_{en} is computed by using the EMAX model (6), (7) and (8):

$$C_{en} = \exp\left(\frac{1}{\gamma}\ln\left(EC_{50}^{\gamma}\frac{\alpha}{1-\alpha}\right)\right) \tag{30}$$

with:

$$\alpha = \frac{BIS_r - BIS_0}{BIS_{\max} - BIS_0} \tag{31}$$

Finally, to compute the nominal input u_n and the nominal state x_n equation (29) is solved to obtain the following solution:

$$x'_n = M^{-1}N \tag{32}$$

where $x'_n = \begin{bmatrix} C_{1n} & C_{2n} & C_{3n} & u_n \end{bmatrix}^T$ and:

$$M = \begin{bmatrix} A_{11} & A_{12} & A_{13} & B_1 \\ A_{21} & A_{12} & A_{23} & B_2 \\ A_{31} & A_{32} & A_{33} & B_3 \\ A_{41} & A_{42} & A_{43} & B_4 \end{bmatrix} \tag{33}$$

$$N = -\begin{bmatrix} A_{14}C_{en} \\ A_{24}C_{en} \\ A_{34}C_{en} \\ A_{44}C_{en} \end{bmatrix} \tag{34}$$

In Fig. 15, a simulation of the BIS in a patient with only this nominal input (u_n) is presented.

As can be observed, the BIS tends to the nominal value (BIS_r=50) if only this input is applied. In practice, several considerations have to be taken into account. The first one is related to the modeling errors in the patient dynamics. In the simulation presented here no modeling errors were considered. In the real implementation, a deviation of the response of the system with respect to this ideal trajectory will be observed. On the other hand, as can be observed, the response exhibits a sluggish behavior that in real practice is undesirable. That is why this action is complemented with an additional term that tries to correct the deviations of the system from the nominal trajectory and also improves the transient response of the BIS curve.

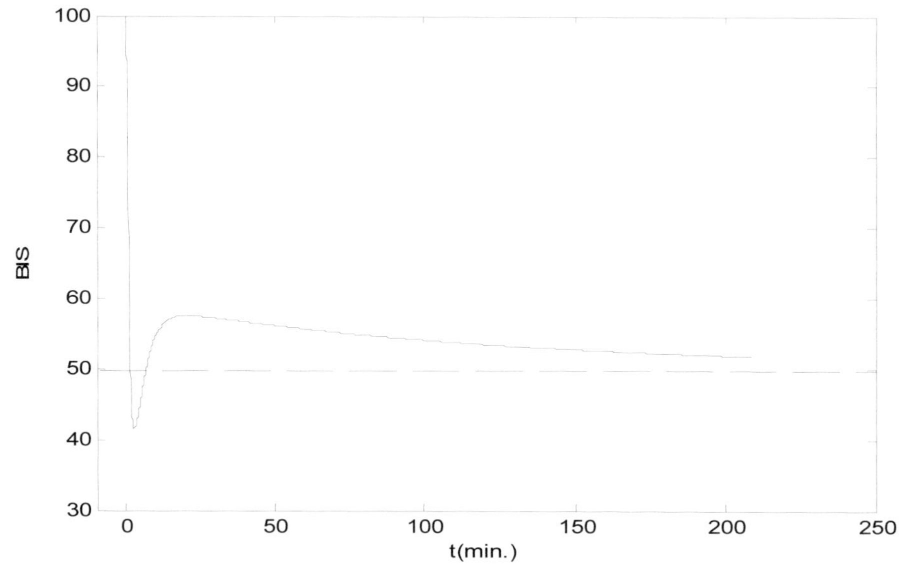

Fig. 15. Simulation of the BIS in a patient applying only the nominal input u_n.

This action is computed considering that the deviations of the BIS from the nominal value can be described by a linear approximation:

$$\delta\dot{x} = A\delta x + B\delta u \tag{35}$$

$$\delta BIS = C\delta x + D\delta u \tag{36}$$

where $\delta x = x - x_n$ and $\delta BIS = BIS - BIS_r$.

Then the control law δu_k can be obtained from an optimization problem (model based predictive controller). The problem can be formulated as obtaining the control law δu_k so that a specified cost function is minimized under a receding horizon strategy. Consider for example the following index:

$$J_k = \sum_{j=1_1}^{N} \gamma(j)\left[w(k+j) - \hat{y}(k+j\,|\,t)\right]^2 + \sum_{j=1}^{NU} \lambda(j)\left[\delta u(k+j-1)\right]^2 \tag{37}$$

where N is the prediction horizon and NU is the control horizon. The problem is to find the sequence δu_{k+j} so that J_k is minimized. Assuming a receding horizon strategy, only the first value of the sequence is applied and the procedure is repeated at k+1. In this optimization, constraints can also be included, although the computational complexity is greatly increased.

Figure 16 shows a simulation of this strategy. Initial condition was BIS=39. As can be observed, the response of the system is now much faster than that observed in figure 14 and achieves a very acceptable error quite soon.

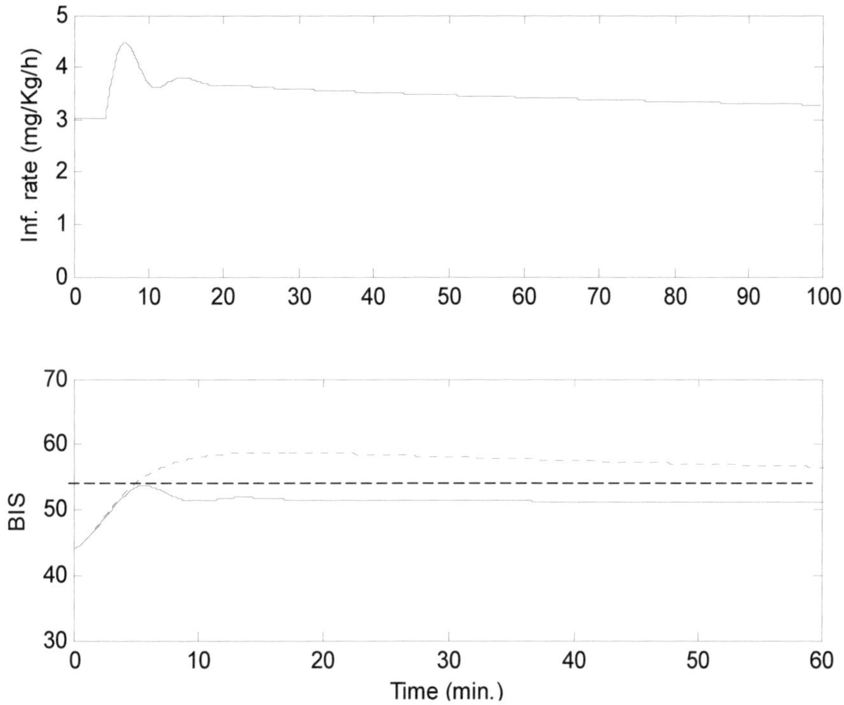

Fig. 16. Simulation of the model-based controller of figure 14 on a patient. Nominal input (dashed line) and nominal+predictive controller (solid line).

8. Conclusion

In this chapter both results on modelling and control of patients under general anaesthesia with propofol is presented. First results presented refer to the synthesis of linear models for use in model-based controllers. The anaesthetic process was segmented into several phases, according to the state of the surgery (consciousness, hypnosis, intubation, incision, etc.). The propofol infusion rate in ml/h was used as the input variable *u(t)*, while the BIS represented the output. Validation of the proposed model was done with real data patients.

For simulation purposes a PK/PD model based on compartmental approaches as obtained. The model was adjusted using information of real data from patients. The obtained model was used to simulate the response of the patients with the different controllers.

Concerning hypnosis control, this chapter presents a review of the state of the art of the closed-loop control of anaesthesia. Then, a description of approaches based on signal feedback and model based controllers are presented.

The chapter proposed an advanced PI controller with several important features. First, an adaptive module is included that adapts the controller to the specific patient behaviour. On the other hand, the controller incorporates a dead-time compensation system that improves notably the performance of the controller. The performance of this compensation is improved by self-adapting the approximation of the patient model used in the Smith Predictor scheme.

The last part of the chapter is devoted to the design of model-based controllers. In particular, a model-based predictive controller is presented that corrects efficiently the transient evolution of the BIS, offering a smooth evolution of this signal to the reference value.

9. Acknowledgment

This work is under the auspicious of the Research Project DPI2010-18278 supported by "Ministerio de Educación y Ciencia" of the Spanish Government.

10. References

Absalom, A.R., Sutcliffe, Kenny, G.N.C., (2002a). *Closed-loop Control of Anesthesia Using Bispectral Index. Performance Assessment in Patients Undergoing Major Orthopedic Surgery under Combined General and Regional Anesthesia.* Anesthesiology; 96. pp.67–73.

Absalom, A.R.; Leslie, K.; Kenny, G.N.C. (2002b). *Closed loop control of sedation for colonoscopy using the Bispectral Index.* Anaesthesia, 57. pp. 690–709.

Absalom, A.R.; Kenny, G.N.C. (2003). *Closed-loop control of propofol anaesthesia using bispectral indexTM: performance assessment in patients receiving computer controlled propofol and manually controlled remifentanil infusions for minor surgery.* British Journal of Anaesthesia 90, No. 6. pp. 737-741.

Åström, K.J.; Wittenmark, B. (1994). *Adaptive Control (2nd ed.).* Addison-Wesley Publishing Company, Inc.

Bressan, N.; Moreira, A.P.; Amorim, P.; Nunes, C.S. (2009). *Target controlled infusion algorithms for anesthesia: Theory vs practical implementation.* Engineering in Medicine and Biology Society, EMBC 2009. Annual International Conference of the IEEE, pp. 6234-6237.

Dumont, G.A.; Martinez, A.; Ansermino, J.M. (2009). *Robust control of depth of anesthesia.* International Journal of Adaptive Control and Signal Processing, No. 23. pp. 435–454.

Furutani, E.; Sawaguchi, Y.; Shirakami, G.; Araki, M.; Fukuda, K. (2005). *A hypnosis control system using a model predictive controller with online identification of individual parameters.* Proceedings of the 2005 IEEE Conference on Control Applications. Toronto, Canada, August, pp. 28-31.

Gil, F.G. (2004). *Sistema de ayuda a la toma de decisiones mediante logica fuzzy en anestesia intravenosa: modelo farmacocinetico/farmacodinamico del propofol.* PhD. Thesis, Universidad de Murcia, España.

Ionescu, C.M.; De Keyser, R.; Torrico, B.C.; De Smet, T.; Struys, M.M.; Normey-Rico, J.E. (2008). *Robust Predictive Control Strategy Applied for Propofol Dosing Using BIS as a Controlled Variable During Anesthesia.* IEEE Transactions On Biomedical Engineering, Vol. 55, No. 9, pp. 2161-2170.

Kazama, T.; Ikeda, K.; Morita, K.; Kikura, M.; Doi, M.; Ikeda, T.; Kurita, T.; Nakajima, Y. (1999). *Comparison of the Effect-site keO s of Propofol for Blood Pressure and EEG Bispectral Index in Elderly and Younger Patients*. Anesthesiology, Vol. 90, No. 6, June, pp. 1517-1527.

Liu, N.; Chazot, T.; Genty, A.; Landais, A.; Restoux, A.; McGee, K.; Laloë, P.A.; Trillat, B.; Barvais, L.; Fischler, M. (2006). *Titration of Propofol for Anesthetic Induction and Maintenance Guided by the Bispectral Index: Closed-loop versus Manual Control. A Prospective, Randomized, Multicenter Study*. Anesthesiology, No. 104. pp. 686–695.

Marsh, B. ; White, M. ; Morton N. ; Kenny, G.N.C. (1991). *Pharmacokinetic model driven infusion of propofol in children*. Br J Anaesth., Vol. 67, pp. 41-48.

Morley, A., Derrick, J., Mainland, P., Lee, B. B. and Short, T. G. (2000). *Closed loop control of anaesthesia: an assessment of the bispectral index as the target of control*. Anaesthesia, 55. pp. 953-959.

Niño J.; De Keyser, R.; Syafiie, S.; Ionescu, C.; Struys, M.M. (2009). *EPSAC-controlled anesthesia with online gain adaptation*. International Journal of Adaptative Control and Signal Processing, No. 23, pp. 455–471.

Sawaguchi, Y.; Purutani, E.; Shirakami, G.; Araki, M.; Fukuda, K. (2003). *A model predictive sedation control system under total intravenous anesthesia*. Proceedings of the IEEE EMBS Asian-Pacific Conference on Biomedical Engineering, pp. 358- 359.

Sakai, T.; Matsuki A.; White P.F.; Giesecke A.H. (2000). *Use of an EEG-bispectral closed-loop delivery system for administering propofol*. Anaesthesiologica Scandinavica, 44. pp. 1007-1010.

Schnider, T.W.; Minto, C.F.; Gambus, P.L.; Anderson, C.; Goodale, D.B.; Shafer S.L.; Youngs, E.J. (1998). *The Influence of method of administration and covariates on the pharmacokinetics of propofol in adult volunteer*. Anesthesiology, Vol. 88, pp. 1170–1182.

Sigl, J.C.; Chamoun, N.G. (1994). *An introduction to bispectral analysis for the electroencephalogram*. Journal of Clinical Monitoring, Vol. 10, No.6, pp. 392-404.

Smith, C. (1972). *Digital Computer Process Control*. Intext Education Publishers. Scranton PA.

Sreenivas, Y.; Samavedham, L.; Rangaiah, G. P. (2008). *Advanced Regulatory Controller for Automatic Control of Anesthesia*. Proceedings of the 17th World Congress of The International Federation of Automatic Control, Seoul, Korea, July, pp. 6-11.

Sreenivas, Y.; Samavedham, L. Rangaiah, G. P. (2009). *Advanced Control Strategies for the Regulation of Hypnosis with Propofol*. Ind. Eng. Chem. Res., No. 48, pp. 3880–3897.

Struys, M.M.; De Smet, T.; Depoorter, B.; Versichelen, L.F.; Mortier, E.P.; Dumortier, F.J.; Shafer, S.L.; Rolly, G. (2000). *Comparison of plasma compartment versus two methods for effect compartment-controlled target controlled infusion for propofol*. Anesthesiology, Vol. 92, No. 2, pp. 399–406.

Struys, M.M.; De Smet, T.; Versichelen, L.F.; Van De Velde, S.; Van den Broecke, R.; Mortier, E.P. (2001). *A Comparison of Closed-loop Controlled Administration of Propofol Using Bispectral Index as the Controlled Variable versus "Standard Practice" Controlled Administration*. Anesthesiology, No. 95. pp. 6–17.

Syafiie, S.; Niño, J.; Ionescu, C.; De Keyser, R. (2009). *NMPC for Propofol Drug Dosing during Anesthesia Induction*. L. Magni et al. (Eds.): Nonlinear Model Predictive Control, LNCIS, No. 384, pp. 501-509.

Part 6

Ethnopharmacology and Toxicology

The Influence of Displacement by Human Groups Among Regions in the Medicinal Use of Natural Resource: A Case Study in Diadema, São Paulo - Brazil

Daniel Garcia and Lin Chau Ming
Universidade Estadual Paulista – Faculdade de Ciências Agronômicas
Brazil

1. Introduction

The migration of human groups around the world and the cultural mix of these people has instigated more researches in the field of ethnobotany/ethnopharmacology in recent years (Pieroni & Vandebroek, 2007). Brazil is an example of blending traditional knowledge combined with the use of natural resources to the cure of various diseases and, therefore, have been the subject of several surveys including ethnobotanical and ethnopharmacological. Given the enormous biological diversity and biochemistry in the several biomes around the world and also in Brazil, it is very difficult to find randomly a molecule on which it is possible to develop a competitive drug, acting on a mechanism known and has significant pharmacological properties (FAPESP, 2011). Therefore, the ethnobotany/ethnopharmacology are among the main strategies used for selecting plants to be investigated in laboratorial studies, those with great chances of success (Spjut & Perdue, 1976; Balick, 1990 as cited in Rodrigues, 2005), and is one of the fastest ways to obtain a safe product and pharmacologically active (Giorgetti et al., 2007).

The ethnobotany looks at how people incorporate the plants in their cultural traditions and folk practices (Balick & Cox, 1997) or, according to Alcorn (1995), is the study of the interrelationships between humans and plants in dynamical systems (as cited in Rodrigues et al., 2005).

The ethnopharmacology was originally defined as a science that sought to understand the universe of natural resources (plants, animals and minerals) as drugs used in the view of human groups (Schultes, 1988). However, over time this discipline has evolved and is defined by the INTERNATIONAL SOCIETY FOR ETHNOPHARMACOLOGY as:

"Interdisciplinary study of the physiological actions of plants, animals and others substances used in indigenous medicines of past and present cultures".

This concept is also currently applied in the case of medicinal substances from non-indigenous people, thus expanding the diversity of information generated in studies ethnopharmacological. The relationship of the biological wealth of the world's diverse ecosystems, sometimes aided by the traditional knowledge of people who directly depend on these places to survive, is ancient for an extensive possibilities of discovering medicinal formulas for curing various diseases. The multiple possibilities resulting from this combination, natural biodiversity and cultural diversity, give richness and complexity in terms of knowledge about the flora and their therapeutic potential, some studies as: Pieroni & Vandebroek (2007) and Garcia et al., (2010) show that this relationship is even more intrinsic when there is displacement of human groups to a new environment.

Brazil offers a favourable environment for studies focused on migration and medicinal plants/animals because it possesses a large area of 8,514,876.599 km^2 (IBGE, 2011) and boasts high indices of cultural and biological diversity. In Brazil, the use of herbs for medicinal purposes is a common practice and very diverse, result of intense mixing that occurred during colonization (Europeans and Africans - sixteen to the eighteen century), added with the ancient knowledge of indigenous people, who ever inhabited these lands (Giorgeti et al., 2007).

Brazil is inhabited by mestizo groups derived from the miscegenation of Indian, Black, European and Asiatic people, 232 indigenous ethnic groups (Instituto Socioambiental, 2011) and 1,342 Quilombola groups (descendants of Afro-Brazilian people) (Fundação Cultural Palmares, 2011). Brazil has the richest flora in the world, with nearly 56.000 species of plants (Ribeiro, 1996; Schultes, 1990). For these and other reasons Brazil may be considered a laboratory *in situ* for a variety of processes that are studied by researchers from diverse fields, including the development of pharmaceutical drugs (Rodrigues, 2007).

However, at present moment, marked by the destruction of natural ecosystems, not only the biodiversity of plants and animals are affected, but also human groups that depend of environments to survive (Davis, 1995).

According to Simões and Lino (2004), the original Atlantic Forest covered approximately 1.3 million km^2, spanning 17 Brazilian states from south to northeast; however, it currently covers only 14 states, and its area has been reduced to 65,000 km^2. Despite alarming fragmentation, the Atlantic Forest still contains more than 20,000 plant species (8,000 endemic) and 1,361 animal species (567 endemic). It is the richest forest in the world in wood plants per unit area; the southern Bahia, for example, holds a record of 454 different species/ha (IBAMA, 2011).

Because of this reality, ethnobotanical and ethnopharmacological surveys make an important role in collecting and valuing traditional knowledge of people about the medicinal use of biodiversity in which they live. This assumption, undoubtedly, is the key to preserve the biodiversity of these sites, as well as cultural traditions, once the ignorance on the potential pharmacological importance for the society becomes absent. While migration has become an integral part of modern globalization is as old as human society (Thomas et al., 2009; Waldstein, 2008). There are many reasons why people decide to leave home and live somewhere else, some having reasons within the place of origin, others with perceived opportunities available from the new environment (Findley & De Jong, 1985; Suzuki, 1996). Whatever the reason for the displacement, the migrants experience some difficulties and opportunities due to its displacement to a new location that those who stay behind may not experience (Lacuna-Richman, 2006). Numerous studies have related information on medicinal plants from human groups who migrated from Haiti to Cuba (Volpato et al., 2009); from Mexico to the U.S.A. (Waldstain, 2006, 2008); from Africa to South America

(Voeks, 2009); from Africa to Brazil (Carney & Voeks, 2003); from Suriname to the Netherlands (van Andel & Westers, 2010); from Colombia to London (Ceuterick et al., 2008); from Germany to eastern Italy (Pieroni et al., 2004); from Albania to southern Italy (Pieroni et al., 2002a, 2002b); and from Europe and Africa to eastern Cuba (Cano & Volpato, 2004; Pieroni & Vandebroek, 2007). However, few studies have focused on migration within a country, such as that described by Rodrigues et al. (2005) and Garcia et al. (2010) regarding migrants from northeastern Brazil who currently occupy the southeast.

Migration between regions encourages contact with the rich biological and cultural diversity and allows interpersonal interactions that contribute to the transformation of local medicinal therapies. As described by Garcia et al. (2010), where the influence of displacement of people from the Northeast and Southeast Brazil to Diadema (São Paulo) resulted in: maintenance, incorporation, replacement and/or discontinued use of natural resources in their medicinal pharmacopoeia. Migrants bring along their traditions, lifestyles, world and health views, such your supporting systems, including knowledge about the use of natural resources to health care and nutrition. These attitudes and practices are held to different ways in the host society (e.g., Nguyen, 2003) and may fall into partial or total disuse, depending of the availability of raw material (Garcia et al., 2010).

This chapter is an attempt to demonstrate the importance that the field ethnobotanist/ethnopharmacological meets in search of new bioactive molecules and how the knowledge about the medicinal use of natural resources can be more diverse and enriched after the displacement of human groups between regions. More broadly and generally, this chapter will also address details of the work done by Garcia et al. (2010) where the authors tried to understand, and comprehend more clearly the extent to which the displacement of people within a country can influence the traditional knowledge about medicinal use of natural resources. We hope this work can contribute significantly to future multidisciplinary research to develop new drugs.

2. Brazilian biodiversity and cultural richness

The Brazilian Atlantic Forest region (Figure 1) was the first to be occupied by European settlers in post-Columbian times (Rodrigues et al., 2008). "Ipe-roxo" (Tabebuia heptaphylla), "cidrão" (*Hedyosmum brasiliensis*), "marcela" (*Achyrocline satureioides*), "estévia" (*Stevia rebaudiana*), "hortelã-do-mato" (*Peltodon radicans*), "espinheira-santa" (*Maytenus* spp), "pata-de-vaca" (*Bauhinia forficata*), "carqueja" (*Baccharis trimera*), "guaco" (*Mikania* spp) and "erva-baleeira" (*Cordia verbenacea*) are some plant species with high chemical and pharmacological potential of the Atlantic Forest biome.

Brazil is very rich in biodiversity, endemism and traditional communities. Is inhabited by diverse ethnic groups, including: Indigenous Ethnic Groups, Quilombo communities, Mestizos, Caiçaras, Fishermen, Rafters, Rubber Tappers, Raizeiros, among other, and the mostly the result of interbreeding between native Indians, Europeans and African elements (Giorgetti et al., 2007).

Native inhabitants of the Atlantic Forest, including non-indigenous, are still in this region, for example, the Caiçaras: people of mixed origin, descendants of European and Native Americans (Rodrigues and Carlini, 2006; Hanazaki et al., 2009). Descendants of Europeans, Africans and Asians settled in Brazil during the colonization and this culminated with cultural miscegenation of many Brazilian communities and ethnic groups, enriching them culturally. All of these groups have traditionally relied on human resources to treat their illnesses and have at their disposal a rich flora.

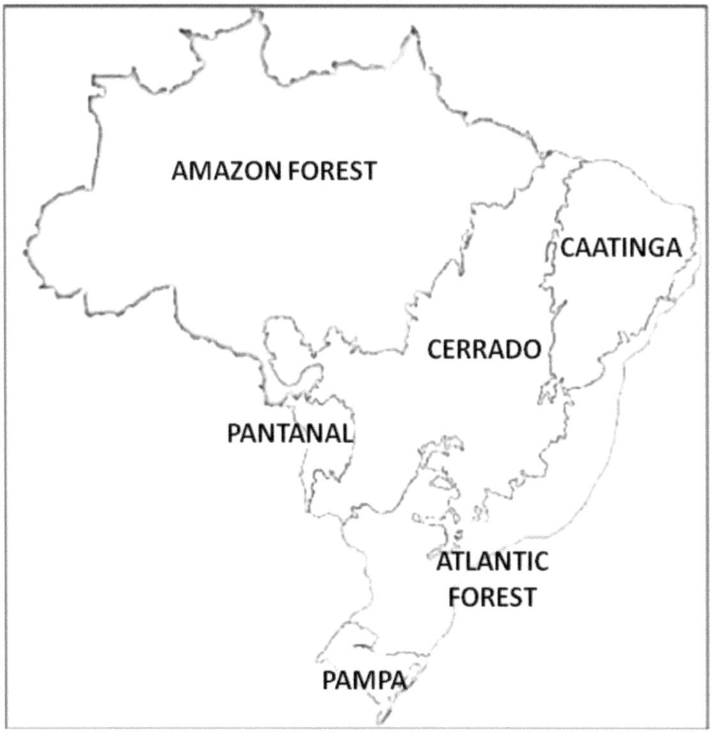

Fig. 1. The six main biomes of Brazil, (IBAMA, 2011)

According to Rodrigues (2005), human groups that live in the forests are still substitutes for laboratory animals, especially in regions where medical treatment is lacking.

The cultural diversity that exists in Brazil is the result of the migration process and miscegenation that begun in the sixteenth century. In this period, were made the first records of the Brazilian medicinal flora (Camargo, 2000; Giulietti et al., 2005; Rodrigues et al., 2008). Little was known about Brazil at the time of the discoveries. The first Jesuits, explorers, scientists, and settlers who arrived in Brazil, reported a lot of characteristics observed on the new environment (Kury, 2001 as cited in Giorgetti et al., 2007).

The first European explorers that arrived in Brazil found a large number of medicinal plants used by indigenous tribes who lived here. Knowledge of local flora was merged those brought from Europe. Those that migrated from Africa (1530-1888) play an important role in traditional popular knowledge in Brazil until today (Rodrigues, 2007). The Africans who came to Brazil adapted your traditions to the new environment (Rodrigues, 2007).

Due the fusion among human groups from different sites of the world and because of the colonization of the Americas, some plants of temperate climate were brought and introduced in tropical locations (Rodrigues et al., 2008), which made these regions, especially South America, a biologically rich and diverse field, with emphasis on the Brazilian forests. This mixture of traditions associated with the weight of diversity vegetal has led to a traditional medicine and herbal treatment methods and of different researchers (e.g., such as Garcia et al., 2010; Ming, 1995; Pio Correa, 1926).

Sometimes, researchers focus on ethnobotanical knowledge and practices at one moment in time, where little attention has been given to the "drivers" of change over time, and thus the migration becomes widely accepted as one of the principle means by which vegetal genetic material, associated knowledge and practices are diffused on the globe (Carney, 2001; Carrier, 2007; Niñez, 1987 as cited in Volpato et al., 2008).

In this context, the main forces that guide the changes in the traditional medicinal knowledge, as cited by Volpato (2009) are: (a) the adaptation of the original knowledge to the new (host) environment; and (b) the development of strategies to obtain the original remedies (Pieroni et al., 2005b; Volpato et al., 2007).

3. Displacement of human groups

Ethnomedicine/ethnopharmacology normally does not cease to carry with the changes in a new social context, and it can continue to influence the choices of care and health practices. The life experiences of migrants in new land, in general, and their professional life in particular, significantly influence in their attitudes and care about the range of health care seeking (Han & Ballis, 2007).

People, who move from their region of origin to live in somewhere else, are subject to various factors that may influence their health and pharmacopoeias. For example, a group of people moving from the Northeast to the Southeast of Brazil were faced with a new routine of life, different customs, new diseases and most importantly, a distinct vegetation. This last factor induces the need to seek pharmacological learning about local natural biodiversity, which can enrich the knowledge of the information ethnopharmacological.

Bharat et al. (2008) mentions that before Lepcha tribe get in Sikim southwest of Tibet, they migrated to Thailand, Burma, Bhutan and Assam during the course of migration, they could collect important information along the way, which was about the use of wild plants available in these sites and important pharmacological characteristics of plants associated with the welfare of humanity local as well as the efficiency that these drugs had to save his life. In turn, in Sikkim, they encountered many new plant species and developed their pharmacological knowledge about them.

As cited by Ososki et al. (2007), ethnobotanical knowledge is dynamic and may evolves with the exchange, transfer and ownership of information among people adapted to new environments (Lee et al., 2001; Voeks and Leony, 2004). There is often an exchange of knowledge, medicinal plants and cultural traditions when human groups migrate between urban and rural settings (Ososki et al., 2007). Knowledge about the use of medicinal plants is sometimes the only option for many human groups in the treatment of diseases.

Some substances become even promising when they are constantly used by human groups, considering the distances travelled and the consequent exposure to different cultures and vegetal resources(Lee et al. 2001; Ososki et al. 2007).

4. Ethnopharmacological survey among migrants living in the Southeast Atlantic Forest of Diadema, São Paulo, Brazil – A case of study (Adapted of Garcia et al., 2010)

4.1 Methodology

4.1.1 Fieldwork

One of the authors (D. Garcia) spent 14 months (September 2007 to November 2008) in the municipality of Diadema, São Paulo, SP, Brazil (23°41′10"S, 46°37′22"W), selecting, observing and interviewing migrants living in the Atlantic Forest remnants. Diadema is occupied by 394.266 inhabitants (IBGE, 2011), most of whom are migrants from other regions of Brazil. The Atlantic Forest remnants found in this city are rich in plants that are either native or introduced by the influence of those migrants present both in urban and rural areas. Migrants who had relevant knowledge regarding the use of plants and animals for medicinal purposes were selected for interviews following the purposive sampling method (Bernard, 1988). After identifying potential interviewees, the researcher visited them to determine whether they did indeed possess knowledge on medicinal plants and whether they wanted to take part in this study. This ethnopharmacological study was approved by the Ethics Committee of Universidade Federal de São Paulo (UNIFESP's Ethics Committee on Research 1969/07) and Conselho de Gestão do Patrimônio Genético (No. 02000.001 049/2008-71). The interviewees also signed consent forms granting permission to access their knowledge and collect botanical and zoological material. Personal and ethnopharmacological data from the interviewees were obtained through informal and semistructured interviews (Bernard, 1988) that addressed the following topics: personal details and migration history (name, sex, age, religion, marital status, place of birth, migration, main occupation, grade of schooling) as well as ethnopharmacology (name of natural resource, use, part used, formula, route of administration, contraindications, dosages, restrictions of use). Each medicinal plant was collected in the presence of the person who described it during the interviews, in accordance with the methods suggested by Lipp (1989). The plants' scientific names were determined by specialists from the Instituto de Botânica do Estado de São Paulo (IB), and vouchers were deposited at the Herbário Municipal de São Paulo (PMSP). The animals collected were placed in glass vials containing 70% ethyl alcohol, and their subsequent identification and deposit were performed by zoologists from the Museum of Zoology, Universidade de São Paulo (MZUSP) and the Bioscience Institute from Universidade de São Paulo (IB-USP). When interviewees cited plants and animals that were used only in their cities of origin, i.e., not available in Diadema, photos from the literature and other information (e.g., popular name, habits and habitat) were used to identify them to at least the genus level. These organisms are marked with asterisks throughout the text and in Table 1. The Herpetofauna of the Northeast Atlantic Forest (Freitas & Silva, 2005) and The Herpetofauna of Caatingas and Altitudes Areas of the Brazilian Northeast (Freitas & Silva, 2007) were used as identification guides. For plants, the authors also consulted Medicinal Plants in Brazil - Native and Exotic (Lorenzi & Matos, 2008).

4.1.2 Database survey

For the plants and animals identified to the species level, the authors searched the bibliographic databases PUBMED (2011) and SCIFINDER (2011) to determine whether they had been targets of previous pharmacological studies. To determine the origin of each plant species, was consulted the Dictionary of Useful Plants: exotic and native (Pio Corrêa, 1926).

4.1.3 Dynamics of use

During the field work, the authors made an effort to understand the dynamics of use for each resource and classified them into the following four categories: maintenance of use (resource used for the same purpose in the migrant's city of origin and in Diadema), replacement (resources that were replaced when migrants arrived in Diadema because the original product was not available in Diadema or was less effective than the new resource), incorporation (resources used for the first time in Diadema to treat diseases common to larger cities, such as hypertension, diabetes and anxiety, which were not common in their homeland), and finally discontinued use (resources that are no longer used in Diadema, usually because they are not available).

4.1.4 Data analysis

The level of homogeneity between plant information provided by different migrants was calculated using the Informants' Consensus Factor, Fic (Trotter & Logan, 1986). This term is calculated as Fic = Nur - Nt /(Nur - 1), where Nur is the number of use reports from informants for a particular plant-usage category and Nt is the number of taxa or species used for that plant usage category across all informants. Values range between 0 and 1, with 1 indicating the highest level of informant consent. For instance, if certain taxa are consistently used by informants, then a high degree of consensus is reached and medicinal traditions are viewed as well-defined (Heinrich, 2000).

4.2 Results and discussion

4.2.1 Migrant interviews

Despite the fact that Diadema is composed by thousands of migrants, the authors could observed that only a few had retained traditional knowledge pertaining to medicinal plants and animals. During this time the authors observed that in many cases, this knowledge has fallen into disuse because of: a) a cultural adaptation to the new city, b) the ease of conventional medical care, c) forest degradation, which restricts use of local plants and animals, furthermore d) many migrants have shown concern to participate in the study, since in the past they suffered persecution from government agencies and physicians, who eventually restrained their medical practice. The five selected interviewees migrated from northeast and southeast Brazil and established themselves in Diadema in the 1940s. Three were born in the northeast: two in Pernambuco state (coded as PE1 and PE2) and one in Sergipe state (SE1). The two remaining migrants were born in the southeast: one in Minas Gerais state (MG1) and one in inland São Paulo state (SP1) (Figure 2). All interviewees were Catholic, married and retired, with the exception of PE1 and PE2 who sell medicinal plants. Their average age was approximately 68 years old (ranging from 53 to 80 years old), and their level of education was semi-illiterate to illiterate. They learned about the medicinal uses of plants and animals from their parents and grandparents (Brazilian natives, European and African descendants) in their homelands. All interviewees arrived in the city of

Diadema as adults, and some had migrated through different regions of Brazil, accumulating knowledge on natural resources from human and biological sources. In Diadema, they acquired knowledge from neighbours, books, media (radio, television, magazines), and personal experiences.

4.2.2 Plants: Dynamics of use

The migrants described their knowledge of 85 plant specimens. As can be seen in Table 1, 78 of them were available in Diadema and were collected, resulting in 65 plant species, the remaining 13 could only be identified to the generic level. The plants belong to 37 taxonomic families, with Asteraceae (16 species), Lamiaceae (8) and Euphorbiaceae (7) as the most common. Previous studies have shown that Asteraceae species are the group most commonly reported to have potential pharmacological properties, not only in the Atlantic Forest (Almeida & Albuquerque, 2002; Begossi et al., 1993; Di Stasi et al., 2002) but also in other Brazilian biomes such as the Amazon Forest (Rodrigues, 2006) the pantanal wetlands (Rodrigues & Carlini, 2004) and the cerrado savannahs (Rodrigues & Carlini, 2005). In a review focusing on plants with possible action/ effects on the central nervous system that were indicated by 26 Brazilian indigenous peoples occupying different Brazilian biomes (Rodrigues et al., 2005), Asteraceae was the second most commonly cited family. The same

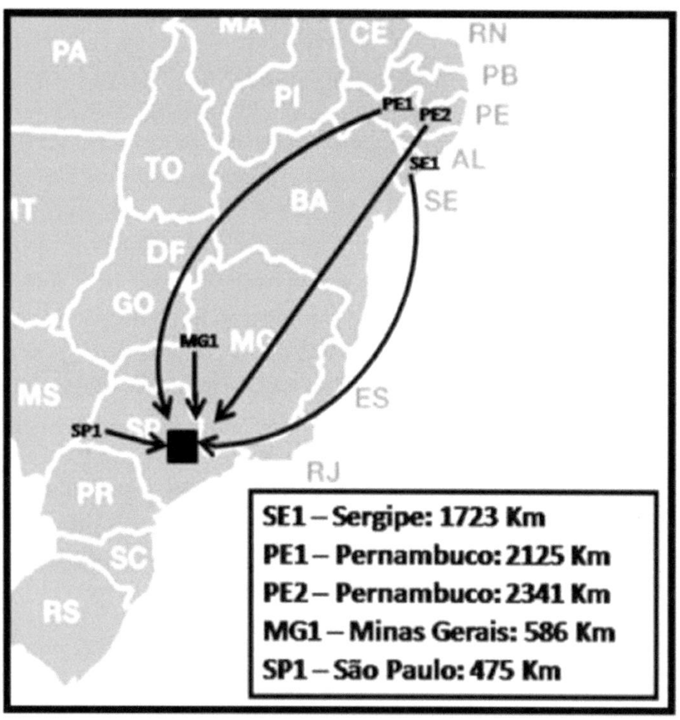

Fig. 2. Location of the Municipality of Diadema, in São Paulo state, southeastern Brazil (black square). Interviewees' migration from their cities of origin to Diadema, being PE (Pernambuco state), SE (Sergipe), MG (Minas Gerais) and SP (São Paulo), and the distance of the displacement (in Km) in each case (adapted of Garcia et al., 2010).

pattern has been detected in other countries, such as Mexico (Díaz, 1977). One factor that may explain the common use of this taxonomic family is the large number of species belonging to it - about 20,000 (Woodland, 1997). Asteraceae also has a wide geographical distribution, both in Brazil and throughout the world (Schultes & Raffaulf, 1990), which facilitates its use by various cultures. From the 65 species identified, it was observed that 33 are native to Brazil while the other 32 are exotic, demonstrating the great floral diversity of the region, which was influenced by European and African people during the civilizing process in Brazil. Furthermore, of the 78 specimens recorded, 54% (42) are spontaneous or were already available in Diadema when interviewees arrived there, while 46% (36) were grown by the migrants, acquired in free markets, or brought from other regions of the country during migration. Below, the authors describe the four 'dynamics of use' categories observed during this study.

4.2.3 Maintenance of use

According to the interviewees, 68 of the 78 specimens cited in the present study, were used in their homelands (highlighted with □ in Table 1). The maintenance of their uses was possible since most of them were available in Diadema, though some were brought from their homelands. SE1 brought four plants from Aquidabã - Sergipe state, for pain relief because they are not available or are more potent than the ones found in Diadema: "bálsamo" (*Sedum* sp.), "anador" (*Alternanthera* sp.), "eucalipto/vick" (*Eucalyptus globulus* Labill.) and "novalgina" (*Achillea millefolium* L.).

4.2.4 Incorporation of use

Fourteen of the 78 specimens listed in Table 1 came to be used by migrants when they arrived in Diadema (highlighted with Δ in Table 1). These incorporations occurred in several ways: through information given by neighbours; through local media, e.g., television, radio, magazines; or through personal efforts, guided by plant organoleptic properties or even by the theory of signatures. This theory, formulated by Paracelsus (XVI century), assumes that characteristics and virtues of herbs can be recognised by their external appearance or "signature" (picture, shape, colour). Finally, observing the relationship between animals and plants can be a valuable guide. PE1 noted that dogs consume "sete-sangria" (*Cuphea carthagenensis* (Jacq.) J. F. Macbr.) when they have diarrhoea; and because it seemed to alleviate their symptoms, he started to use this plant for the same purpose. The migrants incorporated several plants after their arrival in Diadema to treat typical diseases of larger cities: "cipó-cruz" (*Serjania* sp.) to combat high cholesterol; and "guanxuma" (*Sida rhombifolia* L.) and "guiné" (*Petiveria alliaceae* L.) for anxiety. Also included in this category was knowledge concerning local toxic plants, e. g., alamanda-amarela (*Allamanda cathartica* L.) and azaléia (*Rhododendron simsii* Planch.), detailing the risks associated with their consumption.

Similar results were recorded by Volpato et al. (2009), where the use of some plants have been incorporated in Cuban pharmacopoeia by the Haitians. This occurred, according to the authors, as a result of factors such as cultural contact and exchange of information between migrants and host, and personal experimentation or imitation of local practices by migrants. The same authors conclude that Haitians contributed to what is today considered as traditional Cuban medicine by introducing into the dominant Cuban community practices and uses of plants.

Specimen (family) Voucher code	Popular(s) name(s) (migrant) dynamic of use	Origin –geographical distribution - cultivated (C) or spontaneous (S)	Use (part)	Formula and route of administration	Pharmacological studies
Acanthospermum australe (Loefl.) Kuntze (Asteraceae) Garcia 052	Carrapicho (SE1#, MG1□)	Native – Brazilian territory (S)	Wounds in the body (roots)	Medicinal wine - ingestion	Antimalarial activity (Carvalho & Krettli, 1991) and antifungal activity (Portillo et al., 2001)
Achillea millefolium L. (Asteraceae) Garcia 015	Novalgina (MG1, SE1)□	Exotic - south and southeast Brazil (C)	Sedative (leaves)	In natura - ingestion	Antioxidant and antimicrobial activity (Candan et al., 2003)
Ageratum conyzoides L. (Asteraceae) Garcia 010	Mentrasto (PE1)□	Native - southeast to northeast Brazil (S)	Bronchitis* (leaves) Rheumatism* (whole plant)	Infusion - Ingestion Infusion - bath	Anti-inflammatory (Moura et al., 2005), toxic (Singh et al., 2006), antibacterial (Chah et al., 2006) and insecticidal activity (Moreira et al., 2007)
Allamanda cathartica L. (Apocynaceae) Garcia 076	Alamanda-amarela (SE1□, PE1Δ)	Native – Brazilian territory (C)	Toxic (whole plant)	Any oral dose is dangerous	Healing activity (Nayak et al., 2006)
Alpinia zerumbet (Pers.) B.L. Burtt & R.M. Sm. (Zingiberaceae) Garcia 018	Brinco-deprincesa (SE1)Δ	Exotic – Brazilian territory (C)	Sedative (flowers)	Infusion - ingestion	Antihypertensive effects (De Moura et al., 2005), antinociceptive (De Araújo et al., 2005), anti-amoebic activity (Sawangjaroen, 2006) and hepatoprotector (Lin et al., 2008)
Alternanthera sp. (Amaranthaceae) Garcia 039	Anador (SE1)□	No data (C)	Soothing, headache, pain in the body (leaves)	Infusion - ingestion	Not consulted
Artemisia absinthium L. (Asteraceae) Garcia 049	Losna (SP1, SE1, PE2)□	Exotic - Brazilian territory (S)	Laxative (aerial parts)	Infusion - ingestion	Acaricidal properties (Chiasson et al., 2001), antifungal and antibacterial (Kordali et al., 2005) and antioxidant activities (Lopes-Lutz et al., 2008)
Artemisia canphorata Vill. (Asteraceae) Garcia 045	Cânfora (MG1, PE1, SE1)□	Exotic - Brazilian territory (C)	Muscle pain (whole plant)	Decoction - massage	No data found
Asclepias curassavica L. (Apocynaceae) Garcia 037	Algodão-domato (MG1, PE2)□	Exotic - Brazilian territory (S)	Toxic* (whole plant)	Any oral dose is dangerous	Cancer and warts treatment (Kupchan et al., 1964) and poisoning (Radford et al., 1986)
Baccharis dracunculifolia DC (Asteraceae) Garcia 021	Alecrim-docampo (SE1)□	Native - central Brazil (S)	Soothing (aerial parts)	Smoking - inhalation	Bactericidal activity (Orsi et al., 2005), cytotoxic (Fukuda et al., 2006), antiulcerogenic (Klopell et al., 2007), antimicrobial and antifungal (Da Silva et al., 2008) and anti-inflammatory (Paulino et al., 2008)
Baccharis trimera (Less) DC (Asteraceae) Garcia 027	Carqueja (MG1)□	Native - south and southeast Brazil (C)	Diabetes* (whole plant)	Macerate - ingestion	Antihepatotoxic properties (Soicke et al., 1987), anti-inflammatory and analgesic activity (Gené et al., 1996), relaxant effect (Torres et al., 2000), antiproteolytic and anti-hemorrhagic properties (Januário et al., 2004), antioxidant compounds (Simões-Pires et al., 2005), antidiabetic activity (Oliveira et al., 2005) and for losing weight (Dickel et al., 2007)
Bidens pilosa L. (Asteraceae) Garcia 020	Picão-preto (MG1, PE1)□, Picão-branco (SP1)□	Native - tropical America (S)	Blood purifier (whole plant), Healing wounds* (whole plant), Wounds in the body* (roots)	Infusion – Ingestion In natura – Plaster Medicinal wine - ingestion	Hypotensive effects (Dimo et al., 1999), anti-inflammatory activity (Chang et al., 2005), anticancer and antipyretic activity (Sundararajan et al., 2006), antimicrobial (Rojas et al., 2006) and antitumor potential (Kviecinski et al., 2008)

Specimen (family) Voucher code	Popular(s) name(s) (migrant) dynamic of use	Origin -geographical distribution - cultivated (C) or spontaneous (S)	Use (part)	Formula and route of administration	Pharmacological studies
Bryophyllum pinnatum (Lam.) Oken (Crassulaceae) Garcia 040	Folha-santa, folha-da-fortuna (MG1, SP1, PE1)□	Exotic - Brazilian territory (C)	Lumbar pain* (leaves) Sedative* (leaves)	In natura - Plaster In natura - plaster	Antibacterial activity (Obaseiki-Ebor, 1985), anti-ulcer (Pal et al., 1991), antimicrobial (Akinpelu, 2000), antinociceptive, anti-inflammatory and antidiabetic (Ojewole, 2005) and neurosedative and muscle relaxant activities (Yemitan et al., 2005)
Cajanus cajan (L.) Millsp. (Fabaceae s.l.) Garcia 003	Feijão-guandu (SP1)□	Exotic - Brazilian territory (C)	Bronchitis (leaves)	Infusion - ingestion or inhalation	Treatment of postmenopausal osteoporosis (Zheng et al., 2007), antileishmanial and antifungal activity (Braga et al., 2007) and hypocholesterolemic effect (Luo et al., 2008)
Calea sp. (Asteraceae) Garcia 036	Picão (MG1)□	No data (S)	Diuretic (leaves)	Infusion - ingestion	Not consulted
Carica papaya L. (Caricaceae) Garcia 062	Mamão-papaia (PE1)□	Exotic - Brazilian territory (C)	Bronchitis* (powder fruit)	Syrup - ingestion	Abortive (Gopalakrishnan & Rajasekharasetty, 1978), antibacterial activity (Emeruwa, 1982), diuretic (Sripanidkulchai et al., 2001) and healing and abortive effects (Anuar et al., 2008)
Cecropia pachystachya Tréc. (Cecropiaceae) Garcia 068	Embaúba (MG1, SE1)□	Native - south to northeast Brazil (S)	Bronchitis* (powder fruit) Toxic (sap)	Syrup – ingestion Any oral dose is angerous	Antioxidative activity (Velásquez et al., 2003), cardiotonic and sedative effects (Coonsolini et al., 2006) and anti-inflammatory (Schinella et al., 2008)
Chenopodium ambrosioides L. (Chenopodiaceae) Garcia 006	Mentruz, erva-de- santa-maria (PE1#, SE1□)	Native - south and southeast Brazil (S)	Muscle pain (aerial parts) Lesions in bone (aerial parts) Worm* (aerial parts) Bronchitis (aerial parts)	Decoction - Massage In natura - Plaster Infusion - Ingestion Syrup - ingestion	Insecticidal properties (Chiasson et al., 2004), antifungal, antiaflatoxigenic and antioxidant activity (Kumar et al., 2007) and mosquito repellent activity (Gillij et al., 2008)
Cissus sp. (Vitaceae) Garcia 053	Sofre-do-rimquem-qué (MG1)#	No data (S)	Kidney stone (leaves)	Infusion - ingestion	Not consulted
Citrus aurantifolia (Christm.) Swingle (Rutaceae) Garcia 063	Limão (MG1)□	Exotic - Brazilian territory (C)	Fever (leaves)	Infusion - ingestion	Mosquito repellent activity (Das et al., 2003)
Coffea arabica L. (Rubiaceae) Garcia 030	Café (MG1)□	Exotic - Brazilian territory (C)	Diabetes (ripe fruits) Sinusitis (powder fruit)	Infusion Infusion	Antioxidant (Berson, 2008)
Costus spiralis (Jacq.) Roscoe (Costaceae) Garcia 019	Cana-do-brejo (SP1, PE2)□	Native - northeast and southeast Brazil (S)	Laxative and Rheumatism (leaves)	Infusion or decoction - ingestion	Antiurolithiatic (Araújo et al., 1999)
Croton fuscescens Spreng (Euphorbiaceae) Garcia 013	Velando (SE1)□	Native - Brazilian territory (S)	Inhibits the growth of skin stains/wounds in the body (resin)	In natura - topic	No data found

Specimen (family) Voucher code	Popular(s) name(s) (migrant) dynamic of use	Origin –geographical distribution - cultivated (C) or spontaneous (S)	Use (part)	Formula and route of administration	Pharmacological studies
Cuphea carthagenensis (Jacq.) J. F. Macbr. (Lythraceae) Garcia 007	Sete-sangria (MG1□, SP1□, SE1Δ)	Native - Brazilian territory (S)	Intestinal infections and heart problems* (aerial parts)	Infusion - ingestion	Antiinflammatory and antinociceptive activities (Schapoval et al., 1998), vasorelaxant properties (Schuldt et al., 2000), treat high levels of cholesterol and triglycerides (Biavatti et al., 2004)
Cymbopogon citrates DC. - Stapf. (Poaceae) Garcia 026	Capim-limão (MG1, SE1, PE2)□	Exotic - tropical countries (C)	Bronchitis* (leaves) Sedative* (leaves)	Syrup – ingestion Infusion - ingestion	Anxiolytic (Palmieri, 2000), larvicidal activity (Cavalcanti et al., 2004), antibacterial (Wannissorn et al., 2005), antimalarial activity (Tchoumbougnang et al., 2005), insect repellent (Moore et al., 2007), hypoglycemic and hypolipidemic effects (Adeneye et al., 2007) and antimicrobial activity (Nogueira et al., 2008)
Dieffenbachia sp. (Araceae) Garcia 071	Comigo-ninguém- pode (PE1)□	No data (C)	Toxic (whole plant)	Any oral dose is dangerous	Not consulted
Equisetum arvensis L. (Equisetaceae) Garcia 051	Cavalinha (MG1)□	Exotic (C)	Diuretic (leaves)	Infusion - ingestion	No data found
Eucalyptus globulus Labill. (Myrtaceae) Garcia 055	Eucalipto, vick (MG1□, PE1Δ, PE2Δ, SE1□)	Exotic (C)	Sinusitis* (leaves)	Infusion - inhalation	Antihyperglycemic actions (Gray & Flatt, 1998), analgesic and anti-inflammatory effects (Silva et al., 2003), antimicrobial activity (Takahashi et al., 2004) and antibacterial effects (Salari et al., 2006)
Euphorbia heterophylla L. (Euphorbiaceae) Garcia 047	Amendoim-bravo, burra-leiteira (MG1, SP1, SE1, PE1, PE2)□	Native - Americas (S)	Toxic* (whole plant)	Any oral dose is dangerous	Cytotoxic properties (De Almeida Barbosa et al., 2006)
Euphorbia tirucalli L. (Euphorbiaceae) Garcia 046	Avelóz (PE1, PE2)□	Exotic - Brazilian territory (C)	Toxic* (whole plant) Breast cancer* (latex)	Restricted use (reports of blindness) Macerate - ingestion	Anti-tumour activity (Valadares et al., 2006), cause eye injury (Shlamovitz et al., 2007) and effect against arthritis diseases (Bani et al., 2007)
Fevillea passiflora Vell. (Cucurbitaceae) Garcia 022	Pucunã (SE1)□	Native - North and southeast Brazil (S)	Toxic - abortive (seeds)	In natura - ingestion	No data found
Foeniculum vulgare Mill. (Apiaceae) Garcia 064	Erva-doce, funcho (MG1, SP1, PE1, PE2)□	Exotic -Brazilian territory (C)	Sedative (whole plant) Bronchitis* (whole plant) Laxative (whole plant)	Infusion - Ingestion Infusion - Inhalation Infusion or macerate - ingestion	Antimicrobial activity (Aridoğan et al., 2002), antiinflammatory, analgesic and antioxidant activities (Choi et al., 2004), acaricidal activity (Lee, 2004), antifungal effect (Ozcan et al., 2006), antithrombotic activity (Tognolini et al., 2007) and larvicidal activity of the mosquito *Aedes aegypti* (Pitasawat et al., 2007)
Gossypium sp. (Malvaceae) Garcia 066	Algodão (MG1)□	No data (C)	Anti-inflammatory (leaves)	Infusion - inhalation	Not consulted
Hypochoeris sp. (Asteraceae) Garcia 009	Almeirão-boca-de- leão (SE1)Δ	No data (S)	pain (leaves)	In natura - ingestion	Not consulted
Hyptis sp. (Lamiaceae) Garcia 041	Samba-caitá (SE1)□	No data (S)	y ache (leaves)	In natura - ingestion	Not consulted

Specimen (family) Voucher code	Popular(s) name(s) (migrant) dynamic of use	Origin –geographical distribution - cultivated (C) or spontaneous (S)	Use (part)	Formula and route of administration	Pharmacological studies
Impatiens hawkeri W. Bull. (Balsaminaceae) Garcia 044	Impatiens (PE1)^Δ	Exotic - Brazilian territory (C)	Toxic (whole plant)	In closed environment causes tearing, allergy and headache	No data found
Jacaranda sp. (Bignoniaceae) Garcia 011	Salsa-parreira (SE1)□	No data (S)	External allergies, wounds in the body and purifier (leaves)	Decoction - bath	Not consulted
Jatropha gossypiifolia L. (Euphorbiaceae) Garcia 017	Pinhão-roxo (SP1)□	Native - southeast to northeast Brazil (S)	Laxative (powder fruit)	In natura - ingestion	Antimalarial effects (Gbeassor et al., 1989), hypotensive and vasorelaxant effects (Abreu et al., 2003)
Leonurus sibiricus L. (Lamiaceae) Garcia 002	Rubim (MG1, SP1)□	Exotic - Brazilian territory (C)	Healing wounds* (aerial parts)	In natura - plaster	Stimulating action on the uterus (Shi et al., 1995), analgesic and anti-inflammatory activity (Islam et al., 2005) and antibacterial activity (Ahmed et al., 2006)
Lippia alba (Mill.) N. E. Br. (Verbenaceae) Garcia 005	Erva-cidreira (MG1, SE1, PE2)□	Native - almost all Brazilian territory (S)	Expectorant* (aerial parts) Sedative* (aerial parts)	Infusion - Inhalation Infusion or decoction - ingestion	Treatment of respiratory diseases (Cáceres et al., 1991), antiulcerogenic activity (Pascual et al., 2001), sedative and anticonvulsant effects (Zétola et al., 2002), antiviral and antiherpes (Andrighetti-Fröhner et al., 2005)
Ludwigia sp. (Onagraceae) Garcia 078	Erva-de-bicho (SE1)□	No data (S)	Hemorrhoid (whole plant)	Decoction - bath	Not consulted
Malva sylvestris L. (Malvaceae) Garcia 059	Malva-decheiro (MG1)□	Exotic - south and southeast Brazil (S)	Wounds in the body (roots)	Medicinal wine - ingestion	Skin anti-aging property (Talbourdet et al., 2007)
Manihot esculenta Crantz (Euphorbiaceae) Garcia 050	Mandioca (SE1)□	Native - Brazilian territory (C)	conjunctivitis/sty* (dew on the leaves)	In natura - topic	Analgesics and anti-inflammatory effects (Adeyemi et al., 2008)
Mentha arvensis L. (Lamiaceae) Garcia 031	Hortelã (MG1, PE1)□	Exotic - Brazilian territory (C)	Bronchitis* (leaves) Laxative (leaves)	Syrup – ingestion Infusion - ingestion	Antifungal property (Tiwari et al., 1998), vasodilatory actions (Runnie et al., 2004), antioxidative activity (Ka et al., 2005), antibacterial properties (Wannissorn et al., 2005) and insect repellents and fumigants (Moore et al., 2007)
Mentha pulegium L. (Lamiaceae) Garcia 029	Poejo (MG1, PE2)□	Exotic - Brazilian territory (C)	Bronchitis (leaves)	Syrup - ingestion	Larvicidal activity (Cetin et al., 2006), acaricidal effects (Rim et al., 2006) and insecticidal properties (Pavela, 2008)
Mikania glomerata Spreng. (Asteraceae) Garcia 032	Guaco (PE1□, PE2□, SE1^Δ)	Native - northeast to southeast Brazil (S)	Bronchitis* (leaves)	Syrup - ingestion	Analgesic and anti-inflammatory activities (Ruppelt et al., 1991), bronchodilator activity (Soares et al., 2002) and antiophidian properties (Maiorano et al., 2005)
Mimosa pudica L. (Fabaceae s.l.) Garcia 069	Dormideira (SE1)□	Exotic - Brazilian territory (C)	Healing wounds (aerial parts)	In natura - plaster	Antidepressant activity (Molina et al., 2005), antitoxin of the snake Naja kaouthia (Mahanta et al., 2001), anticonvulsant (Ngo et al., 2004) and for reproductive problems (Lans, 2007)
Mirabilis jalapa L. (Nyctaginaceae) Garcia 065	Maravilha (SP1, PE2)□	Native - Brazilian territory (C)	Healing wounds* (aerial parts)	Infusion - plaster	Antibacterial effect (Kusamba et al., 1991) and antimicrobial (Shao et al., 1999)

Specimen (family) Voucher code	Popular(s) name(s) (migrant) dynamic of use	Origin –geographical distribution - cultivated (C) or spontaneous (S)	Use (part)	Formula and route of administration	Pharmacological studies
Ocimum basilicum L. (Lamiaceae) Garcia 061	Manjericão (MG1)□	Exotic - Brazilian territory (C)	Bronchitis* (leaves)	Syrup - ingestion	Antibacterial (Nguefack et al., 2004), mosquito repellent activity (Ntonifor et al., 2006), antimicrobial activity (Viyoch et al., 2006), antigiardial activity (De Almeida et al., 2007) and decreases cholesterol (Bravo et al., 2008)
Ocimum selloi Benth. (Lamiaceae) Garcia 033	Alfavaca (SP1)□	Native - northeast to south Brazil (C)	Soothing (aerial parts) Bronchitis (leaves)	Infusion - inhalation p - ingestion	Mosquito repellent activity (Padilha de Paula et al., 2003)
Petiveria alliaceae L. (Phytolaccaceae) Garcia 004	Guiné (SE1)△	Native - north Brazil (S)	Sedative (aerial parts) Muscle pain* (leaves)	Environment purifier - inhalation Decoction - massage	Antimicrobial substance (Von Szczepanski et al., 1972), antimitotic action (Malpezzi et al., 1994), anti-inflammatory and analgesic effects (Lopes-Martins et al., 2002), antibacterial and antifungal activity (Kim et al., 2006) and antioxidant (Okada et al., 2008)
Phyllanthus caroliniensis Walter (Euphorbiaceae) Garcia 024	Quebra-pedra (SP1, PE1, PE2, SE1)□	Native - USA to Brazil (S)	Kidney stone* (aerial parts)	Infusion or decoction - ingestion	Antinociceptive action (Cechinel Filho et al., 1996)
Piper umbellatum L. (Piperaceae) Garcia 072	Pariparoba (MG1)□	Native - Tropical America (S)	Belly ache and liver pain (leaves)	Infusion - ingestion	Antioxidant (Agbor et al., 2007) and antifungal activity (Tabopda et al., 2008)
Plantago sp. (Plantaginaceae) Garcia 008	Tanchagem (SP1, PE2)□	No data (S)	Anti-inflammatory - mouth and throat (leaves)	Decoction - gargling	Not consulted
Plectranthus amboinicus (Lour.) Spreng. (Lamiaceae) Garcia 073	Hortelã-grande (PE1)□	Exotic - Brazilian territory (C)	For digestion and urine with blood (leaves) Cough (leaves)	Infusion - Ingestion Syrup - ingestion	Scorpion venon antidote (Ka et al., 2005) and antimicrobial activity (Nogueira et al., 2008)
Pluchea sagittalis (Lam.) Cabrera (Asteraceae) Garcia 042	Quitoco (SE1)□	Native - south and southeast Brazil (S)	Diuretic (aerial parts)	Infusion - ingestion	Anti-inflammatory activity (Pérez-Garcia et al., 1996)
Porophyllum ruderale (Jacq.) Cass. (Asteraceae) Garcia 075	Arnica (PE1)□	Native - Brazilian territory (S)	Muscle pain* (aerial parts)	Decoction - massage	Anti-inflammatory (Souza et al., 2004)
Psidium guajava L. (Myrtaceae) Garcia 058	Goiaba (SE1)□	Native - Mexico to Brazil (S)	Heartburn (leaves) Diarrhea (fruit)	Infusion or in natura - ingestion In natura - ingestion	Antibacterial activity (Anas et al., 2008; Cheruiyot et al., 2009; Rahim et al., 2010) and hepatoprotective activity (Roy & Das, 2010)
Rhododendron simsii Planch. (Ericaceae) Garcia 043	Azaléia (PE1)△	Exotic - Brazilian territory (C)	Toxic (whole plant)	Any oral dose is dangerous	Antioxidative (Takahashi et al., 2001)
Rosmarinus officinalis L. (Lamiaceae) Garcia 060	Alecrim (MG1)□	Exotic - all countries with temperate climate (C)	Muscle pain* (leaves)	Decoction - massage	Antibacterial effects (Fu et al., 2007), antimicrobial effect (Weckesser et al., 2007), anti-inflammatory and antitumor effects (Peng et al., 2007), cause reduction of reproductive fertility in male rats (Nusier et al., 2007), antinociceptive effect (González-Trujano et al., 2007), mosquito repellent activity (Gillij et al., 2008), antidiabetic and antioxidant properties (Bakirel et al., 2008)

Specimen (family) Voucher code	Popular(s) name(s) (migrant) dynamic of use	Origin –geographical distribution - cultivated (C) or spontaneous (S)	Use (part)	Formula and route of administration	Pharmacological studies
Ruta graveolens L. (Rutaceae) Garcia 028	Arruda (MG1, PE1, PE2)□	Exotic – Brazilian territory (C)	Earache and conjunctivitis/styl* (leaves) Muscle pain (leaves)	In natura – topic Decoction - massage	Antifertility (Gandhi et al., 1991), fungicide (Oliva et al., 2003), cytotoxic (Ivanova et al., 2005), abortive (De Freitas et al., 2005), anti-tumour (Preethi et al., 2006), anti-inflammatory (Raghav et al., 2006), antiarrhythmic (Khori et al., 2008) and antimicrobial (Nogueira et al., 2008)
Sambucus canadensis L. (Caprifoliaceae) Garcia 025	Sabugueiro (MG1)□	Native - Brazilian territory (S)	Bronchitis* (flowers)	Syrup - ingestion	Infectious diseases and antioxidant activity (Holetz et al., 2002)
Schinus terebinthifolius Raddi (Anacardiaceae) Garcia 035	Aroeira (MG1)□	Native - northeast to south Brazil (S)	Diuretic (leaves)	Infusion - ingestion	Antifungal activity (Schmourlo et al., 2005) and antibacterial (De Lima et al., 2006)
Scoparia dulcis L. (Scrophulariaceae) Garcia 014	Vassourinha (SE1, PE2)□	Native - Brazilian territory (S)	Hip pain/kidneys (leaves	Decoction - bath	Antitumor-promoting activity (Nishino et al., 1993), antioxidant (Ratnasooriya et al., 2005), antimicrobial and antifungal activities (Latha et al., 2006)
Sedum sp. (Crassulaceae) Garcia 038	Bálsamo (MG1, SP1, PE1, SE1)□	No data (C)	Earache (leaves) Laxative (aerial parts)	In natura – topic In natura - ingestion	Not consulted
Senna pendula (Humb. & Bonpl. Ex Willd.) H.S. Irwin & Barneby (Fabaceae s. l.) Garcia 034	Fedegoso (MG1)□	Native - Brazilian territory (S)	Osteoporosis prevention (roots)	Medicinal wine - ingestion	No data found
Serjania sp. (Sapindaceae) Garcia 012	Cipó-cruz (SE1, PE2)Δ	No data (S)	Reduces cholesterol and diarrhea (leaves) External allergies, wounds in the body and detoxifying (leaves)	Macerate - Ingestion Infusion - bath	Not consulted
Sida rhombifolia L. (Malvaceae) Garcia 067	Guanxuma (SE1)Δ	Exotic - Brazilian territory (S)	Sedative (aerial parts)	Infusion - ingestion or inhalation	Cytotoxicity, antibacterial activity (Islam et al., 2003) and antioxidant (Dhalwal et al., 2007)
Solanum americanum L. (Solanaceae) Garcia 070	Maria-pretinha (MG1)□	Native - Americas (S)	Sore throat* (aerial parts)	Infusion - gargle	Treatment of protozoal infections (*American trypanosomes*) (Cáceres et al., 1998) and moderate antioxidant activity (Iwalewa et al., 2005)
Solanum variabile Mart. (Solanaceae) Garcia 056	Jurubeba (MG1, SE1, PE2)□	Native - southeast and south Brazil (S)	Sedative (leaves) Laxative (powder fruit)	Infusion - Ingestion In natura - ingestion	Antiulcerogenic activity (Antonio et al., 2004)
Sonchus oleraceus L. (Asteraceae) Garcia 016	Serralha (PE1)□	Exotic - Brazilian territory (S)	Diabetes (leaves)	In natura - ingestion	Larvicidal potential (Shama et al., 2006)
Stachytarpheta cayennensis (Rich.) Vahl (Verbenaceae) Garcia 054	Gervão (MG1)□	Native - Brazilian territory (S)	Laxative (aerial parts)	Infusion or decoction - ingestion	Anti-inflammatory and anti-ulcerogenic properties (Penido et al., 2006) and hypoglycaemic constituents (Adebajo et al., 2007)

Specimen (family) Voucher code	Popular(s) name(s) (migrant) dynamic of use	Origin –geographical distribution - cultivated (C) or spontaneous (S)	Use (part)	Formula and route of administration	Pharmacological studies
Synadenium grantii Hook. F. (Euphorbiaceae) Garcia 074	Jarnaúba (PE1)Δ	Exotic - southeast to northeast Brazil (C)	Toxic (whole plant) Stomach cancer (latex)	Restricted use Macerate - ingestion	Healing action and anti-hemorrhagic (Rajesh et al., 2007)
Tropaeolum majus L. (Tropaeolaceae) Garcia 057	Capuchinha (SP1, MG1)Δ	Exotic - south and southeast Brazil (C)	Ulcer and laxative (aerial parts)	Infusion or in natura - ingestion	Antitumor activity (Pintão et al., 1995)
Vernonia condensata Baker (Asteraceae) Garcia 001	Boldo-do-Chile, figatil (PE1□, SE1Δ)	Exotic - northeast to southeast Brazil (C)	Liver pain* (leaves)	Infusion - ingestion	Anti-ulcerogenic (Frutoso et al., 1994) and analgesic and anti-inflammatory (Valverde et al., 2001)
Vernonia sp. (Asteraceae) Garcia 048	Assa-peixe (MG1, SE1)□	No data (S)	Chitis (leaves) Expectorant (leaves) Healing wounds (leaves)	Infusion - Ingestion Infusion - Inhalation infusion - plaster	Not consulted
Waltheria indica L. (Sterculiaceae) Garcia 077	Malva-branca (SE1)□	Native - Brazilian territory (S)	Gingivitis* (leaves) Inflammation in the mouth and/or throat* (leaves)	Infusion - gargling	Anti-inflammatory activities (Rao et al., 2005)
Zea mays L. (Poaceae) Garcia 023	Milho (SE1)□	Exotic - Brazilian territory (C)	Bronchitis (flowers) Blood purifier and diuretic (flowers)	Syrup – ingestion Infusion - ingestion	No data found

* their popular and scientific names, geographical origin and distribution, if cultivated or spontaneous, uses, parts utilized, formula, route of administration and pharmacological studies. Marked by (□) the 68 plants whose use had been maintained by the respective migrant, while 14, marked by (Δ) are those whose applications have been incorporated by migrants, finally, 3 (#) are replacements. The matches between the uses proclaimed by the interviewees and pharmacological data have been posted by (*).

Table 1. The 78 plant specimens used by five Diadema's migrants (MG1, SP1, PE1, PE2, SE1)* (adapted of Garcia et al., 2010).

4.2.5 Replacement of use

Three plants used by migrants in their cities of origin were replaced because they were not available or were less effective than plants present in Diadema (highlighted with # in Table 1). Most of these replacements were made according to the criteria listed in the previous section. The interviewee MG1 explained that in his homelands, he used "quebra-pedra"* (*Phyllanthus* cf. *caroliniensis* Walter - Euphorbiaceae) for kidney stone disturbance, but when he arrived in Diadema, he found another plant, "sofre-do-rim-quem-qué" (*Cissus* sp.), that seemed to have a stronger effect.

Another interviewee, PE1, reported that the bark and seeds of "amburana-de-cheiro"* (*Amburana* cf. *cearensis* (Allemão) A.C. Sm. - Fabaceae s.l.) were widely used for anti-inflammatory therapy in Pernambuco state but had to be replaced by "mentruz" (*Chenopodium ambrosioides* L.) because the former was not found in Diadema. In addition, SE1 had to replace "pau-de-sapo"* (*Pouteria* cf. *melinoniana* Boehni - Sapotaceae), whose leaves were used for chronic wounds, with "carrapicho" (*Acanthospermum australe* (Loefl.) Kuntze). The vernacular names of some plants are registered trademarks of allopathic medicines and active ingredients, e.g., Novalgina® (*Achillea millefolium*) and Vick® (*Eucalyptus globulus*) for sinusitis, and Anador® (*Alternanthera* sp.), which is used as a sedative and for general pain. Contact between migrants and allopathic medicine thus led to the 'baptisms' of these plants, following the observation that both, the commercially available products and herbal source have similar effects, as reported by Pires et al., (2009).

Biocultural adaptation, negotiation and cultural identity are key-issues for issues anthropological in the displacement of human groups between regions (Belliard & Ramírez-Johnson, 2005; Janes & Pawson, 1986). Research in culturally homogeneous places and/or non-urban has shown that to follow the pattern of changes in traditional knowledge and use of plant among migrants must involve the degree the process of acculturation (Bodeker et al., 2005; Nesheim et al., 2006 as cited in Pieroni & Vandebroek, 2007). This dynamic interaction between migrants and host societies may result in changes pharmacopeial adapted with plants exchanged(Pieroni & Vandebroek, 2007).

4.2.6 Discontinued use

According to MG1, the following plants used in his homeland fell into disuse because they were not found in Diadema, although he tried to acquire them from local commercial sources: "quina"* (*Strychnos* cf. *pseudoquina* A. St. Hil - Loganiaceae), whose root is used to combat pain in the stomach and intestine; bark oil of "jatobá"* (*Hymenaea* cf. *courbaril* L. - Fabaceae s.l.), used for combat wounds; "batata-de-purga"* (*Operculina* cf. *macrocarpa* (L.) Urb - Convolvulaceae), whose tuber is ingested as a purgative and to clean the blood; bark and leaf of "jalapa"* (*Mirabilis* cf *jalapa* L. - Nyctaginaceae), used to clean the blood; tea of "junco"* (*Cyperus* cf. *esculentus* L. - Cyperaceae), whose root is used for inflammation; bark or seed of "emburana"* (*Amburana* cf. *cearensis* - Fabaceae s.l.), used for migraine and sleeping; and bark of "angico"* (*Anadenanthera* cf. *colubrine* (Vell.) Brenan - Fabaceae s.l.), prepared as a tea for pain in the body and fever. These plants were not described in Table 1, since they could not be collected and identified as well.

In a study performed by Waldstein (2008), it became clear that there is great influence of the host culture (USA) on the lifestyles of immigrants (Mexicans). The study reports that immigrants go through an intense process of acculturation and loss of traditional knowledge over the years, adopting the lifestyle of the host country. One of the problems that can affect traditional knowledge is the possibility of loss due to migration of people to industrialized regions (Pieroni et al., 2005). Due to contact with a new routine of life and, often, different environments (flora, fauna, culture, food, language, religion) people moving between regions, usually adapt more to the new location (those more culturally flexible) or not (those culturally less flexible) variable which makes the loss or incorporation of traditional knowledge about medicinal use of natural resources. For newcomers to the host country, it seems that the adoption of values, language, beliefs, traditions of the dominant group are constant, but, alternatively, some groups reject this and maintain their traditional customs(Ceuterick et al., 2007). The use of traditional foods, for example, is often seen as a symbol of maintenance ethnic identity and a cultural trait very resistant to change (Nguyen, 2003 as cited in Ceuterick et al., 2007).

4.2.7 Plants used for therapeutic purposes

Of the 78 plants, 10 carry some restrictions, as they can be toxic depending on the dose, route or part utilized (Table 1). The uses described in Table 1 are written just as they were reported by the interviewees. The 68 plants used exclusively for medicinal purposes were cited for 41 complaints, which were grouped into 12 functional categories according to bodily system, as detailed in Table 3. Thus, gastrointestinal disturbances include the following complaints (numbers of medicinal plants reported): endoparasitosis (1), ulcer (1), diarrhoea (1), bellyache (2), heartburn (1), intestinal infections (1), liver pain (3). This category also includes plants used to improve digestion (1), to treat tables of haemorrhoid (1), as laxatives (10) and to purify the stomach (2), comprising a total of 24 plants employed in 44 formulas. The most relevant categories of use, measured by number of species employed, were gastrointestinal disturbances (30.8% of plants), inflammatory processes (24.4%) and respiratory problems (23.1%). As seen in Table 4, the group of illnesses representing immunological problems obtained the highest informant consensus factor value (Fic = 0.66), while the other categories presented Fic values lower than 0.5. These low values reflect the diversity of knowledge displayed by migrants, which can probably be attributed to different cultural influences during their migrations through Brazilian territory. Furthermore, the small number of interviewees may have resulted in low values of Fic. The parts of the plants most often used in the formulas were leaves (45.4%) and other aerial parts (22.7%). The most common formula was the infusion (37.8%), followed by in natura (17.6%) and syrup (10.1%). The most cited route of administration was ingestion (51.3%), followed by inhalation (8.4%) and topical (3.4%).

4.2.8 Plants with restrictions on use and/or toxic

Among the 10 specimens with restrictions on use, 6 were designated as only toxic: "alamanda-amarela" (*Allamanda cathartica*), "algodão-do-mato" (*Asclepias curassavica* L.), "amendoim-bravo/burra-leiteira" (*Euphorbia heterophylla* L.), "azaléa" (*Rhododendron simsii*), "comigo-ninguém-pode" (*Dieffenbachia* sp.) and "impatiens" (*Impatiens hawkeri*). The interviewees explained that depending on the dose, the latex of "alamanda- amarela" and "amendoim-bravo" can cause discomfort or even blindness. According to Oliveira et al. (2003), the leaves of *Dieffenbachia picta* Schott contain calcium oxalate, which damages the oral mucosa and provokes pain and oedema, while the leaves of *Allamanda cathartica* contain cardiotonic glycosides and induce intense gastrointestinal disturbances. Although reported as toxic, the latex of two other plants can be used at low doses to treat breast and stomach cancer: "avelóz" (*Euphorbia tirucalli* L.) and "jarnaúba" (*Synadenium grantii* Hook. F.), respectively. The sap of "embaúba" (*Cecropia pachystachya* Tréc.) was indicated as toxic, but its fruits are used to combat bronchitis. Finally, the seeds of "pucunã" (*Fevillea passiflora* Vell.) are toxic, being indicated as abortive. In a recent study, Rodrigues (2007) also described plants with restrictions of use as reported by three Brazilian cultures: the Krahô Indians use two plants as abortives in a single prescription: "aprytytti" (*Acosmium dasycarpum* (Vogel) Yakovlev) and "ahkryt" (*Anacardium occidentale* L.) (Anacardiaceae); their barks are boiled, and the beverage is ingested in at dawn. It is an extremely bitter beverage, rich in tannin and therefore extremely astringent.

4.2.9 Pharmacological data

As can be seen in Table 1, 57 species (73.1%) were featured in previous pharmacological studies. For 30 of these species (52.6%), the uses cited by the migrants showed some similarity to the investigated effects/actions, demonstrating concordance between popular knowledge and academic science (marked with an asterisk in Table 1).

4.2.10 Animals used for therapeutic purposes and dynamics of use

From the five interviewees, only one (PE2) offered knowledge on the medicinal uses of 12 animals. They belong to four taxonomic classes: Reptilia (6 species), Insects (3), Mammalia (2) and Amphibia (1). However, the interviewee has used only two animals since he arrived in Diadema, the other ten animals fell into disuse because they are not available in this city. The two animals were collected, identified and deposited in the Museum of Zoology-USP: ant (*Atta sexdens* L.) and cockroach (*Periplaneta americana* L.). These species belong to the maintenance of use category (highlighted with □ in Table 2). The other ten species therefore belong to the discontinued use category (highlighted with ○ in Table 2) which could not be collected. Their identifications were made by PE2 through consulting images from books (as described in Methodology). For three animals (snake, alligator and giant water bug) PE2 could only hesitantly confirm their identity, probably due to the great diversity of these animals in Brazil. Therefore, they are denoted in Table 2 as probably belonging to one of three possible genera. The animals were used in 14 different medicinal formulas, with the skin most commonly used (33.3%), followed by whole animal (20.0%), bone (13.4%), fat (6.7%), rattle (6.7%), tooth (6.7%), anthill (6.7%) and turtleshell (6.7%). Some studies conducted in Brazil show that concomitant data corroborate and sustain these uses (Alves, 2009; Costa-Neto, 2005; Ferreira et al., 2009; Santos-Fita & Costa-Neto, 2007; Torres et al., 2009). The formulas were cited for the treatment of nine complaints, which were grouped into six functional categories, as shown in Table 5. The most commonly cited formula was powder (66.7%), followed by in natura (20%). The most frequent route of administration was ingestion (78.6%). The most common complaint involved respiratory problems (58.4%; 7 animals) followed by central nervous system (8.3%), inflammatory processes (8.3%),

Scientific name or only genus (family/class) Voucher	Popular name dynamic of use	Complaint (part used) - formula - route of administration
Abedus sp., *Belostoma* sp. or *Diplonychus* sp. (Belostomatidae/Insecta)*	Water cockroach (barata d'água)°	Bronchitis and asthma (whole animal) - powder - ingested
Atta sexdens L. (Formicidae/Insecta) Garcia 001	Ant (formiga) ϒ	Epilepsy (anthill) - in natura - ingested
Chironius sp., *Liophs* sp. (Colubridae/Reptilia)* or *Bothops* sp. (Viperidae/Reptilia)*	Snake (cobra)°	Bronchitis (skin) - powder - ingested
Crocodilus sp., *Cayman* sp. or *Paleosuchus* sp. (Alligatoridae/Reptilia)*	Alligator (jacaré)°	Apoplexy (skin) - syrup of skin powder - ingested Bronchitis (bone) - powder - ingested
Crotalus cf. *durissus* L. (Viperidae/Reptilia)*	Rattlesnake (cascavel)°	Back pain (fat) - in natura - ingested Bronchitis (rattle) - tie it in the neck - topic Heart problems (tooth) - put it in the pocket of shirt
Geochelone sp. (Testudinidae/Reptilia)*	Turtle (tartaruga)°	Bronchitis and asthma - (turtleshell) - powder - ingested
Hydrochoerus cf. *hydrochaeris* L. (Hydrochaeridae/ Mammalia)*	Capybara (capivara)°	Bronchitis and asthma - (skin) - powder - ingested
Iguana cf. iguana L. (Iguanidae/Reptilia)*	Iguana (iguana)°	Osteoporosis and rheumatism (bone) - powder - ingested
Periplaneta americana L. (Blattidae/Insecta) Garcia 002	Cockroach (barata) ϒ	Bronchitis and asthma (whole animal) - powder - ingested
Placosoma sp. (Gymnophthalmidae/Reptilia)*	Lizard (calango)°	Wounds in the body (skin) - powder - ingested
Rhinella sp. (Bufonidae/Amphibia)*	Cururu frog (sapocururu)°	Cancer of skin (whole animal) - in natura: tie it on the cancer for some time each day - topic
Tolypeutes sp. (Dasypodidae/Mammalia)*	Armadillo-ball (tatubola)°	Wounds in the body (skin) - powder - ingested

Marked by (ϒ) the two animals whose use had been maintained, while 10, marked by (°) are those whose uses have fallen into disuse. * Animals that couldn't be collected because were not available in Diadema.

Table 2. The 12 animals indicated by migrant PE2, their popular and scientific names, complaints (part used), formula and route of administration (adapted of Garcia et al., 2010).

Category of use	Complaints (number of plants cited)	Total number of plants
1- Gastrointestinal disturbances	To combat worms (1), ulcer (1), diarrhoea (1), bellyache (2), heartburn (1), intestinal infections (1), liver pain (3), to improve digestion (1), hemorrhoid (1), as laxative (10) and for stomach purify (2)	24
2- Inflammatory processes	As anti-inflammatory (3) and healing (6), to treat sty/conjunctivitis (2), inflammation in the mouth/throat (3), rheumatism (2), sinusitis (2) and gingivitis (1)	19
3- Respiratory problems	To combat cough (1), bronchitis (15) and as expectorant (2)	18
4- Anxiolytic/ hypnotics	As sedative (11)	11
5-Osteomuscular problems	To ease back pain (1), muscles pain (6), hip pain (1), prevent osteoporosis (1) and to treat lesions in bone (1)	10
6- Dermatological problems	To combat external allergies (2), wounds in the body (5) and inhibits the growth of skin stains (1)	8
7- Genitourinary disturbances	As diuretic (5), to combat kidney stone (2) and treating urine with blood (1)	8
8- Endocrine system	To reduce cholesterol (1) and diabetes (3)	4
9- Cardiovascular problems	Treat heart problems (1) and as blood purifier (2)	3
10- Immunological problems	To combat breast cancer (1) and stomach cancer (1)	2
11- Analgesics	Earache (2)	2
12- Fever	To combat fever (1)	1
Total		110*

*Some plants have been cited for more than one complaint, so the total number of plants above (110) is higher than the ones indicated by the interviewees.

Table 3. The 12 categories of use comprising the 41 complaints, their total and partial number of plants cited by the five migrants (adapted of Garcia et al., 2010).

dermatological problems (8.3%), analgesics (8.3%), cardiovascular problems (8.3%) as shown in Table 5. The high humidity of the region (with annual rainfall between 1.000 and 1750 mm) (IBAMA, 2011) is known to lead to bronchitis, cough and asthma. This may explain why so many plants and animals were used to treat respiratory disturbances in Diadema, which has been shown in studies of the Sistema Único de Saúde (2011) to be the second largest cause of death in Diadema - 14,4%. Many animals have been used for medical purposes since antiquity (Antonio, 1994; Conconi & Pino, 1988; Gudger, 1925; Weiss, 1947). Despite the existence of several ethnopharmacological studies suggesting the bioactive potential of Brazilian fauna (Alves & Delima, 2006; Alves & Dias, 2010; Alves & Rosa, 2005; Costa-Neto, 2002, 2006; Hanazaki et al., 2009; Rodrigues, 2006), only marine animals have been investigated by chemical and pharmacological methods (Berllink et al., 2004; Gray, 2006; Kossuga, 2009). No pharmacological data was found in the literature for the five animals identified in the present study: rattlesnake (*Crotalus* cf. *durissus* L.), capybara (*Hydrochoerus* cf. *hydrochaeris* L.), iguana (*Iguana* cf. *iguana* L.), ant (*Atta sexdens*) and cockroach (*Periplaneta americana*). The lack of information available on medicinal animal products leads us to conclude that this is a largely unexplored topic in Brazil and that future pharmacological studies should confirm the potential therapeutic value of these species.

SN	Category of use	Plant specimen	% All Species	Use citation	% All use citation	Fic
1	Gastrointestinal disturbances	24	30.77	44	25.29	0.46
2	Inflammatory processes	19	24.36	28	16.09	0.33
3	Respiratory problems	18	23.07	31	17.82	0.43
4	Anxiolytic/hypnotics	11	14.10	19	10.92	0.44
5	Osteomuscular problems	10	12.82	13	7.47	0.25
6	Dermatological problems	8	10.26	11	6.32	0.3
7	Genitourinary disturbances	8	10.26	13	7.47	0.41
8	Endocrine system	4	5.13	5	2.87	0.25
9	Immunological problems	2	2.56	4	2.30	0.66
10	Cardiovascular problems	3	3.84	3	1.72	0
11	Analgesics	2	2.56	2	1.15	0
12	Fever	1	1.28	1	0.57	0

Table 4. Values of Informant consensus factor (Fic) for each category of use, considering the plants cited by the five Diadema's migrants (adapted of Garcia et al., 2010).

Category of use	Complaints (number of animals)
1-Respiratory problems	bronchitis (7), asthma (4)
2-Central nervous system	epilepsy (1)
3-Inflammatory processes	rheumatism (1)
4-Dermatological problems	wounds in the body (1), skin cancer (1)
5-Analgesics	back pain (1)
6-Cardiovascular problems	treat heart problems (1), hemorrhage (1)
Total	18*

* some animals have been cited for more than one complaint, so their total number above (18) is higher than the number of animals indicated: 12.

Table 5. The 6 categories of use comprising the 9 complaints, their respective number of animals mentioned by the migrant PE2 (adapted of Garcia et al., 2010).

5. Conclusion

The ethnobotanical/ethnopharmacological survey among migrants becomes important in that it rescues the knowledge and values that are rapidly disappearing with the death of older migrants and destruction of biomes around the world (Ososki et al. 2007; Reyes-Garcia et al. 2005).

The studies that rescue a large number of uses for different categories (for exemple: gastrointestinal disorders, inflammation, fever and others), can expand several lines of pharmacological and phytochemical investigations. In addition, it may be more important for the development of new drugs with large pharmacological/phytochemicals effects and safer, as well some therapeutic uses mentioned by the migrants were confirmed by previous studies in the literature.

The study of case in Diadema (São Paulo - Brazil) the migrant interviewees demonstrated a large knowledge about the toxic and medicinal properties of some plants and animals. Migration contributed to increase of knowledge regarding the use of natural resources, mainly through the processes of incorporation and/or resource replacement.

The seven plants [*Impatiens hawkeri* W. Bull., *Artemisia canphorata* Vill., *Zea mays* L., *Equisetum arvensis* L., *Senna pendula* (Humb. & Bonpl. ex Willd.) H.S. Irwin & Barneby, *Fevillea passiflora* Vell. and *Croton fuscescens* Spreng] showed maintenance of use among migrants and have not been studied by pharmacologists yet. These species should be highlighted in further investigations because the maintenance of use during human migrations can be indicative of bioactive potential.

The interviewed migrants had passed through several Brazilian cities and were exposed to distinct vegetation and cultures. In this migration, they have passed on and incorporated knowledge in an intensive exchange where formulas and uses are mixed and re-invented as a result of contact between cultures.

This chapter is an attempt to demonstrate based on some scientific papers, the importance of the field (ethnobotanical/ethnopharmacological) in search of new bioactive molecules and how the information about the use of natural resources for health promotion may be more diverse and enriched when human groups displace among regions. We hope this text can assist as a basis for future multidisciplinary research to development new drugs.

6. Acknowledgment

We thank the interviewees for their hospitality, help, and mainly for providing us with information for the purpose of this study in the city of Diadema - São Paulo - Brazil. We are grateful to Julino Assunção Rodrigues Soares Neto and Valéria Basti. We also appreciate the help of FAPESP (Fundação de Amparo à Pesquisa do Estado de São Paulo), FIC (Faculdade Integral Cantareira), AFIP (Associação Fundo de Incentivo à Psicofarmacologia), FUNDUNESP (Fundação para o Desenvolvimento da UNESP) and Herbário Municipal de São Paulo (PMSP), which provided financial support which made this research possible. We thank Dr. Lúcia Rossi and Prof. Dr. Hussam El Dine Zaher, for conducting the botanical and animal identification, respectively. Finally, we really like to thank Prof. Eliana Rodrigues and Prof. Marcus Vinicius Domingues for their participation and orientation.

7. References

Abreu, I.C.; Marinho, A.S.; Paes, A.M.; Freire, S.M.; Olea, R.S.; Borges, M.O. & Borges, A.C. (2003). Hypotensive and vasorelaxant effects of ethanolic extract from Jatropha gossypiifolia L. in rats. *Fitoterapia*, vol.74, pp.650-657.

Adebajo, A.C.; Olawode, E.O.; Omobuwajo, O.R.; Adesanya, S.A.; Begrow, F.; Elkhawad, A.; Akanmu, M.A.; Edrada, R.; Proksch, P.; Klaes, M. & Verspohl, E.J. (2007). Hypoglycaemic constituents of Stachytarpheta cayennensis leaf. *Planta Med*, vol. 7, pp. 3241-3250.

Adeneye, A.A. & Agbaje, E.O. (2007). Hypoglycemic and hypolipidemic effects of fresh leaf aqueous extract of Cymbopogon citratus Stapf. in rats. *J Ethnopharmacol*, vol. 25, pp.440-444.

Adeyemi, O.O.; Yemitan, O.K. & Afolabi, L. (2008). Inhibition of chemically induced inflammation and pain by orally and topically administered leaf extract of Manihot esculenta Crantz in rodents. *J Ethnopharmacol*, vol. 2, pp. 6-11.

Agbor, G.A.; Vinson, J.A.; Oben, J.E. & Ngogang, J.Y. (2007). In vitro antioxidant activity of three Piper species. *J Herb Pharmacother*, vol. 7, pp. 49-64.

Ahmed, F.; Islam, M.A. & Rahman, M.M. (2006). Antibacterial activity of Leonurus sibiricus aerial parts. *Fitoterapia*, vol. 77, pp.316-317.

Akinpelu, D.A. (2000). Antimicrobial activity of Bryophyllum pinnatum leaves. *Fitoterapia*, vol. 71, pp.193-194.

Alcorn, J.B. (1995). The scope and aims of ethnobotany in a developing world. In: R.E. Schultes & S.V. Reis (eds.). Ethnobotany: evolution of a discipline. Timber Press, Cambridge, pp. 23-39.

Almeida, C. & Albuquerque, U.P. (2002). Uso e conservação de plantas e animais medicinais no estado de Pernambuco (nordeste do Brasil): um estudo de caso. *Interciencia*, vol. 27 pp.276-285.

Alves, R.R.N. (2009). Fauna used in popular medicine in Northeast Brazil. *J Ethnobiol Ethnomed*, vol. 5.

Alves, R.R.N. & Delima, Y.C.C. (2006). Snakes used in ethnomedicine in northeast Brazil environment, development and sustainability. *CAB Abstr Lite*, vol.9, pp.455-464.

Alves, R.R.N. & Dias, T.L.P. (2010). Usos de invertebrados na medicina popular no Brasil e suas implicações para conservação. *Tropical Conservation Science*, vol. 2, pp.159-174.

Alves, R.R.N. & Rosa, I.L. (2005). Why study the use of animal products in traditional medicines? *J Ethnobiol Ethnomed*, vol. 30, pp.1-5.

Anas, K. Jayasree, P.R.; Vijayakumar, T. & Manish Kumar, P.R. (2008). In vitro antibacterial activity of Psidium guajava Linn. leaf extract on clinical isolates of multidrug resistant Staphylococcus aureus. *Indian J Exp Biol*, vol.46, pp.41-46.

Andrighetti-Fröhner, C.R.; Sincero, T.C.; da Silva, A.C.; Savi, L.A.; Gaido, C.M.; Bettega, J.M.; Mancini, M.; de Almeida, M.T.; Barbosa, R.A.; Farias, M.R.; Barardi, C.R. & Simões, C.M. (2005). Antiviral evaluation of plants from Brazilian Atlantic Tropical Forest. *Fitoterapia*, vol.76, pp.374-378.

Antonio, J.M.; Gracioso, J.S.; Toma, W.; Lopez, L.C.; Oliveira, F. & Brito, A.R. (2004). Antiulcerogenic activity of ethanol extract of Solanum variabile (false "jurubeba"). *J Ethnopharmacol*, vol.93, pp.83-88.

Antonio, T.M.F. (1994). Insects as remedies for illnesses in Zaire. *The Food Insects Newsletter*, vol.7, pp. 4-5.

Anuar, N.S.; Zahari, S.S.; Taib, I.A. & Rahman, M.T. (2008). Effect of green and ripe Caricapapaya epicarp extracts on wound healing and during pregnancy. *Food Chem Toxicol*, vol.46, pp.2384-2389.

Araújo, V.T.; Diogo, D.C.; da Silva, M.A.P.; Riggio, L.M.T.; Lapa, A.J. & Souccar, C. (1999). Evaluation of the antiurolithiatic activity of the extract of Costus spiralis Roscoe in rats. *J Ethnopharmacol*, vol.66, pp.193-198.

Aridoğan, B.C.; Baydar, H.; Kaya, S.; Demirci, M.; Ozbaşar, D. & Mumcu, E. (2002). Antimicrobial activity and chemical composition of some essential oils. *Arch Pharm Res*, vol.25, pp.860-864.

Atlas de Desenvolvimento Humano/PNUD, 2011, Avaiable from: <http://www.pnud.org.br/atlas/>.

Bakirel, T.; Bakirel, U.; Keles, O.U.; Ulgen, S.G. & Yardibi, H. (2008). In vivo assessment of antidiabetic and antioxidant activities of rosemary (Rosmarinus officinalis) in alloxan-diabetic rabbits. *J Ethnopharmacol*, vol. 28, pp.64-73.

Balick, M. J. (1990). Ethnobotany and the identification of therapeutic agents from the rainforest. In: CIBA Foundation Symposium on Bioactive Compounds from Plants. Bangkok: CIBA, pp. 22-39,

Balick, M.J. & Cox, P.A. (1997). Plants, people and culture. New York: Scientific American Library.

Bani, S.; Kaul, A.; Khan, B.; Gupta, V.K.; Satti, N.K.; Suri, K.A. & Qazi, G.N. (2007). Anti-arthritic activity of a biopolymeric fraction from Euphorbia tirucalli. *J Ethnopharmacol*, vol.1, pp.92-98.

Begossi, A.; Leitão-Filho, H.F. & Richerson, P.J. (1993). Plant uses a Brazilian coastal fishing community (Búzios Island). *J Ethnobiol Ethnomed*, vol.13, pp.233-256.

Belliard, J.C. & Ramirez-Jhonson, J. (2005). Medical pluralism in the life of Mexican immigrant woman. *Hispanic Journal of Behavioral Science*, vol. 27, pp.267-285.

Berlink, R.G.S.; Hajdu, E.; Rocha, R.M.; Oliveira, J.H.L.L.; Hernandez, I.L.C.; Seleghim, M.H.R.; Granato, A.C.; Almeida, E.V.R.; Nunnez, C.V.; Muricy, G.; Peixinho, S.; Pessoa, C.; Moraes, M.O.; Cavalcanti B.C.; Nascimento, G.G.F.; Thiemann. O;H. & Silva, M. (2004). Challenges and Rewards of Research in Marine Natural Products Chemistry in Brazil. *J Nat Prod*, vol.67, pp.510-522.

Bernard, R.H. (1988). Research methods in cultural anthropology, Sage publications: London.

Berson, D.S. (2008). Natural antioxidants. *J Drugs Dermatol*, vol.7, pp.7-12.

Bharat, K. P. & Badola, K.H. (2008). Ethnomedicinal plant use by Lepcha tribe of Dzongu valley, bordering Khangchendzonga Biosphere Reserve, in North Sikkim, India. *Journal of Ethnobiology and Ethnomedicine*, vol. 4.

Biavatti, M.W.; Farias, C.; Curtius, F.; Brasil, L.M.; Hort, S.; Schuster, L.; Leite, S.N. & Prado, S.R. (2004). Preliminary studies on Campomanesia xanthocarpa (Berg.) and Cuphea carthagenensis (Jacq.) J.F. Macbr. aqueous extract: weight control and biochemical parameters. *J Ethnopharmacol*, vol.93, pp.385-389.

Bodeker, G.C.; Neumann, P.; Lall, Z. & Min, O.O. (2005). Tradicional medicine use and health worker training in a refugee setting at the Thai-Burma border. *Journal of Refugee Studies*, vol.18, pp. 76-99.

Braga, F.G.; Bouzada, M.L.; Fabri, R.L. de O.; Matos, M.; Moreira, F.O.; Scio, E. & Coimbra, E.S. (2007). Antileishmanial and antifungal activity of plants used in traditional medicine in Brazil. *J Ethnopharmacol,* vol. 4, pp.396-402.

Bravo, E.; Amrani, S. & Aziz, M. (2008). Ocimum basilicum ethanolic extract decreases cholesterol synthesis and lipid accumulation in human macrophages. *Fitoterapia,* vol.79, pp.515-523.

Cáceres, A.; Alvarez, A.V.; Ovando, A.E. & Samayoa, B.E. (1991). Plants used in Guatemala for the treatment of respiratory diseases. Screening of 68 plants against gram-positive bacteria. *J Ethnopharmacol,* vol. 31, pp.193-208.

Cáceres, A.; López, B.; González, S.; Berger, I.; Tada, I. & Maki, J. (1998). Plants used in Guatemala for the treatment of protozoal infections. I. Screening of activity to bacteria, fungi and (protozoário) American trypanosomes of 13 native plants. *J Ethnopharmaco,* vol. 62, pp.195-202.

Camargo, M.T.L. de A. (2000). Trabalhos de Antropologia e Etnologia. vol.15, pp.179-187.

Candan, F.; Unlu, M.; Tepe, B.; Daferera, D.; Polissiou, M.; Sökmen, A. & Akpulat, H.A. (2003). Antioxidant and antimicrobial activity of the essential oil and methanol extracts of Achillea millefolium subsp. millefolium Afan. (Asteraceae). *J Ethnopharmacol,* vol. 87, pp.215-220.

Cano, J.H. & Volpato, G. (2004). Herbal mixtures in the traditional medicine of Eastern Cuba. *J Ethnopharmacol,* vol. 90, pp. 293-316.

Carney, J. A. (2001). African Plants in the Columbian Exchange. *Journal of African History,* vol.42, pp.377-396.

Carney, J. & Voeks, R.A. (2003). Landscape legades of the African Diaspora in Brazil. *Prog Hum Geogr,* pp.27-6.

Carrier, N. (2007). In Pieroni, A., and Vandebroek, I. (eds.), A Strange Drug in a Strange Land. Traveling Plants and Cultures. The Ethnobiology and Ethnopharmacy of Migrations. Berghahn, Oxford, pp. 186–203.

Carvalho, L.H. & Krettli, A.U. (1991). Antimalarial chemotherapy with natural products and chemically defined molecules. *Mem Inst Oswaldo Cruz,* vol. 2, pp.181-184.

Cavalcanti, E.S.; Morais, S.M.; Lima, M.A. & Santana, E.W. (2004). Larvicidal activity of essential oils from Brazilian plants against Aedes aegypti L. *Mem Inst Oswaldo Cruz,* vol. 99, pp.541-544.

Cechinel Filho, V.; Santos, A.R.; De Campos, R.O.; Miguel, O.G.; Yunes, R.A.; Ferrari, F.; Messana, I. & Calixto, J.B. (1996). Chemical and pharmacological studies of Phyllanthus caroliniensis in mice. *J Pharm Pharmacol,* vol. 48, pp.1231-1236.

Cetin, H.; Cinbilgel, I.; Yanikoglu, A. & Gokceoglu, M. (2006). Larvicidal activity of some Labiatae (Lamiaceae) plant extracts from Turkey. *Phytother Res,* vol. 20, pp.1088-1090.

Ceuterick, M.; Vandebroek, I.; Torry, B. & Pieroni, A. (2007). The use of home remedies for health care and well-being by Spanish-speaking latino immigrants in London: a reflection on acculturation, pp.145-165.

Ceuterick, M.; Vandebroek, I.; Torry, B. & Pieroni, A. (2008). Cross-cultural adaptation in urban ethnobotany: the Colombian folk pharmacopoeia in London. *J Ethnopharmacol,* vol.120, pp.342-359.

Chah, K.F.; Eze, C.A.; Emuelosi, C.E. & Esimone, C.O. (2006). Antibacterial and wound healing properties of methanolic extracts of some Nigerian medicinal plants. J Ethnopharmacol, vol. 8, pp.164-167.

Chang, C.L.; Kuo, H.K.; Chang, S.L.; Chiang, Y.M.; Lee, T.H.; Wu, W.M.; Shyur, L.F. & Yang, W.C. (2005). The distinct effects of a butanol fraction of Bidens pilosa plant extract on the development of Th1-mediated diabetes and Th2-mediated airway inflammation in mice. *J Biomed Sci*, vol.12, pp.79-89.

Cheruiyot, K.R.; Olila, D. & Kateregga, J. (2009). In-vitro antibacterial activity of selected medicinal plants from Longisa region of Bomet district, Kenya. *Afr Health Sci*, vol.1, pp.42-46.

Chiasson, H.; Bélanger, A.; Bostanian, N.; Vincent, C. & Poliquin, A. (2001). Acaricidal properties of Artemisia absinthium and Tanacetum vulgare (Asteraceae) essential oils obtained by three methods of extraction. *J Econ Entomol*, vol.94, pp.167-171.

Chiasson, H.; Bostanian, N.J. & Vincent, C. (2004). Insecticidal properties of a Chenopodium-based botanical. *J Econ Entomol*, vol.97, pp.1373-1377.

Choi, E.M. & Hwang, J.K. (2004). Antiinflammatory, analgesic and antioxidant activities of the fruit of Foeniculum vulgare. *Fitoterapia*, vol.75, pp.557-565.

Conconi, J.R. & Pino, J.M. (1988). The utilization of insects in the empirical medicine of ancient Mexicans. *J Ethnobiol Ethnomed*, vol.8, pp.195-202.

Consolini, A.E.; Ragone, M.I.; Migliori, G.N.; Conforti, P. & Volonté, M.G. (2006). Cardiotonic and sedative effects of Cecropia pachystachya Mart. (ambay) on isolated rat hearts and conscious mice. *J Ethnopharmacol*, vol.15, pp.90-96.

Costa-Neto, E.M. (2002). The use of insects in folk medicine in the state of Bahia, northeastern Brazil, with notes on insects reported elsewhere in Brazilian folk medicine. *Hum Ecol*, vol. 30, pp.245-263.

Costa-Neto, E.M. (2005). Animal-based medicines: biological prospection and the sustainable use of zootherapeutic resources. *Annals of the Brazilian Academy of Sciences*, vol. 77, pp.33-43.

Costa-Neto, E.M. (2006). Os moluscos na zooterapia: medicina tradicional e importância clínico-farmacológica. *Biotemas*, vol. 19, pp.71-78.

Da Silva Filho, A.A.; de Sousa, J.P.; Soares, S.; Furtado, N.A.; Andrade e Silva, M.L.; Cunha, W.R.; Gregório, L.E.; Nanayakkara, N.P. & Bastos, J.K. (2008). Antimicrobial activity of the extract and isolated compounds from Baccharis dracunculifolia D. C. (Asteraceae). *Z Naturforsch C J Biosci*, vol. 63, pp.40-46.

Das, N.G.; Baruah, I.; Talukdar, P.K. & Das, S.C. (2003). Evaluation of botanicals as repellents against mosquitoes. *J Vector Borne Dis*, vol.40, pp.49-53.

Davis, E.W. (1995). Ethnobotany: an old practice, a new discipline. In: Schultes, R.E. & von Reis, S. (eds.). *Ethnobotany: evolution of a discipline*. Dioscorides Press, Portland.

De Almeida Barbosa, L.C.; de Alvarenga, E.S.; Demuner, A.J.; Virtuoso, L.S. & Silva, A.A. (2006). Synthesis of new phytogrowth-inhibitory substituted aryl-pbenzoquinones. *Chem Biodivers*, vol.3, pp.553-567.

De Almeida, I.; Alviano, D.S.; Vieira, D.P.; Alves, P.B.; Blank, A.F.; Lopes, A.H.; Alviano, C.S. & Rosa, M.S. (2007). Antigiardial activity of Ocimum basilicum essential oil. *Parasitol Res*, vol. 101, pp.443-452.

De Araújo, P.F.; Coelho-de-Souza, A.N.; Morais, S.M.; Ferreira, S.C. & Leal-Cardoso, J.H. (2005). Antinociceptive effects of the essential oil of Alpinia zerumbet on mice. *Phytomedicine*, vol.12, pp.482-486.

De Freitas, T.G.; Augusto, P.M. & Montanari, T. (2005). Effect of Ruta graveolens L. on pregnant mice. *Contraception*, vol.71, pp.74-77.

De Lima, M.R.; de Souza Luna, J.; dos Santos, A.F.; de Andrade, M.C.; Sant'Ana, A.E.; Genet, J.P.; Marquez, B.; Neuville, L. & Moreau, N. (2006). Anti-bacterial activity of some Brazilian medicinal plants. *J Ethnopharmacol*, vol.21, pp.137-147.

De Moura, R.S.; Emiliano, A.F.; de Carvalho, L.C.; Souza, M.A.; Guedes, D.C.; Tano, T. & Resende, A.C. (2005). Antihypertensive and endothelium-dependent vasodilator effects of Alpinia zerumbet, a medicinal plant. *J Cardiovasc Pharmacol*, vol. 46, pp. 288-294.

Dhalwal, K.; Deshpazde, Y.S. & Purohit, A.P. (2007). Evaluation of in vitro antioxidant activity of Sida rhombifolia (L.) ssp. retusa (L.). *J Med Food*, vol.10, pp.683-688

Di Stasi, L.C.; Oliveira, G.P.; Carvalhares, M.A.; Queiroz-Junior, M.; Tien, O.S.; Kakinami, S.H.; & Reis, M.S. (2002). Medicinal plants popularly used in the Brazilian Tropical Atlantic Forest. *Fitoterapia*, vol. 73, pp.69-91.

Díaz, J.L. (1977). Ethnopharmacology of sacred psychoactive plants used by the Indians of Mexico. *Pharmacol Toxicol*, vol.17, pp.647-675.

Dickel, M.L.; Rates, S.M. & Ritter, M.R. (2007). Plants popularly used for loosing weight purposes in Porto Alegre, South Brazil. *J Ethnopharmacol*, vol. 3, pp.60-71.

Dimo, T.; Nguelefack, T.B.; Kamtchouing, P.; Dongo, E.; Rakotonirina, A. & Rakotonirina, S.V. (1999). Hypotensive effects of a methanol extract of Bidens pilosa Linn on hypertensive rats. *C R Acad Sci Gen*, vol. 322, pp.323-329.

Emeruwa, A.C. (1982). Antibacterial substance from Carica papaya fruit extract. *J Nat Prod*, vol. 45, pp.123-127.

FAPESP (2011). Avaiable from: <http://agencia.fapesp.br/14176>.

Ferreira, F.S.; Brito, S.V.; Ribeiro, S.C; Saraiva, A.A.F.; Almeida, W.O. & Alves, R.R.N. (2009). Animal-based folk remedies sold in public markets in Crato and Juazeiro do Norte, Ceará, Brazil. *BMC Complement Altern Med*, vol. 9.

Findley, S. E, De Jong G.F. (1985). Community and family factors influencing family migration in Ilocos Norte. *Philippine Population Journal*, vol.1 pp.18-44.

Freitas, M.A. & Silva, T.F.S. (2005). A herpetofauna da Mata Atlântica nordestina. USEB, Pelotas.

Freitas, M.A. & Silva, T.F.S. (2007). A herpetofauna das caatingas e áreas de altitudes do nordeste Brasileiro. USEB, Pelotas.

Frutuoso, V.S.; Gurjão, M.R.; Cordeiro, R.S. & Martins, M.A. (1994). Analgesic and antiulcerogenic effects of a polar extract from leaves of Vernonia condensata. *Planta Med*, vol. 60, pp. 21-25.

Fu, Y.; Zu, Y.; Chen, L.; Efferth, T.; Liang, H.; Liu, Z. & Liu, W. (2007). Investigation of antibacterial activity of rosemary essential oil against Propionibacterium acnes with atomic force microscopy. *Planta Med*, vol.73, pp.1275-1280.

Fukuda, M.; Ohkoshi, E.; Makino, M. & Fujimoto, Y. (2006). Studies on the constituents of the leaves of Baccharis dracunculifolia (Asteraceae) and their cytotoxic activity. *Chem Pharm Bull*, vol. 54, pp.1465-1468.

Fundação Cultural Palmares (2011). Avaiable from: <http://palmares.gov.br/>.

Gandhi, M.; Lal, R.; Sankaranarayanan, A. & Sharma, P.L. (1991). Post-coital antifertility action of Ruta graveolens in female rats and hamsters. *J Ethnopharmacol,* vol.34, pp.49-59.

Garcia, D.; Domingues, M.V. & Rodrigues, E. (2010). Ethnopharmacological survey among migrants living in the Southeast Atlantic Forest of Diadema, São Paulo, Brazil. *J Ethnobiol Ethnomed,* vol. 6, pp. 29-48.

Gbeassor, M.; Kossou, Y.; Amegbo, K.; de Souza, C.; Koumaglo, K. & Denke, A. (1989). Antimalarial effects of eight African medicinal plants. *J Ethnopharmacol,* vol.25, pp.115-118.

Gené, R.M.; Cartaña, C.; Adzet, T.; Marín, E.; Parella, T. & Cañigueral, S. (1996). Antiinflammatory and analgesic activity of Baccharis trimera: identification of its active constituents. *Planta Med,* vol. 62, pp.232-235.

Gillij, Y.G.; Gleiser, R.M. & Zygadlo, J.A. (2008). Mosquito repellent activity of essential oils of aromatic plants growing in Argentina. *Bioresour Technol,* vol.99, pp.2507-2415.

Giorgetti, M.; Negri, G. & Rodrigues, E. (2007). Brazilian plants with possible action on the central nervous system—A study of historical sources from the 16th to 19th century. *Journal of Ethnopharmacology,* vol.109, pp.338–347.

Giulietti, A.M.; Harley, R.M.; Queiroz, L.P. de.; Wanderley, M. das G. & van den Berg, C. (2005). Biodiversidade e conservação das plantas no Brasil. *Megadiversidade,* vol.1, pp. 52-61.

González-Trujano, M.E.; Peña, E.I.; Martínez, A.L.; Moreno, J.; Guevara-Fefer, P.; Déciga-Campos, M. & López-Muñoz, F.J. (2007). Evaluation of the antinociceptive effect of Rosmarinus officinalis L. using three different experimental models in rodents. *J Ethnopharmacol,* vol. 22, pp.476-482.

Gopalakrishnan, M. & Rajasekharasetty, M.R. (1978). Effect of papaya (Carica papaya Linn) on pregnancy and estrous cycle in albino rats of Wistar strain. *Indian J Physiol Pharmacol,* vol.22, pp.66-70.

Gray, A.M. & Flatt, P.R. (1998). Antihyperglycemic actions of Eucalyptus globulus (Eucalyptus) are associated with pancreatic and extra-pancreatic effects in mice. *J Nutr,* vol.128, pp.2319-2323.

Gray, C.A.; Lira, S.P.; Silva, M.; Pimenta, E.F.; Thiemann, O.H.; Oliva, A.G.; Hajdu, E.; Andersen, R.J. & Berlink, R.G.S. (2006). Sulfated Meroterpenoids from the Brazilian Sponge Callyspongia sp. are Inhibitors of the Antileishmaniasis Target Adenosine Phosphoribosyl Transferase. *J Org Chem,* vol. 71, pp.8685-8690.

Gudger, E.W. (1925). Stitching wounds with the mandibles of ants and beetles. *J Am Med Assoc,* vol. 84, pp.1861-1864.

Han, G. S. & Ballis, H. (2007). Ethnomedicine and dominant medicine in multicultural Australia: a critical realist reflection on the case of Korean-Australian immigrants in Sydney. *Journal of Ethnobiology and Ethnomedicine,* vol. 3.

Hanazaki, N.; Alves, R.R.N. & Begossi, A. (2009). Hunting and use of terrestrial fauna used by Caiçaras from the Atlantic Forest coast (Brazil). *J Ethnobiol Ethnomed,* vol. 5, pp. 5-36.

Heinrich, M. (2000). Ethnobotany and its role in drug development. *Phytother Res,* vol.14, pp.479-488.

Holetz, F.B.; Pessini, G.L.; Sanches, N.R.; Cortez, D.A.; Nakamura, C.V. & Filho, B.P. (2002). Screening of some plants used in the Brazilian folk medicine for the treatment of infectious diseases. *Mem Inst Oswaldo Cruz*, vol.97, pp.1027-1031.

IBAMA (2011). Avaiable from: <http://ibama.gov.br/ecossistemas/mata_atlantica.htm>.

IBGE (2011). Avaiable from: <http://www.ibge.gov.br/home/>.

Instituto Socioambiental (2011). Avaiable from: <http://www.socioambiental.org/>.

Islam, M.A.; Ahmed, F.; Das, A.K. & Bachar, S.C. (2005). Analgesic and anti-inflammatory activity of Leonurus sibiricus. *Fitoterapia*, vol.76, pp.359-362.

Islam, M.E.; Haque, M.E. & Mosaddik, M.A. (2003): Cytotoxicity and antibacterial activity of Sida rhombifolia (Malvaceae) grown in Bangladesh. *Phytother Res*, vol. 17, pp. 973-975.

Ivanova, A.; Mikhova, B.; Najdenski, H.; Tsvetkova, I. & Kostova, I. (2005). Antimicrobial and cytotoxic activity of Ruta graveolens. *Fitoterapia*, vol. 3, pp.344-347.

Iwalewa, E.O.; Adewunmi, C.O.; Omisore, N.O.; Adebanji, O.A.; Azike, C.K.; Adigun, A.O.; Adesina, O.A. & Olowoyo, O.G. (2005). Pro- and antioxidant effects and cytoprotective potentials of nine edible vegetables in southwest Nigeria. *J Med Food*, vol. 8, pp.539-544.

Janes, C. R. & Pawson, I.G. (1986). Migration and biocultural adaptation: Samoans in California. *Social Science & Medicine*, vol. 22, pp. 821-834.

Januário, A.H.; Santos, S.L.; Marcussi, S.; Mazzi, M.V.; Pietro, R.C.; Sato, D.N.; Ellena, J.; Sampaio, S.V.; França, S.C. & Soares, A.M. (2004). Neo-clerodane diterpenoid, a new metalloprotease snake venom inhibitor from Baccharis trimera (Asteraceae): anti-proteolytic and anti-hemorrhagic properties. *Chem Biol Interact*, vol.7, pp.243-251.

Ka, M.H.; Choi, E.H.; Chun, H.S. & Lee, K.G. (2005). Antioxidative activity of volatile extracts isolated from Angelica tenuissimae roots, peppermint leaves, pine needles, and sweet flag leaves. *J Agric Food Chem*, vol. 18, pp.4124-4129.

Khori, V.; Nayebpour, M.; Semnani, S.; Golalipour, M.J. & Marjani, A. (2008). Prolongation of AV nodal refractoriness by Ruta graveolens in isolated rat hearts. Potential role as an anti-arrhythmic agent. *Saudi Med J*, vol.29, pp.357-363.

Kim, S.; Kubec, R. & Musah, R.A. (2006). Antibacterial and antifungal activity of sulfurcontaining compounds from Petiveria alliacea L. *J Ethnopharmacol*, vol. 8, pp.188-192.

Klopell, F.C.; Lemos, M.; Sousa, J.P.; Comunello, E.; Maistro, E.L.; Bastos, J.K. & de Andrade, S.F. (2007). Nerolidol, an antiulcer constituent from the essential oil of Baccharis dracunculifolia DC (Asteraceae). *Z Naturforsch C J Biosci*, vol. 62 pp.537-542.

Kordali, S.; Kotan, R.; Mavi, A.; Cakir, A.; Ala, A. & Yildirim, A. (2005). Determination of the chemical composition and antioxidant activity of the essential oil of Artemisia dracunculus and of the antifungal and antibacterial activities of Turkish Artemisia absinthium, A. dracunculus, A. santonicum, and A. spicigera essential oils. *J Agric Food Chem*, vol. 30, pp.9452-9458.

Kossuga, M.H.; Lira, S.P.; Mchugh, S.; Torres, Y.R.; Lima, B.A.; Veloso, K.; Ferreira Antonio, G.; Rocha, R.M. & Berlink, R.G.S. (2009). Antibacterial Modified Diketopiperazines from two Ascidians of the Genus Didemnum. *J Braz Chem Soc*, vol. 20, pp.704-711.

Kumar, R.; Mishra, A.K.; Dubey, N.K. & Tripathi, Y.B. (2007). Evaluation of Chenopodium ambrosioides oil as a potential source of antifungal, antiaflatoxigenic and antioxidant activity. *Int J Food Microbiol*, vol.10, pp.159-164.

Kupchan, S.M.; Knox, J.R.; Kelsey, J.E. & Saenzrenauld, J.A. (1964). Calotropin, a cytotoxic principle isolated from Asclepias curassavica L. *Science*, vol. 25, pp.1685-1686.

Kury, L. (2001). Viajantes-naturalitas no Brasil oitocentista: experiencia, relato e imagem. *História, Ciência, Saúde-Manguinhos*, vol. 8, pp. 863–880.

Kusamba, C.; Byamana, K. & Mbuyi, W.M. (1991). Antibacterial activity of Mirabilis jalapa seed powder. *J Ethnopharmacol*, vol. 35, pp.197-199.

Kviecinski, M.R.; Felipe, K.B.; Schoenfelder, T.; de Lemos Wiese, L.P.; Rossi, M.H.; Gonçalez, E.; Felicio, J.D.; Filho, D.W. & Pedrosa, R.C. (2008). Study of the antitumor potential of Bidens pilosa (Asteraceae) used in Brazilian folk medicine. *J Ethnopharmacol*, vol.17, pp.69-75.

Lacuna-Richman, C. (2006). The use of non-wood forest products by grants in a new settlement: experiences of a Visayan community in Palawan, Philippines. *Journal of Ethnobiology and Ethnomedicine*, pp. 2:36.

Lans, C. (2007). Ethnomedicines used in Trinidad and Tobago for reproductive problems. *J Ethnobiol Ethnomed*, vol.15, pp.3-13.

Latha, M.; Ramkumar, K.M.; Pari, L.; Damodaran, P.N.; Rajeshkannan, V. & Suresh, T. (2006). Phytochemical and antimicrobial study of an antidiabetic plant: Scoparia dulcis L. *J Med Food*, vol.9, pp. 391-394.

Lee, H.S. (2004). Acaricidal activity of constituents identified in Foeniculum vulgare fruit oil against Dermatophagoides spp. (Acari: Pyroglyphidae). *J Agric Food Chem*, vol.19, pp.2887-2889.

Lee, R.A.; Balick, M.J.; Ling, D.L.; Sohl, F.; Brosi, B.J. & Raynor, W. (2001). Cultural dynamism and change in Micronesia. *Economic Botany*, vol. 55, pp.9-13.

Lin, L.Y.; Peng, C.C.; Yeh, W.T.; Wang, H.E.; Yu, T.H. & Peng, R.Y. (2008). Alpinia zerumbet potentially elevates high- density lipoprotein cholesterol level in hamsters. *J Agric Food Chem*, vol. 25, pp. 4435-4443.

Lipp, F.J. (1989). Methods for ethnopharmacological field work. *J Ethnopharmacol*, vol. 25, pp.139-150.

Lopes-Lutz, D.; Alviano, D.S.; Alviano, C.S. & Kolodziejczyk, P.P. (2008). Screening of chemical composition, antimicrobial and antioxidant activities of Artemisia essential oils. *Phytochemistry*, vol.69, pp.1732-1738.

Lopes-Martins, R.A.; Pegoraro, D.H.; Woisky, R.; Penna, S.C. & Sertié, J.A. (2002). The anti-inflammatory and analgesic effects of a crude extract of Petiveria alliacea L. (Phytolaccaceae). *Phytomedicine*, vol. 9, pp. 245-248.

Lorenzi, H. & Matos, de A. F.J. (2008). Plantas medicinais do Brasil: nativas e exóticas cultivadas. Instituto Plantarum: São Paulo.

Luo, Q.F.; Sun, L.; Si, J.Y.; Chen, D.H. & Du, G.H. (2008). Hypocholesterolemic effect of stilbene extract from Cajanus cajan L. on serum and hepatic lipid in diet-induced hyperlipidemic mice. *Yao Xue Xue Bao*, vol. 43, pp.145-149.

Mahanta, M. & Mukherjee, A.K. (2001). Neutralisation of lethality, myotoxicity and toxic enzymes of Naja kaouthia venom by Mimosa pudica root extracts. *J Ethnopharmacol*, vol.75, pp.55-60.

Maiorano, V.A.; Marcussi, S.; Daher, M.A.; Oliveira, C.Z.; Couto, L.B.; Gomes, O.A.; França, S.C.; Soares, A.M. & Pereira, O.S. (2005). Antiophidian properties of the aqueous extract of Mikania glomerata. *J Ethnopharmacol*, vol. 1, pp. 364-370.

Malpezzi, E.L.; Davino, S.C.; Costa, L.V.; Freitas, J.C.; Giesbrecht, A.M. & Roque, N.F. (1994). Antimitotic action of extracts of Petiveria alliacea on sea urchin egg development. *Braz J Med Biol Res,* vol. 27, pp.749-754.

Manila University Press, Quezon City, Philippines. pp. 38-48.

Ming, L.C. (2006). Levantamento de plantas medicinais na Reserva Extrativista "Chico Mendes". UNESP-Botucatu, pp.160.

Molina, M.; Contreras, C.M. & Tellez-Alcantara, P. (1999). Mimosa pudica may possess antidepressant actions in the rat. *Phytomedicine,* vol. 6, pp.319-323.

Moore, S.J.; Hill, N.; Ruiz, C. & Cameron, M.M. (2007). Field evaluation of traditionally used plant-based insect repellents and fumigants against the malaria vector Anopheles darlingi in Riberalta, Bolivian Amazon. *J Med Entomol,* vol.44, pp.624-630.

Moreira, M.D.; Picanço, M.C.; Barbosa, L.C.; Guedes, R.N.; Barros, E.C. & Campos, M.R. (2007). Compounds from Ageratum conyzoides: isolation, structural elucidation and insecticidal activity. *Pest Manag Sci,* vol.63, pp.615-621.

Moura, A.C.; Silva, E.L.; Fraga, M.C.; Wanderley, A.G.; Afiatpour, P. & Maia, M.B. (2005). Antiinflammatory and chronic toxicity study of the leaves of Ageratum conyzoides L. in rats. *Phytomedicine,* vol.12, pp.138-142.

Nayak, S.; Nalabothu, P.; Sandiford, S.; Bhogadi, V. & Adogwa, A. (2006). Evaluation of wound healing activity of Allamanda cathartica. L. and Laurus nobilis. L. extracts on rats. *BMC Complement Altern Med,* vol.12, pp.138-142.

Nesheim, I.; Dhillion, S.S. & Stolen, K.A. (2006). What happens to traditional knowledge and use of natural resourceswhen people migrate? *Human Ecology,* vol. 34, pp. 99-131.

Ngo Bum, E.; Dawack, D.L.; Schmutz, M.; Rakotonirina, A.; Rakotonirina, S.V.; Portet, C.; Jeker, A.; Olpe, H.R. & Herrling, P. (2004). Anticonvulsant activity of Mimosa pudica decoction. *Fitoterapia,* vol. 75, pp.309-314.

Nguefack, J.; Budde, B.B. & Jakobsen, M. (2004). Five essential oils from aromatic plants of Cameroon: their antibacterial activity and ability to permeabilize the cytoplasmic membrane of Listeria innocua examined by flow cytometry. *Lett Appl Microbiol,* vol. 39, pp.395-400.

Nguyen, M. (2003). Comparison of food plant knowledge between urban Vietnamese living in Vietnam and in Hawai'i. *Economic Botany,* vol.57, pp. 47-80.

Niñez, V. K. (1987). Household gardens: theoretical and policy considerations. *Agricultural Systems,* vol.23, pp.167-186.

Nishino, H.; Hayashi, T.; Arisawa, M.; Satomi, Y. & Iwashima, A. (1993). Antitumorpromoting activity of scopadulcic acid B, isolated from the medicinal plant Scoparia dulcis L. *Oncology,* vol.50, pp.100-103.

Nogueira, J.C.; Diniz, M. de F. & Lima, E.O. (2008). In vitro antimicrobial activity of plants in Acute Otitis Externa. *Braz J Otorhinolaryngo,* vol.74, pp.118-124.

Ntonifor, N.N.; Ngufor, C.A.; Kimbi, H.K. & Oben, B.O. (2006). Traditional use of indigenous mosquito-repellents to protect humans against mosquitoes and other insect bites in a rural community of Cameroon. *East Afr Med J,* vol.83, pp.553-558.

Nusier, M.K.; Bataineh, H.N. & Daradkah, H.M. (2007). Adverse effects of Rosemary (Rosmarinus officinalis L.) on reproductive function in adult male rats. *Exp Biol Med,* vol.232, pp.809-813.

Obaseiki-Ebor, E.E. (1985). Preliminary report on the in vitro antibacterial activity of Bryophyllum pinnatum leaf juice. *Afr J Med Med Sci,* vol.14, pp.199-202.

Ojewole, J.A. (2005). Antinociceptive, anti-inflammatory and antidiabetic effects of Bryophyllum pinnatum (Crassulaceae) leaf aqueous extract. *J Ethnopharmacol*, vol. 13, pp.13-19.

Okada, Y.; Tanaka, K.; Sato, E. & Okajima, H. (2008). Antioxidant activity of the new thiosulfinate derivative, S-benzyl phenylmethanethiosulfinate, from Petiveria alliacea L. *Org Biomol Chem*, vol.21, pp.1097-1102.

Oliva, A.; Meepagala, K.M.; Wedge, D.E.; Harries, D.; Hale, A.L.; Aliotta, G. & Duke, S.O. (2003). Natural fungicides from Ruta graveolens L. leaves, including a new quinolone alkaloid. *J Agri Food Chem*, vol. 12, pp.890-896.

Oliveira, A.C.; Endringer, D.C.; Amorim, L.A.; das Graças, L.; Brandão, M. & Coelho, M.M. (2005). Effect of the extracts and fractions of Baccharis trimera and Syzygium cumini on glycaemia of diabetic and non-diabetic mice. J Ethnopharmacol, vol. 1, pp. 465-169.

Oliveira, R.B.; Godoy, S.A.P. & Costa, F.B. (2003). Plantas Tóxicas: Conhecimento e prevenção de acidentes Holos. São Paulo.

Orsi, R.O.; Sforcin, J.M.; Funari, S.R.; & Bankova, V. (2005). Effects of Brazilian and Bulgarian propolis on bactericidal activity of macrophages against Salmonella typhimurium. *Int Immunopharmacol*, vol. 5, pp.359-368.

Ososki, A.L.; Balick, M.J & Daly, D.C. (2007). Medicinal plants and cultural variation across dominican rural, urban, and transnational landscapes. In. Pieroni, A. & Vandebroek, I. *Traveling cultures and plants: the ethnobiology and ethnopharmacy of human migrations* (Berghahn Books), ISBN-13: 978-1-84545-373-2, New York.

Ozcan, M.M.; Chalchat, J.C.; Arslan, D.; Ates, A. & Unver, A. (2006). Comparative essential oil composition and antifungal effect of bitter fennel (Foeniculum vulgare ssp. piperitum) fruit oils obtained during different vegetation. *J Med Food*, vol.9, pp.552-561.

Padilha de Paula, J.; Gomes-Carneiro, M.R. & Paumgartten, F.J. (2003). Chemical composition, toxicity and mosquito repellency of Ocimum selloi oil. *J Ethnopharmacol*, vol. 88, pp.253-260.

Pal, S. & Nag Chaudhuri, A.K.(1991). Studies on the anti-ulcer activity of a Bryophyllum pinnatum leaf extract in experimental animals. *J Ethnopharmacol*, vol.33, pp. 97-102.

Palmieri MMB: Efeitos sobre o Sistema Nervoso Central de extratos de plantas popularmente citadas como anticonvulsivantes. MsD thesis Universidade Estadual Paulista, Ribeirão Preto; 2000.

Pascual, M.E.; Slowing, K.; Carretero, M.E. & Villar, A. (2001). Antiulcerogenic activity of Lippia alba (Mill.) N. E. Brown (Verbenaceae). *Farmaco*, vol. 56, pp.501-504.

Paulino, N.; Abreu, S.R.; Uto, Y. Koyama, D.; Nagasawa, H.; Hori, H.; Dirsch, V.M.; Vollmar, A.M.; Scremin, A. & Bretz, W.A. (2008). Anti-inflammatory effects of a bioavailable compound, Artepillin C, in Brazilian propolis. *Eur J Pharmacol*, vol.10, pp.296-301.

Pavela, R. (2008). Insecticidal properties of several essential oils on the house fly (Musca domestica L.). *Phytother Res*, vol. 22, pp. 274-278.

Peng, C.H.; Su, J.D.; Chyau, C.C.; Sung, T.Y.; Ho, S.S.; Peng, C.C. & Peng, R.Y. (2007). Supercritical fluid extracts of rosemary leaves exhibit potent antiinflammation and anti-tumor effects. *Biosci Biotechnol Biochem*, vol. 71, pp.2223-2232.

Penido, C.; Costa, K.A.; Futuro, D.O.; Paiva, S.R.; Kaplan, M.A.; Figueiredo, M.R. & Henriques, M.G. (2006). Anti-inflammatory and anti-ulcerogenic properties of Stachytarpheta cayennensis (L.C. Rich) Vahl. *J Ethnopharmacol*, vol. 8, pp.225-233.

Pérez-García, F.; Marín, E.; Cañigueral, S. & Adzet, T. (1996). Anti-inflammatory action of Pluchea sagittalis: involvement of an antioxidant mechanism. *Life Sci*, vol. 59, pp.2033-2040.

Pieroni, A., Nebel, C., Quave, C.L., Münz, H. & Heinrich, M. (2002a). Ethnopharmacology of Liakra, traditional weedy vegetables of the Arbëreshë of the Vulture área in southern Italy. *J Ethnopharmacol*, vol. 81, pp.165-185.

Pieroni, A.; Quave, C.L.; Nebel, S. & Heinrich, M. (2002b). Ethnopharmacy of ethnic Albanians (Arbëreshë) in northern Basilicata (southern Italy). *Fitoterapia*, vol.73, pp.217-241.

Pieroni, A.; Quave, C.L.; Villanelli, M.L.; Mangino, P.; Sabbatini, G. & Santini, L. (2004). Ethnopharmacognostic survey on the natural ingredients used in folk cosmetics, cosmeceuticals and remedies for healing skin diseases in the inland Marches, Central-Eastern Italy. *J Ethnopharmacol,* vol 91, pp. 331-344.

Pieroni, A. & Quave, C.L. (2005a). Traditional pharmacopoeias and medicines among Albanians and Italians in southern Italy: a comparison. *J Ethnopharmacol,* vol.101, pp.258-270.

Pieroni, A.; Münz, H.; Akbulut, M.; Baser, K.H.C. & Durmuskahya, C. (2005b). Traditional phytotherapy and transcultural pharmacy among Turkish immigrants living in Cologne, Germany. *Journal of Ethnopharmacology*, vol.102, pp. 69-88.

Pieroni, A. & Vandebroek, I. (2007). *Traveling cultures and plants: the ethnobiology and ethnopharmacy of human migrations* (Berghahn Books), ISBN-13: 978-1-84545-373-2, New York.

Pintão, A.M.; Pais, M.S.; Coley, H.; Kelland, L.R. & Judson, I.R. (1995). In vitro and in vivo antitumor activity of benzyl isothiocyanate: a natural product from Tropaeolum majus. *Planta Med*, vol. 61, pp.233-236.

Pio Corrêa, M. (1926). Dicionário das plantas úteis do Brasil e das exóticas cultivadas. Imprensa Nacional, pp. 747, Rio de Janeiro.

Pires, J.M.; Mendes, F.R.; Negri, G.; Duarte-Almeida, J.M. & Carlini, E.A. (2009). Antinociceptive peripheral effect of Achillea millefolium L. and Artemisia vulgaris L.: Both plants known popularly by Brand Names of analgesic drugs. *Phytother Res*, vol. 23, pp.212-219.

Pitasawat, B.; Champakaew, D.; Choochote, W.; Jitpakdi, A.; Chaithong, U.; Kanjanapothi, D.; Rattanachanpichai, E.; Tippawangkosol, P.; Riyong, D.; Tuetun, B. & Chaiyasit, D. (2007). Aromatic plant-derived essential oil: an alternative larvicide for mosquito control. *Fitoterapia*, vol.78, pp.205-210.

Portillo, A.; Vila, R.; Freixa, B.; Adzet, T. & Cañigueral, S. (2001). Antifungal activity of Paraguayan plants used in traditional medicine. *J Ethnopharmacol*, vol. 76, pp.93-98.

Preethi, K.C.; Kuttan, G. & Kuttan, R. (2006). Anti-tumour activity of Ruta graveolens extract. *Asian Pac J Cancer Prev*, vol. 7, pp. 439-443.

Prefeitura de Diadema (2011). Avaiable from: <http://www.diadema.sp.gov.br/apache2-default/>.

PUBMED (2010). Avaiable from: <http://www.ncbi.nlm.nih.gov/pubmed>.

Radford, D.J.; Gillies, A.D.; Hinds, J.A. & Duffy, P. (1986). Naturally occurring cardiac glycosides. *Med J Aust*, vol.12, pp.540-544.

Raghav, S.K.; Gupta, B.; Agrawal, C.; Goswami, K. & Das, H.R. (2006). Anti-inflammatory effect of Ruta graveolens L. in murine macrophage cells. *J Ethnopharmacol*, vol. 8, pp.234-239.

Rahim, N.; Gomes, D.J.; Watanabe, H.; Rahman, S.R.; Chomvarin, C.; Endtz, H.P. & Alam, M. (2010). Antibacterial activity of Psidium guajava leaf and bark against multidrug-resistant Vibrio cholerae: implication for cholera control. *Jpn J Infect Dis*, vol.63, pp.271-274.

Rajesh, R.; Shivaprasad, H.V.; Gowda, C.D.; Nataraju, A.; Dhananjaya, B.L. & Vishwanath, B.S. (2007). Comparative study on plant latex proteases and their involvement in hemostasis: a special emphasis on clot inducing and dissolving properties. *Planta Med*, vol. 73, pp.1061-1067.

Rao, Y.K.; Fang, S.H. & Tzeng, Y.M. (2005). Inhibitory effects of the flavonoids isolated from Waltheria indica on the production of NO, TNF-alpha and IL-12 in activated macrophages. *Bio Pharm Bull*, vol. 28, pp. 912-915.

Ratnasooriya, W.D.; Jayakody, J.R.; Premakumara, G.A. & Ediriweera, E.R. (2005). Antioxidant activity of water extract of Scoparia dulcis. *Fitoterapia*, vol. 76, pp. 220-222.

Ribeiro, D. (1996). O povo brasileiro: A formação e o sentido do Brasil. *Companhia das Letras*, São Paulo, Brasil.

Rim, I.S. & Jee, C.H. (2006). Acaricidal effects of herb essential oils against Dermatophagoides farinae and D. pteronyssinus (Acari: Pyroglyphidae) and qualitative analysis of a herb Mentha pulegium (pennyroyal). Korean J Parasitol, vol. 44, pp.133-138.

Rizzini, C.T. (1968). Problemas relacionados com o estudo da distribuição geográfica e identificação das plantas medicinais brasileiras. *Arquivos do Instituto Biológico*, vol. 35, pp. 10-14.

Rodrigues, E. & Carlini, E.A. (2003). Possíveis Efeitos sobre o Sistema Nervoso Central de Plantas Utilizadas por Duas Culturas Brasileiras (quilombolas e índios). *Arquivos Brasileiros de Fitomedicina Científica*, vol.1.

Rodrigues, E. & Carlini, E.A. (2004). Plants used by a Quilombola group in Brazil with potential central nervous system effects. *Phytother Res*, vol.18, pp.748-753.

Rodrigues, E. (2005). A parceria Universidade - Empresa privada na produção de fitoterápicos no Brasil. *Revisa Fármacos e Medicamentos*, Vol. 37, year IV, pp. 30-39.

Rodrigues, E. & Carlini, E.A. (2005). Ritual use of plants with possible action on the central nervous system by the Kraho indians, Brazil. *Phytother Res*, vol.19, pp.129-135.

Rodrigues, E.; Mendes, F.R. & Negri, G. (2005). Plants indicated by Brazilian Indians to Central Nervous System disturbances: a bibliographical approach. *Curr Med Chem*, vol.6, pp.211-244.

Rodrigues, E. (2006). Ethnopharmacology in the Jaú National Park (JNP), state of Amazonas, Brazil. *Phytother Res*, vol. 5, pp.378-391.

Rodrigues, E.; Mendes, F. R. & Negri, G. (2006). Plants indicated by Brazilian Indians to Central Nervous System disturbances: A bibliographical approach. *Current Medicinal Chemistry* - Central Nervous System Agents, Vol. 6, pp. 211-244.

Rodrigues, E and Carlini, E.A. (2006). Use of South American plants for the treatment of neuropsychiatric disorders. *Bulletin of the Board of International Affairs of the Royal College of Psychiatrists,* vol. 3.

Rodrigues, E. (2007). Plants of restricted use indicated by three cultures in Brazil (Caboclo-river dweller, Indian and Quilombola). *Journal of Ethnopharmacology,* Vol. 111, pp. 295–302.

Rodrigues, E.; Tabach, R.; Galduroz, J.C.F. & Negri, G. (2008). Plants with possible anxiolytic and/or hypnotic effects indicated by three Brazilian cultures - Indians, Afrobrazilians, and River-dwellers. *Studies in Natural Products Chemistry,* vol. 35, 549-595.

Rojas, J.J.; Ochoa, V.J.; Ocampo, A.S. & Muñoz, J.F. (2006). Screening for antimicrobial activity of ten medicinal plants used in Colombian folkloric medicine: a possible alternative in the treatment of non-nosocomial infections. *BMC Complement Altern Med,* vol.6.

Roy, C.K. & Das, A.K. (2010). Comparative evaluation of different extracts of leaves of Psidium guajava Linn. for hepatoprotective activity. *Pak J Pharm Sci,* vol. 23, pp.15-20.

Runnie, I.; Salleh, M.N.; Mohamed, S.; Head, R.J. & Abeywardena, M.Y. (2004). Vasorelaxation induced by common edible tropical plant extracts in isolated rat aorta and mesenteric vascular bed. *J Ethnopharmacol,* vol. 92, pp.311-316.

Ruppelt, B.M.; Pereira, E.F.; Gonçalves, L.C. & Pereira, N.A. (1991). Pharmacological screening of plants recommended by folk medicine as anti-snake venom-I. Analgesic and anti-inflammatory activities. *Mem Inst Oswaldo Cruz,* vol. 2, pp.203-205.

Salari, M.H.; Amine, G.; Shirazi, M.H.; Hafezi, R. & Mohammadypour, M. (2006). Antibacterial effects of Eucalyptus globulus leaf extract on pathogenic bacteria isolated from specimens of patients with respiratory tract disorders. *Clin Microbiol Infect,* vol.12, pp.194-196.

Santos-Fita, D. & Costa-Neto, E.M. (2007). As interações entre os seres humanos e os animais: a contribuição da etnozoologia. *Biotemas,* vol.20, pp.99-110.

Sawangjaroen, N.; Phongpaichit, S.; Subhadhirasakul, S.; Visutthi, M.; Srisuwan, N. & Thammapalerd, N. (2006). The anti-amoebic activity of some medicinal plants used by AIDS patients in southern Thailand. *Parasitol Res,* vol. 98, pp. 588-592.

Schapoval, E.E.; Vargas, M.R.; Chaves, C.G.; Bridi, R.; Zuanazzi, J.A. & Henriques, A.T. (1998). Antiinflammatory and antinociceptive activities of extracts and isolated compounds from Stachytarpheta cayennensis. *J Ethnopharmacol,* vol. 60, pp.53-59.

Schinella, G.; Aquila, S.; Dade, M.; Giner, R.; Recio Mdel, C.; Spegazzini, E.; de Buschiazzo, P.; Tournier, H. & Ríos, J.L. (2008). Anti-inflammatory and apoptotic activities of pomolic acid isolated from Cecropia pachystachya. *Planta Med,* vol.74, pp.215-220.

Schmourlo, G.; Mendonça-Filho, R.R.; Alviano, C.S. & Costa, S.S. (2005). Screening of antifungal agents using ethanol precipitation and bioautography of medicinal and food plants. *J Ethnopharmacol,* vol. 15, pp.563-568.

Schuldt, E.Z.; Ckless, K.; Simas, M.E.; Farias, M.R. & Ribeiro-Do-Valle, R.M. (2000). Butanolic fraction from Cuphea carthagenensis Jacq McBride relaxes rat thoracic aorta through endothelium-dependent and endothelium- independent mechanisms. *J Cardiovasc Pharmacol,* vol.35, pp.234-239.

Schultes, R.E. & Raffaulf, R.F. (1990). In The Healing Forest. Medicinal and Toxic Plants of the Nortwest Amazonia. vol. 2. Dioscorides Press: Oregon.

Schultes, R.E. (1988). Ethnopharmacological conservation: a key to progress in medicine. *Acta Botanica*, vol.18, pp. 393-406.

SCIFINDER (2011) Avaiable from: <http://www.cas.org/products/sfacad/index.html>.

Shao, F.; Hu, Z.; Xiong, Y.M.; Huang, Q.Z.; Wang, C.G.; Zhu, R.H. & Wang, D.C. (1999). A new antifungal peptide from the seeds of Phytolacca americana: characterization, amino acid sequence and cDNA cloning. *Biochim Biophys Acta*, vol.19, pp.262-268.

Sharma, P.; Mohan, L. & Srivastava, C.N. (2006). Phytoextract-induced developmental deformities in malaria vector. *Bioresour Technol*, vol. 97, pp.1599-1604.

Shi, M.; Chang, L. & He, G. (1995). Stimulating action of Carthamus tinctorius L., Angelica sinensis (Oliv.) Diels and Leonurus sibiricus L. on the uterus. *Zhongguo Zhong Yao Za Zhi*, vol.20, pp.173-175.

Shlamovitz, G.Z.; Gupta, M. & Diaz, J.A. (2007). A case of acute keratoconjunctivitis from exposure to latex of Euphorbia tirucalli (Pencil Cactus). *J Emerg Med*, vol. 36, pp. 239-241.

Silva, J.; Abebeb, W.; Sousa, S.M.; Duarte, V.G.; Machado, M.I.L. & Matos, F.J.A. (2003). Analgesic and anti-inflammatory effects of essential oils of Eucalyptus. *J Ethnopharmacol*, vol.89, pp. 277-283.

Simões, L.L. & Lino, C.F. (2004). Sustentável Mata Atlântica: a exploração de seus recursos florestais. *SENAC*, São Paulo.

Simões-Pires, C.A.; Queiroz, E.F.; Henriques, A.T. & Hostettmann, K. (2005): Isolation and on-line identification of antioxidant compounds from three Baccharis species by HPLC-UV-MS/MS with post-column derivatisation. *Phytochem Anal*, vol.16, pp.307-314.

Singh, H.P.; Batish, D.R.; Kaur, S.; Kohli, R.K. & Arora, K. (2006). Phytotoxicity of the volatile monoterpene citronellal against some weeds. *Z Naturforsch*, vol. 61, pp.334-340.

Sistema Único de Saúde (2010). Avaiable from: <http://tabnet.datasus.gov.br/tabdata/cadernos/ cadernosmap.htm>.

Soares de Moura, R.; Costa, S.S.; Jansen, J.M.; Silva, C.A.; Lopes, C.S.; Bernardo-Filho, M.; Nascimento da Silva, V.; Criddle, D.N.; Portela, B.N.; Rubenich, L.M.; Araujo, R.G. & Carvalho, L.C. (2002). Bronchodilator activity of Mikania glomerata Sprengel on human bronchi and guinea-pig trachea. *J Pharm Pharmacol*, vol. 54, pp.249-256.

Soicke, H. & Leng-Peschlow, E. (1987). Characterisation of flavonoids from Baccharis trimera and their antihepatotoxic properties. *Planta Med*, vol. 53, pp.37-39.

Souza, M.C.; Siani, A.C.; Ramos, M.F.; Menezes-de-Lima, O.J. & Henriques, M.G. (2004). Evaluation of anti-inflammatory activity of essential oils from two Asteraceae species. *Pharmazie*, vol. 58, pp.582-586.

Spjut, R.W. & Perdue, J.R. (1976). Plant folcklore: a tool for predicting sources of antitumor activity? *Cancer Treatment Reports*, Vol. 60, pp. 979-985.

Sripanidkulchai, B.; Wongpanich, V.; Laupattarakasem, P.; Suwansaksri, J. & Jirakulsomchok. (2001). Diuretic effects of selected Thai indigenous medicinal plants in rats. *J Ethnopharmacol*, vol.75, pp.185-190.

Sundararajan, P.; Dey, A.; Smith, A.; Doss, A.G.; Rajappan, M. & Natarajan, S. (2006). Studies of anticancer and antipyretic activity of Bidens pilosa whole plant. *Afr Health Sci*, vol.6, pp.27-30.

Suzuki, N. (1996). Investing for the future: education, migration and intergenerational conflict in South Cotabato, the Philippines. In Binisaya nga kinabuhi (Visayan life). Edited by Ushijima, Iwao, Cynthia Neri Zayas. Visayas Maritime Anthropological Studies, College of Social Sciences and Philosophy, University of the Philippines, pp. 43-58, Quezon City, Philippines.

Tabopda, T.K.; Ngoupayo, J.; Liu, J.; Mitaine-Offer, A.C.; Tanoli, S.A.; Khan, S.N.; Ali, M.S.; Ngadjui, B.T.; Tsamo, E.; Lacaille-Dubois, M.A. & Luu, B. (2008). Bioactive aristolactams from Piper umbellatum. *Phytochemistry*, vol.69, pp.1726-1731.

Takahashi, H.; Hirata, S.; Minami, H. & Fukuyama, Y. (2001). Triterpene and flavanone glycoside from Rhododendron simsii. *Phytochemistry*, vol. 56, pp.875-879.

Takahashi, T.; Kokubo, R. & Sakaino, M. (2004): Antimicrobial activities of eucalyptus leaf extracts and flavonoids from Eucalyptus maculata. *Lett Appl Microbiol*, vol.39, pp.60-64.

Talbourdet, S.; Sadick, N.S.; Lazou, K.; Bonnet-Duquennoy, M.; Kurfurst, R.; Neveu, M.; Heusèle, C.; André, P.; Schnebert, S.; Draelos, Z.D. & Perrier, E. (2007). Modulation of gene expression as a new skin anti-aging strategy. *J Drugs Dermatol*, vol.6, pp.25-33.

Tchoumbougnang, F.; Zollo, P.H.; Dagne, E. & Mekonnen, Y. (2005). In vivo antimalarial activity of essential oils from Cymbopogon citratus and Ocimum gratissimum on mice infected with Plasmodium berghei. *Planta Med*, vol.7, pp.20-23.

Thomas, E.; Vandebroek, I.; Sanca, S. & Van Damme, P. (2009). Cultural significance of medicinal plant families and species among Quechua farmers in Apillapampa, Bolivia. *Journal of Ethnopharmacology*, vol. 122, pp.60-67.

Tiwari, T.N.; Varma, J.; Dubey, N.K.; Chansouria, J.P. & Ali, Z. (1998). Pharmacological evaluation of some bioactive plant products on albino rats. *Hindustan Antibiot Bull*, vol.40, pp.38-41.

Tognolini, M.; Ballabeni, V.; Bertoni, S.; Bruni, R.; Impicciatore, M. & Barocelli, E. (2007). Protective effect of Foeniculum vulgare essential oil and anethole in na experimental model of thrombosis. *Pharmacol Res*, vol. 56, pp.254-260.

Torres, D.F.; de Oliveira, E.S.; Alves, R.R.N. & Vasconcellos, A. (2009). Etnobotânica e etnozoologia em unidades de conservação: uso da biodiversidade na APA de Genipabu, Rio Grande do Norte, Brasil. *Interciencia*, vol. 34, p.623-629.

Torres, L.M.; Gamberini, M.T.; Roque, N.F.; Lima-Landman, M.T.; Souccar, C. & Lapa, A.J. (2000). Diterpene from Baccharis trimera with a relaxant effect on rat vascular smooth muscle. *Phytochemistry*, vol. 55, pp.617-619.

Trotter, R.T. & Logan, M.H. (1986). Informant consensus: a new approach for identifying potentially effective medicinal plants. In Plants in indigenous medicine and diet: biobehavioral approachs. Edited by: Etkin NL. New York: Redgrave Publishing, pp.91-112.

Valadares, M.C.; Carrucha, S.G.; Accorsi, W. & Queiroz, M.L. (2006). Euphorbia tirucalli L. modulates myelopoiesis and enhances the resistance of tumour-bearing mice. *Int Immunopharmacol*, vol.6, pp.294-299.

Valverde, A.L.; Cardoso, G.L.; Pereira, N.A.; Silva, A.J. & Kuster, R.M. (2001). Analgesic and antiinflammatory activities of vernonioside B2 from Vernonia condensata. *Phytother Res*, vol. 15, pp. 263-264.

van Andel, T.R. & Westers P. (2010). Why Surinamese migrants in the Netherlands continue to use medicinal herbs from their home country. *J Ethnopharmacol*, vol.127pp.694-701.

Velázquez, E.; Tournier, H.A.; de Buschiazzo, P.; Saavedra, G. & Schinella, G.R. (2003). Antioxidant activity of Paraguayan plant extracts. *Fitoterapia*, vol.74, pp.91-97.

Viyoch, J.; Pisutthanan, N.; Faikreua, A.; Nupangta, K.; Wangtorpol, K. & Ngokkuen, J. (2006). Evaluation of in vitro antimicrobial activity of Thai basil oils and their micro-emulsion formulas against Propionibacterium acnes. *Int J Cosmet Sci*, vol. 28, pp.125-133.

Voeks, R.A. & Leony, A. (2004). Foegetting the forest: Assessing medicinal plant erosion in Eastern Brazil. *Economic Botany*, vol. 58.

Voeks, R.A. (2009). Traditions in transition: African diaspora ethnobotany in lowland South America. In Mobility and Migration in Indigenous Amazonia: Contemporary Ethnoecological Perspectives. Edited by: Alexiades, M., pp.275-294, London: Berghahn.

Volpato, G.; Ahmadi, A.; Lamin, S.M.; Broglia, A. & Di Lello, S. (2007). Procurement of traditional remedies and transmission of medicinal knowledge among Sahrawi people displaced in Southwestern Algerian refugee camps. In Traveling Plants and Cultures The Ethnobiology and Ethnopharmacy of Migrations Edited by: Pieroni A, Vandebroek I.; pp. 245-269 Oxford: Berghahn

Volpato, G.; Godínez, D. & Beyra, A. (2008). Migration and Ethnobotanical Practices: The Case of *Tifey* Among Haitian Immigrants in Cuba. *Human Ecology*, vol.37, pp. 43–53.

Volpato, G.; Godínez, D.; Beyra, A. & Barreto, A. (2009). Uses of medicinal plants by Haitian immigrants and their descendants in the Province of Camagüey, Cuba. *Journal of Ethnobiology and Ethnomedicine*, pp.5-16.

Von Szczepanski, C.; Zgorzelak, P. & Hoyer, G.A. (1972). Isolation, structural analysis Arzneimittelforschung vol. 22, pp.1975-1976.

Waldstein, A. (2006): Mexican migrant ethnopharmacology: pharmacopoeia, classification of medicines and explanations of efficacy. *J Ethnopharmacol*, vol. 108, pp.299-310.

Waldstein, A. (2008). Diaspora and Health? Traditional Medicine and Culture in a Mexican Migrant Community. *International Migration*, vol. 46, pp.95-117.

Wannissorn, B.; Jarikasem, S.; Siriwangchai, T. & Thubthimthed, S. (2005). Antibacterial properties of essential oils from Thai medicinal plants. *Fitoterapia*, vol.76, pp. 233-236.

Weckesser, S.; Engel, K.; Simon-Haarhaus, B.; Wittmer, A.; Pelz, K. & Schempp, C.M. (2007). Screening of plant extracts for antimicrobial activity against bacteria and yeasts with dermatological relevance. *Phytomedicine*, vol.14, pp. 508-516.

Weiss, H.B. (1947). Entomological medicaments of the past. *Journal of the New York Entomological Society*, vol.55, pp.155-168.

Woodland, D.W. (1997). Contemporary plant systematics Andrews University Press, London.

Yemitan, O.K. & Salahdeen, H.M. (2005). Neurosedative and muscle relaxant activities of aqueous extract of Bryophyllum pinnatum. *Fitoterapia*, vol. 76, pp.187-193.

Zétola, M.; De Lima, T.C.; Sonaglio, D.; González-Ortega, G.; Limberger, R.P.; Petrovick, R. & Bassani, V.L. (2002) CNS activities of liquid and spray-dried extracts from Lippia alba-Verbenaceae (Brazilian false melissa). *J Ethnopharmacol*, vol. 82, pp.207-215.

Zheng, Y.Y.; Yang, J.; Chen, D.H. & Sun, L. (2007). Effects of the stilbene extracts from Cajanus cajan L. on ovariectomy-induced bone loss in rats. *Yao Xue Xue Bao*, vol. 42, pp.562-565.

Unconventional Raw Natural Sustainable Sources for Obtaining Pharmacological Principles Potentially Active on CNS Through Catalytic, Ecologically Clean, Processes

Yanier Nuñez Figueredo[1], Juan E. Tacoronte Morales[2], Alicia Lagarto Parra[1], Olinka Tiomno Tiomnova[2], Jorge Tobella Sabater[3] and Jorge Leyva Simeon[2]
[1]*Center for Research and Development of Pharmaceuticals, CIDEM, Cerro, Ciudad Habana,*
[2]*Center for Engineering and Chemical Researches, CIIQ, Cerro, Ciudad Habana*
[3]*Pharmaceutical Laboratories MEDSOL, La Lisa, Ciudad Habana, Cuba*

1. Introduction

Natural products have been the most successful source of drugs ever (Tulp & Bohlin, 2005). Historically, the most important natural sources have been plants. Research progressed along two mayor lines: ethnopharmacology and toxicology. These strategies have produced many valuable drugs and are likely to continue to produce hit-lead compounds. However, actually exist numerous unconventional natural sources, ecologically sustainable, of potentially medicinal compounds without research.

The development of pharmaceutical and fine chemistry in Cuba and the synthetic or natural product-oriented generation of new pharmacological and molecular entities, in the II decade of XXI century, it´s sustained in several basic conceptual and methodological principles:

- Structure (including isosteric perception) of compounds generates and define properties, which in their order, determinate application and functionality in the related chemical-pharmacological space (SPAF)
- Sustainability - Scalability (scaling-up facilities) –Applicability in real time (SSA-r_t)
- Maximum of atomic efficiency (*click* and *green* chemistry); maximum of analytical efficiency and maximum of environmental efficiency (MAE^3)
- Chemical bioprospecting of the Cuban biodiversity oriented to discovery of new *ecological* molecular fragments-templates with interesting pharmacological properties for their application in therapeutical treatments of several pathologies of CNS including neuroprotection, neuroregeneration after stroke and ischemia.

- Integration of *in silico* screen to natural products or their mixtures with minimal complexity

Taking this into account, in Cuba (2008-2011) it has been attempted, starting from natural products of the forest industry and raw renewable materials ecologically sustainable, such as rosin, colophony and resinic acids isolated from endemic botanic species belonging to gen. *Pinus* (Pinaceae) the development and application of new heterogeneous catalytic procedures, optimization of design and synthesis of new pharmacological agents structurally based on sodium resinate and dehydroabietic acid (DHAA), with a great added value, as therapeutics for medical treatment of pathologies of CNS, including GABA agonist-antagonists, cannabinoid analogues and sedative molecular systems.

Cuban resin acids, an ecological sustainable natural product, derived form Cuban forestry industry, have been shown to have broad and highly active biological properties, potent microbiocidal and fungicidal actions and potential neuroprotective effects on central nervous system (CNS). In this communication, we studied this novel ecologically sustainable source of potentially therapeutic compounds using, as starting raw material, resins from endemic Cuban *Pinus* specie and show their effect on central nervous system in rodents.

2. Materials and methods

2.1 Chemicals and drugs

2.1.1 Oleoresin, colophony and starting resin acids

The Cuban oleoresin, was milked and collected by incision of the bark from mature trees (*Pinus caribbaea* 7-13 years) planted in Viñales Forestry Station, 168 Km West of Havana, serpentine soil) located in the Western zone of the Cuban archipelago. It was submitted to distillation as reported previously (Franich & Gadgil, 1983). The main components, a mixture of colophony (resin acids), turpentine oils and neutral fraction were separated. The acid fraction was submitted to identification of abietane acids (mixture of abietic, dehydroabietic, levopimaric & pimaric acid) and directly used in pharmacological tests.

For the preparation of extracts, approximately 500 mg of colophony were grinding in an agate mortar into 2-mm pieces, extracted with 4 ml methanol, filtered through glass wool, and the extracts stored at −10°C. Extracts were filtered through 0.45-μm Teflon syringe filters prior to HPLC and used in the next steep for obtaining the sodium salt.

The sodium salt (sodium resinate-SR) was prepared as reported in: CU/2006-0144 patent. Crystallized from a mixture of water: ethanol (8: 2 v/v)

2.2 Chromatography conditions

Analytical HPLC-PDA (Kanuer Smart Line-2005): Column: LichroCART 250 x 0.44 cm RP-18, 5μm particle size (Lichropher 100); mobile phase: acetonitrile-water in gradient conditions (40% to 100%) during 45 min, held at 100% for further 2 min; temperature: 25 ^{0}C; flow rate: 1mL/min; sample injection 10 μL; detection: 200 nm to 505 nm. Data were analyzed with ChromGate 3.1 (Germany) for LC 3D software.

2.3 Structural elucidation

The structural elucidation was based on FTIR spectroscopy (spectrophotometer FT-IR Jasco, FT/IR-460 Plus, Japan, in a range of 280-7200 cm^{-1} with a sensibility of 0,1 cm^{-1}) and NMR spectrometry (^1H y ^{13}C) at room temperature, using a spectrometer Brucker AC-250 MHz, at 28 ^0C in DMSO-d_6 ,using as internal reference TMS, given all the signals in ppm (δ).

Diazepam (DZP, Quimefa, Cuba), pentylenetetrazole (PTZ, Sigma, USA, CAS), picrotoxin (PTX, Sigma, USA, CAS), haloperidol (Esteve S.A, España), amphetamine-sulphate (Sigma, USA, CAS), were used in this study. Solvents were analytical grade and were purified by distillation before used. All drugs and their solutions were prepared immediately before use.

2.4 Synthesis of dehydroabietic acid (DHAA)

2.4.1 Catalytic disproportion of colophony using piritic ash as catalyst (0,5 % (m/m) at 230 ^0C)

500 grams of previously hydrothermally treated colophony is heated during 30 min (130 ^0C) in a glass pyrex reactor (750 mL) equipped with thermometer and stirrer. 1,0 gram of pyritic ash is added and the reaction temperature increased to 230 ^0C. The reaction mixture is maintained at this temperature during 3 h under intense stirring (1500 rpm). (The residual concentration of abietic acid is 0,5–0,8 %). 100 grams of disproportionated colophony in 100 mL of alcohol is filtered through SiO_2-Al_2O_3. The solution is heated to 70 ^0C and then added 18 grams of 2-aminoethanol, and 250 mL of hot water (60-90^0C). The resulting solution is kept at 70 ^0C during 10 min., under gentle stirring, then the reaction mixture is extracted with iso-octane, toluene or a mixture of heptane/ciclohexanone 7/3 v/v (3v x 75 mL). The selective crystallization of the quaternary ammonium salt dehydroabietic acid-2-aminoethanol starts at 50 ^0C. The solution is cooled to 4 ^0C, collecting crystals which are soluble in cool 50 % ethanol (250 mL) Yield: 51,0 grams with 89,5 % of purity related to dehydroabietic acid (98,5 % overall purity). The obtained salt is dissolved 160 mL of hot ethanol and acidified with aqueous HCl (12 %, pH 4-5) and allowed to stand during 8h at room temperature. The pure dehydroabietic acid is collected, washed, re-crystallized from a mixture of 75 % ethanol/water v/v. and dried 3 h. Yield 39,3 % (overall 98,2 %)

2.5 Animals

2.5.1 Pharmacological studies

Male albino mice (Swiss, 18–22 g) in anticonvulsant activity, elevated plus-maze, amphetamine and thiopental-induced sleep, open field activity and aggressive behaviour test and male rats (Wistar, 150–200 g) in amphetamine-induced behavioural stereotypy test were used.

2.5.1.1 Acute toxicity study

Six female rats (Wistar, 150–200 g) were used for evaluating the acute toxicity of test compounds.

All animals (Laboratory of Biological Control. CIDEM, Havana, Cuba) were housed in groups of five under standard laboratory conditions of temperature, humidity and lighting (12:12-h light/dark). Animals had free access to food and water, except during experiment.

They were deprived of food but not water 6 h before the drug administration and each group consisted of ten animals. All experiments were carried out between 8:00 am and 11:00 am in accordance with the Institutional Animal Ethical Committee approved the study and animal care was in conformity with Canadian Council for Animal Care guidelines

SR was administrated in three doses levels (100, 200 y 400 mg/Kg) in all experiment except the elevated plus-maze behaviour test (50, 100 y 150 mg/Kg). The volume of injection in mouse was 0.4 ml/20 g and in rat was 1 ml/100 g. The SR was dissolved in distilled water and administered orally.

2.5.2 Pharmacological and toxicity evaluation

2.5.2.1 Open field activity

Thirty minutes after the administration of vehicle or test compound a mouse was placed in the centre of a round open field of 30 cm diameter and 25 cm high and the open field activity were measured during 6 minutes recording how many times the animal stay in the centre of cage and the number of rising (Sukma et al., 2002; Tyler, 1982).

2.5.2.2 Aggressive behavior

A group of animal was isolated in individually cage and other group remained grouped during six week. The aggressive behaviors were evaluated through an intruder mouse into the isolated mice's home cage and were recorder the aggressive activity (biting attacks and wrestling) in isolated mice was measure as total fighting time during a 20 min period (Tyler, 1982).

2.5.2.3 Thiopental-induced sleep

Animals were divided into three groups: control (distilled water), diazepam (1 mg/kg)-treated and SR-treated groups. Thiopental sodium (30 mg/kg) was injected intraperitoneally 30 min after administration of vehicle or test compound. An animal was placed on its back on a warmed (35 °C) pad. The number of sleeping animals and the duration of loss of righting reflex were recorded. The duration from loss of righting reflex until a mouse regained its righting reflex was measured (Carlini et al., 1986).

2.5.2.4 Drug-induced convulsion

Mice were divided in groups of ten each. The animals were pre-treated with SR 30 min before the administration of PTZ (85 mg/kg, s.c.) or PTX (10 mg/kg, s.c.). The anticonvulsive effect was assessed by measuring the numbers of convulsing mice and deaths, and the latency of the appearance of the first episode of clonic seizure. The cut off time was set as 30 min. after the convulsant administration (Costa & Greengard, 1975; Fischer & Vander, 1998).

2.5.2.5 Elevated plus-maze behavior

The elevated plus-maze consisted of two closed arms (30_/5_/15 cm) and two open arms (30_/5 cm) emanating from a common central platform (5_/5 cm). The two pairs of identical arms were opposite each other. The entire apparatus was elevated to a height of 54 cm above floor level. Thirty minutes after test compound administration, the mouse was placed at the centre of the maze with its head facing an open arm and allowed to explore the maze for 5 min. Entry into an arm was defined as placement of all four paws into an arm and were recorded: number of entries into each type of arm, the percentage of time spent and the percentage of arm entries in open arms (Sukma et al., 2002).

2.5.2.6 Amphetamine-induced behavioral stereotypy

Amphetamine (1.5 mg/Kg) was injected subcutaneously 30 min after administration of vehicle or test compound in rats and the animals were collocated in individually cage to recorder the behavioral stereotypy each 5 min during 1 h. (Kuczenski et al., 1999).

2.5.2.7 Amphetamine -induced sleep in mice

Mice were divided in four groups of ten each. The animals were pre-treated with SR 30 min before the administration of amphetamine 5 mg/Kg (p sc). An animal was placed on its back on a warmed (35 °C) pad and the number of sleeping animals and the duration of loss of righting reflex were recorded.

2.5.2.8 Acute oral toxicity study

A single dose of SR (2000 mg/kg) or distilled water was administered orally (10 mL/Kg) in equal number female (n=3) animals; and rats were returned to an *ad libitum* diet immediately after dosing. All animals were monitored continuously for 12 h after dosing for signs of toxicosis and daily for changes additional behavioural or clinical signs. The animal weights were recorded weekly. Rats were euthanized on day 14 by ether inhalation, and selected organs removed and examined macroscopically for toxicant-induced changes (OECD, 2001).

2.5.2.9 Statistics

Drug effects were assessed by single factor analysis of variance followed by the Student-/Newman-/Keuls post-hoc test. The level of significance was set at $p<0.05$.

3. Results and discussion

The Cuban pine oleoresin, was milked and collected by incision of the bark from mature trees *Pinus caribbaea*. After distillation the main components and mixture of colophony (resinic acids), turpentine oils and neutral fraction were separated and hydrothermally treated to minimize the amount of fatty lineal and branched acids. Colophony was analyzed, treated with stecheometrical amount of NaOH, to obtain the desired sodium resinate and submitted directly, after crystallization from a mixture water: ethanol (30:70 v/v), to neuropharmacological evaluations.

The oleoresin collected from *Pinus caribbaea* is hydrothermally treated and purified through redox-acid/base protocols described in (Cuban patents CU 20060144 & CU20060252), generating a practically pure mixture of rosin-colophony as a mixture of resinic acids (RA, FTIR- cm^{-1}: 3426(γO-H), 2931(C_{sp3}-H y C_{sp2}-H), 2869 (ν^{s} CH_2) y 2929 (ν^{as} CH_2), 1694(γC=O), 1385-1366(δ_s-CH_3), 1450(δ_{as}-CH_3), 1150-1180 isopropyl system, zone 950-970 olefinic fragments, 830-770 trisubstituted olefins; NMR,δ,ppm: 6 zones observed: *0.5-0,8* methyl groups, *1.0-1.2* methyl groups, *1.3-2.0* methylenic groups, *5.0-6.0* olefinic zone exo- and endocyclic bonds, *6.8-7.3* aromatic protons, *11.9-12.5* COOH) that was used directly in the evaluation of its neuropharmacological profile. This mixture (50-52 % of abietic acid), without further purification, was used for obtaining dehydroabietic acid (DHAA) by heterogeneous catalytic disproportionation-aromatization treatment of colophony with pyritic ash ($Fe_2O_3/FeS/Ba^{2+}/SiO_2$, 230ºC, stirring, air, 95%) and the selective precipitation of the 2-aminoethanol salt of DHAA (molar ratio 1:1, 50ºC, 89 %) in aqueous ethanol solution. The pure DHAA was obtained after acidification (pH 4-5; 98%, TLC: Silicagel G_{60}-254, eluent: n-hexane/ethyl acetate 7:3 v/v, 2 drops of isopropanol; chromophoric agent vainilline/H_2SO_4, mp. 171.5-172.3ºC and applied column chromatography; NMR,ppm,δ ^{1}H-^{13}C selected signals: 9,78-OH/184,32-COOH; 7,15 C-11H/C-11 124,90; 6,95 C-12H/C-12 124,20; 6,88 C-14H/C-14 127,0).

The most widely protocol used for resin acid analysis and their derivatives is gas chromatography (GC) of the methyl esters (Zinkel & Engler, 1977) with detection by flame ionization (FID) or mass spectrometry (MS). However, this method has disadvantages for us, including instability of the derivatized samples (Latorre et al., 2003), hazards of methylating reagents (potentially explosive and carcinogenic), and tedious work-up of raw biological material required.

Taking this in consideration, in our laboratory, have been developed a simple analytical methodology for resin acid analysis by high-performance liquid chromatography (HPLC) in gradient conditions. We report a simple protocol for the analysis of abietanes derivatives by reversed-phase HPLC with several advantages including: (1) no sample derivatization is required; (2) extraction and chromatographic conditions are mild, (3) all components of the HPLC mobile (acetonitrile and water) phase are volatile and therefore recovery of compounds from fractionated sample is simplified. These benefits are particularly advantageous in biological studies that require rapid analysis of abietane acid mixtures and screenings for neuroprotective bioactivity.

The results are shown in Fig. 1

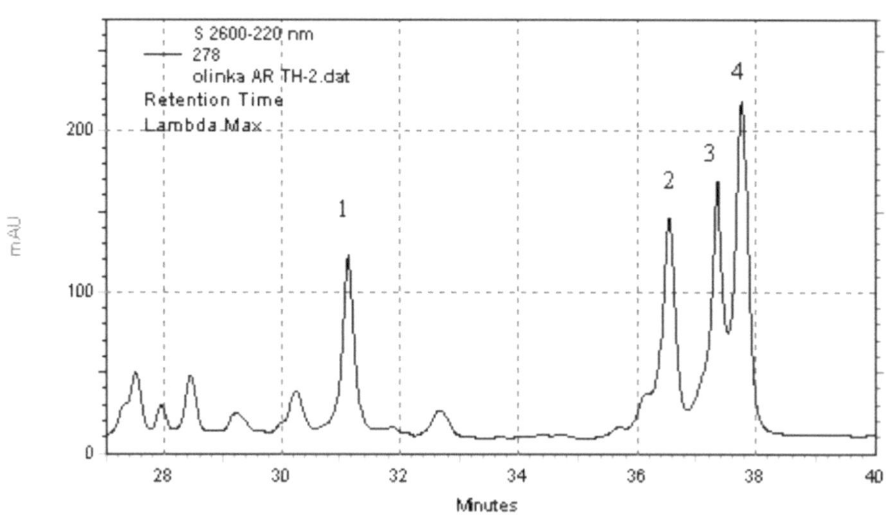

Fig. 1. Abietanes (resin acids present in the Cuban colophony) HPLC analysis of methanol extract obtained from distilled oleoresin. 1= Levopimaric, 2= Palustric, 3= Abietic, 4= Dehydroabietic

The fundamentals (conceptual and methodological) for the analytical technique described here rely on both the optimal combination of wavelengths for detection and the chromatographic resolution of the peaks. Abietanes have distinctive spectra that we used here, together with chromatographic separation, to distinguish and quantify the resin acids by HPLC. The spectra (220-540 nm) of the individual chromatographically separated components (Fig.1), show λ_{max} values of 255 nm (levopimaric), 251 nm (palustric), 266 nm (abietic), and 269, 278 nm (dehydroabietic). The information related is shown in Fig. 2.

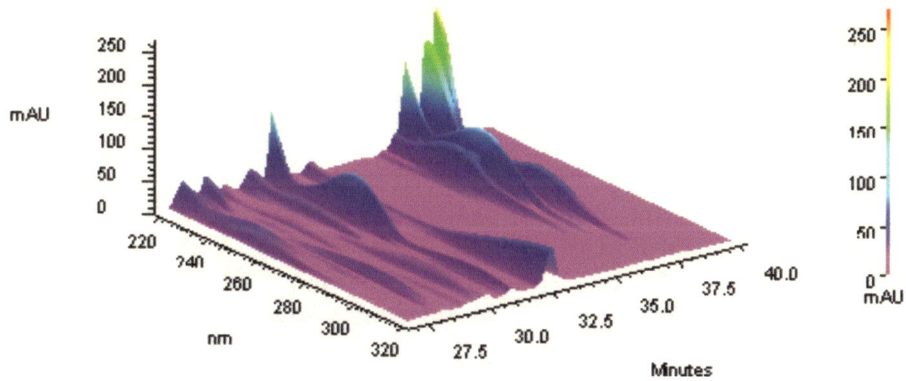

Fig. 2. Spectral chromatogram of analyzed mixture of resin acids present in Cuban colophony

The developed HPLC analysis revealed the main components of the Cuban colophony, a starting raw material for preparing sodium resinate (Fig. 3).

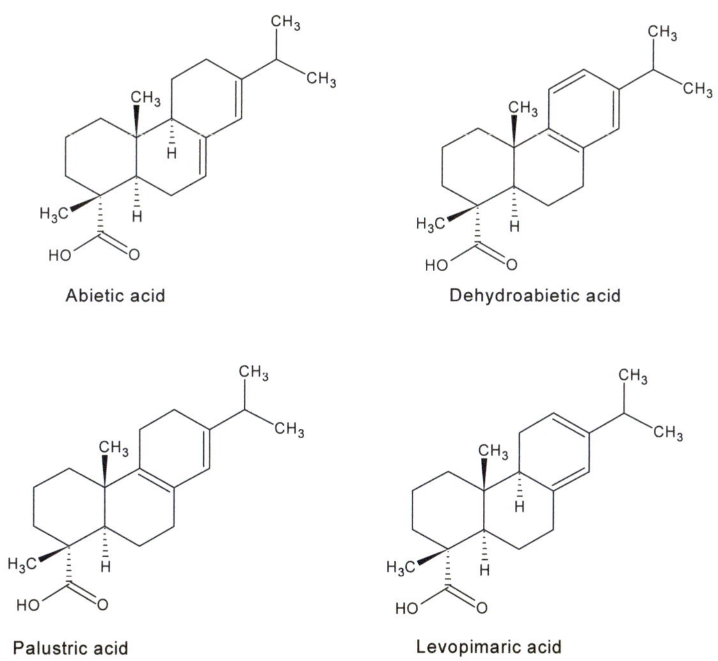

Fig. 3. Main resin acids present in the Cuban colophony. (abietic acid 40 %; dehydroabietic acid 22 %; palustric acid 18 %; levopimaric acid 18-20 %).

The colophony was administered in 3 dosis levels (100, 200 y 400 mg/Kg) in all experiments, except in the case of bioassay of labyrinth in cross (50, 100 y 150 mg/Kg). The DHAA dosis levels were 50, 100 and 200 mg/Kg. The injection volume of administration in mice was 0.4 ml/20 g and 1mL/100 g in rats. The colophony (sodium salt-SR) was dissolved in distillated water and administered orally.

3.1 Open field activity

SR (100, 200 and 400 mg/kg, po.) reduced locomotor activity and rearing in a dose-dependent manner during the observation period. The observations are given in Table 1. Doses of 400 mg/Kg of SR showed similar behaviour to diazepam (DZP) 1 mg/Kg (standard anxiolytic drugs).

The present study demonstrated that SR prepared from natural and pre-treated (hydro-thermally and by acid-basic reaction) resin extracted from Cuban *Pinus* reduced spontaneous locomotor activity in mice. Usually the rodents show an exploratory behaviour when they are collocated in a novel place. However, if the animals are pre-treated with depressant central nervous system drugs, the locomotor activity is decreased. This result is typical for sedative drugs.

Tested groups	mean±S.E.M
Distilled water	24,5 ± 4,20a
SR 100 mg/Kg.	20,2 ± 3,38 b
SR 200 mg/Kg.	19,6 ± 2,22 b
SR 400 mg/Kg.	12,9 ± 4,48 c
DZP 1 mg/Kg.	10,5 ± 3,39 c

Table 1. Effects of SR (100, 200 and 400 mg/kg, po.) on spontaneous locomotor activity. Groups with unequal letters differ to each other for $p < 0.05$.

3.2 Aggressive behavior

Social isolation induces aggressive behavior in several strains of mice. The isolation-induced aggression is proposed to be useful as an animal model for assessing inhibitory activity on central nervous system. Different neurotransmitters such as serotonin, noradrenaline, dopamine and gamma-aminobutyric acid (GABA) are considered to be involved in mediating aggressive behaviour; there are conflicting results on brain neurotransmitter metabolism (Matsuda et al., 2001; Sakaue et al., 2001). Table 2. shows the effects of SR on aggressive behaviour in isolated mice. Test compound reduces an aggressive behaviour in a dose-dependent manner. A similar result to open field test in between 400 mg/Kg of SR and diazepam 1 mg/Kg doses was obtained. This behaviour was reported by Valzelli in 1973 as a classic pattern for central nervous system depressor (Valzelli, 1973). Our results show an anti-aggressive behaviour in orally SR-treated mice. This result can be mediated by inhibitory effects on brain biogenic amines action or excitatory neurotransmitter release and suggests the inhibitory effect of SR on the central nervous system.

Tested groups	mean±S.E.M
Distilled water	24.90 ± 4.15 a
SR 100 mg/Kg.	17.60 ± 3.38 b
SR 200 mg/Kg.	16.75 ± 2.94 b
SR 400 mg/Kg.	12.90 ± 4.48 c
DZP 1 mg/Kg.	10.50 ± 3.39 c

Table 2. Effects of SR (100, 200 and 400 mg/kg, po.) on aggressive behaviour (biting attacks and wrestling) in isolated mice Groups with unequal letters differ to each other for $p<0.05$.

3.3 Thiopental-induced sleep

SR as well as diazepam, a standard reference drug, increased the number of sleeping animals and prolonged the thiopental-induced sleeping time in mice.

All SR doses increase the number of sleeping animals (Table 3) compared with the control, doses of 200 and 400 mg/Kg caused sleep in all animals.

SR (400 mg/Kg) and diazepam (1 mg/Kg) prolonged thiopental induced sleep in the similar manner (Table 4).

Tested groups	Percentage of sleeping animal
Distilled water	12.50
SR 100 mg/Kg.	56.25
SR 200 mg/Kg.	100
SR 400 mg/Kg.	100
DZP 1 mg/Kg.	100

Table 3. Effect of SR on percentage of sleeping animal.

Tested groups	mean±S.E.M
Distilled water	2,25 ± 6.16 a
SR 100 mg/Kg.	8,25 ± 8.65 b
SR 200 mg/Kg.	33,75 ± 8.83 c
SR 400 mg/Kg.	40,00 ± 0 d
DZP 1 mg/Kg.	40,00 ± 0 d

Table 4. Effect of SR on sleeping time (min). Groups with unequal letters differ to each other for $p<0.05$.

3.4 Drug-induced convulsion

Numerous excitatory drugs such as PTZ and PTX, can induce convulsion *via* GABA receptor antagonism, due to, the anxiolytic-like drugs (ex. diazepam) might be inhibit the drug-induced convulsion via inhibition of GABA-ergic inter-neurons.

To further investigate the inhibitory effect of SR on the central nervous system, drugs that can excite or block excitation in the central nervous system were used. Diazepam (4 mg/kg, po.) was highly effective in delaying the occurrence of clonic convulsion (Table 5 and 6) even in protecting animals against convulsion induced by PTX and PTZ. However the different doses of SR tested were unable to protect animals against convulsion and death, and unable to increase the latency of the clonic convulsion induced by pro-convulsivant drugs. Our findings show an ineffective action of SR to avoid the PTZ and PTX-induced convulsion. These results suggest that the sedative effects of test compound might not be mediated via GABA or glycine systems.

Tested groups	Latency of first convulsion	Latency of first clonic convulsion	Time of death	Percentage of animals with clonic convulsion	Percentage of death
PTX 5 mg/Kg + Distilled water	12.0 ± 1.94a	20.66 ± 4.55a	22.66 ± 5.03a	80	30
PTX 5 mg/Kg + SR 100 mg/Kg.	12.0 ± 6.00a	17.0 ± 4.36a	23.0 ± 8.48a	70	20
PTX 5 mg/Kg + SR 200 mg/Kg.	15.90 ± 8.60a	20.2 ± 4.76a	26.0 ± 1.41a	80	20
PTX 5 mg/Kg + SR 400 mg/Kg.	16.8 ± 6.37a	21.62 ± 5.70a	24.0 ± 2.91a	80	20
PTX 5 mg/Kg + DZP 4 mg/Kg	23.0 ± 3.21b	26.0 ± 3.80b	28.1 ± 2.12b	20	0

Table 5. Effect of SR on clonic convulsion induced by PTX. Groups with unequal letters differ to each other for $p<0.05$.

Tested groups	Latency of first convulsion	Latency of first clonic convulsion	Time of death	Percentage of animals with clonic convulsion	Percentage of death
PTZ 85 mg/Kg + Distilled water	7.30 ± 1.66 a	11.66 ± 3.07 a	14.80 ± 3.83 a	60	50
PTZ 85 mg/Kg + SR 100 mg/Kg	6.00 ± 2.45 a	11.50 ± 1.52 a	13.17 ± 3.97 a	60	60
PTZ 85 mg/Kg + SR 200 mg/Kg	7.27 ± 1.35 a	13.16 ± 2.23 a	13.0 ± 3.16 a	60	40
PTZ 85 mg/Kg + SR 400 mg/Kg	7.90 ± 2.28 a	11.50 ± 3.45 a	13.33 ± 1.86 a	60	40
PTZ 85 mg/Kg + DZP4 mg/Kg	25.0 ± 2.18 b	27.1 ± 3.26 b	29.0 ± 1.18 b	20	0

Table 6. Effect of SR on clonic convulsion induced by PTZ. Groups with unequal letters differ to each other for $p<0.05$.

3.5 Elevated plus-maze behavior

Rodents usually avoid open arms and prefer enclosed arms in an elevated plus-maze. Time spent in open arms and numbers of entries into open arms are indexes of neophobic anxiety in animals. Standard anxiolytic drugs such as diazepam increase open-arm exploration, as reflected by increases in the time spent and the number of entries into the open arms (Pellow, 1985).

Diazepam exhibited the conventional profile of anxiolytics in the elevated plus-maze test; it increased the percentage of open arm entries and time spent in open arms (Table 7). However, SR did not significantly modify the percentage of either time spent or arm entries in open arms at any of the doses tested.

Tested groups	Time spent in open arms	Time spent in close arms	Open arm entries (%)	Open close entries (%)	Number of open arm entries (counts)	Number of closed arm entries (counts)
Distilled water	8.2 ± 8.02 a	198.9 ± 44.70 a	14.81 ± 12.45 a	85.18 ± 12.45 a	1.80± 1.62 a	8.9± 2.33 a
SR 50 mg/Kg	9.12 ± 7.07 a	112.56 ± 30.25 a	16.23 ± 14.36 a	87.26 ± 10.25 a	1.93± 0.98 a	8.03± 2.15 a
SR 100 mg/Kg	9,6 ± 14,35 a	85.4 ± 42,77 a	18,68 ± 23,70 a	81,31 ± 23,70 a	1.50± 2.01 a	7.6± 3.60 a
SR 150 mg/Kg	10.08 ± 8.23 a	93.15 ± 29.15 a	17.59 ± 9.23 a	83.26 ± 15.15 a	1.75± 1.29 a	7.98± 2.23 a
DZP 0.5 mg/Kg	55.23 ± 5.56 b	70.18 ± 7.83 b	65,17 ± 12.18 b	34,83 ± 6.65 b	19.05± 2.15 b	10.18± 1.98 a

Table 7. Effect of SR on the elevated plus-maze test in mice (see Table 6). Groups with unequal letters differ to each other for $p<0.05$.

3.6 Amphetamine-induced behavioral stereotypy

Psycho stimulants (such as, amphetamine a simpatic-mimetic amine) administration in rats increase dopamine levels in different brain zones, induce stereotyped behaviours, characterized by repetitive sniffing, biting, grooming, and head movements. The dopamine receptor antagonist or sedative drugs can be reducing its behaviour (Ralph et al. 2001). Table 8 shows behavioral stereotypy after subcutaneously administration of amphetamine, 1.5 mg/Kg (p.sc). Rats treated with SR reduced its behaviour in a dose-dependent manner compared with the water-treated group and amphetamine. The observed results reveal that colophony decreases the stimulant effect either for an antagonism of dopaminergic transmission, inhibition of dopamine releasing, blocking of its post-synaptic receptor or by an activation of some inhibitory transmission with the decrease of excitation caused by the dosis of employed amphetamine. The data suggest that the colophony has not a characteristic profile of active antidepressants. It was confirmed by the evaluation of amphetamine (5 mg/Kg)-induced sleeping and its extension in time.

Tested groups	mean±S.E.M
Distilled water	10.45 ± 3.70a
SR 100 mg/Kg. + amphetamine 1,5 mg/Kg.	22,71 ± 4.90b
SR 200 mg/Kg. + amphetamine 1,5 mg/Kg.	23,92 ± 5,75b
SR 400 mg/Kg. + amphetamine 1,5 mg/Kg.	20,70 ± 5,85b
Distilled water + amphetamine 1,5 mg/Kg.	31,64 ± 5,98c
Haloperidol 5 mg/Kg. + amphetamine 1,5 mg/Kg.	12,28 ± 2,56a

Table 8. Effect of SR on behavioural stereotypy induced by amphetamine. Groups with unequal letters differ to each other for $p<0.05$.

3.7 Amphetamine -induced sleep in mice

Mice treated with different doses of SR exhibited similar behaviour against amphetamine -induced sleep in mice compare with water-treated group (Table 9).

Tested groups	Media ± D.S
Distilled water + amphetamine 5 mg/Kg	189.90 ± 9.65
SR 100 mg/Kg. + amphetamine 5 mg/Kg	190.00 ± 11.51
SR 200 mg/Kg. + amphetamine 5 mg/Kg	195.86 ± 5.05
SR 400 mg/Kg. + amphetamine 5 mg/Kg	190.22 ± 7.07

Table 9. Effect of SR on sleep induced by amphetamine in mice.

Although SR showed a sedative effect in evaluated tests (thiopental-induced sleep, open field activity, aggressive behaviours and amphetamine-induced behavioral stereotypy). The interaction of SR with convulsant drugs, confirms that the sedative effect of test compound might not be related via the GABA or glycine systems.

In this context, recently our group found that abietic and dehydroabietic acids might be responsible of the sedative effects of the SR (Unpublished result).

3.8 Acute oral toxicity study

The death of any animal was not observed during the study. The major adverse effects were related with CNS depression (motor impairment and sedation), but these symptoms disappeared within 4 h. With this exception, no outward behavioral abnormalities were noted during the 2-week post-treatment period. The body weight gains were observed in the similar manner in both groups (Figure 4). Macroscopic alterations were not observed in selected organs and tissues removed (stomach, liver, kidney, brain, spleen and lungs). The administration of SR didn't cause significant toxic symptoms for what classifies in 5 category of the GHS or not classified (mortality> 2000 mg/kg).

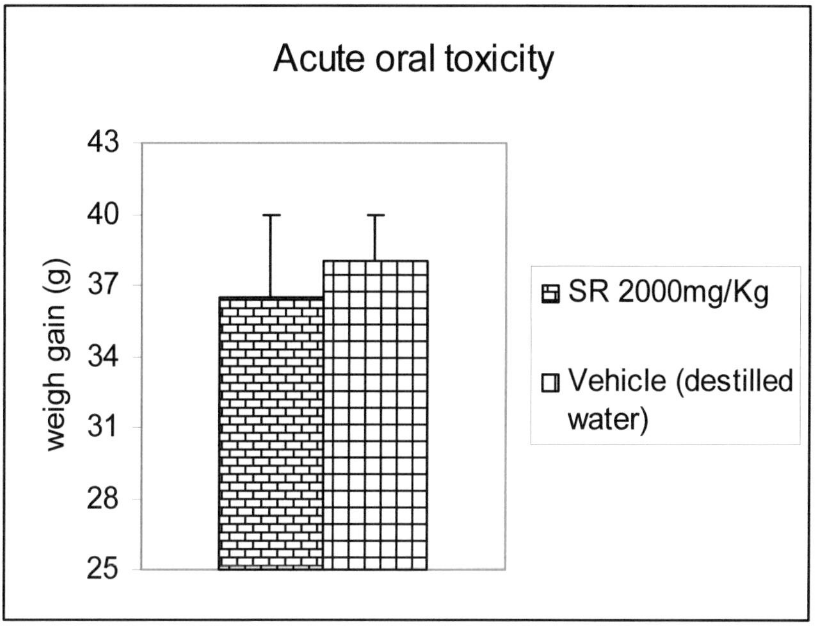

Fig. 4. Effect of SR 2000 mg/Kg on acute oral toxicity test.

Taking into consideration the structural similarity, *grosso modo,*(molecular modeling are underway and are unpublished results yet) between secondary metabolites, DHAA, related derivatives and cannabinoids, the observed pharmacological effects could be attribute to a potential antagonism with glutamate receptors and/or inhibition of noradrenalin-dopamine releasing. The acute toxicity study revealed that no toxic effects were observed, and any symptom (increase of cleaning-up behavior, exploration, decreasing of frequency of movement, etc) disappeared after 4 hrs. In the autopsy were not detected any macroscopic or anatomic effect on organs.

In the case of dehydroabietic acid (DHAA) generated by disproportionation-aromatization of resinic acids the results reveal a dosis depending effect on decreasing of exploratory activity, typical for sedative pharmaceutical compositions. It co-administration (50 mg/Kg) with thiopental, at experimental dosis, increase the number of sleeping animals (65%), a typical depressing action on CNS. The administration of DHAA, at all dosis evaluated, didn't protect animals for PTZ induced convulsions. The experimental data obtained in the Labyrinth in cross model didn't show any relevant results. In the Amphetamine-induced stereotipia model DHAA decreases the stimulant action produced by the subcutaneously administration of 1,5 mg / Kg of amphetamine, in the hypothetically pathways described above. The acute toxicity (DL_{50} > 5000 mg/Kg) study showed that DHAA had not any toxic effects at dosis concentrations used and could be classified in the GSH in the 5 category.

It is noteworthy that synthetic DHAA has a sedative action on CNS and could be employed as starting raw material for designing of new molecular and pharmacological entities potentially useful in the development of formulation for therapy of CNS pathologies where de sedative effect is needed.

Topological studies for determining any QSAR correlation between colophony and derivatives and cannabinoids are underway.

4. Conclusion

The oleoresin, a raw material isolated from Cuban Pinacea (gen. *Pinus, Pinus caribbaea*), constitutes a sustainable resource for developing potentially useful pro-drugs and pharmacologically active substances as resínic acids, sodium resinate (SR) and dehydroabietic acid. The analytical protocol developed (*all in one* wavelengths-retention time) for common abietanes present in Cuban colophony is simple, time-saving, eco-friendly, employing robust reversed-phase HPLC and offer the possibility to determine and quantify the main diterpenic acids (resínico acids) in the natural and modified mixture. The catalytic synthesis of dehydroabietic acid (DHAA) as a principal active pharmaceutical component from colophony for the potential treatment of neuro-psiquiatric dysfunctions and generation of exogenic cannabinoid analogues has been developed under ecological conditions using piritic ash as re-usable catalyst (disproportionation-aromatization) at meso-scale with minimal environmental impact. The neuropharmacological profile (including acute oral toxicity) of SR in rodent behavioural tests was determined; SR reduced spontaneous locomotor activity and aggressive behaviour, increased the number of sleeping animals and prolonged the thiopental-induced sleeping time indicating a the sedative effect of test compound and it might not be related via the GABA or glycine systems. The SR is unable to protect animals against convulsion and death induced by pentylenetetrazole and picrotoxin. The SR (2000 mg/Kg p.o) didn't cause significant toxic symptoms in rats. This finding indicates that the SR can constitute a non conventional source of pharmacological molecular entities with central nervous system depressant activity. The synthetic DHAA has a sedative action on CNS and its acute toxicity (DL_{50} > 5000 mg/Kg) reveals that DHAA had not any toxic effects at dosis concentrations used and could be employed as starting design structural point for developing molecular entities and series leads with potentially remarkable pharmacological properties.

5. References

Carlini, E.A., Contar, J.D.P., Silva, A.R., Silveira- Filho, N.G., Frochtengarten, M.L., Bueno, O.F.A. (1986). Pharmacology of lemongrass (Cymbopogon citratus Stapf). I. Effects of teas prepared from the leaves on laboratory animals. *J. Ethnopharmacol.* 17, 37-64.

Costa, E., Greengard, P. (1975). Mechanism of action of benzodiazepines. New York: *Adv Biochem Psychopharmacol,* Raven Press, pp. 14.

CU Patent 20060144, (2006). Tacoronte J.E et al. Disproportionation of Cuban colophony with piritic ash and obtention of dehydroabietic acid.

CU Patent 20060252, (2006). Tacoronte J.E et al. Natural cannabinoid precursors with pharmacological action on CNS.

Franich R A, Gadgil, P. D. (1983). Fungistatic effects of *Pinus radiata* needle epicuticular fatty and resin acids on *Dothistroma pini. Physiol. Plant Pathol.* 23:183-195.

Fischer, W., Vander, H. (1998). Effect of clobenpropit, a centrally acting histamine H3-receptors antagonist, on electroshock and pentilenetetrazol-induced seizures in mice. *J-Neural-transm.* 105(6-7), 587-99.

Kuczenski, R., Segal, D.S. (1999). Sensitization of amphetamine-induced stereotyped behaviors during the acute response. *J-Pharmacol-Exp-Ther.* 288(2), 699-709.

Latorre A, Rigol A, Lacorte S, Barcelo D. (2003). Comparison of gas chromatography-mass spectrometry and liquid chromatography-mass spectrometry for the determination of fatty and resin acids in paper mill process waters. *J. Chromatogr.* A 991:205-215.

Matsuda, T., Sakaue, M., Ago, Y., Sakamoto, Y., Koyama, Y., Baba, A. (2001). Functional Alteration of Brain Dopaminergic System in Isolated Aggressive Mice, *Jpn. J. Neuropsychopharmacol.* 21, 71-76.

OECD Guideline For Testing Of Chemical "Acute Oral Toxicity - Acute Toxic Class Method" N° 423 Adopted 20 December 2001.

Pellow, S. (1985). Validation of open: closed arm entries in an elevated plus-maze as a measure of anxiety in the rat. *Journal of Neuroscience* Method 14, 149-167.

Ralph, R.J., Paulus, M.P., Fumagalli, F., Caron, M.G., Geyer, M.A. (2001). Prepulse Inhibition Deficits and Perseverative Motor Patterns in Dopamine Transporter Knock-Out Mice: Differential Effects of D1 and D2 Receptor Antagonists. *Journal of Neuroscience.* 21(1), 305-313.

Sakaue, M., Ago, Y., Murakami, C., Sowa, C., Sakamoto, Y., Koyama, Y., Baba, A., Matsuda, T. (2001). Involvement of benzodiazepine binding sites in an antiaggressive effect by 5-HT1A receptor activation in isolated mice. *European Journal of Pharmacology.* 432, 163-166.

Sukma, M., Chaichantipyuth, C.H., Murakami, Y., Tohda, M., Matsumoto, K., Watanabe, H. (2002). CNS inhibitory effects of barakol, a constituent of Cassia siamia Lamk. *J. Ethnopharmacology.* 83, 87:94.

Tulp M, Bohlin L. (2005) Rediscovery of known natural compounds: Nuisance or goldmine? *Bioorganic & Medicinal Chemistry.* 13 5274–5282

Tyler, C. B.; K. A. (1982) Miczed: effects of phencyclidine on aggressive behavior in mice. *Pharmacol Biochem Behav* 17: 503-10.

Valzelli, L. (1973) The isolation syndrome in mice. *Psychopharmacology 31:305-20.*

24

Elucidating the Role of Biliverdin Reductase in the Expression of Heme Oxygenase-1 as a Cytoprotective Response to Stress

James R. Reed
Department of Pharmacology,
Louisiana State University Health Sciences Center, New Orleans, LA, USA

1. Introduction

Hemin is a cofactor in which an atom of iron is coordinated to the nitrogens of four pyrrole groups that make up the protoporphyrin IX ring (see figure below).

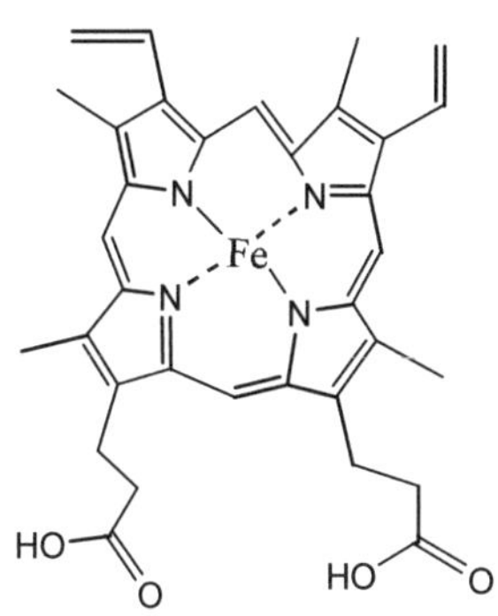

Hemin

Many types of enzymes in living systems use hemin as a prosthetic group to catalyze oxidation/reduction reactions or for the binding/transport of reactive molecules (e.g. oxygen). For instance, several cytochromes of the mitochondrial electron transport chain are "heme" enzymes as are the major drug/xenobiotic-metabolizing enzymes of the endoplasmic reticulum, the cytochromes P450 (CYP or P450). The heme group of the P450s allows these enzymes to use redox chemistry to bind molecular oxygen and cleave the O-O bond, thus forming a reactive, high-valent oxygen species that can insert oxygen into otherwise stable carbon-hydrogen bonds of drugs/xenobiotics (White and Coon, 1980). The unfavorable thermodynamics of this type of reaction has caused the P450s to be likened to "catalytic blowtorches" (Schlichting et al., 2000), and the process is essential for the elimination and clearance of many lipophilic compounds ingested from the environment. Catalase is an important protective heme enzyme that is responsible for degrading hydrogen peroxide. Furthermore, the heme enzymes, nitric oxide synthase and cyclooxygenase, have important signaling roles in the regulation of various cellular processes such as inflammation. However, in terms of the sheer abundance in higher living systems, hemoglobin is the most important heme enzyme as it uses the cofactor to transport oxygen in blood circulation to facilitate oxidative/phosphorylation and energy generation in distal tissues. Because the heme proteins interact with reactive oxygen species (ROS), they are susceptible to ROS-mediated damage, which in turn, results in the accumulation of free or unused heme.

1.1 The toxicity of heme

The reactive nature of hemin does not come without a cost. The free (not enzyme bound) form of the cofactor has been shown *in vitro* to increase the peroxidation of lipids and the fragmentation and cross-linking of DNA and protein resulting from oxidative stress (Kumar and Bandyopadhyay, 2005;Vincent, 1989). One likely explanation for these findings can be drawn from two of the basic reactions of reactive oxygen chemistry, the Fenton reaction and the Haber-Weiss reaction. In the Fenton reaction (below), superoxide anion reduces free molecular iron.

$$O_2^- + Fe^{+3} \longrightarrow O_2 + Fe^{+2} \qquad \text{(Fenton Reaction)}$$

In the Haber-Weiss reaction, the reduced iron can interact with hydrogen peroxide, resulting in cleavage of the O-O bond to form hydroxyl anion and hydroxyl radical (Vincent, 1989).

$$Fe^{+2} + H_2O_2 \longrightarrow Fe^{+3} + HO^- + HO \qquad \text{(Haber-Weiss Reaction)}$$

Using the Haber-Weiss system as an analogy, it is likely that the free hemin functions in a manner similar to that of free iron as a means to produce hydroxyl radical. The hydroxyl radical has been shown to be much more destructive to proteins and DNA than both hydrogen peroxide and superoxide (Davies et al., 1987;Jackson et al., 1987).

It also has been proposed that hemin interacts with hydrogen peroxide to form a putative, hypervalent iron-oxygen species analogous to the reactive intermediate of peroxidase enzymes referred to as Compound I (Vincent, 1989).

$$Fe^{+2} + H_2O_2 \longrightarrow Fe^{+3}{:}O\cdot + H_2O \qquad \text{(Peroxidase-like Reaction)}$$

Because hemin is much more lipophilic than free iron, the oxidative stress associated with free hemin is more destructive to membrane lipids and organelles (Balla et al., 1991). In this respect, the putative iron-oxo species resulting from the reaction of hemin and hydrogen peroxide could be even more deleterious than hydroxyl radical as suggested by the fact that free radical scavengers of hydroxyl radical (e.g. dimethyl sulfoxide) did not protect lipids and proteins from damage when incubated with hemin and hydrogen peroxide (Vincent, 1989). Understandably, the propensity of hemin to damage lipid mixtures causes it to be extremely harmful to cellular membranes and organelles. Free hemin also has been shown to promote inflammatory reactions that have been associated with hepatic, renal, neuronal, and vascular injury (Kumar and Bandyopadhyay, 2005). In particular, several studies have demonstrated the contribution of hemin to the pathogenesis associated with atherosclerosis and ischemia/reperfusion (Wagener et al., 2001).

1.2 The regulation of cellular heme levels

Because of the harmful effects of free heme accumulation, the synthesis and catabolism of heme in living systems is highly regulated. The rate-limiting enzyme for heme synthesis is α-aminolevulinic acid synthetase, and its expression and activity is highly regulated by a variety of agents and stress signals (Ponka, 1997). Heme catabolism is carried out by two enzymatic reactions. The rate-limiting step of heme catabolism is catalyzed by heme oxygenase (HO). This enzyme catalyzes a complicated, multi-step reaction that uses molecular oxygen and electrons (received from a separate redox partner, the cytochrome P450 reductase) to cleave the α-meso bridge of the protoporphyrin IX ring and form ferrous iron, CO, and biliverdin in the process (Kikuchi et al., 2005;Liu et al., 1997;Liu and Ortiz de Montellano, 2000) (see figure below).

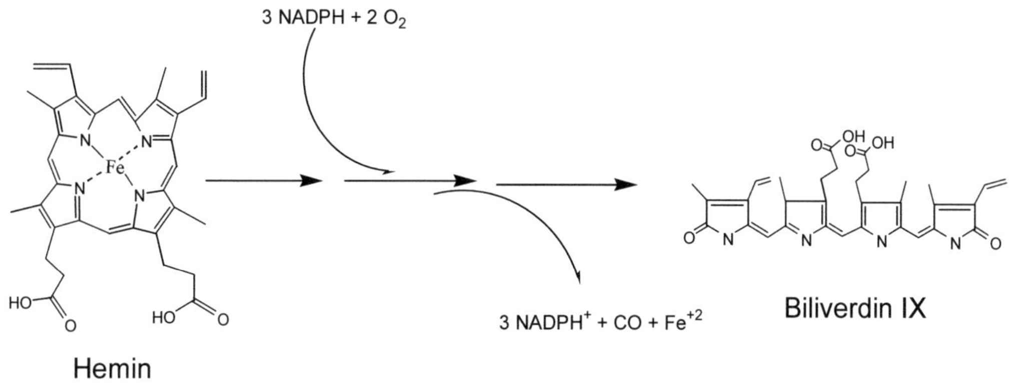

(HO Reaction)

The final step of heme catabolism involves the reduction of the biliverdin formed by HO to bilirubin. This enzymatic step (below) is catalyzed by the biliverdin reductase (BVR). BVR has dual cofactor specificity as both NADH and NADPH can provide electrons to the enzyme. NADPH is the preferred cofactor under basic conditions, whereas NADH is more favorable at lower pH (< 7.0) (Noguchi et al., 1979). The activities of both HO and BVR are highly regulated to effectively coordinate heme catabolism with its synthesis under different conditions.

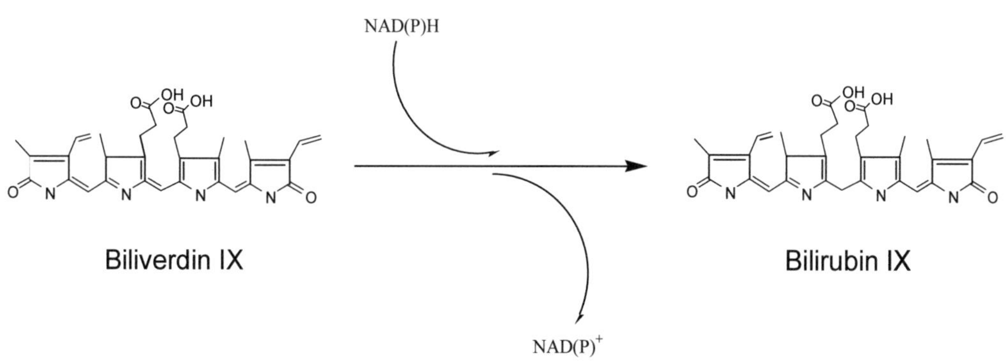

(BVR Reaction)

2. Cellular functions of HO-1 and HO-2

There are two isoforms of HO, known as HO-1 and HO-2 that are expressed through two different genes and are immunologically distinct (Maines et al., 1986;Maines, 1988). The two enzymes are approximately 40% homologous as both have in common a catalytic region of about 24 amino acids (Rotenberg and Maines, 1991) and a hydrophobic, C-terminal tail that serves to anchor the enzymes to the endoplasmic reticulum. HO-1, which is 33 kDa, is highly inducible by a multitude of stimuli and compounds and is constitutively expressed in liver and spleen. HO-2 is constitutively expressed in most tissues, and is highly expressed in brain, kidney, and testes. The HO-2 protein is 36 kDa as it contains additional regulatory sequences (e.g. extra heme-binding sites) which affect its activity in a tissue-specific manner and which might also be regulated by CO and NO binding (Ryter et al., 2006).

2.1 Functions of HO-2

It is generally believed that the main role of HO-2 might be to maintain homeostatic levels of heme during normal cellular metabolism. In one study, HO-2 knockout mice only displayed mild phenotypes and did not show evidence of altered iron maintenance (Poss et al., 1995). The study did show that the mice displayed ejaculation abnormalities (in males) and increased susceptibility to hyperoxic lung damage. Illustrating the importance of HO-2 to brain heme metabolism, these mice also showed dramatically reduced levels of HO activity in the brain. In addition, another study did demonstrate oxygen toxicity and iron accumulation in the lungs of HO-2 knockout mice (Dennery et al., 1998). Thus, HO-1 cannot completely compensate for the absence of HO-2 in terms of cellular function and the regulation of heme levels.

In brain, testes, and cardiovascular tissue, HO-2 activity plays a critical role in function by generating CO which functions as a tissue-specific signaling messenger that acts mainly through activation of guanylyl cyclase. In smooth muscle and endothelial tissue, CO mimics the effects of NO by causing relaxation and vasodilatation, respectively (Hangai-Hoger et al., 2007;Patel et al., 1993). CO also has anti-apoptotic and anti-inflammatory effects mediated through mitogen-activated protein kinases (MAPK) and not guanylyl cyclase (Piantadosi and Zhang, 1996). These signaling relationships will be discussed in more detail below in the chapter. CO also has been postulated to play a role in inhibiting P450 enzymes since the ferrous form of this type of heme protein forms a tight-binding complex with CO.

2.2 Functions of HO-1

Whereas HO-2 seems to be important in managing heme levels during normal cellular metabolism, HO-1 serves to maintain homeostatic levels of heme under conditions of cellular stress. Oxidative stress is associated with increased rates of heme protein damage and in turn, free heme accumulation. Early studies with HO-1 speculated on a cytoprotective role for this enzyme given the following: 1) It was identified as a 32 kDa heat shock protein (Keyse and Tyrrell, 1989) induced by a variety of stressors that included direct oxidative stress; 2) it metabolized a compound (hemin) that was known to be harmful to cells at high concentrations (Kutty and Maines, 1984); and 3) it was induced (greater than 40-fold in some instances (Wright et al., 2006)) in virtually all tissues following exposure to a variety of cellular stressors including oxidative stress, UV radiation, hyperoxia, hypoxia, hyperthermia, heavy metals, metal porphyrins, tumor factors, insulin, endotoxin, and sulfhydryl-reactive compounds (Keyse and Tyrrell, 1989) (reviewed in (Ryter et al., 2006)). Because most of the HO-1-inducing agents also cause elevated levels of oxidative stress, it has been postulated that HO-1 induction represents an early, "sentinel-type" response by the cell to counteract the deleterious effects of oxidative stress (Otterbein et al., 2000;Poss and Tonegawa, 1997b).

3. Experimental evidence for the cytoprotective role of HO-1

3.1 In vitro evidence for the cytoprotective role of HO-1

Most of the in vitro/in vivo evidence for HO-1 playing a cytoprotective role has examined the effects of inducers and inhibitors of HO-1 when cells/animals are dosed with a stressor. These types of studies are described in the paragraphs below. More sophisticated lines of in vivo evidence using gene knockout/therapy to modulate HO-1 levels will be referred to separately. Metal porphyrins and heavy metals are often used alternately in studies to implicate a function of HO in a cellular process. Whereas in most cases, both types of compounds induce the HO-1 gene (a major exception is tin mesoporphyrin which inhibits HO-1 induction) and elevate protein expression, the metal porphyrins will often bind to the HO active site resulting in the inhibition of enzyme activity.

Both in vitro and in vivo studies have demonstrated that the elevated expression and activity of HO-1 is associated with a greater tolerance to various types of stress. It was already mentioned how an in vitro study was used to demonstrate that HO-1 was a 32 kDa heat shock protein which was induced by cellular stress and protected cells from toxicities related to these stressors (Keyse and Tyrrell, 1989). Another interesting in vitro study used HepG2 cells that were transfected to constitutively express CYP2E1 to demonstrate the protective role of HO-1 during CYP2E1-mediated metabolism and oxidative stress (Gong et al., 2004). Of the P450 enzymes, CYP2E1 is especially prone to the breakdown of its monoxygenase catalytic cycle with the concomitant release of superoxide, hydrogen peroxide, and excess water (Gorsky et al., 1984). A previous study by the same lab used these cells to show that the oxidative stress associated with CYP2E1-mediated metabolism could be cytotoxic, especially after prior cellular depletion of glutathione by treatment with L-buthionine-(*S,R*)-sulfoximine (Chen and Cederbaum, 1998). In the study examining the role of HO-1, the cytotoxicity associated with the CYP2E1-mediated metabolism of arachidonic acid was not observed when HO-1 expression was up-regulated by transfection of the cells with an adenovirus containing the cDNA for human HO-1 (Gong et al., 2004). Furthermore, when the cells were treated with chromium mesoporphyrin, which acts as an inhibitor of HO-1, the CYP2E1-related toxicity was potentiated. The in vitro study also implicated CO but not bilirubin in the protective effects of HO-1, probably through the CO-related inhibition of P450 activity (discussed below).

In another in vitro study, the protective effect of the flavonoid, quercetin, on the hepatotoxicity of ethanol was attributed to its induction of HO-1 in hepatocytes because the effects of quercetin were abrogated by treatment with zinc mesoporphyrin (Yao et al., 2009). Addition of free iron increased the damage caused by ethanol, whereas CO treatment protected the cells from ethanol-induced toxicity. Thus, it was thought that the protection afforded by HO-1 induction was in part caused by the inhibition of P450-mediated activation of ethanol by CO. Another study by this group indicated that HO-1 was induced through the MAPK/Nrf2 pathways of signal transduction (Yao et al., 2007). The in vitro studies of course are critical in elucidating the signaling pathways involved in heme metabolism. These pathways are discussed more completely below. Interestingly, the second enzyme responsible for heme metabolism, BVR has a very active role in the signaling required to modulate HO-1 levels with the ever-changing levels of heme in the cell.

3.2 In vivo evidence for the cytoprotective role of HO-1

Many in vivo studies have also tested for the protective role of HO-1 after exposure to toxins. Acetominophen is a widely-used analgesic that unfortunately has a narrow therapeutic index, and overdosing results in liver failure. Cytochrome P450-mediated metabolism is responsible for the harmful effects of acetaminophen as it converts the compound to a reactive quinone-imine that alkylates cellular protein and DNA. Interestingly, cellular glutathione effectively scavenges the reactive intermediate and protects against cytotoxicity. However, when an overdose occurs, the intracellular glutathione gets depleted resulting in the destruction of critical proteins that are necessary for cell function (Gibson et al., 1996). Several studies have tested for the ability of HO-1 to protect against acetaminophen toxicity in rats. In one of these studies, acetaminophen treatment resulted in HO-1 induction. To test whether the HO-1 expression was cytoprotective, the rats were treated with hemin to induce HO-1 prior to exposure to acetaminophen. These rats were indeed protected from acetaminophen hepatotoxicity compared to animals that were not pretreated with hemin. The study also found that biliverdin pretreatment was able to protect the rats from acetaminophen-induced hepatotoxicity (Chiu et al., 2002).

HO-1 induction was also shown to be protective from liver damage caused by carbon tetrachloride (Nakahira et al., 2003) and halothane (Odaka et al., 2000). Both of these compounds can be activated to free radical species by P450-mediated metabolism. Treatment with hepatotoxic doses of these compounds resulted in the rapid accumulation of intracellular free heme which was followed by HO-1 induction. It was found that when the rats were pre-treated with hemin (to induce HO-1) before halothane administration, hepatotoxicity was not observed. Similarly, when rats were treated with tin porphyrin 1 hour before administration of carbon tetrachloride to inhibit HO-1 activity, the carbon tetrachloride-induced liver injury was exacerbated (Nakahira et al., 2003). The findings of these studies suggest that free heme accumulation, presumably derived from the destruction of P450 enzymes, may be the main source of toxicity by these compounds. Thus, HO-1 induction was proposed to be an adaptive response that was critical for recovery from the toxic insults.

Many studies have investigated the ability of HO-1 to protect against endotoxin exposure. Endotoxin is a lipopolysaccharide produced by gram negative bacteria. Tissue exposure to endotoxin results in inflammatory injury and oxidative stress (Murphy et al., 1998) (McCord, 1993). In two separate studies, HO-1 induction in rats by hemin (Wen et al., 2007) and hemoglobin (Otterbein et al., 1995) pretreatment was protective against the deleterious effects of a subsequent (otherwise lethal) dose of endotoxin. In contrast, the rats were more susceptible to endotoxin toxicity, and the protective effects of HO-1 induction were ablated when the animals were treated with metal porphyrins that inhibited the HO-1 activity.

In vivo studies also demonstrated the ability of HO-1 induction to protect against acute renal failure in rats following ischemia/reperfusion (Toda et al., 2002) and exposure to mercuric chloride (Yoneya et al., 2000). Ischemia/reperfusion involves exposing the tissue to a sequence of oxygen deprivation followed by reoxygenation. Reoxygenation is associated with high levels of oxidative stress. Thus, it is a good model to examine the protective role of HO-1. The kidney ischemia/reperfusion study used tin chloride to induce the HO-1. Tin chloride induces HO-1 in a tissue-specific manner and does not induce HO-1 in the liver but does induce it in the kidney, demonstrating the complicated regulation of the HO-1 gene (discussed below). The fundamental role of HO-1 in mediating renal protection was demonstrated by showing that treatment with tin mesoporphyrin, an inhibitor of HO-1, did not prevent renal injury in the rats (Toda et al., 1995).

3.3 Gene knockout/therapy evidence for the cytoprotective role of HO-1

Over the last 10-15 years, novel research studies and interesting clinical findings have confirmed the cytoprotective role for HO-1. One of the seminal studies to demonstrate the protective role of HO-1 examined embryonic fibroblasts from HO-1 knockout mice and compared their attributes to those from normal wild-type animals (Poss and Tonegawa, 1997b). The cells from the knockout mice produced higher levels of ROS and also were less resistant to toxicity caused by hydrogen peroxide, paraquat, heavy metals, and heme exposure. The effects of HO-1 in the protection from free hemin exposure were quite dramatic offering 50% survival at a hemin concentration (200 µM) that was completely toxic to the cells from knockout mice. Another study from the same group, also compared the response of wild-type and HO-1 knockout mice to an intraperitoneal injection of endotoxin (Poss and Tonegawa, 1997a). Because the adult HO-1 knockout mice had a variety of health issues including anemia, iron-overloading, and chronic inflammation, younger mice (6 to 9 weeks) that did not display these phenotypes were used to study the effects of endotoxin. In terms of survival, the knockout mice were significantly more sensitive to endotoxin treatment and demonstrated higher levels of hepatic injury including increased serum liver enzyme levels and liver vacuolization. Interestingly, the hepatic injury seemed to be spatially and temporally related to iron loading malfunctions in both Kupffer cells and hepatocytes. Iron also accumulated in renal proximal cortical tubules.

Gene therapy studies to upregulate HO-1 have also been instrumental in proving that HO-1 is protective against cellular stress. In a study to demonstrate the role of HO-1 in vascular protection, a retroviral vector was used to transfect the human HO-1 gene into rat lung microvessel endothelium (Yang et al., 1999). Cells transfected with the retrovirus had over a 2-fold increase in HO-1 expression and activity. Furthermore, cGMP levels (probably regulated by CO activation of guanyly cyclase was almost 3-fold higher. These endothelial cells were significantly more resistant than untransfected cells to toxicity resulting from hydrogen peroxide and heme exposure. This protection was abolished upon treatment with stannic mesoporphyrin indicating the role of HO-1.

In another gene therapy study to investigate the ability of HO-1 to protect against the exposure of endotoxin in lung, an adenovirus encoding HO-1 was directly inoculated into rat trachea (Inoue et al., 2001). As a result, HO-1 was upregulated in both airway epithelium and alveolar macrophages. This therapy was found to be as effective as HO-1 induction by hemin pretreatment in preventing the inflammatory reaction caused by aerosolized endotoxin exposure. Furthermore, the protection conferred by increased HO-1 expression seemed to be related to higher endogenous levels of Interleukin-10 production by the macrophages.

Gene therapy was also used to compare the oxidative stress resistance of cerebellar granular neurons isolated from wild type and transgenic, homozygous mice that were engineered to overexpress HO-1 (Chen et al., 2000) The transgenic mice overexpressing HO-1 generated lower levels of ROS and were more resistant to oxidative stress resulting from either glutamate or hydrogen peroxide treatment.

3.4 Clinical evidence for the cytoprotective role of HO-1

Finally, in a tragic clinical example, the protective role of HO-1 was profoundly demonstrated by an individual who did not have a functional HO-1 gene (Kawashima et al., 2002). The six-year old male patient presented with growth retardation, anemia, elevated levels of ferritin and heme in serum, low serum bilirubin, intravascular hemolysis, and hyperlipidemia. In contrast to the HO-1 knockout mice showing toxicity from iron overloading, the endothelial tissue of the human patient was more severely affected causing a spectrum of cardiovascular maladies. A lymphoblastoid-derived cell line from this patient was also extremely sensitive to hemin-induced oxidative stress (Yachie et al., 1999).

3.5 Therapeutic potential of HO-1 modulation

On the basis of these scientific and clinical findings, the role of HO-1 in maintaining homeostasis and protecting against cellular stress is now well established. In conjunction, the enzyme has been shown to be protective in various types of disease/injury models including the following: 1) inflammation (sepsis, atherosclerosis), 2) lung injury (pulmonary fibrosis, ventilator-induced injury), 3) cardiovascular injury/disease (myocardial infarction, hypertension), 4) ischemia/reperfusion, and 5) organ transplantation/rejection. There are now several excellent reviews that discuss the pharmacologic potential of HO-1 induction (Abraham and Kappas, 2008;Mancuso and Barone, 2009;Ryter et al., 2006). Unfortunately, this type of therapy is not straightforward as it has been observed that over-expression of HO-1 can be harmful from the accumulation of reactive iron (Suttner and Dennery, 1999) and the bilirubin that results from HO-1-mediated heme catabolism (Claireaux et al., 1953). Thus, HO-1 expression in this type of therapeutic treatment would need to be highly regulated to prevent over-expression of the enzyme.

4. Mechanisms of cellular protection by HO-1

Originally, it was thought that the sole mechanism by which HO-1 protected cells was through the catabolism of free heme and the elimination of its prooxidant activities (discussed at the beginning of the chapter). Ironically, it was originally thought that the other products of the HO-1 reaction were useless (or even toxic) by-products. Now, it is known that CO and biliverdin play multiple roles in protection and that there are actually several mechanisms by which HO-1 performs its cytoprotective functions. It is very likely that there are more mechanisms yet to be identified.

4.1 Protective roles of CO: Cell signaling mediated by CO

The most definitive proof for the protective effects of CO has been derived from studies using CO-releasing molecules (Motterlini et al., 2003) as a surrogate for HO-1-derived CO. As indicated above, the CO formed by HO-1 has been shown to activate guanylyl cyclase to mediate the relaxation and dilation responses of smooth muscle and vascular endothelial cells, respectively (Cardell et al., 1998;Christodoulides et al., 1995). In vascular tissue, CO has also been shown to stimulate relaxation of endothelial smooth muscle cells by activation of calcium-dependent potassium channels (Williams et al., 2004) via a poorly-understood mechanism that does not involve guanylyl cyclase. CO has been shown to serve as a partial agonist to nitric oxide synthetase (NOS) and thus, may down-regulate the level of NOS-dependent signaling (Hangai-Hoger et al., 2007;Ishikawa et al., 2005).

Interestingly, it also was reported that cGMP-dependent signaling was able to induce HO-1 through the cAMP responsive element in its promoter by a mechanism that was not elucidated (Immenschuh et al., 1998a). Logically, these cGMP-related effects may be initiated by HO-1-generated CO. Of course, the cAMP promoter element also allows HO-1 to be induced directly through cAMP-dependent signaling and activation of protein kinase A (Immenschuh et al., 1998b).

Many of the details about other types of signaling involving CO are poorly understood as it appears to be both cell type- and stressor-specific (Song et al., 2003a){Song, 2003 2563 /id}. Most studies have implicated the ability of CO (and CO-releasing molecules) to activate the P38 MAPK pathway in carrying out its anti-apoptotic and anti-inflammatory effects (Brouard et al., 2000;Dérijard et al., 1995;Keum et al., 2006;Otterbein et al., 2000).

The MAPK pathways have been shown to regulate processes such as inflammation, differentiation, tumor promotion, proliferation, apoptosis, stress response, and ion channels (reviewed in (Shen et al., 2005;Wada and Penninger, 2004)). Two of the three arms of the MAPK pathway (JNK and p38) have been implicated in the cellular stress response. Downstream activation of the MAPK pathway, and specifically the JNK arm, leads to the dimerization and DNA binding of the stress response factors, c-Jun and c-fos. CO dramatically inhibited JNK MAPK signaling in murine macrophages exposed to endotoxin which resulted in lower production of inflammatory cytokine, IL-6 (Morse et al., 2003). Furthermore, c-Jun activation has been linked to cellular proliferation (Yoshioka et al., 1995) so this would explain part of the role of CO in mediating proliferation/transformation.

The p38 arm of the MAPK kinase activates ATF-2 which competes with c-fos for binding to c-Jun. This heterodimer binds with greater affinity to the HO-1 promoter than the c-fos/c-Jun heterodimer (Kravets et al., 2004). Furthermore, ATF-2 dimers can bind and directly activate the cyclic AMP responsive element (CRE) in the promoter region of HO-1 (Lee et al., 2002). ATF-2 activation may play a role in the activation of transcription factor, NFκB (Kaszubska et al., 1993). NFκB plays an essential role in the response to both apoptotic and inflammatory stimuli and regulates the expression of cytokines, growth factors, and cell cycle effector proteins (reviewed in (Bonizzi and Karin, 2004;Shen et al., 2005)). ATF-2 involvement in the activation of NFκB could explain the anti-apoptotic/anti-inflammatory affects of CO (see below for more details). In support of the idea that ATF-2 and c-Jun oppose one another in the protective gene expression associated with HO-1 induction, c-Jun has been shown to inhibit activation of NFκB (Tan et al., 2009).

The ERK 1/2 MAPK regulates cellular growth and differentiation. Stimulation of the pathway has been shown to be protective against apoptosis (Wada and Penninger, 2004). However, overstimulation of ERK appears to be the major mechanism by which some oncogenes transforms cells (e.g. Ha-Ras (Hibi et al., 1993)). In one study of human airway smooth muscle cells, CO-mediated affects on guanylyl cyclase led to inhibition of ERK1/2 MAPK (Song et al., 2003b). Thus, this effect of CO on ERK 1/2 MAPK would serve to prevent overstimulation of this pathway and in turn, the uncontrolled proliferation of cells. ERK has been shown to phosphorylate the inhibitory protein of NFκB and thus facilitate activation of the transcription factor (Chun et al., 2003).

It has also been postulated that CO can activate transcription factors indirectly by mitochondrial-driven ROS production (Piantadosi, 2008). More specifically, it is known that CO is a potent inhibitor of the complex III-mediated terminal step of oxidative phosphorylation. The inhibition of this step of the mitochondrial electron transport chain results in excess ROS production which in turn, reacts with critical thiol groups of the phosphatases that turn off activated transcription factors. In this regard, CO-mediated, mitochondrial ROS production has been implicated in the prolonged activation of the phosphoinositide-3-kinase (PI3 kinase)/Akt pathway (Piantadosi, 2008;Pischke et al., 2005). Numerous studies have implicated this pathway in the protective effects of plant-derived antioxidants (that include induction of HO-1) by ultimately leading to the activation of the transcription factors, Nrf2 (Martin et al., 2004;Park et al., 2011;Pugazhenthi et al., 2007). Nrf2 is a member of the Cap-N-Collar/basic leucine zipper family of transcription factor that responds directly and indirectly to oxidative stress to mediate cytoprotective gene transcription through the antioxidant response elements (ARE) of gene promoters (reviewed in (Itoh et al., 1997;Itoh et al., 2003;Kwak et al., 2004)). Thus, CO-mediated activation of PI3 kinase/Akt provides anti-oxidative protection.

4.2 Regulation of important enzymes by HO-1

It was also discussed how the CO released from HO-1 can inhibit various enzyme activities. The ability of the molecule to inhibit cyclooxygenase may provide an anti-inflammatory effect by preventing the synthesis of inflammatory prostaglandins from arachidonic acid. CO also inhibits cytochromes P450. This action could be cytoprotective because unproductive P450-mediated metabolism results in the release of hydrogen peroxide and/or superoxide from the P450 active site. This activity is an unavoidable consequence of metabolism by these enzymes, and the amount of ROS produced in this manner is dependent on the substrate being metabolized and the specific type of P450 carrying out the reaction (Gorsky et al., 1984;Gruenke et al., 1995;Reed and Hollenberg, 2003). Furthermore, it has been reported that P450-mediated metabolism can generate destructive hydroxyl radicals under certain circumstances (Paller and Jacob, 1994;Terelius and Ingelman-Sundberg, 1988). The oxidative stress generated by P450-mediated metabolism is significant as it has been estimated that the rate of ROS formation by the endoplasmic reticulum can be as much as 30% of that by mitochondria during oxidative phosphorylation (Zangar et al., 2004).

In an idea originally proposed at the turn of the century, HO-1 may provide cytoprotection by indirectly inhibiting P450 activity (and its associated production of ROS) through its competition with P450 for binding to the P450 reductase (Emerson and LeVine, 2000). Both P450s and HO-1 obtain electrons needed for their respective reactions by binding to the P450 reductase. One of the odd aspects of the stoichiometry of these enzymes in the endoplasmic reticulum is that the amount of P450 enzymes far outnumber the amount of P450 reductase (with estimates as high as 25 P450s for every P450 reductase (Peterson et al., 1976). Thus, P450-mediated metabolism in the liver endoplasmic reticulum is extremely limited by the amount of available P450 reductase. Although the level of HO-1 in unstressed liver is very low, it can be induced to an amount that is comparable to that of P450s (Reed et al., 2011). Therefore, it seems likely that the induction of HO-1 would attenuate the rate of P450-mediated metabolism by limiting the ability of P450 to interact with P450 reductase. A preliminary investigation from our lab has provided support for this effect of HO-1 induction (Reed et al., 2011). Furthermore, recent studies in which cells were protected from oxidative stress by the transfection and induction of a mutant HO-1 which was not able to catalyze heme degradation also provides support for this type of indirect mechanism of cytoprotection (Lin et al., 2007;Lin et al., 2008). However as discussed below, the results with the shortened, inactive mutant could be explained if the mutant serves as a heme-carrier to shuttle heme to the nucleus in order to directly modulate gene transcription.

Although far from proven, HO-1 also might actually interact with P450 enzymes to accelerate the degradation of the P450s. Several studies, including a few that were cited above (Nakahira et al., 2003;Odaka et al., 2000), have postulated that HO-1 induction following a stress event coincides with a rapid accumulation of free heme which presumably originates from damaged P450 enzymes. Evidence also was derived by observing a dramatic increase in the rate of degradation of labeled heme from P450 enzymes after HO-1 was induced by either hemin or endotoxin treatment (Bissell and Hammaker, 1976). More specifically, the data suggested that HO-1 increased the degradation of the P450 and not just the catabolism of the heme released from the P450. Again, it is not possible to ascertain whether the damaged P450 releases the heme or the HO-1 binds to the P450 to scavenge and catabolize its heme group. More direct evidence of this putative effect of HO-1 was reported in a study finding that the incubation of purified P450s with either HO-1 and HO-2 caused the heme of the P450 enzymes to be degraded to biliverdin in essentially a 1 to 1 ratio (Kutty et al., 1988). The results also were consistent with the interaction of HO-1 and P450 causing one P450 (two were studied in the publication) to degrade to an inactive form.

Surprisingly, the research supporting the idea that HO-1 facilitates degradation of P450s is decades old but has not been followed up on and confirmed. One reason for this is the fact that the full-length HO-1 is very unstable and susceptible to truncation that generates an inactive, soluble form (28 kDa). The C-terminal part of the protein that is cleaved causes the HO-1 to interact with membrane lipids, and its removal alters the manner by which the enzyme interacts with potential membrane binding partners (Huber, III et al., 2009;Huber, III and Backes, 2007). Most in vitro studies of HO-1 have expressed and purified a modified, but active, 30 kDa form of the enzyme that lacks the C-terminal membrane-binding sequence and is soluble as a result. Our lab has recently modified the amino acid sequence of full-length HO-1 to remove a thrombin cleavage site in the C-terminal tale of HO-1 (Huber, III and Backes, 2007). This mutant is full-length and binds to lipid vesicles. The full-length HO-1 mutant also binds much tighter to the P450 reductase and has much higher catalytic efficiency than the active, soluble form of the enzyme (Huber, III et al., 2009). Thus, studies with this mutant will finally enable researchers to understand the enzymatic capability of HO-1 with respect to those of the other potential binding partners in the endoplasmic reticulum. The putative interaction of HO-1 with P450 may allow for very efficient inhibition of the P450 by the HO-1-generated CO, providing a cytoprotective role by effectively removing the P450 as a contributor to cellular, oxidative stress.

4.3 Protective role of biliverdin/bilirubin

Originally biliverdin and the bilirubin formed by the BVR-catalyzed reduction of biliverdin were thought to be cellular waste products. However, it is apparent that both compounds have antioxidant properties and elicit various cytoprotective effects. Early studies implicated the antioxidant effects of these compounds by showing that they reacted with enzymatically generated superoxide in vitro (Galliani et al., 1985;Robertson, Jr. and Fridovich, 1982). Subsequent studies showed bilirubin to be a more potent antioxidant than α-tocopherol with respect to scavenging lipid peroxides (Neuzil and Stocker, 1993). In fact, both biliverdin and bilirubin were found to interact synergistically with vitamin E to prevent lipid peroxidation by an azo compound (Stocker and Peterhans, 1989). The fact that both of these bile pigments are lipophilic, especially bilirubin, makes them typically more effective than water soluble antioxidants in preventing the damage of membranes and organelles. Bilirubin bound to albumin was also shown to be an effective antioxidant in plasma by protecting the oxidation of low density lipoproteins (Stocker et al., 1987). In addition to its ability to scavenge ROS, bilirubin also inhibits the superoxide-generating NADPH oxidase (Kwak et al., 1991).

Evidence for cytoprotection mediated by the bile pigments comes from several studies. Bilirubin was shown to protect both neuronal cultures (Dore et al., 1999) and HeLa cells (Baranano et al., 2002) from hydrogen peroxide-induced toxicity. Furthermore, when cellular bilirubin was depleted by incubation of the cells with short antisense RNA to BVR, preventing the expression of BVR and in turn, its catalyzed conversion of biliverdin to bilirubin, intracellular levels of ROS increased and promoted apoptotic death of neuronal and HeLa cells (Baranano et al., 2002). It was found that the effects of bilirubin depletion had a greater pro-oxidant effect than depletion of cellular glutathione. In another study, pretreatment of cultured endothelial cells with bilirubin also protected cultured endothelial cells from pro-inflammatory responses after challenge by oxidized LDL and TNF-α (Kawamura et al., 2005). The level of protection of the endothelial cells was comparable to that achieved by preinduction of HO-1 with hemin. Interestingly, CO treatment of the cells did not protect them from these responses.

Bilirubin and biliverdin have also been shown to be protective in animal studies. Injection of bilirubin into rats prevented glutathione depletion following administration of cadmium chloride (Ossola and Tomaro, 1995). The two bile pigments also have been shown to be effective in various models of ischemia/reperfusion injury (Clark et al., 2000;Fondevila et al., 2004). Biliverdin treatment was as effective as hemin-mediated HO-1 induction in protecting rats from acetaminophen toxicity (Chiu et al., 2002). Bilirubin treatment also protected rats challenged with endotoxin by preventing an inflammatory response in the animals (Wang et al., 2004). Biliverdin and bilirubin also react with reactive nitrogen species such as nitric oxide and peroxynitrite. Thus, the compounds can attenuate NO signaling, and this was believed to be the cause of the anti-inflammatory effect in the endotoxin study (Wang et al., 2004). Another anti-nitrosative effect of HO-1 recently discovered is the finding that increased HO-1 expression was associated with induction of endothelial cell superoxide dismutase (Kruger et al., 2005). This, in turn, would lower the amount of superoxide available to react with NO to form peroxynitrite.

Biliverdin also inhibits activation of NF-κB in HEK293 cells (Gibbs and Maines, 2007). The effect was observed to be specific for biliverdin and not bilirubin. In fact, overexpression of BVR, which converts the biliverdin to bilirubin, overcame the biliverdin-mediated inhibition of NF-κB. Thus, part of the anti-inflammatory effect of biliverdin may be caused by preventing activation of NF-κB. Biliverdin has also been shown to be a potent inhibitor of c-Jun N-terminal kinase and AP-1 pathway (Tang et al., 2007), and this effect has been associated with pro-inflammatory and pro-apoptotic responses. Bilirubin has been shown to modulate ERK1/2 signaling pathways (Taillé et al., 2003). Furthermore, it has now been shown that both biliverdin and bilirubin activate the aryl hydrocarbon receptor to induce expression of a spectrum of genes including CYP1A1 (Phelan et al., 1998). At this point, it is not fully appreciated how these cell-signaling effects mediated by biliverdin and bilirubin relate to cytoprotection.

In summary, the effects of biliverdin and bilirubin are complex and are poorly understood. Protection by these compounds seems to derive from antioxidant properties of the compounds as well as anti-nitrosative effects from scavenging NO. However, many more mechanisms may be involved to explain their effects. In fact, the effects of these compounds on cell signaling pathways are only beginning to be elucidated. It should also be mentioned that the balance between cytoprotection and toxicity is delicate in the case of bilirubin. High concentrations of this compound are neurotoxic and pro-oxidative (Claireaux et al., 1953;Stocker and Ames, 1987) adding to the complexity and importance of cellular heme regulation.

4.4 Ferrous iron release: The participation of ferritin and HO-1

You can put a rose on a herring, but it will still stink and be red. The same analogy can be used when trying to argue the protective "benefits" of HO-1-mediated ferrous iron production. Free ferrous iron will be a "smelly, red herring" with regards to oxidative/reductive homeostasis in the cell. As mentioned at the beginning of the chapter, the metal is prone to generating highly destructive hydroxyl radicals. Thus, it is a powerful pro-oxidant which would cause it to potentiate oxidative stress. In fact, a study which over-expressed HO-1 through a tetracycline-inducible vector found that the mutant cells were much more prone to deleterious iron-overload (Suttner and Dennery, 1999). Thus, HO-1 expression had a negative effect on cell survival in this instance. Presumably, HO-1 over-expression also could have a negative health impact from the potential build-up of bilirubin levels, as described above.

On the other hand, the metal is essential for the synthesis of heme and in turn, for all of the functions carried out by the heme proteins. Thus, HO-1 does provide a way for the iron in free heme or heme attached to damaged enzymes (which may act as even more potent pro-oxidants than free iron) to be recycled for future heme synthesis in the cell, so its activity does have a net positive effect on cellular health. Furthermore, heme induction also activates expression of the iron-storage protein, ferritin (Eisenstein et al., 1991). Thus, during heme-related stress, both ferritin and HO-1 are coordinately regulated (Tsuji et al., 2000). Ferritin is an iron storage protein that allows for the controlled release of iron to coincide with the metabolic needs of the cell (Ponka, 1997).

Interestingly, it has been suggested that there are *at least* two types of HO-1 inducing agents, heme-dependent and heme-independent (Bauer and Bauer, 2002). Subsequently, it was shown that heme-independent HO-1 induction did not necessarily induce ferritin (Sheftel et al., 2007). However, HO-1 will only produce excess free iron when there is an abundant supply of heme, so the ferritin will be induced in the cell when it is needed. In the study cited above (Suttner and Dennery, 1999) indicating iron over-load in cells overexpressing HO-1, the cells were transfected with an expression vector. Thus, hemin was not involved in the induction of HO-1 and consequently, ferritin was not induced enough to protect against iron overload from catalytically active HO-1.

Although it has not been proven definitively, it has been speculated that the location of HO-1 in the endoplasmic reticulum may facilitate the migration of free iron to the extracellular space and in turn, help maintain iron blood levels (Poss and Tonegawa, 1997a). Whether or not this putative role of HO-1 exists, the activity of the enzyme and the co-ordinate regulation of ferritin when HO-1 is induced through its cognate promoter give the cell a protective way to recycle iron and manage its levels in the cell.

5. Mechanisms of cellular protection by BVR

5.1 BVR-catalyzed redox cycle with lipid peroxides

The anti-oxidant effects and other positive health benefits of bilirubin, that are attributable to catalysis by BVR, are obviously important means of BVR-mediated cytoprotection. The antioxidant effects of this compound were discussed above, but the reason for its potency involves metabolism by BVR. In a study examining the cytoprotective effects of bilirubin in neuronal cells, it was found that as little as 10 nM bilirubin (physiologic levels) protected against 10,000-fold higher concentrations of hydrogen peroxide (Baranano et al., 2002). From these results, it was postulated that BVR participates in a redox cycle with lipid peroxides in which bilirubin is oxidized by the lipid peroxides to biliverdin which, in turn, is reduced by BVR to reform bilirubin (Figure 1). Thus, BVR may have an important role in extending the antioxidant potency of bilirubin. It should be noted that a recent study concluded that the cytoprotective role of this redox cycle was limited as BVR overexpression and inhibition of BVR expression with antisense RNA did not seem to influence hydrogen peroxide-mediated cytotoxicity (Maghzal et al., 2009).

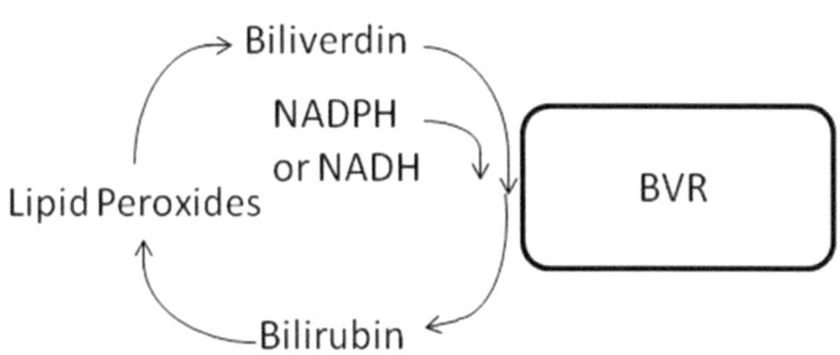

Fig. 1. BVR-catalyzed redox cycle with lipid peroxides. See text for details

5.2 BVR-mediated modulation of cell signaling

BVR may be the most versatile protein known. Research over the last decade has revealed new functions for the enzyme that have broadened its role in the cytoprotective response to cellular stress signals. It is now known that BVR also functions as a dual-specific kinase of serine/threonine and tyrosine residues in proteins, and in this capacity, BVR affects the signaling and cellular responses to a variety of stimuli (Reviewed in (Kapitulnik and Maines, 2009)). Kinases capable of phosphorylating both threonine and tyrosine residues have been identified as those regulating upstream events in signal transduction pathways (Pawson and Scott, 2005). The discovery of this function of BVR was preceded by finding that its ability to metabolize biliverdin was dependent on protein phosphorylation and that the enzyme could catalyze autophosphorylation of this residue (Salim et al., 2001).

Subsequently, it was shown that BVR is regulated by insulin/insulin growth factor stimulation through receptor-mediated tyrosine phosphorylation (Lerner-Marmarosh et al., 2005). BVR binding to this receptor competes with insulin receptor substrates (IRS) 1 and 2 for binding to the receptor. BVR phosphorylates serine residues of the IRS which attenuates their affinity for the insulin receptor kinase, essentially inactivating them. Phosphorylated BVR can activate two protein kinase C proteins, βII and ζ, which are involved in cross-talk between the upstream components of the MAPK and phosphatidylinositol 3-kinase pathways, respectively. Protein kinase C βII also can activate BVR which partly contributes to the activation of BVR by stress signals (Maines et al., 2007). The activation of protein kinase C βII by BVR leads to activation of all three arms of the MAPK signaling. Thus, all of the effects of CO caused by its activation of the P38 MAPK (discussed above) also apply to the activation of this pathway by BVR.

BVR-mediated signaling appears to play a critical role in the recruiting transcription factor, NFκB to the HO-1 promoter (Gibbs and Maines, 2007). Furthermore, NFκB has been shown to be activated by protein kinase Cζ which in turn, is directly activated by BVR (Lerner-Marmarosh et al., 2007). As described in detail below, the involvement of NFκB appears to be important in mediating the anti-apoptotic, anti-inflammatory, and anti-proliferative effects associated with expression of HO-1.

BVR has the ability to form protein complexes with itself and other proteins, and serves to shuttle activated transcription factors to the nucleus. The ability of BVR to function as a dual cofactor enzyme with different pH optima expands its range of function in the cell (Kapitulnik and Maines, 2009). In addition to the activation of the ERK MAPK pathway by BVR through protein kinase C βII, BVR has been shown to play a critical role in shuttling the activated ERK to the nucleus to influence gene transcription (Lerner-Marmarosh et al., 2008).

Interestingly, BVR also binds to NFκB (Gibbs and Maines, 2007). This is intriguing because the HO-1 promoter does not have a prototypical response element for NFκB, and it has been conjectured that it must be recruited to the promoter by other transcription factors (Alam and Cook, 2007). Thus, through this interaction, BVR also may play a role in allowing NFκB to influence HO-1 gene transcription.

In another transport capacity, BVR also complexes with heme and shuttles it to the nucleus where the heme can bind to regulatory elements that influence gene transcription. In fact, heme-mediated gene induction has been shown to be dependent on BVR in renal cells (Tudor et al., 2008). Interestingly, although HO-1 is most typically observed in the endoplasmic reticulum, instances of it being located in other parts of the cell including the plasma membrane (where it localizes to caveolae rafts (Kim et al., 2004)), mitochondria

(Converso et al., 2006), and even as a shortened, soluble component in the nucleus have been reported (Lin et al., 2007). The significance of these findings has yet to be elucidated, but they may indicate that HO-1 also can transport heme to the nucleus (discussed below) and may be involved in targeting BVR to different organelles to mediate signaling or the biliverdin/BVR redox cycle to scavenge ROS from the mitochondria (discussed above).

5.3 BVR-mediated modulation of gene transcription through DNA binding

Although the kinase-dependent activity described above ultimately results in the modulation of gene transcription, BVR also has the capacity to bind to DNA and directly influence gene expression through a basic leucine zipper-binding motif. BVR binds to AP-1/CRE sites in DNA which are typically bound by c-Jun/fos heterodimers to mediate the stress response (Ahmad et al., 2002). In this capacity, BVR binds as homo- and hetero-dimers to recruit or block the binding of other transcription factors and thus, BVR can enhance or inhibit gene expression directly. At this point, BVR-mediated gene transcription has been shown to induce ATF-2 (Kravets et al., 2004). ATF-2 has also been shown to be capable of binding to and activating NFκB (Kaszubska et al., 1993).

Thus, with regards to the role of BVR in recruiting NFκB to the HO-1 promoter, BVR can facilitate its binding directly or through the upregulation and activation of ATF-2. However, it is likely that NFκB would bind to the promoter in different 5'-flanking regions when bound to BVR and ATF-2. Most of the specific effects of BVR-DNA binding on gene expression have not been elucidated. But the enzyme has been shown to translocate to the nucleus of HeLa cells (Tudor et al., 2008) after hemin induction and in rat kidney after exposure of animals to nephrotoxins (Maines et al., 2001). In fact, HeLa, heme-mediated induction of HO-1 expression was shown to be dependent on BVR expression (Tudor et al., 2008).

6. Assessing the dependence of HO-1-mediated cytoprotection on BVR

Given the diverse abilities of BVR to regulate cellular processes, it has been postulated that the HO-1 cytoprotective response is completely dependent on BVR. The hypothesis proposes that the increased expression of HO-1 caused by the wide variety of inducing agents is mediated by the signaling and DNA binding activities of BVR. Furthermore, in a study examining the catalytic steps of the HO-1 reaction, it was determined that binding of BVR and HO-1 was required to increase the rate of release of biliverdin from the HO-1 active site. The study found that in the absence of BVR, biliverdin release was the rate-limiting step of the HO-1 reaction, and its presence dramatically increased turnover by HO-1. In showing that even the catalytic activity of the enzyme was dependent on BVR, the study supported the idea that the HO-1 cytoprotective response was totally dependent on BVR. However, finding that HO-1 activity was dependent on BVR was counter-intuitive because the level of HO-1 can be induced many-fold by cellular exposure to stress signals (Wright et al., 2006). In contrast, the expression level of BVR is typically unchanged after stress (although it may be inducible in kidney (Maines et al., 2001)). Thus, it would seem to be unproductive for the cell to induce HO-1 and have its activity be limited by the supply of BVR. Such a situation also would allow little opportunity for biliverdin to accumulate in cells. Yet, studies show that biliverdin has completely different cytoprotective roles than bilirubin (see above). Thus, the enzymatic data showing that BVR regulated HO-1 enzymatic activity were baffling.

More recent enzymatic studies measuring steady state metabolism by HO-1 showed that BVR had no effect on the rate of HO-1-mediated catalysis (Reed et al., 2010). In fact, this study showed that the rates of HO-1-mediated heme catabolism measured by the formation of both biliverdin and a ferrozene:ferrous iron complex in the absence of BVR were slightly higher than that measured by bilirubin formation in the presence of BVR. The earlier results finding that HO-1 activity was dependent on BVR were attributed to the unusual conditions required to monitor the individual catalytic steps (namely anaerobic with limiting concentrations of NADPH).

The question still remains whether the HO-1-related gene response following exposure to stress signals is completely dependent on BVR. The HO-1 promoter contains a variety of responsive elements that includes two AP-1 sites, a CRE, a Maf recognition domain (binding partner to Nrf2), and a partial site for NFκB binding (Alam and Cook, 2007). Understanding how these responsive elements recruit transcription factors to influence gene transcription is complicated by the fact that many of the response elements overlap and thus, may inhibit or enhance DNA binding by factors to adjacent elements. The transcription factors that activate the HO-1 promoter will vary with the types of stress to which the cell is exposed (reviewed in (Alam and Cook, 2007). Furthermore, studies have shown that the signaling pathways activated by the same stress signals also can vary in different cell types (Ryter et al., 2006). As a result, the transcription factors mediating a specific cytoprotective response can vary in different cell types. Thus, a type of HO-1-mediated cytoprotection may depend on BVR in some cell types but not others. Because of these considerations, the discussion pertaining to the dependence of HO-1 expression on BVR will be a generalization based on the typical roles of the implicated transcription factors in cellular processes.

6.1 Anti-oxidant protection

With this perspective in mind, the various protective roles of cell signaling and gene transcription associated with HO-1 induction are mediated largely through activation of either Nrf2 or NFκB. Certainly one of the first evolutionary roles needed for survival of a cell would have been to develop a defense system for the oxidative stress associated with the activity of heme enzymes. Heme oxygenase is the only enzyme that uses its heme cofactor as a substrate. Furthermore, as discussed below, HO-1 can be induced directly by heme interaction with the HO-1 gene repressor Bach-1. Therefore, it is the only known eukaryotic enzyme that has a substrate that regulates a transcription factor needed for its expression. This scenario would suggest that heme oxygenase represents a very old link in the evolutionary chain. By the same line of reasoning used above to rationalize the evolutionary role of HO-1 function, Nrf2/anti-oxidant response must represent an early evolutionary adaptation to allow living organisms to survive oxidative stress. Interestingly, Bach-1 is an effective repressor of the HO-1 gene because it blocks Nrf2 from binding to the HO-1 promoter. Because heme metabolism is intimately connected to reductive/oxidative homeostasis in the cell, it seems plausible that Nrf2 can mediate HO-1 expression independently from BVR as a response (initially at least) to oxidative stress.

One caveat to the hypothesis that the anti-oxidative response is independent of BVR is dictated by whether or not the shuttling of heme to the nucleus by BVR is the only mechanism by which this can occur (discussed above). As alluded to above, Bach 1 blocks the binding of Nrf2 to the antioxidant response element when Bach 1 is not bound to heme

(Sun et al., 2002). In support of the idea that an anti-oxidant response can be mediated directly by Nrf2 without involvement of BVR, HO-1 was found to be constitutively expressed in Bach 1 knockout mice (Sun et al., 2002). Thus, it is proposed that nuclear heme localization and functional Nrf2 are the essential components of the initial gene response to oxidative stress. In some instances, BVR has been shown to be critical for heme translocation to the nucleus. However, the results are mixed and may be cell type-specific. For instance, the same laboratory has shown that inhibition of BVR expression with small interference (antisense) RNA blocked the hemin-mediated induction of HO-1 cells in HeLa cells (Tudor et al., 2008) but had no effect in COS cells (Ahmad et al., 2002).

Recent studies showing that shortened HO-1 also translocates to the nucleus may serve as another mechanism by which hemin is transported to the nucleus to directly influence gene transcription (Lin et al., 2007). This would allow the shuttling role of BVR to be bypassed in some cells and would explain results showing that increased expression of a catalytically inactive mutant was also able to up-regulate HO-1 expression (Lin et al., 2008). Another way that cells could possibly bypass BVR-mediated heme shuttling can be postulated from the results of a study showing that heme bound to and stabilized Nrf2 (Alam et al., 2003). This led to activation of Nrf2 and the heme-responsive element in the HO-1 promoter. Thus, Nrf2 could also transport heme to the nucleus to influence gene transcription during oxidative stress. Therefore, it does seem necessary to require BVR to transport heme to the nucleus for most cell types.

There also are several general experimental findings that support this inutitive argument. First, Nrf2 is believed to be the primary transcription factor activated directly by oxidative stress, and its activation is associated with induction of phase II and antioxidant enzymes (Bellezza et al., 2010;Ishii et al., 2002;Shen et al., 2005). A multitude of studies have implicated Nrf2 in the induction of HO-1 during oxidative stress (Alam et al., 2003;Gong and Cederbaum, 2006a;Gong and Cederbaum, 2006b;Sun Jang et al., 2009). Finally, in two studies looking at the effects of oxidative stress (by hydrogen peroxide treatment), it was found that cell viability was only marginally affected (Baranano et al., 2002) or not affected at all (Maghzal et al., 2009) by silencing BVR (with interference RNA). The latter study also showed that BVR induction and over-expression also did not provide protection to the cells exposed to hydrogen peroxide. Thus, it may not be a coincidence that studies have not yet implicated a connection between BVR actions and Nrf2. In fact, the binding site for Nrf2 in the HO-1 promoter overlaps with one of the AP-1 sites to which BVR can bind (Alam and Cook, 2007). Differences between antioxidant response elements and AP-1 binding sites have been distinguished previously (Yoshioka et al., 1995). Thus, it appears Nrf2 binding and AP-1 binding by BVR might be somewhat competitive with Nrf2 binding occurring initially after oxidative stress and BVR replacing the transcription factor from the antioxidant response element after prolonged oxidative stress.

In addition, to the demonstration of constitutive HO-1 expression in Bach-1 knockout mice, there appears to be a unique aspect of the HO-1 promoter which allows Nrf2 to initiate transcription without recruitment of other transcription factors. It has been found that the chromatin remodeling protein, BRG1, interacts with Nrf2 to form a Z-DNA structure which permits access for RNA polymerase II to initiate transcription of the HO-1 gene (Zhang et al., 2006). This interaction between BRG-1 and Nrf2 was exclusive to the HO-1 gene (but not other Nrf2-regulated genes) by virtue of a series of TG repeats that are present in the HO-1 promoter. In fact, genetic polymorphisms affecting this region have been shown to correspond to susceptibility to oxidative stress-related diseases (Ishii et al., 2000).

Thus, the right panel of Figure 2 is drawn to indicate the BVR-independent activation of HO-1 gene transcription after exposure to oxidative stress. ROS can activate Nrf2 directly by oxidizing Keap-1 which is responsible for binding Nrf2 in the cytoplasm and facilitating its degradation (Itoh et al., 2003). Oxidation of critical cysteine residues in Keap-1 releases Nrf2, allowing it to translocate to the nucleus and activate gene transcription (reviewed in (Kwak et al., 2004)). In addition, CO inhibits mitochondrial electron transport resulting in ROS production which inhibit phosphatases needed to inactivate PI3K. Prolonged activation of PI3K results in stimulation of Akt which can phosphorylate Nrf2 (Piantadosi, 2008). Phosphorylation causes Keap-1 to release and activate Nrf2. ROS can also lead to activation of JNK MAPK. It has been shown that JNK target, c-Jun, can bind to Nrf2 (Shen et al., 2005). Thus, c-Jun/fos dimers binding to the AP-1 site facilitate the recruitment of Nrf2 to bind to the overlapping Maf-recognition element and induce HO-1 transcription. Previous binding by the c-Jun/fos dimer may help facilitate the binding of Nrf2 if Nrf2 can exchange with fos for binding to c-Jun. BVR is shown in this panel to serve as a heme transporter to the nucleus. That putative role is also indicated for the shortened form of HO-1 that has been identified in the nucleus (Lin et al., 2007) and for Nrf2. One additional role that BVR could play in the prolonged anti-oxidant response is to modulate the initial response by increasing or decreasing the anti-oxidant response depending on the needs of the cell.

6.2 Anti-apoptotic/proliferation protection

For the reasons below, it is postulated that BVR plays an integral role in the signaling responsible for anti-proliferative, anti-inflammatory, and anti-apoptotic responses by facilitating the interaction of NFκB with the HO-1 promoter and by modulating the activity of the transcription factor. As mentioned above, NFκB regulates the expression of cytokines, growth factors, and cell cycle effector proteins (Du et al., 1993;Hayden and Ghosh, 2011;Peng et al., 1995). As a result, the factor regulates important physiological processes such as immune response and apoptosis, and overstimulation or dysregulation of this factor is associated with inflammation, transformation, and proliferation of cells (Bubici et al., 2006). Thus, the cytoprotective role of HO-1 induction for processes such as inflammation, apoptosis, and proliferation would logically involve mechanisms affecting NFκB function. Scientific studies have shown that NFκB and Nrf2 are oppositely and variably regulated by different types of cellular stress (Bellezza et al., 2010). Nrf2 is typically activated by low or moderate levels oxidative stress, whereas NFκB is turned on by inflammatory signals or very high levels of oxidative stress. Thus, with regards to the HO-1 promoter and various cytoprotective responses mediated by enzyme induction, stress signals will specifically alter the relative levels of cellular transcription factors and in turn, will determine whether Nrf2 or NFκB binds to activate transcription of the HO-1 gene. The JNK MAPK target, c-Jun has been shown to bind to Nrf2 (Shen et al., 2005), and inhibit NFκB (Tan et al., 2009). However, the P38 MAPK target, ATF-2 has been shown to bind to NFκB (Kaszubska et al., 1993). The model below proposes that the relative levels of c-Jun and ATF-2 play a major role in different cytoprotective responses mediated by HO-1 induction.

One essential role that BVR may play in modulating cytoprotective gene expression associated with HO-1 induction is the activation and recruitment of NFκB to the HO-1 promoter (Gibbs and Maines, 2007). It is proposed that this function is the main determinant in mediating the anti-apoptotic response associated with HO-1 induction. NFκB activation has been associated with prevention of apoptosis following treatment with cytokines and tumor promoters (Papa et al., 2006;Sen et al., 1996). Biliverdin inhibits activation of NFκB (Gibbs and Maines, 2007), and BVR reverses this affect by metabolizing biliverdin to bilirubin and by promoting PKCζ-mediated phosphorylation and activation of the transcription factor (Lerner-Marmarosh et al., 2007).

The importance of BVR in mediating the apoptotic response has been demonstrated repeatedly. When BVR was over-expressed in HEK 293 and MCF-7 cells, the cells were arrested in G_1/G_0 stage (Gibbs and Maines, 2007). Furthermore, over-expression of BVR also protected cells from NFκB-mediated proliferation after stimulation with TNF-α (Gibbs et al., 2010). These findings are consistent with a number of studies that have used various cell types (HEK293 (Miralem et al., 2005), HeLa (Ahmad et al., 2002), cardiomyocytes (Pachori et al., 2007) and renal epithelial cells (Young et al., 2009)) to show that the inhibition of BVR expression using interference RNA resulted in apoptosis after the cells were challenged with arsenite, hydrogen peroxide, hypoxia/reoxygenation, and angiotensin II, respectively. Thus, repression of BVR expression consistently leads to apoptosis after cells are challenged with various types of stressors. Most importantly, with regards to protection from apoptosis, NFκB has been shown to be a necessary factor for the activation of the tumor suppressor protein, P53 (Ryan et al., 2000). Consistent with the role of BVR in preventing apoptosis, bilirubin also has been shown to have anti-apoptotic effects in a variety of studies (Bulmer et al., 2008;Kim et al., 2006;Parfenova et al., 2006). In addition, activation of ERK MAP kinases (mediated by BVR (Lerner-Marmarosh et al., 2008)) has been shown to favor anti-apoptotic responses (Wada and Penninger, 2004) which would also be consistent with the anti-apoptotic role of BVR. For these reasons, it seems probable that the BVR-mediated recruitment and activation of NFκB are essential for anti-apoptotic HO-1 induction.

It is speculated that BVR also plays another important role in the anti-apoptotic signal. Studies have shown that BVR induces expression of P38 MAPK target, ATF-2 (Kravets et al., 2004). ATF-2 is constitutively expressed and not induced by environmental stimuli (unlike c-Jun) (Angel and Karin, 1991;Herdegen and Leah, 1998). Furthermore, it can form mixed dimers with c-Jun, and this hetero-dimer binds with much tighter affinity to AP-1 sites than c-Jun/fos dimers (Benbrook and Jones, 1990). Furthermore, ATF-2 dimerizes with itself and binds to the CRE response element instead of the AP-1 stress response element. Most importantly with respect to anti-proliferative, anti-inflammatory, and anti-apoptotic cytoprotection, ATF-2 also has been shown to dimerize with NFκB (Kaszubska et al., 1993). It is proposed in the mechanism below that these functions of ATF-2 along with the participation of BVR mediate HO-1-related cytoprotection from apoptotic, inflammatory, and hyper-proliferative stimuli.

The left panel of Figure 2 shows cell signaling cascades that may mediate the general anti-apoptotic HO-1 response. It seems likely that apoptotic/anti-apoptotic specificity involves a change in gene expression mediated by c-Jun/fos dimerization to one mediated by ATF-2 homo-dimerization. The critical events in this transition are BVR-mediated activation of NFκB (by direct phosphorylation and metabolism of biliverdin (BV in figure) to bilirubin (BR) and amplification of P38 MAPK relative to the c-Jun arm of MAPK). As mentioned above, biliverdin has been shown to be an inhibitor of NFκB (Gibbs and Maines, 2007). The amplification of P38 MAPK relative to JNK and ERK MAPKs would be consistent with the effects of CO as the molecule activates P38 but inhibits JNK/ERK MAPKs (summarized above). In addition, biliverdin has been shown to be a potent inhibitor of JNK MAPK (Tang et al., 2007). Furthermore, c-Jun activation has been linked to cellular proliferation (Yoshioka et al., 1995) so switching from c-Jun-driven to ATF-2-driven transcription would be protective against proliferation/transformation. To show attenuation of the JNK MAPK pathway, the JNK arm of MAPK is shown as a dashed arrow in the figure panel to show that its activation is attenuated relative to that of P38 kinase. Because BVR has been shown to activate ERK MAPK (Lerner-Marmarosh et al., 2008), the arrow from ERK is a mixed dash/dot symbol to show moderate activation. Activation of ERK MAPK has been shown to facilitate anti-apoptotic responses (Wada and Penninger, 2004), and this might be related to the ability of ERK proteins to catalyze phosphorylation of the NFκB-inhibitory protein that keeps NFκB in the cytosol (for review of NFκB activation see (Shen et al., 2005)). As described above, signaling and DNA transcription mediated by BVR also lead to activation and increased expression of the P38 target, ATF-2, so this is another factor that increases the relative activation and concentration of ATF-2 (note the arrow from BVR to ATF-2 in the panel). Furthermore, BVR activates PKCβII (the latter can also activate BVR so a double headed arrow connects the two kinases in the panel) which serves to activate all three arms of MAPK signaling.

As ATF-2 concentrations and its level of activation increases relative to c-Jun and fos, c-Jun/fos hetero-dimerization would be replaced with c-Jun/ATF-2 dimerization at the AP-1 site. Because a P38-mediated pathway leading to activation of Nrf2 has been reported as a cytoprotective response in a cell line derived from human bronchial epithelial cells that were exposed to CeO2 nanoparticles, it is possible that the c-Jun/ATF-2 dimer serves as a more potent transcription factor in the recruitment of Nrf2 to the HO-1 promoter (Eom and Choi, 2009). Further increases in the concentration of ATF-2 would favor homo-dimerization of the transcription factor at the CRE site instead of the AP-1 site. ATF-2 has been shown to bind to NFκB (Kaszubska et al., 1993), and it has been shown that P38-mediated phosphorylation of Nrf2 promotes its association with the inhibitory protein, Keap1 (Keum et al., 2006). Both of these aspects of P38 pathway activation would favor activation of NFκB over Nrf2. Thus, it is proposed that the ATF-2 dimerization is the key signal that recruits NFκB to bind to the HO-1 promoter to induce expression of the gene. As proposed in the anti-oxidant response with the c-Jun/fos dimer facilitating recruitment of Nrf2 to the promoter, the ATF-2 dimer would allow NFκB to bind to the promoter as it exchanges with one of the ATF-2 units of the dimer. Another consistent aspect of the transition from the binding of c-Jun to that of ATF-2 in the recruitment of NFκB is the finding that c-Jun has been shown to inhibit NFκB activation (Tan et al., 2009).Thus, in the left panel of figure 2, the role of ATF-2 is represented by having its arrow point towards that for NFκB in the nucleus. Consistent with studies showing that Nrf2 and NFκB are co-regulated in opposite directions in response to stress signals (Bellezza et al., 2010), binding by NFκB is proposed to displace Nrf2 from the HO-1 promoter. The change in binding to the CRE site also may be critical in this regard because the AP-1 site overlaps more with the Nrf2 binding site than the CRE site. Thus, there would be less competition between Nrf2 and NFκB for binding to the HO-1 promoter. Because BVR can bind to both CRE and NFκB (Gibbs and Maines, 2007;Kravets et al., 2004), it may also serve to recruit NFκB to bind near the CRE.

In addition to activating NFκB, BVR also binds to the transcription factor in a manner that modulates its activity to favor protective gene expression relative to harmful pro-apoptotic, pro-inflammatory and pro-proliferative targets (Gibbs et al., 2010). Consistent with the possibility that BVR regulates the activity of NFκB, TNF-α-mediated stimulation caused NFκB to act as a repressor of BVR expression which demonstrates that BVR is competitive with the inflammation process mediated by TNF-α through activation of NFκB. Because of the BVR-mediated modulation of NFκB, the arrow from NFκB is drawn as a dash in the panel.

6.3 Anti-inflammatory protection

It appears that the anti-inflammatory effects associated with HO-1 induction (middle panel of figure 2) might be mediated by both BVR-dependent and BVR-independent processes. ROS formation (produced by immune cells) is a big component of inflammation. Thus, it seems unlikely that the anti-inflammatory response is totally regulated by BVR (middle panel of figure 2). Thus, for the reasons given in the preceding paragraph, Nrf2 will be activated independently of BVR, probably as an initial response to inflammatory stimuli. Another implication of the role of Nrf2 in the HO-1-related anti-inflammatory response has come from studies with plant-derived, phenolic diterpenes that elicit both anti-oxidant and anti-inflammatory responses. Not coincidentally, these compounds also mediate HO-1 induction through Nrf2 following stimulation of phosphatidylinositol 3-kinase (PI3-kinase)/Akt signaling (Martin et al., 2004;Pugazhenthi et al., 2007). The Akt protein kinase activated by PI3K is distinct from the PKCζ that is known to be activated by BVR (Lerner-Marmarosh et al., 2007). As described above, CO has been implicated in mediating signaling through Akt (Piantadosi and Zhang, 1996). Thus, this pathway of Nrf2 activation appears to be related directly to the catalytic activity of HO-1. These mechanisms activating Nrf2 contribute to the anti-inflammatory effects associated with HO-1 induction.

An appealing hypothesis, that seems consistent with research findings, proposes that BVR-independent processes activate Nrf2 at the early stages of inflammation, whereas BVR-mediated MAPK and NFκB activation play critical roles in the cellular response at later stages of inflammation. In support of this idea, NFκB signaling typically opposes Nrf2 mediated signaling as a later event in response to many stress events (Bellezza et al., 2010). The putative ability of BVR to bind and modulate the activity of NFκB is important in the latter response because agonist binding to immune receptors cause potent activation of NFκB. It is important to emphasize that this modulating role is not the only way BVR would protect cells from NFκB-mediated stress. By replacing NFκB with Nrf2 at the HO-1 promoter, BVR would be diverting NFκB from promoting harmful gene expression while freeing up Nrf2 to activate protective gene expression. The anti-inflammatory effects of CO generated by HO-1 activity also would act independently of BVR (described above). A recent study demonstrated that HO-1 activity (as opposed to merely BVR-related cell signaling and DNA binding) was essential for the anti-inflammatory effects following treatment with endotoxin (Tamion et al., 2006). The anti-inflammatory response demonstrated by the treated animals was explained by both the inhibition of tumor necrosis factor-α production and the elevation of interleukin-10. Because the anti-inflammatory effects required catalytic activity by the induced HO-1 (activity was inhibited by treatment with tin mesoporphyrin), it can be assumed that either BVR-mediated signaling/DNA-binding was dependent on HO-1 activity or the effects were caused by bilirubin/CO. Either premise dictates that BVR effects occurred secondary to those mediated by HO-1 activity. For these reasons, it seems that the anti-inflammatory response is pleiotropic and depends on both BVR-dependent and BVR-independent signaling and gene transcription.

In the middle panel, the anti-inflammatory signaling that results in the later-staged recruitment of NFκB to the HO-1 promoter is represented. The scheme for Nrf2 activation preceding NFκB activation is shown in the far right panel. In the anti-inflammatory response, CO formed by HO-1 inhibits the JNK and ERK MAPK pathways. The CO-mediated inhibition of c-Jun protects against uncontrolled proliferation. However, BVR modulates ERK to protect against apoptosis through activation of NFκB. Initially, c-Jun inhibits NFκB activation which is shown as the red block line. Eventually, ERK activity and ATF-2 dimerization at the HO-1 promoter will favor gene transcription mediated by NFκB. BVR also modulates NFκB activity to favor protective gene expression, so the arrow from NFκB is dashed. In addition, as mentioned above, diversion of NFκB to stimulate the protective induction of HO-1 limits its ability to stimulate inflammatory gene expression and allows more Nrf2 to activate transcription of other anti-oxidant genes.

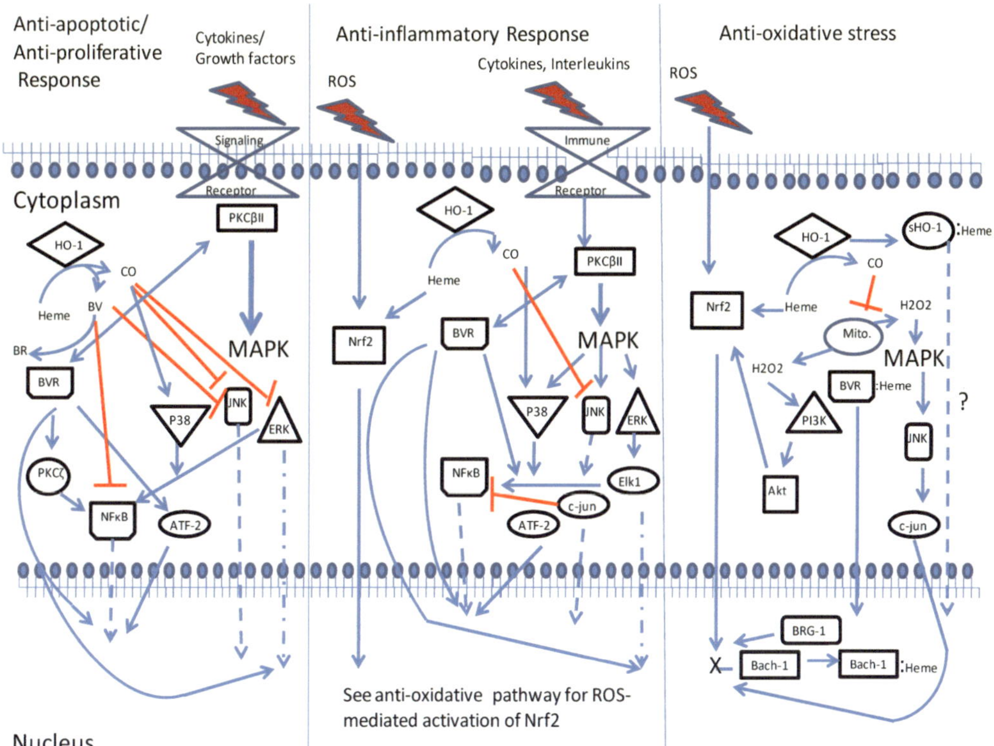

Fig. 2. Signal transduction regulation of the HO-1 protective response to cellular stress signals. The schematic diagram shows the putative signaling pathways responsible for gene induction/repression following different types of cellular stress (apoptotic signals, inflammatory stimuli, and oxidative stress). Arrows ending in the cytoplasm point at downstream kinases or transcription factors activated by the stimuli at the base of the arrow. Arrows ending in the nuclei represent the binding of transcription factors to gene promoters to affect expression and mediate the cytoprotective responses. Double-headed arrows represent kinase reactions that can occur in both directions (see text for details). Dashed arrows indicate attenuated activation, and arrows directed to the same point either have a role in binding together at the promoter or modulating the activity of one another.

7. Conclusions

Hemin is an essential cofactor for heme proteins that carry out a multitude of vital oxidative and oxygen transport-related functions in the cell. Unfortunately, hemin is also reactive and extremely harmful to cells when accumulated in the free form. A highly regulated system has evolved to control the levels of cellular heme. HO-1 and BVR catalyze the steps involved in heme catabolism. Interestingly, the enzymes are also involved in a host of cytoprotective functions mediating anti-oxidant, anti-apoptotic, anti-proliferative, and anti-inflammatory responses that have been proven to be therapeutic in many clinical disease models. HO-1 directly mediates most anti-oxidant effects through the following mechanisms: 1) the removal of heme in coordination with the up-regulation of the iron storage protein, ferritin; 2) the production of a lipophilic, anti-oxidant, biliverdin; 3) the regulation of both cell signaling and gene expression; and 4) the regulation of the cytochrome P450 system. Gene transcription mediated by Nrf2 largely mediates the cellular response to oxidative stress. BVR contributes to the antioxidant response by catalyzing a redox cycle that involves the BVR-mediated conversion of the potent antioxidant, bilirubin. In addition to catalyzing the second step of heme catabolism, BVR also acts as an upstream activator of MAPK and phosphatidylinositol-3-kinase pathway; directly binds to DNA; and participates in the transactivation of AP-1 sites in the HO-1 promoter. The anti-apoptotic effects associated with HO-1 induction are most often caused by BVR-mediated cell signaling and DNA-binding that leads to NFκB activation, but signaling effects related to HO-1-catalyzed CO production work in concert with the effects of BVR to protect against inflammation. Much remains to be learned about the specifics of cytoprotection via BVR-mediated signaling and gene transcription in addition to the roles of biliverdin and bilirubin in altering gene transcription. Similarly, because most in vitro studies of the enzymology of HO-1 have used a shortened mutant that does not bind to membrane or interact with membrane binding partners in the same manner as full length HO-1, almost nothing is known about how interactions between HO-1, BVR, and cytochrome P450 reductase are regulated to influence cell signaling, gene expression, the metabolism by HO-1, and oxidative stress related to P450-mediated, metabolism.

8. References

Abraham NG and Kappas A (2008) Pharmacological and clinical aspects of heme oxygenase. *Pharmacol.Rev.* 60:79-127.

Ahmad Z, Salim M, and Maines MD (2002) Human biliverdin reductase is a leucine zipper-like DNA-binding protein and functions in transcriptional activation of heme oxygenase-1 by oxidative stress. *J.Biol.Chem.* 277:9226-9232.

Alam J and Cook JL (2007) How many transcription factors does it take to turn on the heme oxygenase-1 gene? *Am.J.Respir.Cell Mol.Biol.* 36:166-174.

Alam J, Killeen E, Gong P, Naquin R, Stewart D, Ingelfinger JR, and Nath KA (2003) Heme activates the heme oxygenase-1 gene in renal epithelial cells by stabilizing Nrf2. *Am.J.Physiol.Renal Physiol.* 284:F743-F752.

Angel P and Karin M (1991) The role of Jun, Fos and the AP-1 complex in cell-proliferation and transformation. *Biochim.Biophys.Acta.* 1072:129-157.

Balla G, Vercellotti GM, Muller-Eberhard U, Eaton J, and Jacob HS (1991) Exposure of endothelial cells to free heme potentiates damage mediated by granulocytes and toxic oxygen species. *Lab Invest.* 64:648-655.

Baranano DE, Rao M, Ferris CD, and Snyder SH (2002) Biliverdin reductase: a major physiologic cytoprotectant. *Proc.Natl.Acad.Sci.USA* 99:16093-16098.

Bauer M and Bauer I (2002) Heme oxygenase-1: Redox Regulation and Role in the Hepatic Response to Oxidative Stress. *Antioxid.Redox.Signal.* 4:749-758.

Bellezza I, Mierla AL, and Minelli A (2010) Nrf2 and NF-κB and their concerted modulation in cancer pathogenesis and progression. *Cancers* 2:483-497.

Benbrook DM and Jones NC (1990) Heterodimer formation between CREB and JUN proteins. *Oncogene* 5:295-302.

Bissell DM and Hammaker LE (1976) Cytochrome P-450 Heme and the regulation of hepatic heme oxygenase activity. *Arch.Biochem.Biophys.* 176:91-102.

Bonizzi G and Karin M (2004) The two NF-kappaB activation pathways and their role in innate and adaptive immunity. *Trends Immunol.* 25:280-288.

Brouard S, Otterbein LE, Anrather J, Tobiasch E, Bach FH, Choi AM, and Soares MP (2000) Carbon monoxide generated by heme oxygenase 1 suppresses endothelial cell apoptosis. *J.Exp.Med.* 192:1015-1026.

Bubici, C., Papa, S., Dean, K., and Franzoso, G. Mutual cross-talk between reactive oxygen species and nuclear factor-kappa B: molecular basis and biological significance. Oncogene 25(51), 6731-6748. 2006.

Bulmer AC, Ried K, Blanchfield JT, and Wagner KH (2008) The anti-mutagenic properties of bile pigments. *Mutat.Res.* 658:28-41.

Cardell LO, Ueki IF, Stjärne P, Agusti C, Takeyama K, Lindén A, and Nadel JA (1998) Bronchodilatation in vivo by carbon monoxide, a cyclic GMP related messenger. *Br.J.Pharmacol.* 124:1065-1068.

Chen K, Gunter K, and Maines MD (2000) Neurons overexpressing heme oxygenase-1 resist oxidative stress-mediated cell death. *J.Neurochem.* 75:304-313.

Chen Q and Cederbaum AI (1998) Cytotoxicity and apoptosis produced by cytochrome P450 2E1 in Hep G2 cells. *Mol.Pharmacol.* 53:638-648.

Chiu H, Brittingham JA, and Laskin DL (2002) Differential induction of heme oxygenase-1 in macrophages and hepatocytes during acetaminophen-induced hepatotoxicity in the rat: effects of hemin and biliverdin. *Toxicol.Appl.Pharmacol.* 181:106-115.

Christodoulides N, Durante W, Kroll MH, and Chafer AI (1995) Vascular smooth muscle cell heme oxygenases generate guanylyl cyclase-stimulatory carbon monoxide. *Circulation* 91:2306-2309.

Chun KS, Keum.Y.S., Han SS, Song YS, Kim SH, and Surh YJ (2003) Curcumin inhibits phorbol ester-induced expression of cyclooxygenase-2 in mouse skin through suppression of extracellular signal-regulated kinase activity and NF-kappaB activation. *Carcinogenesis* 24:1515-1524.

Claireaux AE, Cole PG, and Lathe GH (1953) Icterus of the brain in the newborn. *Lancet* 265:1226-1230.

Clark JE, Foresti R, Sarathchandra P, Kaur H, Green CJ, and Motterlini R (2000) Heme oxygenase-1-derived bilirubin ameliorates postischemic myocardial dysfunction. *Am.J.Physiol.Heart Circ.Physiol.* 278:H643-H651.

Converso DP, Taillé C, Carreras MC, Jaitovich A, Poderoso JJ, and Boczkowski J (2006) HO-1 is located in liver mitochondria and modulates mitochondrial heme content and metabolism. *FASEB J.* 20:1236-1238.

Davies KJ, Delsignore ME, and Lin SW (1987) Protein damage and degradation by oxygen radicals. II. Modification of amino acids. *J.Biol.Chem.* 262:9902-9907.

Dennery PA, Spitz DR, Yang G, Tatarov A, Lee CS, Shegog ML, and Poss KD (1998) Oxygen toxicity and iron accumulation in the lungs of mice lacking heme oxygenase-2. *J.Clin.Invest.* 101:1001-1011.

Dérijard B, Raingeaud J, Barrett T, Wu IH, Han J, Ulevitch RJ, and Davis RJ (1995) Independent human MAP-kinase signal transduction pathways defined by MEK and MKK isoforms. *Science* 267:682-685.

Dore S, Takahashi M, Ferris CD, Zakhary R, Hester LD, Guastella D, and Snyder SH (1999) Bilirubin, formed by activation of heme oxygenase-2, protects neurons against oxidative stress injury. *Proc.Natl.Acad.Sci.U.S.A* 96:2445-2450.

Du W, Thanos D, and Maniatis T, (1993) Mechanisms of transcriptional synergism between distinct virus-inducible enhancer elements. *Cell* 74:887-898.

Eisenstein RS, Garcia-Mayol D, Pettingell W, and Munro HN (1991) Regulation of ferritin and heme oxygenase synthesis in rat fibroblasts by different forms of iron. *Proc.Natl.Acad.Sci.USA* 88:688-692.

Emerson MR and LeVine SM (2000) Heme oxygenase-1 and NADPH cytochrome P450 reductase expression in experimental allergic encephalomyelitis: an expanded view of the stress response. *J.Neurochem.* 75:2555-2562.

Fondevila C, Shen XD, Tsuchiyashi S, Yamashita K, Csizmadia E, Lassman C, Busuttil RW, Kupiec-Weglinski JW, and Bach FH (2004) Biliverdin therapy protects rat livers from ischemia and reperfusion injury. *Hepatology* 40:1333-1341.

Galliani G, Monti D, Speranza G, and Manitto P (1985) Biliverdin as an electron transfer catalyst for superoxide ion in aqueous medium. *Experientia* 41:1559-1560.

Gibbs PE and Maines MD (2007) Biliverdin inhibits activation of NF-kappaB: reversal of inhibition by human biliverdin reductase. *Int.J.Cancer* 121:2567-2574.

Gibbs PE, Miralem T, and Maines MD (2010) Characterization of the human biliverdin reductase gene structure and regulatory elements: promoter activity is enhanced by hypoxia and suppressed by TNF-alpha-activated NF-kappaB. *FASEB J.* 24:3239-3254.

Gibson JD, Pumford NR, Samokyszyn VM, and Hinson JA (1996) Mechanism of Acetaminophen-Induced Hepatotoxicity: Covalent Binding versus Oxidative Stress. *Chem.Res.Toxicol.* 9:580-585.

Gong P and Cederbaum AI (2006a) Nrf2 is increased by CYP2E1 in rodent liver and HepG2 cells and protects against oxidative stress caused by CYP2E1. *Hepatology* 43:144-153.

Gong P and Cederbaum AI (2006b) Transcription factor Nrf2 protects HepG2 cells against CYP2E1 plus arachidonic acid-dependent toxicity. *J.Biol.Chem.* 281:14573-14579.

Gong P, Cederbaum AI, and Nieto N (2004) Heme Oxygenase-1 Protects HEPG2 Cells against Cytochrome P450 2E1-dependent Toxicity. *Free Radical Biology and Medicine* 36:307-318.

Gorsky LD, Koop DR, and Coon MJ (1984) On the stoichiometry of the oxidase and monooxygenase reactions catalyzed by liver microsomal cytochrome P-450. Products of oxygen reduction. *J.Biol.Chem.* 259:6812-6817.

Gruenke LD, Konopka K, Cadieu M, and Waskell L (1995) The Stoichiometry of the Cytochrome P-450-catalyzed Metabolism of Methoxyflurane and Benzphetamine in the Presence and Absence of Cytochrome b(5). *J.Biol.Chem.* 270:24707.

Hangai-Hoger N, Tsai AG, Cabrales P, Suematsu M, and Intaglietta M (2007) Microvascular and systemic effects following top load administration of saturated carbon monoxide-saline solution. *Crit.Care Med.* 35:1123-1132.

Hayden MS and Ghosh S (2011) NF-κB in immunobiology. *Cell Res.* 21:223-244.

Herdegen T and Leah JD (1998) Inducible and constitutive transcription factors in the mammalian nervous system: control of gene expression by Jun, Fos and Krox, and CREB/ATF proteins. *Brain Res.Brain Res.Rev.* 28:370-490.

Herr I, van Dam H, and Angel P (1994) Binding of promoter-associated AP-1 is not altered during induction and subsequent repression of the c-jun promoter by TPA and UV irradiation. *Carcinogenesis* 15:1105-1113.

Hibi M, Lin A, Smeal T, Minden A, and Karin M (1993) Identification of an oncoprotein- and UV-responsive protein kinase that binds and potentiates the c-Jun activation domain. *Genes Dev.* 7:2135-2148.

Huber WJ, III and Backes WL (2007) Expression and characterization of full-length human heme oxygenase-1: the presence of intact membrane-binding region leads to increased binding affinity for NADPH cytochrome P450 reductase. *Biochem.* 46:12212-12219.

Huber WJ, III, Scruggs B, and Backes WL (2009) C-Terminal Membrane Spanning Region of Human Heme Oxygenase-1 Mediates a Time Dependent Complex Formation with Cytochrome P450 Reductase. *Biochem.* 48:190-197.

Immenschuh S, Hinke V, Ohlmann A, Gifhorn-Katz S, Katz N, Jungermann K, and Kietzmann T (1998a) Transcriptional activation of the haem oxygenase-1 gene by cGMP via a cAMP response element/activator protein-1 element in primary cultures of rat hepatocytes. *Biochem.J.* 334:141-146.

Immenschuh S, Kietzmann T, Hinke V, Wiederhold M, Katz N, and Muller-Eberhard U (1998b) The rat heme oxygenase-1 gene is transcriptionally induced via the protein kinase A signaling pathway in rat hepatocyte cultures. *Mol Pharmacol* 53:483-491.

Inoue S, Suzuki M, Nagashima Y, Suzuki S, Hashiba T, Tsuburai T, Ikehara K, Matsuse T, and Ishigatsubo Y (2001) Transfer of heme oxygenase 1 cDNA by a replication-deficient adenovirus enhances interleukin 10 production from alveolar macrophages that attenuates lipopolysaccharide-induced acute lung injury in mice. *Hum.Gene Ther.* 12:967-979.

Ishii T, Itoh K, Takahashi S, Sato H, Yanagawa T, Katoh Y, Bannai S, and Yamamoto M (2000) Transcription factor Nrf2 coordinately regulates a group of oxidative stress-inducible genes in macrophages. *J.Biol.Chem.* 275:16023-16029.

Ishii T, Itoh K, and Yamamoto M (2002) Roles of Nrf2 in activation of antioxidant enzyme genes via antioxidant responsive elements. *Methods Enzymol.* 348:190.

Ishikawa M, Kajimura M, Adachi T, Makino N, Goda N, Yamaguchi T, Sekizuka E, and Suematsu M (2005) Carbon monoxide from heme oxygenase-2 Is a tonic regulator against NO-dependent vasodilatation in the adult rat cerebral microcirculation. *Circ.Res.* 97:e104-e114.

Itoh K, Chiba T, Takahashi S, Ishii T, Igarashi K, Katoh Y, Oyake T, Hayashi N, Satoh K, Hatayama I, Yamamoto M, and Nabeshima Y (1997) An Nrf2/small Maf heterodimer mediates the induction of phase II detoxifying enzyme genes through antioxidant response elements. *Biochem.Biophys.Res.Commun.* 236:313-322.

Itoh K, Wakabayashi N, Katoh Y, Ishii T, O'Connor T, and Yamamoto M (2003) Keap1 regulates both cytoplasmic-nuclear shuttling and degradation of Nrf2 in response to electrophiles. *Genes Cells* 8:379-391.

Jackson JH, Schraufstatter IU, Hyslop PA, Vosbeck K, Sauerheber R, Weitzman SA, and Cochrane CG (1987) Role of hydroxyl radical in DNA damage. *Trans.Assoc.Am.Physicians* 100:147-157.

Kapitulnik J and Maines MD (2009) Pleiotropic functions of biliverdin reductase: cellular signaling and generation of cytoprotective and cytotoxic bilirubin. *Cell* 30:129-137.

Kaszubska W, Hooft van Huijsduijnen R, Ghersa P, DeRaemy-Schenk AM, Chen BP, Hai T, DeLamarter JF, and Whelan J (1993) Cyclic AMP-independent ATF family members interact with NF-kappa B and function in the activation of the E-selectin promoter in response to cytokines. *Mol.Cell Biol.* 13:180-190.

Kawamura K, Ishikawa K, Wada Y, Matsumoto H, Kohro T, Itabe H, Kodama T, and Maruyama Y (2005) Bilirubin from heme oxygenase-1 attenuates vascular endothelial activation and dysfunction. *Arterioscler.Thromb.Vasc.Biol.* 25:155-160.

Kawashima A, Oda Y, Yachie A, Koizumi S, and Nakanishi I (2002) Heme oxygenase-1 deficiency: the first autopsy case. *Hum.Pathol.* 33:125-130.

Keum YS, Yu S, Chang PP, Yuan X, Kim JH, Xu C, Han J, Agarwal A, and Kong AN (2006) Mechanism of action of sulforaphane: inhibition of p38 mitogen-activated protein kinase isoforms contributing to the induction of antioxidant response element-mediated heme oxygenase-1 in human hepatoma HepG2 cells. *Cancer Res.* 66:8804-8813.

Keyse SM and Tyrrell RM (1989) Heme oxygenase is the major 32-kDa stress protein induced in human skin fibroblasts by UVA radiation, hydrogen peroxide, and sodium arsenite. *Proc.Natl.Acad.Sci.U.S.A* 86:99-103.

Kikuchi G, Yoshida T, and Noguchi M (2005) Heme oxygenase and heme degradation. *Biochem.Biophys.Res.Commun.* 338:558-567.

Kim HJ, So HS, Lee JH, Park C, Park SY, Kim YH, Youn MJ, Kim SJ, Chung SY, Lee KM, and Park R (2006) Heme oxygenase-1 attenuates the cisplatin-induced apoptosis of auditory cells via down-regulation of reactive oxygen species generation. *Free Radic.Biol.Med.* 40:1810-1819.

Kim HP, Wang X, Galbiati F, Ryter SW, and Choi AM (2004) Caveolae compartmentalization of heme oxygenase-1 in endothelial cells. *FASEB J.* 18:1080-1089.

Kravets A, Hu Z, Miralem T, Torno MD, and Maines MD (2004) Biliverdin reductase, a novel regulator for induction of activating transcription factor-2 and heme oxygenase-1. *J.Biol.Chem.* 279:19916-19923.

Kruger AL, Peterson S, Turkseven S, Kaminski PM, Zhang FF, Quan S, Wolin MS, and Abraham NG (2005) D-4F induces heme oxygenase-1 and extracellular superoxide dismutase, decreases endothelial cell sloughing, and improves vascular reactivity in rat model of diabetes. *Circulation* 111:3126-3134.

Kumar S and Bandyopadhyay U (2005) Free heme toxicity and its detoxification systems in human. *Toxicol.Lett.* 157:175-188.

Kutty RK, Daniel RF, Ryan DE, Levin W, and Maines MD (1988) Rat liver cytochrome P-450b, P-420b, and P-450c are degraded to biliverdin by heme oxygenase. *Arch.Biochem.Biophys.* 260:638-644.

Kutty RK and Maines MD (1984) Hepatic heme metabolism: possible role of biliverdin in the regulation of heme oxygenase activity. *Biochem.Biophys.Res.Commun.* 122:40-46.

Kwak JY, Takeshige K, Cheung BS, and Minakami S (1991) Bilirubin inhibits the activation of superoxide-producing NADPH oxidase in a neutrophil cell-free system. *Biochim.Biophys.Acta.* 1076:369-373.

Kwak MK, Wakabayashi N, and Kensler TW (2004) Chemoprevention through the Keap1-Nrf2 signaling pathway by phase 2 enzyme inducers. *Mutat.Res.* 555:133-148.

Lee MY, Jung CH, Lee K, Choi YH, Hong S, and Cheong J (2002) Activating transcription factor-2 mediates transcriptional regulation of gluconeogenic gene PEPCK by retinoic acid. *Diabetes* 5:3400-3407.

Lerner-Marmarosh N, Miralem T, Gibbs PE, and Maines MD (2007) Regulation of TNF-alpha-activated PKC-zeta signaling by the human biliverdin reductase: identification of activating and inhibitory domains of the reductase. *FASEB J.* 21:3949-3962.

Lerner-Marmarosh N, Miralem T, Gibbs PE, and Maines MD (2008) Human biliverdin reductase is an ERK activator; hBVR is an ERK nuclear transporter and is required for MAPK signaling. *Proc.Natl.Acad.Sci.USA* 105:6870-6875.

Lerner-Marmarosh N, Shen J, Torno MD, Kravets A, Hu Z, and Maines MD (2005) Human biliverdin reductase: a member of the insulin receptor substrate family with serine/threonine/tyrosine kinase activity. *Proc.Natl.Acad.Sci.USA* 102:7109-7114.

Lin Q, Weis S, Yang G, Weng YH, Helston R, Rish K, Smith A, Bordner J, Polte T, Gaunitz F, and Dennery PA (2007) Heme oxygenase-1 protein localizes to the nucleus and activates transcription factors important in oxidative stress. *J.Biol.Chem.*

Lin QS, Weis S, Zhuang T, Abate A, and Dennery PA (2008) Catalytic inactive heme oxygenase-1 protein regulates its own expression in oxidative stress. *Free Radic.Biol.Med.* 44:847-855.

Liu Y, Moenne-Loccoz P, Loehr TM, and Ortiz de Montellano PR (1997) Heme oxygenase-1, intermediates in verdoheme formation and the requirement for reduction equivalents. *J.Biol.Chem.* 272:6909-6917.

Liu Y and Ortiz de Montellano PR (2000) Reaction intermediates and single turnover rate constants for the oxidation of heme by human heme oxygenase-1. *J.Biol.Chem.* 275:5297-5307.

Maghzal GJ, Leck MC, Collinson E, Li C, and Stocker R (2009) Limited role for the bilirubin-biliverdin redox amplification cycle in the cellular antioxidant protection by biliverdin reductase. *J.Biol.Chem.* 284:2925-29259.

Maines MD (1988) Heme oxygenase: function, multiplicity, regulatory mechanisms, and clinical applications. *FASEB J.* 2:2557-2568.

Maines MD, Ewing JF, Huang TJ, and Panahian N (2001) Nuclear localization of biliverdin reductase in the rat kidney: response to nephrotoxins that induce heme oxygenase-1. *J.Pharmacol.Exp.Ther.* 296:1091-1097.

Maines MD, Miralem T, Lerner-Marmarosh N, Shen J, and Gibbs PE (2007) Human biliverdin reductase, a previously unknown activator of protein kinase C betaII. *J.Biol.Chem.* 282:810-822.

Maines MD, Trakshel GM, and Kutty RK (1986) Characterization of two constitutive forms of rat liver microsomal heme oxygenase. Only one molecular species of the enzyme is inducible. *J.Biol.Chem.* 261:411-419.

Mancuso C and Barone E (2009) The heme oxygenase/biliverdin reductase pathway in drug research and development. *Curr.Drug Metab.* 10:579-594.

Martin D, Rojo AI, Salinas M, Diaz R, Gallardo G, Alam J, De Galarreta CM, and Cuadrado A (2004) Regulation of heme oxygenase-1 expression through the phosphatidylinositol 3-kinase/Akt pathway and the Nrf2 transcription factor in response to the antioxidant phytochemical carnosol. *J.Biol.Chem.* 279:8919-8929.

McCord JM (1993) Oxygen-derived free radicals. *New Horiz.* 1:70-76.

Miralem T, Hu Z, Torno MD, Lelli KM, and Maines MD (2005) Small interference RNA-mediated gene silencing of human biliverdin reductase, but not that of heme oxygenase-1, attenuates arsenite-mediated induction of the oxygenase and increases apoptosis in 293A kidney cells. *J.Biol.Chem.* 280:17084-17092.

Morse D, Pischke SE, Zhou Z, Davis RJ, Flavell RA, Loop T, Otterbein SL, Otterbein LE, and Choi AM (2003) Suppression of inflammatory cytokine production by carbon monoxide involves the JNK pathway and AP-1. *J.Biol.Chem.* 278:36993-36998.

Motterlini R, Mann BE, Johnson TR, Clark JE, Foresti R, and Green CJ (2003) Bioactivity and pharmacological actions of carbon monoxide-releasing molecules. *Curr.Pharm.Des.* 9:2525-2539.

Murphy K, Haudek SB, Thompson M, and Giroir BP (1998) Molecular biology of septic shock. *New Horiz.* 6:181-193.

Nakahira K, Takahashi T, Shimizu H, Maeshima K, Uehara K, Fujii H, Nakatsuka H, Yokoyama M, Akagi R, and Morita K (2003) Protective role of heme oxygenase-1 induction in carbon tetrachloride-induced hepatotoxicity. *Biochem.Pharmacol.* 66:1091-1105.

Neuzil J and Stocker R (1993) Bilirubin attenuates radical-mediated damage to serum albumin. *FEBS Lett.* 331:281-284.

Noguchi M, Yoshida T, and Kikuchi G (1979) Purification and properties of biliverdin reductases from pig spleen and rat liver. *J.Biochem.* 86:833-848.

Odaka Y, Takahashi T, Yamasaki A, Suzuki T, Fujiwara T, Yamada T, Hirakawa M, Fujita H, Ohmori E, and Akagi R (2000) Prevention of halothane-induced hepatotoxicity by hemin pretreatment: protective role of heme oxygenase-1 induction. *Biochem.Pharmacol.* 59:871-880.

Ossola JO and Tomaro ML (1995) Heme oxygenase induction by cadmium chloride: evidence for oxidative stress involvement. *Toxicology* 104:141-147.

Otterbein L, Sylvester SL, and Choi AM (1995) Hemoglobin provides protection against lethal endotoxemia in rats: the role of heme oxygenase-1. *Am.J.Respir.Cell Mol.Biol.* 13:595-601.

Otterbein LE, Bach FH, Alam J, Soares M, Tao LH, Wysk M, Davis RJ, Flavell RA, and Choi AM (2000) Carbon monoxide has anti-inflammatory effects involving the mitogen-activated protein kinase pathway. *Nat.Med.* 6:422-428.

Pachori AS, Smith A, McDonald P, Zhang L, Dzau VJ, and Melo LG (2007) Heme-oxygenase-1-induced protection against hypoxia/reoxygenation is dependent on biliverdin reductase and its interaction with PI3K/Akt pathway. *J.Mol.Cell Cardiol.* 43:580-592.

Paller MS and Jacob HS (1994) Cytochrome P-450 mediates tissue-damaging hydroxyl radical formation during reoxygenation of the kidney. *Proc.Natl.Acad.Sci.USA* 91:7002-7006.

Papa S, Bubici C, Zazzeroni F, Pham CG, Kuntzen C, Dean K, and Franzoso G (2006) The NF-kappaB-mediated control of the JNK cascade in the antagonism of programmed cell death in health and disease. *Cell Death Differ.* 13:712-729.

Parfenova H, Basuroy S, Bhattacharya S, Tcheranova D, Qu Y, Regan RF, and Leffler CW (2006) Glutamate induces oxidative stress and apoptosis in cerebral vascular endothelial cells: contributions of HO-1 and HO-2 to cytoprotection. *Am.J.Physiol.Cell Physiol.* 290:C1399-C1410.

Park SY, Lee SW, Baek SH, Lee SJ, Lee WS, Rhim BY, Hong KW, and Kim CD (2011) Induction of heme oxygenase-1 expression by cilostazol contributes to its anti-inflammatory effects in J774 murine macrophages. *Immunol.Lett.* 136:138-145.

Patel VC, Yellon DM, Singh KJ, Neild GH, and Woolfson RG (1993) Inhibition of nitric oxide limits infarct size in the in situ rabbit heart. *Biochem.Biophys.Res.Commun.* 194:234-238.

Pawson T and Scott JD (2005) Protein phosphorylation in signaling--50 years and counting. *Trends Biochem.Sci.* 30:286-290.

Peng HB, Libby P, and Liao JK (1995) Induction and stabilization of I kappa B alpha by nitric oxide mediates inhibition of NF-kappa B. *J.Biol.Chem.* 270:14214-14219.

Peterson JA, Ebel RE, O'Keeffe DH, Matsubara T, and Estabrook RW (1976) Temperature dependence of cytochrome P-450 reduction. A model for NADPH-cytochrome P-450 reductase:cytochrome P-450 interaction. *J.Biol.Chem.* 251:4010-4016.

Phelan D, Winter GM, Rogers WJ, Lam JC, and Denison MS (1998) Activation of the Ah receptor signal transduction pathway by bilirubin and biliverdin. *Arch.Biochem.Biophys.* 357:155-163.

Piantadosi CA (2008) Carbon monoxide, reactive oxygen signaling, and oxidative stress. *Free Radic.Biol.Med.* 45:562-569.

Piantadosi CA and Zhang J (1996) Mitochondrial generation of reactive oxygen species after brain ischemia in the rat Mitochondrial generation of reactive oxygen species after brain ischemia in the rat. *Stroke* 27:327-31; discussion 332.

Pischke SE, Zhou Z, Song R, Ning W, Alam J, Ryter SW, and Choi AM (2005) Phosphatidylinositol 3-kinase/Akt pathway mediates heme oxygenase-1 regulation by lipopolysaccharide. *Cell Mol.Biol.* 51:461-470.

Ponka P (1997) Tissue-specific regulation of iron metabolism and heme synthesis: distinct control mechanisms in erythroid cells. *Blood* 89:1-25.

Poss KD, Thomas MJ, Ebralidz AK, O'Dell TJ, and Tonegawa S (1995) Hippocampal long-term potentiation is normal in heme oxygenase-2 mutant mice. *Neuron.* 15:867-873.

Poss KD and Tonegawa S (1997a) Heme oxygenase 1 is required for mammalian iron reutilization. *Proc.Natl.Acad.Sci.U.S.A.* 94:10919-10924.

Poss KD and Tonegawa S (1997b) Reduced stress defense in heme oxygenase-1 deficient cells. *Proc.Natl.Acad.Sci.U.S A.* 94:10925-10930.

Pugazhenthi S, Akhov L, Selvaraj G, Wang M, and Alam J (2007) Regulation of heme oxygenase-1 expression by demethoxy curcuminoids through Nrf2 by a PI3-kinase/Akt-mediated pathway in mouse beta-cells. *Am.J.Physiol.Endocrinol.Metab.* 293:E645-E655.

Reed JR, Cawley GF, and Backes WL (2011) Inhibition of cytochrome P450 1A2-mediated metabolism and production of reactive oxygen species by heme oxygenase-1 in rat liver microsomes. *Drug Metab Lett.* 5:6-16.

Reed JR and Hollenberg PF (2003) Comparison of substrate metabolism by cytochromes P450 2B1, 2B4, and 2B6: relationship of heme spin state, catalysis, and the effects of cytochrome b5. *Journal of Inorganic Biochemistry* 93:152-160.

Reed JR, Huber WJ, III, and Backes WL (2010) Human heme oxygenase-1 efficiently catabolizes heme in the absence of biliverdin reductase. *Drug Metab Dispos.* 38:2060-2066.

Robertson P, Jr. and Fridovich I (1982) A reaction of the superoxide radical with tetrapyrroles. *Arch.Biochem.Biophys.* 213:353-357.

Rotenberg MO and Maines MD (1991) Characterization of a cDNA-encoding rabbit brain heme oxygenase-2 and identification of a conserved domain among mammalian heme oxygenase isozymes: possible heme-binding site? *Arch.Biochem.Biophys.* 290:336-344.

Ryan KM, Ernst MK, Rice NR, and Vousden KH (2000) Role of NF-kappaB in p53-mediated programmed cell death. *Nature* 404:892-897.

Ryter SW, Alam J, and Choi MK (2006) Heme oxygenase-1/carbon monoxide: From basic science to therapeutic applications. *Physiol.Rev.* 86:583-650.

Salim M, Brown-Kipphut BA, and Maines MD (2001) Human biliverdin reductase is autophosphorylated, and phosphorylation is required for bilirubin formation. *J.Biol.Chem.* 276:10929-10934.

Schlichting I, Berendzen J, Chu K, Stock AM, Maves SA, Benson DE, Sweet RM, Ringe D, Petsko GA, and Sligar SG (2000) The catalytic pathway of cytochrome p450cam at atomic resolution. *Science* 287:1615-1622.

Sen CK, Traber KE, and Packer L (1996) Inhibition of NF-kappa B activation in human T-cell lines by anetholdithiolthione. *Biochem.Biophys.Res.Commun.* 218:148-153.

Sheftel AD, Kim SF, and Ponka P (2007) Non-heme induction of heme oxygenase-1 does not alter cellular iron metabolism. *J.Biol.Chem.* 282:10480-10486.

Shen G, Jeong WS, Hu R, and Kong AN (2005) Regulation of Nrf2, NF-kappaB, and AP-1 signaling pathways by chemopreventive agents. *Antioxid.Redox.Signal.* 7:1648-1663.

Song R, Kubo M, Morse D, Zhou Z, Zhang X, Dauber JH, Fabisiak J, Alber SM, Watkins SC, Zuckerbraun BS, Otterbein LE, Ning W, Oury TD, Lee PJ, McCurry KR, Choi AM. (2003a) Carbon monoxide induces cytoprotection in rat orthotopic lung transplantation via anti-inflammatory and anti-apoptotic effects. *Am.J.Pathol.* 163:231-242.

Song R, Ning W, Liu F, Ameredes BT, Calhoun WJ, Otterbein LE, and Choi AM (2003b) Regulation of IL-1beta -induced GM-CSF production in human airway smooth muscle cells by carbon monoxide. *Am.J.Physiol.Lung Cell Mol.Physiol.* 284:L50-L56.

Stocker R and Ames BN (1987) Potential role of conjugated bilirubin and copper in the metabolism of lipid peroxides in bile. *Proc.Natl.Acad.Sci.USA* 84:8130-8134.

Stocker R, Glazer AN, and Ames BN (1987) Antioxidant activity of albumin-bound bilirubin. *Proc.Natl.Acad.Sci.USA* 84:5918-5922.

Stocker R and Peterhans E (1989) Synergistic interaction between vitamin E and the bile pigments bilirubin and biliverdin. *Biochim.Biophys.Acta.* 1002:238-244.

Sun Jang J, Piao S, Cha YN, and Kim C (2009) Taurine Chloramine Activates Nrf2, Increases HO-1 Expression and Protects Cells from Death Caused by Hydrogen Peroxide. *J.Clin.Biochem.Nutr.* 45:37-43.

Sun J, Hoshino H, Takaku K, Nakajima O, Muto A, Suzuki H, Takahashi S, Shibahara S, Alam J, Taketo MM, Yamamoto M, and Igarashi K (2002) Hemoprotein Bach1 regulates enhancer availability of heme oxygenase-1 gene. *EMBO J.* 21:5216-5224.

Suttner DM and Dennery PA (1999) Reversal of HO-1 related cytoprotection with increased expression is due to reactive iron. *FASEB J.* 13:1800-1809.

Taillé C, Almolki A, Benhamed M, Zedda C, Mégret J, Berger P, Lesèche G, Fadel E, Yamaguchi T, Marthan R, Aubier M, and Boczkowski J (2003) Heme oxygenase inhibits human airway smooth muscle proliferation via a bilirubin-dependent modulation of ERK1/2 phosphorylation. *J.Biol.Chem.* 278:27160-27168.

Tamion F, Richard V, Renet S, and Thuillez C (2006) Protective effects of heme-oxygenase expression against endotoxic shock: inhibition of tumor necrosis factor-alpha and augmentation of interleukin-10. *J.Trauma* 61:1078-1084.

Tan J, Kuang W, Jin Z, Jin F, Yu Q, Kong L, Zeng G, Yuan X, and Duan Y (2009) Inhibition of NFkappaB by activated c-Jun NH2 terminal kinase 1 acts as a switch for C2C12 cell death under excessive stretch. *Apoptosis* 14:764-770.

Tang LM, Wang YP, Wang K, Pu LY, Zhang F, Li XC, Kong LB, Sun BC, Li GQ, and Wang XH (2007) Exogenous biliverdin ameliorates ischemia-reperfusion injury in small-for-size rat liver grafts. *Transplant.Proc.* 39:1338-1344.

Terelius Y and Ingelman-Sundberg M (1988) Cytochrome P-450-dependent oxidase activity and hydroxyl radical production in micellar and membranous types of reconstituted systems. *Biochem.Pharmacol.* 37:1383-1389.

Toda K, Yang LX, and Shizuta Y (1995) Transcriptional regulation of the human aromatase cytochrome P450 gene expression in human placental cells. *J.Steroid Biochem.Mol.Biol.* 53:181-190.

Toda N, Takahashi T, Mizobuchi S, F ujii H, T akahira K, N akahashi S, amashita M, M orita K, H irakawa M, and A kagi R (2002) Tin chloride pretreatment prevents renal injury in rats with ischemic acute renal failure. *Crit.Care Med.* 30:1512-1522.

Tsuji Y, Ayaki H, Whitman SP, Morrow CS, T orti SV, and T orti FM (2000) Coordinate transcriptional and translational regulation of ferritin in response to oxidative stress. *Mol.Cell Biol.* 20:5818-5827.

Tudor C, Lerner-Marmarosh N, Engelborghs Y, Gibbs PE, and Maines MD (2008) Biliverdin reductase is a transporter of haem into the nucleus and is essential for regulation of HO-1 gene expression by haematin. *Biochem.J.* 413:405-416.

Vincent SH (1989) Oxidative effects of heme and porphyrins on proteins and lipids. *Semin.Hematol.* 26:105-113.

Wada T and Penninger JM (2004) Mitogen-activated protein kinases in apoptosis regulation. *Oncogene* 23:2838-2849.

Wagener FADTG, Eggert A, Boerman OC, Oyen WJ, Verhofstad A, Abraham NG, Adema G, van Kooyk Y, de Witte T, and Figdor CG (2001) Heme is a potent inducer of inflammation in mice and is counteracted by heme oxygenase. *Blood* 98:1802-1811.

Wang WW, Smith DL, and Zucker SD (2004) Bilirubin inhibits iNOS expression and NO production in response to endotoxin in rats. *Hepatology* 40:424-433.

Wen T, Wu ZM, Liu Y, Tan YF, Ren F, and Wu H (2007) Upregulation of heme oxygenase-1 with hemin prevents D-galactosamine and lipopolysaccharide-induced acute hepatic injury in rats. *Toxicology* 237:184-193.

White RE and Coon MJ (1980) Oxygen activation by cytochrome P-450. *Annu.Rev Biochem.* 49:315-356.

Williams SE, Wootton P, Mason HS, Bould J, Iles DE, Riccardi D, Peers C, and Kemp PJ (2004) Hemoxygenase-2 is an oxygen sensor for a calcium-sensitive potassium channel. *Science* 306:2093-2097.

Wright MM, Schopfer FJ, Vidyasagar V, Powell P, Chumley P, Iles KE, Freeman BA, and Agarwal A (2006) Fatty acid transduction of nitric oxide signaling: nitrolinoleic acid potently activates endothelial heme oxygenase 1 expression. *Proc.Natl.Acad.Sci.* 103:4299-4304.

Yachie A, Niida Y, Wada T, Igarashi N, Kaneda H, Toma T, Ohta K, Kasahara Y, and Koizumi S (1999) Oxidative stress causes enhanced endothelial cell injury in human heme oxygenase-1 deficiency. *J.Clin.Invest* 103:129-135.

Yang L, Quan S, and Abraham NG (1999) Retrovirus-mediated HO gene transfer into endothelial cells protects against oxidant-induced injury. *Am.J.Physiol.* 277:127-133.

Yao P, Hao L, Nussler N, Lehmann A, Song F, Zhao J, Neuhaus P, Liu L, and Nussler A (2009) The protective role of HO-1 and its generated products (CO, bilirubin, and Fe) in ethanol-induced human hepatocyte damage. *Am.J.Physiol.Gastrointest.Liver Physiol.* 296:G1318-1323.

Yao P, Nussler A, Liu L, Hao L, Song F, Schirmeier A, and Nussler N (2007) Quercetin protects human hepatocytes from ethanol-derived oxidative stress by inducing heme oxygenase-1 via the MAPK/Nrf2 pathways. *J.Hepatol.* 47:253-261.

Yoneya R, Ozasa H, Nagashima Y, Koike Y, Teraoka H, Hagiwara K, and Horikawa S (2000) Hemin pretreatment ameliorates aspects of the nephropathy induced by mercuric chloride in the rat. *Toxicol.Lett.* 116:223-229.

Yoshioka K, Deng T, Cavigelli M, and Karin M (1995) Antitumor promotion by phenolic antioxidants: inhibition of AP-1 activity through induction of Fra expression. *Proc.Natl.Acad.Sci.USA* 92:4972-4976.

Young SC, Storm MV, Speed JS, Kelsen S, Tiller CV, Vera T, Drummond HA, and Stec DE (2009) Inhibition of biliverdin reductase increases ANG II-dependent superoxide levels in cultured renal tubular epithelial cells. *Am.J.Physiol.Integr.Comp.Physiol.* 297:R1546-R1553.

Zangar RC, Davydov DR, and Verma S (2004) Mechanisms that regulate production of reactive oxygen species by cytochrome P450. *Toxicol.Appl.Pharmacol.* 199:316-331.

Zhang J, Ohta T, Maruyama A, Hosoya T, Nishikawa K, Maher JM, Shibahara S, Itoh K, and Yamamoto M (2006) BRG1 interacts with Nrf2 to selectively mediate HO-1 induction in response to oxidative stress. *Mol.Cell Biol.* 26:7942-7952.

25

Antibothropic Action of *Camellia sinensis* Extract Against the Neuromuscular Blockade by *Bothrops jararacussu* Snake Venom and Its Main Toxin, Bothropstoxin-I

Yoko Oshima-Franco et al.*
University of Sorocaba/UNISO, Brazil

1. Introduction

Snake bite envenoming, a serious public health problem in rural areas of tropical and subtropical countries, was included in 2007 as a neglected disease by the World Health Organization (WHO, 2007). Under this geographical perspective Africa, Asia, Oceania and Latin America are the most vulnerable countries to this kind of accident, but also shared by many developing countries (Harrison et al., 2009; Warrel, 2010). An excellent meta-analytic approach about the subject was described by Chippaux (2011), who analysed more than 3,000 references for estimating the burden of snakebites in sub-Saharan Africa. Brazil encloses both requirements, as a developing and a tropical country, and needs to strengthen measures against venomous snake accidents, since, according to Lima et al. (2009), it is the country with the major number of accidents (about 20,000 cases/year), followed by Peru (4,500), Venezuela (2,500-3,000), Colombia (2,675), Ecuador (1,200-1,400) and Argentina (1,150-1.250) (Warrel, 2004).

As mentioned by Nicoleti et al. (2010), venomous snakes in Brazil are represented by *Bothrops, Bothropoides, Bothriopsis, Bothrocophias, Rhinocerophis, Crotalus, Lachesis, Leptomicrurus* and *Micrurus* (see the new taxonomic arrangement proposed by Fenwick et al., 2009). Envenoming by the first five genera produce similar toxic manifestations and treatment assessment are quite the same. They represent 86.9% of accidents, whereas 8.7% were caused by *Crotalus*, 3.6% *Lachesis* and 0.8% by *Leptomicrurus* and *Micrurus* (Ministério da Saúde, 2004).

Bothrops jararacussu snake belongs to the Viperidae family and its venom is able to induce severe signs of local and systemic envenoming, such as necrosis, shock, spontaneous

---

*Luana de Jesus Reis Rosa[1], Gleidy Ana Araujo Silva[1], Jorge Amaral Filho[1], Magali Glauzer Silva[1], Patricia Santos Lopes[2], José Carlos Cogo[3], Adélia Cristina Oliveira Cintra[4] and Maria Alice da Cruz-Höfling[5]
[1]*University of Sorocaba/UNISO, Brazil*
[2]*Federal University of São Paulo/UNIFESP, Brazil*
[3]*University of Vale do Paraiba/UNIVAP, Brazil*
[4]*University of São Paulo/USP, Brazil*
[5]*University of Campinas/UNICAMP/I.B./D.H.E., Brazil*

systemic bleeding and renal failure, incoagulable blood and death (Milani et al., 1997); its venom also blocks *in vitro* the contractile skeletal muscle response (Rodrigues-Simioni et al., 1983). Two myotoxins are responsible for myonecrosis: bothropstoxin-I (Homsi-Brandeburgo et al., 1988), the first myotoxin isolated from the venom that reproduces the effects of the crude venom (Heluany et al., 1992), further characterized as a phospholipase A_2-Lys49 (Cintra et al., 1993); and bothropstoxin-II, a phospholipase A_2 (Gutiérrez et al., 1991), further characterized as an Asp49-PLA_2 myotoxin with low catalytic activity (Pereira et al., 1998), although phylogenetically it is more related to Lys49-PLA_2s than to other Asp49-PLA_2s (dos Santos et al., 2011).

Snake antivenom immunoglobulins (antivenoms) are the only specific treatment for envenoming by snakebites. They are produced by fractionation of plasma usually obtained from large domestic animals hyper-immunized against relevant snake venoms. When injected into an envenomed human patient, antivenom will neutralize any of the effects of the venoms used in its production, and in some instances will also neutralize effects of venoms from closely related species (WHO, 2011a). However, the antibothropic serum effectiveness against the local effects of *Bothrops jararacussu* venom (one of the bothropic venoms used in the serum production) has been debated since the 80's decade (see Correa-Neto et al., 2010). A possible explanation for the lack of effectivenes was given by Battellino et al. (2003) through the use of intravital microscopy after intravenous administration of antibothropic antivenom (BAv), labeled with fluorescein isothiocyanate (FITC). They observed that the antivenom neutralized the systemic effects, but did not efficiently reverse the local effects due to an impaired and/or delayed venom:antivenom interaction at the site of injury. Considering that local effect of venomous snakebites are poorly prevented by specific antivenom, that the access to public health services by people of distant rural regions in tropical and subtropical countries is in general difficult, the use of medicinal plants as a local solution has been a practice of natives of those regions.

Medicinal plants represent a sophisticated biotechnological laboratory that is able to produce a multitude of pharmacologically bioactive substances, with a wide variety of effects (Mahmood et al., 2005). The second beverage (next to water) of major consumption in the world, in its green, black and oolong forms, is the tea from *Camellia sinensis* L. leaves Compounds as polyphenols, polysaccharides, aminoacids, vitamins (Crespy & Williamson, 2004), caffeine and a very small amout of methylxanthines (Yang et al., 1998) can be found in the plant. Catechins, the major component of green tea (fresh leaves are steamed to prevent fermentation, yielding a dry, stable product), and represent the low-molecular-weight polyphenols consisting mainly of flavanol (flavan-3-ol) monomers, such as epicatechin, epicatechin-3-gallate, epigallocatechin and the major, 50-80% of the total catechin, epigallocatechin-3-gallate (Graham, 1992; Khan & Mukhtar, 2007). Catechins account for 6-16% (Zhu & Chen, 1999) up to 30-40% (Phithayanukul et al., 2010) of the dry green tea leaves. The fermentation or semifermentation stage (when the withered leaves are rolled and crushed) during the manufacture of black or oolong tea, respectively, converts catechins to theaflavins (theaflavin, theaflavin-3-gallate, theaflavin-3'-gallate and theaflavin-3,3'-digallate, accounting for 3-6% of solid extract) and thearubigins (accounting for 12-18% of solid extract) (Leung et al., 2001; Khan & Mukhtar, 2007), which are complex polyphenols of poorly-defined chemical structures formed during fermentation of polymerization of theaflavins (Hazarika et al., 1984).

The literature describing the medicinal benefits of tea is extensive, but the report about its consumption to alleviate post game fatigue in players and sportsmen (Krishnamoorthy, 1991) inspired further studies on the mammalian skeletomotor apparatus (Das et al., 1994; 1997). For example, Basu et al. (2005) attributed to theaflavin, but not thearubigin, the facilitatory effect induced at the skeletal myoneural junction. This experimental model has been traditionally used for the pharmacological characterization of snake venoms, and the association between *C. sinensis* and snake venoms was a natural consequence. Thus, results showing the inhibitory effect of tea polyphenols on local tissue damage induced by snake venoms (Pithayanukul et al., 2010), and the inhibitory effect of *Camellia sinensis* leaves extracts against the neuromuscular blockade of *Crotalus durissus terrificus* venom (de Jesus Reis Rosa et al., 2010) were recently published. Here, using the same experimental procedure, the antivenom property of *Camellia sinensis* leaves extract was assayed against *Bothrops jararacussu* venom and its main myotoxin, bothropstoxin-I. Commercial theaflavin (from black tea) and epigallocatechin gallate (from green tea), known to be part of the *C. sinensis* extract, were also tested.

2. Materials and methods

2.1 Hydroalcoholic extract from leaves of *Camellia sinensis*

The leaves of *C. sinensis* were harvested from plants growing in an orchard at the University of Sorocaba - UNISO (Sorocaba, SP, Brazil). A voucher specimen was deposited in the Instituto Agronômico de Campinas (IAC, number 50.469) herbarium (http://herbario.iac.sp.gov.br) after identification by L.C. Bernacci. Briefly, sixty-four grams of leaves powder were macerated along with 150 mL of 70° GL ethanol, over 3 days. After this period, the resulting suspension was placed into a percolator with 50 mL of 70° GL ethanol, and left for a further 3 days. The macerated drug was percolated and a 20% hydroalcoholic extract was obtained (de Jesus Reis Rosa et al., 2010). The solvent was evaporated until dryness, and the dried extract was then protected from light and humidity at room temperature until the assays.

2.2 Pharmacological study

2.2.1 Animals

Male Swiss white mice (26-32 g) were supplied by the Anilab - Animais de Laboratório (Paulínia, São Paulo, Brazil). The animals were housed at 25 ± 3°C on a 12-h light/dark cycle with access to food and water *ad libitum*. This study was approved (protocol number A077/CEP2007) by the Committee for Ethics in Research from the University of Vale do Paraiba (UNIVAP) and all experiments were performed according to the guidelines of the Brazilian College for Animal Experimentation.

2.2.2 Venom and toxin

The crude venom was obtained from adult *Bothrops jararacussu* (Bjssu) snakes (Serpentário do Centro de Estudos da Natureza) and certified by Prof. Dr. Jose Carlos Cogo, University of Vale do Paraiba (Univap), São Jose dos Campos, SP, Brazil. Bothropstoxin-I (BthTX-I) was obtained under the conditions described by Homsi-Brandeburgo et al. (1988).

2.2.3 Mouse phrenic-nerve diaphragm muscle (PND) preparation

The PND was obtained from mice anesthetized with halothane and sacrificed by exsanguination. The diaphragm was removed (Bülbring, 1946) and mounted under a tension of 5 g in a 5 mL organ bath containing continuous-aerated Tyrode solution (control) with the following composition: 137 mM NaCl, 2.7 mM KCl, 1.8 mM $CaCl_2$, 0.49 mM $MgCl_2$, 0.42 mM NaH_2PO_4, 11.9 mM $NaHCO_3$, and 11.1 mM glucose. After stabilization with 95% O_2/5% CO_2, the pH was 7.0. The PND myographic recording was performed according to Melo et al. (2009). Briefly, preparations were stimulated indirectly with supramaximal stimuli (4 x threshold, 0.06 Hz, 0.2 ms) delivered from a stimulator (model ESF-15D, Ribeirão Preto, SP, Brazil) to the nerve through bipolar electrodes. Isometric twitch tension was recorded with a force displacement transducer (cat. 7003, Ugo Basile), coupled to a 2-Channel Recorder Gemini physiograph (cat. 7070, Ugo Basile) via a Basic Preamplifier (cat. 7080, Ugo Basile). PND was allowed to stabilize for at least 20 min before addition of the following substances: BthTX-I alone at 20 µg/mL (n=11); Bjssu alone at 40 µg/mL (n=5); 20 µg/mL BthTX-I + 0.05 mg/mL *C. sinensis* extract (n=5); 40 µg/mL Bjssu + 0.05 mg/mL *C. sinensis* extract (n=3); 40 µg/mL Bjssu + 0.025 mg/mL epigallocatechin gallate (n=3, Sigma-Aldrich, SP, Brazil); 40 µg/mL Bjssu + 0.05 mg/mL theaflavin (n=3); and the controls nutritive Tyrode solution (n=7) and 0.05 mg/mL *C. sinensis* extracts (n=7). The plant extract or commercial phytochemicals concentrations were chosen based on the minor changes obtained in comparison with the basal response of PND incubated with Tyrode nutritive solution (control).

2.3 Quantitative histological study

At least three preparations (n=3) resulting from pharmacological assays were analyzed by quantitative morfometry. Preparations used in the controls, nutritive Tyrode solution and *C. sinensis* hydroalcoholic extract (0.05 mg/mL) were compared to BthTX-I (20 µg/mL), or *C. sinensis* (0.05 mg/mL) + BthTX-I (20 µg/mL) groups, or Bjssu (40 µg/mL), or *C. sinensis* (0.05 mg/mL) + Bjssu venom (40 µg/mL) after fixation in Bouin solution and submission to routinely morphological techniques. Cross-sections (5 µm thick) of diaphragm muscle embedded in paraffin were stained with Hematoxylin-Eosin for microscopy examination. Tissue damage was expressed in percentage (number of damaged muscle cells divided by the total number of cells in three non-overlapping, non-adjacent areas of each preparation) according to Cintra-Francischinelli et al. (2008).

2.4 Thin layer chromatography (TLC)

Aliquots of *C. sinensis* hydroalcoholic extract were spotted onto 0.2 mm thickness silica gel $60F_{254}$ on aluminum plates, 20.10 cm, (Merck, Germany) and developed with ethyl acetate:methanol:water (100:13.5:10, v/v) in a pre-saturated chromatographic chamber along with appropriate phytochemical standards (Simões et al., 2004). These standards (theaflavin and epigallocatechin gallate, Sigma-Aldrich® - USA) were solubilized in methanol (1 mg/mL). The separated spots were visualized (under UV light at 360 nm) with NP/PEG as follows: 5% (v/v) ethanolic NP (diphenylboric acid 2-aminoethyl ester, Sigma Chemical Co., St. Louis, MO, USA) followed by 5% (v/v) ethanolic PEG 4000 (polyethylene glycol 4000, Synth Chemical Co., São Paulo, SP, Brazil). The retention factor (Rf) of each standard was compared with spots exhibited by *C. sinensis* extracts.

2.5 Statistical analysis

Each pharmacological protocol was repeated at least three times. Results were expressed as the mean ± standard error of the mean (SEM). The Student's *t*-test or repeated measures ANOVA were used for statistical comparison of the data. The significance level was set at 5%.

3. Results

3.1 Pharmacological assays

3.1.1 BthTX-I neutralization

Figure 1 shows the PND blockade activity of BthTX-I (20 µg/mL, n=11), which was irreversible even after washing (W) of preparations with fresh nutritive Tyrode solution. However, the previous incubation of the toxin with 0.05 mg/mL *Camellia sinensis* extract totally (100%) prevented the characteristic neurotransmission blockade, showing a better functional outcome of neuromuscular preparation after washing. The 0.05 mg/mL of *Camellia sinensis* extract was chosen in all protocols since it induced minor changes compared with the basal response of PND.

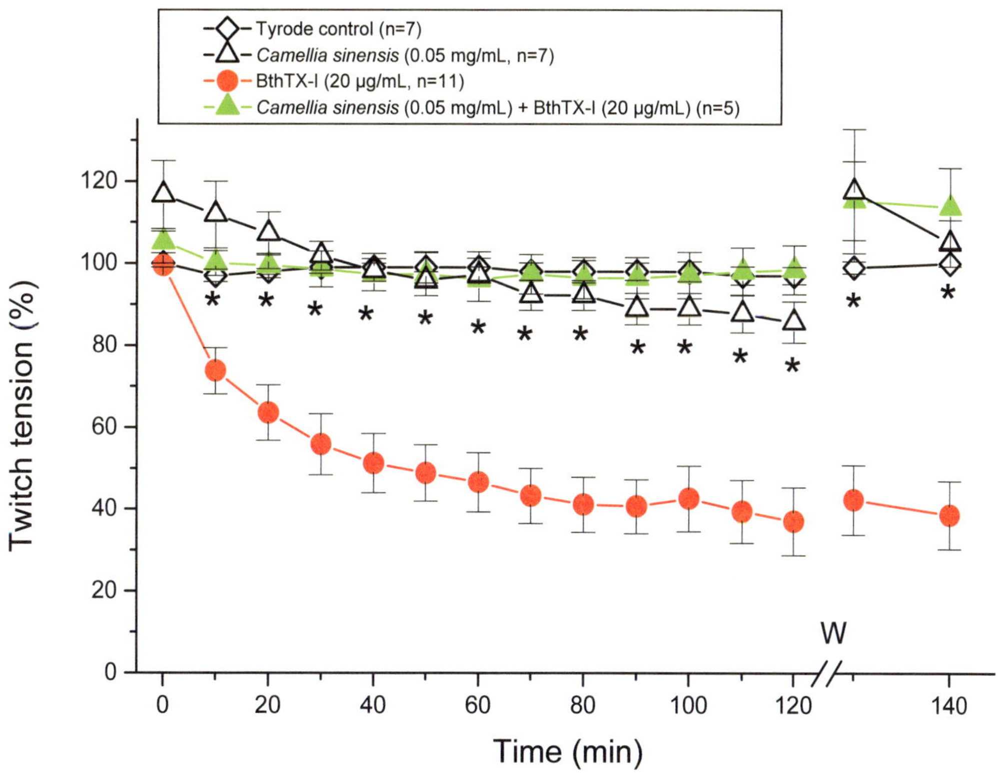

Fig. 1. Isolated mouse phrenic nerve-diaphragm preparations under indirect stimuli. Note the total efficacy of C. sinensis extract in protecting the neuromuscular blockade induced by BthTX-I. Each point represents the mean ± SEM. * = p<0.05 in comparison with the bothropstoxin-I (BthTX-I); W, washing.

3.1.2 Bjssu neutralization

Figure 2 shows the PND blockade activity by Bjssu crude venom. There was no contraction recovery of PND after washing the preparation. *C. sinensis* extract was 78 ± 12 % able to neutralize the venom that, in turn, differently of its myotoxin, contains several constituents.

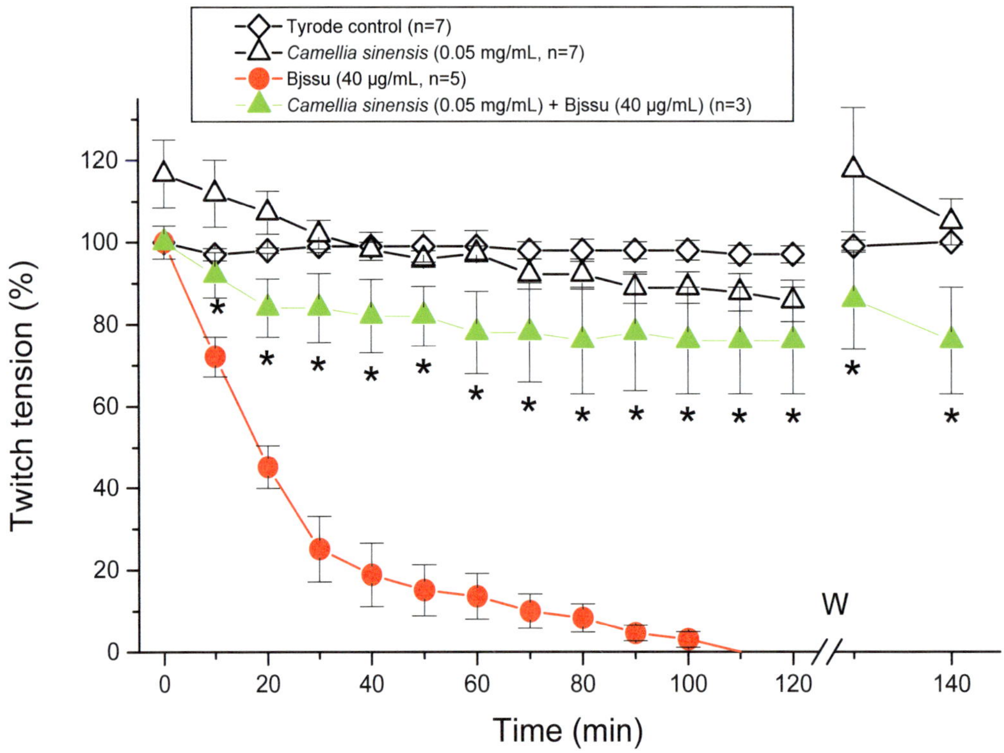

Fig. 2. Isolated mouse phrenic nerve-diaphragm preparations under indirect stimuli. Note the partial efficacy of *C. sinensis* extract in protecting the neuromuscular blockade induced by Bjssu. Each point represents the mean ± SEM. * = $p<0.05$ in comparison with the venom. W, washing. Bjssu, *Bothrops jararacussu* venom.

3.2 Quantitative histological study

Figure 3 shows neuromuscular preparations exposed either to Tyrode (Fig. 3A) or *C. sinensis* extract (Fig. 3B): the muscle fibers were well-preserved, showing changes not significantly different between each other of 15.9 ± 0.8 % or 25.3 ± 1.1 % damaged fibers, respectively. These changes were related mainly to loss of the typical cell cross-sectional polygonal profile. Differently, BthTX-I (Fig. 3C, 66.6 ± 2.3 %) and venom (Fig. 3E, 75.1 ± 1.1 %) alone clearly showed in transversal sections characteristic signals of myonecrosis (m), edematous cells (e), loss of polygonal profile, sarcolemma disruption, delta lesion (arrow), "ghost" cells (g), and nuclei (n) dispersed in the tissue. These changes were already extensively described in the scientific literature. Panel 3D and 3F show cross-sections of PND muscle fibers after *in vitro* neutralization by *C. sinensis* extract of BthTX-I (23.4 ± 1.3 % of lesioned fibers, $p<0.05$) and of Bjssu (27.8 ± 0.9 % of lesioned fibers, $p<0.05$), respectively.

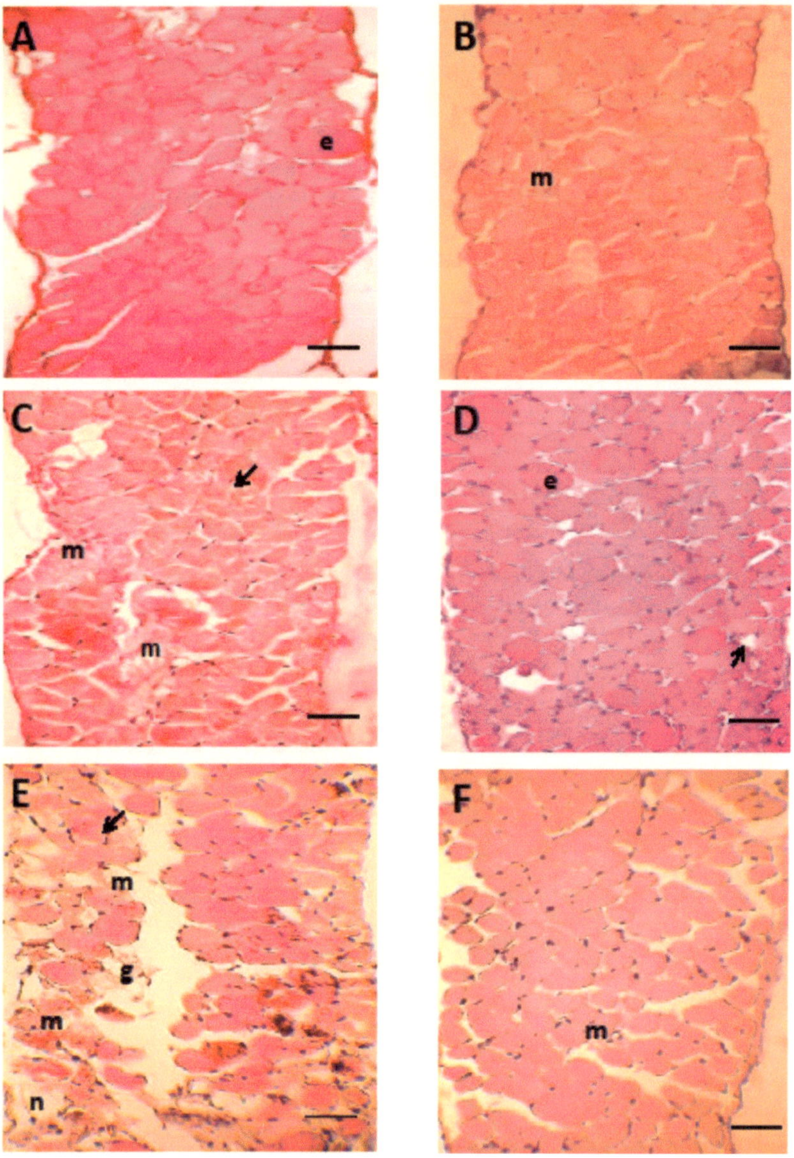

Fig. 3. Cross-sections (5 µm thick) of diaphragm embedded in paraffin and stained with Hematoxylin-Eosin. (A) Control-sham diaphragm preparation (15.9 ± 0.8 %). (B) Neuromuscular preparation exposed to 0.05 mg/mL Camellia sinensis extract (25.3 ± 1.1 %). (C) Muscle incubated with 20 µg/mL BthTX-I (66.6 ± 2.3 %). (E) Muscle incubated with 40 µg/mL Bjssu venom (75.1 ± 1.1 %). The main fibers damage are lettered as follows: myonecrosis (m), edema (e), delta lesion (arrow), sarcolemmal disruption with nuclei (n) dispersion, "ghost" cells (g) visualized by spaces optically empty. Note that area with extensive myonecrosis has a hyaline aspect. Muscles incubated with 0.05 mg/mL Camellia sinensis extract (D and F) shows fibers maintaining its characteristic polygonal profile in despite of a number of them being edematous (e). A slow percentage of them • 23.4 ± 1.3 % for BthTX-I (D); 27.8 ± 0.9 % for Bjssu (F) • • showed myonecrosis (m). Bars = 50 µm.

3.3 Efficacy of commercial phytochemicals against Bjssu venom

Figure 4 shows the effect of commercial 0.05 mg/mL theaflavin and 0.025 mg/mL epigallocatechin gallate from *C. sinensis* on twitch blockade induced by 40 µg/mL Bjssu venom. This paralysis was completely blocked (n=3, *p<0.05 compared to the venom, but did not show statistical differences with *C. sinensis* extract). In addition, following washing out of treated preparation with fresh physiological salt solution, twitch height was re-established (not shown).

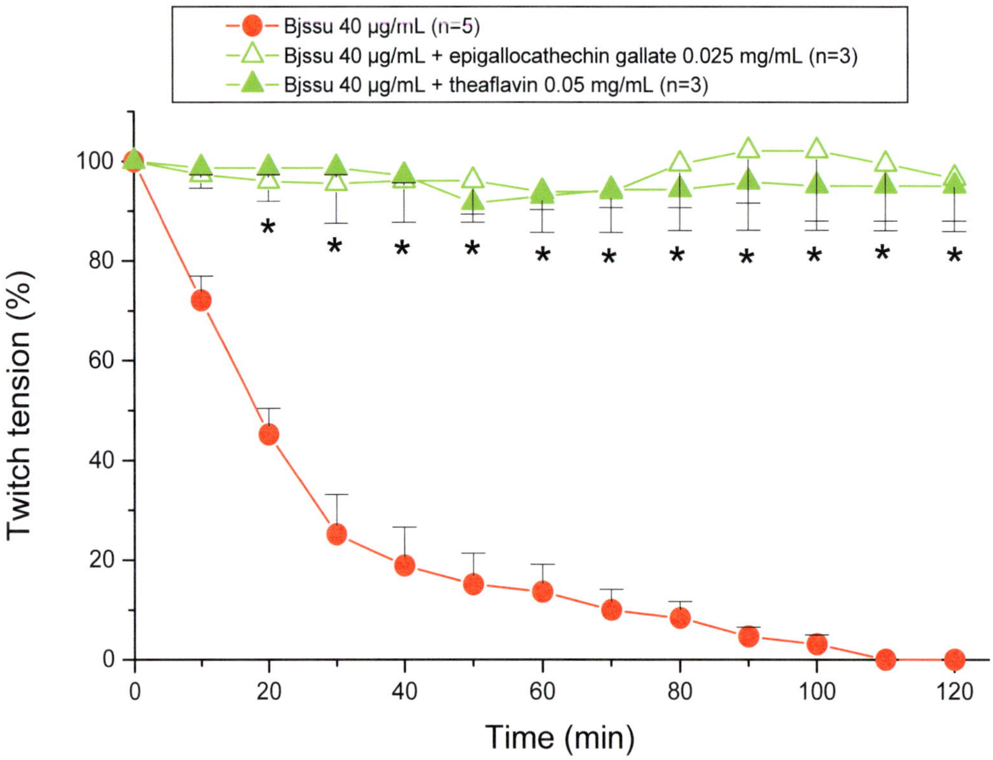

Fig. 4. Isolated mouse phrenic nerve-diaphragm preparations under indirect stimuli. Antibothropic action of commercial phytochemicals from Camellia sinensis. Note total protection against the paralysis of Bjssu (Bothrops jararacussu) venom. Each point represents the mean ± SEM. * = p<0.05 in comparison with the crude venom.

3.4 Thin layer chromatography (TLC)

Figure 5 shows a chromatoplaque of *C. sinensis* leaves extract obtained by TLC exhibiting a complex variety of compounds including theaflavin and epigallocatechin as confirmed by Rf of these commercial phytochemicals. Panel A is the chromatoplaque exposed only to a UV light at 360 nm, whereas Panel B is the same plaque after NP/PEG chromogenic agent pulverization.

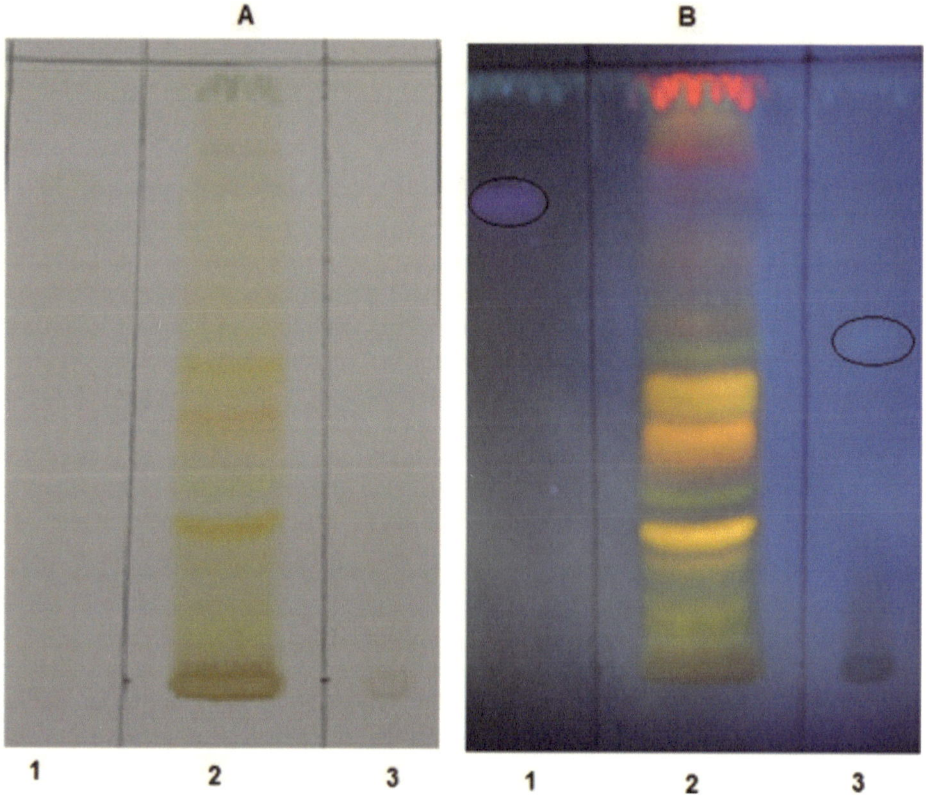

Fig. 5. Thin Layer Chromatography performed by using ethyl acetate:methanol:water (100:13.5:10) solvent/Developer: NP/PEG. Phytochemical standards: 1 - Epigallocatechin gallate (Rf=0.80); 2 – Cs, Camellia sinensis leaves extract; 3 – Theaflavin (Rf=0.56). Panel A: chromatoplaque exposed to UV light at 360 nm. Panel B: is the same plaque after NP/PEG chromogenic agent pulverization. Cs spots are suggestive of several flavonoids (yellow/orange fluorescence) and phenolic constituents (blue fluorescence), including epigallocatechin gallate and theaflavin, respectively. Comparative Rf values between phytochemicals and extract are highlighted in the circle. Rf, retention factor.

4. Discussion

Although the only specific treatment for envenoming by snakebites is immunoglobulins (antivenoms), since it can prevent or reverse most of the systemic effects and hence minimizing mortality and morbidity (WHO, 2011a), any alternative strategy aiming to interrupt or neutralize the steps of envenoming process can be effective for snakebite local effects. The clinical features of the bites of venomous snakes reflect the effects of these venom components that vary between species to species, but can broadly be divided into categories which include i) cytotoxins, causing local swelling and tissue damage, ii) haemorrhagins, which disturb the integrity of blood vessels, iii) compounds, which lead to incoagulable blood, iv) neurotoxins, causing neurotoxicity and iv) myotoxins, which cause muscle breakdown (WHO, 2011b). *Bothrops jararacussu* venom encloses all of them, except *in vivo* neurotoxicity (Milani et al., 1997), but it causes an *in vitro* neuromuscular blockade (Rodrigues-Simioni et al., 1983).

As snake accidents occur by bites and venoms are commonly injected in the subcutaneous muscle tissue, the use of muscle preparations as model for the study of the pharmacological effects of snake venom and toxins is very relevant. Besides, the use of snake venom and toxins as tools to study neuromuscular blockade *in vitro* (Gallacci & Cavalcante, 2010) is very useful given the excitation-contraction coupling process starts with transmission of electrical impulses from nerves towards muscle fibers via release of acetylcholine (ACh) (Hughes et al., 2006).

On the other hand, the plant kingdom represents a rich resource of new molecules able to counteract the venom effects, mainly when the plant is as worldwide as *Camellia sinensis*, an evergreen Asiatic shrub of the Theaceae family. Polyphenols from black or green tea has been shown to be powerful antioxidants with a potent inhibitory effect on low density lipoprotein (LDL) oxidation *in vitro* (Miura et al., 2000), exert anti-carcinogenic (Lambert & Yang, 2003) and anti-inflammatory (Arab & Il'yasova, 2003) effects; act as antibacterial and antiviral agents (Friedman, 2007), and are able to reduce the incidence of coronary heart disease and diabetes (Crozier et al., 2009), among other effects (see Khan & Mukhtar, 2007). Despite its health benefits, there are few studies using *C. sinensis* addressed to snake venom.

Hung et al. (2004) showed an antagonistic effect of 3 mg per mouse of melanin extracted from black tea (MEBT), an unhydrolyzed complex of tea polyphenols (Sava et al., 2001), against *Agkistrodon contortrix laticinctus* (broadbanded copperhead), *Agkistrodon halys blomhoffii* (Japanese mamushi), and *Crotalus atrox* (western diamondback rattlesnake) snake venoms, when administered i.p. immediately after venom administration in the same place of venom injection. Authors demonstrated correlation between antivenom activity of melanin and PLA_2 inhibition as a possible explanation for the protective effect.

Tea polyphenols have been shown to interact with hydrolytic enzymes from *Naja naja kaouthia* Lesson (Elapidae) and *Calloselasma rhodostoma* Kuhl (Viperidae) venoms, inhibiting inflammation and local tissue damage. This effect was attributed to complexation and chelation among the venom proteins and the phenolic contents of the extract. According to the authors, the *Camellia sinensis* extract also inhibited phospholipase A_2, proteases, hyaluronidase and L-amino acid oxidase by *in vitro* neutralization and the hemorrhagic and the dermonecrotic activities of the venoms *in vivo* (Pithayanukul et al., 2010).

Satoh et al. (2002 a,b) reported the protective effect of thearubigin from black tea extract against the neuromuscular blockade caused by botulin neurotoxins and tetanus toxin in synaptosomal membrane preparations. Recently, de Jesus Reis Rosa et al. (2010) reiterate the protective effect of C. sinensis leaves extracts which prevented in vitro the irreversible neuromuscular blockade typical of Crotalus durissus terrificus venom, more specifically caused by crotoxin, the main component of the crude venom (Slotta & Fraenkel-Conrat, 1983). We suggest that the target for C. sinensis protective effect is the motor nerve terminal, since the blockade caused by crotoxin, botulin toxin and tetanus toxin occurs by the inhibition of the neurotransmitter release, differently, from motor nerve terminals (Habermann et al., 1980).

Based on research findings suggesting an effective anti-cancer property attributed mainly to epigallocathechin-3-gallate (Fig. 6A) found primarily in green tea, and theaflavin (Fig. 6B) from black tea, both equally effective antioxidants (Leung et al., 2001), these two compounds were also assayed against *Crotalus durissus terrificus* venom (de Jesus Reis Rosa et al., 2010). Curiously, commercial theaflavin, but not epigallocathechin gallate, maintained partial muscular activity in the presence of 5 µg/mL venom. Coincidently, Basu et al. (2005) showed that only the theaflavin fraction from black tea was able to produce a facilitatory effect at the skeletomotor site, being this facilitation modulated by calcium and nitric oxide signaling.

Concerning the modulation of synaptic nerve-muscle interaction, it was found that ACh and glutamate are co-released from synaptosomes of *Torpedo electric* organ (Vyas & Bradford, 1987), also demonstrated in rat motor nerve terminals (Waerhaug & Ottersen, 1993). Glutamatergic receptors such as N-methyl-D-aspartate (NMDA) have been identified at the postsynaptic membrane in neuromuscular junction of adult rats (Urazaev et al., 1998; Grozdanovic & Gossrau, 1998). Glutamate released from nerve endings probably activates NMDA-receptor mediated Ca^{2+} entry into the sarcoplasm followed by activation of NO (Urazaev et al., 1998). Nonquantal ACh acting through M1-cholinergic receptors (Urazaev et al., 2000; Malomouzh et al., 2007), activates synthesis of NO to serve as a trophic message from motoneurones that keeps the Cl^- transport inactive in the innervated sarcolemma (Urazaev et al., 1999). For a better understanding of the synaptic nerve-muscle modulation, see also the study of Rubem-Mauro et al. (2009) that corroborates the nitric oxide role at the neuromuscular junction.

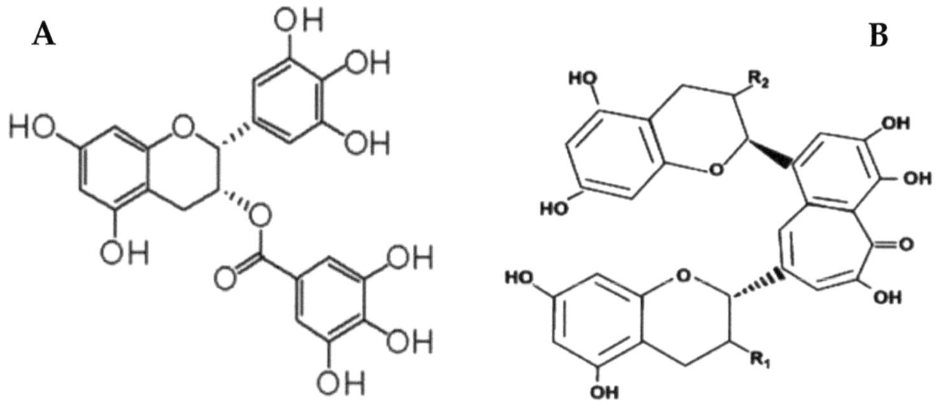

Fig. 6. Structures of major components of *Camellia sinensis*. A, epigallocatechin gallate (Zhu et al., 2008). B, theaflavin (Khan & Mukhtar, 2007).

The well-successful experience between *C. sinensis* leaf extract and presynaptic neurotoxins, and while bothropstoxin-I (BthTX-I) isolated from *Bothrops jararacussu* venom exhibits an earlier presynaptic action (Oshima-Franco et al., 2004) before its well-known myotoxic effect, the same experimental procedure was carried out using *C. sinensis* extract, which protected 100% the neuromuscular blockade (Fig. 1).

Different mechanisms have been proposed for BthTX-I myotoxic effect such as altering the bilayer membrane integrity (Lomonte et al., 2003), binding to the Ca^{2+} -binding region in the pore of Ca^{2+} channels (Oshima-Franco et al., 2004), activating membrane acceptors (Cintra-Francischinelli et al., 2009) or causing a general membrane-destabilizing (Gallacci & Cavalcante, 2009). In order to explain the rationale of this study more details will be given about these mechanisms.

BthTX-I represents a distinct group of PLA_2 homologue myotoxins containing Lys49 instead of Asp49 residue, with consequent loss of Ca^{2+}-binding and enzymatic activity, the segment 115-129 of the C-terminal region, which includes a variable combination of positively charged and hydrophobic/aromatic residues, has the ability to alter the bilayer membrane integrity (Lomonte et al., 2003), a possible way by which *C. sinensis* extract could exert its protection against the toxic effect of BthTX-I.

Oshima-Franco et al. (2004) have shown that BthTX-I, at a concentration that does not produce neuromuscular blockade (0.35 mM) caused the appearance of giant miniature endplate potentials, without affecting the resting membrane potential. The authors suggested that the toxin would act through Ca^{2+} channels, since Mn^{2+} antagonized both neurotoxic and myotoxic actions of the myotoxin and are related to Ca^{2+}fluxes. Mn^{2+} is thought to bind to the Ca^{2+} -binding region in the pore of Ca^{2+} channels, thereby preventing the passage of calcium ions (Nachshen, 1984). The influence of the earlier presynaptic action of BthTX-I is relevant from the pharmacological point of view, as shown here using *C. sinensis* leaves extract, although clinically the bothropic envenomation shows no signs of neurotoxicity. However, *C. sinensis* extract also protected against the myotoxic effects of BthTX-I (Fig. 3D), showing a parallelism between neurotoxic and myotoxic effects of the myotoxin.

Cintra-Francischinelli et al. (2009) excluded the possibility that the inactive Lys49 toxins act by binding to a membrane channel, thus increasing its permeability to Ca2+. The authors have shown that the action of myotoxins from snake venoms on muscle cells begins with the activation of membrane acceptors coupled to intracellular Ca^{2+} stores, which is rapidly followed by the toxin dependent alteration of membrane permeability to ions (and other molecules). By this mechanism, *C. sinensis* is able to inactivate the acceptors signalization.

Gallacci & Cavalcante (2010) proposed a hypothetical mechanism for the *in vitro* neuromuscular blockade induced by snake venom Lys49 PLA_2 homologues (Fig. 7): the binding of the Lys49 PLA_2 homologues to hydrophobic domains in muscle plasma membrane promotes a non-enzymatic alteration of the membrane structure. As a consequence, there is a colapse of the ionic gradient and depolarization of both muscle fiber and nerve terminal, mainly due to re-equilibration of sodium and potassium ions concentration. The persistent cell depolarization could inactivate voltage-dependent sodium channels in the peri-junctional zone. Consequently, the threshold of excitability of the muscle fiber rises out of the reach of the endplate potential; no action potential is triggered and the neuromuscular transmission is blocked. The depolarization of nerve terminal could increase the spontaneous release of acetylcholine, i.e. the frequency of miniature endplate potentials. The action potentials superimposed on the background level of nerve depolarization are reduced since the membrane potential is already shifted nearer to the sodium equilibrium potential. The reduced action potentials promote a decreased calcium influx and consequently a reduction of releasing of evoked acetylcholine. The muscle fiber membrane disruption induced by Lys49 PLA_2 homologues also promotes an increase in the concentration of cytosolic calcium that initiates a complex series of degenerative effects on muscle fiber. By this mechanism, *C. sinensis* extract efficiently did avoid the initial trigger.

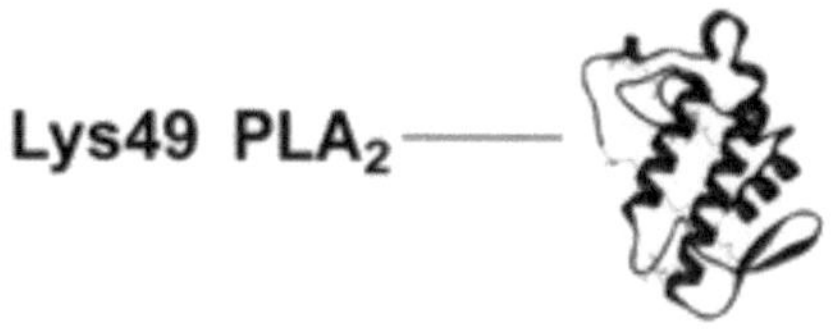

Fig. 7. Molecular structure of snake venom Lys49 PLA_2 homologue (Gallacci & Cavalcante, 2010).

Basu et al. (2005) showed that the theaflavins-induced facilitation was dependent on the calcium concentration of the physiological solution pointing to an involvement of calcium in the facilitatory action of theaflavins. It is evident that the skeletal muscle can contract in the absence of external calcium, but under physiological conditions, when calcium is present in the medium, it induces the release of stored calcium from the sarcoplasmic reticulum in order to maintain the optimal integrity of the contractile mechanism (Endo, 1985). Considering that *C. sinensis* extract totally prevent the neuromuscular blockade induced by the myotoxin and calcium seems to be involved in the toxic mechanism of BthTX-I, by different proposed mechanisms as already discussed, the explanation of Basu et al. (2005) that *C. sinensis*, produces a facilitatory effect, via theaflavin, acting presynaptically as calcium modulating factor is also other possibility.

In spite of the hypothesis discussed here, the actual molecular mechanism involving the *C. sinensis* extract and the BthTX-I interaction remains to be cleared.

Here, when the efficacy of *C. sinensis* extract was assayed against the crude venom, 80% of the contractile response was found preserved even after two hours of the venom exposure (Fig. 2), a promising result, since venom has a complex composition, differently from BthTX-I. Histological analyses clearly showed the protective effect of *C. sinensis* extract against the myotoxic action of venom (Fig. 3E), showing the same positive correlation between neurotoxicity and myotoxicity induced by the venom and the myotoxin.

Whereas only the commercial theaflavin protected against the neuromuscular blockade of *Crotalus durissus terrificus* (de Jesus Reis Rosa et al., 2010), here, both theaflavin and epigallocatechin gallate, totally protected against the paralysis by *Bothrops jararacussu* venom (Fig. 4), a result better than that produced by *C. sinensis* extract, since the amount of these phytochemicals in the extract (as shown in Fig. 5) is lesser than that used in the neutralization assays. However, the *C. sinensis* extract contains a multitude of other compounds, which real participation against the toxic effects of venom must be assayed, hence using an *in vivo* model simulating the cronically black or green tea consumption (by humans) followed by subcutaneous injection of the venoms. A comparison between the treatment with commercial antivenom alone and commercial antivenom plus theaflavin or epigallocatechin gallate is also interesting.

It is well-known that *C. durissus terrificus* and *B. jararacussu* venoms act differently in inducing clinical symptoms as well as *in vitro* paralysis at skeletomotor apparatus. Considering that venoms were previously incubated with each commercial phytochemical, and that epigallocatechin gallate, the major catechin in green tea, totally inhibited the toxic compounds of *B. jararacussu* venom, but did not do so against the rattlesnake venom, it is reasonable to suggest that theaflavin inhibits both presynaptic and postsynaptic venom effects, whereas epigallocatechin gallate inhibits mainly postsynaptic venom effects of these snake venoms, a question that remains to be cleared.

5. Conclusion

Camellia sinensis leaves extract possesses inhibitory effect against the neuromuscular blockade induced by *Bothrops jararacussu* venom and also bothropstoxin-I, by an unclear mechanism of action. Altogether, the data suggest that theaflavin and epigallocatechin gallate have a strong participation on these protective effects.

6. Acknowledgment

This work was supported by a research grant from São Paulo Research Foundation [FAPESP, Proc. 04/09705-8, 07/53883-6, 08/52643-4]. L.J.R.R. is a student of Post-Graduation Course in Pharmaceutical Sciences (Master level) from UNISO. G.A.A.S. had a scholarship (I.C.) from PROBIC/UNISO.

7. References

Arab, L. & Il'yasova, D. (2003). The epidemiology of tea consumption and colorectal cancer incidence. *The Journal of Nutrition* Vol 133, No. 10, (October 2003), pp. 3310S–3318S, ISSN 1541-6100

Basu, S., Chaudhuri, T., Chauhan, S.P.S., Das Gupta, A.K., Chaudhury, L. & Vedasiromoni, J.R. (2005). The theaflavin fraction is responsible for the facilitatory effect of black tea at the skeletal myoneural junction. *Life Sciences*, Vol.76, No.26, (May 2005), pp. 3081–3088, ISSN 1879-0631

Battellino, C., Piazza, R, da Silva, A.M., Cury, Y. & Farsky, S.H. (2003). Assessment of efficacy of bothropic antivenom therapy on microcirculatory effects induced by *Bothrops jararaca* snake venom. *Toxicon*, Vol.41, No.5, (April 2003), pp. 583-593, ISSN 0041-0101

Bülbring, E. (1946). Observation on the isolated phrenic nerve diaphragm preparation of the rat. *British Journal of Pharmacology and Chemotherapy*, Vol.1, (May 1946), pp. 38-61, ISSN 0366-0826

Chippaux, J.P. (2011). Estimate of the burden of snakebites in sub-Saharan Africa: a meta-analytic approach. *Toxicon*, Vol.57, No.4, (March 2011), pp. 586-599. ISSN 0041-0101

Cintra, A.C., Marangoni, S., Oliveira, B. & Giglio, J.R. (1993). Bothropstoxin-I: amino acid sequence and function. *Journal of Protein Chemistry*, Vol.12, No.1, (February 1993), pp. 57-64, ISSN 0277-8033

Cintra-Francischinelli, M., Silva, M.G., Andréo-Filho, N., Gerenutti, M., Cintra, A.C., Giglio, J.R., Leite, G.B., Cruz-Höfling, M.A., Rodrigues-Simioni, L. & Oshima-Franco, Y. (2008). Antibothropic action of *Casearia sylvestris* Sw. (Flacourtiaceae) extracts. *Phytotherapy Research*, Vol.22, No.6, (June 2008), pp. 784-790, ISSN 0951-418X

Cintra-Francischinelli, M., Pizzo, P., Rodrigues-Simioni, L., Ponce-Soto, L.A., Rossetto, O., Lomonte, B., Gutiérrez, J.M., Pozzan, T. & Montecucco, C. (2009). Calcium imaging of muscle cells treated with snake myotoxins reveals toxin synergism and presence of acceptors. *Cellular and Molecular Life Science*, Vol.66, No.10, (March 2009), pp. 1718–1728, ISSN 1420-682X

Correa-Netto, C., Teixeira-Araujo, R., Aguiar A.S., Melgarejo, A.R., De-Simone, S.G., Soares, M.R., Foguel, D. & Zingali, R.B. (2010). Immunome and venome of *Bothrops jararacussu*: a proteomic approach to study the molecular immunology of snake toxins. *Toxicon*, Vol.55, No.7, (June 2010), pp. 1222-1235, ISSN 0041-0101

Crespy, V. & Williamson, G. (2004). A review of the health effects of green tea catechins *in vivo* animal models. *The Journal of Nutrition*, Vol.134, No.12, (December 2004), pp. 3431S-3440S, ISSN 1541-6100

Crozier, A., Jaganath, I.B. & Clifford, M.N. (2009). Dietary phenolics: chemistry, bioavailability and effects on health. *Natural Product Reports*, Vol.26, No.8, (May 2009), pp. 1001–1043, ISSN 0265-0568

Das, M., Vedasiromoni, J.R., Chauhan, S.P.S. & Ganguly, D.K. (1994). Effect of the hot-water extract of black tea (*Camellia sinensis*) on the rat diaphragm. *Planta Medica*, Vol.60, No.5, (October 1994), pp. 470–471, ISSN 0032-0943

Das, M., Vedasiromoni, J.R., Chauhan, S.P.S. & Ganguly, D.K. (1997). Effect of green tea (*Camellia sinensis*) extract on the rat diaphragm. *Journal of Ethnopharmacology*, Vol.57, No.3, (August 1997), pp. 197–201, ISSN 0378-8741

De Jesus Reis Rosa, L., Silva, G.A.A., Amaral Filho, J., Silva, M.G., Cogo, J.C., Groppo, F.C. & Oshima-Franco Y. (2010). The inhibitory effect of *Camellia sinensis* extracts against the neuromuscular blockade of *Crotalus durissus terrificus* venom. *Journal of Venom Research*, Vol.1, No.7, (September 2010), pp. 1-7, ISSN 2444-0324

dos Santos, J.I., Cintra-Francischinelli, M., Borges, R.J., Fernandes, C.A., Pizzo, P., Cintra, A.C., Braz, A.S., Soares, A.M. & Fontes, M.R. (2011). Structural, functional, and bioinformatics studies reveal a new snake venom homologue phospholipase A_2 class. *Proteins*, Vol.79, No.1, (September 2010), pp. 61-78, ISSN 0887-3585

Endo, M. (1985). Calcium release from sarcoplasmic reticulum. In: Bronner, F. (Ed.), *Current Topics in Membrane and Transport*, 25, Academic Press, London, pp. 181-230

Fenwick, A.M., Gutberlet-Jr, R.L., Evans, J. & Parkinson, C.L. (2009). Morphological and molecular evidence for phylogeny and classification of South American pitvipers, genera *Bothrops*, *Bothriopsis*, and *Bothrocophias* (Serpentes: Viperidae). *Zoological Journal of the Linnean Society*, Vol.156, No.3, (March 2009), pp. 617-640, ISSN 0024-4082

Friedman, M. (2007). Overview of antibacterial, antitoxin, antiviral, and antifungal activities of tea flavonoids and teas. *Molecular Nutrition & Food Research*, Vol.51, No.1, (January 2007), pp. 116-134, ISSN 1613-4125

Gallacci, M. & Cavalcante, W.L.G. (2010). Understanding the in vitro neuromuscular activity of snake venom Lys49 phospholipase A2 homologues. *Toxicon*, Vol.55, No.10, (October 2009), pp. 1–11, ISSN 0041-0101

Graham, H. N (1992). Green tea composition, consumption, and polyphenol chemistry. *Preventive Medicine*, Vol.21, No.3, (May 1992), pp. 334-350, ISSN 0091-7435

Grozdanovic, Z. & Gossrau, R. (1998). Co-localization of nitric oxide synthase I (NOS I) and NMDA receptor subunit 1 (NMDAR-1) at the neuromuscular junction in rat and mouse skeletal muscle. *Cell and Tissue Research*. Vol.291, No.1, (January 1998), pp.57-63, ISSN 0302-766X

Gutiérrez, J.M., Núñez, J., Díaz, C., Cintra, A.C., Homsi-Brandeburgo, M.I. & Giglio, J.R. (1991). Skeletal muscle degeneration and regeneration after injection of bothropstoxin-II, a phospholipase A2 isolated from the venom of the snake *Bothrops jararacussu*. *Experimental and Molecular Pathology*, Vol.55, No.3, (December 1991), pp. 217-229, ISSN 0014-4800

Habermann, E., Dreyer, F. & Bigalke, H. (1980). Tetanus toxin blocks the neuromuscular transmission *in vitro* like botulinum A toxin. *Naunyn-Schmiedeberg's Archives of Pharmacology*, Vol.311, No.1, (February 1980), pp. 33-40, ISSN 0028-1298

Harrison, R.A., Hargreaves, A., Wagstaff, S.C., Faragher, B & Lalloo, D.G (2009). Snake envenoming: a disease of poverty. *PLoS Neglected Tropical Diseases*, Vol.3, No.12, (December 2009), pp. e569-e575, ISSN 1935-2735

Hazarika, M., Chakravarty, S. K. & Mahanta, P. K. (1984). Studies on thearubigin pigments in black tea manufacturing systems. *Journal of the Science of Food and Agriculture,* Vol.35, No.11, (November 1984), pp. 1208-1218, ISSN 0022-5142

Heluany, N.F., Homsi-Brandeburgo, M.I., Giglio, J.R., Prado-Franceschi, J. & Rodrigues-Simioni, L. (1992). Effects induced by bothropstoxin, a component from *Bothrops jararacussu* snake venom, on mouse and chick muscle preparations. *Toxicon,* Vol.30, No.10, (October 1992), pp. 1203-1210, ISSN 0041-0101

Homsi-Brandeburgo, M.I., Queiroz, L.S., Santo-Neto, H., Rodrigues-Simioni, L. & Giglio, J.R. (1988). Fractionation of *Bothrops jararacussu* snake venom: partial chemical characterization and biological activity of bothropstoxin. *Toxicon,* Vol.26, No.7, (July 1988), pp. 615-627, ISSN 0041-0101

Hughes, B.W., Kusner, L.L. & Kaminski, H.J. (2006). Molecular architecture of the neuromuscular junction. *Muscle & Nerve,* Vol. 33, No.4, (October 2005), pp. 445–461, ISSN 0148-639X

Hung, Y-C., Sava, V., Hong, M-Y. & Huang, G.S. (2004). Inhibitory effects on phospholipase A_2 and antivenin activity of melanin extracted from *Thea sinensis* Linn. *Life Sciences,* Vol.74, No.16, (March 2004), pp. 2037-2047, ISSN 1879-0631

Khan, N. & Mukhtar, H. (2007). Tea polyphenols for health promotion. *Life Sciences,* Vol.81, No.7, (July 2007), pp. 519-533, ISSN 1879-0631

Krishnamoorthy, K.K. (1991). The nutritional and therapeutic value of tea. In: Yamanishi, T. (Ed.), *Proceedings of the International Symposium on Tea Science,* Japan, pp. 6–11, LC Control Number 92188482

Lambert, J.D. & Yang, C.S. (2003). Mechanisms of cancer prevention by tea constituents. *The Journal of Nutrition,* Vol.133, No.10, (October 2003), pp. 3262S-3267S, ISSN 0022-3166

Leung, L.K., Su, Y., Chen, R., Zhang, Z., Huang, Y. & Chen, Z-Y. (2001). Theaflavins in black tea and catechins in green tea are equally effective antioxidants. *The Journal of Nutrition,* Vol.131, No.9, (September 2001), pp. 2248-2251, ISSN 0022-3166

Lima, A.C.S.F., Campos, C.E.C. & Ribeiro, J.R. (2009). Epidemiological profile of snake poisoning accidents in the State of Amapá. *Revista da Sociedade Brasileira de Medicina Tropical,* Vol.42, No.3, (May-June 2009), pp. 329-335, ISSN 0037-8682

Lomonte, B., Angulo, Y. & Calderón, L. (2003). An overview of lysine-49 phospholipase A2 myotoxins from crotalid snake venoms and their structural determinants of myotoxic action. *Toxicon,* Vol. 42, No. 8, (December 2003), pp. 885–901, ISSN 0041-0101

Mahmood, A., Ahmad, M., Jabeen, A., Zafar, M. & Nadeem, S. (2005). *Pharmacognostic studies of some indigenous medicinal plants of Pakistan,* 26.07.2011, Available from: http://www.siu.edu/~ebl/leaflets/abid.htm

Malomouzh, A.I., Mukhtarov, M.R., Nikolsky, E.E. & Vyskocil, F. (2007). Muscarinic M1 acetylcholine receptors regulate the non-quantal release of acetylcholine in the rat neuromuscular junction via NO-dependent mechanism. *Journal of Neurochemistry,* Vol.102, No.6, (September 2007), pp. 2110-2117, ISSN 0022-3042

Melo, R.F., Farrapo, N.M., Rocha Junior, D.S., Silva, M.G., Cogo, J.C., Dal Belo, C.A., Rodrigues-Simioni, L., Groppo, F.C. & Oshima-Franco, Y. (2009). Antiophidian mechanisms of medicinal plants, In: *Flavonoids: Biosynthesis, Biological Effects and Dietary Sources,* R. B. Keller. (Ed.), 249-262, Nova Science Publishers, ISBN 978-1-60741-622-7, New York, United States of America

Milani Júnior, R., Jorge, M.T., de Campos, F.P., Martins, F.P., Bousso, A., Cardoso, J.L., Ribeiro, L.A., Fan, H.W., França, F.O., Sano-Martins, I.S., Cardoso, D., Ide Fernandez, C., Fernandes, J.C., Aldred, V.L., Sandoval, M.P., Puorto, G., Theakston, R.D. & Warrell, D.A. (1997). Snake bites by the jararacuçu (*Bothrops jararacussu*):

clinicopathological studies of 29 proven cases in São Paulo State, Brazil. *The Quarterly Journal of Medicine*, Vol.90, No.5, (May 1997), pp. 323-334, ISSN 0033-5622

Ministério da Saúde. (2004). Secretaria de Vigilância em Saúde. Sistema de Informação de Agravos de Notificação (SINAN), 07.05.2010, Available from: <http://dtr2004.saude.gov.br/sinanweb/index.php>

Miura, Y., Chiba, T., Miura, S., Tomita, I., Umegaki, K., Ikeda, M. & Tomita, T. (2000). Green tea polyphenols (flavan 3-ols) prevent oxidative modification of low density lipoproteins: an *ex vivo* study in humans. *The Journal of Nutricional Biochemistry*, Vol.11, No.4, (April 2000), pp. 216–222, ISSN 0955-2863

Nachshen, D.A. (1984). Selectivity of the Ca binding site in synaptosome Ca channels: inhibition of Ca influx by multivalent metal cations. *The Journal of General Physiology*, Vol.83, No.6, (June 1984), pp. 941–967, ISSN0022-1295

Nicoleti, A.F., de Medeiros, C.R., Duarte, M.R. & de Siqueira França, F.O. (2010). Comparison of *Bothropoides jararaca* bites with and without envenoming treated at the Vital Brazil Hospital of the Butantan Institute, State of São Paulo, Brazil. *Revista da Sociedade Brasileira de Medicina Tropical*, Vol.43, No.6, (December 2010), pp. 657-661, ISSN 0037-8682

Oshima-Franco, Y., Leite, G.B., Dal Belo, C.A., Hyslop, S., Prado-Franceschi, J., Cintra, A.C.O., Giglio, J.R., Cruz-Höfling, M.A., & Rodrigues-Simioni, L. (2004). The presynaptic pctivity of bothropstoxin-I, a myotoxin from *Bothrops jararacussu* snake venom. *Basic & Clinical Pharmacology & Toxicology*, Vol. 95, No. 4, (October 2004), pp. 175–182, ISSN 1742-7835

Pereira, M.F., Novello, J.C., Cintra, A.C., Giglio, J.R., Landucci, E.T., Oliveira, B. & Marangoni, S. (1998). The amino acid sequence of bothropstoxin-II, an Asp-49 myotoxin from *Bothrops jararacussu* (Jararacuçu) venom with low phospholipase A2 activity. *Journal of Protein Chemistry*, Vol.17, No.4, (May 1998), pp. 381-386, ISSN 0277-8033

Pithayanukul, P., Leanpolchareanchai, J. & Bavovada, R. (2010). Inhibitory effect of tea polyphenols on local tissue damage induced by snake venoms. *Phytotherapy Research*, Vol.24, No.S1, (July 2009), pp. S56–S62, ISSN 0951-418X

Rodrigues-Simioni, L., Borgese, N. & Ceccarelli, B. (1983). The effects of *Bothrops jararacussu* venom and its components on frog nerve-muscle preparation. *Neuroscience*, Vol.10, No.2, (October 1983), pp. 475-489, ISSN 0306-4522

Rubem-Mauro, L., Rocha Jr, D.S., Barcelos, C.C., Costa-Varca, G.H., Andréo-Filho, N., Barberato-Filho, S., Oshima-Franco, Y. & Vila, M.M.D.C. Phenobarbital pharmacological findings on the nerve-muscle basis. *Latin American Journal of Pharmacy, Vol.* 28, No.2, (February 2009), pp. 211-218, ISSN 0326-2383

Satoh, E., Ishii, T., Shimizu, Y., Sawamura, S. & Nishimura, M. (2002a). The mechanism underlying the protective effect of the thearubigin fraction of black tea (*Camellia sinensis*) extract against the neuromuscular blocking action of botulinum neurotoxins. *Pharmacology & Toxicology*, Vol.90, No.4, (April 2002), pp. 199-202, ISSN 0901-9928

Satoh, E., Ishii, T., Shimizu, Y., Sawamura, S. & Nishimura, M. (2002b). A mechanism of the thearubigin fraction of black tea (*Camellia sinensis*) extract protecting against the effect of tetanus toxin. *The Journal of Toxicological Sciences*, Vol.27, No.5, (December 2002), pp. 441-447, ISSN 0388-1350

Sava, V., Yang, S-M., Hong, M-Y., Yan, P-C. & Huang, G.S. (2001). Isolation and characterization of melanic pigments derived from tea and tea polyphenols. *Food Chemistry*, Vol.73, No.2, (March-April 2001), pp. 177–184, ISSN 0308-8146

Simões, C.M.O., Schenkel, E.P., Gosmann, G., Mello, J.C.P., Mentz, L.A. & Petrovick, P.R. (2004). In: *Farmacognosia: da Planta ao Medicamento*, C.M.O. Simões, E.P. Schenkel,

G. Gosmann, J.C.P. Mello, L.A. Mentz, & P.R. Petrovick, (Eds.), UFRGS/UFSC, ISBN 85-7025-682-5, Porto Alegre/Florianópolis, Brazil

Slotta, K.H., Fraenkel-Conrat, H. (1938). Schlangengiffe, III: Mitteilung Reiningung und crystallization des klappershclangengiffes. *Berichte der Deutschen Chemischen Gesellschaft*, Vol.71, pp.1076-1081, ISSN 0365-9488

Urazaev, A.K., Naumenko, N.V., Nikolsky, E.E. & Vyskocil, F. (1999). The glutamate and carbachol effects on the early post-denervation depolarization in rat diaphragm are directed towards furosemide-sensitive chloride transport. *Neuroscience Research*, Vol.33, No.2, (February 1999), pp. 81-86, ISSN 0168-0102

Urazaev, A.Kh., Naumenko, N.V., Poletayev, G.I, Nikolsky, E.E., Vyskocil, F. (1998). The effect of glutamate and inhibitors of NMDA receptors on postdenervation decrease of membrane potential in rat diaphragm. *Molecular and Chemical Neuropathology*, Vol.33, No.3, (April 1998), pp. 163-174, ISSN 1044-7393

Urazaev, A., Naumenko, N., Malomough, A., Nikolsky, E. & Vyskocil, F. (2000). Carbachol and acetylcholine delay the early postdenervation depolarization of muscle fibres through M1-cholinergic receptors. *Neuroscience Research*,Vol.37, No.4, (August 2000), pp.255-263, ISSN 0168-0102

Vyas, S. & Bradford, H.F. (1987). Co-release of acetylcholine, glutamate and taurine from synaptosomes of Torpedo electric organ. *Neuroscience Letters*, Vol.82, No.1, (November 1987), pp. 58-64, ISSN 0304-3940.

Waerhaug, O. & Ottersen, O.P. (1993). Demonstration of glutamate-like immunoreactivity at rat neuromuscular junctions by quantitative electron microscopic immunocytochemistry. *Anatomy and Embryology*, Vol.188, No.5, (November 1993), pp. 501-513, ISSN 0340-2061

Warrel, D.A. (2004). Snakebites in Central and South America: epidemiology, clinical features, and clinical management. In: *The venomous reptiles of the Western Hemisphere*, J.A. Campbell, W.W. Lamar (Eds.), 709-715, Cornell University Press, ISBN 978-080-1441-41-7, New York, United States of America

Warrell, D.A. (2010). Snake bite. *The Lancet*, Vol. 375, No. 9708, (January 2010), pp. 77–88, ISSN 0099-5355

WHO - World Health Organization. (2007). Rabies and envenomings: a neglected public health issue, 25.10.2011, Available from: <http://www.who.int/bloodproducts/animal_sera/Rabies.pdf>

WHO - World Health Organization. (2011a). Guidelines for the production control and regulation of snake antivenom immunoglobulins, 27.07.2011, Available from: <http://www.who.int/bloodproducts/snake_antivenoms/SnakeAntivenomGuideline.pdf>.

WHO - World Health Organization. (2011b). Neglected tropical diseases, 24.07.2011, Available from:\ <http://www.who.int/neglected_diseases/diseases/snakebites/en/>.

Yang, C.S., Chen, L., Lee, M.J., Balentine, D., Kuo, M.C. & Schantz, S.P. (1998). Blood and urine levels of tea catechins after ingestion of different amounts of green tea by human volunteers. *Cancer Epidemiology, Biomarkers &Prevention*, Vol.7, No.4, (April 1998), pp. 351-354, ISSN 1055-9965

Zhu, Q.Y. & Chen, Z.Y. (1999) Isolation and analysis of green tea polyphenols by HPLC. *Analytical Laboratory*, Vol. 18, pp. 70–72, ISSN 1000-0720

Zhu, S., Li, W., Li, J., Sama, A.E. & Wang H. (2008). Caging a beast in the inflammation arena: use of Chinese Medicinal herbs to inhibit a late mediator of lethal sepsis, HMGB1. *International Journal of Clinical and Experimental Medicine*, Vol.1, No.1, (January 2008), pp. 64-75, ISSN 1940-5901.

26

The Effects of *Viscum album* (Mistletoe) QuFrF Extract and Vincristine in Human Multiple Myeloma Cell Lines – A Comparative Experimental Study Using Several and Different Parameters

Eva Kovacs
Cancer Immunology Research
Switzerland

1. Introduction

1.1 Multiple myeloma

Multiple myeloma (MM) is a haematological disorder of malignant plasma cells. B lymphocytes start in the bone marrow and move to the lymph nodes.

When they are activated to secrete antibodies, they are known as plasma cells, which are crucial part of the immune system. Due to the fundamental nature of the system affected, multiple myeloma manifests systemic symptoms that make it difficult to diagnose. Multiple myeloma is characterised by slow proliferation of the tumour cells, mainly in the bone marrow, by production of large amounts of immunoglobulins and osteolytic lesions. Multiple myeloma is a generally incurable disease at present, but remissions may be induced with stem cells transplants, steroids, chemotherapy and treatment with vincristine + doxorubicin + dexamethasone or thalidomide + dexamethasone or bortezomib based regimens or lenalidomide. The different therapeutic modalities have different "target location".

1.2 Epidemiology of multiple myeloma

Multiple myeloma mainly affects older adults, but its causes and other risk factors are unknown. Yearly incidence is 3-6/100 000 worldwide, accounts for 1-2 % of all human cancer. Median survival is 50–55 months.

1.3 The role of cytokines in the growth, progression and dissemination of multiple myeloma

Cytokines are soluble proteins, peptides or glycoproteins that are released by cells. Cytokines can affect the cells via an autocrine and/or paracrine regulation mechanisms. In case of an autocrine regulation mechanism the endogenous produced cytokine affects the same type of cell. In case of a paracrine regulation mechanism the target cell is near to the cytokine produced cell. Cytokine binds to a specific receptor and causes a change in function or in development (differentiation) of the target cell. In both cases, i.e. autocrine and paracrine regulation mechanisms the expression of the membrane receptor is altered.

1.3.1 Interleukins are a group of cytokines which are produced by a wide variety of body cells. The majority of interleukins are synthesized by helper CD4+ T lymphocytes, monocytes/macrophages and by endothelial cells. If the produced cytokine is released, then it is measurable in the supernatant, if not then the cytokine is measurable only intracellular.

Interleukin-6 (IL-6) originally defined as a B cell differentiation factor is produced by different cell types and certain tumour cells. Interleukin-6 acts as a pro-inflammatory and an anti-inflammatory cytokine. As a pro-inflammatory cytokine regulates inflammatory reactions either directly or indirectly. As an anti-inflammatory cytokine Interleukin-6 reduces the inflammatory reactions. IL-6 exits in three molecular weights, i.e. 21-30 kDa, 150-200 or 450 kDa. The biological activity of IL-6 depends on binding to its specific receptors. These membrane receptors composed the glycoprotein gp80 Interleukin-6 receptor alpha (IL-6R, also called CD126) and a signal-transducing component gp130 (also called CD 130). The complex IL-6+IL-6R+gp130 initiate a signal transduction cascade through JAKs (Janus kinases) and STATs (Signal Transducer-Activator of Transcription). The membrane receptors are released from the cells as soluble receptor proteins (sIL-6R and sgp130). As agonist, sIL-6R enhances the biological activity of IL-6 and sgp130 is an antagonist against the complex IL-6+sIL-6R.

Interleukin-6 is a major proliferative factor for the malignant plasma cells (multiple myeloma cells). This cytokine produces by the plasma cells and it affects the cells by an autocrine regulation mechanism with an additional paracrine signalling. IL-6 in a concentration of 2pg/ml can induce 50% proliferation in myeloma cells.

The multiple myeloma cells can be classified into three groups depending on exogenous IL-6: (a) both proliferation and survival of the cells are dependent on IL-6, (b) only proliferation of the myeloma cells is affected by IL-6, (c) the cells are dependent on IL-6 only for survival, but not for proliferation. However there are also some cell lines that are independent of IL-6 both for survival and proliferation. The serum values of IL-6 in 35% or in 97% or in 42% of multiple myeloma patients were significantly higher than in healthy persons (Nachbour et al., 1991; DuVillard et al., 1995; Wierzbowska et al., 1999).

Because about 70% of the secreted IL-6 forms a complex with sIL-6R (Gaillard et al., 1987), the amount of the free IL-6 in serum is low. Therefore the serum level of the sIL-6R is an important parameter in the evaluation and in the progression of multiple myeloma (Papadaki et al., 1997; Wierzbowska et al., 1999).

Interleukin-10 (IL-10) is known as a human cytokine synthesis inhibitory factor (CSIF). It produces by Thelper2 cells, monocytes/macrophages, by B lymphocytes and some tumour cells. Interleukin-10 has (1) immunosuppressive effect and (2) immunostimulatory effect. It down-regulates the expression of Thelper1 cytokines, MHC class II antigens and co-stimulatory molecules on macrophages. Interleukin-10 is a pleiotropic cytokine which increases Bcl-2 levels and protects cells from steroid or doxorubicin-induced apoptosis.

How might the presence of IL-10 contribute to a poor prognosis for some cancer? One possibility: Interleukin-10 is a growth factor for tumour cells. Second possibility: Interleukin-10 suppresses the anti-tumour immune responses.

Interleukin-10 enhances the survival and proliferation of B cells. IL-10 is a growth factor for myeloma cells (Kovacs, 2010a), enhances the proliferation of freshly explanted myeloma cells in a short-term bone marrow culture (Lu et al., 1995). Three out of seven human myeloma cell lines produce IL-10. Elevated IL-10 levels were detected in serum from about 50% of patients having multiple myeloma showing a relation to the clinical manifestation (Otsuki et al., 2000; 2002). Interleukin-6 leads to a marked production of Interleukin-10 in several human multiple myeloma cells. Interleukin-10 is an Interleukin-6 related growth factor for these tumour cells (Kovacs, 2010a).

1.4 Cytostatic effect and cytocidal effect

Cytocidal effect: It is known that there are two important pathways against tumours: To inhibit the tumour cell proliferation (**cytostatic effect**) and/or to induce the death of the tumour cells **(cytocidal effect)**. **Cytocidal effect**: apoptosis or necrosis.

The apoptosis is a physiological process in the life of healthy cells, whereas necrosis is a pathological process for tumour cells. **Cytotoxicity** is the quality of being toxic to cells. There are a **direct** and an **indirect** (cell-mediated) **cytotoxicity.** In case of direct cytotoxicity the cells are treated with cytotoxic compounds leading to necrosis.

1.5 Viscum album (VA) extract

Viscum album (VA) extract from **European mistletoe** plants has fermented and non-fermented preparations. Active components of VA extracts include mistletoe lectins (I, II, III) and viscotoxin, additionally aminoacids, polysaccharides and lipids. The fermented preparations are used either alone or in combination with chemo/radiotherapy in the treatment of tumour patients.

The Viscum album QuFrF (VAQuFrF) is an aqueous and unfermented extract of mistletoe plants growing in the oak tree. It contains 1 µg lectin and 6 µg viscotoxin in 5 mg/ml or 2 µg lectin and 10 µg viscotoxin in 10 mg/ml. The extract is an experimental drug that is not yet used in the treatment of tumour patients.

1.6 Vincristine

Vincristine is a vinca alkaloid. As a chemotherapeutic agent is used mainly in combination with other chemotherapeutic substances in the therapy of multiple myeloma. Vincristine inhibits the proliferation of these tumour cells and as a CCS blocker (El Alaoui, 1997; Lin et al., 1998; Mastberger et al., 2000) arrests the cell cycle phase G2/M by blocking the mitotic spindle formation (Harmsma et al., 2004).

2. Aim

2.1 Comparison of the effects of Viscum album QuFrF extract with those of Vincristine.

2.2 Mode of action of Viscum album QuFrF extract and Vincristine.

2.3 To assess the effective doses of Viscum album QuFrF extract and to transfer these doses to the in vivo situation.

3. Materials and methods

3.1 Test substances

Viscum album QuFrF (VAQuFrF) extract was obtained from the Hiscia Institute (Arlesheim, Switzerland). According to the manufacturer the aqueous unfermented solution of extract 10 mg/ml contains 2 µg lectin and 10 µg viscotoxin. Vincristine sulfate salt was obtained from Sigma GmbH (Schnelldorf Germany, No 8879). Recombinant human interleukin-6 (rh IL-6) was obtained from R & D Systems (No. 206-IL, United Kingdom) and reconstituted in phosphate-buffered saline with 0.18% bovine serum albumin.

3.2 Cells and culture condition

Human myeloma cell lines (MOLP-8, LP-1, RPMI-8226, OPM-2, U-266, COLO-677, KMS-12-BM, were obtained from DSMZ (Braunschweig, Germany). Five cell lines derived from blood, COLO-677 from lymph node, KMS-12-BM from bone marrow. The cells were cultivated in RPMI 1640 supplemented with 10-20% foetal calf serum, 2mM L-glutamine and 1 % gentamicin in a humidified atmosphere with 5% $C0_2$ at 37°C. The doubling times of tumour cell lines were between 35 and 96 hours. For the measurement of the parameters the cell cultures were used within 4-6 weeks after thawing.

3.3 Treatment of cells with VAQuFrF extract or vincristine

a. To measure viability, cytokine production, membrane expression of IL-6 receptor, cell cycle phases and apoptosis /necrosis the cells were cultured at a density of $0.5\text{-}0.7\times10^6$ cells/ml, except for COLO-677 (0.2×10^6 cells/ml). After 24 hours the cells were incubated with VAQuFrF extract or Vincristine (doses: 0, 10, 50 or 100 µg/10^6 cells/ml). The parameters were measured after 24, 48 and 72 hours.
b. To measure proliferation the cells were cultured at a density of $0.5\text{-}0.7\times10^5$ cells/100 µl, except for COLO-677 (0.2×10^5 cells/100 µl). After 24 hours the cells were incubated with VAQuFrF extract or Vincristine (doses: 0, 1, 5, 10 µg/10^5 cells/100µl). The parameter was measured after 24, 48 and 72 hours.

3.4 Treatment of cells with Interleukin-6

a. To measure viability, cytokine production, membrane expression of IL-6 receptor, cell cycle phases and apoptosis /necrosis the cells were cultured at a density of $0.5\text{-}0.7\times10^6$ cells/ml, except for COLO-677 (0.2×10^6 cells/ml). After 24 hours the cells were incubated with IL-6 (dose: 5 ng/10^6cells/ml). The parameters were measured after 24, 48 and 72 hours.
b. To measure proliferation the cells were cultured at a density of $0.5\text{-}0.7\times10^5$ cells/100 µl, except for COLO-677 (0.2×10^5 cells/100 µl). After 24 hours the cells were incubated with IL-6 (dose: 0.5 ng/10^5cells/100µl). The parameter was measured after 24, 48 and 72 hours.

3.5 Measurement of viability

The viabilities of the cultivated tumour cells were determined by 7-aminoactinomycin D (7-AAD), to exclude the non-viable cells in flow cytometric assays. The values are given in %.

3.6 Measurement of cytokine production

The IL-6 production or IL-10 production in the supernatant of the cultured cells was determined by chemiluminescent immunometric assay. The lowest detectable level was 2 pg/ml or 5 pg/ml.

3.7 Measurement of membrane expression of IL-6 receptor

For immunofluorescence staining $3x10^5$ cells/100 µl were incubated with 20 µl phycoerithrin (PE) conjugated monoclonal antibody (CD 126, Immunotech, France) for 30 min at 4 °C. Then the cells were washed, sedimented and analysed in the FACSCalibur flow cytometer. For the expression of the membrane IL-6R (CD 126) the signal intensity (geometric mean of the fluorescence intensity x counts) was used as parameter. The signal intensity of the treated samples was compared with that of untreated samples, which were taken as 100%.

3.8 Measurement of the cell cycle phases

The cell cycle phases GO/GI, S, G2/M were assessed using the cycle test plus DNA reagent kit on a flow cytometer (BD, BioSciences, San Jose, USA No 340242). Briefly: 5x105 cells were incubated at room temperature with trypsin buffer and additionally with trypsin inhibitor+RNAse buffer. The values are expressed in percentage of total viable cell number (100%).

3.9 Measurement of apoptosis and necrosis

Apoptosis was measured using Annexin V-FITC (BD Biosciences Pharmingen, San Diego, USA No 556 570). Necrosis was measured using propidium iodide (PI). Briefly: $1x10^5$ cells were incubated with Annexin V-FITC or PI at room temperature in the dark. Thereafter the samples were analysed in a flow cytometer. Apoptotic cells: Annexin V-FITC positive and PI negative. Necrotic cells: Annexin V-FITC positive and PI positive. The values are given in percent of total cell number.

3.10 Measurement of the proliferation

The proliferation was assessed using cell proliferation reagent WST-1 (Roche, Mannheim, Germany, No 1644 807). The colorimetric assay is based on the reduction of the tetrazolium salt WST-1 by viable cells. The reaction produces the soluble formazan salt. The quantity of the formazan dye is directly correlated to the number of the metabolically active cells. The proliferation rate was measured 1, 2 and 4 h after incubation with the reagents at time points 24, 48 and 72 h. The upper limit of the absorbance was 2.0–2.1. The intra-sample variance of the untreated cells was <10% (3–8%).

3.11 Statistical analysis

Three to four independent measurements were carried out. For the evaluation of the parameters the Mann-Whitney U-test was used. The limit of significance was taken as $P<0.05$.

4. Results

4.1 Production of Interleukin-6 in supernatant of human multiple myeloma cells

Objectives: (a) spontaneous production, (b) production after treatment with VAQuFrF or Vincristine.

Table 1 presents the values of IL-6 in myeloma cell line MOLP-8, LP-1, RPMI-8226, OPM-2, COLO-677. None of the five multiple myeloma cell lines produced Interleukin-6 spontaneously. This means that all the investigated cell lines are IL-6 independent or have **autocrine/paracrine** regulation mechanisms. In case of an **autocrine** regulation mechanism the cytokine is produced endogenously and affects its membrane receptor directly. In case **of paracrine** regulation mechanism the exogenous cytokine also affects the membrane receptor. In two cell lines (RPMI-8226 and OPM-2) exogenous IL-6 led to a high expression of membrane IL-6R and enhanced levels of sIL-6R in the supernatant (Kovacs, 2003; and results are not shown) indicating a paracrine regulation mechanism.

Cell lines	Spontaneous	After treatment with	
		VAQuFrF	Vincristine
MOLP-8	ND	ND	ND
LP-1	ND	ND	ND
RPMI-8226	ND	ND	ND
OPM-2	ND	ND	ND
COLO-677	ND	ND	ND

Maeasurements at 24 and 48 hours after tretment with VAQufrF extractor Vincristine. Dose=50 μg/10^6 cells in both cases.ND = not detectable.

Table 1. Production of Interleukin-6 in human multiple myeloma cell lines.

Treatment with VAQuFrF extract (dose: 50 μg/10^6 cells) and with Vincristine (dose: 50 μg/10^6 cells) also did not lead to IL-6 production in the five multiple myeloma cell lines. These results confirm the findings of previous studies (Kovacs et al., 2006; Kovacs, 2010b).

4.2 Production of interleukin-10 in supernatant of human multiple myeloma cells

Objectives: (a) spontaneous production, (b) production after treatment with IL-6 (dose: 5ng/10^6 cells), (c) production after treatment with VAQuFrF or Vincristine (dose: 50 μg/10^6 cells for both substances), (d) after treatment with IL-6+VAQuFrF or IL-6+Vincristine (doses: 5 ng/10^6 cells +50 μg/10^6 cells in each case). For the combined treatment IL-6 was added 2 hours before the test substances.

Table 2 presents the production of Interleukin-10 in five human multiple myeloma cell lines. Spontaneous IL-10 production was found in 4/5 cell lines: MOLP-8, LP-1, RPMI-8226, COLO-677, however the cell lines MOLP-8 and COLO-677 secreted IL-10 not every time confirming the findings of previous study (Kovacs, 2010a). IL-6 led to a marked increase of

IL-10 production (up to 946 pg/ml) in 5/5 cell lines. VAQuFrF extract and Vincristine reduced the spontaneous IL-10 production in MOLP-8, LP-1 and COLO-677 to non-detectable amounts.

With IL-6+VAQuFrF or IL-6+Vincristine the values were markedly lower after addition of IL-6 but higher than without IL-6 treatment. VAQuFrF and Vincristine reduced the induced IL-10 production to the same degree in cell lines RPMI-8226 and LP-1. In the cell lines OPM-2, MOLP-8, COLO-677 the extract of VAQuFrF inhibited the IL-10 production weaker than Vincristine.

Cell lines	No treatment	After treatment with			IL-6 + VAQuFF	IL-6 + Vincristine
		IL-6	VAQuFrF	Vincristine		
MOLP-8	ND-18	453-862	ND	ND	35-73	8-40
LP-1	10-22	34-95	ND	ND	25-53	31-44
RPMI-8226	32-124	510-946	36-14	15-27	290-334	370-404
OPM-2	ND	8-33	ND	ND	6-14	ND
COLO-677	ND-30	26-105	ND-11	ND	10-32	ND

Maesurements at 24 and 48 hors after tretment. IL-6:5ng/10^6 cells.VAQuFrF and Vincristine: 50 μg/10^6 cells. Range of 4 independent measurements. ND=not detectable

Table 2. Production of Interleukin-10 (pg/ml)in human multiple myeloma cell lines.

No treatment	After treatment with		
	IL-6	VAQuFrF	Vincristine
55-60	49-62	11-17	16-20
82-83	80-85	58-71	30-48
70-72	69-75	30-47	29-53
47-56	49-57	46-55	13-21
67-68	70-81	41-59	21-32

The values are presented in percentage. Range of four independent measurements.

Table 2.A. Viability of human multiple myeloma cells (cell lines see Table 2).

The IL-10 production was measured at 24 and 48 after incubation with IL-6. The results show that in tumour cell lines MOLP-8 and RPMI-8226 the IL-10 production was high during the two days. In the other three cell lines the production decreased slightly at 48 h.

Table 2/A. presents the range of cell viability without treatment and after treatment with the test substances: L-6, VAQuFrF extract and Vincristine. The viability of the untreated MM cells was different: LP-1>RPMI-8226>COLO-677>MOLP-8>OPM-2. The both test substances impaired the viability to different degrees.

IL-6 does not alter the viability, confirming the findings of previous investigations (Kovacs, 2006b, 2010a). It was reported that IL-6 enhances survival of the myeloma cells because it inhibits apoptosis of induction of the anti-Fas (Nordan & Potter, 1986; Hata et al., 1995).

Summarised: The results indicate that the effect of the both test substances on the IL-10 production is due to their apoptotic/necrotic effects. It is possible that VAQuFrF and Vincristine could also impair the membrane expression of IL-10 receptor. To explain this hypothesis further experiments are necessary.

4.3 The effect of Interleukin-6, VAQuFrF and IL-6+VAQuFrF on the membrane expression of Interleukin-6 receptor in human multiple myeloma cells

Objectives: (a) in untreated cells, (b) after treatment with IL-6 (dose: 5 ng/10^6cells), (c) after treatment with VAQuFrF (dose: 50 µg/10^6 cells), (d) after treatment with IL-6+ VAQuFrF(dose: 5 ng/10^6 cells+50 µg/10^6 cells). For the combined treatment IL-6 was added 2 hours before the test substance. For the expression of the membrane IL-6R the signal intensity (geometric mean of the fluorescence intensity x counts) was used as parameter. This parameter was measured at 24 and 48 hours after incubation. The signal intensity of the treated samples, expressed in percentage was compared with that of untreated samples, which were taken as 100%.

Table 3 presents the mean values of the membrane expression of Interleukin -6 receptor in the cell lines LP-1, RPMI-8226 and OPM-2.

Cell lines	No treatment	Treatment with			No treatment	Treatment with		
		IL-6	VAQuFrF	IL-6 + VAQuFrF		IL-6	VAQuFrF	IL-6 + VAQuFrF
LP-1	100	128[a]	28[a]	77[ab]	100	168[a]	34[a]	81[b]
RPMI-8226	100	191[a]	61[a]	81[b]	100	134[a]	42[a]	67[ab]
OPM-2	100	148[a]	94	116[b]	100	104	92	85

Measurements at 24 h after treatment. Measurements at 48 h after treatment.

The mean values of three independent measurementa are expressed in percentage of untreated samples (100). a=p<0.05 vs.untreated samples, b=p<0.05 vs. with IL-6 treated samples.

Table 3. Membrane expression of Interleukin-6 receptor in human multiple myeloma cell lines.

The surface expressions of IL-6R in untreated cells of all three cell lines were in the similar range (results are not shown). Exogenous IL-6 increased the membrane expression its receptor significantly ($P<0.05$). VAQuFrF reduced the membrane expression markedly in LP-1 and RPMI-8226 ($P<0.05$), it had no effect in OPM-2. With IL-6+VAQuFrF the values were lower than with IL-6 ($P<0.05$), but higher than after treatment with VAQuFrF.

In cell lines MOLP-8, COLO-677 and KMS-12-BM exogenous IL-6 led to down-regulation of its receptor, signalling the possible process of endocytosis (results are not shown). It is interesting that all three cell lines in which IL-6 upregulated its membrane receptor sourced from blood. To investigate of the membrane expression of IL-6 receptor in the cell lines MOLP-8, COLO-677 and KMS-12-BM additional experiments are planned.

4.4 Inhibition of proliferation of multiple myeloma cells (cytostatic effect). Induction of apoptosis and necrosis in multiple myeloma cells (cytocidal effect)

Figure 1 and **Figure 2** present the mean values of the proliferation and those of apoptosis/necrosis in six human multiple myeloma cell lines treated with IL-6 or VAQuFrF or Vincristine. The cell lines MOLP-8, LP-1, RPMI-8226, OPM-2 sourced from blood, COLO-677 which is a derivative of RPMI-8226 from lymph node, KMS-12-BM from bone marrow.

To measure the proliferation the following doses were applied (1) IL-6: 0.5 ng/10^5 cells, (2) VAQuFrF or Vincristine: 1, 5, 10 μg/10^5 cells. To measure apoptosis/ necrosis (1) IL-6: 5 ng/10^6 cells, (2) VAQuFrF or Vincristine; 10, 50, 100 μg/10^6 cells. The parameters were measured at 24, 48 and 72 hours after incubation with the test substances.

Proliferation: The values of the treated samples are expressed as percentages of the untreated samples and are the average of four independent experiments. Significance was assessed versus untreated samples (100%).

Apoptosis/necrosis: The values are expressed as percentage of total cell numbers and are the average of four independent experiments. In the untreated samples the percentage of apoptotic cells lay in the range of 5-38%, that of necrotic cells 10-35% during 72 hours. There were big differences between the tumour cell lines.

4.4.1 MOLP-8

Proliferation: IL-6 increased the proliferation on average up to 130-155%. Comparison of VAQuFrF with Vincristine: 24 and 48 hours after incubation VAQuFrF at the dose of 5 and 10 μg/10^5 cells was more effective than Vincristine. 72 hours after there was no difference between the substances in any dose.

Apoptosis/necrosis: In the untreated tumour cells the values of apoptosis lay either in the range of necrosis or above them. IL-6 treatment did not impair either the apoptosis or necrosis. To measure the effects of the two substances on the apoptosis/necrosis we applied ten times less doses. VAQuFrF increased the apoptosis and necrosis at 5 and 10 μg/10^6 cells ($P<0.05$ and $P<0.01$). Vincristine had the same effect as VAQuFrF.

MOLP-8

%	Proliferation IL-6 NO	Proliferation IL-6 YES	Apoptosis IL-6 NO	Apoptosis IL-6 YES	Necrosis IL-6 NO	Necrosis IL-6 YES
	100	155	31	25	18	13
	100	140	20	17	20	17
	100	130	21	23	19	11
	0.5 ng 10^5			5 ng 10^6 cells		

LP-1

%	Proliferation IL-6 NO	Proliferation IL-6 YES	Apoptosis IL-6 NO	Apoptosis IL-6 YES	Necrosis IL-6 NO	Necrosis IL-6 YES
	100	162	16	11	9	4
	100	154	5	10	7	5
	100	128	9	12	10	9
	0.5 ng 10^5			5 ng 10^6 cells		

RPMI-8226

%	Proliferation IL-6 NO	Proliferation IL-6 YES	Apoptosis IL-6 NO	Apoptosis IL-6 YES	Necrosis IL-6 NO	Necrosis IL-6 YES
	100	105	10	6	21	22
	100	133	5	4	19	16
	100	141	3	3	28	22
	0.5 ng 10^5			5 ng 10^6 cells		

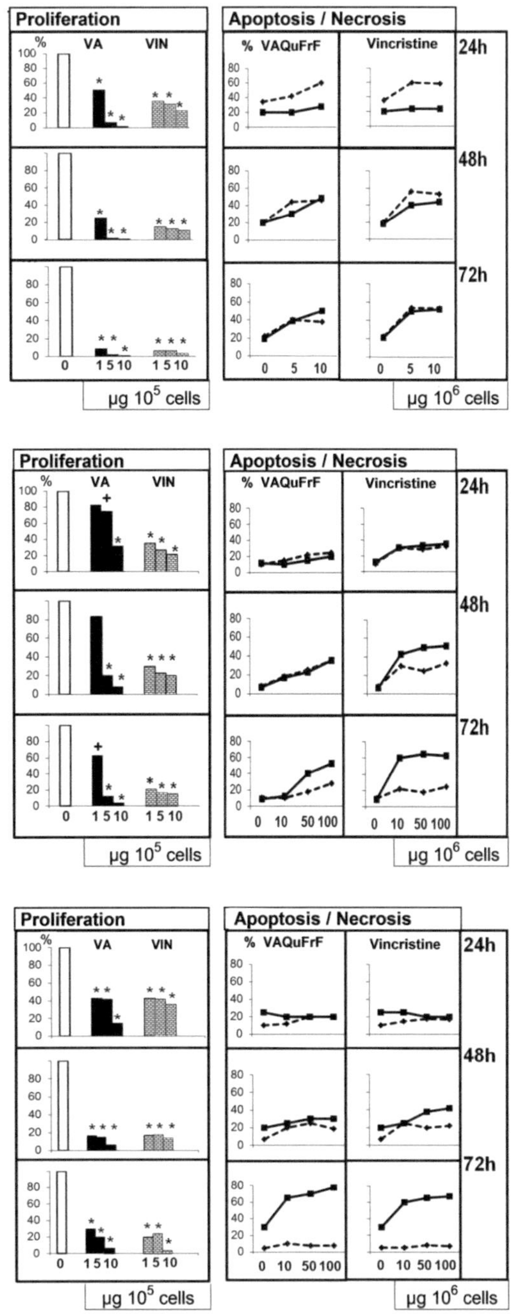

Fig. 1. The effects of IL-6, VAQuFrF extract and Vincristine on the proliferation and on apoptosis/necrosis in human multiple myeloma cell lines MOLP-8, LP-1 and RPMI-8226. The mean values of four independent experiments are expressed as percentage of untreated samples (100%). Proliferation=105 cells. Apoptosis/necrosis=106 cells. ●- - -● apoptotic cells, ●—● necrotic cells. +P<0.05, *P<0.01 compared with untreated samples (Mann-Whitney U-test).

4.4.2 LP-1

Proliferation: With IL-6 the proliferation rate lay on average between 128-162% during 72 hours. VAQuFrF at the dose of 10 μg/10^5 cells inhibited the proliferation more effectively ($P<0.01$) than Vincristine.

Apoptosis/necrosis: In the untreated cell the values of apoptosis lay in the range of necrosis. There was no difference between the values of untreated and with IL-6 treated cells. VAQuFrF did not greatly alter the apoptosis during the investigation time. There was a necrotic effect with a dose dependence from 50 up to 100 μg/10^6 cells ($P<0.05$). Vincristine increased the number of apoptotic cells and that of necrotic cells ($P<0.05$), however without dose dependence. The number of necrotic cells was higher than that of apoptotic cells at each dose after 48 and 72 hours ($P<0.05$ and $P<0.01$).

4.4.3 RPMI-8226

Proliferation: IL-6 increased the proliferation on average up to 105-141%.

The test substances inhibited the proliferation: After 24 and 48 hours VAQuFrF in dose of 10 μg/10^5 cells was more effective than Vincristine ($P<0.01$). In lower doses (5 μg/10^5 cells and 1 μg/10^5 cells) VAQuFrF had the same effect as Vincristine.

Apoptosis/necrosis: The values of apoptosis in untreated cells lay below the necrosis. There were no differences between the values of cells treated with IL-6 and that those of untreated cells.

VAQuFrF and Vincristine did not alter the apoptosis. At 72 hours after treatment with both substances he numbers of necrotic cells was higher than those of apoptotic cells at each dose ($P<0.05$ and $P<0.01$).

4.4.4 OPM-2

Proliferation: IL-6 increased the proliferation on average between 110-130%. Comparison of VAQuFrF with Vincristine: The inhibitory effect of VAQuFrF was weaker than that of Vincristine at each dose and at investigated time point. Additional investigation indicate that higher doses increase the effect of VAQuFrF (results are not presented).

Apoptosis/necrosis: In the untreated cells the values of apoptosis lay in the range of necrosis. IL-6 did not impair either the apoptosis or necrosis of the cells. None of the test substances altered the apoptosis. Vincristine increased markedly the number of necrotic cells between 10 and 100 μg/10^6 cells without dose dependence after 72 hours of treatment. VAQuFrF was ineffective.

4.4.5 COLO-677

Proliferation: With IL-6 the values of proliferation lay on average between 110-115%.

The inhibitory effect of VAQuFrF was weaker than that of Vincristine in doses of 1 and 5 μg/10^5 cells. At the dose of 10 μg/10^5 cells the anti-proliferative effects of VAQuFrF and Vincritine was the same at each investigated time point.

OPM-2

Proliferation		Apoptosis		Necrosis	
% IL-6		IL-6		IL-6	
NO	YES	NO	YES	NO	YES
100	110	22	17	20	23
100	130	38	35	35	28
100	120	30	27	27	32

0.5 ng/10^5 cells | 5 ng/10^6 cells

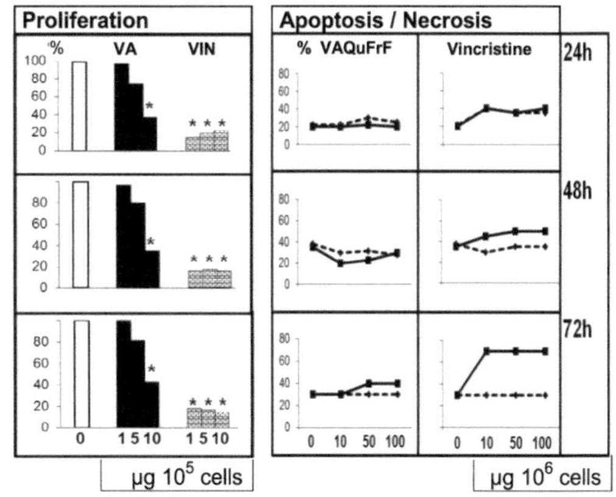

COLO-677

Proliferation		Apoptosis		Necrosis	
% IL-6		IL-6		IL-6	
NO	YES	NO	YES	NO	YES
100	110	8	12	22	18
100	115	18	13	20	25
100	114	10	9	28	30

0.5 ng/10^5 cells | 5 ng/10^6 cells

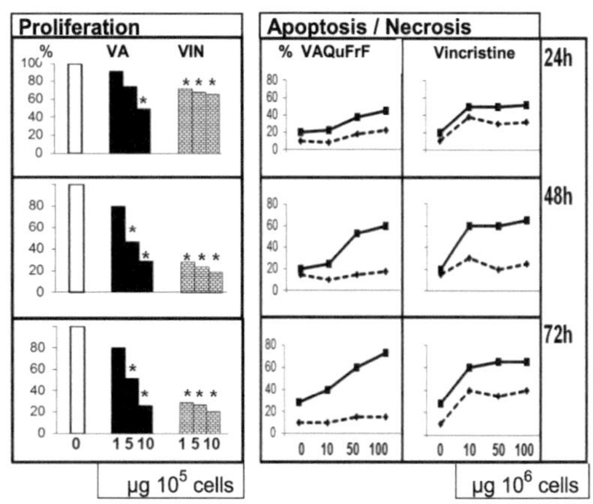

KMS-12-BM

Proliferation		Apoptosis		Necrosis	
% IL-6		IL-6		IL-6	
NO	YES	NO	YES	NO	YES
100	135	21	17	12	15
100	130	19	22	14	16
100	108	24	21	18	21

0.5 ng/10^5 cells | 5 ng/10^6 cells

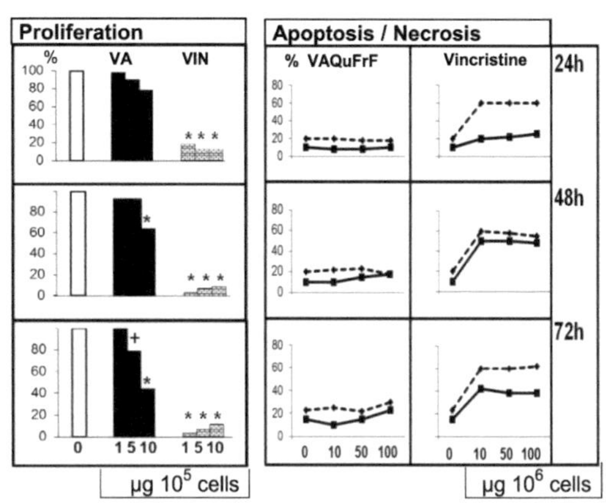

Fig. 2. The effects of IL-6, VAQuFrF extract and Vincristine on the proliferation and on the apoptosis/necrosis in human multiple myeloma cell lines OPM-2, COLO-677 and KMS-12-BM. The mean values of four independent experiments are expressed as percentage of untreated samples (100%). Proliferation=105 cells. Apoptosis/necrosis=106 cells. •- - -• apoptotic cells, •—• necrotic cells. +P<0.05, *P<0.01 compared with untreated samples (Mann-Whitney U-test).

Apoptosis/necrosis: In the untreated tumour cells the values of apoptosis lay either in the range of necrosis or below them. There was no alteration after treatment with IL-6. VAQuFrF did not alter the apoptosis. There was a necrotic effect with a dose dependence (from 50 up to 100 μg/10^6 cells) ($P<0.05$). Vincristine increased the number of apoptotic cells ($P<0.05$). The number of necrotic cells was higher than that of apoptotic at each dose and at each time point ($P<0.05$ and $P<0.01$). The apoptotic /necrotic effects of Vincristine were not dose-dependent.

4.4.6 KMS-12-BM

Proliferation: IL-6 increased the proliferation on average between 108 and 135%. VAQuFrF inhibited the proliferation only in dose of 10 μg/10^5 cells after 48 and 72 hours. Vincristine inhibited the proliferation markedly however without dose dependence at each dose and at each investigated time point.

Apoptosis/necrosis: The values of apoptosis in untreated cells lay above the values of necrosis. IL-6 did not alter the apoptosis and necrosis. VAQuFrF did not impair either the apoptosis or the necrosis in this cell line. Vinristine was effective in KMS-12-BM: The number of apoptotic/necrotic cells was significantly higher ($P<0.01$) at each time point, but without dose dependence.

It was reported that that inhibition of cell proliferation is a stronger prognostic indicator than the apoptosis (Stokke et al., 1998). There is a quantitative correlation between the inhibition of proliferation and apoptosis in lymphoma cells (Leoncini, et al., 1993).

Chemotherapeutic agents influence apoptosis through a mitochondrial pathway (Oancea, et al., 2004). Multiple myeloma cells overexpress Bcl-2, a mitochondrial membrane protein which suppresses apoptosis (Chanen-Khan, 2004; Tsujimoto & Shimizu, 2007). VAQuFrF decreases the levels of Bcl-2 in B and T lymphocytes (Duong Van Huyen et al., 2001).

Summarised: In this study the apoptotic/necrotic effect of Vincristine was more marked than its proliferative effect in all cell lines. There was no dose dependence between 10, 50 or 100 μg/10^6 cells/ml in both parameters. It is possible that Vincristine impairs the proliferation and apoptosis/necrosis with dose dependence only in a lower dose range.

VAQuFrF first inhibits the proliferation and then the cells die by apoptosis and/or necrosis in the MM cell lines LP-1, RPMI-8226 and COLO-677, confirming the findings with RPMI-8226 presented in a previous study (Kovacs et al., 2006a). The inhibitory effect of VAQuFrF was markedly weaker than that of Vincristine in cell lines OPM-2 and KMS-12-BM at each dose and at investigated time point.

4.5 The effect of VAQuFrf on the proliferation of cells with high proliferation rate

The effect of VAQuFrF with doses of 5 and 10μg/10^5 cells was investigated in cell line RPMI-8226 with high proliferation rate, which remained unaltered during 2-3 days. VAQuFrF was more effective in cells having high proliferation rates than in those with low proliferation rates (Kovacs et al., 2006a). Recently the same findings were observed in cell lines LP-1 and OPM-2 (results are not shown).

4.6 The effect of combined treatment with Interleukin-6+VAQUFrF on the proliferation in human multiple myeloma cells

The cell lines MOLP-8, LP-1, RPMI-8226 and COLO-677 were treated with Interleukin-6+VAQuFrF for 24, 48 and 72 hours. To measure the proliferation the following doses were used: 0.5 ng/10^5 cells + 1, 5, 10 µg/10^5 cells. For the combined treatment IL-6 was added to the cell cultures 2 hours before VAQuFrF. For comparison the cell lines were treated only with IL-6 or only with VAQuFrF.

Figure 3 presents the range of values expressed in percentage compared with untreated samples (100%). As expected, VAQuFrF inhibited the spontaneous proliferation markedly in all cell lines. The effect was dose-dependent. IL-6 led to enhanced proliferation in each case. We expected that with the combined treatment the values will be lower than after single treatment of IL-6, but higher than after single treatment of VAQuFrF. This situation has been found only in cell lines MOLP-8 and LP-1 for dose 1µg/10^5 cells. It is suggested that the 2 hours pre-treatment with IL-6 is too short.

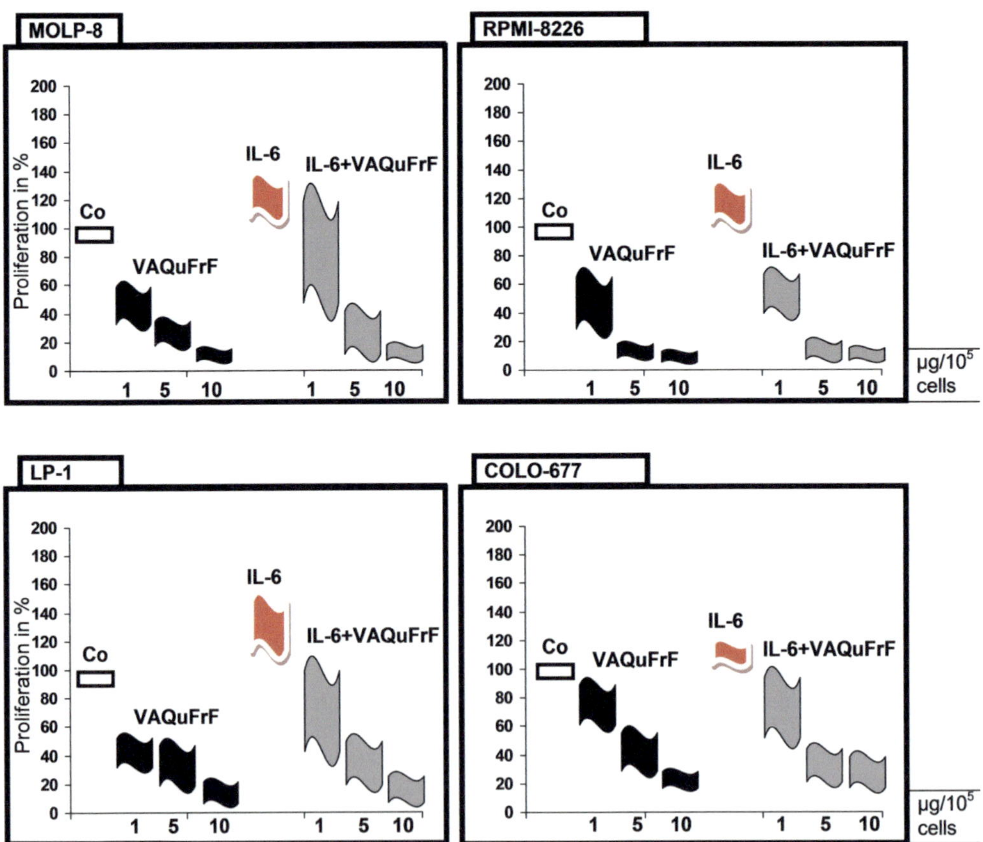

Measurements after 24, 48, 72 hours treatment. Range of values of three independent experiments. ▭ = control

Fig. 3. The effect of combined treatment with IL-6 + VAQuFrF on the proliferation in human multiple myeloma cells. IL-6=0.5 ng/105 cells.

4.7 Investigation of cell cycle phases in human multiple myeloma

Cell division consists of mitosis (M) and interphase, which divides into phases G1, G2, and S. Non dividing cells are in the stable resting phase, called the G0 phase. The blockade in the cell division leads to an arrest in the different cycle phases. This arrest appears as an accumulation of the tumour cells.

The following cell lines: were investigated: MOLP-8, LP-1, RPMI-8226, OPM-2, U-266, COLO-677, KMS-12-BM. The myeloma cells were treated (a) with IL-6 (dose: 5 ng/10^6 cells) (b) with VAQuFrF and with Vincristine (doses: 10, 50, 100 μg/10^6 cells). The investigation was carried out 24, 48 and 72 hours after treatment.

Table 4 presents the range of the values of untreated cells in different cell cycle phases in percentage in the total viable cell number (100%) 24 hours after treatment. **Table 5** presents the mean values resp. the accumulation of treated cells 24 hours after treatment. For the cell lines RPMI-8226, OPM-2 and U-266 the presented values signalize the effects 48 and 72 hours after treatment with VAQuFrF or Vincristine. For a significant increase or decrease, the percentage of the cell number of treated samples was compared with those of untreated samples.

CELL LINES	G0/G1	S	G2/M
MOLP-8	41 - 52	26 - 44	17 - 23
LP-1	50 - 63	27 - 37	8 - 12
RPMI-8226	60 - 78	13 - 28	8 - 15
OPM-2	51 - 62	20 - 38	10 - 19
U-266	48 - 59	17 - 25	9 - 21
COLO-677	36 - 49	42 - 50	10 - 21
KMS-12-BM	45 - 53	39 - 48	3 - 10

Measurements at 24 hour after incubation. Values are expressed in percentage of total viable cell number (100%). Range of four independent experiments.

Table 4. Values of untreated human multiple myeloma cells in different cell cycle phases.

Phases GO/G1: IL-6 did not affect this cell cycle phase. VAQuFrF led to an accumulation of cells in cell line MOLP-8, LP-1 and in KMS-12-BM ($p < 0.05$ and $p < 0.01$). Vincristine had effect in the cell lines MOLP-8 and LP-1 ($p < 0.05$). The both substances were effective at each time point.

Phase S: With IL-6 the number of cells was increased markedly in all cell lines during 72 hours except with OPM-2 and KMS-12-BM. In these cell lines there was no effect at 72 hours. VAQuFrF increased the cell number ($p < 0.01$) in RPMI-8226 and U-266 ($p<0.05$), Vincristine in RPMI-8226, OPM-2 and U-266 ($p < 0.01$ and $p < 0.05$). Both substances were effective only at 48 and 72 hours after incubation.

CELL LINES	G0/G1 IL-6 (5 ng 10⁶ / cells)	G0/G1 VAQuFrF (10 50 100)	G0/G1 Vincristine (10 50 100)	S IL-6 (5 ng 10⁶ / cells)	S VAQuFrF (10 50 100)	S Vincristine (10 50 100)	G2/M IL-6 (5 ng 10⁶ / cells)	G2/M VAQuFrF (10 50 100)	G2/M Vincristine (10 50 100)
MOLP-8	no effect	↑↑ 46 65	↑↑↑ 51 59 64	↑ 55	no effect	no effect	no effect	no effect	no effect
LP-1	no effect	↑↑ 68 72	↑↑ 78 70	↑ 40	no effect	no effect	no effect	no effect	no effect
RPMI-8226	no effect	no effect	no effect	↑ 37	↑↑ 25 33	↑↑↑ 20 42 45	no effect	no effect	↑↑↑ 49 52 50
OPM-2	no effect	no effect	no effect	↑ 45	no effect	↑↑↑ 30 31 39	no effect	no effect	no effect
U-266	no effect	no effect	no effect	↑ 39	↑↑ 22 31	↑↑↑ 23 23 28	no effect	no effect	no effect
COLO-677	no effect	no effect	no effect	↑ 58	no effect	no effect	no effect	↑↑ 18 22	↑↑↑ 54 62 68
KMS-12-BM	no effect	↑ 54	no effect	↑ 53	no effect	no effect	no effect	no effect	↑↑↑ 44 56 70

Treatment with IL-6(5ng/106 cells) or VAQuFrF or Vincristine(10,50,100 µg/106 cells); The investigation was carried out 24, 48 and 72 hours after treatment. Evaluation of three or four independent experiments ↑=accumulation. The numbers present the mean values in percentage.

Table 5. Accumulation of human multiple myeloma cells in different cell cycle phases.

Phases G2/M: IL-6 treatment led to accumulation of cells in LP-1, RPMI-8226 and OPM-2 after 48 and 72 hours. VAQuFrF was effective in COLO-677 ($p < 0.05$). Vincristine led to marked increase of the cell numbers in cell lines RPMI-8226, COLO-677 and KMS-12-BM ($p < 0.01$).

With IL-6 the cell number of each cell line was enhanced in the S phase and in some cell lines in the G2/M phase too. This means that either the DNA synthesis of the cells is increased or the cells are arrested in these cell cycle phases. In this investigation IL-6 led to high proliferation in all cell lines indicating an increased DNA synthesis. This could lead with to arrest in the cycle phase G2/M. In fact we found the accumulation of cells 48 and 72 hours after treatment in some cell lines.

Vincristine blocks the mitotic process by binding to tubulin leading to an arrest of the cycle phase in G2/M (El Alaaoui et al., 1997; Lin et al., 1998). In this study Vincristine led to an accumulation of the cells in cycle phase G2/M in only three out of seven multiple myeloma cell lines. It was effective in S and in G0/G1 phases of five cell lines, indicating that Vincristine also affects these cycle phases. It is interesting that it was effective both in the S and in G2/M cycle phases of the cell line RPMI-8226. VAQuFrF extract had the same effects as Vincristine in five out of seven tumour cell lines; however in a higher dose range. We postulated that different tumour cell lines from the same disorder (multiple myeloma) show a different sensitivity to Vincristine or VAQuFrF.

The inhibition of the G0/G1 phases in different malignancies correlates with anti-proliferative substances (El-Sherbiny et al., 2000; Pellizaro et al., 2008). In fact VAQuFrF blocked the cells in the G0/G1 phases in cell lines MOLP-8 and LP-1 and also inhibited the cell proliferation.

5. Summary and conclusion

In this experimental study we compared **Viscum album (Mistletoe) extract** and **Vincristine** in several human multiple myeloma cell lines using the parameters: (a) the IL-6 production, (b) the IL-10 production, (c) the expression of membrane IL-6 receptor, (d) the proliferation, (e) the apoptosis/necrosis, (f) the cell cycle phases. The following parameters were measured in a "package" i.e. they measured simultaneously: (a) the IL-6 production, (b) the IL-10 production, (c) the proliferation, (d) the apoptosis/necrosis.

The parameters were measured at different times (24, 48 and 72 hours) after incubation with VAQuFrF and Vincristine. Interleukin-6 is a major proliferative factor for the malignant plasma cells (multiple myeloma cells). Therefore this cytokines was measured parallel to the test substances.

Viscum album QuFrF (VAQuFrF) is an experimental drug that is not yet used in the treatment of tumour patients. For this reason it was necessary and important to compare with a well-known clinic-substance. Vincristine is used mainly in combination with other chemotherapeutic substances in the therapy of multiple myeloma.

5.1 Key results

a. Interleukin-6 leads to a markedly increased IL-10 production. Interleukin--6 upregulates markedly the expression of its membrane receptor (IL-6R). IL-6 increases the proliferation and it is effective in the S cell cycle phase. IL-6 does not affect the apoptosis/ necrosis.
b. Neither VAQuFrF nor Vincristine produce IL-6 or lead to an enhanced IL-10 production in any cell line. VAQuFrF and Vincristine inhibits the spontaneous IL-10 production. Both substances **counteract** the increased IL-10 production induced by IL-6. The effects of the two substances are comparable. The results indicate that the effect of the both test substances on the IL-10 production is due to their apoptotic/necrotic effects.
c. VAQuFrF **inhibits** the membrane expression of IL-6 receptor. VAQuFrF **counteracts** the enhanced membrane expression of this receptor induced by IL-6.
d. The **cytocidal effect** of Vincristine is more marked than its **cytostatic** effect in all cell lines.
   The effect of VAQuFrF focuses on the inhibition of proliferation (**cytostatic effect**). VAQuFrF first inhibits the proliferation and then the cells die by apoptosis and/or necrosis.
e. VAQuFrF inhibits the proliferation in cells with **high proliferation** rate **more effectively** than in those with **low growth** rate.
f. **Cell cycle phases:** VAQuFrF extract has the same effect as Vincristine in five out of seven tumour cell lines, however in a higher dose range.

The findings indicate that VAQuFrF extract could be a novel drug in the therapy of multiple myeloma.

To assess the effective doses of Viscum album QuFrF extract and to transfer these doses to the in vivo situation.

The Viscum album QuFrF (VAQuFrF) is an aqueous and unfermented extract of mistletoe plants growing in the oak tree. It contains 2 µg lectin and 10 µg viscotoxin in 10 mg/ml. It was tested in dose range of 10, 50, 100 μg/10^6 cells. 10 μg extract contains 0.002 μg lectin + 0.01 μg viscotoxin, 50 μg extract contains 0.01 μg lectin + 0.05 μg viscotoxin, 100 μg extract contains 0.02 μg lectin + 0.1 μg viscotoxin.

Dosage of Vincristine in the therapy for multiple myeloma: In combination with other chemotherapeutic agents as a part of the VAD regimen 0.4 mg/day intravenously (400 μg/day). In these experimental studies Vincristine was applied in dose range of 10, 50, 100 μg/10^6 cells. The effects of Vincristine on the proliferation and the apoptosis/necrosis were in each cell line without dose dependence. This means that these doses lay in a saturation range. It is planned to investigate the effects of Vincristine in a lower dose range.

The efficient dose range for VAQuFrF lies between 50 and 100 μg/10^6 cells (0.01μg lectin + 0.05 μg viscotoxin and 0.02 μg lectin + 0.1 μg viscotoxin). These date concern the cell lines LP-1, RPMI-8226 and COLO-677. For cell lines OPM-2, KMS-12-BM the dose range lies higher. In MOLP-8 cell line VAQuFrF inhibits the proliferation more effectively than Vincristine.

Our findings suggest that the in vivo effective (active) dose for VAQuFrF will be about 10-20 times higher than that of Vincristine.

6. Future research

1. **Viscum album** (VA) QuFrF extract contains two active components: mistletoe lectins (I, II, III) and viscotoxins.
   Question: Which component is responsible for the effects of this extract? Is this the **lectin(s)** or **viscotoxin** or **both?** Further study is planned to clarify this **question.**
   The non-fermented preparation from VAQuFrF extract contains 2 μg lectin and 10 μg viscotoxin in 10 mg/ml **(ratio between lectin and viscotoxin: 0.2).**
   The **ratio between lectin and viscotoxin from the fermented preparations is 0.06** respectively **0.08.** The fermented preparations are used either alone or in combination with chemo /radiotherapy in the treatment of tumour patients. The extract presented in this study is an experimental drug that is not yet used in the treatment of tumour patients.
2. The results presented in this study indicated that VAQuFrF could effect the membrane expression of IL-6 receptor by antagonism. **Question:** Is this substance a competitive- or a non-competitive antagonist? Additional experiments will give answer to this (important) **question.**
3. To investigate more human multiple myeloma cell lines.
   To investigate **tumour cells isolated from bone marrow** of patients with multiple myeloma.
4. To investigate the anti-proliferative and apoptotic/necrotic effects of Vincristine in a lower dose range, respectively the anti-proliferative and apoptotic/necrotic effects of VAQuFrF extract in a higher dose range.

7. Acknowledgements

The measurements of the parameters were carried out in the laboratory of the Society of Cancer Research (Arlesheim, Switzerland). The idea of this study is based on the findings of the author. As principal investigator she wrote the study protocol and co-ordinated the study. The evaluation of the results, the writing and the completion of this manuscript were not supported from the Society of Cancer Research and from any foundation.

8. References

Chanen-Khan, AA. (2004) Bcl-2 antisense therapy in multiple myeloma. *Oncology* Supplement, 21-24.

Duong Van Huyen, JP., Sooryanarayana Delignat, S., Bloch, MF., Kacatchkine, MD., Kaveri, SV. (2001) Variable sensitivity of lymphoblastoid cells to apoptosis induced by Viscum album QuFrF, a therapeutic preparation of mistletoe lectin. *Chemotherapy* 47, 366-376.

DuVillard, L., Guiguet, M., Casasnovas RO., Caillot, D., Monnier-Zeller, V., et al. (1995) Diagnostic serum level of IL-6 in monoclonal gammopathies. *Brit J Haematol* 89, 243-249.

E1 Alaoui, S., Lawry, J., Griffan, M. (1997) The cell cycle and induction of apoptosis in a hamster fibrosarcoma cell line treated with anti-cancer drugs: its importance to solid tumour chemotherapy. *J Neurol* 31, 195-207.

El-Sherbiny, YM., Cox, MC., Ismail, CA., Shamsuddin, AM., Vucenik, I. (2001) G0/G1 arrest and Sphase inhibition of human cancer cell lines by inositol hexaphosphate (IP6). *Anticancer Research* 21, 2393-2403.

Gaillard, JP., Liautard, J., Klein, P.,Brochier, J. (1997) Major role of the soluble interleukin- 6, interleukin-6 receptor complex for the proliferation of interleukin-6-dependent human myeloma cell lines. *Eur J Immunol* 27, 332-3340.

Harmsma, M., Gromme, M., Ummelen, M., Dignef, W., Tusenius, KJ., et al. (2004) Differential effects of Viscum album extract Iscador^R Qu on cell cycle progression and apoptosis in cancer cells. *Int J Oncol* 125, 1521-1529.

Hata, H., Matsuzaki, H., Takeya, HM., Yoshida, M., Sonoki, T., et al. (1995) Expression of Fas/Apo-1 (CD95) and apoptosis in tumor cells from patients with plasma cell disorders. *Blood* 86, 1939-1945.

Kovacs, E. (2003). How does interleukin-6 affect the membrane expressions of interleukin-6 receptor and gp130 and the proliferation of the human myeloma cell line OPM-2? *Biomed Pharmacother* 57, 489–94.

Kovacs, E., Link, S., Toffol-Schmidt, U. (2006a). Cytostatic and cytocidal effects of mistletoe (Viscum album L.) Quercus extract Iscador. *Drug Research* 56, 467-473.

Kovacs, E. (2006b) Multiple myeloma and B cell lymphoma. Investigation of IL-6, IL-6 receptor antagonist (IL-6RA) and gp130 antagonist (gp130A) in an in vitro model. *The Scientific World Journal* 6, 888-898.

Kovacs, E. (2010a) Interleukin-6 leads to interleukin-10 production in several human multiple myeloma cell lines. Does interleukin-10 enhance the proliferation of these cells? *Leukemia Research* 34, 912-916.

Kovacs, E. (2010b) Investigation of the proliferation, apoptosis/necrosis and cell cycle phases in several human multiple myeloma cell lines. Comparison of Viscum album QuFrF extract with Vincristine in an in vitro model. *The Scientific World Journal* 10, 311-320.

Leoncini, L., Vecchio, MTD., Megha, T., Barbini, P., Galieni, P., et al. (1993) Correlation between apoptotic and proliferative indices in malignant non-Hodgkin's lymphoma. *Am J Pathol* 142, 755-762.

Lin, Ch-KE., Nguyen, TT., Morgan, TL., Mei, RL., Kaptein, JS., et al. (1998) Apoptosis may be either suppressed or enhanced with strategic combinations of anti-neoplastic drugs or anti-IgM. *Experimental Cell Research* 244, 1-13.

Lu, ZY., Zhang, XG., Rodriguez, C., Wijdenes, J., Gu, ZJ., et al. (1995) Interleukin-10 is a proliferation factor but not a differentiation factor for human myeloma cells. *Blood* 85, 2521–27.

Mastberger, SC., Duivenvoorden, 1., Versteegh, RT., Geldof, AA. (2000) Cell cycle arrest and clonogenic tumour cell kill by divergent chemotherapeutic drugs. *Anticancer Research* 20, 1833-1838.

Nachbaur, DM., Herold, M., Maneschg, A., Huber, H. (1991) Serum levels of interleukin-6 in multiple myeloma and other hematological disorders: correlation with disease activity and other prognostic parameters. *Ann Hematol* 62, 54-58.

Nordan, R., & Potter, M. (1986) A macrophage-derived factor required by plasmocytomas for surivival and proliferation in vitro. *Science* 233, 566-569.

Oancea, M., Mani, A., Hussein, MA., Almasan, A. (2004) Apoptosis of multiple myeloma. *Int JHematol* 8, 224-231.

Otsuki, T., Yamada, O., Yata, K., Sakaguchi, H., Kurebayashi, J., et al. (2000) Expression and production of interleukin 10 in human myeloma cell lines. *Br J Haematol* 111, 835–42.

Otsuki, T., Yata, K., Sakaguchi, H., Uno, M., Fujii, T., et al. (2002) IL-10 in myeloma cells. *Leuk Lymphoma* 43, 969–74.

Papadaki, H., Kyriakou, D., Foudoulakis, A., Markidoum F., Alexandrakis, M. (1997) Serum levels of interleukin-6 receptor in multiple myeloma as indicator of disease activity. *Acta Haematologica* 97, 191-195.

Pellizzaro, C., Speranza, A., Zorzet, S., Crucil, I., Sava, G., et al. (2008) Inhibition of human pancreatic cell line MIA PaCa2 proliferation byHA-But, a hyaluronic butyric ester: a preliminary report. *Pancreas* 36, 15-23.

Shinwari, Z., Manogaran, PS., Alrokayan, SA., Al-Hussein, KA., Aboussekhra, A. (2007) Vincristine and Iomustine induce apoptosis and p21 (WAF1) up-regulation in medulloblastoma and normal human epithelial and fibroblast cells. *Neurooncol* 87, 123-132.

Stokke, T., Holte, H., Smedshammer, L., Smeland, EB., Kaalhus, O., et al. (1998) Proliferation and apoptosis in malignant and normal cells in B-cell non-Hodgkin's lymphomas. *Br J Cancer* 77, 1832-1838.

Tsujimoto, Y. & Shimizu, S. (2007) Role of mitochondrial membrane permeability transition in cell death. *Apoptosis* 12, 835-840.

Wierzbowska, A., Urbanska, H., Robak T. (1999) Circulating IL-6 type cytokines and sIL-.6R in patients with multiple myeloma. *Brit J Haematol* 105, 412-419.

27

Ethanol Toxicity in the Brain: Alteration of Astroglial Cell Function

Metoda Lipnik-Štangelj
University of Ljubljana, Faculty of Medicine,
Department of Pharmacology and Experimental Toxicology
Slovenia

1. Introduction

Ethanol consumption has for a long time been associated with brain damage. Experimental studies and necropsy examinations of chronic alcoholics have shown a variety of structural and functional alterations in the neurons as well as in the glial cells. Such alterations are seen also in children with the alcoholic foetal syndrome. Ethanol is known to be a teratogen. Its abusage can result as dysfunction of the central nerve system (CNS), growth deficiency and facial malformation in the fetus, and behavioural, learning, sensory and motor disabilities (Barret et al., 1996; González & Salido, 2009; Šarc & Lipnik-Štangelj, 2009a). Chronic ethanol consumption in the adult is also intimately associated with brain atrophy. Accumulating evidence indicates that ethanol-induced neurobehavioral dysfunctions may be related to disruptions in the patterns of neuronal and glial developments such as depression of neurogenesis, aberrant migration of neurons and alterations in late gliogenesis and neurogenesis. These changes can further reduce the populations of cortical neurons and glial cells, trigger the biochemical alterations in glial cells and deleterious consequences for neuronal-glial interactions, and eventually lead to damage or apoptosis of these cells (González & Salido, 2009; Šarc & Lipnik-Štangelj, 2009b; Sofroniew & Vinters, 2010).

As the most abundant type of glial cells in the brain, astrocytes provide metabolic and trophic support to neurons, modulate synaptic activities and have a strong capacity to scavenge oxidants and suppress cellular apoptosis. However, when the capacity of cells to eliminate the oxidants is overwhelmed, overproduction of reactive oxygen species (ROS) can cause morphological and functional alterations in the cells, including cellular Ca^{2+} homeostasis and some active molecules tightly associated with neuronal activity (Allansson et al., 2001; Halassa et al., 2007; Sofroniew & Vinters, 2010).

Although astrocytes are more resistant than neurons to the oxidative and neurotoxic stresses and to the chemical and toxic damages in the surrounding environment, any impairment of astrocytes can dramatically affect neuronal functions. The ethanol-induced detrimental alterations of astrocytes would lead to perturbances in neuron–astroglia interactions and developmental defects of the brain (González & Salido, 2009; Šarc & Lipnik-Štangelj, 2009b). Given this important role of astroglial cells in neuronal functioning, they have become a significant object of toxicological evaluation.

2. Astrocytes in the central nerve system

Central nerve system is a complex network, constitutes from several types of cells. Besides neuronal cells, where the information is received, integrated and sent as an output signal, there are several other cell types in the CNS. Oligodendrocytes are specialized for the myelin formation, astrocytes have multiple support functions to neurons, and microglial cells play an important role in defence and inflammation, and act as scavengers when tissue is destroyed. Some other types of cells in the CNS are ependimal cells, which are epithelial cells that line brain ventricles and central canal of spinal and assist in secretion and circulation of cerebral spinal fluid, and endothelial cells which create a blood-brain barrier (González & Salido, 2009).

Glial cells were discovered by the pathologist Rudolf Virchow in 1856. They represent the majority cell population in the CNS. There is a number between 12 and 15 billion neurons in cerebral cortex and about a billion neurons in spinal cord, whereas there are 10 to 50 times more glial cells than neurons in the CNS. When they were discovered, glial cells have been recognised as brain glue. They surround neurons and hold them in place. Later it has been realized that glial cells play a number of other functions in the brain. Astrocytes are the most abundant type of glial cells, and present numerous projections that anchor neurons to their blood supply (Braet et al., 2001; González & Salido, 2009; Grafstein et al., 2000; Haydon, 2001).

2.1 Molecular aspects of astrocyte function

Astrocytes signal each other using Ca^{2+} ions (Verkhratsky et al., 1998). This type of cell-to cell communication has been termed "calcium excitability" that occurs as transient or prolonged elevations in intracellular concentration of Ca^{2+} ions. It can be spontaneous or triggered in response to specific neurotransmitters (Araque et al., 2001; Cornell-Bell et al., 1990). The membrane potential of glia is relatively stable, and although they can express voltage-gated channels (Verkhratsky et al., 1998), they exhibit little or no fluctuation in membrane potential.

Astrocytes respond to a variety of extracellular stimuli by raising intracellular concentration of Ca^{2+} ions that modulates different intracellular processes like differentiation, cytoskeleton reorganisation, and secretion of neuroactive molecules (Araque et al., 1998; Sofroniew & Vinters, 2010; Verkhratsky & Kettenmann, 1996). A rise in intracellular concentration of Ca^{2+} ions, localize to one part of an astrocyte can propagate through-out the entire cell, and Ca^{2+} resposes may be transmitted from one astrocate to others, leading to regenerative Ca^{2+} signal that spread within astrocyte networks (Cornell-Bell et al., 1990; Fam et al., 2000). This cell-to-cell communication could effectively signal to neurons, endothelial or other cell type in the CNS. Obviously, Ca^{2+} signalling in astrocytes is complementary to and interacts with signalling in vascular brain cells (Leybaert et al., 2004) and electrical signalling in neurons (Araque et al., 1999; Parpura et al., 1994). Besides calcium excitability, there are also other mechanisms for transmitting signals between astrocytes, such as releasing of diffusible extracellular messengers. Extracellular release of neurotransmitters like glutamate or adenosine triphosphate (ATP), and consequent activation of specific receptors on neighbouring astrocytes, may also mediate Ca^{2+} wave propagation (Bowser & Khakh, 2007). In addition, astrocytes are able to release other signalling molecules like D-serine and eicosanoids, and more than one of describing mechanisms for neurotransmitter release does operate within astrocytes (Araque et al., 2001; Fellin et al., 2004; Gonzales et al., 2006a; Malarkey & Parpura, 2008; Montana et al. 2006).

Released messengers, in turn, activate Ca^{2+} entry or Ca^{2+} release from intracellular stores by acting on ionotropic and metabotropic receptors, respectively. By this way, ATP and glutamate are the major active neurotransitters involved in the cell-to-cell communication of Ca^{2+} signals in astrocytes and other cell types in the CNS (Bowser & Khakh, 2007; Percea & Araque, 2007). Another putative intercellular signalling molecule for cel-to-cell communication is nitric oxide which is synthesized by enzymatic oxidation of L-arginine by nitric oxide synthase (Willmott et al., 2000). Nitric oxide (NO) activates guanylilcyclase and increases cytoplasmic cyclic guanosine monophosphate (cGMP) signalling cascades (Galione et al, 1993).

Communication between astrocytes thus seems to rely on any communication systems and signalling molecules, which act in parallel or display regional and cellular specialisation. From this point of view, there is a bidirectional signal communication system within the CNS, which might be mainly carried out by extracellular messengers, released from any type of cells. Because of their close apposition to neurons, signalling molecules released by astrocytes can modulate synaptic transmission and neuronal excitability, as well as neuronal plasticity and survival. Even it could be possible that astrocytes could play roles in higher cognitive functions like learning and memory. It is not therefore estrange that an alteration in Ca^{2+} signalling, and hence in the function of astrocytes, could affect synaptic activity and plasticity and bran homeostasis (Gonzalez & Salido, 2009).

2.2 Release of intercellular messengers

Close physical relationship between astrocytes and neurones provides an opportunity for many functional interactions. There is a bidirectional signalling pathway between astrocytes and neurons on one side, and astrocytes and blood vessels on the other, which opens the possibility to an exchange of a huge amount of information in the CNS. There are several mechanisms that have been suggested to underline the release of signalling molecules from astrocytes: reverse operation of glutamate transporters, volume-regulated anion channels, gap-junctional hemichannels, diffusional release through purinergic receptors and Ca^{2+}-dependent exocytosis (Araque et al., 2001; Haydon & Carmignoto, 2006; Montana et al., 2006; Parpura et al., 2004). Among the different molecules released, two major signalling messengers, released by astrocytes, are ATP and glutamate (Gonzalez & Salido, 2009).

The mechanisms, by which astrocytes release ATP, appear to be diverse, employing vesicular release, connexion hemi-channels, cystic fibrosis transmembrane regulator, or the P-glycoprotein (Braet et al., 2004). On the other hand, astrocytic glutamate release can be carried out through connexion hemi-channel, excitatory amino acid transporters (EAAT), anion transporter, via $P2X_7$ receptor channels or exocytosis. Depending on the mechanism employed, ATP and/or glutamate release by astrocytes can be Ca^{2+}-dependent or independent (Bowser & Khakh, 2007; Braet et al., 2004).

Besides the mechanisms for ATP and/or glutamate release from astrocytes, exocytosis constitutes the mechanism that has recently received special attention, since it was initially considered to occur only in neurons (Bowser & Khakh, 2007; Fellin et al., 2006; Gonzalez et al., 2006a; Perea & Araque, 2007).

2.3 The role of astroytes in the central nerve system

2.3.1 Astrocytes and development of central nerve system

The developmental generation of astrocytes tends to occur after the initial production of neurons in many CNS regions (Sofroniew & Vinters, 2010). During development of the brain, astrocytes (radial glia) take part in guiding the migration of developing axons and certain neuroblasts (Powel & Geller, 1999). In addition, substantive evidence is accumulating that astrocytes are essential for the formation and function of developing synapses by releasing molecular signals such as thrombospondin (Barres, 2008; Christopherson et al., 2005). Astrocytes appear also to influence developmental synaptic pruning by releasing signals that induce expression of complement C1q in synapses and thereby tag them for elimination by microglia (Barres, 2008).

2.3.2 Blood-brain barrier and regulation of blood flow

Together with brain microvascular endothelial cells astrocytes create the blood-brain barrier that protects the brain from toxic substances in the blood, supplies the brain tissues with nutrients, and filters harmful substances from the brain back to the bloodstream, enabling the proper environment in the CNS. Astrocytes may regulate endothelial cell metabolism, and vasoconstriction and vasodilatation by producing substances with angiogenic properties, such as endothelial growth factor (Proia et al., 2008), ATP (Leybaert et al., 2004), and arachidonic acid, prostagladins and nitric oxide, (Gabryel et al., 2007; Sofroniew & Vinters, 2010), that can increase or decrease CNS blood vessel diameter and blood flow in a coordinated manner. Moreover, astrocytes may be primary mediators of changes in local CNS blood flow in response to changes in neuronal activity (Koehler et al., 2009). Thus, astrocytes play important functions at the level of arterioles where blood flow is controlled, at the level of capillaries where blood-brain barrier is located and at the level of blood immune cells (Leybaert et al., 2004).

2.3.3 Energy, metabolism and homeostasis

Astrocytes play a number of other functions which are crucial for the maintenance of homeostasis and neuronal function. They provide energy supply to neurons and coordinate metabolic reactions. Astrocytes are the principal storage sites of glycogen granules in CNS. The greatest accumulation of astrocytic glycogen occurs in areas of high synaptic density, and its utilisation can sustain neuronal activity during hypoglicemia and during periods of high neuronal activity (Sofroniew & Vinters, 2010).

Astrocytes regulate the external chemical environment by removing excess ions notably potassium, regulate brain cell volume, and participate in recycling neurotransmitters released during synaptic transmission by expressing high levels of transporters for neurotransmitters such as glutamate, GABA, histamine and glycine, that serve to clear the neurotransmitters from the synaptic space. Astrocytes also represent the major site for the detoxification or bioactivation of neurotoxins (Perdan et al., 2009).

2.3.4 Synapse function

There is accumulating evidence that astrocytes play direct roles in synaptic transmission through the regulated release of synaptically active molecules including glutamate, purines

(ATP and adenosine), gamma-aminobutyric acid (GABA), and D-serine. The release of such gliotransmitters occurs in response to changes in neuronal synaptic activity, involves astrocyte excitability as reflected by increases in intracellular concentration of Ca^{2+} ions, and can alter neuronal excitability (Halassa et al., 2007; Perea et al., 2009). Such evidence has given rise to the 'tripartite synapse', which posits that astrocytes play direct and interactive roles with neurons during synaptic activity in a manner that is essential for information processing by neural circuits (Araque et al., 1999; Halassa et al., 2007; Perea et al., 2009).

2.3.5 Immune response

Astrocytes importantly contribute to creation of immune response in the brain. They are an important source of several cytokines and neurotrophic factors in the CNS that have a crucial immunoregulatory role and also promote neuronal survival and neurite growth (Lipnik-Štangelj, 2006). Moreover, cytokines have an impact on neurotoxicity, synaptic transmission and synaptic plasticity in the brain (Allan & Rothwell, 2001). Activation of astrocytes leads to up-regulation of pro-inflammatory cytokines like interleukin-1 beta (IL-1beta), tumour necrosis factor alpha (TNF-alpha), interleukin-6 (IL-6), and inducible nitric oxide synthase (iNOS), and cyclooxygenase 2 (COX2) (Gonzalez & Salido, 2009; Sofroniew & Vinters, 2010).

Research into the actions of IL-1beta in the brain initially focused on its role in host defence responses to systemic disease. IL-1beta can also elicit an array of responses which could inhibit, exacerbate or induce neuronal damage and death (Gonzalez & Salido, 2009).

TNF-alpha has an important function in neurotoxicity, synaptic transmission and synaptic plasticity. It influences homeostatic synaptic scaling by inducing the insertion of AMPA receptors at post-synaptic membranes (Stellwagen & Malenka, 2006). In addition, TNF-alpha may have a pivotal role in augmenting intracerebral immune responses and inflammatory demyelination due to its diverse functional effects on glial cells, such as oligodendrocytes and astrocytes themselves (Šarc et al., 2011).

Unlike TNF-alpha, which is a prototypical pro-inflammatory cytokine, IL-6 affects inflammation and neuronal regeneration via a number of mechanisms. In this sense, besides its immunoregulatory role, IL-6 can also promote neuronal survival and neurite growth. IL-6 can be induced by a variety of molecules including IL-1beta, TNF-alpha, transforming growth factor-beta and prostaglandins, and many other mediators such as beta-amyloid, interferon-g and IL-4 can potentiate these primary inducers, highlighting the complex nature of IL-6 modulation (Šarc et al., 2011; Gonzalez & Salido, 2009).

2.4 Reactive gliosis and glial scar formation

After brain injury, such as a stroke or trauma, astrocytes become reactive, and can undergo to profound proliferation, forming gliosis near or at the site of damage. Astrocyte activity is marked by hypertrophy, resulting in an expression of protein such as glial fibrillary acidic protein (GFAP), adhesion molecules and antigen presenting capabilities, including major histocompatibility antigens. Reactive astrocytes represent an obstacle preventing establishment of normal neural contact and circuitry. On the other hand, reactive astrocytes produce a myriad of neurotoxic substances in various brain pathologies (Mori et al., 2006).

Although reactive astrogliosis is used widely as a pathological hallmark of diseased CNS tissue, definitions of reactive astrogliosis can vary considerably among authors and there are no widely accepted categories of intensity or severity. Recently proposed definition encompasses four key features: (1) reactive astrogliosis is a spectrum of potential molecular, cellular and functional changes in astrocytes that occur in response to all forms and severities of CNS injury and disease including subtle perturbations, (2) the changes undergone by reactive astrocytes vary with severity of the insult along a gradated continuum of progressive alterations in molecular expression, progressive cellular hypertrophy, and in severe cases, proliferation and scar formation, (3) the changes of reactive astrogliosis are regulated in a context-specific manner by inter- and intracellular signalling molecules, (4) the changes undergone during reactive astrogliosis have the potential to alter astrocyte activities both through gain and loss of function that can impact both beneficially and detrimentally on surrounding neural and non-neural cells. Of particular interest as regards function of reactive astrocytes, is recent evidence that reactive astrogliosis and glial scar formation play essential roles in regulating CNS inflammation (Sofroniew, 2009).

In response to different kind of stimulation, reactive astrocytes can make many different kinds of molecules with either pro- or anti-inflammatory potential (John et al., 2003). There is a normal process of reactive astrogliosis and glial scar formation that exerts various beneficial functions including protecting neural cells and function, restricting the spread of inflammation, and promoting tissue repair.

On the contrary, in a manner analogous to inflammation, reactive astrogliosis also has the potential to exert detrimental effects. For example, reactive astrocytes can be stimulated by specific signalling cascades to gain of detrimental effects such as exacerbating inflammation via cytokine production (Brambilla et al., 2009), producing neurotoxic levels of ROS (Hamby et al., 2006), releasing potentially excitotoxic glutamate (Takano et al., 2005), potential contribution to seizure genesis (Tian et al., 2005), compromising blood brain barrier function due to VEGF-production (Argaw et al., 2009), causing cytotoxic edema during trauma and stroke (Zador et al., 2009), and contributing to chronic pain (Milligan et al., 2009).

2.4.1 Molecular mechanisms of reactive gliosis and scar formation

Many different types of intercellular signalling molecules are able to trigger reactive astrogliosis or to regulate specific aspects of reactive astrogliosis, including large polypeptide growth factors and cytokines such as IL-1, IL6, IL-10, TNF-alpha, tumour growth factor beta (TGF-beta), mediators of innate immunity such as lipopolysaccharide and other Toll-like receptor ligands, neurotransmitters such as glutamate and noradrenalin, purines such as ATP, ROS including nitric oxide (NO), hypoxia and glucose deprivation, products associated with neurodegeneration such as beta-amyloid, molecules associated with systemic metabolic toxicity such as NH4, and regulators of cell proliferation such endothelin-1, as reviewed in detail elsewhere (Sofroniew, 2009). Such molecular mediators of reactive astrogliosis can be released by all cell types in CNS tissue, including neurons, microglia, oligodendrocyte lineage cells, pericytes, endothelia, and astrocytes, in response to all forms of CNS insults, ranging from subtle cellular perturbations that release some of the specific factors just listed, to cell stretching as might be encountered during acceleration/deceleration CNS injury and which releases ATP, to intense tissue injury and cell death that release various intracellular molecules that signal intense tissue damage (Sofroniew, 2009).

It is becoming clear that different molecular, morphological, and functional changes in reactive astrocytes are specifically controlled by inter- and intra-cellular signalling mechanisms that reflect the specific contexts of the stimuli and produce specific and gradated responses of reactive astrogliosis. For a long, reactive gliosis and scar formation have been recognized as the main impediment to functional recovery after CNS injury or disease. This absolutely negative viewpoint of reactive astrogliosis is no longer tenable and it is now clear from many different lines of experimental evidence that there is a normal process of reactive astrogliosis that exerts essential beneficial functions and does not do harm. As reviewed in detail elsewhere, many studies using transgenic and experimental animal models provide compelling evidence that reactive astrocytes protect CNS cells and tissue by uptake of potentially excitotoxic glutamate, protection from oxidative stress via glutathione production (Dringen et al., 2000), neuroprotection via adenosine release (Lin et al., 2008), protection from NH4 toxicity (Rao et al., 2005), neuroprotection by degradation of amyloid-beta peptides (Koistinaho et al., 2004), facilitating blood brain barrier repair, reducing vasogenic edema after trauma (Bush et al., 1999), stroke or obstructive hydrocephalus, stabilizing extracellular fluid and ion balance and reducing seizure threshold (Zador et al., 2009), and limiting the spread of inflammatory cells or infectious agents from areas of damage or disease into healthy CNS parenchyma (Bush et al., 1999; Voskuhl et al. 2009).

3. Ethanol in the central nerve system

The deleterious effects of ethanol in CNS could result either from a direct toxic effect of ethanol or from an indirect effect involving its metabolites and/or ROS generation. Ethanol can induce several cellular reactions which result in a modification of cellular redox status that can severely affect the cell's capacity to be protected against the endogenous production of ROS (Gonthier et al., 2004). The consequences derived from the effects of ethanol on cellular structures would end in a morphological and functional impairment of cellular physiology. Among brain cells, astrocytes seem less vulnerable than neurons, but their impairment can dramatically affect neurons because of their protective role towards neurons.

3.1 Ethanol metabolism in the brain

In the CNS, astrocytes represent the major cellular localisation of ethanol metabolism, and have been postulated to protect neurons from ethanol-induced oxidative stress (Watts et al., 2005). The exact enzymatic mechanism responsible for ethanol oxidation in the brain is not clear yet.

Ethanol is normally metabolised in the liver to acetaldehyde by the alcohol dehydrogenase reaction, and acetaldehyde can be further metabolised to acetic acid via aldehyde dehydrogenase reaction. The last step in the pathway is the conversion of acetic acid to acetyl-Co-A. Although theoretically the activity of the latter enzyme is high enough to cope with the rate at which ethanol is oxidized by alcohol dehydrogenase, there is a limit to the rate at which the reaction can continue and can therefore lead to accumulation of acetaldehyde, which is toxic for most tissues, including CNS. Thus, there is always a build up of acetaldehyde which passes out from the liver into the blood, and this acetaldehyde is responsible or some of the unpleasant symptoms of alcohol excess. Once in the bloodstream, the acetaldehyde can also cross the blood-brain barrier and attack the CNS.

In the brain, ethanol can be metabolized by catalase, cytochrome P450 2E1, and alcohol-dehydrogenase, with catalase, playing a pivotal role among the others (Gonzalez et al., 2007).

On the other hand, ethanol also induces up-regulation of antioxidant defences by increasing the enzymatic activities of superoxide-dismutase, catalase, and glutathione-peroxidase (Eysseric et al., 2000; Rathinam et al., 2006). The expression of heat shock proteins like HSP70 (Russo et al., 2001), which have a protective and stabilizing effect on stress-induced injury, is also induced by ethanol. Altogether, this would confer to astrocytes a survival advantage preventing oxidative damage.

3.2 Ethanol influence on astrocyte function

Ethanol has several targets in astrocytes and other cell types, impairing cellular redox status, cell growth and differentiation, interfering with the stimulatory effect of trophic factors or altering the expression of cytoskeletal proteins. In addition, ethanol induces astroglial activation, associated with up-regulation of several pro-inflammatory cytokines, that contribute to neuroinflammation, neurodegeneration and cell apoptosis (Alfonso-Loeches et al., 2010; Šarc & Lipnik-Štangelj, 2009).

3.2.1 The effects of ethanol on developing central nerve system

Ethanol is a known teratogen and has been implicated in the etiology of human fetal alcohol syndrome, which is characterized by distinct craniofacial abnormalities such as microcephaly, agnathia, and ocular aberrations. Prenatal ethanol exposure induces functional abnormalities during brain development affecting neurogenesis and gliogenesis. Thus, ethanol cases a number of changes in several neurochemical systems. Astrocytes are predominant source of postnatal retinoic acid synthesis in the cerebellum, and this acid shows teratogenic effects responsible for the fetal alcohol syndrome.

McCaffery et al. (2004) showed that ethanol could stimulate retinoic acid synthesis leading to abnormal embryonic concentrations of this morphogen and, thus, ethanol could represent a major cause of fetal alcohol syndrome. Additionally, increased sensitivity of glutamate receptors and enhanced trans-membrane transport of glutamate has been observed in the presence of ethanol. This was in relationship to the increase in the expression of the excitatory amino acid transporters EAAT1 and EAAT2. Thus, glutamatergic system is affected by ethanol, which can be viewed as a maladaptive process that disposes the developing brain to fetal alcohol syndrome (Zink et al. 2004).

Furthermore, ethanol affects the synthesis, intracellular transport, distribution, and secretin of N-glicoproteins in different cell types, including astrocytes and neurons (Braza-Boils t al., 2006). Glicoproteins, such as adhesion molecules and growth factors, participate in the regulation of nervous system development. Thus, the alteration in the glycosylation process induced by ethanol could be a key mechanism involved in the teratogenic effects of ethanol exposure on brain development. Further studies by Martinez et al., (2007) showed that long-term ethanol treatment substantially impairs glycosylation and membrane trafficking in primary cultures of rat astrocytes. Ethanol reduced endogenous levels of acive RhoA due to an increase in the activity of small Rho GTP-ases, reduced phosphoinositides levels and induced changes in the dynamics and organization of the actin cytoskeleton.

Ethanol presents as well morphological effects on the developing adolescent brain. There were clear effects immediately and long after drinking cessation of a chronic ethanol administration on two neurotransmitter systems (the serotoninergic and nitrergic), which decreased, and the astrocytic cytoskeleton and neuron, which increased and decreased, respectively (Evrard et al., 2006). The authors concluded that drinking cessation can partially ameliorate the ethanol-induced morphological changes on neurons and astrocytes but cannot fully return it to the basal state.

3.2.2 The effects of ethanol on cholesterol homeostasis

Cholesterol is an essential component of cell membranes and plays an important rule in signal transduction. There are evidences that cholesterol homeostasis may be affected by ethanol, and this may be involved in neurotoxicity (Guizzetti & Costa, 2007). Indeed, the pathogenesis of Alzheimer's disease has been linked to altered cholesterol homeostasis in the brain. Several functions are carried out by cholesterol and are important for brain development, such as glial cell proliferation, synaptogenesis, neuronal survival and neurite outgrowth. In addition, the brain contains high level of cholesterol, mostly synthesized in situ. Furthermore, astrocytes produce large amounts of cholesterol that can be released by these cells and utilized by neurons to form synapses (Gonzalez & Salido, 2009).

3.2.3 The effects of ethanol on synaptic structure

It has been shown that chronic ethanol consumption affects the synaptic structure. The density of dendritic spines was found lower in the nucleus accumbens, and depicted an up-regulation of a subunit of the NMDA receptor. The up-regulated NMDA receptor subunit is a splice variant isoform which is required for membrane-bound trafficking or anchoring into a spine synaptic site. These changes, evoked by ethanol, demonstrated an alteration of micro circuitry for glutamate reception (Zhou et al., 2007).

Adermark and Loviger (2006) showed that ethanol inhibits a Ca^{2+}-insensitive K^+ channel activity, and affects gap junction coupling, demonstrating that astrocytes play a critical role in brain K^+ homeostasis, and that ethanol effects on astrocytic function could influence neuronal activity.

Finally, despite most of the investigations on the effects of ethanol have been performed following its addition to tissue or cell cultures, an interesting study has shown excessive activation of glutamatergic neurotransmission in the cerebral cortex following ethanol withdrawal and its contribution to significant behavioural disturbances and to alcohol craving. These effects were related to the activity of the enzyme glutamine synthetase, which converts released glutamate to glutamine (Miguel-Hidalgo, 2006).

3.2.4 Ethanol and glial oxidative stress

Brain tissue is particularly vulnerable to oxidative damage, possibly due to its high consumption of oxygen and the consequent generation of high quantities of ROS during oxidative phosphorylation. In addition, several regions of the brain are rich in iron, which promotes the production of ROS. On the other hand, the brain counts wit relatively poor levels of antioxidant enzymes and antioxidant compounds. ROS increase intracellular concentration of Ca^{2+} ions, inhibit response of astrocytes to physiological agonists, and stimulate glutamate secretion, which in excess is neurotoxic (Gonzalez et al., 2006a). Although glutamate is the principal excitatory neurotransmitter in the mammalian brain, high levels of this neurotransmitter lead to excitotoxic neuronal death, mediated by Ca^{2+} influx, principally through NMDA-gated channels (Bambrick et al., 2004).

Ca^{2+} signalling is an important medium for neuron-glia interaction, in the sense that neuronal activity can trigger Ca^{2+} signals in glial cells and vice versa. Due to its critical importance for the cellular functions, resting intracellular concentration of Ca^{2+} ions is tightly controlled, and abnormalities in Ca^{2+} regulation lead to impairment of cellular physiology. Ca^{2+}-ROS interplay can be considered as a push-pull relationship. An elevated level of intracellular concentration of Ca^{2+} ions can lead to excessive ROS production, whereas excessive ROS production can lead to cytosolic Ca^{2+} overload (Gonzalez & Salido, 2009). Acute exposure of astrocytes to ethanol increases intracellular concentration of Ca^{2+} ions, probably due to inhibition of plasma membrane Ca^{2+}-ATPase activity (Sepulveda & Mata, 2004). Other changes, evoked by ethanol are cell swelling, and transformation of actin cytoskeleton (Allansson et al., 2001).

Mitochondria represent the major source of intracellular ROS, and Ca^{2+} uptake into the organelle can lead to ROS generation (Gonzalez et al., 2006b; Granados et al., 2004). Ethanol-evoked ROS production takes place in the mitochondria, and accumulated mitochondrial ROS can be released to the cytoplasm leading to damage of different transport mechanisms, ion channel modification, lipid peroxidation, and DNA damage. Furthermore, damage to mitochondrial metabolism may generate additional damaging radial species, thus activating cellular death pathways (Gonzalez et al., 2006a).

Ethanol evokes a dose-dependent increase in glutamate secretion by an exocytosis mechanism, which was dependent on Ca^{2+} mobilisation. The secretory effect of ethanol is reduced in the presence of antioxidants, therefore indicating the participation of ROS in ethanol-evoked glutamate secretion by astrocytes. Glutamate and the attendant increase in intracellular Ca^{2+} play crucial role in triggering excitotoxic cell death in neighbouring cells (Molz et al., 2008). Because astrocytes are the major regulators of glutamate homeostasis, their death can cause and/or aggravate diseases of the CNS.

3.2.5 Ethanol, inflammation and immune response

Ethanol is able to activate glial cells, which is a critical event in the neuroinflammatory processes. Chronic ethanol intake enhances inflammatory mediators like COX-2, and iNOS in rat cerebral cortex and cultured astrocytes. Astrocytes undergo actin cytoskeleton disorganisation, and there is a stimulation of both, interleukin receptor-associated kinase (IRAK)/extracellular signal-regulated kinases (ERK)/nuclear factor-kappaB (NF-kappaB) pathway and the COX-2 expression, which are associated with the inflammatory responses (Guasch et al., 2007).

Ethanol-induced glial activation is also associated with changes in the expression of inflammatory cytokines like IL-1alpha, TNF-alpha, IL-6. Notably, an increased expression of the pro-inflammatory cytokine MCP-1 (monocyte chemoattractant protein 1) and microglial activation as well as astrogliosis have been demonstrated by postmortem analyses in alcoholic brains (Gonzalez & Salido, 2009; He and Crews, 2008).

Besides ethanol, its primary metabolite acetaldehyde is also able to modulate TNF-alpha and IL-6 secretion from cultured astrocytes. Both compounds showed a biphasic, hormetic effect on the IL-6 secretion after the acute as well as after the long-term exposure. It has been shown that long-term exposure to ethanol and acetaldehyde is more toxic than an acute exposure. The maximum stimulation was reached for 50 mM ethanol and 1 mM acetaldehyde after chronic exposure. In contrast, both compounds reduced the TNF-alpha secretion, where the effect was concentration dependent. Acetaldehyde showed to be more potent toxin than ethanol, and the ethanol's toxicity in the brain is at least partially due to its primary metabolite, acetaldehyde (Šarc et al., 2011).

Inflammation is primarily a protective response of the target organism to a noxis. On the other hand, excessive or long-lasting inflammation is often followed by degenerative processes. The stimulatory effect of ethanol and acetaldehyde on IL-6 secretion seems to be involved in both neuroregenerative and survival processes as well as in neurodegeneration. The obtained hormetic dose-response relationship indicates that higher concentrations and long-term exposure could lead in a neurodegenerative direction whereas low concentrations may act as neuroprotective. Unlike TNF-alpha, which is responsible for the induction of multiple pro-inflammatory genes, IL-6 often fails to induce these genes. Moreover, IL-6 can down-regulate the expression of TNF-alpha, which correlate with the data, where the first significant decrease in the TNF-alpha level was found at the highest level of IL-6 after a long-term exposure to ethanol (Šarc et al., 2011).

3.2.6 Ethanol and glial cell death

Apoptosis or programmed cell death is a form of cell death that occurs in multicellular organisms. Apoptosis is a tightly regulated process which engages multiple cell signalling pathways, and involves the altruistic suicide if individual cells in favour of the organism. This process is desirably during organism development and morphological changes, especially at the embryonic stage, as well as during the activation of the immune system. However, defects in apoptosis can result in cancer, autoimmune diseases and neurodegenerative disorders. Studies on Ca^{2+} signalling in apoptosis showed that ethanol potentiates apoptotic cell death induction by thapsigargin, caffeine, and the protonophore, which separately caused similar increases in Ca^{2+} levels, and also induces similar apoptotic death. These effects of ethanol are concentration and time-dependent (Hirata et al., 2006).

The effect of ethanol on the induction of apoptosis in astrocytes, and the formation of ceramide as apoptotic signal was investigated by Schatter et al. (2005). Ethanol induced nuclear fragmentation and DNA laddering, and inhibited phospholipase D-mediated formation of phosphatidic acid, which is a mitogenic lipid messenger. The authors concluded that ethanol induced glial apoptosis during brain development via formation of ceramide. Further studies have shown that astrocytes exposed to ethanol, undergo morphological changes associated with anoikis, a programmed cell death induced by loss of anchorage. Astrocytes depicted peripheral reorganisation of both, focal adhesions and actin-myosin system, cell contraction, membrane blebbing and chromatin condensation (Gonzalez & Salido, 2009).

Recently, it has been shown that ethanol affect intracellular trafficking. In fact, ethanol could interfere with nucleoplasmic transport in astrocytes, in such a way that ethanol induces a delay in both import and export of proteins to the nucleus (Marin et al., 2008).

Neurodegeneration, brain injury, and neuroinflammation are associated not only with increased cell apoptosis but also with the activation of a key proteolytic enzyme in this process, caspase-3. Immunohistochemical findings in mice, fed chronically with ethanol, reveal that inflammatory processes occur concomitantly with caspase-3 activation, suggesting an increase in programmed cell death. Moreover, it seems that the alcohol-induced toll-like receptor 4 (TLR4) response triggers both, inflammatory processes and apoptosis. A recent study suggests that the TLR4 response can also induce oxidative stress and neuronal injury, which agrees with a role of TLR4 in ethanol-induced brain damage and possibly in neurodegeneration (Alfonso-Loeches et al., 2010).

It has been shown that ethanol can activate or inhibit TLR4 by interacting with membrane lipids. Low/moderate ethanol concentrations (10–50 mM, in the range found in the blood of social drinkers and alcoholics) are capable of promoting translocation and clustering of TLR4 and a surface marker protein CD14, and the signalling molecules, like interleukin receptor-associated kinase (IRAK) and extracellular signal-regulated kinases (ERK), into the lipid rafts (Blanco et al., 2008; Fernandez-Lizarbe et al., 2008). Conversely, high ethanol concentrations or lipid raft-disrupting agents (streptolysin-*O* or saponin) inhibit ethanol-induced activation of the TLR4 signalling pathway (Blanco et al., 2008; Fernandez-Lizarbe et al., 2008). However, the molecular mechanism of ethanol interactions with TLR4 remains unknown.

4. Conclusion

Astrocytes are essential for maintaining a healthy and well-functioning brain. They face the synapses, send end-foot processes that enwrap the brain capillaries, and form an extensive network interconnected by gap junctions. They have the potential to impact on essentially all aspects of neuronal function through regulation of blood flow, provision of energy substrates, or by influencing synaptic function and plasticity. Moreover, astrocytes also protect and aid the brain in the functional recovery from injuries. The activation of glial cells in the CNS is the first defence mechanism against pathological abnormalities that occur in neurodegenerative diseases.

Ethanol has an extensive array of actions on astrocytes, transforming them into activated, potentially injurious cells with negative consequences to neuronal function and survival, and to brain function.

Therefore, it is a pivotal solution to seek molecular mechanisms and molecules that may inhibit or attenuate ethanol-induced neurotoxicity in astrocytes, thus offering an alternative strategy to prevent or treat neurodevelopmental disorders and mental retardation caused by ethanol.

5. Acknowledgment

The work was supported by the grant P3-0067 from the Slovenian Research Agency.

6. References

Adermark, L. & Lovinger, D.M. (2006). Ethanol effects on electrophysiological properties of astrocytes in striatal brain slices. *Neuropharmacology,* Vol.51, No.7-8, (December 2006), pp. 1099-1108.

Alfonso-Loeches, S.; Pascual-Lucas, M.; Blanco, A.M.; Sanchez-Vera, I. & Guerri, C. (2010). Pivotal Role of TLR4 Receptors in Alcohol-Induced Neuroinflammation and Brain Damage. *The Journal of Neuroscience,* Vol. 30, No.24, (June 2010), pp. 8285- 8295.

Allan, S.M. & Rothwell, N.J. (2001). Cytokines and acute neurodegeneration. *Nature Review Neuroscience,* Vol.2, No.10, (October 2001), pp. 734-744.

Allansson, L.; Khatibi, S.; Olsson, T. & Hansson, E. (2001)Acute ethanol exposure induces [Ca2+]i transients, cell swelling and transformation of actin cytoskeleton in astroglial primary cultures. *Journal of Neurochemistry,* Vol.76, No.2, (January 2001), pp. 472-479.

Araque, A.; Parpura, V.; Sanzgiri, R.P. & Haydon, P.G. (1998). Glutamate-dependent astrocyte modulation of synaptic transmission between cultured hippocampal neurons. *European Journal of Neuroscience,* Vol.10, No.6, (June 1998), pp. 2129-2142.

Araque, A.; Parpura, V.; Sanzgiri, R.P. & Haydon, P.G. (1999). Tripartite synapses: glia, the unacknowledged partner. *Trends in Neurosciences,* Vol.22, No.5, (May 1999), pp. 208-215.

Araque, A.; Carmignoto, G. & Haydon, P.G. (2001). Dynamic signaling between astrocytes and neurons. *Annual Review of Physiology,* Vol.63, (2001), pp. 795-813.

Argaw, A.T.; Gurfein, B.T.; Zhang, Y.; Zameer, A. & John, G.R. (2009). VEGF-mediated disruption of endothelial CLN-5 promotes blood-brain barrier breakdown. *Proceedings of the National Academy of Sciences USA,* Vol.106, (2009), pp.1977–1982.

Bambrick, L.; Kristian, T. & Fiskum, G. (2004). Astrocyte mitochondrial mechanisms of ischemic brain injury and neuroprotection. *Neurochemistry Research,* Vol.29, (2004), pp. 601-608.

Barres, B.A. (2008). The mystery and magic of glia: a perspective on their roles in health and disease. *Neuron,* Vol.60, (2008), pp. 430–440.

Barret, L.; Soubeyran, A.; Usson, Y.; Eysseric, H. & Saxod, R. (1996). Characterization of the morphological variations of astrocytes in culture following ethanol exposure. *Neurotoxicology,* Vol.17, No.2, (1996), pp. 497-507.

Blanco, A.M.; Perez-Arago, A.; Fernandez-Lizarbe, S. & Guerri, C. (2008). Ethanol mimics ligand-mediated activation and endocytosis of IL-1RI/TLR4 receptors via lipid rafts caveolae in astroglial cells. *Journal of Neurochemistry,* Vol.106, No.2, (July 2008), pp. 625-639.

Bowser, D.N. & Khakh, B.S. (2007). Vesicular ATP is the predominant cause of intercellular calcium waves in astrocytes. *Journal of General Physiology,* Vol.129, No.6, (June 2007), pp. 485-491.

Braet, K.; Paemeleire, K.; D'Herde, K.; Sanderson, M.J. & Leybaert, L. (2001). Astrocyte-endothelial cell calcium signals conveyed by two signalling pathways. *European Journal of Neuroscience,* Vol.13, No.1, (January 2001), pp 79-91.

Braet, K.; Cabooter, L.; Paemeleire, K. & Leybaert, L. (2004). Calcium signal communication in the central nervous system. *Biology of the Cell,* Vol.94, No.1, (February 2004), pp. 79-91.

Brambilla, R.; Persaud, T.; Hu, X.; Karmally, S.; Shestopalov, V.I.; Dvoriantchikova, G.; Ivanov, D.; Nathanson, L.; Barnum, S.R. & Bethea, J.R. (2009) .Transgenic inhibition of astroglial NF-kappaB improves functional outcome in experimental autoimmune encephalomyelitis by suppressing chronic central nervous system inflammation. *Journal of Immunoloy,* Vol.182, (2009), pp.2628–2640.

Braza-Boïls, A.; Tomás, M.; Marín, M.P.; Megías, L.; Sancho-Tello, M.; Fornas, E. & Renau-Piqueras, J. (2006). Glycosylation is altered by ethanol in rat hippocampal cultured neurons. *Alcohol Alcohol,* Vol.41, No.5, (September-October 2006), pp. 494-504.

Bush, T.G. N.P.; Horner, C.H.; Polito, A.; Ostenfeld, T.; Svendsen, C.N.; Mucke, L.; Johnson, M.H. & Sofroniew. M.V. (1999). Leukocyte infiltration, neuronal degeneration and neurite outgrowth after ablation of scar-forming, reactive astrocytes in adult transgenic mice. *Neuron,* Vol.23, (1999), pp. 297–308.

Christopherson, K.S.; Ullian, E.; Stokes, C.C.; Mullowney, C.E.; Hell, J.W.; Agah, A.; Lawler, J.; Mosher, D.F.; Bornstein, P. & Barres, B.A. (2005). Thrombospondins are astrocyte-secreted proteins that promote CNS synaptogenesis. Cell, Vol.120, (2005), pp. 421–433.

Cornell-Bell, A.H.; Finkbeiner, S.M.; Cooper, M. & Smith S.J. (1990). Glutamate induces calcium waves in cultured astrocytes: long-range glial signaling. *Science,* Vol.26, No.247, (January 1990), pp. 470-473.

Dringen, R.; Gutterer, J.M. & Hirrlinger, J. (2000). Glutathione metabolism in brain metabolic interaction between astrocytes and neurons in the defense against reactive oxygen species. *European Journal of Biochemistry,* Vol.267, No.16, (August 2000), pp. 4912-4916.

Evrard, S.G.; Duhalde-Vega, M.; Tagliaferro, P.; Mirochnic, S.; Caltana, L.R. & Brusco, A. (2006). A low chronic ethanol exposure induces morphological changes in the adolescent rat brain that are not fully recovered even after a long abstinence: an immunohistochemical study. *Experimental Neurology,* Vol. 200, No.2, (August 2006), pp. 438-459.

Eysseric, H.; Gonthier, B.; Soubeyran, A.; Richard, M.J.; Daveloose, D. & Barret, L. (2000). Effects of chronic ethanol exposure on acetaldehyde and free radical production by astrocytes in culture. *Alcohol,* Vol.21, No.2, (June 2000) pp. 117-125.

Fam, S.R.; Gallagher, C.J. & Salter, M.W. (2000). P2Y(1) purinoceptor-mediated Ca(2+) signaling and Ca(2+) wave propagation in dorsal spinal cord astrocytes. *Journal of Neuroscience,* Vol.15, No.20, (April 2000), pp. 2800-2808.

Fellin, T.; Pascual, O.; Gobbo, S.; Pozzan, T.; Haydon, P.G. & Carmignoto, G. (2004). Neuronal synchrony mediated by astrocytic glutamate through activation of extrasynaptic NMDA receptors. *Neuron,* Vol.2, No.43, (September 2004), pp. 729-743.

Fellin, T.; Sul, J.Y.; D'Ascenzo, M.; Takano, H.; Pascual, O. & Haydon, P.G. (2006). Bidirectional astrocyte-neuron communication: the many roles of glutamate and ATP. *Novartis Foundation Symposium,* Vol.276, (2006), pp. 208-217.

Fernandez-Lizarbe, S.; Pascual, M.; Gascon, M.S.; Blanco, A. & Guerri, C. (2008). Lipid rafts regulate ethanol-induced activation of TLR4 signaling in murine macrophages. *Molecular Immunology,* Vol.45, (2008), pp. 2007–2016.

Gabryel, B.; Chalimoniuk, M.; Stolecka, A. & Langfort, J. (2007). Activation of cPLA2 and sPLA2 in astrocytes exposed to simulated ischemia in vitro. *Cell Biology International,* Vol.31, No.9, (September 2007), pp. 958-965.

Galione, A.; White, A.; Willmott, N.; Turner, M.; Potter, B.V. & Watson S.P. (1993). cGMP mobilizes intracellular Ca2+ in sea urchin eggs by stimulating cyclic ADP-ribose synthesis. *Nature,* Vol.365, No.6445, (September 1993), pp. 456-459.

Gonthier, B.; Signorini-Allibe, N.; Soubeyran, A.; Eysseric, H.; Lamarche, F. & Barret, L. (2004). Ethanol can modify the effects of certain free radical-generating systems on astrocytes. *Alcoholism,* Vol.28, (2004), pp. 526-533.

González, A.; Granados, M.P.; Pariente, J.A. & Salido, G.M. (2006). H2O2 mobilizes Ca2+ from agonist- and thapsigargin-sensitive and insensitive intracellular stores and stimulates glutamate secretion in rat hippocampal astrocytes. *Neurochemistry Research,* Vol.31, No.6, (June 2006), pp. 741-750.

González, A.; Núñez, A.M.; Granados, M.P.; Pariente, J.A,. & Salido, G.M. (2006). Ethanol impairs CCK-8-evoked amylase secretion through Ca2+-mediated ROS generation in mouse pancreatic acinar cells. *Alcohol,* Vol.31, No.1, (January 2006), pp. 51-57.

González, A.; Pariente, J.A. & Salido, G.M. (2007). Ethanol stimulates ROS generation by mitochondria through Ca2+ mobilization and increases GFAP content in rat hippocampal astrocytes. *Brain Research,* Vol.31, No.1178, (October 2007), pp. 28-37.

González, A. & Salido G.M. (2009). Ethanol alters the physiology of neuron-glia communication. *Internal review of neurobiology,* Vol.88, (2009), pp. 168-199.

Grafstein, B.; Liu, S.; Cotrina, M.L. & Goldman, S.A. (2000). Nedergaard M. Meningeal cells can communicate with astrocytes by calcium signaling. *Annals of Neurology,* Vol.47, No.1, (January 2000), pp. 18-25.

Granados, M.P.; Salido, G.M.; Pariente, J.A. & González, A. (2004). Generation of ROS in response to CCK-8 stimulation in mouse pancreatic acinar cells. *Mitochondrion,* Vol.3, No.5, (April 2004), pp. 285-296.

Guasch, R.M.; Blanco, A.M.; Pérez-Aragó, A.; Miñambres, R.; Talens-Visconti, R.; Peris, B. & Guerri, C. (2007). RhoE participates in the stimulation of the inflammatory response induced by ethanol in astrocytes. *Experimental Cell Research,* Vol.15, No.313, (October 2007), pp.3779-3788.

Guizzetti, M. & Costa, L.G. (2007). Cholesterol homeostasis in the developing brain: A possible new target for ethanol. *Human and Experimental Toxicology,* Vol.26, (2007), pp. 355-360.

Halassa, M.M.; Fellin, T.; Takano, H.; Dong, J.H. & Haydon, P.G. (2007). Synaptic islands defined by the territory of a single astrocyte. *Journal of Neuroscience,* Vol.27, (2007), pp. 6473–6477.

Hamby, M.E.; Hewett, J.A. & Hewett, S.J. (2006). TGF-beta1 potentiates astrocytic nitric oxide production by expanding the population of astrocytes that express NOS-2. *Glia,* Vol.54, (2006), pp.566–577.

Haydon, P.G. (2001). Glia: listening and talking to the synapse. *Nature Reviews Neuroscience,* Vol.2, (2001), pp. 185-193.

Haydon, P.G. & Carmignoto, G. (2006). Astrocyte control of synaptic transmission and neurovascular coupling. *Physiological Reviews,* Vol.86, (2006), pp. 1009-1031.

He, J. & Crews, F.T. (2008). Increased MCP-1 and microglia in various regions of the human alcoholic brain. *Experimental Neurology,* Vol.210, (2008), pp. 349 -358.

Hirata, H.; Machado, L.S.; Okuno, C.S.; Brasolin, A.; Lopes, G.S. & SmAili, S.S. (2006). Apoptotic effect of ethanol is potentiated by caffeine-iduced calcium release in rat astrocytes. *Neuroscience Letters,* Vol.393, (2006), pp. 136-140.

John, G.R.; Lee, S.C. & Brosnan, C.F. (2003). Cytokines: Powerful regulators of glial cell activation. *Neuroscientist,* Vol.9, (2003), pp. 10–22.

Koistinaho, M.; Lin, S.; Wu, X.; Esterman, M.; Koger, D.; Hanson, J.; Higgs, R.; Liu, F.; Malkani, S.; Bales, K.R. & Paul, S.M. (2004). Apolipoprotein E promotes astrocyte colocalization and degradation of deposited amyloid-beta peptides. *Nature Medicine,* Vol.10, (2004), pp. 719–726.

Leybaert, L.; Cabooter, L. & Braet, K. (2004). Calcium signal communication between glial and vascular brain cells. *Acta Neurologica Belgica,* Vol.104, (2004), pp. 51-56.

Lin, J.H.; Lou, N.; Kang, N.; Takano, T.; Hu, F.; Han, X.; Xu, Q.; Lovatt, D.; Torres, A.; Willecke, K.; Yang, J.; Kang, J. & Nedergaard, M. (2008). A central role of connexin 43 in hypoxic preconditioning. *Journal of Neurosciences,* Vol.28, (2008), pp.681–695.

Lipnik-Štangelj, M. (2006). Multiple role of histamine H1-receptor-PKC-MAPK signalling pathway in histamine stimullated nerve growth factor synthesis and secretion. *Biochemical pharmacology,* Vol.72, No.11, (2006), pp. 1375-1381.

Malarkey, E.B. & Parpura, V. (2008). Mechanisms of glutamate release from atrocytes. *Neurochemistry International,* Vol.52, (2008), pp. 142-154.

Marin, M.P.; Tomas, M.; Esteban-Pretel;, G.; Megias, l.; Lopez-Iglesias, C.; Egea, G. & Renau-Piqueras, J. (2008). Chronic ethanol exposure induces alterations in the nucleocytoplasmic transport in growing astroytes. *Journal of Neurochemistry,* Vol.106, (2008), pp. 1914-1928.

Martinez, S.E.; Lazaro-Dieguez, F.; Selva, J.; Calvo, F.; Piqueras, J.R.; Crespo, P.; Claro, E. & Egea, G. (2007). Lysophosphatidic acid rescues RhoA activation and phosphoinositides levels in astrocytes expoed to ethanol. *Journal of Neurochemistry,* Vol.102, (2007), pp. 1044-1052.

McCaffery, P.; Koul, O.; Smith, D.; Napoli, J.L.; Chen, N. & Ullman, M.D. (2004). Ethanol increases retinoic acid production in cerebellar astrocyes and i cerebellum. *Brain Research. Developmental Brain Research,* Vol.153, (2004), pp. 233-241.

Miguel-Hildago, J.J. (2006). Withdrawal from free-choice ethanol consumption results in increased packing density of glutamine synthetase-immunoreactive astrocytes in the prelimbic cortex of alcohol-preffering rats. *Alcohol Alcoholism,* Vol. 41, (2006), pp. 379-385.

Milligan, E.D. & Watkins, L.R. (2009). Pathological and protective roles of glia in chronic pain. *Nature Reviews Neuroscience,* Vol.10, (2009), pp. 23–36.

Molz, S.; Decker, H.; Dal-Cim, T.; Cremonez, C.; Cordova, F.M.;Leal, R.B. & Tasca, C.I. (2008). Glutamate-induced toxicity in hippocampal slices involves apoptotic features and p38(MAPK) signalling. *Neurochemistry Research,* Vol.33, (2008), pp. 27-36.

Montana, V.; Malarkey, E.B.; Verderio, C.; Matteoli, M. & Parpua, V. (2006).Vesicular transmitter release from astrocytes. *Glia,* Vol.54, (2006), pp. 700-715.

Parpura, V.; Basarsky, T.A.; Liu,F.; Jeftinija, K.; Jeftinija, S. & Haydon P.G. (1994). Glutamate-mediated astrocyte-neuron signaling. *Nature,* Vol.369, (1994), pp. 744-747.

Parpura, V.; Scemes, E. & Spary, D.C. (2004). Mechanisms of glutamate release from astrocytes: Gap junction »hemichanneles«, purinergic receptors and exocytotic release. *Neurochemistry International,*Vol.45, (2004), pp. 259-264.

Percea, G. & Araque, A. (2007). Astrocytes potentiate transmitter release at single hippocampal synapses. *Science,* Vol.317, (2007), pp. 1083-1086.

Perdan, K.; Lipnik-Šangelj, M. & Kržan, M. (2009). The impact of astrocytes in the clearance of neurotransmitters by uptake and inactivation. In: *Advances in planar lipid bilayers and liposomes,* A. Ottova-Leitmannova, H.T. Tien (Eds.), Vol.9, (2009), pp. 211-235, doi: 10.1016/S1554-4516(09)09008-5. Elsevier: Academic Press, Amsterdam.

Perea, G.; Navarrete, M. & Araque, A. (2009). Tripartite synapses: astrocytes process and control synaptic information. Trends in Neurosciences, Vol.32, (2009), pp. t421-t431.

Powell, E.M. & Geller, H.M. (1999). Dissection of astrocyte-mediated cues in neuronal guidance and process extension. *Glia,* Vol.26, (1999), pp. 73-83.

Proia, P.; Schiera, G.; Mineo, M.; Ingrassia, A.M.; Santoro, G.; Savettieri, G. & Di Liegro, I. (2008). Astrocytes shed extracellular vesicles that contain fibroblast growth factor-2 and vascular endothelial growth factor. *International Journal of Molecular Medicine,* Vol.21, (2008), pp. 63-67.

Rao, K.V.; Panickar, K.S.; Jayakumar, A.R. & Norenberg, M.D. (2005). Astrocytes protect neurons from ammonia toxicity. *Neurochemistry Research,* Vol.30, (2005), pp. 1311-1318.

Rathinam, M.L.; Watts, L.T.; Stark, A.A.; Mahimainathan, L.; Stewart, J.; Schenker, S. & Henderson, G.I. (2006). Astrocyte control of fetal cortical neuron glutathione homeostasis: Up-regulation by ethanol. *Journal of Neurochemistry,* Vol.96, (2006), pp. 1289-1300.

Russo, A.; Palumbo, M.; Scifo, C.; Cardil, V.; Barcellona, M.L. & Renis, M. (2001). Ethanol-induced oxidative stress in rat astroytes: Role of HSP70. *Cell Biology and Toxicology,* Vol.17, (2001), pp. 153-168.

Schatter, B.; Jin, S.; Loeffelholz, K. & Klein, J. (2005). Cross-talk between phosphatidic acid and ceramide during ethanol-induced apoptosis in astrocytes. *BMC Pharmacology,* Vol.5, No.3, (2005).

Sepulveda, M.R. & Mata, A.M. (2004). The interaction of ethaol with reconstituted synaptosomal plasma membrane Ca2+-ATPase. *Biochimica et Biophysica Acta,* Vol.1665, (2004), pp. 75-80.

Sofroniew, M.V. & Vinters, H.V. (2010). Astrocytes: biology and pathology. Acta Neuropathol. Vol.119, No.1, (January 2010), pp. 7-35.

Stellwagen, D. & Malenka, R.C. (2006). Synaptic scaling mediated by glial TNF-alpha. *Nature,* Vol.440, (2006), pp. 1054-1059.

Šarc, L. & Lipnik-Štangelj, M. (2009a). Influence of ethanol and its first methabolite acetaldehyde on the central nervous system. *Journal of Slovene Medical Society,* Vol.78, No.2, (2009), pp. 91-96.

Šarc, L. & Lipnik-Štangelj, M. (2009b). Comparison of ethanol and acetaldehyde toxicity in rat astrocytes in primary culture. *Archives of industrial hygiene and toxicology,* Vol.60, No.3, (September 2009), pp. 297-305.

Šarc, L.; Wraber, B. & Lipnik-Štangelj, M. (2011). Ethanol and acetaldehyde disturb TNF-alpha and IL-6 production in cultured astrocytes. *Human and experimental toxicology,* (2011), doi: 10.1177/0960327110388533.

Takano, T.; Kang, J.; Jaiswal, J.K.; Simon, S.M.; Lin, J.H.; Yu, Y.; Li. Y.; Yang, J.; Dienel, G.; Zielke, H.R. & Nedergaard, M. (2005). Receptormediated glutamate release from volume sensitive channels in astrocytes. *Proceedings of the National Academy of Sciences USA,* Vol.102, (2005), pp. 16466-16471.

Tian, G.F.; Azmi, H.; Takano, T.; Xu, Q.; Peng. W.; Lin, J.; Oberheim. N.; Lou, N.; Wang, X.; Zielke, H.R.; Kang, J. & Nedergaard, M. (2005). An astrocytic basis of epilepsy. *Nature Medicine,* Vol.11, (2005), pp. 973–981.

Verkhratsky, A. & Kettenmann, H. (1996). Calcium signalling in glial cells. *Trends in Neurosciences,* Vol.19, (1996), pp. 346-352.

Verkhratsky, A.; Orkland, R.K. & Kettenmann, H. (1998). Glial calcium: Homeostasis and signlling function. *Physiological Rewiev,* Vol.78, (1998), pp. 99-141.

Voskuhl, R.R.; Peterson, R.S.; Song, B.; Ao, Y.; Morales, L.B.; Tiwari-Woodruff, S. & Sofroniew, M.V. (2009). Reactive astrocytes form scar-like perivascular barriers to leukocytes during adaptive immune inflammation of the CNS. *Journal of Neurosciences,* Vol.29, (2009), pp. 11511–11522.

Watts, L.T.; Rathinam, M.L.; Schenker, S. & Henderson, G.I. (2005). Astrocytes protect neurons from ethanol-induced oxidative stress and apoptotic death. *Journal of Neuroscience Research,* Vol.80, (2005), pp. 655-666.

Willmott, N.J.; Wong, K. & Strong, A.J. (2000). A fundamental role for the nitric oxide-G-kinase signalling pathway in mediating intercellular Ca2+ waves in glia. *Journal of Neurosciences,* Vol.20, (2000), pp. 1767-1779.

Zador, Z.; Stiver, S.; Wang, V. & Manley, G.T. (2009). Role of aquaporin-4 in cerebral edema and stroke. *Handbook of Experimental Pharmacology,* Vol.190, (2009), pp.159–170.

Zhou, F.C.; Anthony, B.; Dunn, K.W.; Lindquist, W.B.; Xu, Z.C. & Deng, P. (2007). Chronic alcohol driking alters neuronal dendritic spines in the brain rewardcenter nucleus accumbens. *Brain Research,* Vol.1134, (2007), pp. 148-161.

Zink, M.; Schmitt, A.; Vengeliene, V.; Henn, F.A. & Spanagel, R. (2004). Ethanol induces expression of the glutamate transporters EAAT1 and EAAT2 in organotypic cortical slice cultures. *Alcoholism Clinical and Experimental Research,* Vol.28, (2004), pp. 1752-1757.

Part 7

Future Applications

The Involvement of Purinergic System in Pain: Adenosine Receptors and Inosine as Pharmacological Tools in Future Treatments

Francisney Pinto Nascimento[1,2],
Sérgio José Macedo Jr.[2] and Adair Roberto Soares Santos[1,2]
[1]*Department of Pharmacology;*
[2]*Laboratory of Neurobiology of Pain and Inflammation,*
Department of Physiological Sciences; Universidade Federal de Santa Catarina
Brazil

1. Introduction

During the recent years, the interest in the purinergic system has been gaining importance, and this interest is not accidental. The purinergic system is so far known to be involved in several physiological conditions in mammals, becoming a potential therapeutic target for the treatment of many pathologies and disorders. One of the physiological roles is the control of pain. This chapter will emphasize adenosine receptors (P1) and its activation and inhibition by adenosine and by specific agonists or antagonists in the treatment of pain. Although most of the studies quoted in this chapter were performed in animals, in this chapter we will use the expression *analgesia* instead of *antinociception* (term used to report pain in animals) to simplify our communication. Some drugs that act on adenosine receptors have presented interesting results in clinical studies of pain and other drugs are under investigation. Of note, it has recently been shown that inosine, a metabolite of adenosine, has significant analgesic effects in several pre-clinical models of pain. Thus, the inosine can be an important tool in this area of study or even a molecule of interest for future pharmacological approaches, knowing that such as adenosine, it is produced endogenously and devoid of side effects in normal doses. In addition, new approaches using enzyme inhibitors of the purinergic system or supplies of adenosine suggest alternatives to potentiate and lasting analgesic effects of adenosine or analogs. Moreover, the release of purines and the adenosine A_1 receptor activation are essential to analgesia by acupuncture in mice. Thus, purinergic system will be the target of many future pain-treatment researches. After all, it is indispensable to students and biomedical professionals to know and understand basic concepts about this endogenous system.

2. Involvement of purinergic system in pain

2.1 Purinergic receptors: History and involvement in pain

Purinergic receptors history began when Drury and Szent-Györgi described the potent actions of purines adenine and adenosine on the heart and blood vessels (Drury & Szent-

Györgi, 1929). Later, in 1970 Burnstock presented evidence that ATP acted as a neurotransmitter in nonadrenergic noncholinergic (NANC) nerves supplying the gut, and finally, in 1972, the purinergic neurotransmission hypothesis was proposed (Burnstock, 1972). With these discoveries, the number of publications involving ATP and its metabolites grew quickly and continues to do so (Figure 1).

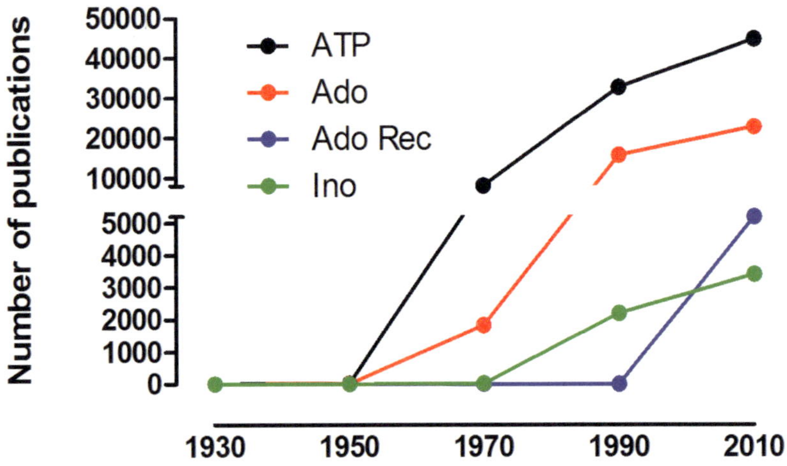

Fig. 1. Total of publications with keywords ATP, Adenosine (Ado), Adenosine Receptors (Ado Rec) and Inosine (Ino) from 1930 until 2010. Source: Pubmed

Afterwards, it was established that the ATP acted as a cotransmitter with classical transmitters in both the peripheral nervous system and in the central and that purines are also powerful extracellular messengers to non-neuronal cells (Burnstock & Knight, 2004). Burnstock, in 1978, provided the basis for the distinction of two classes of purinergic receptors; adenosine-sensitive P1 and ATP-sensitive P2 receptor classes. In 1985, Burnstock and Kennedy proposed a basis for distinguishing two types of P2 purinoceptors, namely, P2X and P2Y. Afterwards, in 1994 Abbracchio and Burnstock through studies of transduction mechanisms and cloning of both P2X and P2Y receptors put forward a new nomenclature system, naming them, P2X ionotropic ligand-gated ion channel receptors and P2Y metabotropic G protein-coupled receptors, respectively. Currently, seven subtypes of P2X receptors ($P2X_1$, $P2X_2$, $P2X_3$, $P2X_4$, $P2X_5$, $P2X_6$, $P2X_7$) and eight subtypes of P2Y receptors ($P2Y_1$, $P2Y_2$, $P2Y_4$, $P2Y_6$, $P2Y_{11}$, $P2Y_{12}$, $P2Y_{13}$, $P2Y_{14}$) are clearly established. P2X and P2Y receptor activation by ATP stimulates cellular excitability, augments the release of excitatory amino acids, and consequently initiates pain responses (Burnstock, 2007; Burnstock & Williams, 2000). In the context of pain neurotransmission, preclinical studies show us that activation of P1 receptors by adenosine decreases pain, inflammation, and cellular excitability (McGaraughty & Jarvis, 2006). During the 80's and 90's research evaluating purinergic system in pain rocketed (Figure 2).

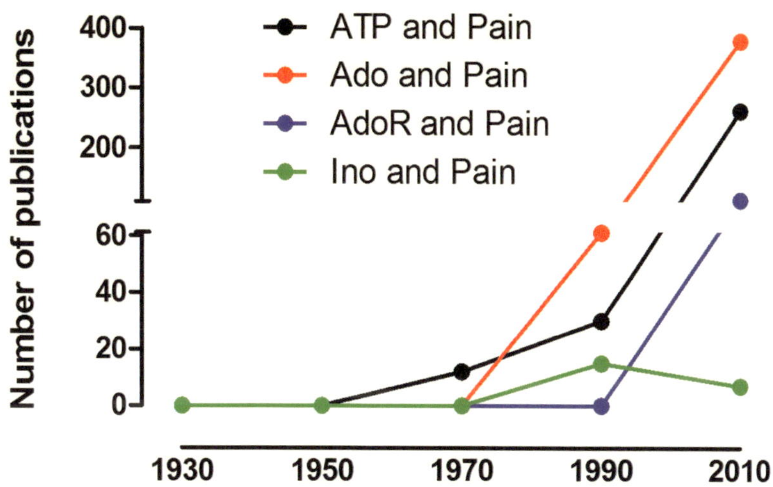

Fig. 2. Total of publications with keywords ATP, Adenosine (Ado), Adenosine Receptors (AdoR) and Inosine (Ino) plus Pain from 1930 until 2010. Source: Pubmed

3. Adenosine receptors and pain

3.1 Adenosine receptors

Adenosine is the natural ligand of P1 receptors, also called adenosine receptors. All these receptors are G-protein coupled and are divided according to pharmacological, biochemical and molecular properties into four subtypes: A_1, A_{2A}, A_{2B} and A_3. Each receptor has a distinct distribution and due to its special features, has distinct roles as well (Burnstock et al., 2011; Fredholm et al., 2011; Ralevic & Burnstock, 1998; Ribeiro et al., 2002; Sawynok & Liu, 2003). Adenosine receptors were cloned and characterized in several mammal species (Burnstock, 2008).

3.2 Distribution of adenosine receptors

Adenosine receptors are present in several species and in distinct tissues. However, their distribution is quite irregular and different among species and mainly among tissues (Fredholm et al., 2011). A_1 receptor (A_{1R}) is a ubiquitous receptor. In the central nervous system, it is distributed in the cerebellum, cerebral cortex, hippocampus, thalamus, spinal cord (substantia gelatinosa), brain stem, olfactory bulb and other central sites. Peripherally A_{1R} distribution is less wide than centrally, but there is a considerable density of A_{1R} in sensory afferent fibers, mainly on C-fibers which are responsible for receiving and conducting the painful stimuli (Dixon et al., 1996; Sawynok, 2009). A_{2A} receptor (A_{2AR})has an even distribution between central and peripheral nervous system, but mainly in central structures as nucleus accumbens, putamen, caudate and in immune tissues, vascular smooth muscle, endothelium, platelets and sensory neurons (Dixon et al., 1996; Fredholm, 1995; Ralevic & Burnstock, 1998; Sawynok, 2009). A_{2B} receptor (A_{2BR}) is also a ubiquitous receptor and it has been found either in many central or peripheral tissues. However, A_{2BR} density is very low and it has been found in great density only in bowel and bladder. A_3 receptors (A_{3R})are widely distributed in several mammals, however, few studies have indicated specific roles for this receptor (Dixon et al., 1996; Ralevic & Burnstock, 1998; Salvatore et al., 1993).

3.3 General adenosine receptor signaling

All adenosine receptors are coupled to G-protein. Nevertheless there are many kinds of G-protein and each one may activate a distinct pathway. Thus, the four adenosine receptors can stimulate or inhibit several pathways and consequently exert many physiological actions (Jacobson & Gao, 2006; Ralevic & Burnstock, 1998). We show below the main signaling characteristics of each adenosine receptor.

3.3.1 A_1 receptor signaling

A_{1R} is coupled to Gi/0 protein family which is pertussis toxin-sensitive. Most of the biological effects induced by A_{1R} activation are due to inhibition of cAMP second messenger (Burnstock, 2007; Jacobson & Gao, 2006; Ralevic & Burnstock, 1998; Sawynok, 1998) (Figure 3 and Table 1).

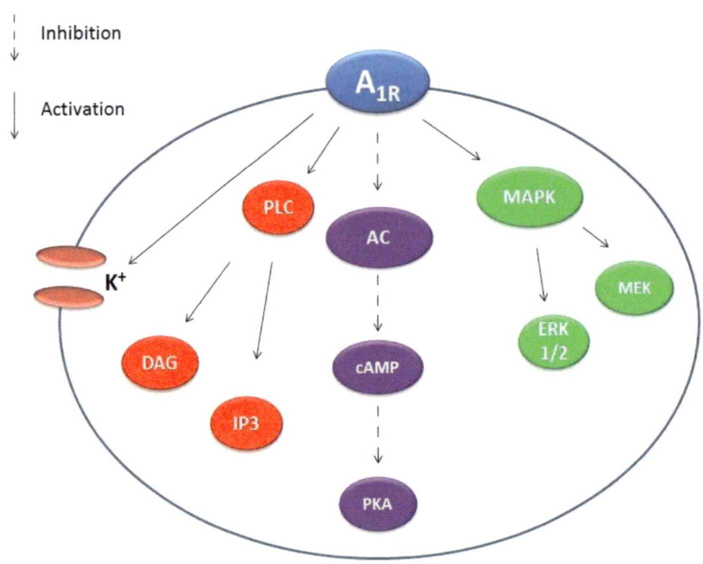

Fig. 3. Adenosine A_1 receptors and its main pathways. A_{1R}, adenosine A_1 receptor; AC, adenylate cyclase; cAMP, cyclic adenosine monophosphate; DAG, diacylglicerol; ERK1/2, extracellular signal-regulated kinases 1 and 2; IP_3, inositol triphosphate; K^+, potassium channels; MAPK, mitogen-activated protein kinase; MEK, MAPK and ERK kinase; PKA, protein kinase; PLC, phospholipase C.

Beta and gamma subunities of $A_{1R,}$ when activated stimulate phospholipase C (PLC). Activation of PLC cleaves phosphatidylinositol 4,5-bisphosphate (PIP_2) into diacylglycerol (DAG) and inositol 1,4,5-trisphosphate (IP_3) leading to increased levels Ca^{+2}. Moreover, the enhancement of intracellular calcium can induce some enzymes such as protein kinase C

(PKC), phospholipase D (PLD), phospholipase A_2 (PLA_2) and others. Furthermore, adenosine or adenosine agonists can activate K^+ channels (Jacobson & Gao, 2006; Megson et al., 1995; Ralevic & Burnstock, 1998). A_{1R} activation can also activate PI3K and MAPK pathways, more specifically ERK1/2 and MEK inducing gene expression changes and glial cell protection (Boison et al., 2010; Shulte & Fredholm, 2003).

3.3.2 A_{2A} receptor signaling

A_{2AR} is coupled to Gs (the most part) and Golf protein (mainly in striatum). The main intracellular event after activation of these proteins is adenylate cyclase activation followed by cAMP production enhancement (Table 1).

Receptor	Adenosine affinity (EC50;nm)	G-protein	cAMP	PKA	PLC	Ca^{+2} channels	K^+ channels
A_1	~70	Gi/Go	Decrease	Inhibits	Activates	Inhibits	Activates
A_{2A}	~150	Gs/Golf	Increase	Activates		Inhibits or Activates	Activates
A_{2B}	~5100	Gs/Gq	Decrease	Activates	Activates		
A_3	~6500	Gi/Go	Increase	Inhibits	Activates		

Table 1. Adenosine receptors signaling. Adapted from Ralevic and Burnstock, 1998; Sawynok and Liu, 2003; Jacobson and Guao, 2006.

The increasing of cAMP stimulates cAMP-dependent kinase (PKA). Thus, PKA becomes able to activate several pathways through PKC, calcium channels, potassium channels, cAMP responsive element-binding (CREB), MAPK, PLC activation (Burnstock, 2007; Cunha et al., 2008; Fredholm et al., 2003, 2007; Jacobson & Gao, 2006; Ralevic & Burnstock, 1998).

3.3.3 A_{2B} receptor signaling

Through Gs and Gq activation A_{2B} receptor induces adenylate cyclase and PLC. In humans, A_{2BR} can increase intracellular calcium by IP_3 activation. Moreover, the arachidonic acid pathway is also involved in A_{2BR} signaling (Feoktistov & Biaggioni, 2011; Jacobson & Gao, 2006; Peakman and Hill, 1994).

3.3.4 A_3 receptor signaling

A_{3R} like A_{1R} is coupled to Gi/0 and also to Gq/11 protein. Its main signaling transduction is the inhibition of adenylate cyclase and stimulation of PLC, IP_3, DAG, PKC and PLD. Also, like other adenosine receptors, A_{3R} activates MAPK pathway, mainly ERK1/2 (Abbracchio et al., 1995; Armstrong & Ganote, 1994; Palmer et al., 1995; Shneyvays et al., 2004).

3.4 A_1 receptors and pain

A_{1R} is the main responsible for inducing analgesia among the adenosine receptors (Burnstock et al., 2011; Sawynok, 1998; Sawynok & Liu, 2003). It has been shown that A_{1R} is widely distributed in the dorsal spinal cord, mainly in lamina II (substantia gelatinosa) (Choca et al., 1988; Horiuchi et al., 2010; Sawynok, 1998). In this site, many afferent sensory nerve have connections with post-synaptic neurons. Also, A_{1R} are localized in the descending projection within dorsal horn (Choca et al., 1988).

3.4.1 Effects of A_1 receptor activation in acute pain

There are several published data showing the important effect of A_{1R} in controlling acute pain (review see Jacobson & Gao, 2006; Sawynok, 1998). Moreover, it has been shown that systemic administration of various A_{1R} agonists can produce analgesic effect in several models of acute pain in animals (Gong et al., 2010; Sawynok, 1998). Probably, these effects are caused by peripheral, supraspinal and mostly by spinal A_{1R}. In mice lacking A_{1R} (knockout animals) a lower pain threshold was observed in hyperalgesia tests (Wu et al., 2005). Further, analgesic effect induced by intrathecal adenosine was abolished as well as the increase of thermal hyperalgesia in A_{1R} knockout mice (Johansson et al., 2001).

Several studies published show that intrathecal injection of A_{1R} agonists cause analgesia in various animal models of acute pain, including tail flick, tail immersion, hot-plate, formalin, acetic acid, capsaicin models and others (Nascimento et al., 2010; Song et al., 2011; Zahn et al., 2007).

A_{1R} is also found in primary afferent neurons and in the cell body and the dorsal root ganglia (Lima et al., 2010; Sawynok, 2009), then it has an important role in modulation of peripheral pain. Many studies have shown that administration of A_{1R} agonists into the paw of animals causes an analgesic effect in several animal models of pain. It has been shown that A_{1R} activation in the periphery inhibits formalin-induced pain and reduces hyperalgesia induced by PGE_2 (Karlsten et al., 1992; Taiwo & Levine, 1990). Further, when the peripheral adenosine A_{1R} is activated, it triggers the NO/cGMP/PKG/K_{ATP} intracellular signaling pathway and then inhibits pain (Lima et al., 2010). Moreover, A_{1R} agonists reduce the thermal hyperalgesia, but not mechanical allodynia, caused by sciatic nerve injury. The thermal hyperalgesia is mediated by C fibers and mechanical allodynia, in turn, is mediated by A fibers, which demonstrates the presence of A_{1R} in C but not in A fibers (Sawynok, 2009).

3.4.2 A_1 receptor and chronic pain

Several authors have shown that different agonists of A_{1R} are able to reduce distinct kinds of chronic pain. The agonist R-PIA inhibits mechanical allodynia induced by spinal nerve ligation in rats (Hwang et al., 2005; Song et al., 2011). In addition, R-PIA also reduces thermal pain threshold in rats that underwent an injury in the spinal cord (Horiuchi et al., 2010). Moreover, other mechanisms are generally involved in analgesic effect in chronic pain induced by A_{1R} activation, such as inhibition of glutamate release. Another A_{1R} agonist, CPA, when given to rats, inhibits pain induced by arthritis and pain induced by neuropathy (Curros-Criado & Herrero, 2005). Also, in experiments with A_{1R} knockout mice it has been observed that these animals present a lower pain threshold than wild-type animals in inflammatory and neuropathic pain models (Wu et al., 2005).

3.4.3 Interactions between A_1 receptor and opioid system

There is a strong relationship between opioidergic and adenosinergic systems in pain modulation. Morphine and other opioids are able to release adenosine (Sawynok et al., 1989; Sweeney et al., 1987a,b; Sweeney et al., 1989). Adenosine or analog administration combined with opioids enhances the analgesic effect of the latter (DeLander & Hopkins, 1986). However, administration of methylxanthines, adenosine receptor antagonists, can augment, decrease or have no effect on analgesic activity of opioids (Sawynok, 2011). In addition, A_{1R} can undergo dimerization with μ receptor in afferents neurons and induce the decrease of cAMP production (Sawynok, 1998).

3.4.4 Interactions among A_1 receptor and other receptors in pain mechanisms

A_{1R} is able to dimerize with alpha-2-adrenergic receptor. Also, it has been shown that serotonin releases adenosine from primary afferents and that A_{1R} receptor antagonist blocks serotonin analgesic actions, suggesting a close involvement between adenosinergic and serotoninergic systems in pain modulation (Sawynok, 1998).

3.4.5 A_1 agonists/antagonists

Methylxanthines (caffeine included) are natural antagonists of adenosine A_{1R} and A_{2AR}. However, the main selective agonists/antagonists to A_{1R} are synthetics. Some of them are listed in Table 2.

Role of drugs	Drug	Chemical name
Agonists A_{1R}	R-PIA	(−)-N^6-(2-Phenylisopropyl)adenosine
	CHA	N6-ciclohexyladenosine
	CPA	N6-cyclopentyladenosine
	CCPA	2-chloro-N6-cyclopentyladenosine
Antagonists A_{1R}	CPT	8-cyclopentyl-1,3-dimethylxanthine
	DPCPX	8-Cyclopentyl-1,3-dipropylxanthine
	8-PT	8-phenyltheophylline

Table 2. Principal adenosine A_1 receptor agonists and antagonists.

3.5 A_{2A} receptors and pain

Taiwo & Levine (1990) demonstrated clear distinct effects of A_{1R} and A_{2AR} activation in peripheral pain. They showed that, in peripheral sites, A_{1R} mediates analgesia while A_{2AR} facilitates painful perception. In addition, other studies also showed that peripheral A_{2AR} activation induced pain (Doak & Sawynok, 1995; Li et al., 2010; Taiwo & Levine, 1990). However, systemically and spinally, the role of A_{2AR} is not entirely clear. Some publications have demonstrated that A_{2AR} activation induces pain (Bastia et al., 2002; Hussey et al., 2007). On the other hand, other authors have showed a reduction of pain when A_{2AR} is activated (By et al., 2011; Borghi et al., 2002; Yoon et al., 2005). These controversial results might be associated with A_{2AR} intracellular signaling. A_{2AR} activation induces cAMP increased production (it can cause pain) and also K^+ channels opening (it can inhibit pain) (Jacobson & Gao, 2006; Regaya et al., 2004; Sawynok, 1998).

A_{2AR} knockout animals are less sensitive to pain, suggesting that A_{2AR} is a pain facilitator in acute (Hussey et al., 2007) and chronic pain (Bura et al., 2008). Bura and coworkers (2008) also demonstrated that microglia and astrocytes expression was higher in wild-type A_{2AR} animals than in A_{2AR} knockout animals. Also, A_{2AR} located in glial cells is responsible for the release of inflammatory mediators that induce and maintain chronic pain (Boison et al., 2010). Thus, A_{2AR} blockade might be an interesting approach for future treatments of neuropathic and chronic pain. Meantime, also in chronic pain exists distinct results about A_{2AR}. A report showed that only one spinal injection of A_{2AR} agonist was able to induce analgesia during several days in rats undergoing neuropathic pain (Loram et al., 2009). After all, it is clear that A_{2AR} is involved in pain modulation. However, more studies are necessary to precisely explain how this receptor works in distinct situations, only then it will be possible to make clinical approaches.

3.6 A_{2B} receptors and pain

Few studies have been evaluating the A_{2BR} role in pain. Most part of these studies showed that A_{2BR} facilitates pain transmission, because A_{2BR} antagonists have reduced pain (Abo-Salem et al., 2004; Bilkei-Gorzo et al., 2008; GodFrey et al., 2006). A_{2BR} antagonist reduced thermal hyperalgesia and was able to potentiate the analgesic effect caused by morphine and acetaminophen (Abo-Salem et al., 2004; Godfrey et al., 2006). Also, the blockade of A_{2BR} presented an analgesic effect in inflammatory pain (Bilkei-Gorzo et al., 2008).

3.7 A_3 receptors and pain

Similar to A_{2BR}, adenosine A_{3R} is not an interesting target to pain relief. However, A_{3R} is implicated in pathological conditions such as ischemic diseases and in inflammation (for review see Borea et al., 2009). Regarding pain, there are few studies evaluating A_{3R} role. Sawynok and colleagues (1997) showed that A_{3R} activation causes pain and paw oedema through release of histamine and serotonin. A_{3R} knockout animals presented an increased pain threshold in some models of pain but not difference in others (Fedorova et al., 2003; Wu et al., 2002). A_{3R} might be an interesting target to inflammatory and autoimmune diseases, but not to pain states.

3.8 Novel approaches in pain management involving adenosine receptors

3.8.1 Management of adenosine receptors by metabolism modulation

The first report showing that adenosine kinase (AK) inhibition reduces behaviour associated to pain was published by Keil and DeLander, 1992. AK inhibitors are able to decrease pain levels when given peripherally or sistemically (Kowaluk et al., 1999; Lynch et al., 1999; Sawynok, 1998). Moreover, these inhibitors are efficacious against acute and chronic pain (Kowaluk et al., 2000; Lynch et al., 1999; McGaraughty et al., 2005; Poon & Sawynok, 1998, 1999; Suzuki et al., 2001). Another enzyme that regulates adenosine level is adenosine deaminase (ADA), that converts adenosine to inosine (Sawynok, 1998). However, the analgesic effect caused by ADA inhibition is not so clear yet. It has been showed that inhibitors of ADA itself are able to cause analgesia in determined animal models (Poon & Sawynok, 1999), but not in others (Keil & DeLander, 1992, 1994).

Coadministration of AK and ADA inhibitors potentiates the analgesic effect of the former (Poon & Sawynok, 1999). Also, adenosine effect is synergically augmented by coadministration of ADA inhibitor (Keil & DeLander, 1994). Distinct effects between AK inhibitors and ADA inhibitors might be because adenosine has a higher affinity by AK than ADA (Arch & Newsholme, 1978). In this point of view, AK seems to be the most important enzyme to regulate adenosine endogenous levels.

3.8.2 Analgesic effect by supply of purinergic substrates

Ecto-5'-nucleotidase (NT5E) is an enzyme located in the cell membrane that catalyzes the extracellular conversion of adenosine monophosphate (AMP) into adenosine in several tissues, included dorsal root ganglia (DRG) and substantia gelatinosa (Zylka, 2011). Recent studies have demonstrated that the analgesic effect of AMP combined with an AK inhibitor halved in NT5E knockout animals and is totally reversed in A_{1R} knockout animals (Sowa et al., 2010a). These results inspired another study that evaluated whether exogenous supply of NT5E (increases supply of adenosine) could induce a long lasting analgesic effect. NT5E presented effects that lasted for 2 days in models of inflammatory and chronic pain. Both effects were dependent on A_{1R} (Sowa, 2010b). Hence, the supply of enzymes that generate adenosine is a new interesting approach that may be used in studies to treat chronic pain.

3.8.3 Involvement of adenosine receptors in acupuncture pain relief

In an elegant study published in 2010, Goldman and colleagues showed that analgesia induced by acupuncture depends on purine release, such as ATP, ADP, AMP and adenosine. In addition, it has been showed that A_{1R} agonist replicates the acupuncture effect. Also, in A_{1R} knockout animals, acupuncture did not present analgesia. Moreover, inhibition of adenosine deaminase prolonged the analgesic effect of acupuncture in mice (Goldman et al., 2010). It is interesting to mention that caffeine, the most widely used drug across the world in beverages such as teas, coffee, *mate*, soft drinks, energy drinks and others is an antagonist of adenosine receptors. Therefore, patients in treatment with acupuncture should not drink these caffeine beverages, because caffeine might reduce the acupuncture analgesic effect (for review see Zylka, 2010).

4. Inosine and pain

4.1 Inosine within of purinergic system

ATP is the main molecule of purinergic system. Inside the cell, ATP may be bi-directionally converted into AMP. AMP is broken down into adenosine. Adenosine may be converted back into AMP through phosphorylation by AK. Moreover, adenosine might leave the cell by nucleoside transporter (NT). Inside the cell, adenosine deaminase is responsible for the conversion from adenosine to inosine. Outside the cell, this conversion is performed by ecto-adenosine kinase or even adenosine deaminase. Inosine is a substrate to purine nucleoside phosphorylase (PNP), leading to hypoxanthines as its products. Hypoxanthines are converted into xanthines and afterwards to uric acid by xanthine oxidase (Figure 4) (See review Sawynok & Liu, 2003).

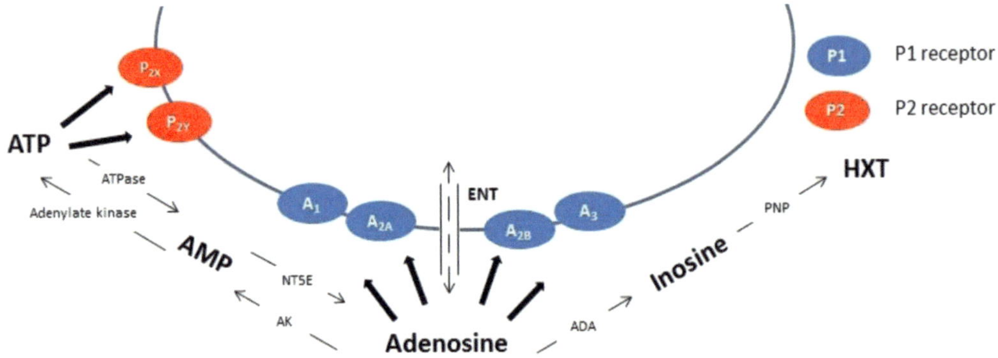

Fig. 4. Purinergic metabolism and its main molecules and enzymes. A_1, adenosine A_1 receptor; A_{2A}, adenosine A_{2A} receptor; A_{2B}, adenosine A_{2B} receptor; A_3, adenosine A_3 receptor ADA, adenosine deaminase; AK, adenosine kinase; AMP, adenosine monophosphate; ATP, adenosine triphosphate; ENT, equilibrative nucleoside transporter; HXT, hypoxanthines; *NT5E, ecto-5'nucleotidase*; P2X, purine P_{2X} receptor; P_{2Y}, purine P_{2Y} receptor; PNP, purine nucleoside phosphorilase.

Thus, inosine is one among many molecules in purinergic system. However, inosine has specific roles in several physiological states, we will show some functions and discuss the role of inosine in pain control in next sections.

4.2 Inosine physiological roles

In recent decades, many physiological roles for inosine have been shown. During the 70's, Aviado demonstrated that inosine exerts cardiotonic actions, such as preventing negative inotropic effect and increasing coronary vasodilatation (Aviado, 1978). Also, inosine presents several effects on axonal growth, such as axon growth induction and damaged neurons stimulation (Benowitz et al., 1999, 2002; Chen et al., 2002). Inosine also induces a regrowth in axotomized retinal ganglion cells in rats (Wu et al., 2003). These data indicate that inosine may constitute a new approach to treat the injured or degenerated nerves in central or peripheral nervous system. Despite of cardiovascular and axonal growth effects, the inflammatory effects of inosine are the most studied. Inosine has significant anti-inflammatory effects in several *in vivo* and *in vitro* models of inflammation (Gomez & Sitkovsky, 2003; Haskó et al., 2000; Marton et al., 2001; Schneider et al., 2006). These effects seem to be mediated by A_{1R}, A_{2R} and A_{3R} (Gomez & Sitkovsky, 2003; Haskó et al., 2000, 2004).

4.3 Inosine effect on acute pain

Inosine has analgesic action when administered by different routes (i.e. intraperitoneal, oral, intrathecal or intracerebroventricular) against pain induced by acetic acid (Nascimento et al., 2010). Of note, inosine also inhibits pain induced by formalin. Formalin test induces 2 distinct types of pain, neurogenic phase (acute pain) and inflammatory phase (inflammatory pain). Inosine is not able to relieve pain in neurogenic phase. However, inosine reduces nearly totally the inflammatory pain in formalin test (Nascimento et al., 2010). The effects of inosine in this model of pain extended the acetic acid data because formalin is a more specific model. Therefore, these results indicate that inosine is able to prevent and reduce pain induced by inflammatory mediators. In this way, inosine may be inhibiting the synthesis or release of several neurotransmitters and mediators involved in pain conditions (Nascimento et al., 2010). We can also conclude that inosine is able to inhibit pain induced by central facilitation. Therefore, inosine increases pain threshold and it may be useful to treat some kinds of pain injury that result from a central sensitization. Adenosine receptors distribution on substantia gelatinosa, mainly A_{1R} and A_{2AR} could explain how inosine acts in this case (Sawynok, 1998; Sawynok & Liu, 2003). Inosine also presents a significant and dose-related inhibition of pain induced by glutamate (acute pain model) injection into the paw of mice (Nascimento et al., 2010).

4.4 Inosine effects on chronic pain

The data described in literature strongly suggests that inosine may have an important effect in controlling chronic pain, since it has anti-inflammatory effect and can reduce acute pain. In fact, Nascimento and colleagues (2010) demonstrated that acute administration of inosine, intraperitoneally, was able to inhibit chronic inflammatory pain induced by CFA in mice, being effective up to 4 hours after administration. The CFA is responsible for inducing chronic inflammation by stimulating the body's immune response, this response is mediated by the synthesis and release of cytokines and inflammatory mediators (Zhang et al., 2011).

In the study published by Nascimento and colleagues (2010), inosine was effective against mechanical and thermal allodynia induced by partial sciatic nerve ligation (PSNL) up to 4 hours after treatment by intraperitoneal route. Further, in another experiment, inosine was given daily for until 22 days and it also presented significant analgesic effect. Pain induced by PSNL is very strong and may last for weeks (Ueda, 2006). Animal models of neuropathic pain induce many functional and biochemical changes in local injury site. After the surgery there is the release of multiple inflammatory and pain mediators which in turn, may also be present in other areas involved and affected by sciatic nerve, as spinal cord and brain (Bridges et al., 2001; Ji & Woolf, 2001; Inoue et al., 2004; Ueda, 2006). Inosine activity in this kind of pain may indicate a promising molecule to new studies, because inosine might have a longer half-life than adenosine and admittedly does not have toxic or side effects.

4.5 Adenosine receptors involved in analgesic effects of inosine

A_{1R} has been considered the main receptor responsible for analgesic effect among adenosine receptors (Burnstock, 2007; Sawynok, 1998). A_{1R} is also the main receptor involved in inosine analgesic effect. Both A_{1R} antagonists DPCPX and 8-PT were able to reverse the inosine action. Inosine in a direct or indirect way activates A_{1R} to induce analgesia (Nascimento et al., 2010). Other studies have showed that adenosine receptor antagonists block *in vivo* and *in vitro* inosine effects (Haskó et al., 2000) and adenosine receptor knockout animals do not present immunoprotective effects of inosine (Gomez & Sitkovsky, 2003). Thus, it is clear that the A_{1R} activation is essential for inosine to exert its effect (Figure 5).

Involvement of A_{2AR} in pain is quite controversial. Some studies show that A_{2AR} blockade leads to analgesic effect (Borghi et al., 2002; Yoon et al., 2005) while other studies demonstrate that the blockade or deletion of A_{2AR} causes pain relief (Bastia et al., 2002; Ledent et al., 1997). Inosine activates A_{2AR} to induce analgesia, at least in the acetic acid model (Nascimento et al., 2010). However, the participation of A_{2AR} receptor in inosine analgesia in other pain animal models might be different or does not exist. Moreover, the A_{2AR} involvement on inosine effect can occur due to its anti-inflammatory profile (Milne & Palmer, 2011) and due to activation of the K^+ channels (Regaya et al., 2004).

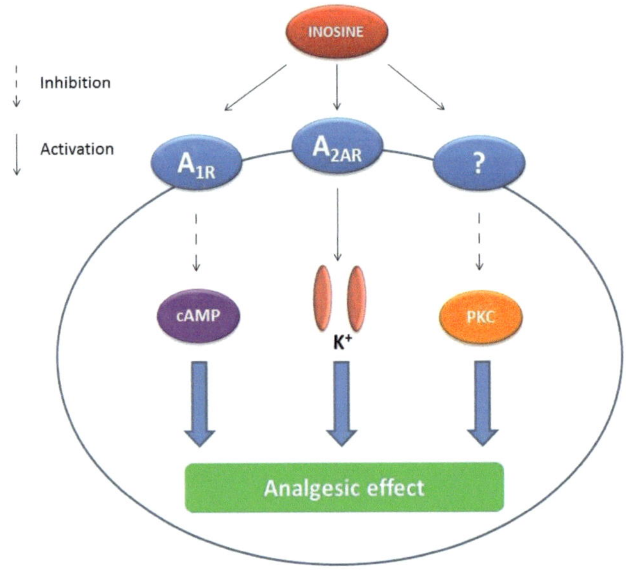

Fig. 5. Principal mechanisms of inosine antinociception. A_{1R}, adenosine A_1 receptor; A_{2AR}, adenosine A_{2A} receptor, cAMP, cyclic adenosine monophosphate; K^+, potassium channels; PKC, protein kinase C.

A_{2BR} and A_{3R} adenosine receptors do not have significant role in pain transmission or modulation (Sawynok, 1998). Although it has been shown that inosine binds to A_{3R}, it seems that A_{2BR} and A_{3R} receptors are not involved in inosine analgesic effect (Nascimento et al., 2010).

4.5.1 Does inosine binds to adenosine receptor?

Few studies have evaluated if inosine binds to adenosine receptor. Jin and co-workers demonstrated that inosine binds to A_{3R} in mast cells, but not to A_{1R} or A_{2AR} (Jin et al., 1997). In 2001, Fredholm's group observed that inosine weakly bound to A_{1R} and A_{3R}, but not to A_{2R} (Fredholm et al., 2001). Fredholm concluded that inosine could not be considered a natural ligand of adenosine receptors. However, because of these few studies and considering *in vivo* studies where adenosine antagonists are able to block inosine effects, it is not is possible to affirm whether inosine is or not a natural ligand or a partial agonist of adenosine receptors. More studies are necessary to elucidate this issue.

4.6 Intracellular signalling involved in analgesic effects of inosine

The intracellular signaling involved in analgesic action of inosine is yet not entirely elucidated. Assuming that inosine effects depend on adenosine receptors, A_{1R} and A_{2AR}, we can consider that adenosine receptors signaling pathways are the major effectors of this effect. As fully mentioned previously, A_{1R} is coupled to Gi/0 protein. A_{1R} signaling causes downstream inhibition of adenylyl cyclase and induction of PLC activity. Further, when A_{1R} is activated it causes potassium channel opening, PI3K and MAPK stimulation. All these pathways might participate in the inosine analgesic effect (Ansari et al., 2009; Jacobson & Gao, 2006; Sawynok, 1998; Schulte & Fredholm, 2003). Inosine inhibits the pain caused by PKC activator. Thus, at least in part, the analgesic action of inosine depends on PKC inhibition (Nascimento et al., 2010), even though it is not clear yet how it happens (Figure 5). Costenla and coworkers showed that an adenosine analog that has preference for A_{2AR} is able to inhibit sodium current in NMDA receptors (Costenla et al., 1999). This signaling occurring *in vivo* could partially explain how A_{2AR} works in analgesia induced by inosine.

4.7 Perspectives

As previously described in this chapter, purinergic system is an important endogenous modulator of pain. Hundreds of pre-clinical studies targeting the adenosine receptors showed analgesic effect in distinct pain models. Inosine, an endogenous modulator of several physiological functions also presents a role in pain transmission. Inosine might be a natural activator of adenosine receptors. Also, it can indirectly increase the release or reduce the uptake of adenosine, potentiating the effect of its precursor. Thus, understanding how inosine acts to induce analgesia may help discover new ways to inhibit pain or new therapeutic targets. Moreover, inosine may be a potential molecule to treat pain, and it has a great advantage to be devoid of toxic or side effects because it has been used clinically for many years for other purposes. Another interesting approach would be to attempt to prolong and potentiate the effect of inosine. For this, a great understanding of purinergic metabolism is necessary in order to correctly and effectively approach this matter.

5. Active drugs on adenosine receptors and their clinical applications

Nowadays there is increasing interest in the therapeutic potential of adenosinergic compounds (including receptor agonists and antagonists, enzyme inhibitors and others), and many adenosine compounds have been evaluated.

5.1 Adenosine receptor ligands and their potential as novel drugs

Adenosine itself, for a long time, was the only adenosine agonist used in humans. It is widely used in the treatment of paroxysmal supraventricular tachycardia (Adenocard®) due to its activation of A_{1R}, and as a diagnostic for myocardial perfusion imaging (Adenoscan®) utilizing its A_{2AR}-activating effects resulting in vasodilation (Müller & Jacobson, 2011). However, other A_{1R}-selective agonists such as Selodenoson, Capadenoson e Tecadenoson have been clinically evaluated for the treatment of paroxysmal supraventricular tachycardia, atrial fibrillation, or angina pectoris (Müller & Jacobson, 2011). Still talking about cardiovascular disorders, selective A_{2AR} agonist, Apadenoson, Binodenoson and Sonedenoson appears as candidates for clinical use (Awad et al., 2006; Desai et al., 2005; Udelson et al. 2004). These agonists are of interest as vasodilator agents in cardiac imaging (Cerqueira, 2006) and inflammation suppressors. Accordingly, Regadenoson is already approved for diagnostic imaging (Iskandrian et al., 2007). A_{3R} selective agonists are also currently in clinical trials and exhibit nanomolar affinity at the receptor, CF101 (Can-Fite Biopharma) and Cl-IB-MECA (CF102) are in trials for autoimmune inflammatory disorders and for liver cancer, respectively. Two other A_{3R} agonists CP-608,039 and its N6-(2,5-dichlorobenzyl) analogue CP-532,903 were previously under development for cardioprotection. MRS3558 (CF502) is in preclinical development for the treatment of autoimmune disease (Avni et al., 2010; Wan et al., 2008).

5.2 Adenosinergic drugs in pain clinical studies and practical

Clinical studies confirm the pre-clinical trials showing that in neuropathic pain patients, adenosine was able to alleviate spontaneous pain, tactile and thermal allodynia, as well as thermal hyperalgesia (Qu et al., 1997). In addition, intravenous infusion of adenosine during breast surgery reduced the postoperative pain (Lynch et al., 2003; Sollevi et al., 1995). Spinal administration of adenosine and adenosine analogs in humans also exhibited analgesic effect. A phase I clinical safety study in healthy volunteers demonstrated that 1000 μg of adenosine given intrathecally lacked side effects and led to a significant decrease in mustard oil-induced inflammatory pain, in tourniquet induced ischemic pain, and decreased areas of secondary allodynia after skin inflammation (Rane et al., 1998).

In another study, a single dose of 0.1 - 0.5 mg/kg of SDZ WAG 994 (adenosine A_{1R} agonist), was evaluated in a phase I clinical study, and this compound was well tolerated. A dose of 1 mg/kg was used in a randomized double-blind clinical trial to determine its efficacy in postoperative dental pain after third molar surgery. However, SDZ WAG 994 did not show significant difference from placebo and was not effective in attenuating postoperative pain after third molar surgery. On the other hand, at higher doses, the compound showed dose-dependent adverse events (Seymour et al., 1999; Wagner et al., 1995; Yan et al., 2003).

Another full high-affinity A_{1R} agonists, GR79236X, was also evaluated in patients with dental pain after third molar extraction. Patients received a 15-min double-blind infusion containing 10 μg/kg of GR79236X, unfortunately, no evidence of efficacy of GR79236X was observed with this compound compared with placebo (Sneyd et al., 2007). Another A_{1R} agonist GW493838 developed by GlaxoSmithKline, was evaluated in phase II clinical trials to determine its analgesic effect in patients with postherpetic neuralgia or peripheral nerve injury caused by trauma or surgery. However, further development of GW493838 has been discontinued (Nelsen et al., 2004; as cited in Elzein & Zablocki, 2008).

Allosteric modulation of A_{1R} function may also be an interesting tool. Accordingly, the A_{1R}-selective allosteric enhancer T-62, given orally was also shown to reduce hypersensitivity in carrageenan-inflamed rats, in addition, phase I clinical trials of T62 have been completed as a treatment for neuropathic pain (Childers et al., 2005). Therewithal, the A_{2AR} agonist BVT.115959 from Biovitrum completed the clinical trials for diabetic neuropathic pain and it was well tolerated but did not significantly improve pain symptoms (Biovitrum, 2005; Zylka, 2011).

6. Conclusion and future directions

This chapter presented a general and updated review about the purinergic system with emphasis in adenosine receptors (P1) and pain. It is possible to conclude that the modulation of this system and its receptors is quite important and interesting for the control of pain. Recent studies have approached this system in new ways and contributed to the development of this research field. Some clinical studies have been carried out with purinergic drugs (adenosine analogs) and some studies have showed quite satisfactory effects, although others haven`t showed statistical difference between treated and non-treated groups. Finally, the possibility of new drugs targeting the purinergic system to treat distinct kinds of pain reaching clinical trials in the next years is clear.

7. References

Abbracchio, MP. & Burnstock, G. (1994). Purinoceptores: are there families of P2X and P2Y purinoceptores? *Pharmacology & Therapeutics,* Vol. 64, No.3, pp. (445-475)

Abbracchio, MP., Brambilla, R., Ceruti, S., Kim, HO., von Lubitz, DK., Jacobson, KA. & Cattabeni, F. (1995). G protein-dependent activation of phospholipase C by adenosine A3 receptors in rat brain. *Molecular Pharmacology,* Vol.48, No. 6, (December, 1995), pp.(1038-1045), ISSN 1038-1045.

Abo-Salem, OM., Hayallah, AM., Bilkei-Gorzo, A., Filipek, B., Zimmer, A. & Müller, CE. (2004). Antinociceptive effects of novel A2B adenosine receptor antagonists. *The Journal of Pharmacology Experimental Therapeutics,* Vol 308, No. 1, (January, 2004), pp. (358-66), ISSN 1521-0103.

Ansari, HR., Teng, B., Nadeem, A., Roush, KP., Martin, KH., Schnermann, J., & Mustafa, SJ. (2009). A(1) adenosine receptor-mediated PKC and p42/p44 MAPK signaling in mouse coronary artery smooth muscle cells. *American Journal of Physiology. Heart and Circulatory Physiology,* Vol. 297, No 3, (September, 2009), pp. (H1032-H1039), ISSN 1522-1539.

Arch, JR. & Newsholme, EA. (1978). Activities and some properties of 5'-nucleotidase, adenosine kinase and adenosine deaminase in tissues from vertebrates and invertebrates in relation to the control of the concentration and the physiological role of adenosine. *The Biochemical Journal,* Vol. 174, No 3, (September, 1978), pp. (965-977).

Armstrong, SC. & Ganote, E. (1994). Adenosine receptor specificity in preconditioning of isolated rabbit cardiomyocytes: evidence of A3 receptor involvement. *Cardiovascular Research,* Vol. 28, No. 7, (July, 1994) pp. (1049-1056).

Aviado, DM. (1978). Effects of fluorocarbons, chlorinated solvents, and inosine on the cardiopulmonary ystem. *Environmental Health Perspectives,* Vol. 26, No. 1, (October, 1978), pp. (207-215).

Avni, HJ., Garzozi, IS., Barequet, F., Segev, F., Varssano, D., Sartani, G., Chetrit, N., Bakshi, E., Zadok, D., Tomkins, O., Litvin, G., Jacobson, KA., Fishman, S., Harpaz, Z., Farbstein, M., Yehuda, SB., Silverman, MH., Kerns, WD., Bristol, DR., Cohn, I. & Fishman, P. (2010). Treatment of dry eye syndrome with orally-administered CF101: data from a phase 2 clinical trial, *Ophthalmology,* Vol. 117, No. 7, (July, 2010), pp. (1287–1293).

Awad, AS., Huang, L., Ye, H., Duong, ET., Bolton, WK., Linden, J. & Okusa, MD. (2006). Adenosine A2A receptor activation attenuates inflammation and injury in diabetic nephropathy. *American Journal of Physiology. Renal Physiology,* Vol. 290, No. 4, (April, 2006), pp. (F828–F837).

Bastia, E., Varani, K., Monopoli, A. & Bertorelli R (2002). Effects of A(1) and A(2A) adenosine receptor ligands in mouse acute models of pain. *Neuroscience Letters,* Vol. 328, No. 3, (August, 2002), pp. (241-244).

Benowitz, LI., Goldberg, DE. & Irwin, N. (2002). Inosine stimulates axon growth in vitro and in the adult CNS. *Progress in Brain Research,* Vol. 137, No. 1, pp. (389-399).

Benowitz, LI., Goldberg, DE., Madsen, JR., Soni, D. & Irwin, N. (1999). Inosine stimulates extensive axon collateral growth in the rat corticospinal tract after injury. *Proceedings of the National Academy Sciences of the United States of America,* Vol. 96, No. 23, (November, 1999), pp. (13486-13490).

Bilkei-Gorzo, A., Abo-Salem, OM., Hayallah, AM., Michel, K., Müller, CE. & Zimmer, A. (2008). Adenosine receptor subtype-selective antagonists in inflammation and hyperalgesia. *Naunyn- Schmiedebergs Archives of Pharmacology,* Vol. 377, No. 1, (March, 2008), pp. (65-76).

Biovitrum, (January, 2008). A Double-Blind, Placebo-Controlled, Randomized, Parallel-Group Study Evaluating the Efficacy and Tolerability of Oral BVT.115959, a Novel A2A Agonist, Versus Placebo in the Treatment of Diabetic Neuropathic Pain, 08.25.2011, Available from http://www.clinicaltrials.gov/ct2/show/NCT00452777?term=Efficacy+and+tolerability+of+novel+A2A+agonist+in+treatment+of+diabetic+neuropathic+pain&rank=1

Boison, D., Chen, JF. & Fredholm, BB. (2010). Adenosine signaling and function in glial cells. *Cell Death Differentiation,* Vol. 17, No. 7, (July, 2010), pp. (1071-1082).

Borea, PA., Gessi, S., Bar-Yehuda, S. & Fishman, P. (2009). A3 adenosine receptor: pharmacology and role in disease. *Handbook of Experimental Pharmacology,* Vol. 193, No. 1, pp. (297-327).

Borghi, V., Przewlocka, B., Labuz, D., Maj, M., Ilona, O. & Pavone, F. (2002). Formalin-induced pain and mu-opioid receptor density in brain and spinal cord are modulated by A1 and A2a adenosine agonists in mice. *Brain Research,* Vol. 956, No. 2, (November, 2002), pp. (339-348).

Bridges, D., Thompson SW. & Rice, AS. (2001). Mechanisms of neuropathic pain. *British Journal of Anaesthesia,* Vol. 87, No. 1, (July, 2001), pp. (12-26), ISSN 1471-67

Bura, SA., Nadal, X., Ledent, C., Maldonado, R. & Valverde, O. (2008). A2A adenosine receptor regulates glia proliferation and pain after peripheral nerve injury. *Pain,* Vol. 140, No. 1, (November, 2008), pp. (95-103).

Burnstock, G. (1972). Purinergic nerves. *Pharmacological Reviews,* Vol. 24, No. 3, (September, 1972), pp. (509–581), ISSN: 1521-0081

Burnstock, G. (1978). A basis for distinguishing two types of purinergic receptor, In: *Cell Membrane Receptors for Drugs and Hormones: A Multidisciplinary Approach,* Straub, RW. & Bolis L., pp. (107–118), Raven Press, New York.

Burnstock, G. (2007). Purine and pyrimidine receptors. *Cellular and Molecular Life Sciences,* Vol. 64, No. 12, (June, 2007), pp. (1471-1483).

Burnstock, G. (2008). Purinergic signalling and disorders of the central nervous system. *Nature Reviews. Drug Discovery,* Vol. 7, No. 7, (July, 2008), pp. (575-590), ISSN: 1474-1784

Burnstock, G. & Kennedy, C. (1985). Is there a basis for distinguishing two types of P2-purinoceptor? *General Pharmacology,* Vol. 16, No. 5, pp. (433–440).

Burnstock, G. & Knight, GE. (2004). Cellular distribution and functions of P2 receptor subtypes in different systems. *International Review of Cytology,* Vol. 240, No.1, pp. (31–304).

Burnstock, G. & Williams, M. (2000). P2 purinergic receptors: modulation of cell function and therapeutic potential. *The Journal of Pharmacology and Experimental Therapeutics*, Vol. (295), No. 3, (December, 2000), pp. (862–869), ISSN 1521-0103

Burnstock, G., Fredholm, BB. & Verkhratsky, A. (2011). Adenosine and ATP receptors in the brain. *Current Topics in Medicinal Chemistry*, Vol.11, No.8, (April, 2011), pp. (973-1011), ISSN: 1568-0266

By, Y., Condo, J., Durand-Gorde, JM., Lejeune, PJ., Mallet, B., Guieu, R. & Ruf, J. (2011). Intracerebroventricular injection of an agonist-like monoclonal antibody to adenosine A(2A) receptor has antinociceptive effects in mice. *Journal of Neuroimmunology*, Vol. 230, No. 1-2, (January, 2011), pp. (178-182).

Cerqueira, MD. (2006). Advances in pharmacologic agents in imaging: new A2A receptor agonists. *Current Cardiology Reports*, Vol. 8, No. 2, (March, 2006), pp. (119–122).

Chen, P., Goldberg, DE., Kolb, B., Lanser, M. & Benowitz, LI. (2002). Inosine induces axonal rewiring and improves behavioral outcome after stroke. *Proceedings of the National Academy of Sciences of the United States of America*, Vol. 99, No. 13, (June, 2002), pp. (9031-9036).

Childers, SR., Li, X., Xiao, R. & Eisenach, JC. (2005). Allosteric modulation of adenosine A1 receptor coupling to G-proteins in brain. *Journal of Neurochemistry*, Vol. 93, No.3, (May, 2005), pp. (715 -723).

Choca, JI., Green, RD. & Proudfit, HK. (1988). Adenosine A1 and A2 receptors of the substantia gelatinosa are located predominantly on intrinsic neurons: an autoradiography study. *Journal of Pharmacology and Experimental Therapeutics*, Vol. 247, No. 2, (November, 1988), pp. (757-764), ISSN: 1521-0103

Costenla, AR., De Mendonca, A., Sebastião, A. & Ribeiro, JA. (1999). An adenosine analogue inhibits NMDA receptor-mediated responses in bipolar cells of the rat retina. *Experimental Eye Research*, Vol. 68, No. 3, (March, 1999), pp. (367-70).

Cunha, RA., Ferre, S., Vaugeois, JM. & Chen, JF. (2008). Potential therapeutic interest of adenosine A2A receptors in psychiatric disorders. *Current Pharmaceutical Design*, Vol. 14, No. 15, (May, 2008), pp. (1512-1524), ISSN: 1381-6128

Curros-Criado, MM. & Herrero, JF. (2005). The antinociceptive effects of the systemic adenosine A1 receptor agonist CPA in the absence and in the presence of spinal cord sensitization. *Pharmacology, Biochemistry and Behaviour*, Vol. 82, No. 4, (December, 2005), pp. (721-726).

DeLander, GE. & Hopkins, CJ. (1986). Spinal adenosine modulates descending antinociceptive pathways stimulated by morphine. *Journal of Pharmacology and Experimental Therapeutics*, Vol.239, No. 1, (October, 1986), pp. (88-93), ISSN 1521-0103

Desai, C., Victor-Veja, S., Gadangi, S., Montesinos, MC., Chu, CC. & Cronstein, BN. (2005). Adenosine A2A receptor stimulation increases angiogenesis by down-regulating production of the antiangiogenic matrix protein thrombospondin 1. *Molecular Pharmacology*, Vol. 67, No. 5, (May, 2005), pp. (1406–1413), ISSN: 1521-0111

Dixon, AK., Gubitz, AK., Sirinathsinghji, DJ., Richardson, PJ. & Freeman, TC. (1996). Tissue distribution of adenosine receptor mRNAs in the rat. *British Journal of Pharmacology*, Vol. 118, No. 6, (July, 1996), pp. (1461-1468).

Doak, GJ. & Sawynok, J. (1995). Complex role of peripheral adenosine in the genesis of the response to subcutaneous formalin in the rat. *European Journal of Pharmacology*, Vol. 281, No. 3, (August, 1995), pp. (311-318).

Drury, AN. & Szent-Györgyi, A. (1929). The physiological activity of adenine compounds with special reference to their action upon the mammalian heart. *The Journal of Physiology*, Vol. 68, No. 3, (November, 1929), pp. (213-237).

Elzein, E. & Zablocki, J. (2008). A1 adenosine receptor agonists and their potential therapeutic applications. *Expert Opinion on Investigational Drugs*, Vol. 17, No. 12, (December, 2008), pp. (1901-1910).

Fedorova, IM., Jacobson, MA., Basile, A. & Jacobson, KA. (2003). Behavioral characterization of mice lacking the A3 adenosine receptor: sensitivity to hypoxic neurodegeneration. *Cellular and Molecular Neurobiology*, Vol. 23, No. 3, (June, 2003), pp. (431-447).

Feoktistov, I. & Biaggioni, I. (2011). Role of adenosine A(2B) receptors in inflammation. *Advaces in Pharmacology*, Vol. 61, No. 1, pp. (115-144).

Fredholm, BB. (1995). Purinoceptors in the nervous system. *Pharmacology & Toxicology*, Vol. 76, No. 4, (April, 1995), pp. (228-239).

Fredholm, BB., Cunha, RA. & Svenningsson, P. (2003). Pharmacology of adenosine A2A receptors and therapeutic applications. *Current Topics in Medicinal Chemistry*, Vol. 3, No. 4, (February, 2003), pp. (413-426), ISSN 1568-0266

Fredholm, BB., Chern, Y., Franco, R. & Sitkovsky, M. (2007). Aspects of the general biology of adenosine A2A signaling. *Progress in Neurobiology*, Vol. 83, No 5, (December, 2007), pp. (263-276).

Fredholm, BB., IJzerman, AP., Jacobson, KA., Linden, J. and Muller, CE. (2011). International Union of Basic and Clinical Pharmacology. LXXXI. Nomenclature and classification of adenosine receptors- an update. *Pharmacological Reviews*, Vol.63, No. 1, (March, 2011), pp. (1-34), ISSN 1521-0081

Fredholm, BB., Irenius, E., Kull, B. & Schulte, G. (2001). Comparison of the potency of adenosine as an agonist at human adenosine receptors expressed in Chinese hamster ovary cells. *Biochemical Pharmacology*, Vol. 61, No. 4, (February, 2001), pp. (443-448).

Godfrey, L., Yan, L., Clarke, GD., Ledent, C., Kitchen, I. & Hourani, SM. (2006). Modulation of paracetamol antinociception by caffeine and by selective adenosine A2 receptor antagonists in mice. *European Journal of Pharmacology*, Vol. 531, No.1-3, (February, 2006), pp. (80-86).

Goldman, N., Chen, M., Fujita, T., Xu, Q., Peng, W., Liu, W., Jensen, TK., Pei, Y., Wang, F., Han, X., Chen, JF., Schnermann, J., Takano, T., Bekar, L., Tieu, K. & Nedergaard, M. (2010). Adenosine A1 receptors mediate local anti-nociceptive effects of acupuncture. *Nature Neuroscience*, Vol. 13, No. 7, (July, 2010), pp. (883-888), ISSN 1546-1726

Gomez, G. & Sitkovsky, MV. (2003). Differential requirement for A2a and A3 adenosine receptors for the protective effect of inosine in vivo. *Blood*, Vol. 102, No. 13, (December, 2003), pp. (4472-4478), ISSN 1528-0020

Gong, QJ., Li, YY., Xin, WJ., Wei, XH., Cui, Y., Wang, J., Liu, Y., Liu, CC., Li, YY. & Liu, XG. (2010). Differential effects of adenosine A1 receptor on pain-related behavior in normal and nerve-injured rats. *Brain Research*, Vol. 1361, (November, 2010), pp. (23-30).

Haskó, G., Kuhel, DG., Németh, ZH., Mabley, JG., Stachlewitz, RF., Virág, L., Lohinai, Z., Southan, GJ., Salzman, AL. & Szabó, C. (2000). Inosine inhibits inflammatory cytokine production by a posttranscriptional mechanism and protects against endotoxin-induced shock. *Journal of Immunology*, Vol. 164, No. 2, (January, 2000), pp. (1013-1019), ISSN 1550-6606

Haskó, G., Sitkovsky, MV. & Szabó, C. (2004). Immunomodulatory and neuroprotective effects of inosine. *Trends in Pharmacological Science*, Vol. 25, No. 3, (March, 2004), pp. (152-157).

Horiuchi, H., Ogata, T., Morino, T. & Yamamoto, H. (2010). Adenosine A1 receptor agonists reduce hyperalgesia after spinal cord injury in rats. *Spinal Cord*, Vol. 48, No. 9, (September, 2010), pp. (685-690), ISSN 1476-5624

Hussey, MJ., Clarke, GD., Ledent, C., Hourani, SM. & Kitchen, I. (2007). Reduced response to the formalin test and lowered spinal NMDA glutamate receptor binding in adenosine A2A receptor knockout mice. *Pain*, Vol. 129, No. 3, (June, 2007), pp. (287-294).

Hwang, JH., Hwang, GS., Cho, SK. & Han, SM. (2005). Morphine can enhance the antiallodynic effect of intrathecal R-PIA in rats with nerve ligation injury. *Anesthesia & Analgesia*, Vol. 100, No 2, (February, 2005), pp. (461-468), ISSN 1526-7598

Inoue, M., Rashid, MH., Fujita, R., Contos, JJ., Chun, J. & Ueda, H. (2004). Initiation of neuropathic pain requires lysophosphatidic acid receptor signaling. *Nature Medicine*, Vol. 10, No. 7, (July, 2004), pp. (712-718), ISSN 1546-170X

Iskandrian, AE., Bateman, TM., Belardinelli, L., Blackburn, B., Cerqueira, MD., Hendel, RC., Lieu, H., Mahmarian, JJ., Olmsted, A., Underwood, SR., Vitola, J. & Wang, W. (2007). Adenosine versus regadenoson comparative evaluation in myocardial perfusion imaging: results of the ADVANCE phase 3 multicenter international trial. *Journal of Nuclear Cardiology*, Vol. 14, No. 5, (September, 2007) pp. (645–658).

Jacobson, KA. & Gao, GZ. (2006). Adenosine receptors as therapeutic targets. *Nature Reviews. Drug Discovery*, Vol. 5, No. 3, (March, 2006), pp. (247-264), ISSN 1474-1784

Ji, RR. & Woolf, CJ. (2001). Neuronal plasticity and signal transduction in nociceptive neurons: implications for the initiation and maintenance of pathological pain. Neurobiology of Disease, Vol. 8, No. 1, (February, 2001), pp. (1-10).

Jin, X., Shepherd, RK., Duling, BR. & Linden, J. (1997). Inosine binds to A3 adenosine receptors and stimulates mast cell degranulation. *The Journal of Clinical Investigation*, Vol. 100, No. 11, pp. (2849-2857).

Johansson, B., Halldner, L., Dunwiddie, TV., Masino, SA., Poelchen, W., Giménez-Llort, L., Escorihuela, RM., Fernández-Teruel, A., Wiesenfeld-Hallin, Z., Xu, XJ., Hardemark, A., Betsholtz, C., Herlenius, E. & Fredholm, BB. (2001). Hyperalgesia, anxiety, and decreased hypoxic neuroprotection in mice lacking the adenosine A1 receptor. *Proceedings of the National Academy of Sciences of the United States of America*, Vol. 98, No. 16, (July, 2001), pp. (9407-9412).

Karlsten, R., Gordh, T. & Post, C. (1992). Local antinociceptive and hyperalgesic effects in the formalin test after peripheral administration of adenosine analogues in mice. *Pharmacology & Toxicology*, Vol. 70, No. 6 Pt 1, (June, 1992), pp. (434-438).

Keil, GJ 2nd. & DeLander, GE. (1992). Spinally-mediated antinociception is induced in mice by an adenosine kinase-, but not by an adenosine deaminase-, inhibitor. *Life Sciences*, Vol. 51, No. 19, pp. (PL171 - PL176).

Keil, GJ 2nd. & DeLander, GE. (1994). Adenosine kinase and adenosine deaminase inhibition modulate spinal adenosine- and opioid agonist-induced antinociception in mice. *European Journal of Pharmacology*, Vol. 271, No. 1, (December, 1994), pp. (37-46).

Kowaluk, EA., Mikusa, J., Wismer, CT., Zhu, CZ., Schweitzer, E., Lynch, JJ., Lee, CH., Jiang, M., Bhagwat, SS., Gomtsyan, A., McKie, J., Cox, BF., Polakowski, J., Reinhart, G., Williams, M. & Jarvis, MF. (2000). ABT-702 (4-amino-5-(3-bromophenyl)-7-(6-morpholino-pyridin- 3-yl)pyrido[2,3-d]pyrimidine), a novel orally effective adenosine kinase inhibitor with analgesic and anti-inflammatory properties. II. In vivo characterization in the rat. *Journal of Pharmacology and Experimental Therapeutics*, Vol. 295, No. 3, (December, 2000), pp. (1165-1174).

Kowaluk, EA., Kohlhaas, KL., Bannon, A., Gunther, K., Lynch, JJ 3rd. & Jarvis, MF. (1999). Characterization of the effects of adenosine kinase inhibitors on acute thermal nociception in mice. *Pharmacology, Biochemitry & Behaviour*, Vol. 63, No. 1, (May, 1999), pp. (83-91).

Ledent, C., Vaugeois, JM., Schiffmann, SN., Pedrazzini, T., El Yacoubi, M., Vanderhaeghen, JJ., Costentin, J., Heath, JK., Vassart, G. & Parmentier, M. (1997). Aggressiveness, hypoalgesia and high blood pressure in mice lacking the adenosine A2a receptor. *Nature*, Vol. 388, No. 6643, pp. (674-678), ISSN 1476-4687

Li, X., Conklin, D., Pan, HL. & Eisenach, JC. (2003). Allosteric adenosine receptor modulation reduces hypersensitivity following peripheral inflammation by a central mechanism. *The Journal of Pharmacology and Experimental Therapeutics*, Vol. 305, No. 3, (June, 2003), pp. (950-955), ISSN 1521-0103

Lima, FO., Souza, GR., Verri, WA Jr., Parada, CA., Ferreira, SH., Cunha, FQ. & Cunha, TM. (2010). Direct blockade of inflammatory hypernociception by peripheral A1 adenosine receptors: involvement of the NO/cGMP/PKG/KATP signaling pathway. *Pain*, Vol. 151, No. 2, (November, 2009), pp. (506-515).

Loram, LC., Harrison, JA., Sloane, EM., Hutchinson, MR., Sholar, P., Taylor, FR., Berkelhammer, D., Coats, BD., Poole, S., Milligan, ED., Maier, SF., Rieger, J. & Watkins, LR. (2009). Enduring reversal of neuropathic pain by a single intrathecal injection of adenosine 2A receptor agonists: a novel therapy for neuropathic pain. *The Journal of Neuroscience*, Vol. 29, No. 44, (November, 2009), pp. (14015-14025), ISSN 1529-2401

Lynch, JJ 3rd., Jarvis, MF. & Kowaluk, EA. (1999). An adenosine kinase inhibitor attenuates tactile allodynia in a rat model of diabetic neuropathic pain. *European Journal of Pharmacology*, Vol. 364, No.2-3, (January, 1999), pp. (141-146).

Lynch, ME., Clark, AJ. & Sawyonk, J. (2003). Intravenous adenosine alleviates neuropathic pain: a double blind placebo controlled crossover trial using an enriched enrollment design. *Pain*, Vol. 103, No. (1-2), (May, 2003), pp. (111 -117).

Marton, A., Pacher, P., Murthy, KG., Németh, ZH., Haskó, G. & Szabó, C. (2001). Anti-inflammatory effects of inosine in human monocytes, neutrophils and epithelial cells in vitro. *International Journal of Molecular Medicine*, Vol. 8, No. 6, (December, 2001), pp. (617-621).

McGaraughty, S. & Jarvis, MF. (2006). Purinergic control of neuropathic pain. *Drug Development Research,* Vol. 67, No. 4, (April, 2006), pp. (376–388).

McGaraughty, S., Cowart, M., Jarvis, MF. & Berman, RF. (2005). Anticonvulsant and antinociceptive actions of novel adenosine kinase inhibitors. *Current Topics Medicinal Chemistry,* Vol. 5, No. 1, pp. (43-58). ISSN: 1568-0266

Megson, AC., Dickenson, JM., Townsend-Nicholson, A. & Hill, SJ. (1995). Synergy between the inositol phosphate responses to transfected human adenosine A1-receptors and constitutive P2-purinoceptors in CHO-K1 cells. *British Journal of Pharmacology,* Vol. 115, No. 8, (August, 1995), pp. (1415-14124).

Milne, GR. & Palmer, TM. (2011). Anti-inflammatory and immunosuppressive effects of the A2A adenosine receptor. *The Scientific World Journal,* Vol. 11, No. 1, (February, 2011), pp. (320-339).

Müller, CE. & Jacobson, KA. (2011). Recent developments in adenosine receptor ligands and their potential as novel drugs. *Biochimica et Biophysica Acta,* Vol. 1808, No. 5, (May, 2011), pp. (1290-1308).

Nascimento, FP., Figueredo, SM., Marcon, R., Martins, DF., Macedo, SJ Jr., Lima, DA., Almeida, RC., Ostroski, RM., Rodrigues, AL. & Santos, ARS. (2010). Inosine reduces pain-related behavior in mice: involvement of adenosine A1 and A2A receptor subtypes and protein kinase C pathways. *The Journal of Pharmacology and Experimental Therapetics,* Vol. 334, No. 2, (May, 2010), pp. (590-598), ISSN: 1521-0101

Palmer, TM., Benovic, JL. & Stiles, GL. (1995). Agonist-dependent phosphorylation and desensitization of the rat A3 adenosine receptor. Evidence for a G-protein-coupled receptor kinase-mediated mechanism. *The Journal of Biological Chemistry,* Vol. 270, No. 49, (December, 1995), pp. (29607-29613), ISSN: 1083-351-X

Peakman, MC. & Hill, SJ. (1994). Adenosine A2B-receptor-mediated cyclic AMP accumulation in primary rat astrocytes. *British Journal of Pharmacology,* Vol. 111, No. 1, (January, 1994), pp. (191-198)

Poon, A. & Sawynok, J. (1999). Antinociceptive and anti-inflammatory properties of an adenosine kinase inhibitor and an adenosine deaminase inhibitor. *European Journal of Pharmacology,* Vol. 384, No. 2-3, (November, 1999), pp. (123-38)

Poon, A. & Sawynok, J. (1998). Antinociception by adenosine analogs and inhibitors of adenosine metabolism in an inflammatory thermal hyperalgesia model in the rat. *Pain,* Vol. 74, No. 2-3, (January, 1998), pp. (235-245)

Qu, X., Cooney, G. & Donnelly, R. (1997). Short-term metabolic and haemodynamic effects of GR79236 in normal and fructose-fed rats. *European Journal of Pharmacology,* Vol. 338, No. 3, (November, 1997), pp. (269 -276)

Ralevic, V. & Burnstock, G. (1998). Receptors for purines and pyrimidines. *Pharmacological Reviews,* Vol. 50, No. 3, (September, 1998), pp. (413-492). ISSN: 1521-0081

Rane, K., Segerdahl, M., Goiny, M. & Sollevi, A. (1998). Intrathecal adenosine administration, a phase 1 clinical safety study in healthy volunteers, with additional evaluation of its influence on sensory thresholds and experimental pain. *Anesthesiology,* Vol. 89, No. 5, (November, 1998), pp. (1108–1115).

Regaya, I., Pham, T., Andreotti, N., Sauze, N., Carrega, L., Martin-Eauclaire, MF., Jouirou, B., Peragut, JC., Vacher, H., Rochat, H., Devaux, C., Sabatier, JM. & Guieu, R. (2004). Small conductance calcium-activated K+ channels, SkCa, but not voltage-gated K+ (Kv) channels, are implicated in the antinociception induced by

CGS21680, a A2A adenosine receptor agonist. *Life Sciences*, Vol. 76, No. 4, (December, 2004), pp. (367-377).

Ribeiro, JA., Sebastiao, AM. & de Mendonça, A. (2002). Adenosine receptors in the nervous system: pathophysiological implications. *Progress in Neurobiology*, Vol. 68, No. 6, (December, 2002), pp. (377-392).

Salvatore, CA., Jacobson, MA., Taylor, HE., Linden, J. & Johnson, RG. (1993). Molecular cloning and characterization of the human A3 adenosine receptor. *Proceedings of the National Academy of Sciences of the United States of America*, Vol. 90, No. 21, (November, 1993), pp. (10365-10369).

Sawynok, J. (1998). Adenosine receptor activation and nociception. *European Journal of Pharmacology*, Vol. 347, No. 1, (April, 1998), pp. (1-11).

Sawynok, J. (2009). Adenosine Receptors, In: *Peripheral Receptor Targets for Analgesia: Novel Approaches to Pain Management*, Brian E Cairns, pp. (137-152), John Wiley and Sons, Inc, ISBN: 978-0-470-25131-7, New Jersey, USA

Sawynok, J. (2011). Methylxanthines and pain, In: *Methylxanthines - Handbook Experimental Pharmacology*, Bertil B Fredholm, Vol. 200, pp. (311-329), Springer Berlin Heidelberg, ISBN: 3642-134424, Berlin, Germany

Sawynok, J. & Liu, XJ. (2003). Adenosine in the spinal cord and periphery: release and regulation of pain. *Progress in Neurobiology*, Vol. 69, No. 5, (April, 2003), pp. (313-340)

Sawynok, J., Sweeney, MI. & White, TD. (1989). Adenosine release may mediate spinal analgesia by morphine. *Trends in Pharmacological Sciences*, Vol. 10, No. 5, (May, 1989), pp. (186-189)

Sawynok, J., Zarrindast, MR., Reid, AR. & Doak, GJ. (1997). Adenosine A3 receptor activation produces nociceptive behaviour and edema by release of histamine and 5-hydroxytryptamine. *European Journal of Pharmacology*, Vol. 333, No. 1, (August, 1997), pp. (1-7)

Schneider, L., Pietschmann, M., Hartwig, W., Marcos, SS., Hackert, T., Gebhard, MM., Uhl, W., Büchler, MW. &Werner, J. (2006). Inosine reduces microcirculatory disturbance and inflammatory organ damage in experimental acute pancreatitis in rats. *American Journal of Surgery*, Vol. 191, No. 4, (April, 2006), pp. (510-514)

Schulte, G. & Fredholm, BB. (2003). Signalling from adenosine receptors to mitogen-activated protein kinases. *Cell Signalling*, Vol 15, No. 9, (September, 2003), pp. (813-827)

Seymour, RA., Hawkesford, JE., Hill, CM., Frame, J. & Andrews, C. (1999). The efficacy of a novel adenosine agonist (WAG 994) in postoperative dental pain. *British Journal of Clinical Pharmacology*, Vol. 47, No. 6, (June, 1999), pp. (675-680)

Shneyvays, V., Zinman, T. & Shainberg, A. (2004). Analysis of calcium responses mediated by the A3 adenosine receptor in cultured newborn rat cardiac myocytes. *Cell Calcium*, Vol. 36, No. 5, (November, 2004), pp. (387-396)

Sneyd, JR., Langton, JA., Allan, LG., Allan, LG., Peacock, JE. & Rowbotham, DJ. (2007). Multicenter evaluation of the adenosine agonist GR79236X in patients with dental pain after third molar extraction. *British Journal of Anaesthesia*, Vol. 98, No. 5, (May, 2007), pp. (672 -676)

Sollevi, A., Belfrage, M., Lundeberg, T., Segerdahl, M. & Hansen, P. (1995). Systemic adenosine infusion: a new treatment modality to alleviate neuropathic pain. *Pain*, Vol. 61, No. 1, (April, 1995), pp. (155–158)

Song, JG., Hahm, KD., Kim, YK., Leem, JG., Lee, C., Jeong, SM., Park, PH. & Shin, JW. (2011). Adenosine triphosphate-sensitive potassium channel blockers attenuate the antiallodynic effect of R-PIA in neuropathic rats. *Anesthesia & Analgesia*, Vol. 112, No. 6, (June, 2011), pp. (1494-1499)

Sowa, NA., Taylor-Blake, B. & Zylka, MJ. (2010a). Ecto-5'-nucleotidase (CD73) inhibits nociception by hydrolyzing AMP to adenosine in nociceptive circuits. *The Journal of Neurosci*, Vol. 30, No. 6, (February, 2010), pp. (2235-2244), ISSN: 1529-2401

Sowa, NA., Voss, MK. & Zylka, MJ. (2010b). Recombinant ecto-5'-nucleotidase (CD73) has long lasting antinociceptive effects that are dependent on adenosine A1 receptor activation. *Molecular Pain*, Vol. 6, No. 20, (April, 2010)

Suzuki, R., Stanfa, LC., Kowaluk, EA., Williams, M., Jarvis, MF. & Dickenson, AH. (2001). The effect of ABT-702, a novel adenosine kinase inhibitor, on the responses of spinal neurones following carrageenan inflammation and peripheral nerve injury. *British Journal of Pharmacology*, Vol. 132, No. 7, (April, 2001), pp. (1615-1623).

Sweeney, MI., White, TD., Jhamandas, KH. & Sawynok, J. (1987b). Morphine releases endogenous adenosine from the spinal cord in vivo. *European Journal of Pharmacology*, Vol. 141, No. 1, (September, 1987), pp.(169-170)

Sweeney, MI., White, TD. & Sawynok, J. (1987a). Involvement of adenosine in the spinal antinociceptive effects of morphine and noradrenaline. *The Journal of Pharmacology and Experimental Therapeutics*, Vol. 243, No. 2, (November, 1987) pp. (657-665)

Sweeney, MI., White, TD. & Sawynok, J. (1989). Morphine, capsaicin and K+ release purines from capsaicin-sensitive primary afferent nerve terminals in the spinal cord. *The Journal of Pharmacology and Experimental Therapeutics*, Vol. 248, No. 1, (January, 1989), pp. (447-454)

Taiwo, YO. & Levine, JD. (1990). Direct cutaneous hyperalgesia induced by adenosine. *Neuroscience*, Vol. 38, No. 3, (March, 1990), pp. (757-762)

Udelson, JE., Heller, GV., Wackers, FJ., Chai, A., Hinchman, D., Coleman, PS., Dilsizian, V., DiCarli, M., Hachamovitch, R., Johnson, JR., Barrett, RJ. & Gibbons, RJ. (2004). Randomized, controlled dose-ranging study of the selective adenosine A2A receptor agonist binodenoson for pharmacological stress as an adjunct to myocardial perfusion imaging. *Circulation*, Vol. 109, No. 4, (February, 2004), pp. (457–464), ISSN: 1524-4539

Ueda, H. (2006). Molecular mechanisms of neuropathic pain-phenotypic switch and initiation mechanisms. *Pharmacology & Therapeutics*, Vol. 109, No. 1-2, (January, 2006), pp. (57-77)

Wagner, H., Milavec-Krizman, M., Gadient, F., Menninger, K., Schoeffter, P., Tapparelli, C., Pfannkuche, HJ. & Fozard, JR. (1995). General pharmacology of SDZ WAG 994, a potent selective and orally active adenosine A1 receptor agonist. *Drug Development Research*, Vol. 34, No. 3, (March, 1995), pp. (276 - 288).

Wan, TC., Ge, ZD., Tampo, A., Mio, Y., Bienengraeber, MW., Tracey, WR., Gross, JG., Kwok, WM. & Auchampach, JA. (2008). The A3 adenosine receptor agonist CP-532,903 [N6-(2,5-dichlorobenzyl)-3′-aminoadenosine-5′-N-methylcarboxamide] protects against myocardial ischemia/reperfusion injury via the sarcolemmal ATPsensitive potassium channel. The *Journal of Pharmacology and Experimental Therapeutics*, Vol. 324, No. 1, (September, 2007), pp. (234–243), ISSN: 1521-0103

Wu, WP., Hao, JX., Halldner, L., Lövdahl, C., DeLander, GE., Wiesenfeld-Hallin, Z., Fredholm, BB. & Xu, XJ. (2005). Increased nociceptive response in mice lacking the adenosine A1 receptor. *Pain*, Vol. 113, No. 3, (February, 2005), pp. (395-404).

Wu, MM., You, SW., Hou, B., Jiao, XY., Li, YY. & Ju, G. (2003). Effects of inosine on axonal regeneration of axotomized retinal ganglion cells in adult rats. *Neuroscience Letters*, Vol. 341, No. 1, (April, 2003), pp. (84-86).

Wu, WP., Hao, JX., Halldner-Henriksson, L., Xu, XJ., Jacobson, MA., Wiesenfeld-Hallin, Z. & Fredholm, BB. (2002). Decreased inflammatory pain due to reduced carrageenan-induced inflammation in mice lacking adenosine A3 receptors. *Neuroscience*, Vol. 114, No. 3, (October, 2002), pp. (523-527)

Yan, L., Burbiel, JC., Maass, A. & Muller, CE. (2003). Adenosine receptor agonists from basic medicinal chemistry to clinical development. *Expert Opinion on Emerging Drugs*, Vol. 8, No. 2, (November, 2003), pp. (537 -576), ISSN: 1472-8214

Yoon, MH., Bae, HB. & Choi, JI. (2005). Antinociception of intrathecal adenosine receptor subtype agonists in rat formalin test. *Anesthesia & Analgesia*, Vol. 101, No. 5, (November, 2005), pp. (1417-1421), ISSN: 1526-7598

Zahn, PK., Straub, H., Wenk, M. & Pogatzki-Zahn, EM. (2007). Adenosine A1 but not A2a receptor agonist reduces hyperalgesia caused by a surgical incision in rats: a pertussis toxin-sensitive G protein-dependent process. *Anesthesiology*, Vol. 107, No. 5, (November, 2007), pp. (797-806)

Zhang, Y., Li, A., Lao, L., Xin, J., Ren, K., Berman, BM. & Zhang, RX. (2011). Rostral ventromedial medulla mu, but not kappa, opioid receptors are involved in electroacupuncture anti-hyperalgesia in an inflammatory pain rat model. *Brain Research*, Vol. 1395, (June, 2011), pp. (38-45)

Zylka, MJ. (2010). Needling adenosine receptors for pain relief. *Nature Neuroscience*, Vol. 13, No. 7, (July, 2010), pp. (783-784), ISSN: 1546-1726

Zylka, MJ. (2011). Pain-relieving prospects for adenosine receptors and ectonucleotidases. *Trends in Molecular Medicine*, Vol. 17, No. 4, (April, 2011), pp. (188-196)

Therapeutic Organometallic Compounds

Beril Anilanmert
Istanbul University, Institute of Forensic Sciences, Turkiye

1. Introduction

Most drugs used today are purely organic compounds. Especially after the enormous success of the cisplatin (Fig 1) in tumor treatment, interest in metal complexes has grown (Allardyce & Dyson, 2006). Synthetic organometallic compounds are generally considered to be toxic or non-compatible with biological systems. Despite this perception, the medicinal properties of organometallic compounds, in particular organo-transition metal compounds, have been probed for a long time and in the last few years the area has grown considerably.

Transition metals have an important place within medicinal biochemistry (Rafique et al, 2010). Transition metals represent the d block element which includes groups 3 - 12 on the periodic table. They have partially filled d-shells in any of their commonly occuring oxidation state. Metal complex or coordination compound is a structure consisting of a central metal atom, bonded to a surrounding array of ligands (molecules or anions), which donate electron pair to the metal. Research has shown significant progress in utilization of transition metal complexes as drugs to treat several human diseases like carcinomas, lymphomas, infection control, anti-inflammatory, diabetes, and neurological disorders. Transition metals exhibit different oxidation states and can interact with a number of negatively charged molecules. This activity of transition metals has started the development of metal-based drugs with promising pharmacological application and may offer unique therapeutic opportunities.

2. Therapeutic applications of some old and new organometallic complexes and discoveries and ongoing studies

Various metal complexes have been tested in anticancer therapy (Meng et al, 2009). The development of metal complexes with platinum central atoms such as cisplatin or carboplatin had an enormous impact on current cancer chemotherapy (Fig 1, 2) (Ott & Gust, 2007). In particular, cisplatin has become one of the most widely used drugs and is highly effective in treating several cancers such as ovarian and testicular cancers (Meng et al, 2009).

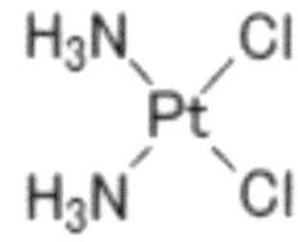

Fig. 1. Molecular structure of cisplatin.

Most of the platinum compounds that entered clinical trials follow the same empirical structure-activity relationships (Abu-Surrah & Kettunen, 2006). A necessary prerequisite for an active Pt-drug seems to be *cis*-coordination by bidentate amine ligands or two amines (at least one -NH group on the amine) and two leaving groups with an intermediate binding strength (e.g. Cl^-, SO_4^{2-}, citrate or oxalate) to platinum. The limitations of cisplatin have stimulated research in the field of platinum antitumor chemistry by giving specific goals. These include reduction in toxicity of cisplatin (nausea, ear damage, vomiting, loss of sensation in hands, and kidney toxicity), acquired drug resistance observed in certain tumors, inefficiency of the drug against some of the commonest tumors (e.g. colon and breast).

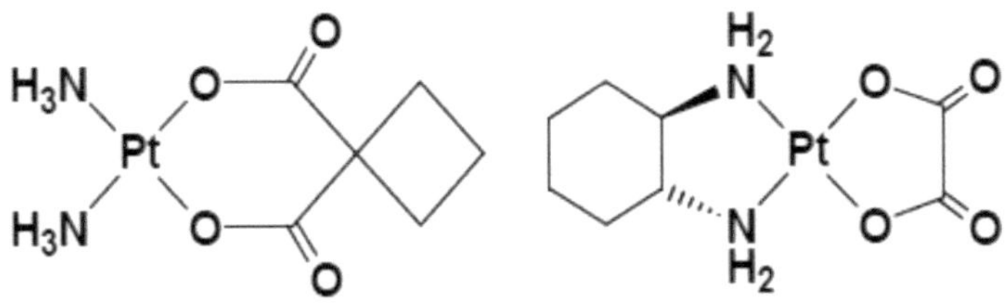

Fig. 2. Structures of carboplatin (left) and oxaliplatin (right) (Hanif, 2010)

Thousands of other platinum complexes have been synthesized and biologically evaluated for their antitumor properties, from which about fourty entered clinical phase I trials but only two carboplatin and oxaliplatin (Fig. 2) have received worldwide approval (Abu-Surrah & Kettunen, 2006). Carboplatin exhibits a tumor inhibiting profile identical to that of cisplatin, however with fewer side effects, whereas oxaliplatin is used in a combination therapy against metastatic colorectal cancer.

Some platinum(II) and palladium(II) complexes with new *trans-l*-dach (1R,2R-cyclohexanediamine) based diamine and diimine donor ligands containing the enantiomerically pure myrtenyl groups as terminal substituents were synthesized in 2008. The anti-proliferative effect of compounds Dichloro[(1R,2R)-(-)-N^1,N^2-bis{(1R)-(-)myrtenyl}-1,2-diamino cyclohexane]-platinum(II).3H_2O, Dichloro[1R,2R)-(-)-N^1,N^2-bis{(1R)-(-) myrtenylidene}-1,2-diamino cyclohexane]-platinum(II) and Dichloro [(1R,2R)-(-)-N^1,N^2-bis{(1R)-(-)myrtenyl}-1,2-diaminocyclohexane]-palladium(II).1.5H_2O together with the commercial drugs cisplatin (Cis-Pt) and oxaliplatin (Ox-Pt) were investigated in L1210 Cell line using 3H-thymidine incorporation (Abu-Surrah et. al., 2008). As shown in Figure 3, the platinum compounds Dichloro[(1R,2R)-(-)-N^1,N^2-bis{(1R)-(-)myrtenyl}-1, 2-diaminocyclo hexane]-platinum(II).3H_2O and Dichloro [1R,2R)-(-)-N^1,N^2-bis{(1R)-(-) myrtenylidene}-1,2-diaminocyclohexane]-platinum(II) suppress proliferation more efficiently than the commercial platinum-based drugs with an IC_{50} of 0.6 and 0.7 µL, respectively. Compound Dichloro[(1R,2R)-(-)-N1,N2-bis{(1R)-(-) myrtenyl}-1,2-diaminocyclohexane]- platinum(II).3H_2O is 17-folds more potent than the commercial oxaliplatin and cisplatin. No significant difference could be observed between the complex that contains the diamine nitrogen ligand and the one holding the corresponding diimine ligand. The authors also synthesized the palladium complex; Dichloro[(1R,2R)-(-)-N^1,N^2-bis{(1R)-(-)myrtenyl}-1,2-diaminocyclohexane]-palladium(II).1.5H_2O, which also suppresses proliferation efficiently with an IC_{50} of 4.2 µL. This is about 2-folds more potent than the commercial oxaliplatin and cisplatin.

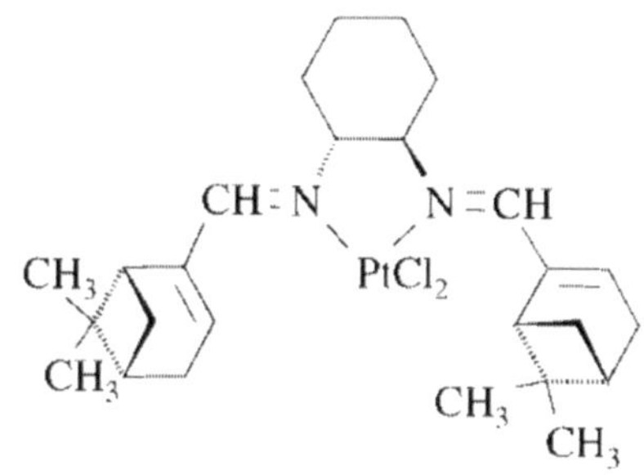

(a) Dichloro[(1R,2R)-(-)-N1,N2-bis{(1R)-(-)myrtenyl}-1,2-diamino cyclohexane]-platinum(II).$3H_2O$

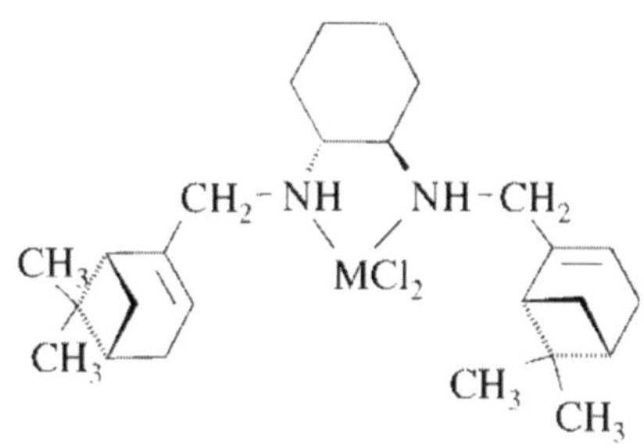

(b) Dichloro[1R,2R)-(-)-N1,N2-bis{(1R)-(-) myrtenylidene}-1,2-diamino cyclohexane]-M(II) M=Pt(II), Pl(II)

Fig. 3. The structure of some platinum(II) and palladium(II) complexes with new *trans-l-*dach based diamine and diimine donor ligands containing the enantiomerically pure myrtenyl groups as terminal substituents (Abu-Surrah & Kettunen, 2006).

In a total look, platinum complexes display, along with other kinds of anticancer drugs, two major drawbacks: (a) severe toxicities (neurotoxicity, nephrotoxicity, etc.) and (b) limited applicability to a narrow range of tumors, as several of them exhibit natural or induced resistance. These unresolved problems in platinum-based anticancer therapy have stimulated increased research efforts in the search for novel non platinum-containing metal species as cytostatic agents. Non-platinum metals may have different chemical behavior (oxidation state, redox potential, coordination geometry, additional coordination sites, binding preferences to biomolecules according to the HSAB [hard and soft (Lewis) acids and bases] principle etc.), rate of hydrolysis or kinetics of ligand exchange reactions and the ability to replace essential metals (Abu-Surrah & Kettunen, 2006). Therefore, it is likely that non-platinum metal-based compounds may have different mechanisms of action, biodistribution and biological activity.

The antitumor properties of a number of different metal ions and their complexes have been evaluated, but only a few non-platinum metal-based drugs are currently in clinical studies, the most promising ones contain ruthenium and gallium ions (Abu-Surrah & Kettunen, 2006). Preclinical and clinical investigations confirmed that the development of new metal agents with modes of action different from cisplatin is possible (Ott & Gust, 2007). Thus, complexes with iron, cobalt, or gold central atoms have shown promising results in preclinical studies and compounds with titanium, ruthenium, or gallium central atoms (as in Fig 4) have already been evaluated in phase I and phase II trials. Other metal complexes that have shown potential anticancer activity are the complexes of Rh(I), Rh(III), Ir(I), Ir(II), Ir(IV), Os(II) and Os(III). Many platinum and non-platinum metal complexes such as palladium, ruthenium, rhodium, copper, and lanthanum, with aromatic N-containing ligands as pyridine, imidazole and 1,10-phenanthroline, and their derivatives (whose donor properties are somewhat similar to the purine and pyrimidine bases), have shown very promising antitumor properties in vitro and in vivo in cisplatin-resistant model systems or against cisplatin-insensitive cell lines (Zhao & Lin, 2005).

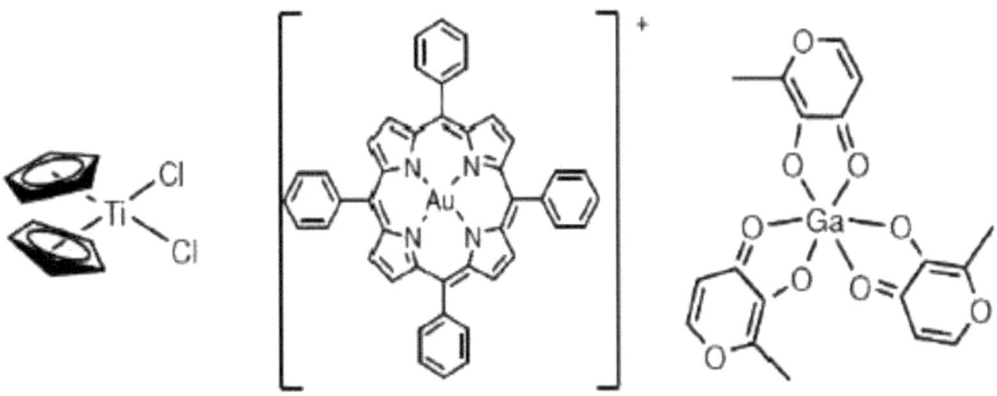

Fig. 4. The chemical structures of titanocene dichloride (a), gold tetraphenylporphyrin (b) and gallium maltolate (c) (Hanif, 2010).

The notable analogy between the coordination chemistry of platinum(II) and palladium(II) compounds has advocated studies of Pd(II) complexes as antitumor drugs (Abu-Surrah & Kettunen, 2006). A key factor that might explain the reason that platinum is most useful, comes from the ligand-exchange kinetics. The hydrolysis of the leaving ligands in palladium complexes is too rapid: 10^5 times faster than their corresponding platinum analogues. They dissociate readily in solution leading to very reactive species that are unable to reach their pharmacological targets. This implies that if an antitumor palladium drug is to be developed, it must somehow be stabilized by a strongly coordinated nitrogen ligand and a suitable leaving group. If this group is reasonably non labile, the drug can maintain its structural integrity *in vivo* long enough. As a way to increase the stability of the palladium(II) complexes, two chelates forming two rings around the central atom were prepared and evaluated. A series of compounds bearing two chelating ligands the N-N and O-O ligand (XO_3: selenite or tellurite) were prepared. The N-N ligand did not influence the activity but the oxygen coordinated leaving group did. Selenite complexes were invariably better cytotoxic agents than tellurite complexes and cisplatin. The complex [bipy)Pd(SeO_3)] (Fig 5) was found to bind to DNA through a coordinate covalent bond. Another study investigated compounds [((1R,2R)-(-)-1,2-diaminocyclohexane)Pd(3-methylorotate)] which gave a high activity for sarcoma 180 but a low one against P388 leukemia and [(1R,2R)-(-)-1,2-diaminocyclohexane)Pd(5-fluroorot)] which also displayed significant antitumor activity. These strong chelating ligands replacing chloro or nitro ligands induce a reduction in the rate of hydrolysis.

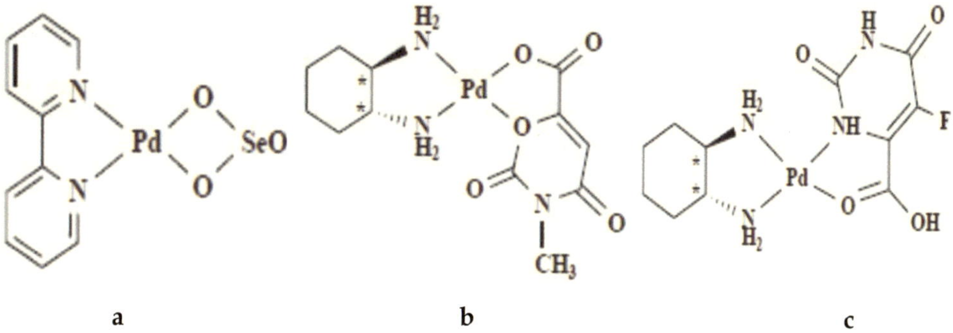

Fig. 5. The geometrical structure of [bipy)Pd(SeO_3)] (a), [((1R,2R)-(-)-1,2-diaminocyclohexane) Pd(3-methylorotate)] (b), [(1R,2R)-(-)-1,2-diaminocyclohexane)Pd(5-fluroorot) (c)] (Abu-Surrah & Kettunen, 2006)

Both ruthenium and osmium, along with iron, are members of group VIIIB and are placed in the fourth, fifth and sixth row of the periodic table, respectively. They are classified as the 'Platinum group' along with rhodium, palladium, iridium and platinum. All these metals often occur together in the same mineral deposits and have closely related physical and chemical properties. The application of iron in group 8 metal complexes in anticancer drug design is the ferrocenyl derivative of tamoxifen (ferrocifen) (Jauen et al, 2006), and two ruthenium containing drug candidates NAMI-A and KP1019 in clinical trials. In trying to find better alternatives to tamoxifen, Jaouen et al. (Top et al, 2001), have investigated tamoxifen analogs that contain an organometallic moiety. The researchers studied the effects of several hydroxy-substituted ferrocifens on the proliferation of two lines of breast cancer cells, one used for tumors mediated by the ERα receptor, and one used for tumors mediated by ERβ. Three of the ferrocifens (Fig 6) exhibited a strong antiproliferative effect in both cell lines while hydroxytamoxifen, as expected, was effective only against the cells having the ERα receptor. Ferrocifenes exhibit anticancer activity against hormone dependent and hormone independent breast cancers (Rafique et al, 2010). The ferrocene derivatives having hydroxyl group in phenyl ring have high affinity for estrogen receptor. Ferrocene by itself had no effect.

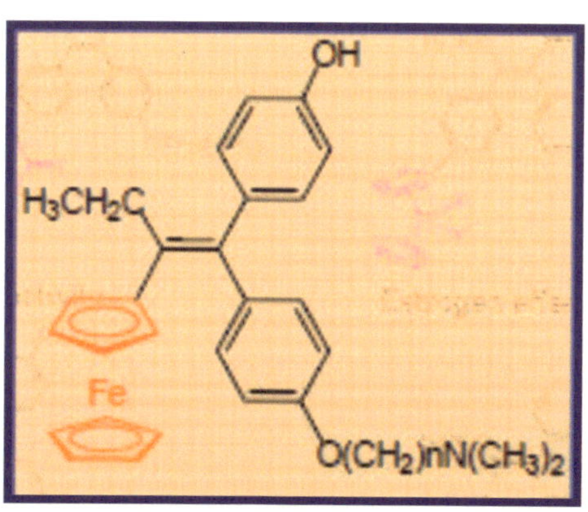

Fig. 6. The main molecular structure of ferrocifenes.

Special attention has been paid to ruthenium compounds because they exhibit cytotoxicity against cancer cells, analogous ligand exchange abilities to platinum complexes, no cross-resistance with cisplatin, and may display reduced toxicity on healthy tissues by using iron transport (Meng et al, 2009). Ruthenium complexes demonstrate similar ligand exchange kinetics to those of platinum(II) antitumor drugs already used in the clinic while displaying only low toxicity (Brabec & Novakova, 2006). This is in part due to the ability of ruthenium complexes to mimic the binding of iron to molecules of biological significance, exploiting the mechanisms that the body has evolved for transport of iron.

Ruthenium complexes tend to accumulate preferentially in neoplastic masses in comparison with normal tissue (Rademaker-Lakhai et al, 2004). They probably use transferrin, for its similarities with iron, to accumulate in the tumor. A transferrin-ruthenium complex can be actively transported into tumor tissues that have high transferrin-receptor densities. Once bound to the transferrin receptor, the complex liberates ruthenium that can be easily internalized in the tumor. Next, ruthenium (III) complexes likely remain in their relatively inactive ruthenium(III) oxidation state until they reach the tumor site. In this environment, with its lower oxygen content and pH than normal tissue, reduction to the more reactive ruthenium(II) oxidation state takes place. This reaction, named "activation by reduction" would provide not only a selective toxicity but also an efficacy toward hypoxic tumors known to be resistant to chemotherapy and/or radiotherapy. Finally, some complexes are more effective against the tumor metastases than against the primary tumor. Due to differing ligand geometry between their complexes, ruthenium compounds bind to DNA affecting its conformation differently than cisplatin and its analogues (Brabec & Novakova, 2006). In addition, non-nuclear targets, such as the mitochondrion and the cell surface, have also been implicated in the antineoplastic activity of some ruthenium complexes. So, ruthenium compounds have a pattern of cytotoxicity and antitumor activity that is different from that of cisplatin tissue (Rademaker-Lakhai et al, 2004). Ruthenium complexes exhibit both nitric oxide release and scavenging functions that can affect vasodilation and synapse firing (Clarke, 2003). Simple ruthenium complexes are unusually effective in suppressing the immune response by inhibiting T cell proliferation. Thus, ruthenium compounds offer the potential over antitumor platinum(II) complexes currently used in the clinic of reduced toxicity, a novel mechanism of action, the prospect of non-cross-resistance and a different spectrum of activity. Although the pharmacological target for antitumor ruthenium compounds has not been completely identified, there is a large body of evidence indicating that the cytotoxicity of many ruthenium complexes correlates with their ability to bind DNA although few exceptions have been reported. One of the first ruthenium compounds described to have anticancer activity was ruthenium red, and further work showed the anticancer potential of ruthenium-containing drugs (Rafique et al, 2010). Since then, several teams have synthesized and characterized new compounds containing ruthenium(II) or ruthenium(III). Ruthenium red and the related Ru360 strongly inhibit calcium ion uptake in the mitochondria (Clarke, 2003).

Ru(II) and Ru(III) complexes have shown very promising properties while the Ru(III) compound NAMI-A (imidazolium *trans*-[tetrachloro(DMSO)(imidazole)ruthenate(III)]) , is the first ruthenium compound that successfully entered phase I clinical trials as an antimetastatic drug candidate (Katsaros & Anagnostopoulou, 2002; Antonarakis & Emadi,

2010). Ruthenium compound KP1019 (indazolium *trans*-[tetrachlorobis(1H-indazole) ruthenate(III)]), as an anticancer drug against colon carcinomas and their metastases has also entered clinical trials so far. It has shown direct antitumor activity against a wide range of primary explants of human tumors by inducing apoptosis (Antonorakis & Emadi, 2010). Both compounds showed relatively little side-effects and better tolerance in clinical phase I trials (Fig. 7). In preclinical studies, NAMI-A has demonstrated inhibitory effects against the formation of cancer metastases in a variety of tumor animal models but appears to lack direct cytotoxic effects (Antonarakis & Emadi, 2010). In case of NAMI-A, DNA is thought to be a less important target, and anti-angiogenic activity based on the NO metabolism has been described (Bharti & Singh, 2009). NAMI-A interaction with the microenvironment involving integrin activation that results in reduced cell invasiveness and migration has been proposed and this may be the reasons for the activity of ruthenium compounds against cisplatin-resistant tumors. Ruthenium compounds ONCO4417 and DW1/2 have been demonstrated to show Pim-1 kinase inhibition in preclinical systems (Sekhon, 2010). A phase I and pharmacokinetic study was also carried out with the new ruthenium complex indazolium trans-[tetrachlorobis(1H-indazole)ruthenate(III)] (KP1019, FFC14A) (Lentz et al, 2009). Seven patients with various types of solid tumours refractory to standard therapy were treated with escalating doses of KP1019 (25-600 mg) twice weekly for 3 weeks. No dose-limiting toxicity occurred. Ruthenium plasma concentration-time profiles after the first dose and under multiple-dose conditions were analysed using a compartmental approach. The pharmacokinetic disposition was characterised by a small volume of distribution, low clearance and long half-life. Only a small fraction of ruthenium was excreted renally.

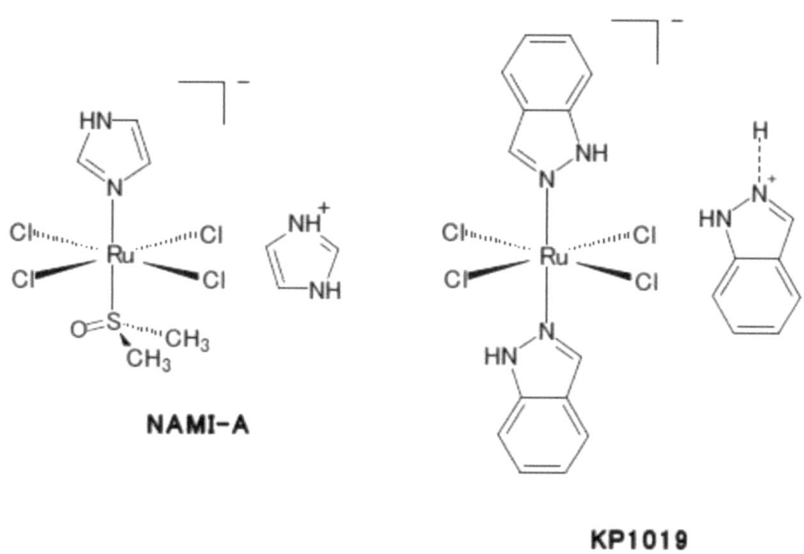

Fig. 7. Structure of ruthenium complexes NAMI-A and KP1019 (Llorca, 2005).

Many biological properties have been attributed to ruthenium complex I (*trans*-[$RuCl_2(nic)_4$]) and ruthenium complex II (*trans*-[$RuCl_2$ (i-nic)$_4$]) including nitric oxide synthase inhibition (Valvassori et al, 2006). However, side effects of the ruthenium compounds should also be evaluated. In the investigation of the pharmacological effects of these complexes on anxiety and memory formation on adult male Wistar rats, no effects were observed in the anxiety parameters and habituation to an open-field while memory impairment was observed. The ruthenium complexes impaired memory retention compared with vehicle group in the inhibitory avoidance, as when administrated 30 min prior as immediately after training. The memory impairment induced by ruthenium complexes may be due to their nitric oxide synthase inhibition capacity.

Rhodium belongs to the same group as platinum and ruthenium. However, rhodium compounds, analogues to the corresponding platinum and ruthenium compounds that possess significant antitumor properties, were found to be less effective as anticancer agents mainly due to their toxic effects. Dimeric mu-Acetato dimers of Rh(II) as well as monomeric square planar Rh(I) and octahedral Rh(III) complexes have shown interesting antitumor properties.

In 2009, Meng et al. have studied both in vitro and in vivo the biological properties of RDC11 (Fig 8), which contain a covalent bond between the ruthenium atom and a carbon. RDC11 inhibited the growth of various tumors implanted in mice more efficiently than cisplatin. Importantly, in striking contrast with cisplatin, RDC11 did not cause severe side effects on the liver, kidneys, or the neuronal sensory system. It was shown to interact poorly with DNA and induced only limited DNA damages compared with cisplatin, suggesting alternative transduction pathways. The target genes of the endoplasmic reticulum stress pathway, such as Bip, XBP1, PDI, and CHOP, were activated in RDC11-treated cells. Activation of CHOP led to the expression of several of its target genes, including proapoptotic genes. Acting through an atypical pathway involving CHOP and endoplasmic reticulum stress, RDC11 is thought to provide an interesting alternative for anticancer therapy (Meng et al, 2009).

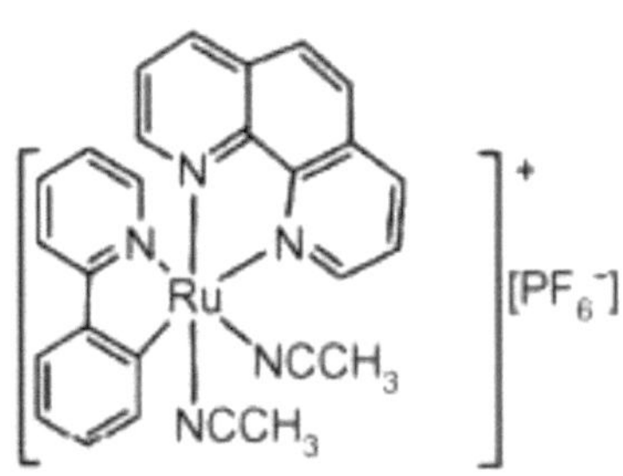

Fig. 8. Molecular structure of RDC11 (Meng et al, 2009).

A class of ruthenium(II)-arene complexes that are weakly cytotoxic in vitro, were also shown to have selective antimetastatic activity in vivo, in the literature (Anga, et. al., 2011). These compounds, [Ru(η6-p-arene)Cl_2(1,3,5-triaza-7-phosphaadamantane)] termed RAPTA, interact strongly with proteins, with the ability to discriminate binding to different proteins, but show a relatively low propensity to bind DNA, which is considered to be the main target of many metal-based drugs. The basic RAPTA structure is quite stable in physiological environments, and studies have shown that aquation of the chloride bonds occurs, it may not be an essential step for anticancer drug activity - direct substitution with biomolecular targets is also possible. Based on the concept of bifunctional radiopharmaceuticals (Ogawa et al, 2007), developed a highly stable ^{186}Remercaptoacetylglycylglycylglycine (MAG3) complex-conjugated bisphosphonate, [[[[(4-hydroxy-4,4-diphosphonobutyl) carbamoylmethyl]carbamoylmethyl]carbamoylmethyl] carbamoylmethane thiolate] oxorhenium (V) (^{186}Re-MAG3-HBP), for the treatment of painful bone metastases. ^{186}Re-MAG3-HBP accumulated at the site where tumor cells were injected in a rat model of bone cancer and significantly inhibited tumor growth and attenuated the allodynia induced by bone cancer without having critical myelosuppressive side effects. The results indicate that ^{186}Re-MAG3-HBP could be useful as a therapeutic agent for the palliation of metastatic bone pain.

Since DNA has often been proposed as the target of these organometallic antineoplastic agents, there is a particular emphasis on those that can interact with nucleic acids (Clarke et al, 1999). Nevertheless, heavy metals are generally toxic by binding to sulfur and nitrogen sites on proteins and, thus, can interfere with a number of modes of metabolism. Several metals also exhibit action through redox activity. Gallium appears to operate through the displacement of metal ions in iron metabolism or bone. In large part, action of gallium complexes seems to be a consequence of the similarity of gallium(III) to iron(III): Gallium interferes with the cellular transport of iron by binding to transferrin, and also interferes with the action of ribonucleotide reductase, which then results in inhibition of DNA synthesis (Hannon, 2007). The key to activity is making gallium(III) bioavailable, and work is focused on ligands which stabilize gallium against hydrolysis and facilitate membrane permeation. Among the developed gallium comounds, tris(8-quinolinolato)gallium(III) (KP46/FFC11) has entered clinical trials (Fig 9).

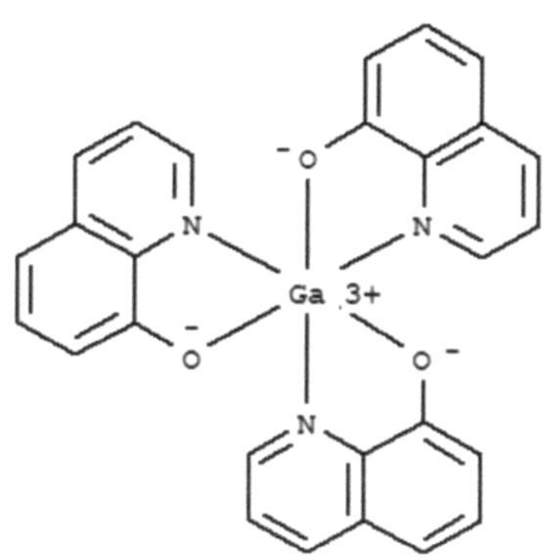

Fig. 9. Molecular structure of Tris(8-quinolinolato)gallium(III)

Gallium-based anticancer chemotherapeutics are appreciably progressing in clinical studies (Timerbaev et al, 2009). The interest of drug developers and clinicians in gallium compounds is due to a proven ability of gallium cations to inhibit tumour growth, and enhanced bioavailability and moderate toxicity provided by the conversion of gallium into chelate complexes. One of the complexes suitable for a more convenient oral administration is tris(8-quinolinolato) gallium(III) (KP46). KP46 is an orally bioavailable gallium complex, which exerts its antitumoral activity via inhibition of ribonucleotide reductase, induction of S phase arrest and apoptosis (Dittrich et al, 2005). In preclinical models KP46 was proved to be a stronger anticancer agent than gallium nitrate and it was effective on a model of tumor-associated hypercalcemia. Nominated from a range of gallium complexes for the clinical stage of development, KP46 has finished phase I trials with the outcome of promising tolerability and evidence of clinical activity in renal cell carcinoma (Timerbaev et al, 2009). The adverse reactions of the complex, observed in a study, where 7 patients were used were neutropenia and anemia, stomatitis and conjunctivitis, dizziness, headache and acne, fatigue and diarrhaea both (Dittrich et al, 2005). In one out of the 4 patients with renal cell carcinoma an unconfirmed partial response has been observed after 8 weeks and in a second patient with renal cell carcinoma the disease was stabilized for 29 weeks. Peak plasma levels were reached 5-7 h after intake and pharmacokinetic analysis revealed a long terminal half-life (28 h). KP46 has been well tolerated with some preliminary evidence of efficacy in renal cell carcinoma.

The low-spin $5d^6$ Ir^{III} organometallic half-sandwich complexes $[(\eta^5\text{-}Cp^x)Ir(XY)Cl]^{0/+}$, Cp^{xph} : tetramethyl(phenyl)cyclopentadienyl, or Cp^{xbiph}: tetramethyl(biphenyl)cyclopentadienyl, XY = 1,10-phenanthroline, 2,2'-bipyridine, ethylenediamine, or picolinate, were investigated at 2011 (Liu et al, 2011). Complexes with N,N-chelating ligands readily form adducts with 9-ethylguanine but not 9-ethyladenine; picolinate complexes bind to both purines. Cytotoxic potency toward A2780 human ovarian cancer cells increases with phenyl substitution on Cp^x: $Cp^{xbiph} > Cp^{xph}$. The hydrophobicity and intercalative ability of Cp^{xph} and Cp^{xbiph} make a major contribution to the anticancer potency of their Ir^{III} complexes.

Among the metallocene dihalide complexes MX_2Cp_2 (where M=Ti, V, Mo, Nb etc., X= halide and Cp = η5-cyclopentadienide), titanocene (Fig 10), $TiCl_2Cp_2$ or MTK4 is the most successful anticancer agent as shown in phase I/II clinical trials (Bharti & Singh,2009). Titanocene dichloride had been recognized as active anticancer drug against breast and gastrointestinal carcinomas. Previously DNA was supposed to be the target of $[TiCl_2Cp_2]$ in a manner similar to cisplatin due to the similarity in Cl---Cl distances. Later, the aqueous chemistry of $[TiCl_2Cp_2]$ showed that DNA is not the site of action for this drug. The anticancer activity of $TiCl_2Cp_2$ is due to inhibition of collagenase type IV activity, which is involved in regulation of cellular proliferation, protein kinase C and DNA topoisomerase II activities. Titanium may also replace iron in transferrin and facilitate cellular uptake into tumor cells. The titanocene dichloride is believed to be accumulated via the transferrin-dependent pathways. Dose limiting toxicities of titanium compounds include nephrotoxicity and elevation of creatinine and bilirubin levels.

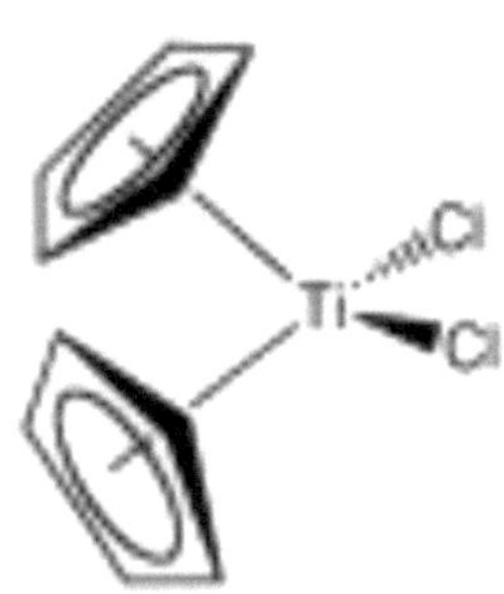

Fig. 10. Molecular structue of titanocene (Hannon, 2007)

Budotitane [cis-diethoxybis(1-phenylbutane-1,3-dionato)titanium (IV)] (Fig 11), was the first non-platinum transition-metal anticancer agent to be tested in clinical trials (Schilling et al, 1995). It is effective against a number of tumors in animals and is well tolerated (Bharti &

Singh, 2009). *In vitro* and *in vivo* experiments with budotitane showed no significant DNA damage. The dose-limiting side effects include cardiac arrhythmia, hepatotoxicity, renal toxicity and a reversible loss of taste (Dabrowiak, 2009; Antonarakis & Emadi, 2010). Ti(IV) compounds are known to inhibit proteases and telomerases. Inhibition of proteases in rapidly growing tumor cells may block the growth of tumor cells. Inhibition of telomerase may control all protein synthesis.

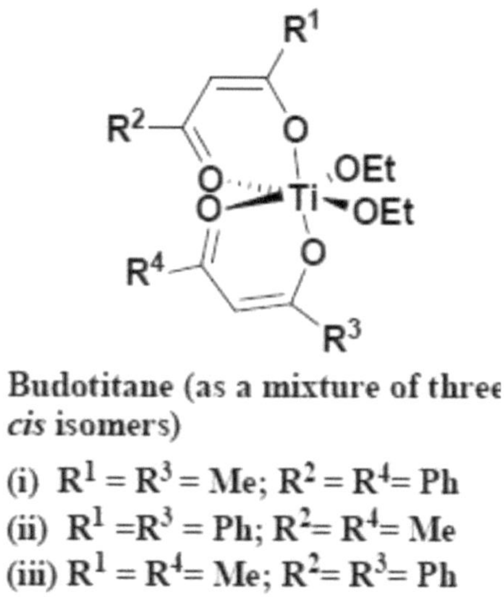

Fig. 11. The molecular structure of budotitane (Bharti & Singh, 2009).

Gold compounds are used for treating arthritis and cancer, they have potential for treating AIDS, malaria and Chagas disease (Dabrowiak, 2009). A property of Au^{+3} that greatly complicates its chemistry is that many of its simple complexes can easily be reduced to Au^{+} by a variety of ligands, including thiols and thioethers found on cysteine and methionine residues of peptides and proteins. Even the disulfide linkage, R-S-S-R′, which is generally considered a poorer ligand than a thiol or a thioether, binds to and reduces Au^{+3} to Au^{+}. Since there are agents in the biological system that can oxidize Au^{+} to Au^{+3}, gold compounds can, in principle, exist in a variety of different coordination states in the biological system. These properties, and the fact that the concentrations of gold compounds normally encountered in therapeutic situations are very low, make it difficult to determine the chemistry of gold in the biological environment. Gold thiolate complexes were found especially effective at slowing the progression of rheumatod arthritis. Sodium aurothiomalate (myochrysine), aurothioglucose (solganol) and aurothiosulfate (sanochrysine) are water-soluble polymeric antiarthritic compounds that are administered to the patient by injection, so-called injectable or parenteral drugs, while auranofin, which is only slightly soluble in water, is given to the patient orally in capsule form. The earlywork on auranofin and its analogs revealed that Au^{+} complexes that have phosphine and thioglucose ligands were effective in killing B16 melanoma and P388 leukemia cells in culture. One compound that showed a significantly broader range of activity than auranofin and one of its analogs against a number of different tumor models implanted in mice was the tetrahedral cation $[Au(dppe)_2]^{+}$, bis[1,2-bis(diphenylphosphino) ethane]gold(I).

$[Au(dppe)_2]^+$ is active alone, and in combination with cisplatin, against P388 leukemia in mice, and it is also active against various sarcomas in mice. The compound aurocyanide, $[Au(CN)_2]^-$, which is a biotransformation product in chrysotherapy, has been found to inhibit proliferation of HIV in a strain of CD_4^+. A gold complex with two attached thioglucose ligands has been shown to protect MT-4 cells from the HIV virus by binding to a specific cysteine residue on a 120 kDa protein, gp120, which is part of the outer envelope of the virus. The compound [bpza][$AuCl_4$], where bpza is the diprotonated-chloride form of a bis-pyrazole ligand, inhibits both reverse transcriptase and HIV-1 protease. Since these enzymes function differently in the life cycle of the HIV virus, inhibiting both with a single compound is unusual. Reverse transcriptase is responsible for converting viral RNA into double-stranded DNA prior to the integration of the latter into genomic DNA of the T cell, and HIV-1 protease controls the maturation and production of infectious virons (virus particles). Since [bpza][$AuCl_4$] is nontoxic to peripheral blood mononuclear cells in the immune system, the compound is thought to have potential as an anti-HIV agent.

A recent report by Sannella et al. (Sanella et al, 2008) showed that auranofin and other gold compounds inhibit the growth of Plasmodium falciparum, a protozoan parasite carried by Anopheles mosquitoes that causes malaria. The researchers suggested that the mechanism by which the gold compounds inhibit the growth of P. falciparum is related to the ability of the complexes to block the function of the enzyme thioredoxin reductase, TrxR.

Nickel is an essential component in different types of enzymes such as urease, carbon monoxide dehydrogenase, and hydrogenase (Abu-Surrah & Kettunen, 2006). Recently, some results showing also apparent potential of this platinum group element in antitumor studies have been reported. For example the cytotoxicity of the nickel (II) complexes containing 1,2-naphtoquinone-based thiosemicarbazone ligands (NQTS) was tested on MCF7 human breast cancer cell line and compared to free ligand and another naphthoquinone, commercial antitumor drug etoposide. According to the reported data, Ni-NQTS complex has the highest antitumor activity with an IC50 of 2.2 μM. The mechanistic study of action showed inhibition of topoisomerase II. Recent studies showed that the corresponding nickel complexes of semicarbazones (Fig 12) have even greater inhibitory effect on MCF7 cell growth. They display IC50 values in 2-5 μM range and also in general they produce lower side effect than thiosemicarbazones.

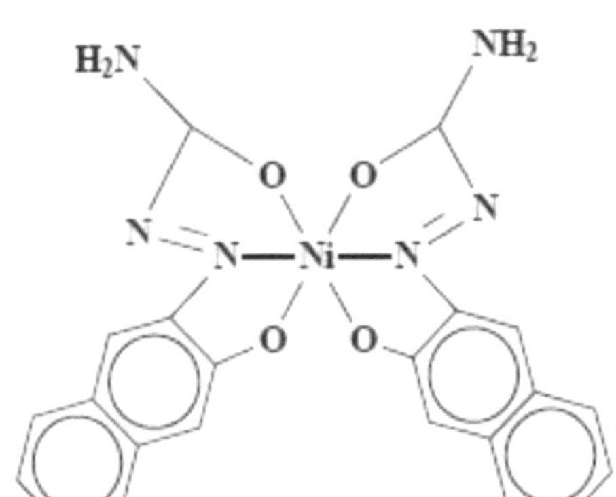

Fig. 12. Structure of a Ni(II)-semicarbazone based antitumor complex (Abu-Surrah & Kettunen, 2006)

In 2010, new methoxy-substituted nickel(II)(salophene) derivatives are synthesized and their anticancer properties were investigated (Lee et al, 2010). It was demonstrated that the most active complex [Ni(II)(3-methoxy-salophene)] (Fig 10) is not necrotic in Burkitt-like lymphoma cells (BJAB) and human B-cell precursor cells (Nalm-6). [Ni(II)(3-methoxy-salophene)] inhibited proliferation and induced apoptosis in a concentration dependent manner, giving evidence for the involvement of CD95 receptor-mediated, extrinsic pathway. Furthermore, [Ni(II)(3-methoxy-salophene)] overcame vincristine drug resistance in BJAB and Nalm-6 cells.

Organometallic compounds like Iron (III)-salophene with selective cytotoxic and antiproliferative properties have also been used in platinum resistant ovarian cancer cells (Rafique et al, 2010).

The low-spin Fe(II) complex sodium nitroprusside (Fig 13) is a clinically used metal-nitrosyl complex (Guo & Sadler, 1999). It is often used to lower blood pressure in humans. Its hypotensive effect is evident within seconds after infusion, and the desired blood pressure is usually obtained within one to two minutes. It is also useful in cases of emergency hypertension, heart attacks, and surgery. Its therapeutic effects depend on release of nitric oxide, which relaxes vascular smooth muscle. Activation in vivo may involve reduction to $[Fe(CN)_5(NO)]^{3-}$, which then releases cyanide to give $[Fe(CN)_4(NO)]^{2-}$ and then nitric oxide.

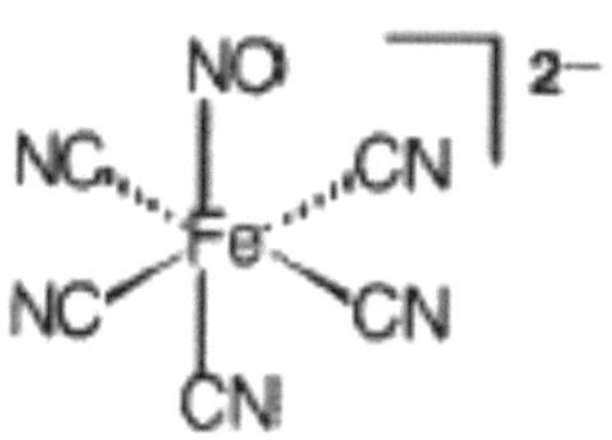

Fig. 13. Fe(II) complex with nitroprusside

The low cytotoxicity of ferrocene, coupled with its lipophilicity ($logP_{octanol/water} = 3.28$) and its electrochemical behaviour (redox potential of the ferrocene/ferrocenium couple, $E^0 = +0.400$ V versus SCE (Saturated Calomel Electrode), suggested that this compound could yield interesting results if incorporated into a known drug (Blackie & Chibale, 2008). The ferrocenyl moiety has several characteristics which make it a good addition to known drug molecules. Its lipophilicity, electron density, relative thermal and chemical stability, and interesting redox behaviour are all favourable in this respect. There are several reported successes of increased efficacy of ferrocenyl analogues of known drugs. Brocard and co-workers, combined Chloroquine and ferrocene in the same molecule by inserting a ferrocenyl group into the side chain of Chloroquine, producing a hybrid compound called Ferroquine (Fig 11), which is more potent than Chloroquine. They have shown that incorporation of a ferrocenyl moiety as an integral part of the side chain of chloroquine between the two nitrogens had superior efficacy to other analogues in which the moiety was terminal on the side chain or bonded to the quinoline nitrogen. Some analogues of the compound were produced bearing different alkyl groups on the terminal tertiary nitrogen. They established that the dimethylamino terminal group was superior in efficacy (Fig 14)

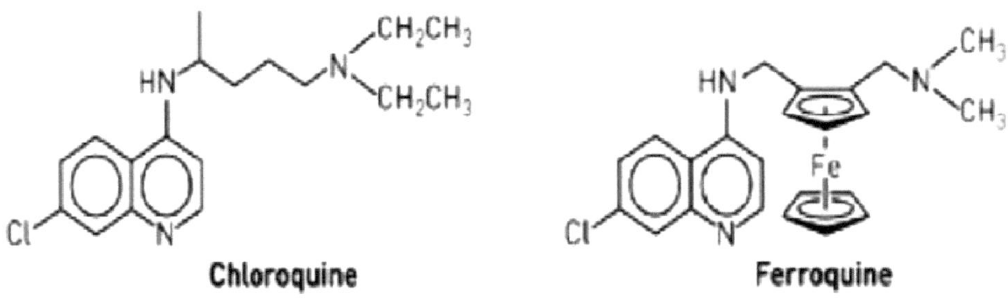

Fig. 14. Molecular structure of Chloroquine and Ferroquine.

The highly established chemistry of ferrocenes that allows an easy and rapid access to a bank of reagents and derivatives has given them a considerable role in the field of analytical chemistry (Rudrangi et al, 2010). Ferrocene-based derivatization of various functional groups and detection techniques is of high interest in particular. The chemistry of ferrocenes is well explored and a wide range of ferrocene derivatives are easily obtained through the established synthetic routes.The ferrocenes allow the use of a large variety of detection techniques like UV/Visible absorption spectroscopy, atomic spectroscopy, atomic absorption spectroscopy (AAS), inductively coupled plasma (ICP) excitation with optical emission spectroscopy (OES) or mass spectrometry (MS), electron impact or electrospray ionization (ESI) MS, and the electrochemical detection (ECD) techniques that include voltammetry or amperometry.

The role of the length of the methylene spacer between the two nitrogens in chloroquine analogues has been shown to have an influence on efficacy in chloroquine resistant strains of *P. falciparum*. Aminoquinolines with short (2-3 carbons) and long (10–12 carbons) methylene side chains are equipotent against chloroquine-sensitive, chloroquineresistant, and multidrug-resistant strains of *P. falciparum*. Whilst aminoquinolines with side chains of intermediate length (4–8 carbons) showed efficacy against chloroquinesensitive strains of *P. falciparum*, they showed a significant decrease in efficacy against chloroquine-resistant strains of *P.Falciparum*. In the chloroquine-sensitive D10 strain, the longer the methylene spacer, the lower the efficacy. It may be that the changes in lipophilicity and *pKa* values and other physicochemical effects of the incorporation of the ferrocenyl moiety into chloroquine are the primary factor in the enhanced efficacy of ferroquine.

As published as a patent application in 2006 (Maurel & Cudennec, 2009), some manganese based organometallic complexes having Mn-SOD like activities, pharmaceutical compositions and dietetic products for use in oxidative stress, including cancer and inflammatory conditions, were also designed. Many human diseases are associated with the overproduction of oxygen free radicals that inflict cell damage (Rafique et al, 2010). Primary reactive oxygen species (ROS) such as superoxide radical, hydrogen peroxide, hydroxyl radicals, and ortho-quinone derivatives of catecholamines exert their cellular effects by modifying DNA, lipids, and proteins to form secondary electrophiles (Zhang & Lippard, 2003). Damage caused by the primary and secondary ROS contributes to the pathogenesis of important human diseases. In particular, one consequence of oxidative metabolism is the generation of superoxide radicals (O_2^-.) which mediate extensive damage to the cellular components of living organisms. The molecular dismutation of O_2^-. to hydrogen peroxide (H_2O_2) and oxygen (O_2) is catalysed by superoxide dismutases (SODs).These enzymes are suggested to form the first line of the cell's defence against oxygen damage. Indeed, mice defective for SOD do not survive and reduction of functional capabilities of this enzyme generates an high increase of oxidative stress in connection with strong mitochondrial disabilities of cells. Fe-containing SODs (FeSOD) are largely confined to prokaryotes and the Cu/Zn enzymes (Cu/ZnSOD) predominantly to eukaryotes. Mn-containing SODs (MnSOD) are universally present. In eukaryotes MnSODs are localised in the mitochondria, while the Cu/ZnSODs reside in the cytosol. SODs from various sources are currently of great interest as potential therapeutic treatments for oxidative damage. SOD has function against certain inflammatory processes (In particular, deficiency in Mn-SOD is supposed to have some significance in the development of rheumatoid arthritis). SOD has also function against inflammatory processes in alcohol-induced liver damage. Additional potential therapeutic effects for SOD include: (i) prevention of oncogenesis, tumour promotion and invasiveness, and UV-induced damage; (ii) protection of cardiac tissue against post-ischemia reperfusion damage; (iii) antiinflamatory effect; (iv) reducing the cytotoxic and cardiotoxic effects of anticancer drugs; (v) endothelial disorders; (vi) degenerative diseases; (vii) coagulation disorders, and; (viii) improving the longevity of living cells. Currently bovine Cu/ZnSOD is being utilised for the treatment of inflamed tendons in horses and for treating osteoarthritis in man. It has been shown that the mitochondrial antioxidant enzyme manganese-containing superoxide dismutase (MnSOD) functions as a tumor suppressor gene and that reconstitution of MnSOD expression in several human cancer cell lines leads to reversion of malignancy.

The use of SOD in therapy is limited by its short plasma half-life (clearance by the kidney) and inability to penetrate cell membranes (i.e., extracellular activity only) (Guo & Sadler, 1999). Low molecular mass mimics of SOD are therefore of much potential pharmaceutical interest. For example, a variety of Mn- and Fe-based porphyrins and macrocyclic complexes exhibit SOD mimic activity.

Among metal complexes (Cu, Fe, Mn) capable of catalyzing dismutation of the superoxide anion, those of manganese are a current focus for developing SOD mimics as drugs because of the low in vivo toxicity of this metal ion (Zhang & Lippard, 2003). Mn(II) and Mn(III) macrocycles appear to be particularly promising (Guo & Sadler, 1999). For example, a manganese (II) complex with bis (cyclohexylpyridine)-substituted macrocyclic ligand has been designed as a functional mimic of SOD which was reported to have a significant of inflammation and reperfusion injury (Aston et al., 2001, Rafique et al, 2010). This complex has remarkably high kinetic and thermodynamic stability with regard to dissociation, is oxidatively stable as well and is excreted intact with no dissociation in vivo This stability profile shows that this is a catalytically active SOD mimic. Manganese complexes have also been used to treat cell and tissue oxidative injuries by acting as superoxide anion scavenger. Nitrogen containing macrocyclic complexes of Manganese (II) have shown anti microbial activity. An octahedral geometry for these complexes has been confirmed by spectroscopic analysis. Many manganese complexes have been screened against a number of pathogenic fungi and bacteria to evaluate their growth and potential. Another example to the therapeutic effects of manganese complexes is Mn(III)5,10,15,20-tetrakis(4-benzoic acid)-porphyrin, which can protect against neurodegeneration and is therefore of potential interest for the treatment of brain diseases such as Parkinson and Alzheimer diseases (Meng et al, 2009). Results from systematic modification of the porphyrin ligand demonstrate that placement of four positively charged ortho-(N-alkyl) pyridyl groups (alkyl: methyl and ethyl) in the meso positions of porphyrin can strongly facilitate the disproportion of O_2^-., owing to favorable electrostatic contributions. SC-52608 (Fig 15) is another complex, able to scavenge superoxide and therefore effectively protect the regionally ischemic and reperfused myocardium from injury. Both complexes reduced oxidative stress injury in vivo and they have high stability and catalytic efficacy (Guo & Sadler, 1999; Zhang & Lippard, 2003). In the search for a lipophilic manganese SOD mimic, a dinuclear manganese(III) complex of biliverdin IX dimethyl ester was discovered to have such activity. In this example O_{2-} . dismutation is effected by a Mn(III)/Mn(IV) redox couple. In addition, the manganese complex does not bind to NO and reacts very slowly with H_2O_2, demonstrating specificity towards O_{2-}..

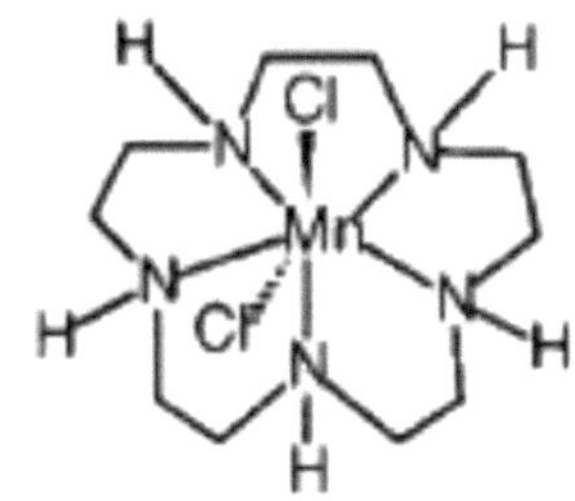

Fig. 15. Molecular structure of SC-52608 (Guo & Sadler, 1999)

The incorporation of manganese into the structure of antioxidants like pyran, pyridine, benzopyran and quinoline i.e., kojic acid, 6-hydroxynicotinic acid, 7-hydroxyflavone, 8-hydroxyquinoline and 8-hydroxyquinoline ethylenediamine, made the complexes possessed the SOD activity and increased radical scavenging activity of antioxidants as expected (Vajgupta et al, 2003). Manganese atom is therefore the essential part for SOD action. 7-hydroxyflavone complex was promising, since it exhibited potent radical scavenging ability and suppressed the MAP-induced hypermotility without reducing the locomotor activity in normal condition, and also improved the impaired learning and memory in transient ischemic mice.

A new approach involves modelling the pharmacological properties of established drugs with organometallic fragments (Ott et al, 2009). The metallocyclic peptide, bacitracin, has an interesting SOD activity. The Mn(II)–bacitracin complex (Piacham et al, 2006) (Fig 16, 17) is potentially useful as an effective agent against oxidative stress (for O_2^-. scavenging). On the other hand, probably this Mn(II)–bacitracin may be involved in the respiratory burst mechanism of white blood cells that could enhance bacterial killing by synergistic process to convert superoxide radical into hydrogen peroxide which is used by enzyme myeloperoxidase to convert normally unreactive halide ions into reactive hypohalous acids that are toxic to bacteria. Also its antibiotic mechanism could be useful for bacterial and oxidative stress treatments.

Bacitracin provides strong affinity to divalent metal ions such as Zn(II), Cu(II), Co(II), and Mn(II) in the formation of 1:1 complex. Structural characterization of metallobacitracin showed that it is composed of a cyclic heptapeptide and a short N-terminal sequence containing a thiazoline ring (Fig 17). The divalent metals interact with the cyclic and the linear peptides to form a strong bending structure that encapsulates the metal inside the coordination sphere. It is interesting to note that the established order of binding affinity of the transition metal ions was found to be inversely correlated with the observed SOD activity reported in this work. The order of metal binding affinity and SOD activity is Cu(II) > Ni(II) > Co(II) ≈Zn(II) >Mn(II) (Brabec & Novakova, 2006) and Mn(II) > Cu(II) > Co(II) > Ni(II), respectively. However, it should be noted that the negative correlation is valid for Mn(II), Co(II), and Ni(II) but not Cu(II).

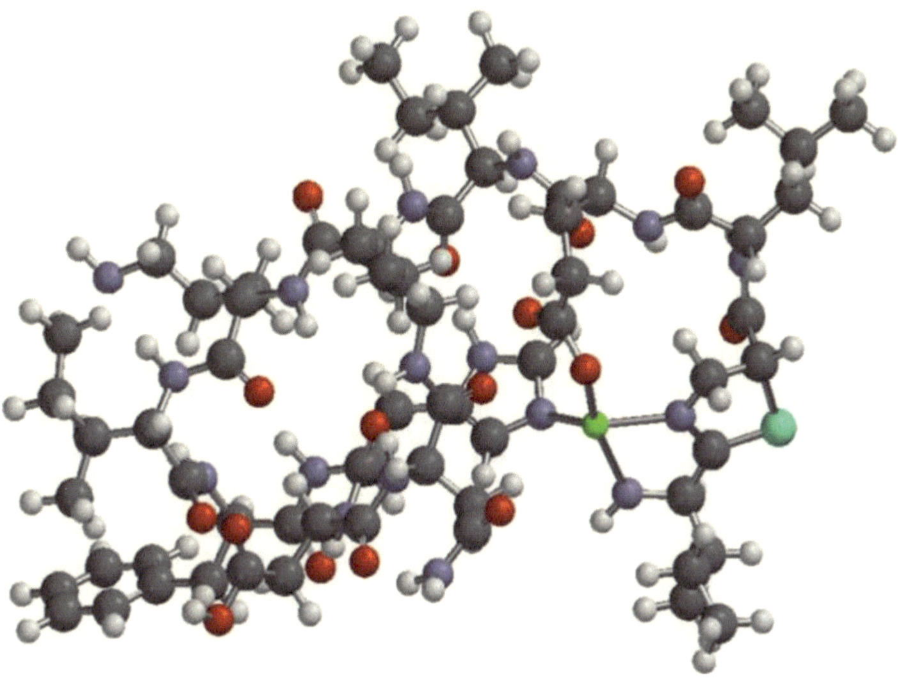

Fig. 16. Molecular modeling of Mn(II)-bacitracin complex (Piacham et al, 2006)

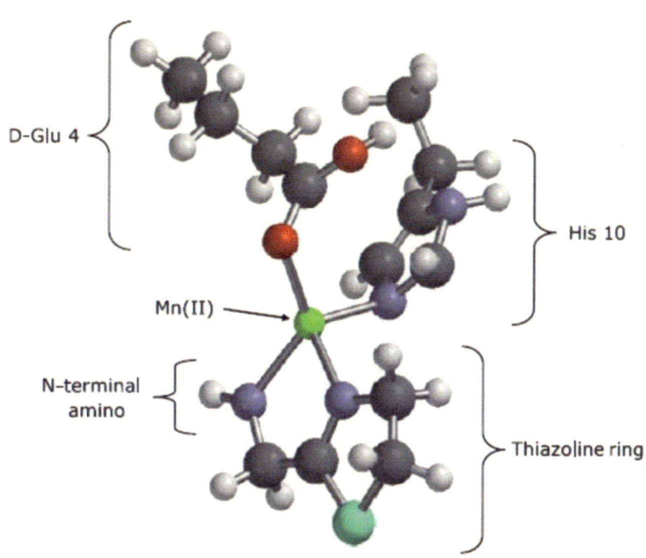

Fig. 17. Mn(II) ligand models derived from metallobacitracin complexes (Piacham et al, 2006)

It is possible that the observed trend, in which Cu(II)-bacitracin did not follow the order of increasing SOD activity with decreasing metal binding affinity, is because Cu(II) takes on a different coordination chemistry from the other divalent metal ions in which Cu(II) forms a tetragonally distorted geometry with two coordinated nitrogens and two coordinated oxygens, particularly, His-10 imidazole nitrogen, thiazoline nitrogen, Glu-4 carboxylate oxygen, and Asp-11 carboxylate oxygen. Proton NMR studies established that Co(II) is coordinated to three nitrogens and one oxygen, namely, His-10 imidazole nitrogen, thiazoline nitrogen, Ile-1 amino nitrogen, and Glu-4 carboxylate oxygen. For the construction of the molecular models of metallobacitracin, it was assumed that Mn(II) and Ni(II) adopt a similar coordination chemistry to that of Co(II) because they all have a vacant d shell.

Cobalt–aspirin complexes are investigated as potential cytostatics (Ott et al, 2009). Aspirin (acetylsalicylic acid) belongs to the family of nonsteroidal antirheumatics (NSAR), which have anti-inflammatory and pain-relieving effects The pharmacological effects of NSARs stem from the inhibition of enzymes in the cyclooxygenase family (COX). Besides the role of NSARs in inflammatory processes, they also seem to be involved in tumor growth. NSARs have thus come into focus as potential cytostatics. It may be possible to improve anti-tumor activity in the case of aspirin by binding it to an organometallic fragment. A hexacarbonyldicobalt–aspirin complex (Fig 18), is shown to inhibit COX activity differently from aspirin. Whereas the effect of aspirin stems from the acetylation of a serine residue in the active center of COX, Co-Aspirin complex does not attack this side chain, but acetylates several other sites instead. This may block access to the active center of the enzyme, resulting in a different activity spectrum for the drug. Experiments with zebra fish embryos showed that in contrast to aspirin, Co-Aspirin inhibits both cell growth and the formation of small blood vessels (angiogenesis). Tumors are dependent on newly formed blood vessels for their nutrients and can be starved out by the inhibition of angiogenesis. In addition, Co-Aspirin modulates other tumor-relevant metabolic pathways. For example, it activates the enzyme caspase, which is involved in processes that lead to apoptosis (programmed cell death).

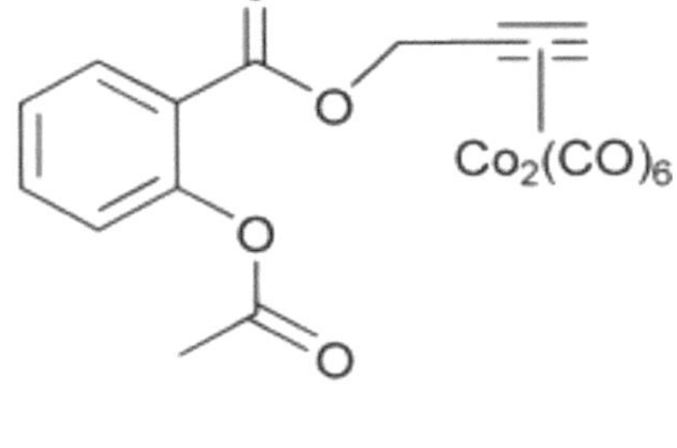

Fig. 18. The structure of hexacarbonyldicobalt–aspirin complex (Ott et al, 2009)

Sadler and coworkers (Meggers, 2007) investigated the binding of metal complexes of 1,4,8,11-tetraazacyclotetradecane (cyclam) macrocycles to the CXCR4 coreceptor and lysozyme as a model protein. In such metallocyclam complexes, the metal is supposed to function by controlling the conformation and configuration of the macrocycle. Additional direct coordinative bonds with the target protein can be formed with the vacant axial coordination sites. One of the most potent members of this family is the xylyl-bicyclam AMD3100 (Fig 19), a CXCR4 receptor inhibitor, which is in clinical trials for the treatment of AIDS. The anti-HIV activity correlates with its binding to the coreceptor protein CXCR4. CXCR4 is a chemokine receptor that transduces signals of its endogenous ligand, CXCL12/stromal cell-derived factor-1 (SDF-1) (Tamamura et al, 2006). CXCR4 is classified into 7TMGPCR and plays a physiologically critical role by the action of CXCL12 in the migration of progenitors during embryologic development of the cardiovascular, hemopoietic, central nervous systems, etc. In addition, CXCR4 was previously identified as a coreceptor that is used by X4-HIV-1 in its entry into T cells and has recently been proven to be involved in several problematic diseases, including HIV infection, metastasis of several types of cancer, leukemia cell progression, rheumatoid arthritis. Thus, CXCR4 is thought to be a great therapeutic target to overcome these diseases, and several inhibitors directed against CXCR4 have been developed to date. Research performed on AMD3100 analogs have revealed that if it is complexed with certain metals it will increase the bonding affinity to CXCR4 by causing the cyclam rings to take on a folded cis configuration (Snell, 2005). When Zn(II)-xylyl-bicyclam binds with acetate, it undergoes a configuration change and becomes *cis* folded. The cyclam ring can function as a tetradentate coordination ring for transition metals, and it has been shown that chelation of such metal ions by the macrocyclic rings of AMD3100 alters its binding affinity to the CXCR4 receptor (Gerlach et al, 2003). Thus, the Zn^{2+} complex of AMD3100 binds with a 10-fold higher affinity to the receptor as compared to AMD3100 alone and has an up to 6-fold increased potency as an anti-HIV agent. Zn^{2+} is located in the center of the cyclam ring, coordinating the four nitrogens in a planar fashion. Since Zn^{2+} does not coordinate in a square planar conformation, it either obtains a square pyramidal or an octahedral geometry with one or two vacant coordination sites. Zn^{2+} has the option to make strong interactions with both histidine and cysteine residues, as well as acidic residues such as aspartates. The CXCR4 receptor does not contain any free extracellular cysteines; however, the main interaction points for AMD3100 are two aspartates, and furthermore, several histidine residues are located in TM-III, TM-V, and TM-VII (TM: transmembrane domain) pointing toward the main ligand binding crevice (Figure 20). Thus, metal ion coordination could either improve the binding mode of AMD3100 to one or more of the two aspartates, Asp171 and Asp262, or it could pick up interaction with one or more of the His residues that potentially could serve as partners in the coordination of Zn^{2+} bound by the bicyclam.

The level of anti-HIV activity expressed by these metal complexes were Zn>Ni>Cu>Co>Pd in decreasing order. The affinity of AMD3100, a symmetrical nonpeptide antagonist composed of two 1,4,8,11-tetraazacyclotetradecane (cyclam) rings connected through a 1,4-dimethylene(phenylene) linker to the CXCR4 chemokine receptor was increased 7, 36, and 50-fold, respectively, by incorporation of Cu^{2+}, Zn^{2+}, or Ni^{2+} into the cyclam rings of the compound. The rank order of the transition metal ions correlated with the calculated binding energy between free acetate and the metal ions coordinated in a cyclam ring. Construction of AMD3100 substituted with only a single Cu^{2+} or Ni^{2+} ion demonstrated that the increase in binding affinity of the metal ion substituted bicyclam is achieved through an enhanced interaction of just one of the ring systems.

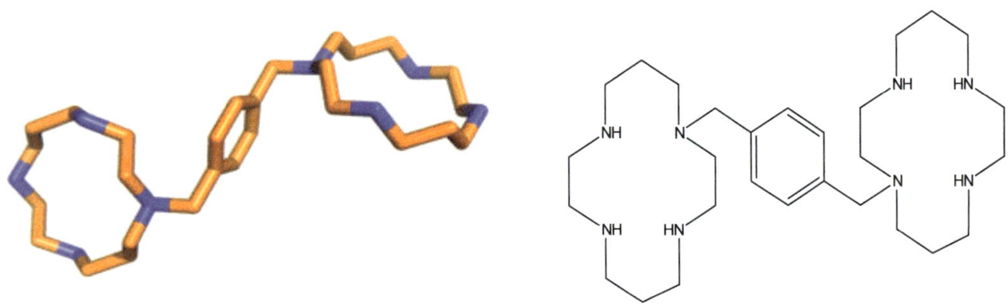

a b

Fig. 19. The 3D (a) and 2D (b) structure of AMD3100 (New Indications for AMD-3100, In: Drug Discovery Opinion, 2008; (Snell, 2005)]

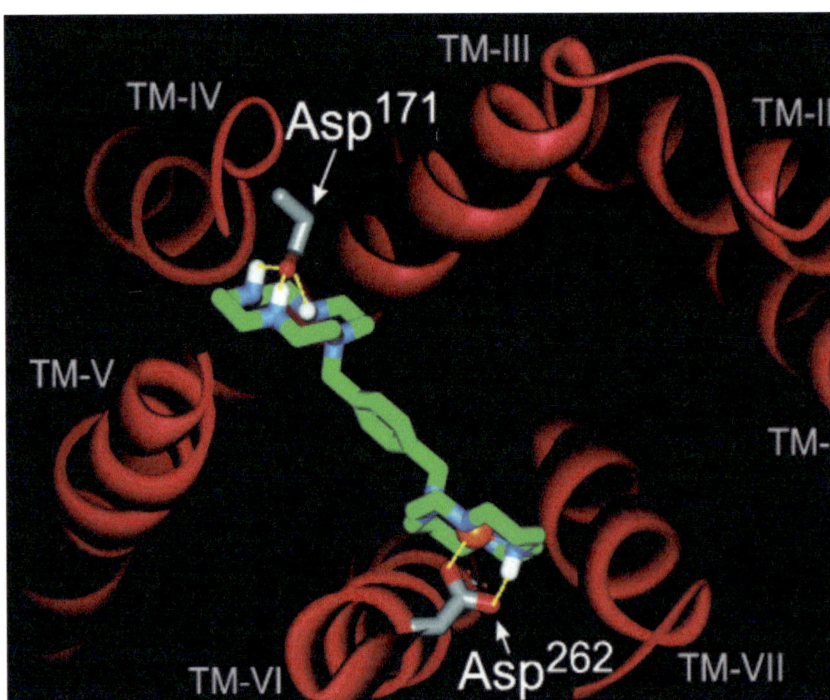

Fig. 20. Molecular model of the main ligand-binding pocket of the CXCR4 receptor with AMD3100(Zn) manually docked into favorable interactions with Asp171 in TM-IV and Asp262 in TM-VI. The receptor model is built over the rhodopsin model of Palcewski et al (Palczewski et al, 2000). The conformation of AMD3100 is based on structural requirements of high antiviral effects of AMD3100 and the crystallographic X-ray structure of 6,6′-spirobis- (1,4,8,11-tetraazacyclotetradecane)-dinickel(II)tetraperchlorate, obtained from the Cambridge Structural Database (Gerlach et al, 2003).

Several low molecular weight nonpeptide compounds having the dipicolylamine-zinc(II) complex structure were also identified as potent and selective antagonists of the chemokine receptor CXCR4 (Tamamura et al, 2006). These compounds showed strong inhibitory activity against CXCL12 binding to CXCR4, and one of them (which has two sets of the [bis(pyridin-2-ylmethyl) amino]methylene unit with zinc(II) complexation at the para-position of benzene) exhibited significant anti-HIV activity.

The use of organometallic complexes are also investigated in the treatment of leishmania. The drugs for treating cutaneous lesions, or, in the case of visceral leishmaniasis (kala-azar), caused by the species L. donovani or L. infantum have traditionally been pentavalent antimonials, aromatic diamidines and fungicides such as amphotericine B (Mesa-Valle et al, 1996). However, these are extremely toxic and cause a great number of side effects. Many recent efforts have been made to synthesize and evaluate alternative compounds for treating these parasites. In the last few years, certain metal complexes have proven anti-tumoral against such protozoan parasites as Trypanosoma cruzi, T. rhodesiense and L. donovani. One property that the tumor cells share with the trypanosomatids is rapid multiplication. Three organometallic complexes which have previously shown in vitro activity against the promastigote forms of L. donovani and have also shown a similar activity against the amastigote like forms, are Cis-Pt(DDH)(Ac.19 2,5-Dihydroxi-benzensulphonic)$_2$ and those of Rh(I): $Rh(CO)_2Cl$(5Cl-2-Methylbenzothiazole), $Rh(CO)_2Cl$(2-Aminobenzothiazole) were investigated by Mesa-Valle et al. (Mesa-Valle et al, 1996). In vitro toxicity of the complexes for the cells of the strain J-774 and the effect exerted on the parasite's biosynthesis of macromolecules were investigated. Only the $Rh(I)(CO)_2Cl$(2-Aminobenzothiazole) complex induced substantial toxicity in the cells. The $Rh(I)(CO)_2Cl$(5-Cl-2-Methylbenzothiazole) complex inhibited DNA, RNA, and protein synthesis. The best candidate, given its slight toxicity for mammal cells and its high activity against Leishmania by inhibiting the synthesis of macromolecules, is found as the complex Rh(I):$Rh(CO)_2Cl$(5-Cl-2-Methylbenzothiazole). Croft et al. investigated the effect of 27 Platinum, Rhodium and Iridium drug complexes against Leishmania donovani amastigotes in mouse peritoneal macrophages in vitro (Croft et al, 1992). Rh(III)-mepacrine, Ir(III) pyrrolidine dithiocarbamate and Ir(III) diethyl dithiocarbamate which showed antileishmanial activity had ED_{50} values of less than 1 μM. The two Iridium complexes produced, respectively, a 50% and 39% suppression of L. donovani amastigotes in the liver of BALB/c mice following the subcutaneous administration of 200 mg/kg for 5 consecutive days. Ultrastructural studies suggest that the amastigote kinetoplast-mitochondrion complex is the primary site of action of the Ir and Rh complexes. Ir-(cycloocta-1,5-diene)-pentamidine tetraphenylborate which has previously been studied on promastigote forms of Leishmania, was investigated for its antileishmanial properties on Leishmania donovani and Leishmania major mouse models, compared with pentamidine used as reference compound in the year 2000 (Loiseau, et al, 2000). In vitro, the iridium complex had the same IC_{50} value on intracellular forms of Leishmania as pentamidine (15 μM). In vivo, the compound could not be injected intravenously due to the DMSO excipient so that the treatments were performed intraperitoneally or subcutaneously. On the L. donovani LV9/Balb/C mouse model, the iridium complex was not toxic after intraperitoneal treatment at 232 mg/kg/day x 5 or

147 μmoles/kg/day x 5, whereas all the mice died within five days when treated at the same dose with pentamidine isethionate. However, only 23% of parasite suppression was observed with the iridium complex. On a L. major MON 74/Balb/C mouse model, susceptible to intravenously administered pentamidine at 6.7 μmoles/kg/day x 5 (54% of parasite suppression), the iridium complex exhibited 32% of parasite suppression after a treatment at 76 μmoles/kg/day x 5 administered subcutaneously. Transmission electron microscopy of amastigotes from infected and treated mice show aggregation of ribosomal material, distension of the nuclear membrane and kDNA depolymerization. The mechanism of action therefore involves several targets: membranes, ribosomes and kDNA. The researchers recommend the Iridium complex as a suitable candidate to be encapsulated in drug carriers such as liposomes or nanoparticles.

Organometallic complexes of Pt, Rh, Ir, Pd, Os, have been synthesized and their trypanocidal activity was studied in vitro and in vivo by Loiseau (Loiseau et al, 1992). Among these, the Ir-(cycloocta-1,5-diene)-pentamidine complex, showed in vitro activity at 60 μg/L on Tripanosoma brucei brucei. Moreover, all infected mice were cured by this compound subcutaneously administered in a single dose at 0.5 mg/kg (0.317 μmol/kg). In the same conditions, pentamidine cured all the mice at 5 μmol/kg. Ir-(cycloocta-1,5-diene)-pentamidine (or P1995) was 16 fold more efficient than pentamidine. Since the chemotherapeutic index of this molecule was 7.5 fold higher than those of pentamidine, the authors recommend P1995 to be considered as a potential trypanocidal drug of the future.

Scientists are looking for alternative approaches for the treatment of diabetes. Several trace elements, such as vanadium and zinc, exert insulin-mimetic effects in in vitro and in vivo systems (Hiromura & Sakurai, 2008). The complexes of these metals and small organic compounds (ligands) improved glucose utilization in both diabetic model animals and human diabetic patients . Both vanadyl and zinc complexes enhanced glucose uptake into the adipocytes without the addition of any hormones. Under the same experimental conditions, these complexes inhibited epinephrine-induced free fatty acid (FFA) release. Because of this insulin-mimetic activity, oxovanadium(IV) (vanadyl) and zinc(II) (zinc) complexes are proposed to be potent antidiabetic agents for both type 1 and type 2 Diabetes Mellitus therapy. New types of insulin-mimetic vanadyl and zinc complexes such as Bis(allixinato)oxovanadium(IV), [VO(alx)2], bis(allixinato)zinc(II) [$Zn(alx)_2$], bis(thioallixin-*N*-methyl)zinc(II) [$Zn(tanm)_2$] (Fig 21), were developed as the potent activators of the insulin signaling pathway. Although these complexes activate Akt/PKB, their critical action sites are slightly different from each other. Different action sites of the metal complexes may depend on the chemical characteristic of the vanadyl and zinc metal ions. The characteristic of ligand is important for the passing through the plasma membrane. $VO(alx)_2$, $Zn(alx)_2$, and $Zn(tanm)_2$ also play unique roles in cells; $VO(alx)_2$ regulates the activation of the FoxO1, while $Zn(alx)_2$ and $Zn(tanm)_2$ regulate the activation of HSL (hormone-sensitive lipase), resulting in the suppression of free fatty acid release. The common mechanism of action of $VO(alx)_2$, $Zn(alx)_2$, and $Zn(tanm)_2$ is their effect on the insulin signaling pathway; this in turn regulates gene transcription and suppresses lipolysis signaling.

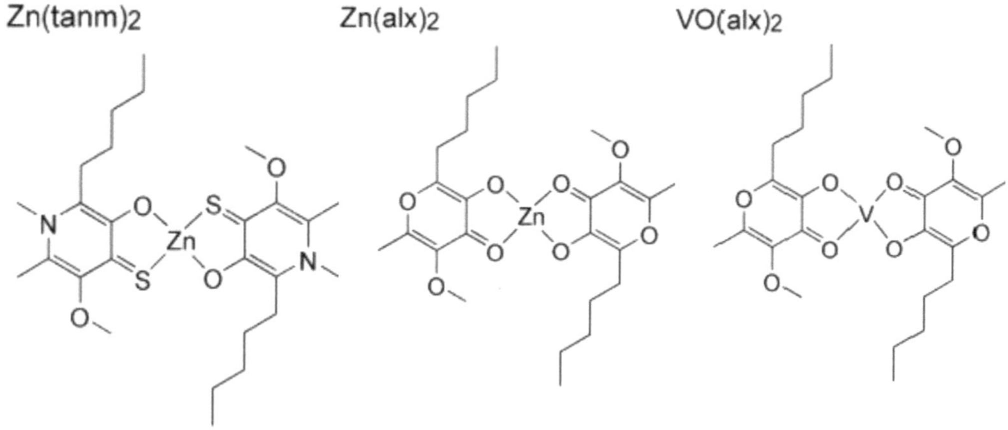

Fig. 21. The molecular structures of $VO(alx)_2$, $Zn(alx)_2$, and $Zn(tanm)_2$ (Hiromura & Sakurai, 2008)

Another application of organometallic complexes is antiinflammatory therapy. Numerous Cu(II) complexes of NSAIDs with enhanced anti-inflammatory activity and reduced gastrointestinal (GI) toxicity compared with their uncomplexed parent drug, were developed (Hiromura & Sakurai, 2008). No Cu(II) anti-inflammatory drug is currently available for oral human use, although an ethanolic gel-base of Cu-salicylate (Alcusal®) is available for topical temporal relief of pain and inflammation in humans (Weder et al, 2002). A Cu(II) dimer of indomethacin (IndoH_/1- (4-chlorobenzoyl)-5-methoxy-2-methyl-1H-Indole-3-acetic acid) with low toxicity is commercially available in Australasia, South East Asia and South Africa in a variety of oral pharmaceutical dosage forms for veterinary use. These low toxicity Cu drugs are of enormous interest, because many of today's anti-inflammatory drug therapies, including the NSAIDs, remain either largely inadequate and/or are associated with problematic side effects, e.g. renal insufficiency and failure, GI ulceration, bleeding or perforation ('NSAID gastropathy'), exacerbation of hypertension and congestive heart failure (CHF). Sorenson reported that Cu(II)-complexes of these antiinflammatory drugs were more active in animal models than either their parent inorganic Cu(II) salt or the parent NSAID . The pharmacological activity was proposed to be due to the inherent physico-chemical properties of the complex itself rather than just that of its constituents, since the amount of Cu(II) in such complexes does not correlate with anti-inflammatory activity. Sorenson reported that a salicylate complex of Cu(II) was ≈30 times more effective than aspirin as an anti-inflammatory agent. In two previous reviews, Sorenson reported over 140 Cu(II) complexes with anti-inflammatory activity. However, limited information is available on the nature of the Cu complexes of NSAIDs in biological matrices and in pharmaceutical formulations. SOD activity, redox behavior, lipophilicity and stability constants may be useful parameters in evaluating the biological activity of these Cu compounds.

The proposed curative properties of Cu-based nonsteroidal anti-inflammatory drugs (NSAIDs) have led to the development of numerous Cu(II) complexes of NSAIDs with enhanced anti-inflammatory activity (Trinchero et al, 2004) Crystalline complexes, Cu(II)–

NSAID (ibuprofen, naproxen, tolmetin, and diclofenac), with a carboxylic function have been studied by means of infrared and Raman spectroscopy. All NSAIDs bind to the metal through the carboxylate group. The spectroscopic data support the formation of dimeric $[Cu_2L_4(H_2O)_2]$ complexes in which the COO^- group behaves as a bridging bidentate ligand. The preparation and properties of the Cu(II) complex $Cu(SAS)_2.H_2O$ are reported for the antiinflammatory drug Salsalate (SAS) (Underhill et al, 1989). The complex is reported to exhibit an increased superoxide dismutase activity compared with the parent drug molecule in the nitroblue tetrazolium assay. Weder and friends synthesized Cu(II) indomethacin complexes (Weder et al, 1999).

Drugs belonging to the non-steroidal anti-inflammatory drug group (NSAID) are not only used as anti-inflammatory and analgesic agents, but also exhibit chemopreventive and chemosuppressive effects on various cancer cell lines (Roy et al, 2006). They exert their anticancer effects by inhibiting both at the protein level and/or at the transcription level. Cu(II) complexes of these NSAIDs show better anti-cancer effects than the bare drugs. UV-Visible spectroscopy was used to characterize the complexation between Cu(II) and two NSAIDs belonging to the oxicam group, piroxicam and meloxicam, both of which exhibit anticancer properties. For the first time, this study shows that, Cu(II)-NSAID complexes can directly bind with the DNA backbone, and the binding constants and the stoichiometry or the binding site sizes have been determined. Thermodynamic parameters from van't Hoff plots showed that the interaction of these Cu(II)-NSAID complexes with ctDNA is an entropically driven phenomenon. Circular dichroism spectroscopy showed that the binding of these Cu(II)-NSAIDs with ctDNA result in DNA backbone distortions which is similar for both Cu(II)-piroxicam and Cu(II)-meloxicam complexes. Competitive binding with a standard intercalator like ethidium bromide (EtBr) investigated by circular dichroism spectroscopy as well as fluorescence measurements indicate that the Cu(II)-NSAID complexes could intercalate in the DNA.

Inspired from Sorenson's studies, new investigations on formation and synthesis of Cu(II) complexes with antiinflammatory drugs were carried out as well as Zn(II) complexes, where some of them are ternary complexes (Anılanmert et al, 2010). The formation conditions and constants of Cu(II)-tryptophan-aspirin and Zn(II)-tryptophan-aspirin ternary complexes in aqueous solutions were determined using potentiometric method to provide chemical data for the synthesis, considering the synergistic capability of aspirin, the antiinflammatory activity of Cu(II), the synergistic effect of tryptophan-aspirin combination in migraine and in diseases which cause immune activation, the stronger analgesic, antiinflammatory and antithrombotic effect of Cu(II)-aspirinate and Zn(II)-aspirinate than aspirin, decreased gastrointestinal toxicity of Cu(II)-aspirinate and Zn(II)-aspirinate than aspirin, the stronger analgesic and antiinflammatory effects of some Cu(II)-amino acid complexes than Cu(II)-aspirinate and the increased bioavailability of Zn(II)-amino acid complexes. The effects of leucine in cancer, wound healing and regulation of glucose in blood, anticancer activity and healing activity of Cu(II) on radiation effects, antiinflammatory effects of Cu(II)-aspirin and Cu(II)-amino acid compounds, sinergistic activity of aspirin and its anticancer effect which was proved in recent years are known (Anılanmert, 2006). Under the light of these effects, the formation of Cu(II)-leucine-aspirin was also investigated using potentiometric and spectrophotometric method. The anticancer action and wound healing effect on skin cancers topically and through injection into tumours should be investigated in the future. These ternary complexes have only been investigated using potentiometry, UV and IR spectrometry, synthesis studies are going on, yet no in vitro and in vivo study is performed, however they are recommended to be investigated for the above therapeutic effects.

3. Conclusion

In this chapter, clinical uses of organometallic complexes and some prominent studies on new therapeutic complexes were mentioned. Developments in explorations of organometallic compounds, in various therapeutic areas continue to be an active and productive area of research. Increasingly powerful tools, notably spectroscopic techniques like time-resolved infrared are used for identifying and structurally characterizing the solid complex, optical spectroscopic and potentiometric methods are used for monitoring intermediates and species in solution. Besides these preclinical and clinical studies are significantly enhancing our knowledge and understanding of the structure and mechanistic aspects of the therapeutic organometallic complexes.

4. References

Abu-Surrah, A.S., Kettunen, M., Leskelä, M., Al-Abed, Y. (2008), Platinum and Palladium Complexes Bearing New (1R,2R)-(-)-1,2-Diaminocyclohexane (DACH)-Based Nitrogen Ligands: Evaluation of the Complexes Against L1210 Leukemia, *Zeitschrift für anorganische und allgemeine Chemie*, Vol.634, No.14, (October 2008), 2655-2658, 1521-3749 DOI: 10.1002/zaac.200800281

Abu-Surrah, A.S., Kettunen, M. (2006), Platinum Group Antitumor Chemistry: Design and development of New Anticancer Drugs Complementary to Cisplatin, *Current Medicinal Chemistry*, Vol.13, 1337-1357, 0929-8673/06.

Allardyce, C. S., Dyson, P.J. (2006) Medicinal Properties of Organometallic Compounds, In: *Bioorganometallic Chemistry (Topics in Organometallic Chemistry)*, Gerard Simonneaux, Volume 17, pp.177-210, Springer-Verlag, 10 3-540-33047-9 , Berlin, Heidelberg DOI:10.1007/3418_001.

Anga, W. H., Casini, A., Sava, G., Dyson, P.J., (2011), Organometallic ruthenium-based antitumor compounds with novel modes of action, *Journal of Organometallic Chemistry*, Vol. 696, No.5, (March 2011), pp. 989-999, 0022-328X.

Anilanmert, B., Pekin, M., Apak, R. (2010), Investigation of the Formation of Copper(II)-Tryptophane-Aspirin Ternary Complexes, *Asian Journal of Chemistry*, Vol.22, No.10, (November-December 2010), 8060-8072, 0970-7077.

Anilanmert, B. (2006), *Determination of the stability constants of the ternary complexes that tryptophan-aspirin, leucine-aspirin ligands and Cu(II) and Zn(II) metals form, using potentiometric method*, doctorate thesis, Marmara University Institute of Health Sciences, 2006, Istanbul.

Antonarakis, E.S., Emadi, A., (2010), Ruthenium-based chemotherapeutics: are they ready for prime time?, *Cancer Chemotherapy and Pharmacology*, Vol.66, No.1, (March 2010), pp.1-9, 1432-0843.

Aston, K. Rath, N., Naik,A., Slomczynska, U., Schall,O. F., Riley, D.P.: Computer-Aided Design (CAD) of Mn(II) Complexes: Superoxide Dismutase Mimetics with Catalytic Activity Exceeding the Native Enzyme, Inorg. Chem. 2001, 40, 1779-1789, 0020-1669

Bharti, S.K., Singh, S.K. (2009) Recent Developments In The Field of Anticancer Metallopharmaceuticals, *International Journal of PharmTech Research*, Vol.1, No.4, (October-December 2009), pp. 1406-1420, 0974-4304.

Blackie, M.A.L., Chibale, K. (2008), Metallocene Antimalarials: The Continuing Quest, *Metal-Based Drugs*, Vol. 2008, Article ID 495123, doi:10.1155/2008/495123, 1687-5486.

Brabec V, Nováková O. DNA binding mode of ruthenium complexes and relationship to tumor cell toxicity. *Drug Resistance Updates*, Vol.9, No.3, (June 2006), pp. 111-22, 1368-7646.

Clarke, M.J., Zhu, F., Frasca, D.R., (1999) Non-Platinum Chemotherapeutic Metallopharmaceuticals, *Chemical Reviews*, Vol. 99, No.9, (July 1999), pp.2511-2533, 1520-6890.

Clarke, M.J. (2003) Ruthenium metallopharmaceuticals, *Coordination Chemistry Reviews*, Vol.236, No.1-2, (January 2010), pp.209-233, 0010-8545.

Croft, S.L., Neal, R.A., Craciunescu, D.G., Certad-Fombona, G. (1992), The activity of platinum, iridium and rhodium drug complexes against Leishmania donovani., *Tropical Medicine and Parasitology*, Vol. 43, No.1, (March 1992), pp.24-28, 0035-9203.

Dabrowiak, J.C. (2009), *Metals in Medicine*, pp.191-214, John Wiley and Sons, Ltd., Ist. Ed., West Sussex, 978-0-470-68196-1.

Dittrich, C., Hochhaus, A., Schaad, S., Salama, C., Jaehde, U., Jakupec, M. A., Hauses, M.,Gneist, M., Keppler, B. K. (2005) Phase I and pharmacokinetic study of the oral tris-(8-quinolinolato) gallium(III) complex (FFC11, KP46) in patients with solid tumors - a study of the CESAR Central European Society for Anticancer Drug Research - EWIV, *Journal of Clinical Oncology, Proceedings of ASCO Annual Meeting.* (June 2005), Vol 23, No. 16S, Part I of II, June 1 Supplement, pp.3205, 0732-183X.

Lentz, F., Drescher, A., Lindauer, A., Henke, M., Hilger, R.A., Hartinger, C.G., Scheulen, M.E., Dittrich, C., Keppler, B.K., Jaehde, U. (2009), Pharmacokinetics of a novel anticancer ruthenium complex (KP1019, FFC14A) in a phase I dose-escalation study, *Anti-Cancer Drugs*, Vol.20, No.2, (February 2009), pp. 97-103, 1473-5741.

Guo, Z., Sadler, P.J. (1999), Metals in Medicine *Angewandte Chemistry International Edition*, Vol.38, No.11, (June 1999), pp. 1512 – 1531, 1521-3773.

Gerlach, L.O., Jakobsen, J.S., Jensen, K.P., Rosenkilde, M.R., Skerlj, R.T., Ryde, U., Bridger, G.J., Schwartz, T.W. (2003), Metal Ion Enhanced Binding of AMD3100 to Asp262 in the CXCR4 Receptor, *Biochemistry*, Vol. 42, No.3, (January 2003),pp. *710-717*, 1520-4995.

Hanif, M. (2010) *From Biomolecules to Organometallic Compounds with Tumor- Inhibiting Properties*, Supervisor: O. Univ.-Prof. Dr. Bernhard K. Kepler, Vienna.

Hannon, M.J., (2007), Metal-based anticancer drugs: From a past anchored in platinum chemistry to a post-genomic future of diverse chemistry and biology, *Pure and Applied Chemistry*, Vol.79, No.12, (January 2007), pp.2243–2261, 1365-3075.

Hiromura, M., Sakurai, H. (2008), Action mechanism of metallo-allixin complexes as antidiabetic agents, *Pure and Applied Chemistry*, Vol.80, No.12, pp. 2727–2733.

Jaouen, G., Top, S., Vessieres, A., (2006), Chap 3, Organometallics targeted to specific biological sites: The development of new therapies, In: *Bioorganometallics: Biomolecules, Labeling, Medicine,* Ed. Jaouen, G., pp 65-95, Wiley-VCH, 9783527607693, Weinheim.

Katsaros, N., Anagnostopoulou, A. (2002) Rhodium and its compounds as potential agents in cancer treatment., *Critical Reviews in Oncology/ Hematology*, Vol.42, No.3, (June 2002), pp. 297-308, 2002, 1040-8428.

Lee, S., Hille, A., Frias, C., Kater, B., Bonitzki, B., Wolf, S., Scheffler, H., Prokop, A., Gust, R. (2010), [NiII(3-OMe-salophene)]: A Potent Agent with Antitumor Activity, *Journal of Medicinal Chemistry*, Vol.53, No.16, (July 2010), pp 6064–6070, 1520-4804.

Liu, Z., Habtemariam, A., Pizarro, A.M., Fletcher, S.A., Kisova, A., Vrana, O., Salassa, L., Bruijnincx, P.C.A., Clarkson, G.J., Brabec, V., Sadler, P.J. (2011), Organometallic Half-Sandwich Iridium Anticancer Complexes, *Journal of Medicinal Chemistry*, Vol.54, No.8, (April 2011), pp.3011- 3026, 1520-4804.

Llorca, C.S.(2005): *New mono- and dinuclear ruthenium complexes containing the 3,5-bis(2-pyridyl)pyrazole ligand, synthesis, characterization and applications*, PhD dissertation, 84-689-2580-2, Girona.

Loiseau, P.M., Mbongo, N., Bories, C., Boulard, Y., Craciunescu, D.G. (2000), In vivo antileishmanial action of Ir-(COD)-pentamidine tetraphenylborate on Leishmania donovani and Leishmania major mouse models, *Parasite*, Vol. 7, No.2, (June 2000), pp.103-108, 1776-1042.

Loiseau, P.M., Craciunescu, D.G., Doadrio-Villarejo, J.C., Certad-Fombona, G., Gayral, P.(1992), Pharmacomodulations on new organometallic complexes of Ir, Pt, Rh, Pd, Os: in vitro and in vivo trypanocidal study against Trypanosoma brucei brucei., *Tropical Medicine and Parasitology*, Vol.43, No.2, (June 1992), pp.110-114, 0003-4983.

Maurel, J.C., Cudennec, C.A., (2009) *Manganese based organometallic complexes, pharmaceutical compositions and dietetic products*, Assignees: MEDESIS PHARMA S.A., IPC8 Class: AA61K3156FI, USPC Class: 514169, Publication date: 10/01/2009, Patent application number: 20090247492.

Meggers, E. (2007), Exploring biologically relevant chemical space with metal complexes, *Current Opinion in Chemical Biology*, Vol.11, No. 3, (June, 2007), pp. 287-292, 1367-5931.

Meng, X., Leyva, M.L., Jenny, M., Gross, I., Benosman, S., Fricker, B., Harlepp, S., He´braud, P., Boos, A., Wlosik, P., Bischoff, P., Sirlin, C., Pfeffer, M., Loeffler, J., Gaiddon, C. (2009) A Ruthenium-Containing Organometallic Compound Reduces Tumor Growth through Induction of the Endoplasmic Reticulum Stress Gene CHOP, *Cancer Research*, Vol.69 , No.13, (July 2009), 5458-5466, 1538-7445.

Mesa-Valle, C.M., Moraleda-Lindez,V., Craciunescu, D., Osuna, A. (1996), Antileishmanial action of organometallic complexes of Pt(II) and Rh(I), *Chemotherapy*, Vol. 91, No.5, (September/October 1996), pp. 625-633, 0009-3157.

New Indications for AMD-3100, In: *Drug Discovery Opinion, DDO Limited, Consultancy for Biotech and Pharma,* 2008, Available from: http://drugdiscoveryopinion.com/2008/08/new-indications-for-amd-3100/

Ogawa, K., Mukai, T., Asano, D., Kawashima, H., Kinuya, S., Shiba, K., Hashimoto, K., Mori, H., Saji, H., (2007), Therapeutic effects of a 186Re-complex-conjugated bisphosphonate for the palliation of metastatic bone pain in an animal model. *Journal of Nuclear Medicine,* Vol. 48, No.1, (January 2007), pp. 122-127, 2159-662X.

Ott, I., Gust R. (2007) Non platinum metal complexes as anti-cancer drugs, *Archive der Pharmazie,* Vol.340, No.3, (March 2007), pp.117-26, 0365-6233

Ott, I., Kircher, B., Bagowski, C.P., Vlecken, D.H.W., Ott, E.B., Will, J., Bensdorf, K., Sheldrick, W.S., Gust, R. (2009) Modulation of the Biological Properties of Aspirin by Formation of a Bioorganometallic Derivative *Angewandte Chemie International Edition*, Vol. 48, No. 6, (January 2009), pp. 1160–1163, 1521-3773

Palczewski, K., Kumasaka, T., Hori, T., Behnke, C. A., Motoshima, H., Fox, B. A., Le, T. I, Teller, D. C., Okada, T., Stenkamp, R. E. , Yamamoto, M., and Miyano, M. (2000) Crystal structure of rhodopsin: A G protein-coupled receptor, *Science*, Vol. 289 , No.5480, (August 2000), pp.739-745, 0036-8075.

Piacham, T., Isarankura-Na-Ayudhya, C., Nantasenamat, C., Yainoy, S., Ye, L., Bülow, L., Prachayasittikul, V. (2006) Metalloantibiotic Mn(II)-bacitracin complex mimicking manganese superoxide dismutase. *Biochemical and Biophysical Research Communications,* Vol.341, No. 4, (March 2006), pp.925-930, 0006-291X.

Rademaker-Lakhai, J.M., van den Bongard, D., Pluim, D., Beijnen, J.M., Schellens, J. H. M. (2004) A Phase I and Pharmacological Study with Imidazolium-trans-DMSO-imidazole-tetrachlororuthenate, a Novel Ruthenium Anticancer Agent, *Clinical Cancer Research,* Vol.10, No.11, (June 2004), pp. 3717-3727, 1557-3265.

Rafique, S., Idrees, M., Nasim, A., Akbar, H., Athar, A. (2010) Transition metal complexes as potential therapeutic Agents *Biotechnology and Molecular Biology Reviews,* Vol. 5, No. 2 (April 2010), pp.38-45, 1538-2273.

Roy S., Banerjee R., Sarkar, M. (2006), Direct binding of Cu(II)-complexes of oxicam NSAIDs with DNA backbone, *Journal of Inorganic Biochemistry,* Vol.100, No.8, (August 2006), pp.1320-1331, 0162-0134.

Rudrangi, S.R.S., Bontha, V.K., Bethi, S., Reddy, V., (2010), Ferrocenes: Legendary Magıc Bullets In Organometallic Chemistry-An Overview, *International Journal of Pharma Research and Development,* Vol.2, No.8, (October 2010), pp.53-61, 0974-9446, Publication Ref No.: IJPRD/2010/PUB/ARTI/VOV-2/ISSUE-8/OCT/008

Sannella, A.R., Casini, A., Gabbiani, C., Messori, L., Bilia, A.R., Vincieri, F.R., Majori, G., Severini, C. (2008), New uses for old drugs. Auranofin, a clinically established antiarthritic metallodrug, exhibits potent antimalarial effects in vitro: mechanistic and pharmacological implications. *FEBS Letters,* Vol.582, No.6, (March 2008), pp.844–847, 0014-5793.

Sekhon, B.S., (2010), Metalloantibiotics and antibiotic mimics - an overview, *Journal of Pharmaceutical Education and Research*, Vol. 1, No. 1, (June 2010), pp.1-20, 0976 - 8238.

Snell, T.L. (2005), Synthesis and Characterization of Cross-Bridged AMD3100 Analogs, *Centaurus*, Vol. 13, pp.27-31, (May 2005), 0008-8994.

Tamamura, H., Ojida, A., Ogawa, T., Tsutsumi, H., Masuno, H., Nakashima, H., Yamamoto, N., Hamachi, I., Fujii, N., (2006), Identification of a New Class of Low Molecular Weight Antagonists against the Chemokine Receptor CXCR4 Having the Dipicolylamine-Zinc(II) Complex Structure, *Journal of Medicinal Chemistry*, Vol.49, No.11, (June 2006), pp. 3412-3415, 1520-4804.

Timerbaev, A.R., (2009), Advances in developing tris(8-quinolinolato)gallium(III) as ananticancer drug: critical appraisal and prospects., *Metallomics*, Vol.1, No.3, (April 2009), pp.193-198, 1756-5901.

T. Schilling, K. B. Keppler, M. E. Heim, G. Niebch, H. Dietzfelbinger, J. Rastetter, A. R. Hanauske (1995), Clinical phase I and pharmacokinetic trial of the new titanium complex budotitane, *Investigational New Drugs* , Vol. 13, No.4, (December 1995), pp.327-332, 1573-0646.

Top, S., Vessières, A., Cabestaing, C., Laios, I., Leclercq, G., Provot, C., Jaouen, G. (2001), Studies on organometallic selective estrogen receptor modulators. (SERMs) Dual activity in the hydroxy-ferrocifen series, *Journal of Organometallic Chemistry*, Vol. 637–639, (December 2001), pp.500-506, 2001, 0022-328X.

Trinchero, A., Bonora, S., Tinti, A., Fini, G. (2004), Spectroscopic behavior of copper complexes of nonsteroidal anti-inflammatory drugs, *Biopolymers*, Special Issue: Selected Papers from the 10th European Conference on the Spectroscopy of Biological Molecules (ECSBM 2003), Vol.74, No.1-2, (October, 2004), pp.120–124, 1097-0102.

Underhill, A.E., Bury, A., Odling, R.J., Fleet, M.B., Stevens, A., Gomm, P.S. (1989), Metal complexes of antiinflammatory drugs. Part VII: Salsalate complex of copper(II) , *Journal of Inorganic Biochemistry*, Vol.37, No.1, (September 1989), pp. 1-5, 0162-0134.

Vajragupta, O., Boonchoong, P., Sumanont, Y., Watanabe, H., Wongkrajang, Y., Kammasud, N. (2003), Manganese-Based Complexes of Radical Scavengers as Neuroprotective Agents, *Bioorganic Medicinal Chemistry*, Vol.11, No.10, (May 2003), pp.2329–2337, 0968-0896.

Valvassori, S.S., Cristiano, M.P., Cardoso, D.C., Santos, G.D., Martins, M.R., Quevedo, J., da Paula, M.M.S. (2006) Pharmacological Activity of Ruthenium Complexes trans-[$RuCl_2(L)_4$] (L = Nicotinic or i-Nicotinic acid) on Anxiety and Memory in Rats, *Neurochemical Research*, Vol.31, No.12, (December, 2006), pp.1457-1462, 0364-3190.

Weder, J.E., Dillon, C.T., Hambley, T.W., Kennedy, B.J, Lay, P.A., Biffin, J.R., Regtop, H.L., Davies, N.M. (2002), Copper complexes of non-steroidal anti-inflammatory drugs: an opportunity yet to be realized, *Coordination Chemistry Reviews*, Vol.232, No.1-2, (October, 2002), pp.95-126, 0010-8545.

Weder, J.E., Hambley, T.W., Kennedy, B.J., Lay, P.A., MacLachlan, D., Bramley, R., Delfs, C.D., Murray, K.S., Moubaraki, B., Warwick, B., Biffin, J.R., Regtop, H.L. (1999),

Anti-Inflammatory Dinuclear Copper(II) Complexes with Indomethacin. Synthesis, Magnetism and EPR Spectroscopy. Crystal Structure of the *N,N*-Dimethylformamide, *Adduct Inorganic Chemistry,* Vol.38 , No.8, (April 1999), pp.1736–1744, 1520-510X.

Zhang, C.X., Lippard, S.J. (2003) New metal complexes as potential therapeutics *Current Opinion in Chemical Biology,* Vol.7, No.4, (August, 2003),.481-489, 1367-5931.

Zhao, G., Lin, H. (2005), Metal complexes with aromatic N-containing ligands as potential agents in cancer tretment. *Current Medicinal Chemistry- Anticancer Agents.* Vol.5, No.2, (March 2005), 137-147, 1568-0118.

30

Aging: Drugs to Eliminate Methylglyoxal, a Reactive Glucose Metabolite, and Advanced Glycation Endproducts

Indu Dhar and Kaushik Desai
Department of Pharmacology, College of Medicine, University of Saskatchewan, Saskatoon, SK, Canada

1. Introduction

The aging process not only affects the whole body, but also affects individual cells. While the age-related changes in the body are popularly recognized as wrinkling of the skin, indicating alterations in basement membrane proteins, the processes of cellular aging are less well defined. The underlying common theme of cellular aging and whole body aging seems to be an increase in oxidative stress. Advanced glycation endproducts (AGEs), which are widely accepted to alter basement membrane proteins, also increase oxidative stress. Reactive dicarbonyls, such as methylglyoxal (MG), formed during glycolysis and other metabolic processes are precursors of AGEs formation and triggers of oxidative stress. MG, AGEs and oxidative stress are very likely to induce DNA damage and be at the root of cellular aging. Thus, a strategy to prevent an elevation of MG, formation of AGEs and the associated oxidative stress has great therapeutic potential to slow the aging process at the cellular and the whole body level.

2. The ageing process

The process of aging is accepted as an inevitable normal part of the life cycle of each and every living organism. Aging can be grossly defined as an overall decline in biological functions. Thus, aging involves gradual changes in the body such as reduced immunity, loss of muscle strength, stiffening of the arterial wall, loss of elasticity and wrinkling of the skin, and decline in memory, all of which result in increasing weakness, risk of developing diseases, and ultimately death. These changes take place at the cellular, organ and the whole organism level. The whole process of aging unfolds very clearly in species with a long life span such as human beings. Cellular aging ultimately translates into whole body aging.

Hayflick et al. [1] first described cellular senescence in the sixties when they showed that normal cells had a limited ability to proliferate in culture. Cellular senescence is believed to be initiated by increased cellular stress [2, 3]. Factors contributing to cellular stress and aging include dysfunctional telomeres (telomere length) [4, 5], DNA damage [6] and mitogenic or oncogenic stimuli and signals [2, 4, 5]. The factors such as age and oxidative stress affect telomere length and telomerase activity which in turn affects cellular senescence [4]. Oxidative stress has been shown to damage DNA and affect life span [7-10]. A controversial view of cellular senescence is that it is an important protective mechanism against transformation of the cell into a malignant phenotype, in which case it would affect only mitotically active cells [2, 3]. The molecular mechanisms involved in cellular senescence are still being unraveled and will not be considered further in this review. The focus of this review will be on MG, a reactive dicarbonyl metabolic intermediate produced in the body, AGEs, and oxidative stress, all of which are interrelated and affect cellular as well as whole body aging. We will discuss some compounds that can scavenge MG, prevent the formation of AGEs (inhibitors) or break the existing AGEs (AGE breakers).

3. Theories of aging

Aging has been attributed to a number of different causes which have been presented in the form of different theories. These theories are based broadly on two different ideas, one of which is programmed life processes (program theories, e.g. Biological Clock theory, Limited Number of Proliferation theory), and the other one is of errors, mainly at the DNA and gene level, in life processes (error theories, e.g. Disease theory, Cross-linking theory, Rate of living theory, Free radical theory). A number of theories of aging are based on the combination of these two ideas, i.e. program theories and error theories [11-14].

Changes at the cellular level ultimately affect the whole body. The cell is a dynamic centre of ongoing metabolic activity driven by almost constant use of oxygen. Reasonably, the metabolic activity may affect survival or the death of the cell. The 'Rate of living theory' implicates the role of metabolism in aging, which is based on the observation that animals with higher metabolic rates often have shorter life spans. Since the metabolic processes and oxygen consumption can also generate oxidative stress, an excess of which is deleterious for the cell, the 'Free radical theory' of aging has become one of the more popular theories. The free radical theory proposes a connection between the metabolic rate and aging through an increased oxidative stress generation.

4. Free radical theory of aging

Max Rubner proposed the 'rate of living theory' early in the 20th century [15]. He observed that larger animals, which generally have slower metabolic rates, live longer than smaller animals with faster metabolic rates [15]. Even though it is now common knowledge that metabolism is associated with the generation of free radicals, it was Commoner *et al.* [16] who discovered the formation of free radicals *in vivo*. Commoner et al. [16] found that an increase in an organism's metabolic activity can increase the concentration of endogenous free radicals. Free radicals are atoms or molecules with an unpaired electron in an orbit, making them highly reactive. The high reactivity of free radicals makes them deleterious for cells because they react with proteins, lipids, DNA and other biomolecules, and disrupt their structure and function. Free radicals can be derived from oxygen mainly in the form of superoxide anions ($O_2^{\bullet -}$) and hydroxyl radicals ($^{\bullet}OH$), which are known as reactive oxygen species (ROS). Free radicals can also be in the form of highly reactive non-radicals which do not have an unpaired electron in their orbit, such as hydrogen peroxide (H_2O_2). Normally, the cells and the body have adequate antioxidant defenses which can neutralize free radicals and prevent the generation of oxidative stress resulting from an excess of free radicals [17-22]. The formation of free radicals and the function of antioxidants have been nicely explained in reviews by Haliwell [20, 21].

The free radical theory of aging was proposed by Denham Harman in 1956 [23]. The free radical theory of aging attributes the aging process to cumulative cellular damage inflicted by the reaction of free radicals with key functional cellular and tissue constituents resulting in impaired function, disease and death [23]. The discovery of an antioxidant enzyme, superoxide dismutase (SOD) [24], which plays a key role to eliminate superoxide anion levels, provided some validity to the free radical theory, which was not initially accepted by many.

The mitochondrial respiratory chain is a major source of free radicals, mainly in the form of superoxide anions, which cause damage to the mitochondria and reduce life span [25, 26]. The damage inflicted by ROS, especially to DNA [7], rather than the metabolic rate, showed a greater correlation with life span [8]. Damage to DNA was formulated into the somatic mutation theory, which states that genetic mutations caused by an excess of free radicals could lead to accelerated aging [7, 9, 10].

The fact that increased production of ROS in the mitochondria can reduce life span was supported by several studies. Thus, Ku *et al.*, [27] showed that the rates of mitochondrial superoxide anion and hydrogen peroxide generation were inversely correlated to maximum life span potential when they compared seven different mammalian species with different life spans ranging from 3.5 to 30 years. Similarly, ROS production was higher in heart mitochondria of the rat, which has a life span of about 4 yrs, than in the long-lived pigeon, which has a longer life span of 35 yrs [28]. Theoretically, therefore, if the free radical production is diminished, the life span should increase. This has been demonstrated in several species. Thus, over expression of SOD and catalase in the worm *Caenorhabditis elegans* (*C. Elegans*) through *age-1* alleles, increases their oxidative defenses and life span by 65% longer on average [29, 30]. Increased activity of SOD and reduced oxidative stress in the transgenic *Drosophila* (*Drosophila melanogaster*) flies also slows the aging process and results in a longer life [31, 32]. Also, over expression of catalase in the peroxisome, the mitochondria or the nucleus in transgenic mice, reduced oxidative damage, hydrogen peroxide production, and delayed the development of cardiac pathology and cataract formation along with an average increase of 5.5 months in the life span [33]. The observation that long-lived animals have lower levels of antioxidant enzymes was explained as being due to a lower rate of production of oxygen radicals [34].

Interestingly, some of the studies in rodents did not produce the expected results. For example, the administration of antioxidants [35], or over expression of CuZn SOD and catalase in mice [36], or SOD in rats [37], did not increase their life spans. In rodents, one reason for the lack of additional protective effects, which are normally associated with an increase in antioxidants, could be their ability to synthesize vitamin C [38], which might already be providing the required protection. This was verified by knocking out the vitamin C synthesizing enzyme, L-gluconolactone oxidase (GLO) in mice, which then have to depend on dietary vitamin C [39]. GLO knockout mice had damaged aortic walls when they were fed a diet low in vitamin C, which underlined the importance of the constitutive antioxidant function of vitamin C in rodents [39]. Thus, studies in rodents do not provide unequivocal support for the free radical theory of aging [40].

Another way of increasing free radical production and oxidative stress is by increasing total caloric intake, which can be easily done be feeding an excess of glucose. A correlation between life span and dietary caloric intake was reported in rats and mice by McCay *et al.* [41]. One quantitative estimate was provided in the study by Weindruch and Walford [42] who showed that a 40% reduction in dietary caloric intake extended maximum life span by one third. A high dietary caloric intake causes an increased rate of DNA damage [43], due to a high metabolic rate which in turn results in higher amounts of superoxide anion, hydrogen peroxide and hydroxyl radical formation [44].

5. Methylglyoxal

Chemically, MG, or pyruvaldehyde, is a highly reactive electrophilic α,β-dicarbonyl compound [45, 46] (Fig. 1). MG has been proposed to be formed mainly during glycolysis, through spontaneous nonenzymatic transformation of triose phosphates [45, 47-49] (Fig. 2). MG synthase has been proposed to convert the triose phosphate intermediate, dihydroxyacetone phosphate (DHAP), into MG, especially when inadequate inorganic phosphate is available [50, 51]. Other sources of MG, which are believed to produce lower amounts of MG, include intermediates of protein and fatty acid metabolism, such as aminoacetone produced from L-threonine and glycine [52, 53], and acetone [54, 55], respectively (Fig. 2). Semicarbazide-sensitive amine oxidase (SSAO) catalyzes the breakdown of aminoacetone [52, 55, 56], while acetone and acetol mono-oxygenase (AMO) converts acetone to acetol and acetol to MG, respectively [54] (Fig. 2). SSAO is found in substantial amounts in the vascular smooth muscle cells and the plasma [55].

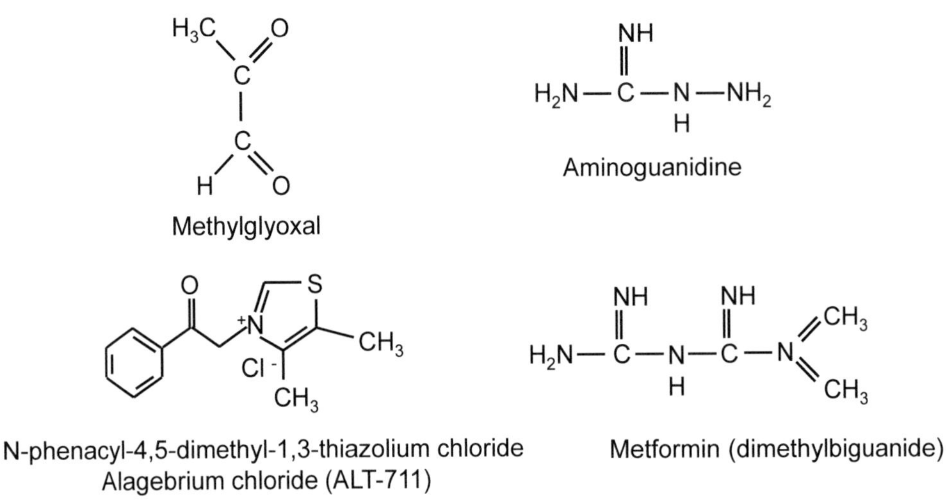

Fig. 1. Structure of methylglyoxal (MG) and three compounds with an ability to bind MG or inhibit the formation of advanced glycation endproducts (AGEs) or break formed AGEs. These compounds are discussed in this review.

After MG is formed, it is rapidly degraded to D-lactic acid by the highly efficient and ubiquitous glyoxalase system, which consists of two key enzymes, glyoxalase I (lactoylglutathione lyase) and glyoxalase II (hydroxyacylglutathione hydrolase) [57-59] (Fig. 2). Reduced glutathione (GSH) plays a key role by binding MG and presenting it to glyoxalase I. Thus, adequate availability of GSH is important in keeping MG levels low in the body. For this reason enzymes involved in the synthesis and recycling of GSH, such as glutathione peroxidase and glutathione reductase are also important in the metabolism of MG [60-62].

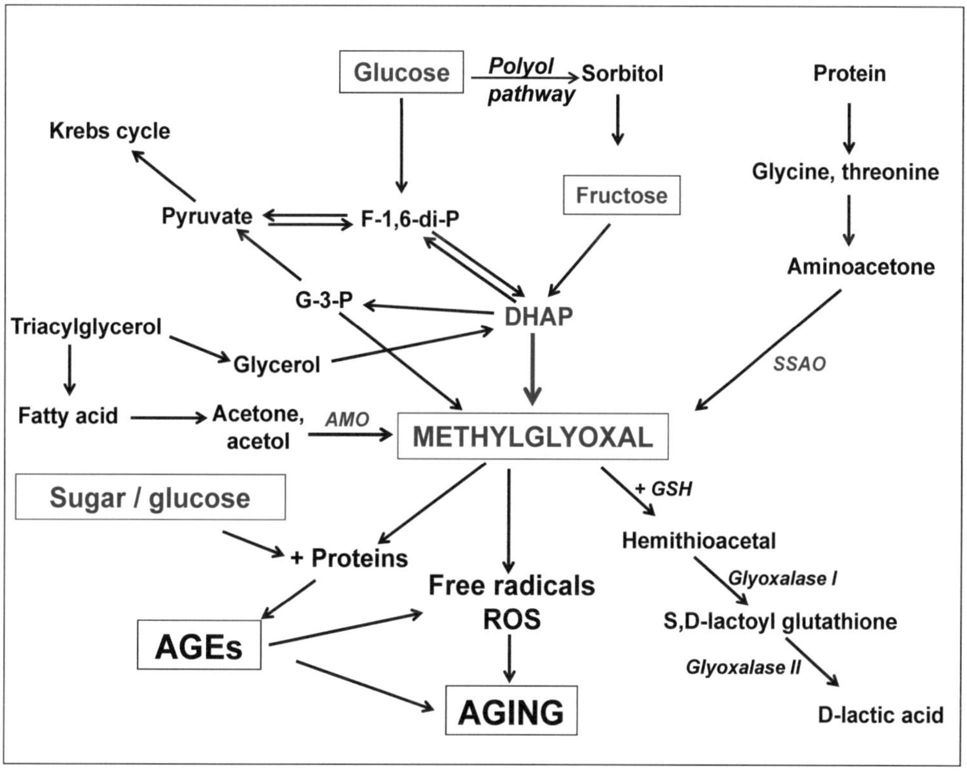

Fig. 2. A schematic of key sources and steps of methylglyoxal (MG) formation from intermediates of glucose, protein and fat metabolism, and its degradation by the glyoxalase enzymes. Abbreviations: AGEs - advanced glycation endproducts; AMO - amine oxidase; DHAP - dihydroxacetone phosphate; FA - fatty acid; F-1-P - fructose-1-phosphate; F-1,6-di-P - fructose-1,6-diphosphate; F-6-P - fructose-6-phosphate; G-3-P - glyceraldehyde-3-phosphate; G-6-P - glucose-6-phosphate; ROS - reactive oxygen species; SSAO - semicarbazide-sensitive acetone/acetol mono-oxygenase; GSH, reduced glutathione.

Despite the efficient glyoxalase system, MG levels can increase significantly in the plasma and different organs such as the aorta and the kidneys [61, 63-66]. We have shown that MG levels are elevated in the plasma, aorta and kidney of fructose-fed Sprague-Dawley rats and spontaneously hypertensive rats (SHR) [61, 63-65]. Patients with type 1 and type 2 diabetes have 2-6 fold higher plasma levels of MG compared to healthy people [67, 68]. MG possibly plays a role in the pathogenesis of insulin resistance and type 2 diabetes as shown by several *in vitro* [69-71], and by our recent *in vivo* study in acute [66] and chronic MG-treated

Sprague-Dawley rats [72]. Elevated MG levels are linked to the development of micro-vascular complications of diabetes such as retinopathy and nephropathy, and other conditions such as atherosclerosis and neurodegenerative diseases [73-77]. MG levels are high in the cerebrospinal fluid of patients with Alzheimer's disease [76].

6. Advanced glycation endproducts

Unwanted chemical modification of physiologic constituent molecules of the body, which leads to the formation of harmful chemical entities, seems to be an unavoidable part of metabolic processes of the body. One type of modification, known as glycation, a nonenzymatic reaction, is a serious hazard of excess glucose availability in the body. The chemical interaction leading to the formation of AGEs starts when a reducing sugar condenses with the amino groups of proteins at their N terminus or on lysyl side chains (ε-amino groups) [78]. This nonenzymatic glycation involves a series of post-translational modifications. Glycation begins with the aldehyde or the ketone carbonyl group of the sugar combining with the protein to form an unstable aldimine intermediate or a Schiff base. Later on the Schiff base undergoes an Amadori rearrangement to form a stable Amadori product, a l-amino-l-deoxyfructose derivative with a stable ketoamine linkage, which can get cyclized to form a ring structure [78-80]. The Amadori product can undergo oxidation, degradation or rearrangement and form AGEs, a heterogenous group of products. Auto oxidation of glucose (Wolff pathway) [81] or of the Schiff bases (Namiki pathway) [82] can lead to formation of reactive diacrbonyls, but these pathways which are readily observed at high glucose concentrations *in vitro*, are not predominant *in vivo* [83]. The Maillard reaction, also known as the "browning reaction", involves oxidation of the glycated product which forms a brown coloured product. Glucose, fructose and glucose-6-phosphate are all involved in glycation, albeit at different rates of reaction with glucose, the most important contributor, reacting at a comparatively slower rate than the other two [6]. Increased glucose levels, as seen in diabetic patients, causes more AGEs formation than in healthy people. These AGEs affect the normal function of several proteins and enzymes, and are responsible for aging [74, 80] and the complications of diabetes such as nephropathy and retinopathy [79]. Another way by which the glycation reaction causes damage is through the formation of reactive α-dicarbonyl compounds, such as MG, glyoxal and 3-deoxyglucosone (3-DG), when the sugar molecule undergoes fragmentation [78].

MG can also cause AGEs formation [78, 79]. In fact, MG and two other dicarbonyl metabolic intermediates, 3-DG and glyoxal, are believed to be major sources of intracellular and plasma AGEs formation [79, 84, 85], which are commonly implicated in the aging process. Any MG which is not degraded by the glyoxalase system or aldose reductase, reacts non-enzymatically with arginine or lysine residues of proteins [45] to form irreversible AGEs. This glycation is not random, but it depends on the structural configuration and (or) physical locations of the target proteins [86, 87]. The AGEs produced by the reaction between MG and arginine are hydroimidazolone Nε-(5-hydro-5-methyl-4-imidazolon-2-yl)-ornithine and argpyrimidine [88], whereas the AGE, Nε-carboxyethyllysine (CEL) [89, 90] is formed when MG reacts with lysine. Further crosslinking of these AGEs produces fluorescent products such as pentosidine and cross-line, and non-fluorescent ones such as argpyrimidine, methylglyoxal-lysine dimer (MOLD), glyoxal-lysine dimer (GOLD) and imidazolones [91, 92]. The presence of these AGEs can be detected immunohistochemically in tissues [93].

7. Methylglyoxal, AGEs, oxidative stress and aging

The damage inflicted by oxidative stress and the formation of intracellular AGEs likely contribute to cellular aging. From this point of view, both increased MG and AGEs would cause accelerated cellular aging. MG would be a double-edged sword because it is a potent inducer of oxidative stress [17, 62, 94, 95], as discussed below, and it is a major precursor of AGEs formation. AGEs also induce oxidative stress.

8. Methylglyoxal and oxidative stress

The role of MG in inducing oxidative stress is well established [17]. Several studies have helped to develop an integrated view of the multiple pathways activated by MG to increase oxidative stress (Fig. 3). The reader is referred to our earlier review on MG and oxidative stress [17]. MG increases the formation of superoxide [94, 96-99], hydrogen peroxide and peroxynitrite [94, 95, 98, 100], proinflammatory cytokines, such as interleukin 1β (IL-1β) [101], interleukin-6 (IL-6), interleukin-8 (IL-8) and tumor necrosis factor-α (TNF-α) [67, 101], in different cell types such as VSMCs [62, 94, 95], endothelial cells [102], rat kidney mesangial cells [97], rat hepatocytes [100], neutrophils [67, 98], platelets [99], cultured neural cells from rat hippocampus [101], cultured cortical neurons [103], and SH-SY5Y neuroblastoma cells [104].

MG has been shown to increase the activity of several prooxidant enzymes such as NADPH oxidase [94, 97] (Fig. 3), p38 MAPK [98, 102], and increase the of expression of JNK and PPAR-α [104].

Excess superoxide can react with nitric oxide (NO) to form peroxynitrite ($ONOO^-$) [105] (Fig. 3). Peroxynitrite is a strong oxidant and nitrating agent. Because of its oxidizing properties, peroxynitrite can damage a wide range of molecules including DNA and proteins in cells [105].

Besides directly increasing free radical production, MG can increase oxidative stress by reducing antioxidants (Fig. 3) such as GSH [104, 106, 107], glutathione peroxidase [108], glutathione reductase [60, 62, 108, 109], and manganese superoxide dismutase (MnSOD) [96], in different cells such as erythrocytes [106, 107], VSMCs [62, 96], and endothelial cells [109]. Reduced antioxidants in turn impair the detoxification of MG, increase its half-life and set up a vicious cycle to cause further oxidant damage. Glutathione peroxidase removes hydrogen peroxide with the help of GSH which in turn is converted to oxidized glutathione (GSSG). Glutathione reductase recycles GSSG to GSH [62, 110] (Fig. 3).

An increased production of ROS was also observed in monocytes treated with MG-modified albumin [111]. Thus, MG induced thrombosis and inflammation by activating monocytes, induced apoptosis of neutrophils, and caused platelet-neutrophil aggregates [112].

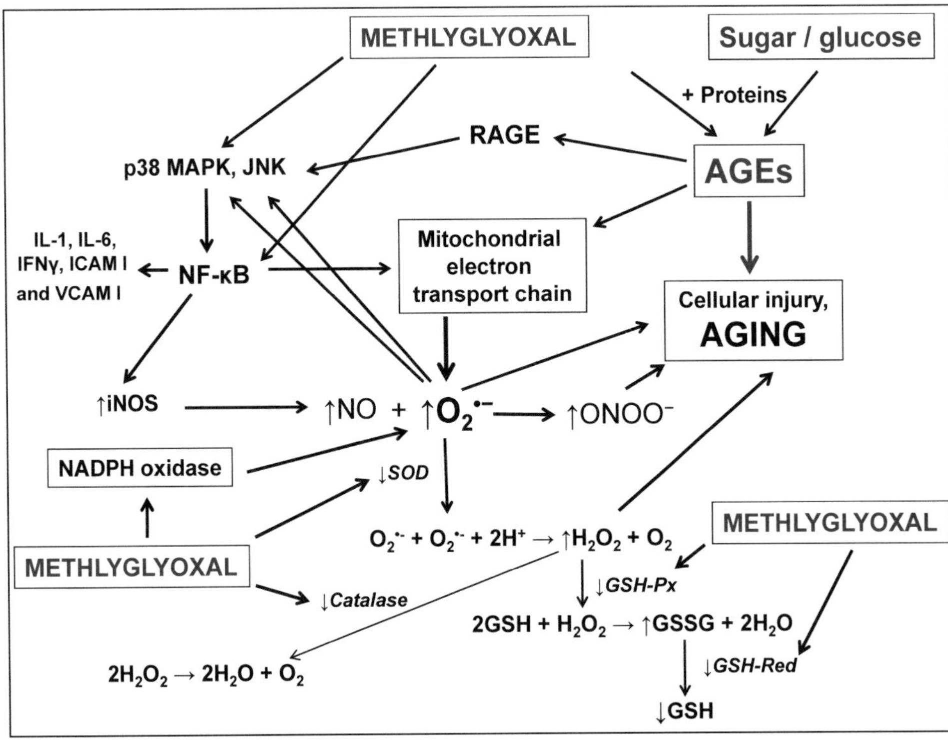

Fig. 3. A schematic of oxidative stress pathways activated by methylglyoxal and advanced glycation endproducts and their implication in aging. Abbreviations: AGEs, advanced glycation end products; GSH-Px, glutathione peroxidase; GSH-Red, glutathione reductase; GSH, reduced glutathione; GSSG, oxidized glutathione; H_2O_2, hydrogen peroxide; ICAM 1, intercellular adhesion molecule 1; IFNγ, interferon γ; IL1, interleukin 1; JNK, JUN N-terminal kinase; MG, methylglyoxal; NF-κB, nuclear factor-kappaB; NO, nitric oxide; $O_2^{\bullet -}$, superoxide anion; $ONOO^-$, peroxynitrite; p38 MAPK, p38 mitogen activated protein kinase; RAGE, receptor for advanced glycation endproduct; SOD, superoxide dismutase; VCAM 1, vascular cell adhesion molecule 1.

Metabolic activity in the mitochondria is at the centre of the free radical theory of aging. Mitochondria, which are the major sites of ATP and energy production in the cell, also generate about 85% of total intracellular superoxide when electrons escape, mainly from complex I and complex III, and react with oxygen [23, 113-116].

MG increases mitochondrial superoxide production [116, 117]. Treatment of rat aortic VSMCs (A-10 cells) with MG (30 μM) significantly increased mitochondrial superoxide production by 69.9% compared with untreated cells. The AGEs cross-link breaker, alagebrium (50 μM), and SOD mimetic 4-hydroxy-tempo (Tempol, 500 μM) significantly decreased MG-induced mitochondrial superoxide production by 57% and 85.8%, respectively. Mitochondrial nitrotyrosine formation was also increased by MG [96].

In *in vivo* studies elevated MG levels are associated with increased oxidative stress. For example, we have shown that in 13 wk old SHR with elevated blood pressure, significantly elevated plasma and aortic MG levels are associated with increased levels of superoxide, and significantly reduced GSH levels, glutathione peroxidase, and glutathione reductase activities, compared with age-matched Wistar Kyoto (WKY) rats [61]. Similarly, in diabetes mellitus and hypertension, increased MG levels are associated with increased oxidative stress [61, 65, 67, 68, 118].

An excess of MG, CEL and CML indicate carbonyl overload and are associated with oxidative stress [73, 79, 119-123].

Glycated proteins and AGEs also induce oxidative stress (Fig. 3) through several mechanisms. AGEs induce production of cytokines and growth factors [124-130]. AGEs bind to the receptor for AGEs (RAGE) and scavenger receptors to induce oxidative stress in various cells including VSMCs, endothelial cells, and mononuclear phagocytes [128, 131]. In endothelial cells AGEs increase expression of vascular cell adhesion molecule-1 (VCAM-1), intercellular adhesion molecule-1 (ICAM-1), and increase activity of NF-κB to increase oxidative stress [126, 132].

9. Methylglyoxal and aging

The accumulation of AGEs in extracellular tissue proteins, such as the basement membrane and matrix proteins of blood vessels and skin, is a well known phenomenon characteristic of aging and age-related diseases. Several studies demonstrate aging associated increase in AGEs. Thus, accumulation of AGEs in the vessel walls results in a gradual loss of elasticity, which makes older subjects more susceptible to cardiovascular diseases [133, 134]. MG-induced AGEs, such as CEL and CML, increased with age in human lens and cause cataract formation [90]. In a study on 172 subjects serum levels of CML, 8-isoprostanes and C-reactive protein, which are markers of oxidative stress, were higher in elderly people (>60 years old) compared with younger people (<45 years old) [135]. One reason why AGEs accumulate during the aging process could be due to an age-related decrease in antioxidant enzymes. Thus, Mailankot et al. [136] reported that the activity and expression of glyoxalase I protein, which is involved in MG degradation, decreased with age in the anterior epithelial cells of human lens, which causes an accumulation of MG. Similarly, an age-dependent decrease in catalase activity in the skin may be responsible for elevated MG and peroxynitrite production [137].

However, it is doubtful whether extracellular AGEs accumulation plays a causative role in aging. On the other hand AGEs formation inside the cell, such as AGE-nucleotides in DNA, may contribute to cellular senescence [6, 60, 74, 80]. DNA integrity is an important determinant of lifespan and errors in DNA repair would lead to substitutions, deletions, insertions, and transpositions of nucleotides, with increased risk of carcinogenesis and reduced life span. Animals with a longer lifespan and more efficient DNA repair have delayed carcinogenesis [80]. In this regard MG-induced DNA damage can have a more direct effect on aging.

Studies directly implicating MG in the aging process are very few and this is one area where there is a knowledge gap. The study by Morcos et al in the worm *C. elegans* highlights the role of MG, glyoxalase I and MG-induced ROS formation in aging and life span [138]. They showed that the activity of glyoxalase I was markedly reduced with age resulting in accumulation of MG-derived adducts and oxidative stress markers, which further inhibited the expression and the activity of glyoxalase I. Over expression of glyoxalase I decreased MG-induced modification of mitochondrial proteins and ROS production, and prolonged the lifespan of *C. elegans*; whereas CeGly knock-out produced the opposite effect [138].

Scheckhuber et al. studied the degradation of MG by the glyoxalase system enzymes and its effect on growth and lifespan in filamentous ascomycete and a model of aging, Podospora anserine (*P. anserina*) [139]. Using genetic manipulation of the two enzymes of the glyoxalase system, they found that up-regulation of both components of the glyoxalase system was effective in increasing lifespan in P. anserina.

Oxidative stress-induced cellular senescence was demonstrated in the study by Sejeresen and Rattan [140]. They treated human skin fibroblasts with MG (400 μM), or glyoxal (1.0 mM), and found the appearance of various senescent phenotypes within three days. These phenotypes showed growth arrest, had increased hydrogen peroxide and the glyoxal-induced AGE, Nε-carboxymethyl lysine (CML) protein levels, and altered SOD and catalase antioxidant enzyme activities [140]. Sejeresen and Rattan proposed this model to study cellular senescence *in vitro* [140].

In this review we have highlighted some important facts that oxidative stress is a major factor in the cellular and whole body aging processes, AGEs are strongly associated with aging and MG is a major precursor of AGEs formation, and both MG and AGEs are potent inducers of oxidative stress. Based on these facts, it is highly likely that MG may have a major role in the aging process through induction of oxidative stress as depicted in the scheme in Fig. 3. In fact, elevated MG levels may be responsible for causing accelerated aging in many tissues and organs of the cardiovascular system, nervous system, and other systems of the human body. A strategy to prevent aging should include targeting MG by reducing excessive formation, inhibit AGEs formation, and remove excessively formed MG and AGEs from the body.

10. Anti-MG and anti-AGEs compounds

The deleterious effects of MG and AGEs can be prevented by compounds that can do one or all of the following: (i) bind and neutralize reactive aldehydes, especially MG, (ii) prevent the formation of AGEs, (iii) neutralize formed AGEs, (iv) break down formed AGEs.

Considering these multiple ways of preventing the effects of MG or AGEs these compounds will be termed as "anti-MG" or "anti-AGE". Unfortunately, specific anti-MG or anti-AGE compounds are not yet available. The ones available are non-specific and have one or more other effects, which limits their usefulness. A number of the available compounds happen to have anti-MG as well as anti-AGE effects.

The possible sites at which anti-AGEs and anti-MG drugs can work are shown in Fig. 4, which outlines the various stages of AGEs formation.

Site 1. The first step in glycation is the binding of a sugar to the free amino groups of a protein. Drugs that bind to the amino group of proteins, such as aspirin, can prevent the binding of the sugar to the amino group. This group of compounds is likely to produce non-specific effects.

Site 2. Compounds can be used to bind aldose and ketose sugars to neutralize them and prevent them from reacting with proteins. E.g. Aminoguanidine reacts with the carbonyl group of glucose and prevents AGEs formation.

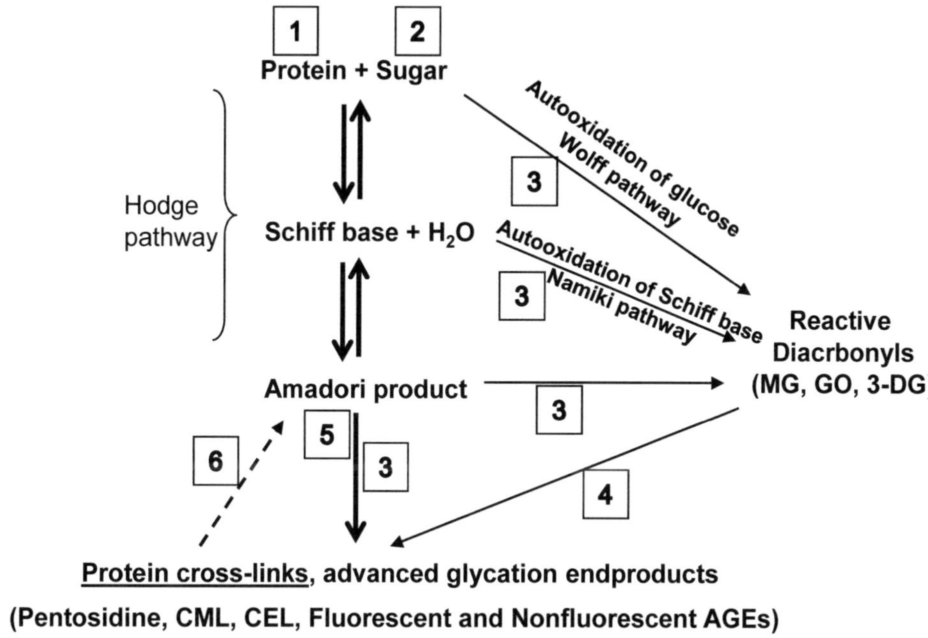

Fig. 4. Stages of formation of advanced glycation endproducts (AGEs) from glycation of proteins. Nonenzymatic glycation of protein leads to reversible formation of Schiff bases, which lead to further reversible formation of Amadori adducts and ultimate formation of stable irreversible AGEs. Solid vertical arrows show these steps which form the classical Hodge pathway of AGEs formation. Auto oxidation of glucose (Wolff pathway) or of the Schiff base (Namiki pathway) forms reactive dicarbonyls such as methylglyoxal (MG), glyoxal (GO) or 3-deoxyglucosone (3-DG) which is mostly seen *in vitro*, rather than *in vivo*. The dicarbonyls, which are also formed from other metabolic pathways, also contribute significantly to AGEs formation, as explained in the text. The various sites at which anti-AGEs and anti-MG compounds can act are indicated by numbers and discussed in the text. Based on the scheme proposed by Khalifah et al. [83]

Site 3. AGEs and reactive aldehydes also generate reactive oxygen species which adds to their damaging effects [17, 141, 142]. Antioxidants such as vitamin C or E [143] and metal chelators such as penicillamine [144] can be used to quench ROS and metal ions.

Site 4. Reactive aldehydes such as MG, glyoxal, glycoaldehyde and glucosones, which are formed during nutrient metabolism and AGEs formation, are a major source of AGEs formation. Reactive aldehydes can be neutralized by compounds such as aminoguanidine [145, 146] and metformin [147, 148].

Site 5. Amadori adducts, formed in the intermediate stages of AGEs formation can either be quenched by compounds such as aminoguanidine, or degraded enzymatically by enzymes such as amadoriase and human fructosamine-3-kinase, which belong to this group [149, 150]. Amadoriases have not been detected in higher organisms [151, 152].

Site 6. The final group of compounds acts on formed AGEs and are therefore, known as AGE breakers or cross-link breakers. E.g. phenacylthiazolium bromide (PTB) [153] and alagebrium (previously known as ALT-711), which are thiazolium compounds. AGEs which do not have cross-links such as pentosidine [154], GOLD and MOLD [155] will not be affected by these drugs.

Some of the more common compounds with anti-MG or anti-AGEs effects are described below.

Aminoguanidine is one of the popular and widely used AGEs inhibitor [145] and MG scavenger. Despite being a guanidine derivative it shares many common properties with hydrazine and is classified as a hydrazine [156]. As described above, aminoguanidine acts at site 2 as well as site 4 (Fig. 4) meaning that it prevents AGEs formation by combining with the carbonyl group of glucose as well as by scavenging reactive dicarbonyls formed during various metabolic processes [146]. The inhibitory effect of aminoguanidine is mainly at the Amadori stage [83]. Aminoguanidine is not a specific AGEs inhibitor or MG scavenger and it has other actions. Aminoguanidine potently inhibits histaminases [157, 158] and prevents deamination of histamine and putrescine. Aminoguanidine also inhibits nitric oxide synthase (NOS) [159, 160] and prevents the formation of nitric oxide (NO), a dynamic signaling molecule in the body [161], from L-arginine. Aminoguanidine also binds to the enzyme S-adenosylmethionine decarboxylase and increases synthesis of polyamines such as spermidine and spermine from ornithine [162]. Aminoguanidine can also bind pyridoxal and cause vitamin B6 deficiency, which in turn can result in adverse reactions to aminoguanidine [163]. A number of *in vitro* and *in vivo* studies have described the inhibitory effects of aminoguanidine on AGEs formation [145, 146, 164-167]. The doses used *in vivo* range from 25 mg/kg/day [145, 166] to 50 mg/kg/day [165] and up to 100 mg/kg/day [167]. Thus, aminoguanidine is far from an ideal MG scavenger and AGEs inhibitor. In clinical trials aminoguanidine was found to be too toxic for use in patients. Two double-masked, multiple-dose, placebo-controlled, randomized clinical trials, ACTION I and ACTION II [168, 169] investigated the therapeutic potential of aminoguanidine in preventing the progression of renal damage in patients with diabetic nephropathy. The ACTION I trial involving 690 participants did not show a statistically significant difference between the placebo group and the combined aminoguanidine dose groups, even though patients treated with aminoguanidine showed a tendency of having a lower risk of doubling of serum creatinine [168]. Due to safety concerns and an apparent lack of efficacy, the External Safety Monitoring Committee for the ACTION II trial involving 599 participants recommended early termination [169]. Patients with diabetes may have impaired red blood cell-deformability, which could cause microvascular and kidney damage. A one year trial with aminoguanidine and erythropoietin on 12 patients on dialysis restored red blood cell-deformability to near-normal levels, an effect attributed to inhibition of AGEs formation by aminoguanidine [170]. As mentioned earlier the toxic effects of aminoguanidine have limited its therapeutic potential. For example, like hydrazine, aminoguanidine may be associated with drug-induced systemic lupus erythematosus and abnormal liver function tests, and it can cause flu-like syndromes and vasculitis [169]. Aminoguanidine can also cause damage to DNA through hydroxyl- and hydrogen peroxide-formation in the presence of Fe^{+3} [171].

Metformin is an oral dimethylbiguanide antihyperglycemic agent, which can also inhibit AGEs formation [172], through its action in the post-Amadori stages [83, 173]. Metformin has also been proposed to have a MG scavenging effect attributed to its guanidino group, which binds with MG to form an inactive product, triazepinone [147, 148, 174, 175]. The MG-scavenging effect of metformin resulted in significantly reduced elevated MG levels in type 2 diabetes patients treated with high doses of metformin, between 1,500 and 2,500 mg/day [172]. We have shown that fructose-fed Sprague-Dawley rats had significantly elevated serum MG and blood pressure, and increased levels of MG, hydrogen peroxide and the MG-derived AGE, CEL, in the aorta, all of which were attenuated by metformin [65]. Metformin has been proposed to protect against MG-induced increased atherogenicity of low density lipoprotein (LDL) [176]. The use of metformin as a MG scavenger and AGEs inhibitor is limited, and hopefully more studies showing its anti-MG, anti-AGEs effectiveness will promote its use for this purpose. Metformin can be considered to have a good therapeutic potential in this regard since it is already in clinical use for type 2 diabetes as an insulin sensitizing agent.

Pioglitazone, a thiazolidinedione, is a peroxisome proliferator-activated receptor gamma (PPARγ) agonist which acts as an insulin sensitizer and is used in type 2 diabetes. Pioglitazone has been proposed to have anti-AGEs effect by inhibiting glycation, AGEs formation and protein cross-linking [177, 178]. Studies employing pioglitazone as an anti-MG or anti-AGEs compound are not forthcoming and more evidence is needed to make definitive statements about the therapeutic potential of pioglitazone in this regard.

N-acetylcysteine (NAC) is a MG scavenging and antioxidant compound [179, 180]. There are good reasons for using NAC as an anti-MG compound: NAC can increase GSH levels [181], which is an efficient MG scavenger and antioxidant [70, 179, 180], NAC is a cysteine containing thiol compound and MG binds with high affinity to cysteine [180, 181], and NAC is already used clinically for other conditions such as acetaminophen overdose [179, 181]. More studies employing NAC as an anti-MG drug should provide interesting results and may help to establish the potential of NAC in this regard.

A widely used class of antihypertensive drugs has been proposed to have anti-AGE effects. Angiotensin receptor blockers (ARBs) and angiotensin converting enzyme inhibitors (ACEIs) have been shown to protect against kidney damage, an effect claimed to be independent of their blood pressure lowering action [182-185], but proposed to be due to an anti-AGE effect. Clinical trials evaluating AGEs lowering effects of ARBs and ACEIs at blood pressure lowering doses can add to the therapeutic utility of these drugs.

A number of compounds have been investigated for anti-AGE effects in limited studies, but have not been widely used as such in experimental studies in animals or humans. These compounds include the cycloxygenase inhibitors, aspirin [186-188], ibuprofen [189], diclofenac [190], xanthine derivative, pentoxifylline [191, 192], which is used for claudication in peripheral vascular disease, metal chelators, D-penicillamine [144] and desferoxamine [83, 144], thiamine pyrophosphate and pyridoxamine [193-195]. Many more studies are necessary for these compounds in order to draw definitive conclusions about their anti-MG or anti-AGE effects.

A number of deglycating enzymes have been discovered, especially in microorganisms, which remove the sugar bound to the protein molecule, and possibly provide these bacteria with energy substrates derived from glycated products [196]. These enzymes, known as amadoriases, include fructosylamine oxidases [197, 198], fructosamine-3-kinase [149, 150], fructoselysine-6-kinase [199], fructoselysine-3-epimerase (FrlC) [200], and glucoselysine-6-

phosphate deglycase [201]. The use of these enzymes or development of stable analogues for deglycation therapy remains speculative .

A number of AGE inhibitors were synthesized and screened for their AGEs inhibitory effects by Rahbar et al. [173, 202, 203]. These are derivatives of aryl ureido and aryl carboxaminido phenoxy isobutyric acids and were derived from some known AGEs inhibitors. These compounds act at multiple stages of the AGEs formation process. Some of these compounds have AGEs breaking properties. More studies are needed for these compounds to establish their specificity and safety for therapeutic use.

11. AGEs breakers

The AGEs which have undergone cross-linking are very stable products and their concentration, especially in long-lived matrix proteins, increases with age. AGEs inhibitors are ineffective against formed AGEs and compounds which can break the cross-links are required. The AGEs breaker compounds can prove invaluable to slow down the aging process, and in the treatment of established stages of diseases such as diabetes, Alzheimer's, atherosclerosis and rheumatoid arthritis.

The first AGEs breaking compound reported was phenacylthiazolium bromide (PTB) in 1996. PTB breaks the covalent cross-links of AGEs [204]. Administration of PTB (10 mg/kg/day, intraperitoneal for 4 wks) reduced the amount of IgG bound to the surface of red blood cells in diabetic rats [153]. However, PTB is not stable.

The search for a stable derivative of PTB resulted in the synthesis of ALT 711 (4,5-dimethylthiazolium) [205]. ALT 711 (now known as alagebrium) reduced arterial stiffness in streptozotocin-induced diabetic rats [205]. In aging rats, ALA (10 mg/kg for 16 weeks) also increased glutathione peroxidase and superoxide dismutase activities and reduced oxidative stress [206]. Alagebrium improved impaired cardiovascular function in older rhesus monkeys [207]. Alagebrium demonstrated promising results and a good safety profile in phase 2 clinical trials. In a clinical study involving 93 subjects, 50 yrs and older, with evidence of vessel stiffness (pulse pressure ≥60 mm Hg, systolic blood pressure ≥140 mm Hg, and large artery compliance ≤1.25 mL/mm Hg), alagebrium (210 mg, once per day for 56 days) improved arterial compliance [208]. In another group of 13 patients aged 65±2 yrs with systolic hypertension (systolic blood pressure > 140 mmHg, diastolic blood pressure <90 mm Hg), alagebrium (210 mg/kg twice a day for 8 weeks) reduced vascular fibrosis and markers of inflammation [209]. Alagebrium (administered for 16 weeks) decreased left ventricular mass and improved left ventricular diastolic filling in another trial in 23 patients with diastolic heart failure [210, 211].

However, in a recent study [212] involving 102 patients (aged 62 ± 11 years) with heart failure (left ventricular ejection fraction (LVEF ≤0.45), alagebrium (400 mg/day/36 wks) did not improve exercise tolerance and systolic dysfunction, and no changes were observed in a number of secondary endpoints. Thus, the authors could not verify the claims that alagebrium has beneficial effects in systolic heart failure [212].

Alagebrium has been reported to be a weak inhibitor of thiamine diphosphokinase and is unlikely to interfere with thiamine metabolism at therapeutic concentrations [213]. However, the authors urge caution when new AGE-crosslink breakers based on thiamine are designed, to make sure they are not potent inhibitors of thiamine diphosphokinase.

In the studies described above alagebrium has been studied mainly for its chronic effects on AGEs as an AGEs breaker. We investigated whether alagebrium also has acute preventive effects against the reactive dicarbonyl, MG, in 12 wk old male Sprague-Dawley rats [66]. Our results showed that alagebrium also has acute (< 6 h) MG scavenging ability [66]. AGEs are formed slowly over a time ranging from 24 h to up to 7 days and more. Therefore, the attenuation of MG-induced acute effects (seen within 6 h of MG administration) is most likely due to scavenging of MG by alagebrium. Thus, alagebrium significantly attenuated the significant increases in MG levels in the plasma, and different organs (measured 2 h after administration), and also attenuated MG-induced impaired glucose tolerance and the reduced insulin-stimulated glucose uptake by adipose tissue. In an *in vitro* assay in which MG (10 μM) was incubated with or without alagebrium (100 μM) for different times at 37° C, alagebrium significantly reduced the amount of detectable MG [66]. Our results strongly indicate an acute MG scavenging effect of alagebrium which can add to its AGEs breaking ability. More direct evidence of interaction of alagebrium and MG using mass spectrometry would be very useful. We have also recently shown that alagebrium significantly attenuated the deleterious effects of chronic MG administration for 4 wks on glucose tolerance and pancreatic islet β-cell function in male Sprague-Dawley rats [72].

In conclusion, MG and AGEs are very likely to be involved in the initiation and or progression of the aging process. Commonly available pharmacological compounds to investigate these roles of MG and AGEs, such as aminoguanidine, are non-specific, whereas some of the newer compounds appear promising in inhibiting AGEs formation at multiple steps in the pathway in *in vitro* studies. However, more *in vivo* studies are required before their therapeutic potential can be established. A more dedicated effort is necessary to identify newer anti-MG and anti-AGEs compounds which are more specific and safer before more can be done about their therapeutic potential.

12. References

[1] Hayflick, L. The limited in vitro lifetime of human diploid cell strains. *Exp. Cell Res.* 37: 614-636; 1965.

[2] Kovacic, J. C.; Moreno, P.; Hachinski, V.; Nabel, E. G.; Fuster, V. Cellular senescence, vascular disease, and aging: Part 1 of a 2-part review. *Circulation* 123:1650-1660; 2011.

[3] Kovacic, J. C.; Moreno, P.; Nabel, E. G.; Hachinski, V.; Fuster, V. Cellular senescence, vascular disease, and aging: Part 2 of a 2-part review: Clinical vascular disease in the elderly. *Circulation* 123:1900-1910; 2011.

[4] Matthews, C.; Gorenne, I.; Scott, S.; Figg, N.; Kirkpatrick, P.; Ritchie, A.; Goddard, M.; Bennett, M. Vascular smooth muscle cells undergo telomere-based senescence in human atherosclerosis: Effects of telomerase and oxidative stress. *Circ. Res.* 99:156-164; 2006.

[5] Campisi, J.; d'Adda di Fagagna, F. Cellular senescence: When bad things happen to good cells. *Nat. Rev. Mol. Cell Biol.* 8:729-740; 2007.

[6] Bucala, R.; Model, P.; Cerami, A. Modification of DNA by reducing sugars: A possible mechanism for nucleic acid aging and age-related dysfunction in gene expression. *Proc. Natl. Acad. Sci. U. S. A.* 81:105-109; 1984.

[7] Beckman, K. B.; Ames, B. N. The free radical theory of aging matures. *Physiol. Rev.*78:547-581; 1998.
[8] Finkel, T.; Holbrook, N. J. Oxidants, oxidative stress and the biology of ageing. *Nature* 408:239-247; 2000.
[9] Barja, G.; Herrero, A. Oxidative damage to mitochondrial DNA is inversely related to maximum life span in the heart and brain of mammals. *FASEB J.* 14:312-318; 2000.
[10] Mandavilli, B. S.; Santos, J. H.; Van Houten, B. Mitochondrial DNA repair and aging. *Mutat. Res.* 509:127-151; 2002.
[11] Vina, J.; Borras, C.; Miquel, J. Theories of ageing. *IUBMB Life*59:249-254; 2007.
[12] Weinert, B. T.; Timiras, P. S. Invited review: Theories of aging. *J. Appl. Physiol.* 95:1706-1716; 2003.
[13] Semsei, I. On the nature of aging. *Mech. Ageing Dev.* 117:93-108; 2000.
[14] Medvedev, Z. A. An attempt at a rational classification of theories of ageing. *Biol. Rev. Camb. Philos. Soc.* 65:375-398; 1990.
[15] [Anonymous]. Max rubner--1854-1932. energy physiologist. *JAMA* 194:86-87; 1965.
[16] Commoner, B.; Townsend, J.; Pake, G. E. Free radicals in biological materials. *Nature* 174:689-691; 1954.
[17] Desai, K. M.; Wu, L. Free radical generation by methylglyoxal in tissues. *Drug Metabol. Drug Interact.* 23:151-173; 2008.
[18] McCord, J. M. The evolution of free radicals and oxidative stress. *Am. J. Med.* 108:652-659; 2000.
[19] Cadenas, E. Biochemistry of oxygen toxicity. *Annu. Rev. Biochem.* 58:79-110; 1989.
[20] Halliwell, B. Antioxidant defence mechanisms: From the beginning to the end (of the beginning). *Free Radic. Res.* 31:261-272; 1999.
[21] Halliwell, B. Reactive oxygen species in living systems: Source, biochemistry, and role in human disease. *Am. J. Med.* 91:14S-22S; 1991.
[22] Gilca, M.; Stoian, I.; Atanasiu, V.; Virgolici, B. The oxidative hypothesis of senescence. *J. Postgrad. Med.* 53:207-213; 2007.
[23] Harman, D. Aging: A theory based on free radical and radiation chemistry. *J. Gerontol.* 11:298-300; 1956.
[24] McCord, J. M.; Fridovich, I. Superoxide dismutase. an enzymic function for erythrocuprein (hemocuprein). *J. Biol. Chem.* 244:6049-6055; 1969.
[25] Harman, D. Aging: Overview. *Ann. N. Y. Acad. Sci.* 928:1-21; 2001.
[26] Gruber, J.; Schaffer, S.; Halliwell, B. The mitochondrial free radical theory of ageing--where do we stand? *Front. Biosci.* 13:6554-6579; 2008.
[27] Ku, H. H.; Brunk, U. T.; Sohal, R. S. Relationship between mitochondrial superoxide and hydrogen peroxide production and longevity of mammalian species. *Free Radic. Biol. Med.* 15:621-627; 1993.
[28] Herrero, A.; Barja, G. Sites and mechanisms responsible for the low rate of free radical production of heart mitochondria in the long-lived pigeon. *Mech. Ageing Dev.* 98:95-111; 1997.
[29] Johnson, T. E.; Tedesco, P. M.; Lithgow, G. J. Comparing mutants, selective breeding, and transgenics in the dissection of aging processes of caenorhabditis elegans. *Genetica* 91:65-77; 1993.
[30] Larsen, P. L. Aging and resistance to oxidative damage in caenorhabditis elegans. *Proc. Natl. Acad. Sci. U. S. A.* 90:8905-8909; 1993.

[31] Tower, J. Transgenic methods for increasing drosophila life span. *Mech. Ageing Dev.* 118:1-14; 2000.

[32] Arking, R.; Burde, V.; Graves, K.; Hari, R.; Feldman, E.; Zeevi, A.; Soliman, S.; Saraiya, A.; Buck, S.; Vettraino, J.; Sathrasala, K.; Wehr, N.; Levine, R. L. Forward and reverse selection for longevity in drosophila is characterized by alteration of antioxidant gene expression and oxidative damage patterns. *Exp. Gerontol.* 35:167-185; 2000.

[33] Schriner, S. E.; Linford, N. J.; Martin, G. M.; Treuting, P.; Ogburn, C. E.; Emond, M.; Coskun, P. E.; Ladiges, W.; Wolf, N.; Van Remmen, H.; Wallace, D. C.; Rabinovitch, P. S. Extension of murine life span by overexpression of catalase targeted to mitochondria. *Science* 308:1909-1911; 2005.

[34] Perez-Campo, R.; Lopez-Torres, M.; Cadenas, S.; Rojas, C.; Barja, G. The rate of free radical production as a determinant of the rate of aging: Evidence from the comparative approach. *J. Comp. Physiol. [B]*.168:149-158; 1998.

[35] Huang, T. T.; Carlson, E. J.; Gillespie, A. M.; Shi, Y.; Epstein, C. J. Ubiquitous overexpression of CuZn superoxide dismutase does not extend life span in mice. *J. Gerontol. A Biol. Sci. Med. Sci.* 55:B5-9; 2000.

[36] Perez, V. I.; Van Remmen, H.; Bokov, A.; Epstein, C. J.; Vijg, J.; Richardson, A. The overexpression of major antioxidant enzymes does not extend the lifespan of mice. *Aging Cell.* 8:73-75; 2009.

[37] Mehlhorn, R. J. *Oxidants and antioxidanrs in aging. in: Physiological basis of aging and geriatrics.* Boca Raton, FL:CRC; 2003.

[38] Linster, C. L.; Van Schaftingen, E. Vitamin C. biosynthesis, recycling and degradation in mammals. *FEBS J.* 274:1-22; 2007.

[39] Maeda, N.; Hagihara, H.; Nakata, Y.; Hiller, S.; Wilder, J.; Reddick, R. Aortic wall damage in mice unable to synthesize ascorbic acid. *Proc. Natl. Acad. Sci. U. S. A.* 97:841-846; 2000.

[40] Muller, F. L.; Lustgarten, M. S.; Jang, Y.; Richardson, A.; Van Remmen, H. Trends in oxidative aging theories. *Free Radic. Biol. Med.* 43:477-503; 2007.

[41] McCay, C. M.; Crowell, M. F.; Maynard, L. A. The effect of retarded growth upon the length of life span and upon the ultimate body size. *J. Nutr.* 10:63-79; 1935.

[42] Weindruch, R.; Walford, R. L. *The retardation of aging and disease by dietary restriction.* Springfield IL: Charles C. Thomas.; 1988.

[43] Simic, M. G.; Bertgold, D. S. *Urinary biomarkers of oxidative DNA base damage and human caloric intake. in: Biological effects of dietary restriction.* New York: Springer-Verlag.; 1991.

[44] Szatrowski, T. P.; Nathan, C. F. Production of large amounts of hydrogen peroxide by human tumor cells. *Cancer Res.*51:794-798; 1991.

[45] Thornalley, P. J. Pharmacology of methylglyoxal: Formation, modification of proteins and nucleic acids, and enzymatic detoxification--a role in pathogenesis and antiproliferative chemotherapy. *Gen. Pharmacol.* 27:565-573; 1996.

[46] Kalapos, M. P. Methylglyoxal in living organisms: Chemistry, biochemistry, toxicology and biological implications. *Toxicol. Lett.* 110:145-175; 1999.

[47] Phillips, S. A.; Thornalley, P. J. The formation of methylglyoxal from triose phosphates. investigation using a specific assay for methylglyoxal. *Eur. J. Biochem.* 212:101-105; 1993.

[48] Sato, J.; Wang, Y. M.; van Eys, J. Methylglyoxal formation in rat liver cells. *J. Biol. Chem.* 255:2046-2050; 1980.

[49] Kalapos, M. P. The tandem of free radicals and methylglyoxal. *Chem. Biol. Interact.* 171:251-271; 2008.

[50] Hopper, D. J.; Cooper, R. A. The regulation of escherichia coli methylglyoxal synthase; a new control site in glycolysis? *FEBS Lett.* 13:213-216; 1971.

[51] Ray, S.; Ray, M. Isolation of methylglyoxal synthase from goat liver. *J. Biol. Chem.* 256:6230-6233; 1981.

[52] Lyles, G. A.; Chalmers, J. The metabolism of aminoacetone to methylglyoxal by semicarbazide-sensitive amine oxidase in human umbilical artery. *Biochem. Pharmacol.* 43:1409-1414; 1992.

[53] Deng, Y.; Yu, P. H. Simultaneous determination of formaldehyde and methylglyoxal in urine: Involvement of semicarbazide-sensitive amine oxidase-mediated deamination in diabetic complications. *J. Chromatogr. Sci.* 37:317-322; 1999.

[54] Casazza, J. P.; Felver, M. E.; Veech, R. L. The metabolism of acetone in rat. *J. Biol. Chem.* 259:231-236; 1984.

[55] Yu, P. H.; Wright, S.; Fan, E. H.; Lun, Z. R.; Gubisne-Harberle, D. Physiological and pathological implications of semicarbazide-sensitive amine oxidase. *Biochim. Biophys. Acta* 1647:193-199; 2003.

[56] Lyles, G. A.; Chalmers, J. Aminoacetone metabolism by semicarbazide-sensitive amine oxidase in rat aorta. *Biochem. Pharmacol.* 49:416-419; 1995.

[57] Vander Jagt D.L. *The glyoxalase system. in: Glutathione: Chemical, biochemical and medical aspects - part A.* John Wiley & Sons Inc.; 1989.

[58] Thornalley, P. J. Glyoxalase I--structure, function and a critical role in the enzymatic defence against glycation. *Biochem. Soc. Trans.* 31:1343-1348; 2003.

[59] Thornalley, P. J. The glyoxalase system in health and disease. *Mol. Aspects Med.* 14:287-371; 1993.

[60] Blakytny, R.; Harding, J. J. Glycation (non-enzymic glycosylation) inactivates glutathione reductase. *Biochem. J.* 288 (Pt 1):303-307; 1992.

[61] Wang, X.; Desai, K.; Chang, T.; Wu, L. Vascular methylglyoxal metabolism and the development of hypertension. *J. Hypertens.* 23:1565-1573; 2005.

[62] Wu, L.; Juurlink, B. H. Increased methylglyoxal and oxidative stress in hypertensive rat vascular smooth muscle cells. *Hypertension* 39:809-814; 2002.

[63] Wang, X.; Chang, T.; Jiang, B.; Desai, K.; Wu, L. Attenuation of hypertension development by aminoguanidine in spontaneously hypertensive rats: Role of methylglyoxal. *Am. J. Hypertens.* 20:629-636; 2007.

[64] Wang, X.; Desai, K.; Clausen, J. T.; Wu, L. Increased methylglyoxal and advanced glycation end products in kidney from spontaneously hypertensive rats. *Kidney Int.* 66:2315-2321; 2004.

[65] Wang, X.; Jia, X.; Chang, T.; Desai, K.; Wu, L. Attenuation of hypertension development by scavenging methylglyoxal in fructose-treated rats. *J. Hypertens.* 26:765-772; 2008.

[66] Dhar, A.; Desai, K. M.; Wu, L. Alagebrium attenuates acute methylglyoxal-induced glucose intolerance in sprague-dawley rats. *Br. J. Pharmacol.* 159:166-175; 2010.

[67] Wang, H.; Meng, Q. H.; Gordon, J. R.; Khandwala, H.; Wu, L. Proinflammatory and proapoptotic effects of methylglyoxal on neutrophils from patients with type 2 diabetes mellitus. *Clin. Biochem.* 40:1232-1239; 2007.

[68] McLellan, A. C.; Thornalley, P. J.; Benn, J.; Sonksen, P. H. Glyoxalase system in clinical diabetes mellitus and correlation with diabetic complications. *Clin. Sci. (Lond)* 87:21-29; 1994.

[69] Jia, X.; Olson, D. J.; Ross, A. R.; Wu, L. Structural and functional changes in human insulin induced by methylglyoxal. *FASEB J.* 20:1555-1557; 2006.

[70] Jia, X.; Wu, L. Accumulation of endogenous methylglyoxal impaired insulin signaling in adipose tissue of fructose-fed rats. *Mol. Cell. Biochem.*306:133-139; 2007.

[71] Riboulet-Chavey, A.; Pierron, A.; Durand, I.; Murdaca, J.; Giudicelli, J.; Van Obberghen, E. Methylglyoxal impairs the insulin signaling pathways independently of the formation of intracellular reactive oxygen species. *Diabetes* 55:1289-1299; 2006.

[72] Dhar, A.; Dhar, I.; Jiang, B.; Desai, K. M.; Wu, L. Chronic methylglyoxal infusion by minipump causes pancreatic beta-cell dysfunction and induces type 2 diabetes in sprague-dawley rats. *Diabetes* 60:899-908; 2011.

[73] Baynes JW Thorpe SR. Role of oxidative stress in diabetic complications: A new perspective on an old paradigm. *Diabetes* 48:1-9; 1999.

[74] Baynes, J. W. From life to death--the struggle between chemistry and biology during aging: The maillard reaction as an amplifier of genomic damage. *Biogerontology* 1:235-246; 2000.

[75] Baynes, J. W.; Thorpe, S. R. Glycoxidation and lipoxidation in atherogenesis. *Free Radic. Biol. Med.* 28:1708-1716; 2000.

[76] Kuhla, B.; Luth, H. J.; Haferburg, D.; Boeck, K.; Arendt, T.; Munch, G. Methylglyoxal, glyoxal, and their detoxification in alzheimer's disease. *Ann. N. Y. Acad. Sci.* 1043:211-216; 2005.

[77] Yu, P. H. Involvement of cerebrovascular semicarbazide-sensitive amine oxidase in the pathogenesis of alzheimer's disease and vascular dementia. *Med. Hypotheses* 57:175-179; 2001.

[78] Singh, R.; Barden, A.; Mori, T.; Beilin, L. Advanced glycation end-products: A review. *Diabetologia*44:129-146; 2001.

[79] Vlassara, H.; Bucala, R.; Striker, L. Pathogenic effects of advanced glycosylation: Biochemical, biologic, and clinical implications for diabetes and aging. *Lab. Invest.* 70:138-151; 1994.

[80] Baynes, J. W. The role of AGEs in aging: Causation or correlation. *Exp. Gerontol.* 36:1527-1537; 2001.

[81] Wolff, S. P.; Bascal, Z. A.; Hunt, J. V. "Autoxidative glycosylation": Free radicals and glycation theory. *Prog. Clin. Biol. Res.* 304:259-275; 1989.

[82] Glomb, M. A.; Monnier, V. M. Mechanism of protein modification by glyoxal and glycolaldehyde, reactive intermediates of the maillard reaction. *J. Biol. Chem.* 270:10017-10026; 1995.

[83] Khalifah, R. G.; Baynes, J. W.; Hudson, B. G. Amadorins: Novel post-amadori inhibitors of advanced glycation reactions. *Biochem. Biophys. Res. Commun.* 257:251-258; 1999.

[84] Kilhovd, B. K.; Giardino, I.; Torjesen, P. A.; Birkeland, K. I.; Berg, T. J.; Thornalley, P. J.; Brownlee, M.; Hanssen, K. F. Increased serum levels of the specific AGE-compound methylglyoxal-derived hydroimidazolone in patients with type 2 diabetes. *Metabolism* 52:163-167; 2003.

[85] Mostafa, A. A.; Randell, E. W.; Vasdev, S. C.; Gill, V. D.; Han, Y.; Gadag, V.; Raouf, A. A.; El Said, H. Plasma protein advanced glycation end products, carboxymethyl

cysteine, and carboxyethyl cysteine, are elevated and related to nephropathy in patients with diabetes. *Mol. Cell. Biochem.* 302:35-42; 2007.

[86] Jana, C. K.; Das, N.; Sohal, R. S. Specificity of age-related carbonylation of plasma proteins in the mouse and rat. *Arch. Biochem. Biophys.* 397:433-439; 2002.

[87] Poggioli, S.; Bakala, H.; Friguet, B. Age-related increase of protein glycation in peripheral blood lymphocytes is restricted to preferential target proteins. *Exp. Gerontol.* 37:1207-1215; 2002.

[88] Shipanova, I. N.; Glomb, M. A.; Nagaraj, R. H. Protein modification by methylglyoxal: Chemical nature and synthetic mechanism of a major fluorescent adduct. *Arch. Biochem. Biophys.* 344:29-36; 1997.

[89] Glomb, M. A.; Rosch, D.; Nagaraj, R. H. N(delta)-(5-hydroxy-4,6-dimethylpyrimidine-2-yl)-l-ornithine, a novel methylglyoxal-arginine modification in beer. *J. Agric. Food Chem.* 49:366-372; 2001.

[90] Ahmed, M. U.; Brinkmann Frye, E.; Degenhardt, T. P.; Thorpe, S. R.; Baynes, J. W. N-epsilon-(carboxyethyl)lysine, a product of the chemical modification of proteins by methylglyoxal, increases with age in human lens proteins. *Biochem. J.* 324 (Pt 2):565-570; 1997.

[91] Chellan, P.; Nagaraj, R. H. Protein crosslinking by the maillard reaction: Dicarbonyl-derived imidazolium crosslinks in aging and diabetes. *Arch. Biochem. Biophys.* 368:98-104; 1999.

[92] Konishi, Y.; Hayase, F.; Kato, K. Novel imidazolones compound formed by the advanced maillard reaction of 3-deoxyglucosone and arginine residues in proteins. *Biosci Biotechnol Biochem* 58:1953-1955; 1994.

[93] Uchida, K.; Khor, O. T.; Oya, T.; Osawa, T.; Yasuda, Y.; Miyata, T. Protein modification by a maillard reaction intermediate methylglyoxal. immunochemical detection of fluorescent 5-methylimidazolone derivatives in vivo. *FEBS Lett.* 410:313-318; 1997.

[94] Chang, T.; Wang, R.; Wu, L. Methylglyoxal-induced nitric oxide and peroxynitrite production in vascular smooth muscle cells. *Free Radic. Biol. Med.* 38:286-293; 2005.

[95] Dhar, A.; Desai, K.; Kazachmov, M.; Yu, P.; Wu, L. Methylglyoxal production in vascular smooth muscle cells from different metabolic precursors. *Metabolism* 57:1211-1220; 2008.

[96] Wang, H.; Liu, J.; Wu, L. Methylglyoxal-induced mitochondrial dysfunction in vascular smooth muscle cells. *Biochem. Pharmacol.* In press; 2009.

[97] Ho, C.; Lee, P. H.; Huang, W. J.; Hsu, Y. C.; Lin, C. L.; Wang, J. Y. Methylglyoxal-induced fibronectin gene expression through ras-mediated NADPH oxidase activation in renal mesangial cells. *Nephrology (Carlton)* 12:348-356; 2007.

[98] Ward, R. A.; McLeish, K. R. Methylglyoxal: A stimulus to neutrophil oxygen radical production in chronic renal failure? *Nephrol. Dial. Transplant.* 19:1702-1707; 2004.

[99] Leoncini, G.; Poggi, M. Effects of methylglyoxal on platelet hydrogen peroxide accumulation, aggregation and release reaction. *Cell Biochem. Funct.* 14:89-95; 1996.

[100] Kalapos, M. P.; Littauer, A.; de Groot, H. Has reactive oxygen a role in methylglyoxal toxicity? A study on cultured rat hepatocytes. *Arch. Toxicol.* 67:369-372; 1993.

[101] Di Loreto, S.; Caracciolo, V.; Colafarina, S.; Sebastiani, P.; Gasbarri, A.; Amicarelli, F. Methylglyoxal induces oxidative stress-dependent cell injury and up-regulation of interleukin-1beta and nerve growth factor in cultured hippocampal neuronal cells. *Brain Res.* 1006:157-167; 2004.

[102] Akhand, A. A.; Hossain, K.; Mitsui, H.; Kato, M.; Miyata, T.; Inagi, R.; Du, J.; Takeda, K.; Kawamoto, Y.; Suzuki, H.; Kurokawa, K.; Nakashima, I. Glyoxal and methylglyoxal trigger distinct signals for map family kinases and caspase activation in human endothelial cells. *Free Radic. Biol. Med.* 31:20-30; 2001.

[103] Kikuchi, S.; Shinpo, K.; Moriwaka, F.; Makita, Z.; Miyata, T.; Tashiro, K. Neurotoxicity of methylglyoxal and 3-deoxyglucosone on cultured cortical neurons: Synergism between glycation and oxidative stress, possibly involved in neurodegenerative diseases. *J. Neurosci. Res.*57:280-289; 1999.

[104] Amicarelli, F.; Colafarina, S.; Cattani, F.; Cimini, A.; Di Ilio, C.; Ceru, M. P.; Miranda, M. Scavenging system efficiency is crucial for cell resistance to ROS-mediated methylglyoxal injury. *Free Radic. Biol. Med.* 35:856-871; 2003.

[105] Pacher, P.; Beckman, J. S.; Liaudet, L. Nitric oxide and peroxynitrite in health and disease. *Physiol. Rev.* 87:315-424; 2007.

[106] Nicolay, J. P.; Schneider, J.; Niemoeller, O. M.; Artunc, F.; Portero-Otin, M.; Haik, G.,Jr; Thornalley, P. J.; Schleicher, E.; Wieder, T.; Lang, F. Stimulation of suicidal erythrocyte death by methylglyoxal. *Cell. Physiol. Biochem.* 18:223-232; 2006.

[107] Beard, K. M.; Shangari, N.; Wu, B.; O'Brien, P. J. Metabolism, not autoxidation, plays a role in alpha-oxoaldehyde- and reducing sugar-induced erythrocyte GSH depletion: Relevance for diabetes mellitus. *Mol. Cell. Biochem.* 252:331-338; 2003.

[108] Park, Y. S.; Koh, Y. H.; Takahashi, M.; Miyamoto, Y.; Suzuki, K.; Dohmae, N.; Takio, K.; Honke, K.; Taniguchi, N. Identification of the binding site of methylglyoxal on glutathione peroxidase: Methylglyoxal inhibits glutathione peroxidase activity via binding to glutathione binding sites arg 184 and 185. *Free Radic. Res.* 37:205-211; 2003.

[109] Paget, C.; Lecomte, M.; Ruggiero, D.; Wiernsperger, N.; Lagarde, M. Modification of enzymatic antioxidants in retinal microvascular cells by glucose or advanced glycation end products. *Free Radic. Biol. Med.* 25:121-129; 1998.

[110] Juurlink, B. H. Management of oxidative stress in the CNS: The many roles of glutathione. *Neurotox Res.* 1:119-140; 1999.

[111] Rondeau, P.; Singh, N. R.; Caillens, H.; Tallet, F.; Bourdon, E. Oxidative stresses induced by glycoxidized human or bovine serum albumin on human monocytes. *Free Radic. Biol. Med.* 45:799-812; 2008.

[112] Gawlowski, T.; Stratmann, B.; Stirban, A. O.; Negrean, M.; Tschoepe, D. AGEs and methylglyoxal induce apoptosis and expression of mac-1 on neutrophils resulting in platelet-neutrophil aggregation. *Thromb. Res.* 121:117-126; 2007.

[113] Chance, B.; Oshino, N.; Sugano, T.; Mayevsky, A. Basic principles of tissue oxygen determination from mitochondrial signals. *Adv. Exp. Med. Biol.* 37A:277-292; 1973.

[114] Turrens, J. F.; Boveris, A. Generation of superoxide anion by the NADH dehydrogenase of bovine heart mitochondria. *Biochem. J.*191:421-427; 1980.

[115] Turrens, J. F. Superoxide production by the mitochondrial respiratory chain. *Biosci. Rep.* 17:3-8; 1997.

[116] Rosca, M. G.; Mustata, T. G.; Kinter, M. T.; Ozdemir, A. M.; Kern, T. S.; Szweda, L. I.; Brownlee, M.; Monnier, V. M.; Weiss, M. F. Glycation of mitochondrial proteins from diabetic rat kidney is associated with excess superoxide formation. *Am. J. Physiol. Renal Physiol.* 289:F420-30; 2005.

[117] Rabbani, N.; Thornalley, P. J. Dicarbonyls linked to damage in the powerhouse: Glycation of mitochondrial proteins and oxidative stress. *Biochem. Soc. Trans.* 36:1045-1050; 2008.

[118] Vander Jagt, D. L. Methylglyoxal, diabetes mellitus and diabetic complications. *Drug Metabol. Drug Interact.* 23:93-124; 2008.

[119] Ando, K.; Beppu, M.; Kikugawa, K.; Nagai, R.; Horiuchi, S. Membrane proteins of human erythrocytes are modified by advanced glycation end products during aging in the circulation. *Biochem. Biophys. Res. Commun.* 258:123-127; 1999.

[120] Li, Y. M.; Steffes, M.; Donnelly, T.; Liu, C.; Fuh, H.; Basgen, J.; Bucala, R.; Vlassara, H. Prevention of cardiovascular and renal pathology of aging by the advanced glycation inhibitor aminoguanidine. *Proc. Natl. Acad. Sci. U. S. A.*93:3902-3907; 1996.

[121] Kilhovd, B. K.; Giardino, I.; Torjesen, P. A.; Birkeland, K. I.; Berg, T. J.; Thornalley, P. J.; Brownlee, M.; Hanssen, K. F. Increased serum levels of the specific AGE-compound methylglyoxal-derived hydroimidazolone in patients with type 2 diabetes. *Metabolism* 52:163-167; 2003.

[122] Degenhardt, T. P.; Thorpe, S. R.; Baynes, J. W. Chemical modification of proteins by methylglyoxal. *Cell. Mol. Biol. (Noisy-Le-Grand)* 44:1139-1145; 1998.

[123] Sugimoto, K.; Nishizawa, Y.; Horiuchi, S.; Yagihashi, S. Localization in human diabetic peripheral nerve of N(epsilon)-carboxymethyllysine-protein adducts, an advanced glycation endproduct. *Diabetologia* 40:1380-1387; 1997.

[124] Lo, T. W.; Westwood, M. E.; McLellan, A. C.; Selwood, T.; Thornalley, P. J. Binding and modification of proteins by methylglyoxal under physiological conditions. A kinetic and mechanistic study with N alpha-acetylarginine, N alpha-acetylcysteine, and N alpha-acetyllysine, and bovine serum albumin. *J. Biol. Chem.* 269:32299-32305; 1994.

[125] Oya, T.; Hattori, N.; Mizuno, Y.; Miyata, S.; Maeda, S.; Osawa, T.; Uchida, K. Methylglyoxal modification of protein. chemical and immunochemical characterization of methylglyoxal-arginine adducts. *J. Biol. Chem.* 274:18492-18502; 1999.

[126] Kikuchi, S.; Shinpo, K.; Takeuchi, M.; Yamagishi, S.; Makita, Z.; Sasaki, N.; Tashiro, K. Glycation--a sweet tempter for neuronal death. *Brain Res. Brain Res. Rev.* 41:306-323; 2003.

[127] Westwood, M. E.; Thornalley, P. J. Induction of synthesis and secretion of interleukin 1 beta in the human monocytic THP-1 cells by human serum albumins modified with methylglyoxal and advanced glycation endproducts. *Immunol. Lett.* 50:17-21; 1996.

[128] Wautier, M. P.; Chappey, O.; Corda, S.; Stern, D. M.; Schmidt, A. M.; Wautier, J. L. Activation of NADPH oxidase by AGE links oxidant stress to altered gene expression via RAGE. *Am. J. Physiol. Endocrinol. Metab.* 280:E685-94; 2001.

[129] Basta, G.; Lazzerini, G.; Massaro, M.; Simoncini, T.; Tanganelli, P.; Fu, C.; Kislinger, T.; Stern, D. M.; Schmidt, A. M.; De Caterina, R. Advanced glycation end products activate endothelium through signal-transduction receptor RAGE: A mechanism for amplification of inflammatory responses. *Circulation* 105:816-822; 2002.

[130] Chen, J.; Brodsky, S. V.; Goligorsky, D. M.; Hampel, D. J.; Li, H.; Gross, S. S.; Goligorsky, M. S. Glycated collagen I induces premature senescence-like phenotypic changes in endothelial cells. *Circ. Res.* 90:1290-1298; 2002.

[131] Thornalley, P. J. Cell activation by glycated proteins. AGE receptors, receptor recognition factors and functional classification of AGEs. *Cell. Mol. Biol. (Noisy-Le-Grand)* 44:1013-1023; 1998.

[132] Bierhaus, A.; Chevion, S.; Chevion, M.; Hofmann, M.; Quehenberger, P.; Illmer, T.; Luther, T.; Berentshtein, E.; Tritschler, H.; Muller, M.; Wahl, P.; Ziegler, R.; Nawroth, P. P. Advanced glycation end product-induced activation of NF-kappaB is suppressed by alpha-lipoic acid in cultured endothelial cells. *Diabetes* 46:1481-1490; 1997.

[133] Asif, M.; Egan, J.; Vasan, S.; Jyothirmayi, G. N.; Masurekar, M. R.; Lopez, S.; Williams, C.; Torres, R. L.; Wagle, D.; Ulrich, P.; Cerami, A.; Brines, M.; Regan, T. J. An advanced glycation endproduct cross-link breaker can reverse age-related increases in myocardial stiffness. *Proc. Natl. Acad. Sci. U. S. A.* 97:2809-2813; 2000.

[134] Scuteri, A. Slowing arterial aging: How far have we progressed? *J. Hypertens.* 25:509-510; 2007.

[135] Uribarri, J.; Cai, W.; Peppa, M.; Goodman, S.; Ferrucci, L.; Striker, G.; Vlassara, H. Circulating glycotoxins and dietary advanced glycation endproducts: Two links to inflammatory response, oxidative stress, and aging. *J. Gerontol. A Biol. Sci. Med. Sci.* 62:427-433; 2007.

[136] Mailankot, M.; Padmanabha, S.; Pasupuleti, N.; Major, D.; Howell, S.; Nagaraj, R. H. Glyoxalase I activity and immunoreactivity in the aging human lens. *Biogerontology* 2009.

[137] Corstjens, H.; Declercq, L.; Hellemans, L.; Sente, I.; Maes, D. Prevention of oxidative damage that contributes to the loss of bioenergetic capacity in ageing skin. *Exp. Gerontol.* 42:924-929; 2007.

[138] Morcos, M.; Du, X.; Pfisterer, F.; Hutter, H.; Sayed, A. A.; Thornalley, P.; Ahmed, N.; Baynes, J.; Thorpe, S.; Kukudov, G.; Schlotterer, A.; Bozorgmehr, F.; El Baki, R. A.; Stern, D.; Moehrlen, F.; Ibrahim, Y.; Oikonomou, D.; Hamann, A.; Becker, C.; Zeier, M.; Schwenger, V.; Miftari, N.; Humpert, P.; Hammes, H. P.; Buechler, M.; Bierhaus, A.; Brownlee, M.; Nawroth, P. P. Glyoxalase-1 prevents mitochondrial protein modification and enhances lifespan in caenorhabditis elegans. *Aging Cell.* 7:260-269; 2008.

[139] Scheckhuber, C. Q.; Mack, S. J.; Strobel, I.; Ricciardi, F.; Gispert, S.; Osiewacz, H. D. Modulation of the glyoxalase system in the aging model podospora anserina: Effects on growth and lifespan. *Aging (Albany NY)* 2:969-980; 2010.

[140] Sejersen, H.; Rattan, S. I. Dicarbonyl-induced accelerated aging in vitro in human skin fibroblasts. *Biogerontology* 10:203-211; 2009.

[141] Chappey, O.; Dosquet, C.; Wautier, M. P.; Wautier, J. L. Advanced glycation end products, oxidant stress and vascular lesions. *Eur. J. Clin. Invest.*27:97-108; 1997.

[142] Gillery, P. Advanced glycation end products (AGEs), free radicals and diabetes. *J. Soc. Biol.* 195:387-390; 2001.

[143] Kutlu, M.; Naziroglu, M.; Simsek, H.; Yilmaz, T.; Sahap Kukner, A. Moderate exercise combined with dietary vitamins C and E counteracts oxidative stress in the kidney and lens of streptozotocin-induced diabetic-rat. *Int. J. Vitam. Nutr. Res.* 75:71-80; 2005.

[144] Wondrak, G. T.; Cervantes-Laurean, D.; Roberts, M. J.; Qasem, J. G.; Kim, M.; Jacobson, E. L.; Jacobson, M. K. Identification of alpha-dicarbonyl scavengers for cellular protection against carbonyl stress. *Biochem. Pharmacol.* 63:361-373; 2002.

[145] Brownlee, M.; Vlassara, H.; Kooney, A.; Ulrich, P.; Cerami, A. Aminoguanidine prevents diabetes-induced arterial wall protein cross-linking. *Science* 232:1629-1632; 1986.

[146] Edelstein, D.; Brownlee, M. Mechanistic studies of advanced glycosylation end product inhibition by aminoguanidine. *Diabetes* 41:26-29; 1992.

[147] Beisswenger, P.; Ruggiero-Lopez, D. Metformin inhibition of glycation processes. *Diabetes Metab.* 29:6S95-103; 2003.

[148] Ruggiero-Lopez, D.; Lecomte, M.; Moinet, G.; Patereau, G.; Lagarde, M.; Wiernsperger, N. Reaction of metformin with dicarbonyl compounds. possible implication in the inhibition of advanced glycation end product formation. *Biochem. Pharmacol.* 58:1765-1773; 1999.

[149] Szwergold, B. S.; Kappler, F.; Brown, T. R. Identification of fructose 3-phosphate in the lens of diabetic rats. *Science* 247:451-454; 1990.

[150] Delpierre, G.; Rider, M. H.; Collard, F.; Stroobant, V.; Vanstapel, F.; Santos, H.; Van Schaftingen, E. Identification, cloning, and heterologous expression of a mammalian fructosamine-3-kinase. *Diabetes* 49:1627-1634; 2000.

[151] Saxena, A. K.; Saxena, P.; Monnier, V. M. Purification and characterization of a membrane-bound deglycating enzyme (1-deoxyfructosyl alkyl amino acid oxidase, EC 1.5.3) from a pseudomonas sp. soil strain. *J. Biol. Chem.* 271:32803-32809; 1996.

[152] Takahashi, M.; Pischetsrieder, M.; Monnier, V. M. Isolation, purification, and characterization of amadoriase isoenzymes (fructosyl amine-oxygen oxidoreductase EC 1.5.3) from aspergillus sp. *J. Biol. Chem.* 272:3437-3443; 1997.

[153] Vasan, S.; Zhang, X.; Zhang, X.; Kapurniotu, A.; Bernhagen, J.; Teichberg, S.; Basgen, J.; Wagle, D.; Shih, D.; Terlecky, I.; Bucala, R.; Cerami, A.; Egan, J.; Ulrich, P. An agent cleaving glucose-derived protein crosslinks in vitro and in vivo. *Nature* 382:275-278; 1996.

[154] Grandhee, S. K.; Monnier, V. M. Mechanism of formation of the maillard protein cross-link pentosidine. glucose, fructose, and ascorbate as pentosidine precursors. *J. Biol. Chem.* 266:11649-11653; 1991.

[155] Frye, E. B.; Degenhardt, T. P.; Thorpe, S. R.; Baynes, J. W. Role of the maillard reaction in aging of tissue proteins. advanced glycation end product-dependent increase in imidazolium cross-links in human lens proteins. *J. Biol. Chem.* 273:18714-18719; 1998.

[156] Nilsson, B. O. Biological effects of aminoguanidine: An update. *Inflamm. Res.* 48:509-515; 1999.

[157] SCHULER, W. The inhibition of histaminase. *Experientia* 8:230-232; 1952.

[158] Ivy, A. C.; Ivy, E. K.; Karvinen, E.; Lin, T. M. Effect of an histaminase inhibitor (aminoguanidine) on the gastric secretory response to exogenous histamine. *Am. J. Physiol.* 186:231-238; 1956.

[159] Corbett, J. A.; Tilton, R. G.; Chang, K.; Hasan, K. S.; Ido, Y.; Wang, J. L.; Sweetland, M. A.; Lancaster, J. R.,Jr; Williamson, J. R.; McDaniel, M. L. Aminoguanidine, a novel inhibitor of nitric oxide formation, prevents diabetic vascular dysfunction. *Diabetes* 41:552-556; 1992.

[160] Laszlo, F.; Evans, S. M.; Whittle, B. J. Aminoguanidine inhibits both constitutive and inducible nitric oxide synthase isoforms in rat intestinal microvasculature in vivo. *Eur. J. Pharmacol.* 272:169-175; 1995.

[161] Moncada, S.; Palmer, R. M.; Higgs, E. A. Nitric oxide: Physiology, pathophysiology, and pharmacology. *Pharmacol. Rev.* 43:109-142; 1991.

[162] Stjernborg, L.; Persson, L. Stabilization of S-adenosylmethionine decarboxylase by aminoguanidine. *Biochem. Pharmacol.* 45:1174-1176; 1993.

[163] Miyata, T.; van Ypersele de Strihou, C. Angiotensin II receptor blockers and angiotensin converting enzyme inhibitors: Implication of radical scavenging and transition metal chelation in inhibition of advanced glycation end product formation. *Arch. Biochem. Biophys.* 419:50-54; 2003.

[164] Sajithlal, G. B.; Chithra, P.; Chandrakasan, G. Advanced glycation end products induce crosslinking of collagen in vitro. *Biochim. Biophys. Acta* 1407:215-224; 1998.

[165] Corman, B.; Duriez, M.; Poitevin, P.; Heudes, D.; Bruneval, P.; Tedgui, A.; Levy, B. I. Aminoguanidine prevents age-related arterial stiffening and cardiac hypertrophy. *Proc. Natl. Acad. Sci. U. S. A.* 95:1301-1306; 1998.

[166] Seyer-Hansen, M.; Andreassen, T. T.; Oxlund, H.; Jorgensen, P. H. The influence of aminoguanidine on borohydride reducible collagen cross-links and wound strength. *Connect. Tissue Res.* 26:181-186; 1991.

[167] Ino-ue, M.; Ohgiya, N.; Yamamoto, M. Effect of aminoguanidine on optic nerve involvement in experimental diabetic rats. *Brain Res.* 800:319-322; 1998.

[168] Bolton, W. K.; Cattran, D. C.; Williams, M. E.; Adler, S. G.; Appel, G. B.; Cartwright, K.; Foiles, P. G.; Freedman, B. I.; Raskin, P.; Ratner, R. E.; Spinowitz, B. S.; Whittier, F. C.; Wuerth, J. P.; ACTION I Investigator Group. Randomized trial of an inhibitor of formation of advanced glycation end products in diabetic nephropathy. *Am. J. Nephrol.* 24:32-40; 2004.

[169] Freedman, B. I.; Wuerth, J. P.; Cartwright, K.; Bain, R. P.; Dippe, S.; Hershon, K.; Mooradian, A. D.; Spinowitz, B. S. Design and baseline characteristics for the aminoguanidine clinical trial in overt type 2 diabetic nephropathy (ACTION II). *Control. Clin. Trials* 20:493-510; 1999.

[170] Brown, C. D.; Zhao, Z. H.; Thomas, L. L.; deGroof, R.; Friedman, E. A. Effects of erythropoietin and aminoguanidine on red blood cell deformability in diabetic azotemic and uremic patients. *Am. J. Kidney Dis.* 38:1414-1420; 2001.

[171] Suji, G.; Sivakami, S. DNA damage by free radical production by aminoguanidine. *Ann. N. Y. Acad. Sci.* 1067:191-199; 2006.

[172] Beisswenger, P. J.; Howell, S. K.; Touchette, A. D.; Lal, S.; Szwergold, B. S. Metformin reduces systemic methylglyoxal levels in type 2 diabetes. *Diabetes*48:198-202; 1999.

[173] Rahbar, S.; Figarola, J. L. Novel inhibitors of advanced glycation endproducts. *Arch. Biochem. Biophys.* 419:63-79; 2003.

[174] Baynes, J. W. Role of oxidative stress in development of complications in diabetes. *Diabetes* 40:405-412; 1991.

[175] Ota, K.; Nakamura, J.; Li, W.; Kozakae, M.; Watarai, A.; Nakamura, N.; Yasuda, Y.; Nakashima, E.; Naruse, K.; Watabe, K.; Kato, K.; Oiso, Y.; Hamada, Y. Metformin prevents methylglyoxal-induced apoptosis of mouse schwann cells. *Biochem. Biophys. Res. Commun.* 357:270-275; 2007.

[176] Rabbani, N.; Godfrey, L.; Xue, M.; Shaheen, F.; Geoffrion, M.; Milne, R.; Thornalley, P. J. Glycation of LDL by methylglyoxal increases arterial atherogenicity: A possible contributor to increased risk of cardiovascular disease in diabetes. *Diabetes* 60:1973-1980; 2011.

[177] Rahbar, S.; Natarajan, R.; Yerneni, K.; Scott, S.; Gonzales, N.; Nadler, J. L. Evidence that pioglitazone, metformin and pentoxifylline are inhibitors of glycation. *Clin. Chim. Acta* 301:65-77; 2000.

[178] Hirasawa, Y.; Matsui, Y.; Ohtsu, S.; Yamane, K.; Toyoshi, T.; Kyuki, K.; Sakai, T.; Feng, Y.; Nagamatsu, T. Involvement of hyperglycemia in deposition of aggregated protein in glomeruli of diabetic mice. *Eur. J. Pharmacol.* 601:129-135; 2008.

[179] Millea, P. J. N-acetylcysteine: Multiple clinical applications. *Am. Fam. Physician* 80:265-269; 2009.

[180] Vasdev, S.; Ford, C. A.; Longerich, L.; Parai, S.; Gadag, V.; Wadhawan, S. Aldehyde induced hypertension in rats: Prevention by N-acetyl cysteine. *Artery* 23:10-36; 1998.

[181] Lauterburg, B. H.; Corcoran, G. B.; Mitchell, J. R. Mechanism of action of N-acetylcysteine in the protection against the hepatotoxicity of acetaminophen in rats in vivo. *J. Clin. Invest.* 71:980-991; 1983.

[182] Forbes, J. M.; Cooper, M. E.; Thallas, V.; Burns, W. C.; Thomas, M. C.; Brammar, G. C.; Lee, F.; Grant, S. L.; Burrell, L. M.; Jerums, G.; Osicka, T. M. Reduction of the accumulation of advanced glycation end products by ACE inhibition in experimental diabetic nephropathy. *Diabetes* 51:3274-3282; 2002.

[183] Izuhara, Y.; Nangaku, M.; Inagi, R.; Tominaga, N.; Aizawa, T.; Kurokawa, K.; van Ypersele de Strihou, C.; Miyata, T. Renoprotective properties of angiotensin receptor blockers beyond blood pressure lowering. *J. Am. Soc. Nephrol.* 16:3631-3641; 2005.

[184] Miyata, T.; van Ypersele de Strihou, C.; Ueda, Y.; Ichimori, K.; Inagi, R.; Onogi, H.; Ishikawa, N.; Nangaku, M.; Kurokawa, K. Angiotensin II receptor antagonists and angiotensin-converting enzyme inhibitors lower in vitro the formation of advanced glycation end products: Biochemical mechanisms. *J. Am. Soc. Nephrol.* 13:2478-2487; 2002.

[185] Nangaku, M.; Miyata, T.; Sada, T.; Mizuno, M.; Inagi, R.; Ueda, Y.; Ishikawa, N.; Yuzawa, H.; Koike, H.; van Ypersele de Strihou, C.; Kurokawa, K. Anti-hypertensive agents inhibit in vivo the formation of advanced glycation end products and improve renal damage in a type 2 diabetic nephropathy rat model. *J. Am. Soc. Nephrol.* 14:1212-1222; 2003.

[186] Rao, G. N.; Lardis, M. P.; Cotlier, E. Acetylation of lens crystallins: A possible mechanism by which aspirin could prevent cataract formation. *Biochem. Biophys. Res. Commun.* 128:1125-1132; 1985.

[187] Lin, P. P.; Barry, R. C.; Smith, D. L.; Smith, J. B. In vivo acetylation identified at lysine 70 of human lens alphaA-crystallin. *Protein Sci.*7:1451-1457; 1998.

[188] Ajiboye, R.; Harding, J. J. The non-enzymic glycosylation of bovine lens proteins by glucosamine and its inhibition by aspirin, ibuprofen and glutathione. *Exp. Eye Res.* 49:31-41; 1989.

[189] Raza, K.; Harding, J. J. Non-enzymic modification of lens proteins by glucose and fructose: Effects of ibuprofen. *Exp. Eye Res.* 52:205-212; 1991.

[190] van Boekel, M. A.; van den Bergh, P. J.; Hoenders, H. J. Glycation of human serum albumin: Inhibition by diclofenac. *Biochim. Biophys. Acta* 1120:201-204; 1992.

[191] Regensteiner, J. G.; Stewart, K. J. Established and evolving medical therapies for claudication in patients with peripheral arterial disease. *Nat. Clin. Pract. Cardiovasc. Med.* 3:604-610; 2006.

[192] Rahbar, S.; Natarajan, R.; Yerneni, K.; Scott, S.; Gonzales, N.; Nadler, J. L. Evidence that pioglitazone, metformin and pentoxifylline are inhibitors of glycation. *Clin. Chim. Acta* 301:65-77; 2000.

[193] Booth, A. A.; Khalifah, R. G.; Hudson, B. G. Thiamine pyrophosphate and pyridoxamine inhibit the formation of antigenic advanced glycation end-products: Comparison with aminoguanidine. *Biochem. Biophys. Res. Commun.* 220:113-119; 1996.

[194] Nagaraj, R. H.; Sarkar, P.; Mally, A.; Biemel, K. M.; Lederer, M. O.; Padayatti, P. S. Effect of pyridoxamine on chemical modification of proteins by carbonyls in diabetic rats: Characterization of a major product from the reaction of pyridoxamine and methylglyoxal. *Arch. Biochem. Biophys.* 402:110-119; 2002.

[195] Stitt, A.; Gardiner, T. A.; Alderson, N. L.; Canning, P.; Frizzell, N.; Duffy, N.; Boyle, C.; Januszewski, A. S.; Chachich, M.; Baynes, J. W.; Thorpe, S. R. The AGE inhibitor pyridoxamine inhibits development of retinopathy in experimental diabetes. *Diabetes* 51:2826-2832; 2002.

[196] Monnier, V. M. Bacterial enzymes that can deglycate glucose- and fructose-modified lysine. *Biochem. J.*392:e1-3; 2005.

[197] Horiuchi, T.; Kurokawa, T.; Saito, N. Purification and properties of fructosylamino acid oxidase from corynebacterium sp. 2-4-1. *Agri Biol Chem* 53:103-110; 1989.

[198] Horiuchi, T.; Kurokawa, T. Purification and properties of fructosylamine oxidase from aspergillus sp. 1005. *Agri Biol Chem* 55:333-338; 1991.

[199] Wiame, E.; Delpierre, G.; Collard, F.; Van Schaftingen, E. Identification of a pathway for the utilization of the amadori product fructoselysine in escherichia coli. *J. Biol. Chem.* 277:42523-42529; 2002.

[200] Wiame, E.; Van Schaftingen, E. Fructoselysine 3-epimerase, an enzyme involved in the metabolism of the unusual amadori compound psicoselysine in escherichia coli. *Biochem. J.*378:1047-1052; 2004.

[201] Wiame, E.; Lamosa, P.; Santos, H.; Van Schaftingen, E. Identification of glucoselysine-6-phosphate deglycase, an enzyme involved in the metabolism of the fructation product glucoselysine. *Biochem. J.* 392:263-269; 2005.

[202] Rahbar, S.; Kumar Yernini, K.; Scott, S.; Gonzales, N.; Lalezari, I. Novel inhibitors of advanced glycation endproducts. *Biochem. Biophys. Res. Commun.* 262:651-656; 1999.

[203] Rahbar, S.; Yerneni, K. K.; Scott, S.; Gonzales, N.; Lalezari, I. Novel inhibitors of advanced glycation endproducts (part II). *Mol. Cell Biol. Res. Commun.* 3:360-366; 2000.

[204] Ulrich, P.; Zhang, X. Pharmacological reversal of advanced glycation end-product-mediated protein crosslinking. *Diabetologia* 40 Suppl 2:S157-9; 1997.

[205] Wolffenbuttel, B. H.; Boulanger, C. M.; Crijns, F. R.; Huijberts, M. S.; Poitevin, P.; Swennen, G. N.; Vasan, S.; Egan, J. J.; Ulrich, P.; Cerami, A.; Levy, B. I. Breakers of advanced glycation end products restore large artery properties in experimental diabetes. *Proc. Natl. Acad. Sci. U. S. A.* 95:4630-4634; 1998.

[206] Guo, Y.; Lu, M.; Qian, J.; Cheng, Y. L. Alagebrium chloride protects the heart against oxidative stress in aging rats. *J. Gerontol. A Biol. Sci. Med. Sci.* 2009.

[207] Vaitkevicius, P. V.; Lane, M.; Spurgeon, H.; Ingram, D. K.; Roth, G. S.; Egan, J. J.; Vasan, S.; Wagle, D. R.; Ulrich, P.; Brines, M.; Wuerth, J. P.; Cerami, A.; Lakatta, E. G. A cross-link breaker has sustained effects on arterial and ventricular properties in older rhesus monkeys. *Proc. Natl. Acad. Sci. U. S. A.* 98:1171-1175; 2001.

[208] Kass, D. A.; Shapiro, E. P.; Kawaguchi, M.; Capriotti, A. R.; Scuteri, A.; deGroof, R. C.; Lakatta, E. G. Improved arterial compliance by a novel advanced glycation end-product crosslink breaker. *Circulation* 104:1464-1470; 2001.

[209] Zieman, S. J.; Melenovsky, V.; Clattenburg, L.; Corretti, M. C.; Capriotti, A.; Gerstenblith, G.; Kass, D. A. Advanced glycation endproduct crosslink breaker (alagebrium) improves endothelial function in patients with isolated systolic hypertension. *J. Hypertens.* 25:577-583; 2007.

[210] Little, W. C.; Zile, M. R.; Kitzman, D. W.; Hundley, W. G.; O'Brien, T. X.; Degroof, R. C. The effect of alagebrium chloride (ALT-711), a novel glucose cross-link breaker, in the treatment of elderly patients with diastolic heart failure. *J. Card. Fail.* 11:191-195; 2005.

[211] Bakris, G. L.; Bank, A. J.; Kass, D. A.; Neutel, J. M.; Preston, R. A.; Oparil, S. Advanced glycation end-product cross-link breakers. A novel approach to cardiovascular pathologies related to the aging process. *Am. J. Hypertens.* 17:23S-30S; 2004.

[212] Hartog, J. W.; Willemsen, S.; van Veldhuisen, D. J.; Posma, J. L.; van Wijk, L. M.; Hummel, Y. M.; Hillege, H. L.; Voors, A. A.; for the BENEFICIAL investigators. Effects of alagebrium, an advanced glycation endproduct breaker, on exercise tolerance and cardiac function in patients with chronic heart failure. *Eur. J. Heart Fail.* 13:899-908; 2011.

[213] Krautwald, M.; Leech, D.; Horne, S.; Steele, M. L.; Forbes, J.; Rahmadi, A.; Griffith, R.; Munch, G. The advanced glycation end product-lowering agent ALT-711 is a low-affinity inhibitor of thiamine diphosphokinase. *Rejuvenation Res.* 14:383-391; 2011.

31

Ethanol Interference on Adenosine System

Silvânia Vasconcelos et al.*
Federal University of Ceará, Department of Physiology and Pharmacology
Brazil

1. Introduction

It is well documented in literature a wide range of behavioral and physiological effects arising from ethanol intake (Spinetta et al., 2008; Soares et al., 2009; Brust, 2010). Because it is a substance that affects differently and simultaneously several neurotransmitter systems, covering different brain areas (Dahchour & De Witte, 2000; Vasconcelos et al., 2008; Vengeliene et al., 2008), it becomes complex to reveal the mechanism of action that governs its effects, being still a challenge for researchers. In addition, ethanol has a biphasic behavioral presenting an excitatory feature in the early stages and a depressant feature in its chronic use.

Among the wide range of pathways in central nervous system that are modified by ethanol, it is important to highlight those that explain ethanol diverse effects, like the ones releasing gamma-amynobutiric acid (GABA), glutamate, dopamine and norepinephrine (Kaneyuki et al., 1991; Vasconcelos et al., 2004). Moreover, another pathway that is rising on researches about ethanol effects is the adenosinergic system (Prediger et al., 2006; Thorsell et al., 2007).

Adenosine was described as a potent depressor of neuronal activity (Dunwiddie & Haas, 1985), and acts mainly via A1 receptor, which is a presynaptic inhibitor of the release of neurotransmitters such as dopamine, GABA, glutamate, acetylcholine and norepinephrine (Fredholm et al., 2001; Dunwiddie & Masino, 2001). Moreover, adenosine is involved in behavioral processes like motor function, anxiety, depression, reward and drug addiction, and human disorders such as Parkinson disease and schizophrenia (Moreau and Huber, 1999).

In addition, there is strong evidence of an involvement of the adenosinergic system on ethanol effects, including the extracellular increase of adenosine after acute exposure to ethanol (Krauss et al., 1993; Nagy et al., 1990), the accentuation or blockade of ethanol-induced motor incoordination provided by adenosine receptor agonists or antagonists, respectively (Dar, 2001; Soares et al., 2009), and the reduction of anxiogenic-like behavior in acute ethanol withdrawal (Prediger et al., 2006). Adenosine antagonists, like caffeine, are implicated in alcohol tolerance (Fillmore, 2003), and retrograde memory impairment caused by ethanol (Spinetta et al., 2008). Thus, adenosine receptors seem to modulate some of the

* Sarah Escudeiro[1], Ana Luíza Martin[1], Paula Soares[1], Antônio Vieira Filho[2], Larissa Silva[2], Kátia Cilene Dias[1], Danielle Macêdo[1], Francisca Cléa Sousa[1], Marta Fonteles[1] and Manoel Cláudio Patrocínio[2]
[1]*Federal University of Ceará, Department of Physiology and Pharmacology, Brazil*
[2]*College of Medicine Christus, Brazil*

pharmacological properties of ethanol, interacting with it by blocking or accentuating its properties.

2. Ethanol and adenosine relation in different neurotransmission systems

It's known in literature that ethanol alone interferes in different neurotransmitter systems, as GABAergic, glutamatergic, dopaminergic, serotonergic, noradrenergic, cholinergic and others, including adenosinic; however, its action on this last system has currently deserved more attention, due to its neuromodulator/neuroprotector action. Thus, in the present topic updates will be discussed on the relationship between ethanol and adenosine and its consequent interference in some systems above.

To better understand the association of ethanol and adenosine on different neurotransmitter systems, it is necessary to explore the likely hypotheses that explain how ethanol interferes with the adenosine system. Carmichael et al. (1991) suggested that a probable mechanism could occur via metabolism of ethanol by acetate, where this would be incorporated into acetyl-coenzyme A with subsequent formation of AMP, thereby directing the synthesis of adenosine.

Another possible mechanism of interaction between these two substances can be related to the fact that ethanol inhibits facilitated diffusion transporters, being the ENT1 (Equilibrative Nucleoside Transporter) an example, increasing the availability of extracellular adenosine (Diamond et al., 1991; Krauss et al., 1993). Finally, ethanol may facilitate the activation of receptors that have adenylate cyclase (AC) as intracellular signaling system (Rabin; Molinoff, 1981; Hoffman; Tabakoff, 1990), which is displayed by adenosine receptors. Therefore, there are different points of possible interference of the increased concentration of extracellular adenosine induced by ethanol on other neurotransmitter systems.

The GABAergic system in the striatum may be modulated by adenosine with regard to the effects of ethanol on motor coordination and sleep, involving cAMP (Meng; Dar, 1995; Meng et al., 1997). It was found that the use of adenosine agonists accentuate the reduction in the motor coordination induced by ethanol, whereas Ro15-4513, a weak partial inverse agonist of the benzodiazepine class of drugs, attenuated by blocking the effect of the first when used in combination (Meng; Dar, 1994, 1995), suggesting a participation via $GABA_A$ by an alteration in the conductance of chloride ions (Meng et al., 1997, Mohler et al., 1984). A mechanism suggested by Londos et al. (1980) and Van Calk et al. (1970) relates ethanol to alterations in the production of cAMP via AC through the A1 receptor, ie, increased availability of adenosine induced by ethanol leads to greater signs of adenosine on your receptor that has a higher affinity, which is related with inhibitory G protein, reducing cAMP production and concomitant modulation of the GABAergic system that increases chloride conductance.

This ratio adenosine/ethanol with the GABAergic system can still be related to opioid system, where ethanol induces the increased availability of β-endorphin which activates μtype receptors, altering the release of GABA in dopaminergic neurons in the ventral tegmental area, an area involved to reward behavior and abuse of ethanol (Mendez et al, 2003; Marinelli et al, 2004; Lam et al, 2008; Jarjour et al, 2009).

Indirectly, this relationship can also occur through ionotropic ATP receptors, that has the function of specific subtypes (P2X4R and P2X2R) inhibited by ethanol (Davies et al., 2002, 2005), altering the modulation of release of different substances such as GABA, glycine and glutamate (Mori et al., 2001; Papp et al., 2004).

Concerning the glutamatergic system, this one demonstrates relationship with the two subtypes of adenosine receptors A_1 and A_{2A}, once these receptors appear hetero-dimerized in glutamatergic nerve terminals in the striatum, modulating the concentration of glutamate in accordance with the availability of adenosine, where a lower concentration activates A_1R inhibiting glutamate release, and a higher concentration activates $A_{2A}R$, stimulating the release of glutamate and greater activation of the NMDA receptor. This regulates the release of dopamine in the nucleus accumbens stimulating higher consumption of ethanol (Ciruela et al., 2006; Quarta et al., 2004).

Another finding that reinforces the relationship ethanol/adenosine/glutamate is the synergic interaction that occurs between A_{2A} and mGluR5 receptors (which is related to the consumption of ethanol in the nucleus accumbens) in the striatum, that is, the co-activation of these receptors increases the phosphorylation of proteins regulated by dopamine and cAMP, increased ethanol consumption (Nishi et al., 2003). In addition, NMDA and A_1 receptors present a cross modulation on the negative effects of ethanol, like a reduction on motor coordination in the cerebellum, striatum and motor cortex (Mitchell; Neafsey; Collins, 2009). This relationship could be involved with the altered activity of Protein Kinase C (PKC) (Othman et al., 2002). This enzyme has a modulating function against the concentration of glycine, GABA internalization, externalization of NMDA expression of 5-HT3 (Chapell et al., 1998; Lan et al., 2001; Zhang et al., 1995; Sun et al., 2003).

Regarding the dopaminergic system, A_{2A} and D_2 receptors (as well as A_1 and D_1) exhibit dimerization between them, relating to the reward system in the striatum probably by modulation of AC activity by ethanol, leading to an increase in the concentration of cAMP and the activity of PKA, desensitizing D_2, and thus leading to an increased consumption of ethanol (Ferre et al., 2008; Mailliard & Diamond, 2004; Yao et al., 2002; 2003). A possible mechanism of the final response of the dimerized activation of these receptors is that ethanol desensitizes receptors linked to the stimulatory G protein (α subunit), modulating the coupling of D_2 with the AC pathway, which may be related to PKA (Yao et al., 2001; Batista et al., 2005). Inoue et al. (2007) found that co-activation of A_{2A} and D_2 mediates the transient interaction between nicotine and ethanol, showing an indirect relationship with the cholinergic system, where the use of antagonists of this co-activation can prevent, mitigate or even reverse the use of smoke and ethanol.

Indirectly, the adenosine system also maintains relation to the dopaminergic system via receptors P2XR which were identified in mesolimbic dopaminergic neurons, modulating their activity and, equivalently, the consumption of ethanol (Heine et al., 2007; Xiao et al., 2008).

Adenosine and serotonin systems are related in regard to ethanol via P2X receptors (P2XR). That is, 5-HT3 and P2XR are functionally coupled and both have their actions modulated by ethanol (inhibits P2X2 and P2X4 and stimulates 5-HT3), besides being involved with other neurotransmitter systems such as glycine, GABA, glutamate (mentioned above) and dopamine in the nucleus accumbens and ventral tegmental area (Davies et al., 2006).

Other neurotransmitters still present a few studies involving ethanol and the adenosine system, such as glycine, where ethanol inhibits their specific receptors probably via PKC (Tao & Ye, 2002), and taurine, which normalizes the activity of ATPases in tissues pretreated with ethanol (Pushpakiran et al., 2005), showing some indirect relationship with the system in focus.

3. Adenosine agonists and antagonists in the responses induced by ethanol

As widely described, ethanol affects several mechanisms of transmission on the central nervous system, bringing a wide range of behavioral and neurochemical responses. To reduce the risks and to prevent the damages arising from ethanol intake, many researches are engaged in finding other substances that could inhibit or reduce the responses of ethanol in the organism. An alternative for this proposition is to study the relationship of the mechanism of action of ethanol effects and substances that may interfere in these pathways. Adenosine system, as already mentioned, interacts with many effects induced by ethanol, affecting their responses as being influenced by them. This system has gained remarkable interest in research because of its neuromodulator/neuroprotective action (Halbach & Dermietzel, 2006; Wardas, 2002), and may bring about a new target for developing drugs that can interfere with the effects caused by ethanol.

Among the wide range of adenosine receptor agonists and antagonists used in experiments involving ethanol treatment, we will focus on the most common substances, like adenosine, N6-[2-(3,5-dimethoxyphenyl)-2-(2-methylphenyl)ethyl]adenosine g(DPMA), 2-chloro-N6-cyclopentyladenosine (CCPA), R(−)-N6-phenylisopropyladenosine (R-PIA) as agonists, and caffeine, theophylline, 1,3-dipropyl-8-cyclopentylxanthine (DPCPX), 3,7-Dimethyl-1-propargylxanthine (DMPX) as antagonists, these last being well described and characterized in a review performed by Muller & Jacobson (2011).

A moderate alcohol intake may not be harmful and has even beneficial effects in prevention of cardiovascular diseases, for example (Di Castelnuovo et al., 2010), but heavy alcohol consumption could be associated with some risks to the body, like reduced brain mass, neuronal loss, neuropathological changes, and impairment of cognitive functions, amnesia, dementia and even a significant increase in mortality. Furthermore, the consumption of significant quantities of ethanol during pregnancy is responsible for the Fetal Alcohol Syndrome (FAS), and prenatal alcohol exposure in humans, as well as in rodents, leads to an impaired cognitive and behavioral function, resulting from damage to the central nervous system (Chen et al., 2003; Riley et al., 2004; Hamilton et al., 2003). Thus, taking into account the substantial importance of this system, studies looking for the lessening of these various damages caused by ethanol intake are strictly necessary.

High amount of experimental studies, involving ethanol administration, use a chronic treatment as methodology protocol; but subchronic and acute treatments are also well used (Soares et al., 2009; Prediger et al., 2006). While acute treatment simulates hangover, chronic treatment usually refers to the withdrawal symptoms and body's adaptive responses to prolonged consumption of ethanol.

Although many studies have consistently demonstrated increases in anxiety-like behavior during the withdrawal period after chronic exposure to ethanol in rodents (Lal et al., 1991; Knapp et al., 1993; Gatch & Lal, 2001), there are limited experimental findings regarding this symptom after a single ethanol challenge dose. Prediger et al. (2006) designed an experimental study of acute ethanol withdrawal (hangover) in mice, in which a time-dependent development of anxiety-like behavior after an intraperitoneal administration of a single dose of ethanol (4 g/kg) in mice was assessed, and the potential of adenosine A_1 and A_{2A} receptor agonists in reducing this behavior was evaluated. They presented evidence that acute administration of 'nonanxiolytic' doses of adenosine (5–10 mg/kg, i.p.) or the selective adenosine A1 receptor agonist CCPA (0.05–0.125 mg/kg, i.p.), but not the adenosine A_{2A} receptor agonist DPMA (0.1–5.0 mg/kg, i.p.), which reduces the anxiety-like behavior during ethanol hangover in mice, as indicated by a significant increase in the exploration of the open arms of the elevated plus maze. In addition, the effect of CCPA (0.05 mg/kg, i.p.) was prevented by the pretreatment with the selective adenosine A_1 receptor antagonist DPCPX (3.0 mg/kg, i.p.), demonstrating that the activation of adenosine A_1 receptors, but not adenosine A_{2A} receptors, reduces the anxiogenic-like behaviour observed during acute ethanol withdrawal in mice.

In general, sensitivity to the adverse effects of ethanol is inversely correlated with alcohol consumption. In a study with mice lacking the A_{2A} receptor, Naassila et al. (2002) showed that these animals are less sensitive to the acute effects of ethanol as hypothermia and sedation, and consume more ethanol in a two-bottle choice paradigm compared with wild-type littermate control mice, demonstrating that the $A_{2A}R$ is involved in the sensitivity to the hypothermic and sedative effects of ethanol playing a role in alcohol-drinking behavior.

Furthermore, caffeine presents an ability to decrease sensitivity to the stumbling and tiredness associated with drinking large quantities of ethanol. Thus, adenosine receptors antagonists also appear to mediate some of the reinforcement effects of ethanol. This reinforcement is in part mediated via $A_{2A}R$ activation and probably associated with intracellular A_2 activation of cAMP/PKA signalling cascades in the nucleus accumbens (Thorsell, et al., 2007; Adams et al., 2008), but the exact mechanism of action remains unclear. Studies in humans examining methylxanthine and ethanol interactions have mostly focused on the influence that caffeine exerts on ethanol intoxication, and have yielded mixed results (Liguori and Robinson 2001; Drake et al. 2003); but a point that needs further attention is the fact that these studies converge upon the point that caffeine consumed in association with ethanol, rather than improving ethanol-induced impairments, would reduce the self-perception of ethanol intoxication (Morelli & Simola, 2011), since human data also show that caffeine enhances tolerance to ethanol (Fillmore, 2003).

In addition to reinforcing effects, adenosine also appears to be related to locomotive effects of ethanol at high dose (6 g/kg) in subchronic treatment during 5 days, as shown in the experimental study of Soares et al. (2009), in which the administration of Aminophylline, a non-selective adenosine receptor antagonist, at low doses (5 and 10 mg/kg) produced some degree of locomotion stimulation, and was able to reverse the depressive effects produced by ethanol on the number of falls and time spent in the bar, in the Rota rod test, suggesting a partial blockage of the action of ethanol. The selective A_1R agonist N^6-cyclohexyladenosine (CHA) has also been found to potentiate, and the antagonist DPCPX attenuates ethanol-induced motor incoordination in mice (Meng et al., 1997).

Chronic ethanol intake leads to several changes in the balance of neurotransmitter pathways and its receptors, being studied oftentimes focusing withdrawal symptoms. Accordingly

Concas et al. (1994), the adenosine receptor agonist CCPA produces inhibition of these symptoms, such as tremors and audiogenically induced seizures in rats treated repeatedly with ethanol (12–18 g/kg daily for 6 days), an effect prevented by DPCPX. Similar results about the specificity of the adenosine receptor in the responses of ethanol effects have been reported by Kaplan et al (1999) in mice receiving a 14-day liquid diet containing ethanol and treated with the adenosine A_1 receptor agonist R-PIA during the withdrawal period, indicating the adenosine A_1R modulate anxiety-like responses in mice, not only in acute, but also in chronic treatment with ethanol.

Thus, adenosine receptor activation seems to be strongly linked with sensitivity and reinforcement properties of ethanol either in A_1, or in $A_{2A}R$, with an opposite relation of activation, whereas the adenosine A_1R agonists reduce sensitivity, $A_{2A}R$ antagonists demonstrate to play this role. Despite A_{2A} knockout mice showed reduced conditioned place preference for ethanol. Houchi et al. (2008) showed that the increased propensity to drink ethanol in A_{2A} knockout mice was associated with an increase in sensitivity to the motor stimulant and anxiolytic effects of ethanol. Contrasting with these findings, the administration of A_{2A} antagonist DMPX reduced ethanol reward and consumption, in a study performed by Thorsell et al. (2007), in which a decreased lever-pressing for ethanol in an operant chamber was observed.

Caffeine and selective adenosine receptor antagonists may also reduce the duration of ethanol-induced loss of the righting reflex (El Yacoubi et al., 2003), reverse deficits in motor coordination induced by ethanol (Barwick & Dar, 1998; Connole et al., 2004) and reverse retrograde memory impairment caused by a high dose of ethanol (3 g/kg) (Spinetta et al., 2008). Indeed, the combination of caffeine and ethanol produces a beneficial effect after experimental traumatism brain injury (Dash et al., 2004), projecting its effect on stroke (Aronowski et al., 2003; Belayev et al., 2004) and indicating the importance of the interaction between caffeine and ethanol.

Beyond neurotransmission/neuromodulation, it is important to give attention to other factors that contribute to the relationship between adenosine system and ethanol effects, as indicated in a review performed by Ruby et al. (2011) about adenosine signalling in anxiety, which underlies the importance of the adenosine transporter ENT1. Many aspects of ethanol-related behaviors and anxiety appear to be involved in genetic factors as polymorphism and in the gene encoding ENT1 could be associated with alcoholism and depression in women (Gass et al., 2010). Further, acute ethanol inhibits ENT1, while chronic ethanol treatment leads to decreased ENT1 expression (Short et al., 2006; Sharma et al., 2010). Also, mice lacking this adenosine transporter displayed a decreased A_1 adenosine tone in the nucleus accumbens and elevated levels of ethanol consumption compared with wild-type mice (Choi et al., 2004). In contrast, it has been shown that ethanol operant self-administration is not altered by an A_1R antagonist while it is bimodally affected by an $A_{2A}R$ antagonist (Arolfo et al., 2004).

4. Conclusion and future prospects

As noted above, there are many different points of adenosine system interference on the effects of ethanol administration. This interaction is of fundamental importance because it could be a new target for developing drugs that may interfere, reducing the damage caused by ethanol.

5. Acknowledgment

This work was sponsored by the Conselho Nacional de Desenvolvimento Científico e Tecnológico - CNPq, Coordenação de Aperfeiçoamento de Pessoal de Nível Superior - CAPES, and Fundação Cearense de Apoio ao Desenvolvimento Científico e Tecnológico FUNCAP Grants.

6. References

Adams CL, Cowen MS, Short JL, & Lawrence AJ. (2008). Combined antagonism of glutamate mGlu5 and adenosine A2A receptors interact to regulate alcohol-seeking in rats. *International Journal Neuropsychopharmacol,* 11: 229-241.

Arolfo MP, Yao L, Gordon AS, Diamond I, & Janak PH. (2004). Ethanol operant self-administration in rats is regulated by adenosine A2 receptors. *Alcohol Clin Exp Res,* 28: 1308–1316.

Aronowski J, Strong R, Shirzadi A, & Grotta JC (2003). Ethanol plus caffeine (caffeinol) for treatment of ischemic stroke: preclinical experience. *Stroke,* 34: 1246-1251.

Barwick VS, & Dar MS. (1998). Adenosinergic modulation of ethanol induced motor incoordination in the rat motor cortex. *Prog. NeuroPsychopharmacol. Biol. Psychiatry,* 22: 587- 607.

Batista LC, Prediger RD, Morato GS, Takahashi RN, (2005). Blockade of adenosine and dopamine receptors inhibits the development of rapid tolerance to ethanol in mice. Psychopharmacology, 181: 714-721.

Belayev L, Khoutorova L, Zhang Y, Belayev A, Zhao W, Busto R, & Ginsberg MD. (2004). Caffeinol confers cortical but not subcortical neuroprotection after transient focal cerebral ischemia in rats. *Brain Res,* 1008: 278-283.

Brust JCM. (2010). Ethanol and Cognition: Indirect Effects, Neurotoxicity and Neuroprotection: A Review. *Int. J. Environ. Res. Public Health,* 7: 1540-1557.

Carmichael FJ, Israel Y, Crawford M, Minhas K, Saldivia V, Sandrin S, Campisi P, Orrego H. (1991). Central nervous system effects of acetate: contribution to the central effects of ethanol. *J Pharmacol Exp Ther,* 259: 403-408.

Chapell R, Bueno OF, Alvarez-Hernandez X, Robinson LC, Leidenheimer NJ. (1998). Activation of protein kinase C induces gamma-aminobutyric acid type A receptor internalization in Xenopus oocytes. *J Biol Chem,* 273: 32595-32601.

Chen WJ, Maier SE, Parnell SE, & West JR. (2003). Alcohol and the developing brain: neuroanatomical studies, *Alcohol Res. Health,* 27: 174–180.

Choi DS, Cascini MG, Mailliard W, Young H, Paredes P, McMahon T, Diamond I, Bonci A., & Messing R.O. (2004). The type 1 equilibrative nucleoside transporter regulates ethanol intoxication and preference. *Nat Neurosci,* 7: 855–861.

Ciruela F, Casado V, Rodrigues R, Lujan R, Burgueno J, Canals M, Borycz J, Rebola N, Goldberg SR, Mallol J, Cortes A, Canela EI, Lopez-Gimenez JF, Milligan G, Lluis C, Cunha RA, Ferre S, Franco R. (2006). Presynaptic control of striatal glutamatergic neurotransmission by adenosine A1-A2A receptor heteromers. *J Neurosci,* 26: 2080-2087.

Concas A, Cuccheddu T, Floris S, Mascia MP, & Biggio G. (1994). 2-Chloro-N6-cyclopentyladenosine (CCPA), an adenosine A1 receptor agonist, suppressed ethanol withdrawal syndrome in rats. *Alcohol Alcohol,* 29: 261–264.

Connole L, Harkin A, & Maginn M. (2004). Adenosine A1 receptor blockade mimics caffeine's attenuation of ethanol induced motor incoordination. *Basic Clin Pharmacol Toxicol,* 95: 299-304.

Dahchour A, & De Witte P. (2000). Ethanol and amino acids in the central nervous system: assessment of the pharmacological actions of acamprosate. *Prog. Neurobiol,* 60: 343-362.

Dar MS. (2001). Modulation of ethano-induced motor incoordination by mouse striatal A1 adenosinergic receptor. Brain Res. Bull, 55: 513–520.

Dash PK, Moore AN, Moody MR, Treadwell R, Felix JL, & Clifton GL. (2004). Post trauma administration of caffeine plus ethanol reduces contusion volume and improves working memory in rats. *J Neurotrauma,* 21: 1573-1583.

Davies DL, Asatryan L, KuO ST, Woodward JJ, King BF, Alkana RL, Xiao C, Ye JH, Sun H, Zhang L, Hu XQ, Hayrapetyan V, Lovinger DM, Machu TK. (2006). Effects of ethanol on adenosine 5'-triphosphate–gated purinergic and 5-hydroxytryptamine3 receptors. *Alcohol Clin Exp Res,* 30: 349-358.

Davies DL, Kochegarov AA, Kuo ST, Kulkarni AA, Woodward JJ, King BF, Alkana RL. (2005). Ethanol differentially affects ATP-gated P2X(3) and P2X(4) receptor subtypes expressed in Xenopus oocytes. *Neuropharmacology,* 49: 243-253.

Davies DL, Machu TK, Guo Y, Alkana RL. (2002). Ethanol sensitivity in ATPgated P2X receptors is subunit dependent. *Alcohol Clin Exp Res,* 26: 773-778.

Diamond I, Nagy L, Mochly-Rosen D, Gordon A. (1991). The role of adenosine and adenosine transport in ethanol-induced cellular tolerance and dependence. Possible biologic and genetic markers of alcoholism. *Ann NY Acad Sci,* 625: 473-487.

Di Castelnuovo A, Costanzo S, Donati MB, Iacoviello L, de Gaetano G. (2010). Prevention of cardiovascular risk by moderate alcohol consumption: epidemiologic evidence and plausible mechanisms. *Intern Emerg Med,* 5(4):291-7.

Drake CL, Roehrs T, Turner L, Scofield HM, Roth T. (2003). Caffeine reversal of ethanol effects on the multiple sleep latency test, memory, and psychomotor performance. *Neuropsychopharmacology,* 28: 371-378.

Dunwiddie TV, & Haas HL. (1985). Adenosine increases synaptic facilitation in the in vitro rat hippocampus: evidence for a presynaptic site of action. *J Physiol,* 369: 365-77.

Dunwiddie TV, & Masino SA. (2001). The role and regulation of adenosine in the central nervous system. *Annu. Rev. Neurosci.,* 24: 31–55.

El Yacoubi M, Ledent C, Parmentier M, Costentin J, & Vaugeois JM. (2003). Caffeine reduces hypnotic effects of alcohol through adenosine A2A receptor blockade. *Neuropharmacology,* 45: 977–985.

Ferre S, Ciruela F, Borycz J, Solinas M, Quarta D, Antoniou K, Quiroz C, Justinova Z, Lluis C, Franco R, Goldberg SR. (2008). Adenosine A1-A2A receptor heteromers: new targets for caffeine in the brain. *Front Biosci,* 13: 2391-2399.

Fillmore MT. (2003). Alcohol tolerance in humans is enhanced by prior caffeine antagonism of alcohol induced impairment. *Exp Clin Psychopharmacol,* 11: 9-17.

Fredholm BB, Ijzerman AP, Jacobson KA, Klotz K, Linden J. (2001). International Union of Pharmacology XXV - Nomenclature and classification of adenosine receptors. *Pharmacol Rev,* 53: 527-52.

Gass N, Ollila HM, Utge S, Partonen T, Kronholm E, Pirkola S, Suhonen J, Silander K, Porkka-Heiskanen T, & Paunio T. (2010). Contribution of adenosine related genes to the risk of depression with disturbed sleep. *J Affect Disord,* 126: 134-139.

Gatch MB, & Lal H. (2001). Animal models of the anxiogenic effects of ethanol withdrawal. *Drug Dev Res,* 54: 95–115.

Halbach OB, & Dermietzel R. (2006). Neuromodulators, In: *Neurotransmitters and neuromodulators.* 2ed, pp. (320-325), WILEY-VCH Verlag GmbH & Co. KGaA, ISBN 978-3-527-31307-5, Weinheim, Germany.

Hamilton DA, Kodituwakku P, Sutherland RJ, Savage DD. (2003). Children with Fetal Alcohol Syndrome are impaired at place learning but not cued-navigation in a virtual Morris water task, Behav. Brain Res. 143: 85– 94.

Heine C, Wegner A, Grosche J, Allgaier C, Illes P, & Franke H. (2007). P2 receptor expression in the dopaminergic system of the rat brain during development. *Neuroscience,* 149:165-181.

Hoffman PL, & Tabakoff B. (1990). Ethanol and guanine nucleotide binding proteins: a selective interaction. *FASEB J,* 4: 2612-2622.

Houchi H, Warnault V, Barbier E, Dubois C, Pierrefiche O, Ledent C, Daoust M, Naassila M (2008). Involvement of A2A receptors in anxiolytic, locomotor and motivational properties of ethanol in mice. *Genes Brain Behavior,* 7(8): 887-98.

Inoue Y, Yao L, Hopf FW, Fan P, Jiang Z, Bonci A, Diamond I. (2007). Nicotine and ethanol activate protein kinase A synergistically via G(i) betagamma subunits in nucleus accumbens/ventral tegmental cocultures: the role of dopamine D(1)/D(2) and adenosine A(2A) receptors. *J Pharmacol Exp Ther,* 322: 23-29.

Jarjour S, Bai L, & Gianoulakis C. (2009). Effect of acute ethanol administration on the release of opioid peptides from the midbrain including the ventral tegmental area. *Alcohol Clin Exp Res,* 33: 1033-1043.

Kaneyuki T, Morimasa T, Okada H, Shohmori T. (1991). The effect of acute and repeated ethanol administration on monoamines and their metabolites in brain regions of rats. *Acta Med Okayama,* 45: 201-8.

Kaplan GB, Bharmal NH, Leite-Morris KA, Adams WR. (1999). Role of adenosine A1 and A2A receptors in the alcohol withdrawal syndrome. *Alcohol,* 19: 157–162.

Knapp DJ, Saiers JA, & Pohorecky LA. (1993). Observations of novel behaviors as indices of ethanol withdrawal-induced anxiety. *Alcohol Alcohol (Suppl),* 2: 489–493.

Krauss SW, Ghirnikar RB, Diamond I, & Gordon AS. (1993). Inhibition of adenosine uptake by ethanol is specific for one class of nucleoside transporters. *Mol Pharmacol,* 44: 1021-1026.

Lal H, Prather PL, Rezazadeh SM. (1991). Anxiogenic behavior in rats during acute and protracted ethanol withdrawal: reversal by buspirone. *Alcohol,* 8: 467–471.

Lam MP, Marinelli PW, Bai L, Gianoulakis, C. (2008). Effects of acute ethanol on opioid peptide release in the central amygdala: an in vivo microdialysis study. *Psychopharmacology,* 201: 261-271.

Lan JY, Skeberdis VA, Jover T, Grooms SY, Lin Y, Araneda RC, Zheng X, Bennett MV, Zukin RS. (2001). Protein kinase C modulates NMDA receptor trafficking and gating. *Nat Neurosci,* 4: 382-390.

Liguori A, & Robinson JH. (2001). Caffeine antagonism of alcohol induced driving impairment. *Drug Alcohol Depend,* 63:123 129.

Londos C, Cooper DMF, & Wolff J. (1980). Subclasses of external adenosine receptors. *Proc Natl Acad Sci USA,* 77: 2551-2554.

Mailliard WS, & Diamond I. (2004). Recent advances in the neurobiology of alcoholism: the role of adenosine. *Pharmacol Ther,* 101:39-46.

Marinelli PW, Quirion R, & Gianoulakis C. (2004). An in vivo profile of beta-endorphin release in the arcuate nucleus and nucleus accumbens following exposure to stress or alcohol. *Neuroscience,* 127: 777-784.

Mendez M, Leriche M, & Carlos Calva J. (2003). Acute ethanol administration transiently decreases [3H]-DAMGO binding to mu opioid receptors in the rat substantia nigra pars reticulate but not in the caudate-putamen. *Neurosci Res,* 47: 153-160.

Meng ZH, Anwer J, & Dar MS. (1997). The striatal adenosinergic modulation of ethanol-induced motor incoordination in rats: possible role of chloride flux. *Brain Research,* 776: 235–245.

Meng ZH, & Dar MS. (1994). Intrastriatal Ro15-4513 functionally antagonizes ethanol-induced motor incoordination and striatal adenosinergic modulation of ethanol-induced motor incoordination in rats. *J Pharmacol Exp Ther,* 271: 524-534.

Meng ZH, & Dar MS. (1995). Possible role of striatal adenosine in the modulation of acute ethanol-induced motor incoordination in rats. *Alcohol Clin Exp Res,* 19: 892-901.

Meng ZH, Pennington SN, & Dar MS. (1998). Rat striatal adenosinergic modulation of ethanol-induced motor impairment: possible role of striatal cyclic AMP. *Neuroscience,* 85: 919-930.

Mitchel RL, Neafsey EJ, & Collins MA. (2009). Essential involvement of the NMDA receptor in ethanol preconditioning-dependent neuroprotection from amyloid-beta in vitro. *J Neurochem,* 111: 580-588.

Mohler H, Sieghart W, Richards JG, & Hunkeler W. (1984). Photoaffinity labeling of benzodiazepine receptors with a partial inverse agonist. *Eur J Pharmacol,* 102: 191-192.

Morelli M, & Simola N. (2011). Methylxanthines and Drug Dependence: A Focus on Interactions with Substances of Abuse, In: *Methylxanthines, Handbook of Experimental Pharmacology,* Ed. Fredholm BB, pp. 483-508, Springer, ISBN 978 3 642 13442 5, London.

Moreau J-L, & Huber G. (1999). Central adenosine A_{2A} receptors: an overview. Brain Res *Brain Res Rev,* 31: 65–82.

Mori M, Heuss C, Gähwiler BH, & Gerber U. (2001). Fast synaptic transmission mediated by P2X receptors in CA3 pyramidal cells of rat hippocampal slice cultures. *J Physiol,* 535: 115-123.

Muller CE, & Jacobson KA. (2011). Xanthines as Adenosine Receptor Antagonists. In: *Methylxanthines, Handbook of Experimental Pharmacology,* Ed. Fredholm BB, pp. 151-200, Springer, ISBN 978 3 642 13442 5, London.

Naassila M, Ledent C, Daoust M. (2002). Low Ethanol Sensitivity and Increased Ethanol Consumption in Mice Lacking Adenosine A2A Receptors. *The Journal of Neuroscience,* 22(23): 10487–10493.

Nagy LE, Diamond I, Casso DJ, Franklin C, Gordon AS. (1990). Ethanol increases extracellular adenosine by inhibiting adenosine uptake via the nucleoside transporter. *J Biol Chem,* 265: 1946–1951.

Nishi A, Liu F, Matsuyama S, Hamada M, Higashi H, Nairn AC, Greengard P. (2003). Metabotropic mGlu5 receptors regulate adenosine A2A receptor signaling. *Proc Natl Acad Sci USA,* 100: 1322-1327.

Othman T, Sinclair CJ, Haughey N, Geiger JD, Parkinson FE. (2002). Ethanol alters glutamate but not adenosine uptake in rat astrocytes: evidence for protein kinase C involvement. *Neurochem Res,* 27: 289-296.

Papp L, Vizi ES, Sperlagh B. (2004). Lack of ATP-evoked GABA and glutamate release in the hippocampus of P2X7 receptor-/- mice. *Neuroreport,* 15: 2387-2391.

Prediger RDS, Silva GE, Batista LC, Bittencourt AL, Takahashi RN. (2006). Activation of Adenosine A1 Receptors Reduces Anxiety-Like Behavior During Acute Ethanol Withdrawal (Hangover) in Mice. *Neuropsychopharmacology,* 31: 2210–2220.

Pushpakiran G, Mahalakshmi K, Viswanathan P, Anuradha CV. (2005). Taurine prevents ethanol-induced alterations in lipids and ATPases in rat tissues. *Pharmacol Rep,* 57: 578-587.

Quarta D, Borycz J, Solinas M, Patkar K, Hockemeyer J, Ciruela F, Lluis C, Franco R, Woods AS, Goldberg SR, Ferre S. (2004). Adenosine receptor-mediated modulation of dopamine release in the nucleus accumbens depends on glutamate neurotransmission and N-methyl-D-aspartate receptor stimulation. *J Neurochem,* 91: 873-880.

Rabin RA, & Molinoff PB. (1981). Activation of adenylate cyclase by ethanol in mouse striatal tissue. *J Pharmacol Exp Ther,* 216: 129-134.

Riley E.P., McGee C.L., Sowell E.R. (2004). Teratogenic effects of alcohol: a decade of brain imaging. *Am. J. Med. Genet.,* 127: 35- 41.9

Ruby CL, Adams CA, Mrazek DA, & Choi D. (2011). Adenosine Signaling in Anxiety, In: *Anxiety Disorders,* Ed. Kalinin VV, pp. 51-68, InTech, ISBN 978-953-307-592-1, Croatia.

Sharma R, Engemann S, Sahota P, & Thakkar MM. (2010). Role of adenosine and wakepromoting basal forebrain in insomnia and associated sleep disruptions caused by ethanol dependence. *Journal of Neurochemistry,* 115: 782-794.

Short JL, Drago J, & Lawrence AJ. (2006). Comparison of ethanol preference and neurochemical measures of mesolimbic dopamine and adenosine systems across different strains of mice. *Alcoholism: Clinical and Experimental Research,* 30: 606-620.

Soares PM, Patrocínio MC, Assreuy AM, Siqueira RC, Lima NM, Arruda MO, Escudeiro SS, de Carvalho KM, Sousa FC, Viana GS, Vasconcelos SM. (2009). Aminophylline (a theophylline-ethylenediamine complex) blocks ethanol behavioral effects in mice. *Behav Pharmacol,* 20: 297-302.

Spinetta MJ, Woodlee MT, Feinberg LM, Stroud C, Schallert K, Cormack LK, Schallert T. (2008). Alcohol-induced retrograde memory impairment in rats: prevention by caffeine. *Psychopharmacology,* 201: 361–371.

Sun H, Hu XQ, Moradel EM, Weight FF, Zhang L. (2003). Modulation of 5-HT3 receptor-mediated response and trafficking by activation of protein kinase C. *J Biol Chem,* 278: 34150-34157.

Tao L, & Ye JH. (2002). Protein kinase C modulation of ethanol inhibition of glycine-activated current in dissociated neurons of rat ventral tegmental area. *J Pharmacol Exp Ther,* 300:967-975.

Thorsell A, Johnson J, & Heilig M. (2007). Effect of the adenosine A2a receptor antagonist 3,7- dimethyl-propargylxanthine on anxiety-like and depression-like behavior and alcohol consumption in Wistar Rats. *Alcoholism: Clinical and Experimental Research*, 31: 1302-1307.

Van Calker D, Müller M, & Hamprecht B. (1978). Adenosine inhibits the accumulation of cyclic AMP in cultured brain cells. *Nature*, 276: 839-841.

Vasconcelos SM, Cavalcante RA, Aguiar LM, Sousa FC, Fonteles MM, Viana GS. (2004). Effects of chronic ethanol treatment on monoamine levels in rat hippocampus and striatum. *Braz J Med Biol Res*, 37: 1839-46.

Vasconcelos SM, Sales GT, Lima NM, Soares PM, Pereira EC, Fonteles MM, Sousa FC, Viana GS. (2008). Determination of amino acid levels in the rat striatum, after administration of ethanol alone and associated with ketamine, a glutamatergic antagonist. *Neurosci Lett*, 444: 48-51.

Vengeliene V, Bilbao A, Molander A, & Spanagel R. (2008). Neuropharmacology of alcohol addiction. *British Journal of Pharmacology*, 154: 299–315.

Wardas J. (2002). Neuroprotective role of adenosine in the CNS. *Pol. J. Pharmacol.*, 54: 313–326.

Xiao C, Zhou C, Li K, Davies DL, Ye JH. (2008). Purinergic type 2 receptors rat GABAergic synapses on ventral tegmental area dopamine neurons are targets for ethanol action. *J Pharmacol Exp Ther*, 327:196-205.

Yao L, Arolfo MP, Dohrman DP, Jiang Z, Fan P, Fuchs S, Janak PH, Gordon AS, Diamond I. (2002). Betagamma Dimers mediate synergy of dopamine D2 and adenosine A2 receptor-stimulated PKA signaling and regulate ethanol consumption. *Cell*, 109:733-743.

Yao L, Asai K, Jiang Z, Ishii A, Fan P, Gordon AS, Diamond I. (2001). Dopamine D_2 receptor inhibition of adenylyl cyclase is abolished by acute ethanol but restored after chronic ethanol exposure (tolerance). *J Pharmacol Exp Ther*, 298: 833-839.

Yao L, Fan P, Jiang Z, Mailliard WS, Gordon AS, Diamond I. (2003). Addicting drugs utilize a synergistic molecular mechanism in common requiring adenosine and Gi-beta gamma dimers. *Proc Natl Acad Sci USA*, 100: 14379-14384.

Zhang L, Oz M, & Weight FF. (1995). Potentiation of 5-HT3 receptor-mediated responses by protein kinase C activation. *Neuroreport*, 6: 1464-1468.